Present Knowledge in Nutrition

Sixth Edition

Myrtle L. Brown, Editor

International Life Sciences Institute
Nutrition Foundation
Washington, D.C.
1990

International Life Sciences Institute–Nutrition Foundation, 1126 Sixteenth Street, N.W., Washington, D.C. 20036

© 1990 International Life Sciences Institute–Nutrition Foundation

First edition published 1953, second edition 1956, third edition 1967, fourth edition 1976, fifth edition 1984, sixth edition 1990

Printed in the United States of America

Library of Congress Catalog Card Number 90-082033
ISBN 0-944398-05-7

Contents

Special Physiological Needs

Chronic Diseases

Evaluation of Nutritional Status

Special Topics

Continuing Issues

Editorial Committee

Contributors

Marvin E. Ament, M.D.
Chief, Division of Pediatric Gastroenterology and
    Nutrition
Chief, Hospital Enteral and Parenteral Nutrition Support
    Services
University of California Medical Center
Los Angeles, CA

Claude D. Arnaud, M.D.
Chief, Division of Gerontology and Geriatric Medicine
Director, Center for Biomedical Research on Aging
University of California
San Francisco, CA 94120

Gary R. Beecher, Ph.D.
Research Chemist
Nutrient Composition Laboratory
Human Nutrition Research Center
Agricultural Research Service
U.S. Department of Agriculture
Beltsville, MD 20705

David R. Bevan, Ph.D.
Associate Professor
Department of Biochemistry and Nutrition
Virginia Polytechnic Institute and State University
Blacksburg, VA 24061

John G. Bieri, Ph.D.
Scientist Emeritus
National Institute of Arthritis, Diabetes, and Digestive
    and Kidney Disease
National Institutes of Health
Bethesda, MD 20892

George A. Bray, M.D.
Director
Pennington Center
Baton Rouge, LA 70808

Myrtle L. Brown, Ph.D.
Professor Emeritus
Department of Biochemistry and Nutrition
Virginia Polytechnic Institute and State University
Blacksburg, VA 24061

Raymond F. Burk, Jr., M.D.
Professor
Division of Gastroenterology
Department of Medicine and Center in Molecular
    Toxicology
Vanderbilt University School of Medicine
Nashville, TN 37232

Faith Sikkema Burnham, M.M.S.
Department of Biochemistry
Emory School of Medicine
Atlanta, GA 30322

Elsworth R. Buskirk, Ph.D.
Marie Underhill Noll Professor of Human Performance
Laboratory for Human Performance Research
Pennsylvania State University
University Park, PA 16802

Betty Ruth Carruth, Ph.D., R.D.
Professor
Department of Nutrition and Food Sciences
University of Tennessee
Knoxville, TN 37996-1900

Thomas W. Castonguay, Ph.D.
Associate Professor
Department of Human Nutrition and Food Science
University of Maryland
College Park, MD 20742

Ann M. Coulston, M.S., R.D.
Research Dietitian
General Clinical Research Center
Stanford University Medical Center
Stanford, CA 94305

Robert J. Cousins, Ph.D.
Boston Family Professor of Nutrition
Director, Center for Nutritional Sciences
University of Florida
Gainesville, FL 32611

Yasmin S. Cypel
Food Consumption Research Branch
Human Nutrition Information Service
U.S. Department of Agriculture
Hyattsville, MD 20782

Peter R. Dallman, M.D.
Professor of Pediatrics
School of Medicine
University of California Medical Center
San Francisco, CA 94143

John T. Devlin, M.D.
Assistant Professor
Metabolic Unit, Department of Medicine
University of Vermont College of Medicine
Burlington, VT 05405

Jacqueline Dupont, Ph.D.
Food and Nutrition Science Consulting
Fort Collins, CO 80524

Marie T. Fanelli-Kuczmarski
Division of Health Examination Statistics
National Center for Health Statistics
U.S. Department of Health and Human Services
Hyattsville, MD 20782

Axel G. Feller, M.D.
Department of Medicine
Chicago Medical School
North Chicago, IL 60033

Gilbert B. Forbes, M.D.
Professor of Pediatrics and Biophysics
University of Rochester School of Medicine
and Dentistry
Rochester, NY 14642

Daniel D. Gallaher, Ph.D.
Assistant Professor
Department of Food Science and Nutrition
University of Minnesota
St. Paul, MN 55108

Philip J. Garry, Ph.D.
Professor
Department of Pathology
University of New Mexico School of Medicine
Albuquerque, NM 87131

Cutberto Garza, M.D., Ph.D.
Professor and Director
Division of Nutritional Sciences
Cornell University
Ithaca, NY 14853

Nora A. Hallquist, M.S.
Department of Nutritional Sciences
Cook College
Rutgers University
New Brunswick, NJ 08903

Alfred E. Harper, Ph.D.
Professor, Biochemistry and Nutritional Sciences
College of Agriculture and Life Sciences
University of Wisconsin
Madison, WI 53706

James M. Hempe, Ph.D.
Research Associate
Food Science and Human Nutrition Department
Center for Nutritional Sciences
University of Florida
Gainesville, FL 32611

Victor Herbert, M.D., J.D.
Professor
Department of Medicine
Mt. Sinai School of Medicine and
  Bronx VA Medical Center
Bronx, NY 10468

Basil S. Hetzel, M.D.
Executive Director
International Council for the Control of Iodine
  Deficiency Disorders (ICCIDD)
CSIRO Division of Human Nutrition
Adelaide 5000, Australia

Clarie B. Hollenbeck, Ph.D.
Research Scientist
Geriatric Research Education and Clinical Center
Veterans Administration Medical Center
Palo Alto, CA 94304, and
Research Coordinator
General Clinical Research Center
Stanford University School of Medicine
Stanford, CA 94305

Neil A. Holtzman, M.D., M.P.H.
Professor of Pediatrics
Johns Hopkins University School of Medicine
Johns Hopkins Hospital
Baltimore, MD 21209

Edward S. Horton, M.D.
Professor and Chairman
Department of Medicine
University of Vermont College of Medicine
Burlington, VT 05405

Robert A. Jacob, Ph.D.
Research Leader, Biochemistry
Western Human Nutrition Research Center
Agricultural Research Service
U.S. Department of Agriculture
Presidio of San Francisco, CA 94129

Herbert F. Janssen, Ph.D.
Associate Professor
Orthopaedic Surgery and Physiology
Texas Tech University Health Sciences Center
Lubbock, TX 79430

Carl L. Keen, Ph.D.
Professor
Department of Nutrition
University of California
Davis, CA 95616

Janet C. King, Ph.D.
Professor and Chair
Department of Nutritional Science
University of California
Berkeley, CA 94720

Saulo Klahr, M.D.
Joseph Friedman Professor of Renal Disease
Director, Renal Division
Washington University School of Medicine
St. Louis, MO 63123

Howard R. Knapp, M.D., Ph.D.
Assistant Professor of Medicine
Division of Clinical Pharmacology
Vanderbilt University
Nashville, TN 37232-6602

Kathleen M. Koehler, Ph.D.
Assistant Professor
Department of Health Promotion, Physical Education
    and Leisure Programs
University of New Mexico *and*
Clinical Nutrition Research Center
University of New Mexico School of Medicine
Albuquerque, NM 87131

David Kritchevsky, Ph.D.
Associate Director
The Wistar Institute of Anatomy and Biology
Philadelphia, PA 19104

Carlos L. Krumdieck, M.D., Ph.D.
Professor and Vice-Chairman
Department of Nutritional Sciences
The University of Alabama at Birmingham
Birmingham, AL 35294

Michael C. Latham, M.D.
Professor and Director
Program in International Nutrition
Division of Nutritional Sciences
Ithaca, NY 14853

Orville A. Levander, Ph.D.
Research Chemist
Vitamin and Mineral Nutrition Center
Human Nutrition Research Center
Agricultural Research Service
U.S. Department of Agriculture
Beltsville, MD 20705

Friedrich C. Luft, M.D.
Professor
Medizinische Klinik IV mit Poliklinik der Universität
    Erlangen-Nürnberg
8520 Erlangen, West Germany

Ruth H. Matthews
Chief
Nutrient Data Research Branch
Human Nutrition Information Service
U.S. Department of Agriculture
Hyattsville, MD 20782

Donald B. McCormick, Ph.D.
Professor and Chairman
Department of Biochemistry
School of Medicine
Emory University
Atlanta, GA 30322

Donald J. McNamara, Ph.D.
Professor
Department of Nutrition and Food Science
University of Arizona
Tucson, AZ 85721

Alfred H. Merrill, Jr., Ph.D.
Associate Professor
Department of Biochemistry
Emory University School of Medicine
Atlanta, GA 30322

Mack C. Mitchell, M.D.
Associate Professor of Medicine
Alcohol Research Center
Johns Hopkins University School of Medicine
Baltimore, MD 21205

Donald M. Mock, M.D., Ph.D.
Director of Pediatric Gastroenterology
Department of Pediatrics
University of Iowa Hospitals and Clinics
Iowa City, IA 52242

Forrest H. Nielsen, Ph.D.
Director, Grand Forks Human Nutrition
    Research Center
Agricultural Research Service
U.S. Department of Agriculture
Grand Forks, ND 58202

Anthony W. Norman, Ph.D.
Professor
Department of Biomedical Sciences and Biochemistry
University of California
Riverside, CA 92521

Boyd L. O'Dell, Ph.D.
Professor Emeritus
Department of Biochemistry
University of Missouri
Columbia, MO 65211

James A. Olson, Ph.D.
Distinguished Professor of Biochemistry
Department of Biochemistry and Biophysics
Iowa State University
Ames, IA 50011

Robert E. Olson, M.D., Ph.D.
Professor of Medicine
Health Sciences Center
State University of New York at Stony Brook
Stony Brook, NY 11794

Robert H. Ophaug, Ph.D.
Associate Professor
School of Dentistry
University of Minnesota
Minneapolis, MN 55455

Eleanor M. Pao, Ph.D.
Chief, Food Consumption Research Branch
Human Nutrition Information Service
U.S. Department of Agriculture
Hyattsville, MD 20782

Daniel Rudman, M.D.
Professor of Medicine
Medical College of Wisconsin
Milwaukee, WI 53295-1000

Sarah D. Sanchez, M.S.
Division of Gerontology and Geriatric Medicine
Department of Medicine
University of California, San Francisco, *and*
Center for Biomedical Research on Aging
San Francisco Institute on Aging
South San Francisco, CA 94080

Howerde E. Sauberlich, Ph.D.
Professor and Director
Division of Experimental Nutrition
Department of Nutrition Sciences
University of Alabama at Birmingham
Birmingham, AL 35294

Barbara O. Schneeman, Ph.D.
Professor and Chairman
Department of Nutrition
University of California
Davis, CA 95616

Adria R. Sherman, Ph.D.
Professor and Chair
Department of Nutritional Sciences
Cook College
Rutgers University
New Brunswick, NJ 08903

Maurice E. Shils, M.D., Sc.D.
Adjunct Professor of Public Health Sciences
    and Medicine (Nutrition)
Bowman Gray School of Medicine
Wake Forest University
Winston-Salem, NC 27103

Helen Smiciklas-Wright, Ph.D.
Professor of Nutrition
Department of Nutrition
College of Health and Human Development
Pennsylvania State University
University Park, PA 16802

MaryFran Sowers, Ph.D.
Assistant Professor
Department of Epidemiology
The University of Michigan
Ann Arbor, MI 48109-2029

Robert D. Steele, Ph.D.
Professor
Department of Nutritional Sciences
University of Wisconsin
Madison, WI 53706

Judith S. Stern, Sc.D.
Professor of Nutrition and of Internal Medicine
Director, Food Intake Laboratory
University of California
Davis, CA 95616

Barbara J. Stoecker, Ph.D., R.D.
Associate Professor
Department of Food, Nutrition and Institution
    Administration
Oklahoma State University
Stillwater, OK 74078

CONTRIBUTORS

John W. Suttie, Ph.D.
Professor
Department of Biochemistry
University of Wisconsin
Madison, WI 53706

Marian E. Swendseid, Ph.D.
Professor and Head, Division of Nutritional Sciences
School of Public Health
University of California
Los Angeles, CA 90024

Béla Szepesi, Ph.D.
Research Chemist
Carbohydrate Nutrition Laboratory
Beltsville Human Nutrition Research Center
Agricultural Research Service
U.S. Department of Agriculture
Beltsville, MD 20705

Jean Weininger, Ph.D.
Research Associate
Department of Nutritional Sciences
University of California
Berkeley, CA 94720

Catherine E. Woteki, Ph.D.
Deputy Director
Division of Health Examination Statistics
National Center for Health Statistics
U.S. Department of Health and Human Services
Hyattsville, MD 20782

Sheri Zidenberg-Cherr
Department of Nutrition
University of California
Davis, CA 95616

Foreword

The International Life Sciences Institute (ILSI) is a nonprofit, worldwide foundation established in 1978 to advance the understanding of scientific issues relating to nutrition, food safety, toxicology, and environmental safety. By bringing together scientists from academia, government, and industry, ILSI seeks a balanced approach to solving problems with broad implications for the well-being of the general public.

ILSI's standards, the quality of the research it supports, and the worldwide as well as regional meetings and symposia it sponsors are recognized by the scientific community throughout the world. Additionally, ILSI is affiliated with the World Health Organization as a "nongovernmental organization" of international significance and has "specialized consultative status" with the Food and Agriculture Organization of the United Nations.

ILSI has branches in Australia, Europe, Japan, and North America, with branches under consideration in Latin America and elsewhere. The North American branch, known as ILSI-Nutrition Foundation, resulted from the merger, in 1985, of ILSI and The Nutrition Foundation, Inc. The latter was formed in 1941 to further the scientific understanding of nutrition, and was known for its active support of nutrition research.

Among The Nutrition Foundation's many programs was the publication of *Present Knowledge in Nutrition*, which first appeared in 1953. ILSI-Nutrition Foundation is pleased to continue the tradition of publishing this nutrition classic, which is used in classrooms, laboratories, and clinics around the world.

Alex Malaspina, President
International Life Sciences Institute

Preface

The first edition of *Present Knowledge in Nutrition* was published in 1953 by The Nutrition Foundation, Inc. That and the two successive editions comprised articles on essential nutrients that were reprinted from *Nutrition Reviews*, also a Nutrition Foundation publication. The fourth edition (1976) contained, in addition to chapters on essential nutrients, several chapters devoted to chronic diseases that were believed to involve a nutrition component. The fifth edition, published in 1984, continued along this line but also included a number of new chapters, none of which had been published previously in *Nutrition Reviews*.

Nutrition Reviews is now published by Springer-Verlag New York under the aegis of the International Life Sciences Institute–Nutrition Foundation, the North American branch of ILSI. No articles from that publication were reprinted here. The current edition of *Present Knowledge in Nutrition* includes only chapters that were written specifically for this volume.

As in the 1984 edition, a number of new chapters are included in this, the sixth edition. Additionally, the publication format was changed to accommodate the growing size of the book. Although we tried to limit the length of each chapter according to guidelines suggested by the Editorial Committee, some authors were unable to conform to the limits of the guidelines. However, we believe that the lack of conformity was, in most cases, justifiable and can be attributed to recent findings in these areas. In many other areas, there was less recent information.

I thank the members of the Editorial Committee for their suggestions on chapters to be included in this publication and on authors to write the chapters. Additionally, I want to express my gratitude to the authors who wrote the 59 chapters herein. I thank Karen Taylor, publications manager at ILSI-NF when this project began, and Roberta Gutman, current publications manager, for their support and assistance in contacting authors. My thanks also to Karen S. Dove, secretary, for her efficient and congenial support. Most especially, I thank Judith H. Dickson, copy editor, for her careful and substantive editing and for her good humor through often trying circumstances. Without their help and encouragement this volume likely would not have been born.

Myrtle L. Brown
Editor

Chapter 1

John T. Devlin and Edward S. Horton

Energy Requirements

Undernutrition remains a leading cause of mortality and morbidity in developing countries worldwide. It has been estimated that over 400 million people worldwide are undernourished,[1] and this number is expected to increase as overpopulation continues. In the United States inadequate nutrition continues to be of concern for many segments of the population, such as pregnant women, young children, elderly adults, and those living below the poverty level. National and international health policies are attempting to address the critical issue of uneven distribution of food supplies among various segments of the population.

In industrialized countries such as the United States, the major nutritional problem is one of surfeit, with excess dietary calories and fat contributing to the disproportionate increase in metabolic diseases prevalent in our society. The gift of "modernization" and technological advancement may, like the Trojan horse, carry the seeds of destruction for societies that traditionally have been free of the diseases of plenitude (obesity, noninsulin-dependent diabetes mellitus, hypertension, and hyperlipidemias). The toll for overindulgence is great both in human and in financial terms.

Energy Needs

Food is required as a fuel for the maintenance of energy-requiring processes that sustain life. Energy is required for maintaining the physiochemical environment of the intact animal, the so-called internal milieu, and for sustaining the electromechanical activities that define the organism. The major body store of energy is adenosine triphosphate (ATP) and other high-energy phosphate bonds. How efficiently a person is able to convert the potential energy available in foodstuffs into body energy stores is subject to individual variation and may explain the propensity toward or resistance to weight gain in different

subjects over a long period of time. The so-called thrifty gene may have had survival value for Native American Indians subject to harsh desert conditions with limited available food sources. However, such metabolic efficiency may be considered maladaptive in present-day America, where food is plentiful and obesity is nearly endemic. Differences between lean and obese individuals in Na^+-K^+ ATPase pump activity, thermogenic responses to various hormonal and environmental stimuli, and possibly in substrate cycle activity may help us understand the biochemical nature of this metabolic efficiency.[2] As emphasized by Sims,[3] any discussion of obesity must acknowledge the heterogeneity present in obese individuals and may help to explain some of the divergent results reported in various studies.

Energy Balance

The first law of thermodynamics, that of conservation of energy, appears to hold for intact living organisms. In the late 18th century, Lavoisier made the landmark discovery that the life-sustaining process of respiration was merely a form of chemical combustion and as such was capable of precise measurement. By the end of the next century, Rubner[4] was measuring the excretion rates of expired carbon dioxide and urinary nitrogen to estimate energy expenditure in human subjects. This method, known as indirect calorimetry, estimates metabolic rate from measurements of oxygen consumption and carbon dioxide production. When urinary nitrogen excretion is measured, the net rates of substrate oxidation also can be calculated by using the tables of Lusk.[5]

For measurements of resting metabolic rate (RMR) in a supine, resting subject, the ventilated-hood system was shown to be capable of high degrees of accuracy (2–5%) with minimal inconvenience to the subject during relatively long-term measurements (several hours).[6] A steady state of carbon dioxide production and respiratory exchange must be reached, and subjects should have normal acid-base balance. For longer time periods, indirect calorimetry chambers have been used for many years. The technique was recently described by Ravussin et al.[7] The chambers are large enough to allow subjects to move freely and perform normal daily activities (i.e., sleeping, eating, and mild exercise) and to allow for precise measurement of energy expenditure over 24 h. An advantage of the chamber is the ability to estimate physical activity with a radar-detection device.

The doubly labeled water technique, using $^2H_2$ and ^{18}O labeled water, has been shown to be capable of accurately measuring energy expenditure in free-living subjects over a period of several weeks.[8] This technique offers the potential for more prolonged studies in subjects engaged in normal daily activities but is not widely available because of cost and the requirement for an isotope ratio mass spectrometry facility.

Direct calorimetry is probably the most accurate method for measuring energy expenditure (capable of only 1–2% error) but also is not widely used because of cost, limited chamber size, and slow response time. In addition, since the time of Atwater and Benedict,[9] many investigators have demonstrated the close correlation between direct and indirect calorimetric measurements. Consequently, the former method is seldom utilized in present-day research studies. A novel version of the direct calorimeter, the space suit described by Webb, is intriguing but is still in the experimental stage.[10]

Energy Intake. Energy intake is a highly variable component of the energy balance equation and may be very important in the causation and maintenance of the obese state (*see* Chapter 3). In addition to total energy intake, Danforth[11] emphasized the importance of the composition of food intake in the pathogenesis of obesity. This factor will be discussed in greater detail below (*Thermic effect of food*).

Energy Expenditure. Energy expenditure includes several components: RMR, the thermic effect of exercise, the thermic effect of food (formerly known as specific dynamic action), and facultative thermogenesis (also known as adaptive thermogenesis). Each of these components will be discussed below.

Resting metabolic rate. RMR is usually the greatest contributor (60–75%) to total daily energy expenditure. RMR is a measurement of the energy expended for maintenance of normal body functions and homeostasis plus a component for activation of the sympathetic nervous system. RMR is measured with the subject in a supine or sitting position in a comfortable environment several hours after the last meal or significant physical activity. The basal metabolic rate (BMR), originally defined by Boothby and San-

diford,[12] is measured in the morning upon awakening, before any physical activity, and 12–18 h after the last meal. It may be slightly lower than RMR, but the difference is small and RMR is now the more commonly used measurement. Several factors are known to influence the RMR, including nutritional state, thyroid function, and sympathetic nervous system activity. Differences in RMR due to differences in body size, sex, or age are largely corrected if the data are related to fat-free mass (FFM).[7] Most studies do not find a difference between lean and obese subjects when RMR is expressed per kg FFM. This lack of difference highlights the importance of accurate body composition measurements (*see* Chapter 2) when comparing different groups of subjects in the ongoing search for clues to explain and correct the obese state. The decrease in RMR with aging is explained largely by decreases in lean body mass. Women also have lower RMRs than men because of smaller body size, although the RMR seems to vary with the menstrual cycle.[13]

It was shown that differences in FFM, age, and sex may account for 83% of the variance in RMR between different individuals.[7] Of great importance, family membership contributes an additional 11% to the variance in RMR per kg FFM. Similar findings of a genetic component to RMR were reported in monozygotic twins[14] and in retrospective studies of adopted children in Denmark.[15] Subjects with lower RMRs appear to be more susceptible to weight gain over the period of followup both in adult[16] and pediatric populations.[17] The authors speculate that weight gain in such subjects would reach a plateau once the increase in lean body mass and energy cost of bodily movement brought subjects into energy balance. This theory suggests one mechanism for positive energy balance and weight gain over a long period of time in genetically susceptible individuals.

RMR is dependent also on thyroid hormone status and sympathetic nervous system (SNS) activity. The major clinical use of energy expenditure measurements during the early part of this century was to diagnose over- and underactivity of the thyroid gland. Recent studies showed a relationship between RMR and rates of norepinephrine turnover by use of infusions of radioactive norepinephrine, which is a better index of SNS activity than is measurement of catecholamine concentration in plasma. Chronic administration (2 wk) of the β-adrenergic agonist terbutaline increases RMR by 8% in humans,[18] whereas pharmacologic blockade of the SNS by the acute administration of α- and β-blocking drugs appears to have little effect on RMR.[19]

Thermic effect of exercise. Thermic effect of exercise (TEE) is the second largest component of energy expenditure. It represents the cost of physical activity above basal levels. In a moderately active individual it comprises 15–30% of total energy requirements. Of all the compartments of energy expenditure, TEE is most variable and, therefore, most amenable to alteration. Increases in energy expenditure 10–15 times above the RMR can be achieved with intense exercise. Few, if any, factors appear to affect TEE except the amount of work done. Several studies have compared TEE in lean and obese subjects, and in most cases no differences in the efficiency of exercise were found when the energy cost of moving the increased body weight of obese subjects was taken into account.[20] Previous exercise may increase metabolic rate for at least 18 h[21] and potentiates the thermic response to insulin-glucose infusions for >14 h.[22]

The degree of spontaneous physical activity appears to be another variable that may allow for positive energy balance and weight gain in subjects prone to obesity. Earlier studies suggested that obese girls were less active during periods of recreation than were their lean schoolmates.[23] Using the indirect calorimetry chamber, Ravussin et al.[7] demonstrated a wide range in spontaneous physical activity, termed *fidgeting*, among individuals. Fidgeting accounted for between 100 and 800 kcal/d in their subjects.

Thermic effect of food. The thermic effect of food (TEF) refers to the increase in energy expenditure above RMR that occurs for several hours after the ingestion of a meal. The earlier term *specific dynamic action* was initially applied to dietary protein, but it is now recognized that ingestion of each macronutrient (protein, fat, and carbohydrate) results in a thermogenic effect. The TEF is the result of energy expended to digest, transport, metabolize, and store food. On average the TEF accounts for ~10% of daily energy expenditure but differs depending on the metabolic fate of ingested substrate. The cost of storing the fat contained in a meal in adipose tissue requires only 3% of the energy content of a meal. If glucose is directly oxidized, all of the available energy is used, whereas if it is first stored directly as glycogen, there is a loss of 7% of the available energy.[24] Evidence suggests that only about one-third of liver glycogen repletion in 24-h starved rats occurs via the direct pathway from glucose; the remainder comes from triose phosphate intermediates and other mechanisms.[25] The cost of this indirect pathway of glycogenesis from triose phosphate intermediates is greater than the cost of direct synthesis of glycogen from glucose.

Theoretically, excess dietary carbohydrate can result in de novo lipogenesis resulting in an increase in adipose tissue stores. However, this process is energy inefficient, requiring 26% of the ingested calories.[24] In addition, it was shown that carbohydrate overfeeding results in very little net lipogenesis over 24 h.[26] Thus, fat balance remains negative at least in the short term after carbohydrate overfeeding, because lipid oxidation continues. These considerations led Danforth[11] to conclude that the composition of the diet is at least as important as the energy content in determining whether a positive fat balance is maintained. Of the three macronutrients, protein produces the greatest TEF.[27] This effect appears to be due to the high energy cost of protein synthesis and degradation, which is ~24% of available energy.

SNS appears to play an important role in TEF, especially after carbohydrate ingestion. Glucose ingestion and intravenous glucose-insulin infusions result in a 5–7% increase in energy expenditure above RMR, and up to 70% of this increase can be inhibited by administration of β-adrenergic blocking drugs such as propranolol.[19,28] Increases in norepinephrine appearance correlate with the thermic response to a meal. Although subjects with insulin resistance demonstrate a decreased TEF, this impairment becomes normal if either insulin or glucose concentrations are increased sufficiently to result in normal rates of glucose disposal.[29] TEF after fructose ingestion, which does not require insulin for cellular uptake, is normal in insulin-resistant subjects, again suggesting that the major determinant of TEF after carbohydrate ingestion is substrate metabolism rather than insulin secretion or action per se. Whether previous studies demonstrated a decreased TEF in obese compared with lean subjects may have depended on the degree of insulin resistance present in the obese group.[30] Insulin is capable of directly stimulating sodium-potassium ATPase pump activity, and may exert thermogenic effects by direct stimulation of insulin-sensitive areas of the hypothalamus.[31]

TEF is highly variable among different individuals, and even repeated measurements in the same individual under the same laboratory and nutrient conditions demonstrate a high degree of variability. Therefore, studies comparing the TEF between different populations, such as lean and obese subjects, must be interpreted cautiously.

Facultative thermogenesis. The final component of energy expenditure, facultative thermogenesis, is readily demonstrable in animals but is less well described in humans. It appears to account for ≤10–15% of total daily energy expenditure but may have significant effects on long-term weight changes. Facultative thermogenesis is the change in energy induced by changes in ambient temperature, food intake, emotional stress, and other factors. The best-described version of facultative thermogenesis is nonshivering thermogenesis in rodents exposed to cold environments, during which heat production is increased via SNS stimulation of brown adipose tissue (BAT). BAT mitochondria have a unique proton conductance mechanism that allows them to reversibly uncouple oxidation from ADP phosphorylation.[32] Under stimulation of the SNS, the intracellular concentration of free fatty acids is increased and proton conductance is uncoupled. Both thyroid hormone and insulin are required for norepinephrine to increase BAT thermogenesis.[33] Glucagon may contribute to thermogenesis directly or indirectly by increasing catecholamine concentrations. The role of BAT in facultative thermogenesis in adult humans is questionable and probably is small in magnitude,[34] although BAT was histologically identified in adults chronically exposed to cold outdoor temperatures.[35] Use of immunocytochemical techniques demonstrated the presence of the mitochondrial uncoupling protein with a molecular weight of 32,000 in adult humans.[36] Intriguingly, elevated catecholamine concentrations in pheochromocytoma were shown to increase thermogenesis in the intraabdominal adipose tissue sites that are the same sites containing BAT in infants.[37]

Another form of facultative thermogenesis that is consistently demonstrated in man occurs with altered levels of nutritional intake. Decreased energy intakes for prolonged periods result in a progressive decrease in RMR that is greater than can be accounted for by decreases in FFM. Associated with decreased energy intake is reduced insulin secretion and reduced activity of 5'-monodeiodinase, which converts the primary thyroid gland secretagogue (3,3',5,5'-tetraiodothyronine, T_4) to the metabolically active thyroid hormone (3,3',5-triiodothyronine, T_3).[38] Dietary carbohydrate is the primary nutrient regulating plasma concentrations of T_3. Recently, Danforth[39] demonstrated that energy balance is more important than the absolute rate of energy intake or expenditure in altering T_3 concentrations. The decrease in T_3 is not entirely responsible for the decreased RMR during fasting, because restoring T_3 concentration to normal does not increase the RMR of starved rats.[40] Both an increase in T_3 and nutrient ingestion are required for the increase in RMR to occur with refeeding. Underfeeding decreases the activity of the SNS, as determined by norepinephrine-turnover studies.[41] The finding that RMR may remain depressed for prolonged periods after dietary stabilization after rapid weight-reduction programs sounds a cautionary note regarding the clinical application of very-low-calorie diets.[42] In obese subjects undergoing a more gradual and conservative weight-loss program, energy expenditure per kg FFM did not diminish.[43]

Experimental overfeeding in man has provided some valuable insights. Neumann[44] first used the term *luxus consumption* in 1902, and in the same year Rubner[4] in studies with dogs described the process whereby overfed lean animals were able to dissipate the increased energy intake through heat loss. Although the convincing demonstration of this process in long-term studies has been difficult, studies yielding negative results have been criticized for inadequate duration or magnitude of overfeeding. As pointed out by Garrow,[45] there appears to be a threshold of ~20,000 kcal for the demonstration of luxus consumption in humans. In a review of earlier studies of overfeeding, Webb[46] concluded that only about half of the weight gain predicted from the composition of increased body weight actually occurred. The Vermont study of experimental overfeeding in prisoners showed that previously lean subjects required approximately twice the daily caloric intake to maintain increased body weight as did the spontaneously obese, although there was a large degree of individual variation.[47] These subjects had little difficulty losing the excess weight when the period of overfeeding ended. As alluded to above, the composition of the diet appears to play an important role in the facility of weight gain, with fat overfeeding resulting in more efficient weight gain than overfeeding a mixed diet.

With regard to the mechanisms of luxus consumption, increases in thyroid hormone concentrations and SNS activity appear to play important roles. As mentioned above, carbohydrate is the major nutrient increasing T_3 production. Current attention is being focused on the activity of substrate cycles, such as the Cori cycle (glucose to lactate to glucose) and glucose (glucose to glucose-6-phosphate) and fructose (fructose-1-phosphate to fructose-1,6-diphosphate) cycles to explain differences in energetics with altered nutritional states. Newsholme[48] points out that such cycles, formerly called futile cycles, are far from futile and probably play important roles in finely regulating substrate fluxes in opposing directions. Recent studies demonstrated increased activity of glucose and fructose cycles in experimental hyperthyroidism[49] and increased activity of the lipid cycle (lipolysis to reesterification) in burn patients.[50] The latter was shown to be partly under the influence of the SNS and was partially inhibited by administration of propranolol. As mentioned above, the sodium-potassium ATPase pump is under the influence of hormonal regulation, with thyroid hormones, insulin, phosphatidylinositol, and possibly norepinephrine exerting effects on pump activity.[51]

The extent to which defective facultative thermogenesis can contribute to or maintain the obese state was briefly commented on in relation to TEF. Impairments in TEF during feeding or insulin-glucose infusions in obesity appear to be largely secondary to insulin resistance and decreased glucose disposal and are improved by treatments such as diet and exercise that improve insulin sensitivity.[52] Whether differences in substrate-cycle activity in either the fasting or postprandial state can explain a tendency toward weight gain in obesity requires further studies. Genetics appears to play an important role in determining the metabolic adaptation as demonstrated by overfeeding of twins by the group of Laval University.[14]

Summary

Although there are large interindividual differences in energy requirements, much of the variance can be accounted for by FFM, age, sex, and the level of physical activity. Genetic factors also appear to play an important role. Determining which factors help to explain the development or perpetuation of the obese state requires further investigation, but greater understanding will likely follow the improvements in technical capabilities and better-designed and controlled long-term studies in obese subjects. Because of an epidemic of the associated metabolic diseases in Western societies, this improved understanding is essential for the health of the population.

References

1. D.M. Hegsted (1984) Energy requirements. In: *Present Knowledge in Nutrition*, 5th ed. (R.E. Olson, H.P. Broquist, C.O. Chichester, W.J. Darby, A.C. Kolbye, Jr., and R.M. Stalvey, eds.), pp. 1–6, The Nutrition Foundation, Washington, DC.
2. M. DeLuise, G.L. Blackburn, and J.S. Flier (1980) Reduced activity of the red-cell sodium-potassium pump in human obesity. *N. Engl. J. Med.* 303:1017–1022.
3. E.A.H. Sims (1982) Characterization of the syndromes of obesity. In: *Diabetes Mellitus and Obesity* (B.N. Brodoff and S.J. Bleicher, eds.), pp. 219–226, Williams and Wilkins, Baltimore, MD.
4. M. Rubner (1902) Die Gesetze des Energieverbrauchs bei der Ernahrung, Deutiche, Leipzig.
5. G. Lusk (1924) Animal calorimetry: analysis of the oxidation of mixtures of carbohydrate and fat. *J. Biol. Chem.* 59:41–42.
6. E. Jequier (1981) Long-term measurement of energy expenditure in man: direct or indirect calorimetry? In: *Recent Advances in Obesity Research III* (G.A. Bray, ed.), pp. 130–135, Newman, London.
7. E. Ravussin, S. Lillioja, T.E. Anderson, L. Christin, and C. Bogardus (1986) Determinants of 24-hour energy expenditure in man: methods and results using a respiratory chamber. *J. Clin. Invest.* 78: 1568–1578.
8. D.A. Schoeller and P. Webb (1986) Five-day comparison of the doubly labelled water method with respiratory gas exchange. *Am. J. Clin. Nutr.* 40:153–158.
9. W.O. Atwater and F.G. Benedict (1905) A respiration calorimeter with appliances for the direct determination of oxygen. Publication 42, Carnegie Institute of Washington, Washington, DC.
10. P. Webb, J.F. Annis, and S.J. Troutman (1980) Energy balance in man measured by direct and indirect calorimetry. *Am. J. Clin. Nutr.* 33:1287–1298.
11. E. Danforth (1985) Diet and obesity. *Am. J. Clin. Nutr.* 41:1132–1145.
12. W.M. Boothby and I. Sandiford (1929) Normal values for standard metabolism. *Am. J. Physiol.* 90:290–291.
13. S.J. Solomon, M.S. Kurzer, and D.H. Calloway (1982) Menstrual cycle and basal metabolic rate in women. *Am. J. Clin. Nutr.* 36: 611–616.
14. C. Bouchard, A. Tremblay, J-P. Despres, et al. (1988) Sensitivity to overfeeding: the Quebec experiment with identical twins. *Prog. Food Nutr. Sci.* 12:45–72.
15. A.J. Stunkard, T.I.A. Sorensen, C. Hanis, et al. (1986) An adoption study of human obesity. *N. Engl. J. Med.* 314:193–198.
16. E. Ravussin, S. Lillioja, W.C. Knowler, et al. (1988) Reduced rate of energy expenditure as a risk factor for body-weight gain. *N. Engl. J. Med.* 318:467–472.
17. S.B. Roberts, J. Savage, W.A. Coward, et al. (1988) Energy expenditure and intake in infants born to lean and overweight mothers. *N. Engl. J. Med.* 318:461–466.
18. K. Scheidegger, M. O'Connell, D.C. Robbins, et al. (1984) Effects of chronic beta-receptor stimulation on sympathetic nervous system activity, energy expenditure, and thyroid hormones. *J. Clin. Endocrinol. Metab.* 58:895–903.
19. R.A. DeFronzo, D. Thorin, J.P. Felber, et al. (1984) Effect of beta and alpha adrenergic blockade on glucose-induced thermogenesis in man. *J. Clin. Invest.* 73:633–639.
20. G.A. Bray, B.J. Whipp, and S.N. Koyal (1974) The acute effects of food intake on energy expenditure during cycle ergometry. *Am. J. Clin. Nutr.* 27:254–259.
21. R. Bielinski, Y. Schutz, and E. Jequier (1985) Energy metabolism during the postexercise recovery in man. *Am. J. Clin. Nutr.* 42: 69–82.
22. J.T. Devlin and E.S. Horton (1986) Potentiation of the thermic effect of insulin by exercise: differences between lean, obese, and non-insulin-dependent men. *Am. J. Clin. Nutr.* 43:884–890.
23. B.A. Bullen, R.B. Reed, and J. Mayer (1964) Physical activity of obese and nonobese adolescent girls appraised by motion picture sampling. *Am. J. Clin. Nutr.* 14:211–223.
24. J.-P. Flatt (1987) Dietary fat, carbohydrate balance, and weight maintenance: effects of exercise? *Am. J. Clin. Nutr.* 45:296–306.
25. J. Katz and J.D. McGarry (1984) The glucose paradox: is glucose a substrate for liver metabolism. *J. Clin. Invest.* 74:1901–1909.
26. K. Acheson, T. Schutz, E. Bessard, et al. (1984) Nutritional influences on lipogenesis and thermogenesis after a carbohydrate meal. *Am. J. Physiol.* 246:E62–70.
27. K.S. Nair, D. Halliday, and J.S. Garrow (1983) Thermic response to isoenergetic protein, carbohydrate or fat meals in lean and obese subjects. *Clin. Sci.* 65:307–312.
28. K. Acheson, E. Jequier, and J. Wahren (1983) Influence of beta-adrenergic blockade on glucose-induced thermogenesis in man. *J. Clin. Invest.* 72:981–986.
29. E. Ravussin, K.J. Acheson, O. Vernet, E. Danforth, and E. Jequier (1985) Evidence that insulin resistance is responsible for the decreased thermic effect of glucose in human obesity. *J. Clin. Invest.* 76:1268–1273.
30. E. Ravussin, K.J. Acheson, O. Vernet, et al. (1985) Evidence that insulin resistance is responsible for the decreased thermic effect of glucose in human obesity. *J. Clin. Invest.* 76:1268–1273.
31. N.K. Rosic, M.L. Standaert, and R.J. Pollet (1985) The mechanism of insulin stimulation of (Na$^+$,K$^+$)-ATPase transport activity in muscle. *J. Biol. Chem.* 260:6206–6212.
32. D.G. Nicholls and R. Locke (1984) Thermogenic mechanisms in brown fat. *Physiol. Rev.* 64:1–64.
33. J. Himms-Hagen (1984) Thermogenesis in brown adipose tissue as an energy buffer. *N. Engl. J. Med.* 311:1549–1558.
34. A.J. Astrup, J. Bulow, J. Madsen, et al. (1985) Contribution of BAT and skeletal muscle to thermogenesis induced by ephedrine in man. *Am. J. Physiol.* 248:E507–E515.
35. J.M. Heaton (1972) The distribution of brown adipose tissue in the human. *J. Anat.* 112:35–39.
36. M.E.J. Lean and W.P.T. James (1983) Uncoupling proteins in hu-

man brown adipose tissue mitochondria: isolation and detection by specific antiserum. *FEBS Lett.* 163:235–240.

37. M.E.J. Lean, W.P.T. James, G. Jennings, et al. (1986) Brown adipose tissue in patients with phaeochromocytoma. *Int. J. Obes.* 10:219–227.

38. A. Burger, M. O'Connell, K. Scheidegger, et al. (1987) Monodeiodination of triiodothyronine and reverse triiodothyronine during low and high calorie diets. *J. Clin. Endocrinol. Metab.* 65:829–835.

39. E. Danforth (1989) Hormonal adaptation to energy balance and imbalance and the regulation of energy expenditure. In: *Hormones, Thermogenesis, and Obesity* (H.A. Lardy and F. Stratman, eds.), pp. 19–32, Elsevier, New York.

40. A.G. Burger, M. Berger, K. Wimpfheimer, et al. (1980) Interrelationships between energy metabolism during starvation in the rat. *Acta Endocrinol.* 93:322–331.

41. J. Bazelmans, P.J. Nestel, K. O'Dea, et al. (1985) Blunted norepinephrine responses to changing energy states in obese subjects. *Metabolism* 34:154–160.

42. C.A. Greissler, D.S. Miller, and M. Shah (1987) The daily metabolic rate of the postobese and the lean. *Am. J. Clin. Nutr.* 45:914–920.

43. M.-U. Yang, S. Heshka, and F.X. Pi-Sunyer (1988) Resting metabolic rate after weight loss in obese patients. *Clin. Res.* 36:774A (abstr).

44. R.O. Neumann (1902) Experimentalle Beitrage zur Lehre von dem taglichen Nahrungsbedarf der Menschen unter besonder Berucksichtigung der notwendigen Eisweissmenge. *Arch. Hyg.* 45:1–2.

45. J.S. Garrow (1978) The regulation of energy expenditure in man. In: *Recent Advances in Obesity Research II* (G.A. Bray, ed.), pp. 200–236, Newman, London.

46. P. Webb (1980) The measurement of energy exchange in man: an analysis. *Am. J. Clin. Nutr.* 33:1299–1310.

47. E.A.H. Sims (1976) Experimental obesity, dietary induced thermogenesis and their clinical implications. *Clin. Endocrinol. Metab.* 5:377–395.

48. E.A. Newsholme (1980) A possible metabolic basis for the control of body weight. *N. Engl. J. Med.* 302:400–405.

49. G.I. Shulman, P.W. Landenson, M.H. Wolfe, et al. (1985) Substrate cycling between gluconeogenesis and glycolysis in euthyroid, hypothyroid, and hyperthyroid man. *J. Clin. Invest.* 76:757–764.

50. R.R. Wolfe, D.N. Herndon, F. Jahoor, et al. (1987) Effect of severe burn injury on substrate cycling by glucose and fatty acids. *N. Engl. J. Med.* 317:403–408.

51. D.A. Simmons, E.F.O. Kern, A.I. Winegrad, et al. (1986) Basal phosphatidylinositol turnover controls aortic Na^+/K^+ ATPase activity. *J. Clin. Invest.* 77:503–513.

52. E. Ravussin, C. Bogardus, R.S. Schwartz, et al. (1983) Thermic effect of infused glucose and insulin in man: decreased response with increased insulin resistance in obesity and non-insulin-dependent diabetes mellitus. *J. Clin. Invest.* 72:893–902.

Chapter 2

Gilbert B. Forbes

Body Composition

The late 19th-century and early 20th-century biochemists realized that neutral fat did not bind water or electrolytes and hence suggested that tissue composition be calculated on a fat-free basis. Under the assumption that the lean body mass (or as some prefer, the fat-free mass) of the entire body has a constant composition, investigators have used modern techniques to estimate the size of the lean body mass (LBM) by assaying the body content of one of its components.[1] We now have methods for determining body fluid volumes, body density, and total body potassium so that estimates of LBM and body fat can be made in a nonhazardous manner. As a result we now have a great deal of information on these two body components for both normal and diseased individuals.

LBM is defined as body weight minus ether-extractable fat and is thus synonymous with fat-free mass (FFM). The structural lipids contained in cell walls and nerve elements are neglected because the amounts of these components are very small in comparison with neutral fat. Body cell mass (BCM) consists of the cellular components of muscle, viscera, blood, and brain, i.e., "the working, energy-metabolizing portion of the human body in relation to its supporting structures."[2] BCM is estimated by multiplying total body potassium by the reciprocal of the average intracellular K concentration:

$$BCM \text{ (kg)} = \text{total K (mmol)} \times 0.00833$$

Neutron-activation techniques can assess total body content of calcium, phosphorus, nitrogen, sodium, and chloride. Recently some additional techniques have been developed that are currently under study: electrical conductivity and impedance, computerized tomography, photon absorptiometry, and nuclear magnetic resonance. Meanwhile anthropometric techniques have been subjected to intense study, and it has been known for a long time that the metabolic balance technique can estimate changes in body content (but not total body content) of a number of elements.[1,3]

Methods

Table 1 lists the currently available techniques for estimating body composition together with the advantages and disadvantages of each. Some are suitable only for the research laboratory. A frequently used technique is that of anthropometry: skinfold thickness (actually a double layer of skin plus subcutaneous tissue) is determined at various sites, most commonly at the triceps and subscapular sites and circumferences of the arm, abdomen, thigh, and buttocks. Although this technique is best suited for field work and for the assessment of large numbers of individuals, the skinfold method suffers from lack of precision and from the basic uncertainty of the ratio of subcutaneous fat to total body fat. Recent observations by computed axial tomography (CAT) scan suggest that the ratio of intraabdominal fat to subcutaneous fat varies considerably in adults[4] and that a large share of total body fat in both men and women is to be found in the trunk and upper legs,[5,6] which are far removed from the triceps and subscapular sites.

The publications of Durnin and Womersley[7] and Pollock et al.[8] contain tables listing body fat content as a function of skinfold thickness (usually the sum of thickness at several sites). Others have used combinations of skinfold thickness, circumferences, and body weight for this purpose. The quantitative relationships between anthropometric measurements and body composition vary somewhat by age and sex and indeed among various investigators.

Because LBM comprises 70–90% of body weight in normal children and adults, it is obvious that LBM and weight will be related, and in subjects of widely varying fat content one can anticipate that body fat and weight will also be related. As will be noted later,

Table 1. Body composition techniques: advantages and disadvantages

	Advantages	Disadvantages
Density	Apparatus inexpensive Estimates LBM and fat simultaneously Nonhazardous Can be repeated frequently	Subject cooperation necessary for underwater weighing technique Unsuitable for young children and elderly people Error from intestinal gas
Dilution methods	Estimate body fluid volumes Inexpensive Great variety: determines Na, K, Cl(Br), H_2O	Radiation exposure (some materials) Blood samples needed (some materials) Incomplete equilibration of Na, K; overestimation by deuterium, tritium; value for extracellular fluid depends on method used; $^{18}O_2$ assay requires elaborate equipment
^{40}K counting	No hazard Minimal subject cooperation needed Can be repeated frequently	Instrument expensive Proper calibration necessary Problem in interpretation in subjects with K deficiency
Metabolic balance	No hazard Suitable for many elements Can detect small changes in body content (<1%)	Measures only *change* in body composition Meticulous subject cooperation required Metabolic ward expensive Error from unmeasured skin losses Many laboratory analyses needed
Creatinine excretion	No hazard Estimate of muscle mass	Meticulous subject cooperation required Influenced by diet Collection time critical Day-to-day variation (c.v. 5–10%)
Anthropometry (skinfold thickness, circumferences)	Inexpensive Direct estimate of body fat and regional muscle	Poor precision in obese subjects, and in those with firm subcutaneous tissue Regional variation in subcutaneous fat layer; uncertainty ratio subcutaneous fat:total fat
CAT scan	Delineates organ size; fat distribution; bone size	Instrument expensive Radiation exposure
Electrical conductivity (TOBEC, EMME)	No hazard Estimate of LBM	Apparatus expensive
Bioelectrical impedance	Apparatus inexpensive No hazard Estimate of LBM	Precision now under investigation
Neutron activation	Minimal subject cooperation needed Body content of Ca, P, N, Na, Cl	Apparatus very expensive Calibration very difficult Radiation exposure
Nuclear magnetic resonance	Delineates organ size, muscle, fat, fat distribution, total body water	Apparatus very expensive
Dual photon absorptiometry	Estimates bone mineral content, total and regional; body fat, soft tissue lean	Expensive Radiation exposure

LBM is a function of stature at all ages. It is obvious that measurements of skinfold thickness and abdominal and buttock circumferences will bear some relationship to body fat and that biacromial, wrist, and knee diameters will vary with LBM. Although the correlations between various anthropometric measurements and LBM or body fat are not very high (r^2 in the range of 0.4–0.8), the simplicity of the techniques means that they can be readily applied to large numbers of individuals in the field.

Cross-sectional areas of the muscle-bone component and the fat component of the arm can be calculated from arm circumference and skinfold thickness, and tables of normal values have been published.[9] However, two recent studies showed that the former area is overestimated (and especially so in obese individuals) compared with CAT-scan measurements.[10,11] Hence such anthropometric measurements are subject to variable degrees of error.

Body Density. Body density is usually determined

by weighing the subject in air and then underwater, with corrections for residual lung volume and an assumed value for intestinal gas. By use of a principle first described by Archimedes, the relative proportions of lean (in adults D = 1.100 g/cm³) and fat (D = 0.900 g/cm³) can be calculated from the observed density of the whole body. It is likely that the density of the LBM in children and in elderly adults differs from that of young and middle-aged adults. The usual formula is

$$\text{Fraction fat} = \frac{4.95}{D} - 4.50$$

Dilution Techniques. Plasma volume can be estimated with Evans blue dye (T-1824) or ^{131}I-labeled albumin, and total erythrocyte mass can be estimated with erythrocytes tagged with ^{32}P, ^{51}Cr, ^{55}Fe, or ^{59}Fe or by carbon monoxide uptake. Materials for extracellular fluid volume are inulin, SCN^-, Br^-, $^{82}Br^-$, $^{35}S_2O_3^-$, or $^{35}SO_4^{2-}$; the estimations varying somewhat among these. Total body water is estimated by deuterium, tritium, or oxygen-18 or by dilution of urea, alcohol, or N-acetyl-4-aminopyrine. Intracellular fluid volume is calculated by difference. Because ~73% of the LBM consists of water, its size can be estimated from total body water; body fat is weight minus LBM.

^{40}K Counting. The body contains enough of this naturally occurring isotope (t½ 1.3×10^9 y, body content 4 kBq) to permit its detection and quantitation by low-background scintillation counters. From the known abundance of ^{40}K (0.012%), one can calculate total body potassium content. Several types of detectors have been used; each instrument demands calibration. Once body potassium content has been determined, lean weight is calculated under the assumption that this body component has a relatively constant potassium content; body fat is the difference between body weight and LBM.

Total body potassium can also be determined by ^{42}K dilution, but because complete equilibration of the administered isotope is not achieved by the end of the usual 24-h equilibration period, it is best to designate the derived quantity as total exchangeable potassium. The very short physical half-life of ^{42}K (12 h) makes for difficulties in using this technique.

By cadaver analysis the potassium content of the LBM is 68 mmol/kg.[1] Some investigators have used this value for adult males and 64.2 for adult females,[1] whereas others use 64.5 and 58 mmol/kg, respectively,[12] or 66.4 and 59.7, respectively.[13] (It should be noted that the composition of the LBM in infants differs from adults: water content is higher, whereas potassium content and density are lower.[1])

Urine Creatinine Excretion. The assumption that urinary creatinine is an index of muscle mass is supported by the work of Schutte et al.[14] in dogs. Studies of human subjects of widely varying body size have also shown a good relationship between creatinine excretion and lean weight.[15] On the basis of human and animal data, fat-free skeletal muscle, on average, makes up 49% of total fat-free weight.[15] However, all of the published regressions of urinary creatinine excretion on LBM have positive intercepts on the y axis, so the Cr:LBM (and hence the Cr:muscle mass) is somewhat lower for individuals who excrete large amounts of creatinine than for those who excrete smaller amounts. The urine collections must be timed accurately, and the excretion rate can be affected by diet. On the basis of individuals consuming a normal diet, the relationship between muscle mass (MM) and creatinine excretion (Cr) is[1]

$$\text{MM (kg)} = 14.3 \text{ Cr (g/d)} + 3.6$$

Metabolic Balance. Although the metabolic-balance technique cannot estimate body content per se, it can detect small changes in body content of a number of elements. For example, a change in body nitrogen content of 16 g, equivalent to 0.5 kg LBM, is easily detected, whereas such a change is well within the error of body composition techniques. The drawbacks are the meticulous cooperation required of the subject, the need for a fore period to allow adjustment to a given diet, the need to estimate cutaneous losses (which are most difficult to measure), and the nonrandom nature of the intake and excretion variables, the result being that positive balances tend to be overestimated and negative balances underestimated, never the reverse.

Other Techniques. These include total-body electrical conductivity (TOBEC; estimates lean weight by electrical conductivity), bioelectrical impedance, dual photon absorptiometry, computerized tomography, and nuclear magnetic resonance (or magnetic resonance imaging). The last three provide certain advantages (which are gained at considerable expense) in that skeletal weight and body fat distribution, both internal and subcutaneous, can be estimated. All are now undergoing extensive trials.

The TOBEC instrument generates an oscillating radio frequency current (5 MHz) in a large solenoidal coil. The degree to which the induced electrical current is perturbed by a subject placed in the coil is proportional to the water content of the subject and thus to lean body weight.[16,17]

The bioelectrical impedance technique consists of passing a weak alternating current (800 µA, 50 kHz) through the body. The observed impedance is an inverse function of total body water; the results are improved by including the square of stature in the calculation.[3,18]

The technique of photon absorptiometry consists

of scanning the body with a radioactive source (gadolinium-153) that emits two gamma rays of differing energy. The attenuation of these rays by body tissues is subjected to computer analysis to yield estimates of total bone mineral, total body soft tissue, and body fat.[1,3] The instrument can also estimate vertebral bone mineral and femoral bone mineral separately if desired. The radiation dose is 0.02–0.1 mSv. The dual photon technique is superior to the technique employing a single photon source (iodine-125 or americium-241), which has been widely used for estimating mineral content of individual bones.

Computerized axial tomography can delineate organ size, regional fat depots, and skeletal size. Multiple cuts are needed to assess the entire body, so the radiation exposure is appreciable.

Neutron activation involves exposing the entire body to a known flux of neutrons and measuring the induced radioactivity. This can yield estimates of total-body calcium, phosphorus, nitrogen, sodium, chlorine, and carbon. The apparatus is intricate, expensive, and difficult to calibrate; there are only a few such instruments in operation in the entire world. Surprisingly, the radiation dose to the subject is rather small, ~0.3 mGy.[1,3]

The principle of nuclear magnetic resonance is beyond the scope of this article. It offers the opportunity of delineating organ size and structure, body fat distribution, total body water, and muscle size, all without radiation exposure. It is, of course, very expensive.

In the process of applying any of the above-mentioned techniques, it must be remembered that all are subject to technical error, variously estimated at 2–6%. None is foolproof, and each one demands practice and attention to detail to achieve worthwhile results.

Variations in LBM and Body Fat

Age and Sex. Table 2 lists average values for selected age groups. The onset of puberty is accompanied by a spurt in LBM, which is more intense in boys, and an increase in body fat especially in girls; the end result is that adult women have only about two-thirds as much LBM as men while having a larger percent body fat. Indeed, in young adults the sex difference in LBM (M:F 1.4) is relatively greater than the difference in stature (ratio 1.08) or in body weight (ratio 1.25). The sex ratio for urinary creatinine excretion (an index of muscle mass) is 1.5. During the later adult years both sexes experience a modest decline in LBM. These are, of course, average values, and it has been established that both LBM and body fat show considerable variability as does body weight.

When subjects of a given age, sex, and height are analyzed, LBM exhibits much less variability than body fat, and hence it is fat that accounts for much of the variability in body weight.

Stature. At all ages thus far examined LBM is a function of stature. On average the regression slope is 0.69 kg LBM/cm in adult males and 0.29 kg/cm in adult females.[1] Skeletal size is also a function of height as is total-body calcium, the regression slope being 20 g calcium/cm height.[1] On the basis of these findings, a 186-cm male would be expected to have ~1370 g calcium in his body and a 154-cm woman to have only 730 g calcium.

Race. Orientals are usually shorter and lighter than Caucasians, so it is to be expected that they would have a smaller lean weight. North American blacks, on the other hand, tend to have a slightly larger LBM than do whites and more total-body calcium. The studies of Cohn et al[19] on adult subjects showed black:white of 1.15 for total body potassium and 1.17 for total body calcium for males; these were, respectively, 1.17 and 1.22 for females, whereas that for stature was only 1.01.

Heredity. It is well known that weight and height are under genetic influence. Studies have shown that the same is true for LBM, total body fat, and skinfold thickness.[20]

Pregnancy. Of the total weight gain during pregnancy, some 12–13 kg on average, the fetus, placenta, and amniotic fluid together comprise ~4.2 kg; the remaining 8 kg is maternal tissue per se. Plasma volume and extracellular and intracellular fluid volumes all increase, and because the ratio of body water to body potassium increases, the increase in extracellular fluid volume is proportionately greater than that of intracellular fluid volume, which is in keeping with the observation that many pregnant women have mild edema. A portion of the weight gain—variously estimated at 2–4 kg—consists of fat.

Table 2. Average values for weight, LBM, and percent fat as a function of age

	Newborn	10-y-old boy	10-y-old girl	15-y-old boy	15-y-old girl	Adult man	Adult woman
Weight (kg)	3.4	31	32	60	54	72	58
LBM (kg)	2.9	27	26	51	40	61	42
Percent fat	14	13	19	13	26	15	28

Some Correlates of Body Composition

Because the adult female has only about two-thirds as much LBM as the male, it is obvious that the requirements for protein and energy are correspondingly less. The Recommended Dietary Allowances of the National Research Council reflect this sex difference.[21] Basal metabolic rate is more closely related to LBM than it is to body weight. It would seem prudent to adjust the dose of certain drugs, i.e., those that do not distribute in body fat, on the basis of LBM rather than body weight.

Body fat stores serve an important function in times of energy deprivation. It is well known that obese individuals can tolerate much longer fasts than can those who are thin. In individuals given 1400–1900 kcal diets, LBM accounted for about half of the total weight loss in those who were thin but only ~20% in those who were obese.[1] Obese individuals preferentially burn fat and so tend to conserve lean tissue when faced with an energy deficit.

Influence of Nutrition

The availability of modern body-composition techniques has made it possible to study the long-term changes in body composition without having to deal with the technical problems inherent in the metabolic-balance method. It is the long-term change, whether it be weight loss or weight gain, that deserves consideration. Of paramount importance to the modern nutritional scene is the matter of energy balance.

Energy Deficit. Generally speaking, the rate of weight loss is proportional to the energy deficit: individuals who fast lose weight more rapidly than those given submaintenance amounts of food. Careful studies of underfed subjects have shown that weight reduction involves a loss of both LBM and fat. The relative contribution of each of these components to the total weight loss depends on two factors: the initial body fat content and the magnitude of the energy deficit. For example, thin individuals who fast lose twice as much nitrogen per kilogram of weight loss as do obese individuals, and as noted earlier thin individuals consuming 1400–1900 kcal diets have a relatively greater loss of LBM per unit weight loss than do obese individuals.[22]

The second factor is equally important: for all categories of initial body fat content studied to date, the $\Delta LBM:\Delta W$ is directly related to the magnitude of the energy deficit.[22] This ratio is highest in those who fast and progressively decreases, i.e., more lean is conserved, as more food is consumed. One searches in vain for well-controlled studies showing that body nitrogen and LBM can be completely preserved on low-energy diets, a conclusion reached many years ago by Calloway and Spector.[23] Such losses do tend to diminish with time, however, and so does the rate of weight loss.

Obese patients subjected to intestinal bypass or gastric stapling operations also lose LBM as they lose weight; in various studies LBM comprises 15–40% of the total weight loss.[22]

Energy Excess. When undernourished individuals are induced to gain weight, both LBM and fat increase. It is important to recognize that the same thing happens when normal individuals are overfed. A compilation of studies from several sources shows that the amount of weight gain experienced during deliberate overfeeding of normal adults is directly proportional to the total excess energy consumed during the overfeeding period.[1] The average energy cost of the weight gain was 8 kcal/g gain. Moreover, about a third of the gain consisted of LBM. It goes without saying that such diets must be adequate in protein and other essentials.

When observations on diet-induced weight loss and weight gain are considered in toto, it is apparent that LBM and fat are in a sense companions; a change in one is accompanied by a change in the other, although not always in the same proportion.

Body Composition in Obesity. Except in rare instances human obesity can develop only in the face of a positive energy balance, so in this sense it is a nutritional disease. Obese children tend to be tall for age, and studies of obese children, adolescents, and adults show that a portion of their excess weight (10–30%) consists of LBM. Such data can only be inter-

Table 3. Reference man and woman: total body content*

Substance	Male	Female
Water	45,000 g (2500 mol)	31,000 g (1700 mol)
Hydrogen, nonaqueous	2,000 g (1000 mol)	—
Oxygen, nonaqueous	2,900 g (90 mol)	—
Carbon	16,000 g (1333 mol)	
Nitrogen	1,800 g (64 mol)	1,300 g (46 mol)
Calcium	1,100 g (27 mol)	830 g (21 mol)
Phosphorus	500 g (16 mol)	400 g (13 mol)
Potassium	140 g (3600 mmol)	100 g (2560 mmol)
Sodium	100 g (4170 mmol)	77 g (3200 mmol)
Chlorine	95 g (2680 mmol)	70 g (2000 mmol)
Sulfur	140 g (4400 mmol)	—
Magnesium	19 g (780 mmol)	—
Silicon	18 g (640 mmol)	—
Iron	4.2 g (75 mmol)	—
Fluorine	2.6 g (140 mmol)	—
Zinc	2.3 g (35 mmol)	—
Copper	0.07 g (1.1 mmol)	—
Manganese	0.01 g (180 μmol)	—
Iodine	0.01 g (79 μmol)	—

* Seventeen additional elements (all < 330 mg) are listed in reference 24. For many the body content is a function of diet.

preted to mean that obese individuals are overnourished. The exceptions are individuals with increased adrenocortical activity and those given diets that are high in energy and very low in protein; under these circumstances body fat increases at the expense of the LBM.

The situation is quite different in animals that become obese after experimentally induced hypothalamic lesions and in Zucker rats. These animals tend to be stunted and to have a smaller LBM than do controls[1] and, hence, cannot serve as proper models for human obesity.

Body Composition in Undernutrition. Patients with anorexia nervosa have a reduction in both body fat and LBM. Generally, extracellular fluid volume tends to be better preserved than intracellular fluid volume in undernourished states so that the ratio of extracellular to intracellular fluid volume is increased. In severe malnutrition, especially when complicated by trauma or infection, body cells have reduced amounts of potassium, phosphorus, and magnesium and increased amounts of sodium.

Other Influences. Physical activity contributes to the stability of the LBM. LBM tends to diminish during bed rest and in the absence of gravity. Vigorous and sustained exercise results in an increase in LBM (though the changes are of modest degree) and a decrease in body fat. The larger LBM and smaller body fat content of many athletes probably represents the combined influences of heredity and prolonged physical training.

The most striking effects are those produced by the administration of anabolic steroids, large doses of which result in greater increases in LBM than any recorded thus far from exercise alone.[1]

Table 3 lists the multitude of elements to be found in the body of a male adult (the so-called reference man) as compiled by the International Committee on Radiation Protection.[24] I have added some values for certain elements for the average woman as determined by body composition assays.

References

1. G.B. Forbes (1987) *Human Body Composition: Growth, Aging, Nutrition, and Activity*, Springer-Verlag, New York.
2. F.D. Moore, K.H. Olesen, J.D. McMurrey, H.V. Parker, M.R. Ball, and C.M. Boyden, eds. (1963) *The Body Cell Mass and Its Supporting Environment: Body Composition in Health and Disease*, W.B. Saunders Co., Philadelphia.
3. H.C. Lukaski (1987) Methods for the assessment of human body composition: traditional and new. *Am. J. Clin. Nutr.* 46:537–556.
4. G.A. Borkan, S.G. Gerzof, A.H. Robbins, D.E. Hults, C.K. Silbert, and J.E. Silbert (1982) Assessment of abdominal fat by computed tomography. *Am. J. Clin. Nutr.* 36:172–177.
5. L. Sjöström, H. Kvist, A. Cederblad, and U. Tylén (1986) Determination of total adipose tissue and body fat in women by computed tomography, ^{40}K and tritium. *Am. J. Physiol.* 250:E736–E745.
6. H. Kvist, B. Chowdhury, L. Sjöström, U. Tylén, and A. Cederblad (1988) Adipose tissue volume determination in males by computed tomography and ^{40}K. *Int. J. Obesity* 12:249–266.
7. J.V.G.A. Durnin and J. Womersley (1974) Body fat assessed from total body density and its estimation from skinfold thickness: measurements on 481 men and women aged from 16 to 72 years. *Br. J. Nutr.* 32:77–97.
8. M.L. Pollock, J.H. Wilmore, and S.M. Fox III (1984) *Exercise in Health and Disease*, W.B. Saunders Co., Philadelphia.
9. A.R. Frisancho (1981) New norms of upper limb fat and muscle areas for assessment of nutritional status. *Am. J. Clin. Nutr.* 34:2540–2545.
10. S.B. Heymsfield, C. McManus, J. Smith, V. Stevens, and D.W. Nixon (1982) Anthropometric measurement of muscle mass: revised equations for calculating bone-free arm muscle area. *Am. J. Clin. Nutr.* 36:680–690.
11. G.B. Forbes, M.R. Brown, and H.J.L. Griffiths (1988) Arm muscle plus bone area: anthropometry and CAT scan compared. *Am. J. Clin. Nutr.* 47:929–931.
12. S.H. Cohn, D. Vartsky, S. Yasumura, et al. (1980) Compartmental body composition based on total-body nitrogen, potassium, and calcium. *Am. J. Physiol.* 239:E524–E530.
13. J. Womersley, K. Boddy, P.C. King, and J.V.G.A. Durnin (1972) A comparison of the fat-free mass of young adults estimated by anthropometry, body density and total body potassium content. *Clin. Sci.* 43:469–475.
14. J.E. Schutte, J.C. Longhurst, F.A. Gaffney, B.C. Bastian, and C.G. Blomqvist (1981) Total plasma creatinine: an accurate measure of total striated muscle. *J. Appl. Physiol.* 51:762–766.
15. G.B. Forbes and G.J. Bruining (1976) Urinary creatinine excretion and lean body mass. *Am. J. Clin. Nutr.* 29:1359–1366.
16. M.D. Van Loan, K.R. Segal, E.F. Bracco, P. Mayclin, and T.B. Van Itallie (1987) TOBEC methodology for body composition assessment: a cross-validation study. *Am. J. Clin. Nutr.* 46:9–12.
17. W.J. Cochran, W.W. Wong, M.L. Fiorotto, H.-P. Sheng, P.D. Klein, and W.J. Klish (1988) Total body water estimated by measuring total-body electrical conductivity. *Am. J. Clin. Nutr.* 48:946–950.
18. K.R. Segal, B. Gutin, E. Presta, J. Wang, and T.B. van Itallie (1985) Estimation of human body composition by electrical impedance methods: a comparative study. *J. Appl. Physiol.* 58:1565–1571.
19. S.H. Cohn, C. Abesamis, I. Zanzi, J.F. Aloia, S. Yasumura, and K.J. Ellis (1977) Body elemental composition: comparison between black and white adults. *Am. J. Physiol.* 232:E419–E422.
20. C. Bouchard, R. Savard, J.-P. Després, A. Tremblay, and C. Leblanc (1985) Body composition in adopted and biological siblings. *Hum. Biol.* 57:61–75.
21. National Research Council (1989) *Recommended Dietary Allowances*, 10th ed., National Academy Press, Washington, DC.
22. G.B. Forbes (1987) Lean body mass-body fat interrelationships in humans. *Nutr. Rev.* 45:225–231.
23. D.H. Calloway and H. Spector (1954) Nitrogen balance as related to caloric and protein intake in active young men. *Am. J. Clin. Nutr.* 2:405–412.
24. International Commission on Radiation Protection (1975) *Report of the Task Force Group on Reference Man*, no. 23, Pergamon Press, Oxford.

Hunger and Appetite

Words such as hunger and appetite have been used with a variety of meanings. To dieters the word hunger may conjure up images of foods recently omitted from the diet. To nutritionists the same word may conjure up images of children in developing nations suffering from marasmus. Although everyone has some basis for an intuitive definition of hunger, the term as it will be used in this chapter will refer specifically to internal signals that stimulate the acquisition and consumption of food. These signals may originate in the brain or in the periphery or may develop as habit. The signal set has many constituent parts that act in concert to initiate feeding. These factors contribute to a control system that helps to regulate caloric balance. Although each factor can be manipulated to promote the initiation of eating, there is not one primary mechanism that can be called the hunger mechanism. Rather, a number of sometimes complex and often redundant events occur that result in the body asking the question, "Is there anything to eat?"

By some accounts the reciprocal state of hunger is satiety. Usually, hunger is experienced in the absence of satiety cues and vice versa. Although they are undoubtedly interactive states, satiety and hunger will be treated in this chapter as separate phenomena.

Appetite commonly implies mild hunger usually directed at a choice of food items and often with expectations of reward. One can have specific hungers or appetites for specific food items. Appetite will be used in this chapter as a term to refer to signals that guide selection and consumption of specific foods and nutrients. Unlike hunger signals, which are usually aversive in nature and are to be avoided, appetite signals are not necessarily aversive. Further, they can arise in the absence of hunger. The signals associated with appetite usually work at a level secondary to those mediating caloric intake and arise in response to the body asking, "What do I want to eat?" These signals promote feeding behaviors that are flexible and readily modifiable on the basis of experience, as well as subject to influences such as palatability and custom.

In this review we will briefly summarize some of the neurological, physiological, psychological, and cultural bases of hunger and appetite. This review is not all inclusive but simply highlights some of the key findings and places them in historical perspective.[1-7] Many additional factors such as emotions, perceptual differences, and eating disorders can play a role in modifying the signals used to initiate feeding. These factors, though interesting in their own right, are not discussed here. The interested reader is referred to several excellent chapters on these phenomena in Silverstone's Dahlem Conference report[3] and in Wurtman and Wurtman's series *Nutrition and the Brain*.[8]

Hunger

Where has the search for the critical signal led us? Speculation about the nature of hunger has a long history.[9] It was in 1929 that Cannon[10] proposed that gastric contractions arising from an empty stomach played a critical role in signaling the brain that it was time once again to eat. Some years later, Morgan and Morgan[11] suggested that other factors, namely insulin, could increase the food intake of hungry rats. The importance of this discovery was the implication that there were blood-borne factors that could alter hunger. At about the same time, Hetherington and Ranson[12] demonstrated that small lesions of the hypothalamus were capable of producing ravenous eating in rats. Almost independent of this movement away from the stomach and into the brain, the pioneer Richter[13-16] developed his concept of self-regulatory behaviors. Since those early starts the central nervous system and the peripheral physiological systems have been studied in the search for a better understanding of the nature of hunger. Some of the highlights of that search are discussed below.

Central Factors. A number of areas in the brain, including several discrete areas of the hypothalamus, amygdala, septum, globus pallidus, zona incerta, hippocampus, nucleus accumbens, and midbrain tegmentum were identified with feeding.[5,7,17] During the last 40 years much of this research focused on the hypothalamus. Mayer[18,19] proposed the existence of a brain center that monitored glucose utilization (his glucostatic hypothesis). He suggested that a decrease in glucose utilization served as the signal used by a hypothalamic center to initiate feeding. Kennedy[20] proposed a hypothalamic feeding mechanism that was sensitive to the concentration of metabolites related to the size of body fat reserves. Mellinkoff et al.[21] proposed the aminostatic hypothesis, which noted a reciprocal relationship between serum amino acid concentrations and food intake in humans. Finally Brobeck[22] proposed that animals eat to keep warm and stop eating to prevent hyperthermia (thermostatic hypothesis). Brobeck went on to postulate that the thermic effects of food could act via the preoptic area, but more recent data indicate that hunger is not reliably associated with brain temperature (Figure 1).[7]

All of these theories had a single factor playing a dominant role in elicitation of hunger. The ultimate outcome of all of this work was the realization that hunger was not the result of a single factor but rather was elicited by a set of factors that were capable of initiating feeding by stimulating what Stellar[9] came to refer to as "a final common path." Today, Cannon's question "What is hunger?" is translated into different questions: What are the physiological, psychological, and cultural factors that determine the initiation of a meal? Are the factors that stimulate

feeding also determinants of the size and frequency of meals? Rather than attempt to detail and critique each of these approaches to the understanding of hunger, let it suffice to review some notable examples. For instance, Mayer's glucostatic theory served as a major framework in the study of brain glucose utilization. The hypothesis that hunger and satiety centers were located in separate nuclei of the hypothalamus[24] was abandoned in the light of impressive anatomical,[25,26] metabolic, and behavioral data.[27] For example, Gold[25] showed that lesions of the fiber tracts that pass by the ventromedial nucleus of the hypothalamus (but not fibers from the structure itself) can produce the ventromedial hypothalamic (VMH) syndrome in rats. Although that work challenged the primacy of the role of the hypothalamus, other evidence suggests that the structure nevertheless is important in controlling feeding. For example, feeding was initiated in rats when 2-deoxy-D-glucose was injected directly into the lateral ventricles, which resulted in decreased glucose utilization of adjacent hypothalamic areas.[28]

Leibowitz[29] suggested that two separate cholinergic mechanisms modulate hunger. The first is under α-noradrenergic control and is located in the medial (paraventricular) hypothalamic region. This mechanism stimulates feeding behavior. It may be influenced by input that originates in the midbrain and ascends through the periventricular region of the diencephalon. The second mechanism involves a second set of receptors (both β-adrenergic and dopaminergic) located in the anterolateral hypothalamic region that receive input from midbrain areas. This second system appears to suppress intake.

Over the past few years several techniques for

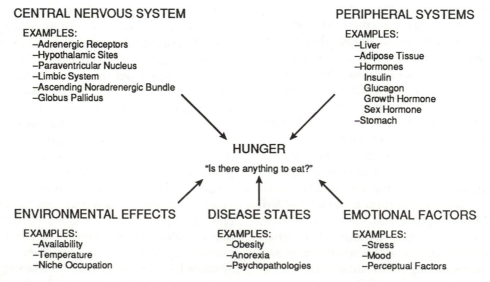

Figure 1. A partial listing of the ever-growing number of factors that are known to influence the onset of hunger. From reference 23.

measuring neurotransmitter concentration in freely moving, conscious animals have greatly enhanced our insights into how the brain controls intake. For example, in vivo intracerebral microdialysis coupled with high-pressure liquid chromatography and electrochemical detection makes it possible to measure the extracellular concentrations of neurotransmitters, their precursors, and the degradation by-products in discrete areas of the brain.[30] Among the most promising results using this technique was the report of Hernandez and Hoebel,[31] who showed that dopamine concentrations in the nucleus accumbens dramatically increase when animals pressed a lever for food reward. This same area of the brain was identified as one of the major reward centers of the brain, suggesting that at least part of the reason that we eat is that eating is rewarding or pleasurable and that the neural mechanism governing this aspect of eating is the same as that governing other rewarding events. This viewpoint has become increasingly popular with the elucidation of the role of endorphins and enkephalins on food intake.[32] These and other neuromodulators may be important determinants of intake under some conditions.[33] What makes them particularly intriguing is that some of these neuromodulators also play a role in the way that the brain experiences pleasure. It is our suggestion that although we eat for more than the pleasure derived from the behavior, certainly the hedonic satisfaction experienced during eating plays a major role in determining not only what we eat but also how much and how often we eat.[34] The roles of the endogenous opiates and their neuroanatomical substrates have not been thoroughly characterized but hold tremendous potential for the near future.[32,33] Similarly, many of the peptides that were identified as likely neurotransmitters in both the central and peripheral nervous systems also were found in regions of the brain that have been shown to play roles in feeding behavior. Some of these (e.g., insulin, cholecystokinin, caerulein, and glucagon) have long been suspected of playing a role in modulating satiety. More recent studies included peptides such as somatostatin, corticotropin releasing factor (CRF), vasoactive intestinal peptide, and neurotensin. All of these peptides were shown to decrease feeding when administered in picomole quantities directly into the brain. By contrast, fewer peptides were successful in stimulating intake. Included in these feeding stimulators are neuropeptide Y, dynorphin, and β-endorphin.[35]

Peripheral Factors. Research on the role of the stomach has moved from one of initiating meals to one of terminating eating.[36] Leading the way in this shift was the observation that people who had undergone surgical removal of their stomachs continued to eat food at regular intervals and reported experiencing hunger.[37] This finding obviously negates the existence of a primary role of the stomach in hunger. Gastrointestinal peptides such as cholecystokinin and bombesin (released into the blood stream during a meal) decrease food intake.[38,39] These peptides, however, are thought to act upon satiety mechanisms. Other theories of hunger have stressed the involvement of the liver. Russek and Racotta[40] theorized that so-called hepatic glucoreceptors respond to the concentration of some metabolite of the glycolytic chain (that is, pyruvate and/or lactate) in the hepatocytes. These metabolites have a hyperpolarizing effect on their membranes "so that . . . hunger would normally arise when liver glycogen levels (and that of the corresponding metabolite acting on the membrane) reach a certain minimum value."[40] Consistent with this hypothesis is that intraperitoneal injections of lactate are more satiating at low doses than are injections of glucose.[41] Further, increases in blood lactate concentrations produced short-term anorexia.[42] Thirdly, hepatic infusions of 2-deoxy-D-glucose result in a rapid onset of feeding; the animals usually begin to eat during the injections.[43] Finally, Stricker et al.[44] reported that hepatic portal vein injections of fructose (which cannot readily cross the blood-brain barrier) and not keto acids (which cannot be used by the liver but can be used by the brain) can dramatically and almost immediately reduce the food intake of hungry, insulin-pretreated rats. Opponents of this theory note that deafferentation of the liver does not measurably alter feeding.[45] Further, diabetic animals are hyperphagic, yet hepatocyte concentrations of pyruvate and lactate are low.

Glucose regulation. The effects of insulin on intake are not clear. Most of the early investigators who studied the problem showed that insulin increases food consumption.[46] In intact rats, for example, exogenous administration of 10 IU/d of protamine zinc insulin (PZI) to intact adult rats (a dose that would result in a marked drop in blood glucose) resulted in a 100% increase in food intake.[47] Subsequent work revealed that a single injection of regular insulin, as opposed to long-acting preparations like PZI, promotes increases in meal frequency within 4–6 h after the injection. The treated animal then compensates for the increased intake by cutting back on subsequent intake, with the net effect that 24-h intake does not differ from controls.[48] By comparison, chronic infusions of regular insulin result in a decrease in intake.[49] Woods et al.[50,51] suggested that fluctuations in plasma insulin were monitored by the brain and formed one basis for hunger. They modified this hypothesis to emphasize the role of insulin in the cerebrospinal fluid (CSF). CSF insulin (~25% of the concentration of plasma) was positively correlated with adiposity. When insulin was injected into the CSF of the lateral ventricles (which bathe the hypothalamus), baboons decreased their food intake and body weight.[51] Figlewicz et al.[52] reported that genetically obese Zucker rats have decreased insulin binding in olfactory bulbs. They also reported that decreased insulin binding is seen in the hypothalamus and olfactory bulbs of Wistar Kyoto fafa rats.[53] They speculated that these findings are consistent with the hypothesis that central insulin does not provide an adequate signal for control of food intake in these genetically obese animals.[53] Thus, Woods and Porte[54] suggested that insulin may be involved indirectly and directly in two systems that have an impact on food intake. First, there is a short-term regulatory system sensitive to fluctuations in blood glucose and, therefore, responsive to the effects of circulating insulin. Thus, when blood glucose decreases, feeding is stimulated. Second, there is a slower-acting system that is sensitive to CSF insulin, independent of blood glucose, directly reflective of adiposity, and inversely related to food intake.

This argument is consistent with recent work reported by Campfield et al.[55] demonstrating that blood glucose concentrations in rats decrease immediately before the onset of meals. These authors also demonstrated that preventing the transient decline in blood glucose by intravenous glucose results in the failure of meal initiation until a subsequent transient decline in circulating glucose takes place. These results, which were preceded by similar reports from Louis-Sylvestre and LeMagnen[56] and Steffens,[57] established a renewed interest in the possibility of a blood-borne signal that is used to initiate eating. These data suggest also that at least one hunger signal is related to glucose metabolism. Other signals have yet to be so elegantly elucidated.

Adipose tissue. A discussion of peripheral factors involved in hunger would be incomplete without a discussion of adipose tissue. The aforementioned lipostatic hypothesis of Kennedy[20] suggested a hypothalamic feeding mechanism that monitored body fat stores via circulating amounts of metabolites. In still another refinement of the original Kennedy lipostatic hypothesis, Greenwood et al.[58] proposed that the activity of lipoprotein lipase (LPL) in adipose tissue can potentiate hunger by altering the availability of circulating metabolites. They based this hypothesis in part on the fact that the hyperphagic, genetically obese Zucker rat (fafa) has increased adipose tissue LPL activity and that this elevation precedes the development of hyperphagia.[59] Furthermore, when progesterone is injected into female rats, increases in adipose tissue LPL activity precede the increases in food intake and subsequent increases in fat cell size and depot weight.[60] The activity of this "gatekeeper" enzyme controls the concentration of triglycerides entering adipose cells and by default removes them from access to other cells. The reduction in availability then triggers further consumption.

Another candidate for an adipose-tissue-derived signal is the protease adipsin. Speigelman and his colleagues[61] reported that the expression of adipsin (which is made by adipocytes and found in the blood) is less in genetically obese ob/ob and db/db mice. More research is needed to establish the physiological significance of these observations.

Meal patterns. Is hunger a determinant of meal size? One of the most interesting predictions stemming from any one of these theories of hunger is that the signals (metabolites) used as cues to stimulate feeding are proportional in magnitude to the deficit experienced. This deficit should intensify as a function of time since the last meal. Thus, a more intense hunger signal is correlated with time since the last meal and should result in larger meal initiation and subsequent alleviation of the deficit. That reasoning led to the prediction that the interval between meals should be strongly correlated with the size of a meal. To test that prediction, LeMagnen and Tallon[62] studied the relationship between the time between meals and the size of the meals. They reported that there was a significant correlation between the size of any meal and the interval immediately following that meal but that the interval immediately preceding a meal was not a predictor of meal size. Several investigators attempted to replicate the observed correlation with varied success. Finally, Panksepp[63] pointed out a statistical flaw in the LeMagnen procedure that in part accounted for the discrepant results. More recently, DeCastro[64] applied a more powerful statistical technique (multiple linear regression analysis) and reported that the premeal interval can predict meal size if one included information about the amount of food eaten during the preceding 2 h as well as information about water intake immediately before and during the meal. Castonguay et al.[65,66] showed that the definition of both the minimum meal size and end-of-the-meal that are used to analyze meal patterns play a major role in determining the statistical relationship between meal size and intermeal interval. Although the association between hunger and meal size is intuitive, the actual relationship is complex.

Environmental factors. In addition to studies of how internal events stimulate feeding, environmental stresses such as temperature, physical activity, and food availability also affect hunger. For example, cold environmental temperatures increased food consumption even if cold exposure was limited to only 3 h/d.[67] In contrast, heat stress reduced food intake, presumably reflecting the decreased energy needed to maintain body temperature.

The relationship between exercise and food intake is not clear. Exercise has been reported to increase, decrease, or have no effect on food intake.[68] The extent of the changes in food intake is dependent upon the intensity, duration, and type of exercise and is influenced by the age and sex of the individual.[69] In adult rats isolated bouts of exercise ranging in duration from 2 to 6 h decreased food intake on the day of the exercise.[70] The decrease was greatest for the longest exercise period. Furthermore, the closer the next meal time was to the termination of the exercise, the greater the anorexia. With chronic exercise this situation was reversed; the rats that exercised the longest had the largest food intake. When energy expenditure was held constant and intensity was varied, the reduction in food intake of male rats was greatest in the high-intensity group within the first 24 h and lasted up to 3 d after exercise.[71] In humans the effects of acute exercise are to decrease food intake immediately after exercise.[69] For moderately active humans, chronic exercise promotes increased caloric intake. For example, middle-aged men and women joggers consumed more calories than sedentary control subjects who were slightly shorter and heavier.[72]

Other studies showed that the effect of exercise is markedly influenced by hormonal status. Male rats placed on an exercise regimen lose weight even though given free access to food, whereas females more closely compensate for the increased caloric demand that accompanies exercise by eating more food.[73] Finally, the cessation of an exercise program results in an increase in food intake within 3 d. This increased intake is preceded by an increase in plasma insulin (by 48 h) and is followed by increases in plasma triglycerides (within 84 h) and activity of adipose tissue LPL (also within 84 h).[65] Additional data suggest that this effect may be mediated in part by changes in the sympathetic nervous system.

Availability. Another environmental approach to the study of hunger is to manipulate the availability of food. Collier et al.[74] argued that animals do not have to use physiological signals to initiate meals but rather feed in anticipation of nutritive and caloric need. They showed that rats will push a small lever an extraordinary number of times if they are rewarded for their efforts by gaining access to a meal. For example, rats will tolerate requirements of up to 5,000 responses per meal of laboratory stock diet. Cats, ferrets, chickens, wild rats, and guinea pigs also will adjust their food intake when required to work for meals.[75] These adjustments take two forms. Typically the number of meals declines as the cost of earning a meal increases. As meal frequency declines, the size of any given meal increases. These adjustments most often compensate for one another with

the net effect that total caloric intake is maintained at a characteristic level and body weight is maintained. Further, animals adjust meal size in relation to the cost of gaining access to food so as to preserve daily caloric intake. Through this series of experiments, Collier et al.[76] suggested that under most circumstances animals learn to eat in anticipation of their nutrient and energy needs rather than in response to the depletion of energy stores. Hunger, then, can be an aversive stimulus, and feeding serves as a learned mechanism to avoid the onset of that stimulus. Qualifying that veiwpoint was a recent paper by Swiergiel and Cabanac,[77] who showed that rats that are required to feed in a cold environment fail to compensate for differences in the caloric density of their diets. Rather, these animals respond to low-calorie diets by eating less and more slowly and as a result maintain lower body weights. By contrast when these animals are given access to a high-calorie (high-fat) diet, they meet their energy requirements by increasing their eating rate. The conclusion that can be drawn from these studies is that the interaction between availability and energy need is not as straightforward as once believed.

Appetite

Because food varies in availability, sensitive and complex systems have developed in many different species to maintain energy balance. Unlike the common need for energy, nutrient demands and ways in which they are met differ from species to species and from one environment to another. Despite these differences animals have adapted to their particular ecological niche. With regard to macronutrient (protein, carbohydrate, and fat) selection, one of three strategies to secure a nutritionally balanced diet is used: (1) an animal eats a diet that is used by its digestive flora as food and in turn uses these as sources of energy and essential nutrients (the herbivorous strategy), (2) the animal feeds on the flesh of animals and secures a balanced diet via some other animal's efforts (the carnivorous strategy), or (3) the animal picks and chooses from both plant and animal food items thereby securing energy and nutrients from a wide variety of sources (the omnivorous strategy). This last strategy, although permissive of a great deal of variation, requires the animal not only to balance intake of the quantity of energy (calories) but also to meet specific nutrient needs (dietary quality) all within the context of caloric regulation. This second type of hunger (the need for specific nutrients) is what most researchers mean when using the term appetite. The cravings experienced by some people are often for specific foods. Unfortunately, little is known about their underlying basis. There is some

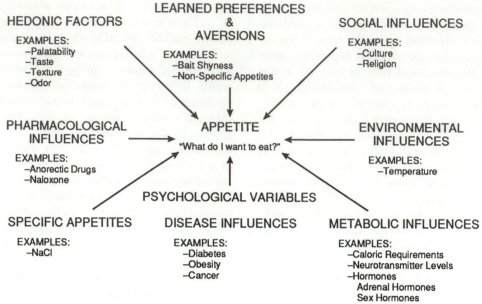

Figure 2. Some of the factors that determine appetite. From reference 23.

evidence that cravings for nonnutritive items (such as clay or dirt) can be symptomatic of deficiencies of specific minerals.[78] It was proposed that such aberrant ingestive behavior may be one beneficial way of defending the body against toxins. Clay or dirt can act as a chelating agent thereby preventing the absorption of some toxins that are found in foods.[79]

The remainder of this section briefly discusses some of the key areas of research that are aimed at a better understanding of the nature of the signals that direct the omnivore's selection of foods.

Macronutrients. In 1915, Evvard[80] demonstrated that pigs could compose a diet from several food sources and actually grow better than controls fed a scientifically formulated standard control composite diet. This first experimental demonstration of dietary selection served as a departure point for the growing interest in the mechanisms that are used to guide food selection. Five years later, Osborne and Mendel[81] reported that laboratory rats selected diets that were nutritionally adequate in preference to similar but protein-deficient diets. In 1929 Davis[82] reported that human infants given a choice of a wide variety of foods selected a diet that met both caloric and nutrient requirements. Although later critiques of that now classic report point out that the food items available to these children were mostly adequate by themselves, Davis's work sparked further research efforts into a better understanding of the selection phenomenon. At about the same time, Richter[13] demonstrated that rats were very sensitive to the quality of their diets and that selection of foods was influenced by bodily need. For example, adrenalectomized rats increase their intake of salt solu-

tions so as to behaviorally adjust for their failure to retain sodium. Similarly, pancreatectomized rats decrease their intake of carbohydrate[14] and increase their intake of fat.[83,84]

Until recently one of the most insightful criticisms leveled at the research into dietary selection was the failure of researchers to go beyond a description of selection into an analysis of the mechanisms that operate to promote appropriate nutrient choice.[84] That void is being filled today by reports of how different neural and metabolic changes are associated with different selection patterns. Some of these systems are outlined in Figure 2. Ashley and Anderson[85] made the still-controversial proposal that circulating tryptophan, one of the rat's essential amino acids (tryptophan competes with the large neutral amino acids to cross the blood-brain barrier), serves as the critical event signaling brain centers to begin to initiate protein meals. Peters and Harper[86,87] recently challenged that hypothesis on the basis of their observation that no consistent correlation was detected between protein consumption and either the ratio of plasma tryptophan to neutral amino acids or brain serotonin concentration. Other researchers have focused their efforts on other neurotransmitters. For example, Leibowitz et al.[88] suggested that protein consumption is under dopaminergic control and that α-adrenergic receptor systems modulate carbohydrate consumption. The mechanism that they proposed includes an antagonistic role for serotonin, in which 5-hydroxytryptophan interacts antagonistically with both norepinephrine and its α-2-noradrenergic receptors that normally function to enhance carbohydrate intake especially at the onset of the feeding cycle. Wurtman and colleagues[89] attempted to develop a theory aimed at understanding the physiological basis for carbohydrate choice ("carbohydrate craving"). Detailed examination of several aspects of the theory that changes in brain serotonin concentration influence carbohydrate-rich food choices has not supported the hypothesis.[90]

Others implicated the prepyriform cortex in the control of protein quality.[91] Rats maintained on a low-protein diet usually refuse to eat a diet missing an essential amino acid. Electrolytic lesions of the prepyriform cortex interfere with that rejection so that lesioned animals readily accept the imbalanced diet.[92]

Although fat is an important part of any diet, little is known about the factors that control dietary fat intake. Genetically obese Zucker rats will, under some conditions, consume three times as much fat as their lean littermates consume.[93] After adrenalectomy, however, the obese rats' fat intake decreased selectively.[94] Much of this work was replicated and extended by Romsos and colleagues.[95,96] We[97] speculated that endogenous opiates may be controlling the intake of dietary fat. Much more work, including the measurement of the endorphins, needs to be done to test this hypothesis. Other investigators have studied how altered metabolic states affect selection. For example, rats housed in a cold environment will selectively increase their intake of carbohydrate rather than protein.[98] Kanarek[99] demonstrated that rats selectively increase carbohydrate consumption when treated with insulin. Finally, obesity can affect selection patterns. For example, we[93] showed that genetically obese Zucker rats will compose a diet that is lower in protein and higher in fat than the diet selected by lean littermates. However, there is no evidence that the diet composition of obese humans differs from that composed by normal-weight individuals.[100] However, there is evidence from our work with experimental animals that "yo-yo" dieting results in an increase in dietary fat selection when reduced rats regain weight.[101] Further, exercise suppresses the increase in fat selection.

Sensory psychologists have added a unique approach to the study of nutrient selection. For example, Young[102] theorized that the palatability of food items determines their consumption and developed a sophisticated approach (isohedonic contours) to the systemic study of the taste properties of foods (principally nutrients in solution). Although Young's original hypothesis about palatability was extensively modified by more recent reports,[103] taste properties play an important role in guiding selection especially under conditions of ample choice.[4]

Specific Appetites. The mechanisms guiding the intake of macronutrients are not the only subjects of experimental attention. For example, it was hoped that the rat's avidity for sodium would serve as a model system for the study of appetites.[104] Sodium appetite, however, appears to be unique so that extensive generalizations into other appetitive systems cannot be made. On the other hand, much information exists about the mechanisms underlying sodium appetite. Naive rats made deficient in sodium will choose solutions of sodium salts in preference to nonsodium salts with a minimum of delay. Nachman[105] made rats sodium deficient by either dietary restriction or adrenalectomy. He then gave the rats access to one of five different sodium-containing solutions. Sodium-deficient rats drank more of the sodium-containing solutions than did controls. The difference in intake was significant within 15 s of first access. No differences were observed when palatable solutions of potassium chloride, calcium chloride, etc. were used. The specificity and the time course for recognition of the sodium ion are two pieces of evidence supporting the hypothesis that rats have a specific appetite for sodium.[106] It is postulated that sodium deficiency changes the taste threshold for that ion. Taste receptors of sodium-deficient rats have a much lower threshold for sodium than do taste receptors of control rats.[107]

The physiological and anatomical adaptation to sodium requirements does not seem to have analogues for other nutrients. Thiamin, calcium, zinc, and other nutrients were carefully examined and rats failed to respond as they did to sodium with regard to specificity or time for recognition. The intake of other nutrients in response to deficiency is probably achieved through the operation of a learning process in which the animal associates particular foods with the alleviation (or avoidance) of deficiencies. For example, Rodgers and Rozin[108] showed that rats made deficient in thiamin show enhanced acceptance of novel diets. Rodgers[109] went on to show that deficient animals prefer a novel thiamin-containing diet. These same animals, when given a choice between two novel diets, one that contains thiamin and one that does not, fail to show a preference for the thiamin-supplemented diet. It was suggested that dietary deficiencies result in the increased acceptance of novel food items and an avoidance of food items that were consumed at the onset of the deficiency. Thus, thiamin-deficient rats choose novel diets, but when given a choice between two novel diets, fail to correctly select the novel diet that also alleviates their deficiency.

Cultural Factors. Any discussion of food-item selection in response to appetite would be incomplete without reference to one of the major factors guiding human food selection—culture. Human societies have developed collective wisdom about the selection and preparation of foods that they transmit from generation to generation.[110,111] Humans eat only a very limited set of food items in response to both availability and custom. Although custom does not change the physiological function of hunger or appetite, it does provide a framework for directing feeding in response to these signals. The cuisine developed by any one culture provides norms for the cultivation, preparation, and sometimes seasonal consumption habits of its members. Readers interested in these phenomena are encouraged to consult any one of several fine review articles.[3,4,110,111]

Conclusion

Some would argue that the terms hunger and appetite can apply only to humans because only humans can say that they are hungry or have a specific appetite.[3] Further, investigators working with laboratory animals can only observe feeding behavior. In contrast, we argue that hunger and appetite, as defined in this paper, have physiological bases and are not solely behavioral phenomena. In the most basic sense they are a set of signals that promote the initiation of feeding and guide the choice of food items. These signals can be measured in theory and in practice. The neurosciences are the wave of the future and will integrate disparate data on metabolism and neurology into a rational whole.

References

1. D. Booth (1978) *Hunger Models: Computable Theory of Feeding Control.* Academic Press, London.
2. D. Novin, M. Wyrwick, and G. Bray, eds. (1976) *Hunger: Basic Mechanisms and Clinical Implications,* Raven Press, New York.
3. T. Silverstone (1976) Introduction. In: *Appetite and Food Intake.* (T. Silverstone, ed.), pp. 11–14, Abakon Verlagsgesellschaft, Berlin.
4. J. Solms, D.A. Booth, R.M. Pangborn, and O. Raunhardt (1987) *Food Acceptance and Nutrition,* Academic Press, New York.
5. J.E. Morley, M.B. Sterman, and J.H. Walsh, eds. (1988) *Nutritional Modulation of Neural Function,* Academic Press, New York.
6. J. LeMagnen (1985) *Hunger (Problems in the Behavioural Sciences),* Cambridge University Press, Cambridge.
7. C.I. Thompson (1980) *Controls of Eating,* SP Medical and Scientific Books, New York.
8. R.J. Wurtman and J.J. Wurtman, eds. *Nutrition and the Brain,* vols. 1–8, Raven Press, New York.
9. E. Stellar (1976) The CNS and appetite: historical introduction. In: *Appetite and Food Intake* (T. Silverstone, ed.), pp. 15–20, Abakon Verlagsgesellschaft, Berlin.
10. W.B. Cannon (1929) *Bodily Changes in Pain, Hunger, Fear and Rage,* Appleton Century, New York.
11. C.T. Morgan and J.P. Morgan (1940) Studies in hunger. I. The effects of insulin upon the rat's rate of eating. *J. Gen. Psychol.* 56:137–147.
12. A.W. Hetherington and S.W. Ranson (1940) Hypothalamic lesions and adiposity in the rat. *Anat. Rec.* 78:149–172.
13. C.P. Richter (1939) Salt taste thresholds of normal and adrenalectomized rats. *Endocrinology* 24:367–371.
14. C.P. Richter and E.C.H. Schmidt (1939) Behavior and anatomical changes produced in rats by pancreatectomy. *Endocrinology* 25:698–706.
15. C.P. Richter (1936) Increased salt appetite in adrenalectomized rats. *Am. J. Physiol.* 115:155–161.
16. C.P. Richter and J.F. Eckert (1937) Increased calcium appetite of parathyroidectomized rats. *Endocrinology* 21:50–54.
17. S.P. Grossman (1972) Neurophysiologic aspects: extrahypothalamic factors in the regulation of food intake. *Adv. Psychosom. Med.* 7:49–72.
18. J. Mayer (1953) Glucostatic mechanism of regulation of food intake. *N. Engl. J. Med.* 249:13–16.
19. J. Mayer (1953) Regulation of energy intake and body weight: the glucostatic theory and the lipostatic hypothesis. *Ann. N.Y. Acad. Sci.* 63:15–43.
20. G.C. Kennedy (1953) The role of depot fat in the hypothalamic control of food intake in the rat. *Proc. R. Soc. London [Biol.]* 140:578–592.
21. S.M. Mellinkoff, M. Frankland, D. Boyle, and M. Greipel (1956) Relation between serum amino acid concentration and fluctuations in appetite. *J. Appl. Psychol.* 8:535–538.
22. J.R. Brobeck (1947) Food intake as a mechanism of temperature regulation. *Yale J. Biol. Med.* 20:545–552.
23. T.W. Castonguay, E.A. Applegate, D.E. Upton, and J.S. Stern (1984) Hunger and appetite: old concepts/new distinctions. In: *Present Knowledge in Nutrition,* 5th ed. (R.E. Olson, H.P. Broquist, C.O. Chichester, W.J. Darby, A.C. Kolbye, Jr., and R.M. Stalvey), pp. 19–34, The Nutrition Foundation, Washington, DC.
24. B.K. Anand and J.R. Brobeck (1951) Hypothalamic control of food intake in rats and cats. *Yale J. Biol. Med.* 24:123–140.
25. R.M. Gold (1973) Hypothalamic obesity: the myth of the ventromedial nucleus. *Science* 182:488–490.
26. J.E. Ahlskog and B.G. Hoebel (1973) Overeating and obesity from damage to a noradrenergic system in the brain. *Science* 182:166–169.
27. M.I. Friedman and E.M. Stricker (1976) The physiological psychology of hunger: a physiological perspective. *Psychol. Bull.* 83:409–431.
28. A.N. Epstein, S. Nicolaidis, and R. Miselis (1975) The glucoprivic theory of feeding behavior. In: *Neural Integration of Physiological Mechanisms and Behavior* (G.J. Mogenson and F.R. Calaresu, eds.), pp. 148–168, University of Toronto Press, Toronto.
29. S. Leibowitz (1976) Brain catecholaminergic mechanisms for control of hunger. In: *Hunger: Basic Mechanisms and Clinical Implications* (D. Novin, W. Wyrwicka, and G. Bray, eds.), pp. 1–18, Raven Press, New York.
30. B.G. Stanley, D.H. Schwartz, L. Hernandez, B.G. Hoebel, and S.F. Leibowitz (1989) Patterns of extracellular norepinephrine in the paraventricular hypothalamus: relationship to circadian rhythm and deprivation-induced eating behavior. *Life Sci.* 45:275–282.
31. L. Hernandez and B.G. Hoebel (1988) Feeding and hypothalamic stimulation increase dopamine turnover in the accumbens. *Physiol. Behav.* 44:599–606.
32. A.S. Levine, J.E. Morley, B.A. Gosnell, C.J. Billington, and T.J. Bartness (1985) Opioids and consummatory behavior. *Brain Res. Bull.* 14:663–672.
33. B.G. Stanley, D. Lanthier, A.S. Chin, and S.F. Leibowitz (in press) Suppression of neuropeptide Y-elicited eating by adrenalectomy and hypophysectomy: reversal with corticosterone. *Brain Res.*
34. B.J. Rolls (1985) Experimental analyses of the effects of variety in a meal on human feeding. *Am. J. Clin. Nutr.* 42:932–939.
35. J. Morley, A.S. Levine, B. Gosnell, and D.D. Krahn (1985) Peptides as central regulators of feeding. *Brain Res. Bull.* 14:511–519.
36. J.A. Deutsch, W.G. Young, and T. Kalogeris (1978) The stomach signals satiety. *Science* 201:165–167.
37. O.H. Wangensteen and H.A. Carlson (1931) Hunger sensations in a patient after total gastrectomy. *Proc. Soc. Exp. Biol. Med.* 28:545–547.

38. J. Gibbs, R.C. Young, and G.P. Smith (1973) Cholecystokinin decreases food intake in rats. *J. Comp. Physiol. Psychol.* 84: 488–495.

39. C.L. McLaughlin and C.A. Baile. Feeding response of weanling Zucker obese rats to cholecystokinin and bombesin. *Physiol. Behav.* 25:341–346.

40. M. Russek and R.A. Racotta (1980) A possible role of adrenaline and glucagon in the control of food intake. *Front. Horm. Res.* 6: 120–137.

41. R. Racotta and M. Russek (1977) Food and water intake of rats after intraperitoneal and subcutaneous administration of glucose, glycerol and sodium lactate. *Physiol. Behav.* 18:267–273.

42. C.A. Baile, W.M. Zinn, and J. Mayer (1970) Effects of lactate and other metabolites on food intake of monkeys. *Am. J. Physiol.* 219:1606–1613.

43. D. Novin, D.A. VanderWeele, and M. Rezek (1973) Infusion of 2 deoxy-d-glucose into the hepatic portal system causes eating: evidence for peripheral glucoreceptors. *Science* 181:858–860.

44. E.M. Stricker, N. Rowland, C.F. Saller, and M.I. Friedman (1977) Homeostasis during hypoglycemia: central control of adrenal secretion and peripheral control of feeding. *Science* 196:79–81.

45. L.L. Bellinger, V.E. Mendel, F.E. Williams, and T.W. Castonguay (1984) The effect of liver denervation on meal patterns, body weight and body composition of rats. *Physiol. Behav.* 33:661–667.

46. M.I. Grossman (1955) Integration of current views on the regulation of hunger and appetite. *Ann. N.Y. Acad. Sci.* 63:76–91.

47. J. Panksepp, A. Pollack, K. Krost, R. Meeker, and M. Ritter (1975) Feeding in response to repeated protamine zinc insulin injections. *Physiol. Behav.* 14:487–493.

48. A.B. Steffens (1970) Plasma insulin content in relation to blood glucose level and meal pattern in the normal and hypothalamic hyperphagic rats. *Physiol. Behav.* 5:147–152.

49. D.A. VanderWeele, F.X. Pi-Sunyer, D. Novin, and M.J. Bush (1980) Chronic insulin infusion suppresses food ingestion and body weight gain in rats. *Brain Res. Bull.* 5(suppl. 4):7–11.

50. S.C. Woods, E. Decke, and J.R. Vasselli (1974) Metabolic hormones and regulation of body weight. *Psychol. Rev.* 81:26–43.

51. S.C. Woods, E.C. Lotter, L.D. McKay, and D. Porte, Jr. (1979) Chronic intracerebroventricular infusion of insulin reduces food intake and body weight of baboons. *Nature* 282:503–505.

52. D.P. Figlewicz, D.M. Dorsa, L.J. Stein, et al. (1985) Brain and liver insulin binding is decreased in Zucker rats carrying the fa gene. *Endocrinology* 117:1537–1543.

53. D.P. Figlewicz, H. Ikeda, T.R. Hunt, et al. (1986) Brain insulin binding is decreased in Wistar Kyoto rats carrying the fa gene. *Peptides* 7:61–65.

54. S.C. Woods and D. Porte, Jr. (1978) The central nervous system, pancreatic hormones, feeding and obesity. *Adv. Metab. Dis.* 9: 283–312.

55. L.A. Campfield, P. Brandon, and F. Smith (1985) On-line continuous measurement of blood glucose and meal pattern in freely feeding rats: the role of glucose in meal initiation. *Brain Res. Bull.* 14:605–616.

56. J. Louis-Sylvestre and J. LeMagnen (1980) A fall in blood glucose level precedes meal onset in free-feeding rats. *Neurosci. Biobehav. Rev.* 4(suppl. 1):13–16.

57. A.B. Steffens (1969) Blood glucose and FFA levels in relation to the meal pattern in the normal rat and the ventromedial hypothalamic lesioned rat. *Physiol. Behav.* 4:215–225.

58. M.R.C. Greenwood, M.P. Cleary, L.S. Steingrimsdottir, and J.R. Vasselli (1981) Adipose tissue metabolism and genetic obesity: the LPL hypothesis. *Int. J. Obes.* 5:718–730.

59. M.P. Cleary, J.R. Vasselli, and M.R.C. Greenwood (1980) Development of obesity in Zucker obese (fafa) rats in absence of hyperphagia. *Am. J. Physiol.* 238:E284–E292.

60. G.N. Wade and J.M. Gray (1979) Gonadal effects on food intake and adiposity: a metabolic hypothesis. *Physiol. Behav.* 22:583–593.

61. J.S. Flier, K.S. Cook, P. Usher, and B.M. Speigelman (1987) Severely impaired adipsin expression in genetic and acquired obesity. *Science* 237:405–408.

62. J. LeMagnen and S. Tallon (1966) La periodicite spontanee de la prise d'aliments ad libitum du rat blanc. *J. Physiol. (Paris)* 58: 323–349.

63. J. Panksepp (1973) Reanalysis of feeding patterns in the rat. *J. Comp. Physiol. Psychol.* 82:78–94.

64. J.M. DeCastro (1978) An analysis of the variance in meal patterning. *Neurosci. Biobehav. Rev.* 2:301–309.

65. T.W. Castonguay, D.E. Upton, P.M.B. Leung, and J.S. Stern (1982) Meal patterns in the genetically obese Zucker rat: a reexamination. *Physiol. Behav.* 28:911–916.

66. T.W. Castonguay, L.L. Kaiser, and J.S. Stern (1986) Meal pattern analysis: artifacts, assumptions, and implications. *Brain Res. Bull.* 17:439–443.

67. C.L. Hamilton (1967) Food and temperature. In: *Handbook of Physiology. Alimentary Canal,* vol. 1 (C.F. Code, ed.), pp. 303–317, American Physiological Society, Washington, DC.

68. L.B. Oscai (1973) The role of exercise in weight control. *Exerc. Sports Med.* 1:103–123.

69. J.S. Stern (1983) Diet and exercise. In: *Contemporary Issues in Clinical Nutrition,* vol. 4 (M.R.C. Greenwood, ed.), pp. 65–84, Churchill Livingston, New York.

70. J.A.F. Stevenson, B.M. Box, V. Feleki, and J.R. Beaton (1966) Bouts of exercise and food intake in the rat. *J. Appl. Physiol.* 21:118–122.

71. V.L. Katch, R. Martin, and J. Martin (1979) Effects of exercise intensity on food consumption in the male rat. *Am. J. Clin. Nutr.* 32:1401–1407.

72. S.N. Blair, N.M. Ellsworth, W.L. Haskell, M.P. Stern, J.W. Farquhar, and P.D. Wood (1981) Comparison of nutrient intake in middle aged men and women and runners and controls. *Med. Sci. Sports Exerc.* 13:310–315.

73. D.M. Nance, B. Bromley, R.J. Barnard, and R.J. Gorski (1977) Sexually dimorphic effects of forced exercise on food intake and body weight in the rat. *Physiol. Behav.* 19:155–158.

74. G. Collier, E. Hirsch, and P.H. Hamlin (1972) The ecological determinants of reinforcement in the rat. *Physiol. Behav.* 9:705–716.

75. G. Collier and C.K. Rovee-Collier (1980) A comparative analysis of optimal foraging behavior: laboratory simulations. In: *Foraging Behavior: Ecological, Ethological and Psychological Approaches* (A.C. Kamil and T. Sargent, eds.), pp. 39–76, Garland Press, New York.

76. G.H. Collier, D. Johnson, W. Hill, and L. Kaufman (1986) The economics of the law of effect. *J. Exp. Anal. Behav.* 146:113–136.

77. A.H. Swiergiel and M. Cabanac (1989) Lack of caloric regulation in rats during short-term feeding. *Am. J. Physiol.* 256:R518–522.

78. C.T. Snowdon (1977) A nutritional basis for lead pica. *Physiol. Behav.* 18:885–893.

79. J.A. Halsted (1968) Geophagia in man: its nature and nutritional effects. *Am. J. Clin. Nutr.* 21:1384–1392.

80. J.M. Evvard (1915) Is the appetite of swine a reliable indication of physiological needs? *Proc. Iowa Acad. Sci.* 22:375–403.

81. T.B. Osborne and L.B. Mendel (1918) The choice between adequate and inadequate diets, as made by rats. *J. Biol. Chem.* 35:19–27.

82. C.M. Davis (1928) Self-selection of diet by newly weaned infants. *Am. J. Dis. Child.* 36:651–679.

83. J. Lat (1967) Self-selection of dietary components. In: *Handbook of Physiology, Alimentary Canal,* vol. 1 (C.F. Code, ed.), pp. 367–386, American Physiological Society, Washington, DC.

84. S.R. Overmann (1976) Dietary self-selection by animals. *Psychol. Bull.* 83:218–235.

85. D.V.M. Ashley and G.H. Anderson (1975) Correlation between the plasma tryptophan to neutral amino acids ratio and protein intake in the self-selecting weanling rat. *J. Nutr.* 105:1412–1421.

86. A.E. Harper and J.C. Peters (1989) Protein intake, brain amino acid and serotonin concentrations and protein self-selection. *J. Nutr.* 119:677–689.

87. J.C. Peters and A.E. Harper (1987) A skeptical view of the role of central serotonin in the selection and intake of protein. *Appetite* 8:206–210.

88. S.R. Leibowitz, G. Shor-Posner, and G.F. Weiss (in press) In: *Serotonin: From Cell to Pharmacology and Therapeutics* (Paoletti R, Vanhoutte PM, eds.), Wolters-Kluwer NV, Norwell, MA.

89. H.R. Lieberman, J.J. Wurtman, and B. Chew (1986) Changes in mood after carbohydrate consumption among obese individuals. *Am. J. Clin. Nutr.* 44:772–778.

90. J.D. Fernstrom (1986) Effects of protein and carbohydrate ingestion on brain tryptophan levels and serotonin synthesis: putative relationship to appetite for specific nutrients. In: *Interaction of the Chemical Senses with Nutrition* (J.G. Brand and M. Kare, eds.), pp. 395–414, Academic Press, New York.

91. P.M.B. Leung and Q.R. Rogers (1971) Importance of prepyriform cortex in food intake response of rats to amino acids. *Am. J. Physiol.* 221:929–935.

92. D. Gietzen, P.M.B. Leung, T.W. Castonguay, W.J. Hartman, and Q.R. Rogers (1986) Time course of food intake and plasma and brain amino acid concentrations in rats fed amino acid imbalanced or deficient diets. In: *Interaction of the Chemical Senses with Nutrition* (J.G. Brand and M. Kare, eds.), pp. 415–456, Academic Press, New York.

93. T.W. Castonguay, W.J. Hartman, E.A. Fitzpatrick, and J.S. Stern (1982) Dietary self-selection and the Zucker rat. *J. Nutr.* 112: 796–800.

94. T.W. Castonguay, M.F. Dallman, and J.S. Stern (1986) Some metabolic and behavioral effects of adrenalectomy on the obese Zucker rat. *Am. J. Physiol.* 251:R923–R933.

95. B.P. Warwick and D.R. Romsos (1988) Energy balance in adrenalectomized ob/ob mice: effects of dietary starch and glucose. *Am. J. Physiol.* 255:R141–R148.

96. H.K. Kim and D.R. Romsos (1988) Adrenalectomy fails to stimulate brown adipose tissue metabolism in ob/ob mice fed glucose. *Am. J. Physiol.* 255:E597–E603.

97. T.W. Castonguay and J.S. Stern (1983) The effect of adrenalectomy on dietary component selection by the genetically obese Zucker rat. *Nutr. Rep. Int.* 28:725–731.

98. A.I. Leshner, G.H. Collier, and R.L. Squibb (1971) Dietary self-selection at cold temperatures. *Physiol. Behav.* 6:1–3.

99. R.B. Kanarek, R. Marks-Kaufman, and B.J. Lipeles (1980) Increased carbohydrate intake as a function of insulin administration in rats. *Physiol. Behav.* 25:779–782.

100. R. Beaudoin and J. Mayer (1953) Food intakes of obese and non-obese women. *J. Am. Diet. Assoc.* 29:29–33.

101. T. Gerrardo-Gettens, G. Miller, M.R.C. Greenwood, K.D. Brownell, and J.S. Stern (1989) Dietary fat selection is altered during weight cycling. *FASEB J.* 3:A448 (abstr.).

102. P.T. Young (1967) Palatability: the hedonic response to foodstuff. In: *Handbook of Physiology. Alimentary Canal,* vol. 1 (C.F. Code, ed.), pp. 353–366, American Physiological Society, Washington, DC.

103. T.W. Castonguay, E. Hirsch, and G.H. Collier (1981) Palatability of sugar solutions and dietary selection? *Physiol. Behav.* 27:7–12.

104. G. Wolf, J.F. McGovern, and L.V. Dicara (1974) Sodium appetite: some conceptual and methodologic aspects of a model drive system. *Behav. Biol.* 10:27–42.

105. M. Nachman (1962) Taste preferences for sodium salts by adrenalectomized rats. *J. Comp. Physiol. Psychol.* 55:1124–1129.

106. E.E. Krieckhaus and G. Wolf (1968) Acquisition of sodium by rats: interaction of innate mechanisms and latent learning. *J. Comp. Physiol. Psychol.* 65:197–201.

107. R.J. Contreras and M. Frank (1979) Sodium deprivation alters neural responses to gustatory stimuli. *J. Gen. Physiol.* 73:569–594.

108. W.L. Rodgers and P. Rozin (1966) Novel food preferences in thiamine-deficient rats. *J. Comp. Physiol. Psychol.* 41:1–4.

109. W.L. Rodgers (1967) Specificity of specific hungers. *J. Comp. Physiol. Psychol.* 64:49–58.

110. P. Rozin (1976) Psychobiological and cultural determinants of food choice. In: *Appetite and Food Intake* (T. Silverstone, ed.), pp. 285–312, Abakon Verlagsgesellschaft, Berlin.

111. F.J. Simoons (1976) Food habits as influenced by human culture: approaches in anthropology and geography. In: *Appetite and Food Intake* (T. Silverstone, ed.), pp. 313–330, Abakon Verlagsgesellschaft, Berlin.

Chapter 4

Obesity

George A. Bray

This chapter will focus on the physiological and nutritional aspects of overweight and will point out that the location of body fat may be more significant than the total amount of fat itself in the health risks associated with obesity. The role of increased food intake, reduced physical activity, and altered thermogenesis as mechanisms for the development of excessive fat deposits will be reviewed. Finally, an approach to treatment for obesity will be discussed using a risk-benefit approach. For more detailed information about various facets of obesity, especially treatment, the reader is referred to several recent monographs.[1–6]

Definition and Measurement of Body Fat and Its Distribution

Because both overweight and fat distribution may be useful predictors of health risks associated with obesity, we need to have a clear definition of these terms. Overweight is an increase of body weight above a standard defined in relation to height. Obesity, on the other hand, is an abnormally high percentage of body fat, which may be generalized or localized. To determine whether an individual is obese or simply overweight because of increased muscle mass, one needs techniques and standards for quantitating body weight, body fat, and distribution of body fat. Several approaches to this problem are listed in Table 1, which also includes an estimate of the cost, ease of use, and accuracy of these methods. (Also *see* chapter 2, Body Composition.)

Anthropometric Measurements. Anthropometric measurements include height and weight; circumferences of the chest, waist, hips, or extremities; and skinfold thickness[6] (Table 1). The tables of "desirable weight" provided by the Metropolitan Life Insurance Company have received widest use. These tables are divided into three subgroups by frame size. However, no direct measures of frame size were made when these data were collected. The upper and lower frame sizes appear to be the upper and lower quarters (quartiles) of the population, with the medium frame representing the middle two quarters. The newest tables, published in 1983, provide a higher weight range than older tables.

Weight and height can also be related in several ways. Of these, the ratio called the body mass index (BMI) or Quetelet index (kg/m^2) is most useful. The correlation of BMI with body fat as measured from body density is between 0.7 and 0.8.[7] Figure 1 is a nomogram for determining BMI. The desirable range for BMI for each height appears to increase slightly with age in women but not in men.[8] These ranges are listed in Table 2. The BMI also can be used to assess health risks associated with overweight, and may also be used as a guide to therapy.

The distribution of BMI in the American population is shown in Figure 2.[9] The peak frequency for women is at a BMI of 21. For men the peak is at 26. Women show a greater skew to the right with a possible bimodal distribution. Men show a narrow and more normal distribution.

The degree of body fat or obesity can be assessed from the thickness of skinfolds.[6] One difficulty with skinfold measurements is that the equations used to estimate body fat vary with age, sex, and ethnic background. Body fat increases with age even though the sum of the skinfold measurements remains constant.[6] This finding implies that with aging, fat accumulates at other than subcutaneous sites.

The ratio of waist or abdominal circumference to the hip or gluteal circumference provides an index of the regional fat distribution and has proven valuable as a guide to health risks. A nomogram for obtaining the abdominal-gluteal ratio (android-gynoid ratio or AGR), or waist-hips ratio (WHR), is shown in Figure 3. The circumference of the waist is obtained at the narrowest area above the umbilicus. The hip circumference is at the maximal gluteal protrusion.

Table 1. Comparison of methods of estimating body fat and its distribution

	Cost*	Ease of use	Accuracy	Regional fat
Height and weight	$	Easy	High	No
Skinfold measurements	$	Easy	Low	Yes
Circumferences	$	Easy	Moderate	Yes
Density				
Immersion	$$	Moderate	High	No
Plethysmograph	$$$	Difficult	High	No
Water (^3H_2O)	$$	Moderate	High	No
(D_2O or $H_2{}^{18}O$)	$$	Moderate	High	No
Potassium (^{40}K)	$$$	Difficult	High	No
Conductivity (TOBEC)	$$$	Moderate	Moderate	No
Impedance	$$	Easy	Moderate	No
Fat-soluble gas	$$	Difficult	High	No
Computed tomography	$$$$	Difficult	High	Yes
Ultrasound	$$$	Moderate	Moderate	Yes
Neutron activation	$$$$	Difficult	High	No
Magnetic resonance	$$$$	Difficult	High	Yes

* $ = low cost, $$ = moderate cost, $$$ = high cost, $$$$ = very high cost.

Abdominal fat (high AGR) is characteristic of males and is referred to as android or upper-body obesity. Fat on the hips (low AGR) is typical of females and

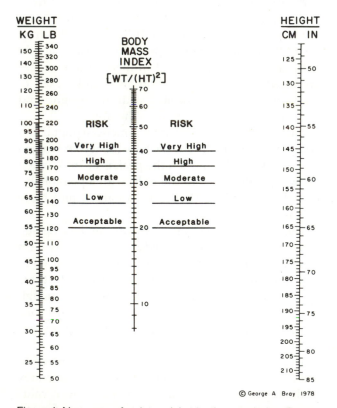

Figure 1. Nomogram for determining body mass index. To use this nomogram, place a ruler or other straight edge between the body weight in kilograms or pounds (without clothes) located on the left-hand line and the height in centimeters or in inches (without shoes) located on the right-hand line. The body mass index is read from the middle of the scale and is in metric units. (Copyright 1978, George A. Bray. Used with permission.)

is referred to as gynoid or lower-body obesity. The percentile values for AGR or WHR for men and women in relation to age are shown in Figure 4. Values above the 10th percentile are at very high risk for adverse health consequences of upper-body obesity as discussed in more detail later.

Isotopic, Chemical, and Other Methods to Measure Body Compartments. Both chemical and isotopic markers can be used to estimate body water, body fat, or potassium.[6,10] Measurement of body density provides a valuable quantitative technique for measuring body fat and fat-free mass. Density is determined from the weight of the body after submersion and out of water using Archimede's principle.[3,6] The technique is relatively easy if appropriate facilities are available, but it remains primarily a research method.

Total body electrical conductivity (TOBEC) also can be used to quantitate lean tissue and fat because of differences in the ability of these components to conduct electromagnetic waves.[11] However, these instruments are expensive.[11] A relatively inexpensive instrument for measuring body fat uses electrical impedance (bioelectric impedance analysis or BIA).[12] Electrodes are applied to one arm and leg and the impedance is measured. Because impedance is related to the aqueous portion of the body, formulas are used to estimate the percentage of fat in the body. The estimation with BIA of body fat in lean subjects has a very high correlation with body fat measured by density. It is also valid and accurate for measuring fat in both lean and obese subjects.

Computerized tomographic scans and nuclear-magnetic-resonance scans can provide quantitative estimates of regional fat and can give a ratio of in-

Table 2. Desirable body mass index range in relation to age*

Age group	Body mass index	
	Women	Men
y	kg/m²	
19–24	19–24	19–24
25–34	20–25	20–25
35–44	21–26	20–25
45–54	22–27	20–25
55–64	23–28	20–25
65+	24–29	20–25

* Body mass index can be determined from the nomogram in figure 1. From reference 8.

traabdominal to extraabdominal fat.[13] Ultrasonic waves applied to the skin will be reflected by the fat, muscle, and other interfaces and can also provide a measure of fat thickness in regional locations.[14] Finally, neutron activation of the whole body can be used to identify chemical components by their emission spectra.[15] This procedure is expensive and available only in a few centers.

In summary, body fat can be estimated in several ways. From a practical point of view, three methods are most useful. Measurements of height and weight, preferably expressed as the BMI, provide an estimate of the degree of overweight. BIA provides a quantitative estimate of total fat. For estimating regional fat distribution, measurement of the circumference of the abdomen or waist and the gluteus or hips expressed as a ratio has been most useful, but the thickness of the subscapular skinfold may also be used.

By use of one or more of these techniques, the major components of the body can be determined. The proportions of fat and nonfat components are depicted for a normal-weight (70 kg) male and an obese (100 kg) male as well as a normal-weight (55 kg) female and an obese (85 kg) female (Figure 5). The extra 30 kg of weight adds ~50% to body weight but increases body energy stored as fat by 200%.

Prevalence of Obesity

At birth the human body contains ~12% fat. This amount is higher than that for any other mammal except the whale. In the newborn period, body fat rises rapidly to reach a peak of ~25% by age 6 mo and then declines to 15–18% in the prepubertal years.[6] At puberty there is a significant increase in the percentage of fat in females and a significant decrease in males. By age 18 y males have ~15–18% body fat and females, 20–25%. Fat increases in both sexes after puberty and during adult life rises to be-

tween 30% and 40% of body weight. Between ages 20 and 50 y, fat content of males approximately doubles and that of females increases by ~50%. Total body weight, however, rises by only 10–15%, indicating that there is a reduction in lean body mass.[6]

The prevalence of obesity in Americans is shown in Figure 6. The percentage of overweight black women is substantially higher than that for white women (Panel B), but these racial differences are minor or reversed in men (Panel A). In both sexes, the prevalence of overweight increases with age.[16]

The percentage of body fat is influenced by the level of physical activity.[17] During physical training, body fat usually decreases and lean tissue increases. After training ends, however, this process is reversed. These shifts between body fat and lean tissue can occur without a change in body weight, but if regular activity is maintained throughout adult life, the increase in body fat may be prevented. Socioeconomic conditions also play an important role in the development of obesity. Excess body weight is 7–12 times more frequent in women from lower social classes than in women from upper social classes.[18] In males social class and race have a much less pronounced relationship to overweight.

By use of the BMI, it is possible to compare the prevalence of obesity in several countries (Table 3).[8] The prevalence of individuals with a BMI of 25–30 kg/m² is almost identical in all of the populations. The higher percentage of men than women in the 25–30 kg/m² range results from the fact that the median BMI for women is 22 kg/m² whereas the median for men is 25 kg/m² (see Figure 2). The prevalence of those with a BMI > 30 kg/m² is, however, higher

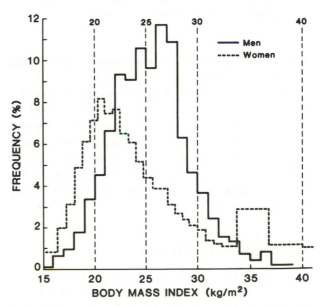

Figure 2. Frequency distribution of body mass index in America for men and women.

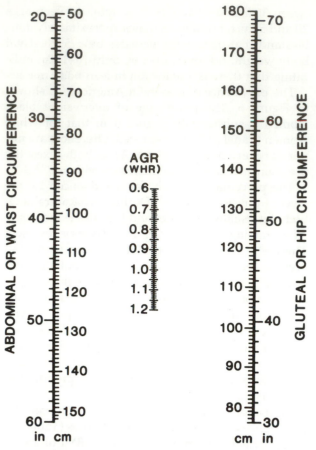

Figure 3. Nomogram for determining the ratio of abdominal (waist) circumference to gluteal (hips) circumference. Place a straight edge between the column for waist circumference and the column for hip circumference and read the ratio from the point where this straight edge crosses the AGR or WHR line. The waist or abdominal circumference is the smallest circumference below the rib cage and above the umbilicus, and the hips or gluteal circumference is taken as the largest circumference at the posterior extension of the buttocks. (Copyright 1987, George A. Bray. Used with permission.)

in both the United States and Canada than in the other three countries.

There are at least three possible explanations for the higher prevalence of obesity in North America. First, the higher proportion of automobiles may significantly reduce energy expenditure more than in other countries. Second, there may be differences in quantity or quality of dietary intake. Third, higher rates of smoking may explain the lower rate of obesity outside North America.

Pathogenesis of Obesity

Nutrient Imbalance. Food intake. Obesity is a problem of nutrient imbalance—more foodstuffs are stored as fat than are used for energy and metabolism. Do obese subjects ingest more food energy than

lean subjects? Based on both cross-sectional and longitudinal studies, the answer appears to be no. Between ages 50 and 60 y, men gained an average of 3.5 kg in the Zutphen study but showed a mean decrease in energy intake.[19] The implication is that energy expenditure had declined more than energy intake. Food intake of obese and lean subjects has been compared in a number of studies (Table 4). In all but one the mean caloric intake was less in the obese group. This difference was statistically significant for most comparisons of lean and obese women but not for comparisons of men. In spite of the reduced caloric intake in overweight subjects, a positive correlation has been reported between BMI and total fat and saturated fatty acid intake.[26]

Energy requirements generally decline with age, and we would anticipate that food intake would show a corresponding decrease.[6] The values for energy intake from three surveys are presented in Figure 7. The peak values occur in the second decade of life followed by a gradual decline in successive decades for both sexes. Thus, the increase in body weight and body fat with age cannot be attributed to increased nutrient intake but must be related to a relatively greater reduction in energy expenditure.

Direct observations of food intake have shown that obese persons choose and/or eat larger meals than do lean persons. In a variety of studies on food choice, Stunkard and Kaplan[27] found relative uniformity in the size of meals chosen in naturalistic settings. The energy content of the meals was strongly affected by eating site, and there was great variability in the amount of food chosen at each site. Thus, the major influence on how much people choose to eat is where they eat it. Eating in a cafeteria led to more food ingestion. The adjustment of energy intake to chronic changes in energy concentration of foods eaten produced a nearly uniform pattern, with obese individuals failing to compensate for changes in energy concentration as well as normal-weight individuals did.[28]

In summary, epidemiological data suggest that food intake may be lower in overweight than in lean subjects. Direct observation of obese subjects, however, tends to support the conclusion that they choose and eat more food and often do so more rapidly than normal-weight subjects. External environmental influences, such as lighting and noise, may modify the quantity and the quality of food eaten by obese individuals more than by lean individuals. Accuracy of energy estimates may be lower in obese individuals.[29] However, weight gain in adult life probably results from greater decrease in energy expenditure rather than any increase in food intake, which actually seems to decline with age. Moreover, large eaters of the same age and body weight as small eat-

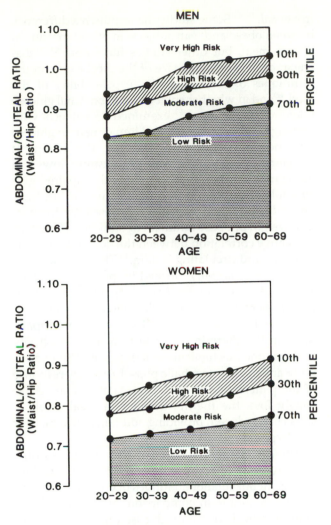

Figure 4. Percentiles for fat distribution. The percentiles for the ratio of abdominal circumference to gluteal circumference (ratio of waist to hips) are depicted for men and women by age groups. The relative risk for these percentiles is indicated based on the available information. (Plotted from tabular data in the Canadian Standardized Test of Fitness Third Edition 1986. Copyright 1987, George A. Bray. Used with permission.)

ers have less body fat and are more active than small eaters.[30]

Energy expenditure. The components of energy expenditure are depicted in Figure 8.

Resting metabolism is defined as the total energy required by the body in the resting state and is influenced by age, sex, body weight, drugs, climate, and genetics.[31] It represents ~70% of total energy expenditure. When corrected for body weight, the highest rate of energy expenditure occurs in infants. There is a gradual decline in childhood and a further slow decline of ~2% per decade in adult life. Metabolic rates for women are usually lower than those for men of comparable height and weight primarily due to the higher body fat level in women. Resting metabolic rate has the best relationship to fat-free body mass, but it is also closely related to surface area and total body weight because heat loss is related to the surface area of the skin. A higher body weight or greater lean body mass is associated with a higher metabolic rate as illustrated for lean and obese men in Figure 9.[31-33] This is due in part to the fact that obese individuals tend to have an expanded lean body mass and, thus, greater resting metabolic rates than lean people of similar heights. Metabolic rate clusters in families. If one individual is below the median for energy utilization, other members of the family also tend to be below the median.[34] A low resting metabolic rate in relation to lean body mass may be a predictor for lower physical activity, higher body fat, and an increased likelihood of becoming obese.[35]

The relationship of physical activity to obesity can be studied by laboratory observations or by observation in the natural environment. In the laboratory, the treadmill and cycle ergometer have been the main tools used to examine the efficiency of exercising muscle in obese subjects. In both obese and lean individuals, the efficiency for coupling energy release to muscular contraction is ~30%.[36] That is, the work of turning the flywheel on a cycle ergometer accounted for 30% of the energy expended during cycling. Thus, there is no evidence to indicate an abnormality in the metabolic coupling of substrate metabolism to the contraction of muscular tissue in moderately or massively obese subjects.[36]

The second approach to studying energy expenditure is observation. Obese individuals often are observed to be less active than normal-weight individuals. A lower level of spontaneous movement, however, does not necessarily imply reduced energy expenditure, because the overweight individual uses more energy for any given movement.[36] In one approach to this problem, Waxman and Stunkard[37] related movement to energy expenditure and found that obese boys expend more energy on the playground but expend similar amounts in the home compared with lean siblings. Thus, spending less time in physical activity does not necessarily result in a reduction of energy expenditure.

In normal-weight individuals, graded increases in physical activity have been reported to increase food intake. In obese individuals, however, changing the level of physical activity has a much smaller effect on food intake.[38] As noted above, large eaters have less fat and are more active than small eaters matched for age, sex, height, and weight.[30] Thus the level of physical activity may modulate food intake and body fat in lean subjects. A disturbance in this system may play a key role in the development of obesity.

When food is eaten, the metabolic rate increases and then returns toward normal. The process requires

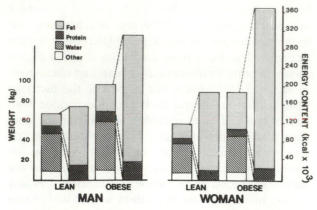

Figure 5. Body composition in obesity. The percentages of fat, protein, water, and other components for a normal 70-kg man and 55-kg woman are shown at the left of each group along with the data for an obese individual who is 30 kg heavier. The contribution of fat and protein to body energy stores is also indicated in the bar to the right of the one for weight. (Copyright 1987, George A. Bray. Used with permission.)

several hours, and during this time the increase in energy expenditure can approximate 10–15% of the total energy value of the ingested food. One explanation for this thermogenic response to a meal is that it results from enhanced activity of the sympathetic nervous system, the effects of which are shown in activity of brown adipose tissue or muscle.[39,40] If this is correct, then a reduction in sympathetic activity of obese subjects compared with lean ones might provide a mechanism for enhanced metabolic efficiency that might allow energy to be stored rather than burned. A loss of these sympathetic nervous system mechanisms might also explain why increasing physical activity does not significantly reduce food intake in obese subjects.

The concept that an altered thermic response to food may serve as a mechanism for the storage of extra calories in human obesity is intriguing and con-

troversial.[41-43] Some studies have shown a difference between obese and lean subjects in energy produced after a meal, but other studies have not. The discrepancy may lie in the size of the meal eaten, in the techniques of recording, in the palatability of the food,[42] and in whether subjects had abnormal glucose tolerance. Golay et al.[43] examined 55 subjects with varying degrees of obesity and impairment in glucose tolerance, including frank diabetes. The increment in energy expenditure was significantly lower in obese nondiabetics and in those with impaired glucose tolerance than in normal volunteers.[43] In turn, obese diabetics had a smaller response than the normal-weight or obese nondiabetic subjects. There was a negative correlation between the degree of thermic response and circulating insulin.[43] The thermic effect of glucose is partially blocked by propranol, a drug that blocks β-receptors. This component of diet-induced thermogenesis is called facultative thermogenesis. These data suggest that there is an impairment in the thermic response to a meal in obesity and that one mechanism associated with this change is the anticipatory (cephalic phase) secretory response of the pancreatic system for releasing insulin. After weight loss, the thermic effect of a meal in obese subjects is reduced, providing additional evidence for this hypothesis.

Adipose Tissue. Over 90% of body energy is stored as triglyceride in adipose tissue.[6,44] Protein provides important but smaller quantities of energy. Glycogen stores are minute in comparison, but glycogen provides a critical source of glucose during exercise or short-term fasting.

Adipose tissue has two principal functions: *1*) synthesis and storage of fatty acids in triacylglycerols and *2*) release of fatty acids as a source of metabolic fuel. It may also serve as a source of information about body energy stores. Triglyceride is stored in fat cells, which differ in number and size between

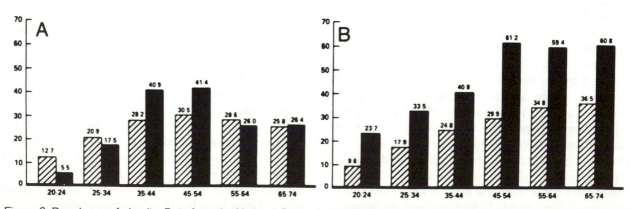

Figure 6. Prevalence of obesity. Data from the National Center for Health Statistics show the percentage of overweight men (A) and women (B) by age and socioeconomic status using the 85th percentile of weights-for-height for ages 20–24 y as the upper limits for weight. ▨ whites, ■ blacks. (Reprinted from reference 18. Used with permission.)

Table 3. Percentage of overweight and obese individuals in several affluent countries*

	Age	Overweight		Obese	
		Males	Females	Males	Females
	y	%		%	
North America					
United States	20–74	31	24	12	12
Canada	20–69	40	28	9	12
Europe					
Great Britain	16–65	34	24	6	8
Netherlands	20+	34	24	4	6
Australia	25–64	34	24	7	7

* Adapted from reference 8.

one region of the body and another. Women generally have more gluteal fat than men. The total number of fat cells is increased in individuals with obesity beginning in childhood.[45] Storage of fat in the first months of life occurs primarily by an increase in the size of already existing fat cells. By the end of the first year, fat-cell size has nearly doubled with little change in the total number of fat cells,[45] either in children who become obese or in those who do not. In children who are lean, the size of the fat cells decreases after the first year of life. Obese children, on the other hand, retain throughout childhood the large fat cells that developed during the first year of life. Fat cells multiply in number throughout the growing years in a process that usually terminates in adolescence. The number of fat cells in obese children increases more rapidly than that in lean children, reaching adult levels by the age of 10–12 y.[45] Current evidence suggests that after puberty acute changes in body fat stores occur primarily by increasing the size of adipocytes that already exist, with little or no change in total number. Acute weight loss is likewise accomplished primarily by a reduction in the size of extant fat cells. However, recent evidence suggests that the number of fat cells also may change in adult life.[46] A chronic increase in body fat may lead to an increase in the number of fat cells; conversely, a prolonged reduction in body fat may possibly lead to a decrease in the number of fat cells.[46]

The size, number, and distribution of fat cells are useful in classifying obesity and in estimating the prognosis with different forms of therapy.[47] Obese individuals who are ≥75% above desirable weight almost always have an increased number of fat cells, whereas those with more modest degrees of overweight may be hypercellular but are much more likely to have only an increase in fat cell size (hypertrophic obesity). The duration of weight loss that follows successful dietary treatment for obesity is shorter and the rate at which weight is regained is

Table 4. Calorie intake of overweight and normal-weight or lean individuals

Author	Normal weight or lean			Overweight			p
	n	Sex	Calorie intake	n	Sex	Calorie intake	
Beaudoin and Mayer[20]	58	F	2198 ± 587*	59	F	1964 ± 594*	<0.05
	20	F	2201 ± 475*	33	F	2829 ± 674*	<0.01
Lincoln[21]	98	M, F	3319	101	M, F	3144	N.S.
Baecke et al.[22]	47	M	3070 ± 105*	27	M	2983 ± 167*	N.S.
	50	F	2280 ± 65*	45	F	2045 ± 64*	<0.05
Kromhout[23]‡	202	M	3193 ± 606*	202	M	2916 ± 652*	<0.001
Braitman et al.[24]§	708	M	2359	79	M	2411	N.S.
	1246	F	1689	245	F	1525	<0.001
Romieu et al.[25]‖	45	F	1684 ± 315†	47	F	1635 ± 340†	N.S.

* $\bar{x}$ ± SEM.
† $\bar{x}$ ± SD.
‡ Comparison of the lowest and highest quartile of BMI.
§ Comparison of <101% of optimum weight vs. >149% optimum weight.
‖ Comparison of the lowest and highest tertile of BMI.

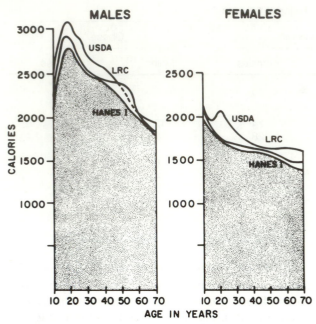

Figure 7. Relation of food intake to age. Data from three studies of food intake in relation to age are plotted for men and women. USDA, U.S. Department of Agriculture; LRC, Lipid Research Clinics; HANES I, first Health and Nutrition Examination Survey. (Copyright 1987, George A. Bray. Used with permission.)

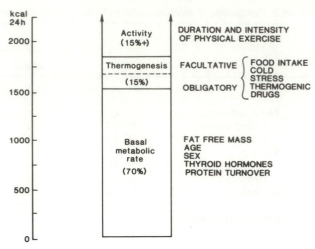

Figure 8. Components of energy expenditure. The energy partition into basal energy needs, thermogenesis, and activity was estimated based on a 2500 kcal/d requirement. The upper end is open, indicating that activity is variable and can be increased for the normal individual. However, this component usually comprises ~30% of total daily energy expenditure. (Copyright 1987, George A. Bray. Used with permission.)

more rapid in individuals with hypercellular obesity than in those with hypertrophic obesity.[47] The identification of adipsin,[48] a peptide secreted by fat cells, may provide a clue about how this might work.

Health Risks Associated with Being Overweight

Overweight and Health Risks. The effects of overweight on health have been evaluated in both prospective and retrospective studies. Studies involving >750,000 subjects each from the life insurance industry,[49] the American Cancer Society,[50] and Norway[51] yielded similar results, which are consistent with many but not all smaller prospective studies.[52] The overall relationship between BMI and excess mortality is shown in Figure 10, which plots relative mortality for various deviations of BMI using the American Cancer Society data.[50] The data show a J-shaped curve, with the minimum mortality for both men and women occurring among individuals with a BMI of 22–25 kg/m². Deviations in BMI above and below this range are associated with an increase in mortality. Individuals with a BMI of 30 kg/m² clearly have increased mortality. As the BMI approaches 40 kg/m², the curve becomes progressively steeper. It is also apparent that mortality increases when BMI falls below 20 kg/m². A recent study examining mortality during 16 y of follow-up in 2381 males and

females in Scotland illustrates the relationship between mortality and BMI.[53] Mortality from lung cancer increased as BMI decreased, whereas mortality from cardiovascular disease increased with increasing BMI. At the two extremes of the J-shaped relationship between BMI and mortality, the causes of death are different. Some cancers and respiratory and digestive diseases comprise the excess mortality associated with low body weights (BMI < 20 kg/m²) whereas cardiovascular diseases, diabetes mellitus, gall bladder disease, and other cancers make up the excess mortality in the overweight (BMI > 30 kg/m²).

Fat Distribution and Health Risks. One of the most important developments in understanding

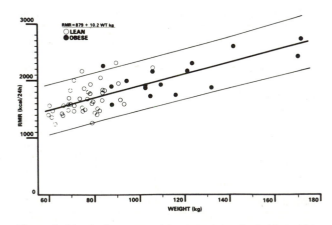

Figure 9. Metabolic rate and body weight. As body weight increases, the metabolic rate increases. The slope of this relationship is approximately 24-h energy expenditure = 750 kcal + 15 kcal/kg. (Reprinted from reference 31. Used with permission.)

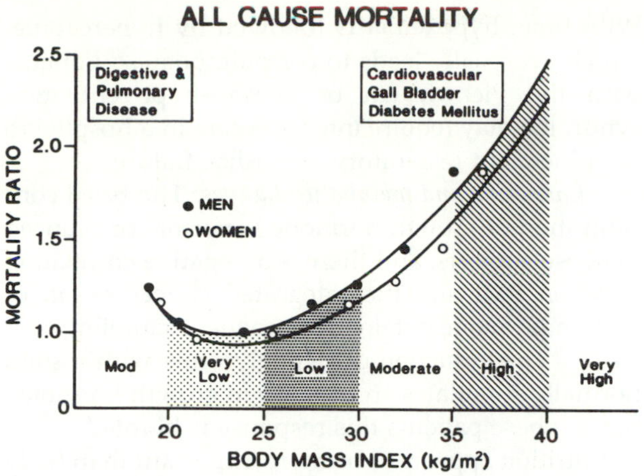

ALL CAUSE MORTALITY

Figure 10. Mortality ratio and body mass index. Data from the American Cancer Society study are plotted for men and women to show relationship of body mass index (BMI) to overall mortality. At a BMI <20 kg/m^2 and >25 kg/m^2 there is an increase in relative mortality. The major causes for this increased mortality are listed along with a division of BMI groupings into various levels of risk. (Adapted from reference 50. Copyright 1987, George A. Bray. Used with permission.)

health risks associated with overweight has come from measurements of body fat distribution. There are two types of fat distribution: (1) the abdominal, android, upper-body, or male type and (2) the gynoid, lower-body, or female type. The former has a higher AGR, or WHR. As early as the 1950s, Vague[54] suggested that a preponderance of abdominal fat increases the risk for diabetes and cardiovascular disease. Five prospective studies have examined the relation of fat distribution to morbidity and mortality.[55-59] Whether the AGR or WHR or the subscapular skinfold measurement or a combination of skin fold measurements were used as the indicator of fat distribution, all studies found a clear-cut and highly significant increase in the risk of death and/or an increased risk of diabetes, hypertension, heart attack, and stroke with increased upper-body obesity. Fat distribution was a more important risk factor for morbidity and mortality than overweight per se and had a relative risk ratio of ≥2.

In the Honolulu Heart Study,[59] BMI and subscapular skinfold thickness were related for thirds (tertiles) of the men under study. There was a graded increase in risk of heart attack with each tertile that was independent of other risk factors. Increased truncal fat was as hazardous as hypertension, smoking, or hypercholesterolemia (Figure 11).

In addition to the prospective data described above, cross-sectional studies have also shown increased prevalence of glucose intolerance, insulin resistance, elevated blood pressure, and elevated blood lipids in both males and females with increased abdominal fat or upper-body obesity.[60,61] It has been suggested

that the abdominal or android fat pattern may represent an increase in the size and/or number of more metabolically active intraabdominal fat cells. These fat cells release free fatty acids directly into the portal circulation, which might interfere with insulin clearance in the liver and thus affect various metabolic processes. It is interesting in this context that a recent study from Japan used abdominal computed tomography scanning of fat distribution to separate intraabdominal or visceral fat from subcutaneous fat and thus defined a visceral-subcutaneous fat ratio (V:SQ). This ratio was correlated inversely with glucose tolerance.[62]

Obesity and Organ Function. Cardiovascular system. The relation of hypertension to obesity has been widely recognized. It is important to use a cuff that encircles 75% of the arm, because smaller cuffs may artificially elevate blood pressure.[63] However, even with the limitations in the techniques of measuring blood pressure by indirect auscultation, the available data almost uniformly indicate the important relationship between body weight and blood pressure and between fat distribution and blood pressure.[64] Upper-body obesity is associated with further elevations in blood pressure (Figure 12).[65]

Increased blood pressure probably results from increased peripheral arteriolar resistance. During and after weight loss there is usually a reduction in blood pressure. Obesity also increases the work of the heart even when blood pressure is normal. This too can be reversed with weight loss.[66] A cardiomyopathy of obesity has been reported and is associated with congestive heart failure.

Diabetes mellitus. Obesity appears to aggravate the development of diabetes, and weight loss appears to reduce the risk of this disease.[67,68] Drenick[67] followed a group of obese men, none of whom were initially diabetic. During 6 y of follow-up, the percentage of those with frank diabetes increased to >50%. An additional 30% showed impaired glucose tolerance, indicating that during the 6 y of follow-up, >80% of the group showed a deterioration in glucose tolerance. The risk of diabetes is worsened with increased abdominal fat and with weight gain.[65] With weight loss, glucose tolerance improves, insulin secretion decreases, and insulin resistance is reduced.[69]

Gallbladder disease. The association of obesity with gallbladder disease has been documented in several studies.[6,65] Obese women aged 20–30 y had a sixfold increase in the risk of developing gallbladder disease compared with normal-weight women. By age 60 y, nearly one-third of obese women can expect to develop gallbladder disease.[6] The relation of gallbladder disease to fat distribution is also evident (see Figure 12). This tendency to gallstones may result

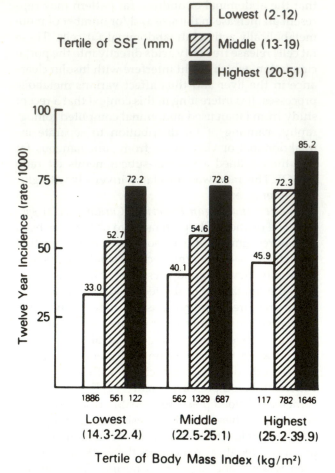

Figure 11. Incidence of heart disease in relation to body mass index (BMI) and skinfold thickness. Men in the Honolulu Heart Study were grouped according to tertiles of BMI and then into tertiles of subscapular skinfold thickness for each tertile of BMI. There is a graded effect of increasing subscapular skinfold on 12-y incidence of heart attack within each of the tertiles of BMI (Adapted from reference 59. Used with permission.)

from increased cholesterol synthesis that is observed in obesity. Approximately 20 mg/d of cholesterol are synthesized for each extra kilogram of stored fat. This in turn results in increased biliary excretion of cholesterol, producing a bile which is more saturated in cholesterol and, thus, increasing the risk of gallstone disease.[6]

Pulmonary function. Measurements of pulmonary function are normal in most obese individuals.[70,71] Only with massive obesity are decreased reserve volumes and lowered arterial oxygen saturation obvious. The most important pulmonary problem in the obese patient is the Pickwickian or obesity-hypoventilation syndrome that, although uncommon, occurs mainly in massively obese individuals. There is a growing body of literature that suggests that the symptoms of this syndrome result largely from sleep apnea.[70]

With time, hypoxemia is followed by hypercapnia, which eventually leads to cor pulmonale.[70] Patients with the Pickwickian or obesity-hypoventilation syndrome may require intensive care in a hospital to treat incipient respiratory or cardiac failure.

Endocrine and metabolic changes. The basal concentration of growth hormone is normal or reduced in obese subjects, and there is a negative correlation between BMI and the integrated concentration of growth hormone obtained by frequent sampling over 24 h.[72] The induction of hypoglycemia with insulin normally stimulates an increase in growth hormone, but in obese patients this response is blunted.[6,73]

Nutrition appears to be more important than body weight per se in determining the circulating concentration of triiodothyronine.[74] During fasting and severe caloric restriction, total thyroxine (T_4) levels remain normal, but the serum concentration of total triiodothyronine (T_3) decreases, and that of reverse T_3 (rT_3) increases. In contrast to starvation, overnutrition is associated with an increase in serum T_3 and a fall in rT_3[74] in both obese and lean subjects.

The diurnal rhythm of cortisol is preserved in patients with simple obesity,[6,73] but afternoon values may be above normal. There is a small but significant negative correlation of cortisol with percent overweight in women but not men. One milligram of dexamethasone at midnight followed by measurement of plasma cortisol the next morning or measurement of urinary free cortisol in a 24-h urine collection is the best screening test to separate obesity from Cushing's syndrome. Obese patients who do not suppress with this test are a small group for whom more complex procedures are needed to exclude the possibility of Cushing's syndrome.

In obese males, the plasma concentration of testosterone is decreased.[73] This reduction in total testosterone is accompanied by a reduction in the level of sex-hormone-binding globulin resulting in a normal level of free testosterone in moderately obese men.[75] However, in massively obese men, there may be a decrease in free testosterone as well.

In obese girls, the onset of menarche occurs at a younger age than in normal-weight girls.[6] The observation that menstruation is initiated when body weight reaches a critical mass provides one explanation for this phenomenon. As the rate of growth accelerates in late childhood, the entrance into this critical weight range may initiate puberty. Because obese girls grow faster and enter this critical mass at a younger age than normal-weight girls do, menstruation usually starts at an earlier age. The obese patient often shows a decrease in the regularity of menstrual cycles and an increase in the frequency of other menstrual abnormalities. In one study, 43% of women with menstrual disorders were overweight.[76]

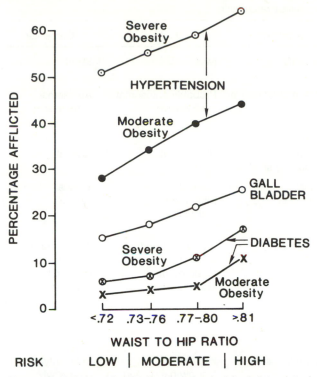

Figure 12. Relationship of ratio of abdominal (waist) to gluteal (hip) circumference to various risks of obesity. These data were adapted from the retrospective studies in reference 65. (Used with permission.)

Does Weight Loss Improve Health? Both the insurance companies[49] and the Framingham study[77] provide data suggesting that weight reduction may be beneficial. In both men and women who successfully lose and maintain a lower weight, mortality was reduced to within the normal limits based on sex and age according to life-insurance statistics. From the data obtained in Framingham, MA, a 10% reduction in relative weight for men was associated with a decrease in serum glucose of 0.14 mmol/L, a decrease in serum cholesterol of 0.292 mmol/L, a decrease in systolic blood pressure of 6.6 mm Hg, and a decrease in serum uric acid of 19.6 μmol/L.[77] For each 10% reduction in the body weight of men, these data predict that there would be an anticipated 20% decrease in the incidence of coronary artery disease.

Clinical Types of Obesity

Genetic Factors in Obesity. In human obesity, genetic factors are expressed in two ways. First, there is a group of rare forms of dysmorphic obesity in which genetic factors are of prime importance. Second, there is a genetic substrate upon which environmental factors interact in the development of obesity.

The dysmorphic forms of obesity are listed in Table

5. In most of them obesity is only of moderate degree, but it may be pronounced particularly in the Prader-Willi syndrome. These forms of obesity are transmitted by both recessive and dominant modes of inheritance. The Prader-Willi syndrome is associated in half or more of the cases with a translocation or deletion on the short arm of chromosome 15.[78]

Family studies show that obesity runs in families, but they do not critically separate environmental from genetic factors.[6] The distinction can be made in studies using adopted children or twins. In the Danish adoption registry, a sample of 800 adoptees showed no relationship between BMI of the adoptive parents and their children.[79] On the other hand, the BMI of the biological parents increased with increasing weight of the children. These data suggest that inheritance plays an important role in the risk of developing obesity and are consistent with most but not all other studies of adopted children.[6,80]

The most definitive evidence for genetic versus environmental factors in the development of obesity comes from the examination of body weight in twins.[6,81,82] Monozygotic twins have identical genetic material whereas dizygotic twins have the genetic diversity of brothers and/or sisters. However, the environmental closeness of monozygotic twins should permit evaluation of these groups of twins along with other siblings and more distant relatives in order to identify genetic factors in obesity. Using BMI as the criterion for obesity, Stunkard et al.[81] compared 1983 male monozygotic and 2104 male dizygotic twins from the Veterans Administration twin registry. Monozygotic twins had a higher correlation between their body weights than did dizygotic twins, and calculations of the heritability for obesity suggested that nearly two-thirds of the variability in BMI was attributable to genetic factors.

Bouchard and his colleagues measured skinfolds and total body fat in various groups of individuals with differing degrees of genetic relationship, including monozygotic and dizygotic twins.[82] In adopted siblings, there is a very low order of correlation. Biological siblings, however, showed a higher correlation, and as might be expected, the correlation was highest among monozygotic twins. Biological siblings had a lower order of correlation for all of the variables than did dizygotic twins, although both groups have the same genetic variability, implying that there was an environmental influence operative in the dizygotic twins that was absent in their biological siblings. On the basis of a technique called path analysis, these data on the genetic and nongenetic components for body fat and BMI can be partitioned into transmissible and nontransmissible components (Figure 13). Approximately half of the

Table 5. Comparison of syndromes of obesity-hypogonadism and mental retardation

Feature	Prader-Willi	Bardet Biedl	Ahlstrom	Cohen	Carpenter
Mental retardation	Mild to moderate		Normal IQ	Mild	Slight
Inheritance	Sporadic two-thirds have defective Chr 15 (q:1.2)	Autosomal recessive	Autosomal recessive	Probably autosomal recessive	Autosomal recessive
Stature	Short	Normal Infrequently short	Normal Infrequently short	Short or tall	Normal
Obesity	Generalized moderate severe Onset: 1–3 y	Generalized Early onset: 1–2 y	Truncal Early onset: 2–5 y	Truncal Midchildhood, age 5 y	Truncal Gluteal
Craniofaces	Narrow bifrontal diameter Almond shaped eyes Strabismus V-shaped mouth High arched palate	Not distinctive	Not distinctive	High nasal bridge Arched palate Open mouth Short philtrum	Acrocephaly Flat nasal bridge High arched palate
Limbs	Small hands and feet Hypotonia	Polydactyly	No abnormalities	Hypotonia Narrow hands and feet	Polydactyly Syndactyly Genu valgum
Reproductive status	Primary hypogonadism	Primary hypogonadism	Hypogonadism in males only	Normal gonadal function or hypogonadotrophic hypogonadism	Secondary hypogonadism
Other features	Enamel hypoplasia				

distribution of body fat is nontransmissible and approximately 25% is genetic.

In summary, single and polygenic inheritance are both involved in the transmission of obesity in man. The best estimates suggest that genetic factors may be of less importance than environmental factors in the determination of total body fat but of more significance in determining its distribution.

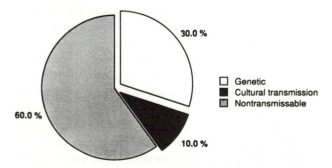

Figure 13. Genetic factors in obesity. The genetic and non-genetic transmission of fat-free mass and the ratio of subcutaneous fat to fat mass are presented from the analysis in reference 82. (Used with permission.)

Classification of Obesity. Obesity can be classified in at least three ways: by the anatomic characteristics and regional distribution of adipose tissue, by etiologic causes, and by the age at onset of obesity.

Anatomic classification. An anatomic classification is based on the number of adipocytes and on fat distribution. In many obese individuals whose problems began in childhood, the number of adipocytes may be increased by two- to fourfold (normal range = 20 to 60 $\times$ 10^9 fat cells). Individuals with increased numbers of fat cells have hypercellular obesity. This is distinguished from other forms of obesity in which the total number of adipocytes is normal, but the size of individual fat cells is increased. In general, all obesity is associated with an increase in the size of adipocytes, but only selected forms have an increase in the total number of such fat cells.

Obesity may also be classified according to body fat distribution (see Figure 4). Both males and females with upper-body obesity have an increased risk of cardiovascular disease, hypertension, and diabetes. On the other hand, lower-body obesity appears to carry a much lower risk to health.

Etiologic classification. There are a number of etiologic causes for obesity. Endocrine diseases may cause obesity, but such cases are rare.[6] Moreover, endocrine diseases usually produce only small increases in body fat. Hyperinsulinism, caused by islet cell tumors or by injection of excess quantities of insulin, results in increased food intake and increased fat storage, but the magnitude of this effect is usually modest. A somewhat more substantial obesity is observed with the increased cortisol secretion of Cushing's syndrome. Obesity may also occur with hypothyroidism. Finally, aberrations in the distribution of body fat are also observed with hypogonadism.

Hypothalamic obesity is a rare syndrome in man[83] but can be regularly produced in animals by injury to the ventromedial region of the hypothalamus. This region is responsible for integrating information about energy stores and regulating the function of the autonomic nervous system. Hypothalamic obesity has been reported in human subjects under a variety of circumstances. The major factors producing hypothalamic damage are trauma, malignancy, and inflammatory disease. Symptoms and signs that accompany the syndrome include those related to intracranial pressure, endocrine alterations, and a variety of neurological and physiological derangements. Treatment of the syndrome requires treating the underlying disease and giving appropriate endocrine support.

Physical inactivity plays an important role in the development of obesity. Gross obesity in rats can be produced by severe restriction of activity. In a modern affluent society, energy-sparing devices also reduce energy expenditure and may enhance the tendency to become fat.[6]

Diet is another etiologic factor in obesity. This is particularly prominent in experimental animals but also may play a role in the development of human obesity. When rodents eat a high-fat diet, drink sucrose-containing solutions, or eat a cafeteria-type diet, most strains are unable to appropriately regulate energy balance and ingest more energy than is needed for weight maintenance. The excess energy is accumulated as fat, and the animals become obese to various degrees. Recent epidemiologic data in women show that overweight women eat more total fat and saturated fatty acids than do normal-weight women.[26] Thus, a high-fat diet may increase the risk of obesity for those who are predisposed.

Classification by age of onset. Progressive childhood obesity is a hypercellular form of obesity.[6] Such individuals develop the abnormality early in life and show a continuing deviation in weight gain thereafter. At this time, none of the forms of obesity, including progressive childhood obesity, can be detected at birth. Birth weights of children who become obese are in general not different from the birth weights of those whose childhood weights are normal. The critical periods for the appearance of progressive childhood obesity are in the first 2 y of life and again between ages 4 and 11 y. The most serious form begins in this latter period and may progress thereafter. Childhood-onset obesity is usually hypercellular, and it may be resistant to therapy. Adult-onset obesity tends to be hypertrophic with large fat cells.

Approaches to Treatment

Goals and Realities of Treatment. Treating individuals with weight problems has many similarities to treating other chronic diseases. Hypertension, for example, can be effectively treated by current medications. Yet, the side effects of treatment and the need to treat individuals who may have no overt symptoms from hypertension lead to high levels of therapeutic failure, including unwillingness of such individuals to seek medical help, unwillingness to maintain treatment once prescribed, and termination of treatment because of some of the side effects of medication. Treatment of obesity has similar problems.

In addition, treatments for overweight individuals are almost always palliative and not curative. In the current state of knowledge, we are usually unable to cure obesity. That is, most treatments for obesity, when terminated, do not produce a permanent remission. A simple analogy is appendectomy, where the patient is cured by surgical removal of the diseased appendix. Comparable results with treatment of overweight patients are rare. One example would be effective treatment for Cushing's syndrome, where the primary presenting symptom is obesity. For most cases of obesity, however, we are seeking palliation and alleviation of symptoms associated with the condition, not a cure.

Recidivism, that is, regaining of lost weight, is a third reality of treatment for obesity. Of those who lose weight on any treatment program, a significant percentage will fail to maintain this weight loss.[84] Identification of those individuals who will be successful in losing weight is at best an inexact procedure. Some suggested techniques for identifying those who are likely to succeed include the initial 1-wk weight loss, frequency and regularity of attendance at a weight-loss program, and the belief that you can control your own weight. However, additional insight is needed before we will be able to identify successful individuals at the beginning of treatment.

The fourth reality of treatment for obesity is its cost. Each year, more than $50 billion are spent on

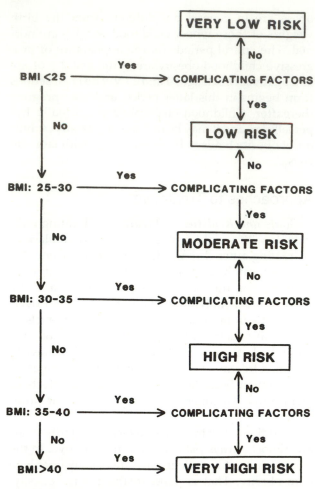

Figure 14. Risk classification algorithm. The patient is first placed into a category based on body mass index. The presence or absence of complicating factors determines the degree of health risk. Complicating factors include elevated abdominal-gluteal ratio (male 0.95, female 0.85), diabetes mellitus, hypertension, hyperlipidemia, male sex, and age < 40 y. (Copyright 1987, George A. Bray. Used with permission.)

efforts to control weight gain or induce weight loss.[85] More than 50% of the expenditure is for diet foods ($30 billion) with the remainder distributed into several other categories. In the discussion below we will try to evaluate the cost and effectiveness of various methods of weight control.

Evaluation of Risk Associated with Obesity. Because all treatments entail some risk, the first essential in deciding whether treatment is appropriate and what that treatment should be is the assessment of the risk associated with adiposity. Two independent variables can be used to assess this risk. The first is the risk associated with the degree of deviation in body weight from normal. Underweight individuals have increased risk for respiratory disease, tuberculosis, digestive disease, and some cancers (see Figure 12). Overweight individuals, on the other hand, are more prone to cardiovascular disease, gallbladder

disease, high blood pressure, and diabetes.[80] Body weights associated with BMI of 20–25 kg/m² have no increased risk from body weight. When BMI is <20 kg/m² or >25 kg/m², risk increases in a curvilinear fashion. Individuals with a BMI of 25–30 kg/m² have low risk, those with a BMI between 30 and 35 kg/m² have moderate risk, those with a BMI between 35 and 40 kg/m² have high risk, and those with a BMI >40 kg/m² have very-high risk from their excess weight.

The distribution of body fat is also a useful guide to risks. The higher the proportion of abdominal or truncal fat, the greater the risk (see Figure 4). The algorithm in Figure 14 provides a means of including both total body fat, as estimated from the body mass index, and the distribution of body fat in making decisions about relative risk from adiposity.[85] At any given level of BMI, the risk to health is increased with abdominal fat. Other factors included in Figure 14 that increase risk from overweight are the presence of medical problems such as diabetes mellitus, hypertension, or hyperlipidemia; age < 40 y with increasing weight; and male sex.[86]

A Risk-benefit Assessment of Treatment. Treatments for obesity can be grouped by their relative risk (Figure 15). They can be further divided by whether they influence nutrient intake or energy loss. In a quantitative sense, treatments that reduce energy intake have a greater potential for acute weight loss than those that increase energy expenditure. Because all of our nutrient energy comes from food, we can reduce energy intake to zero (starvation). Energy expenditure, on the other hand, has a minimum level associated with the energy required to maintain body temperature and to repair tissues and maintain func-

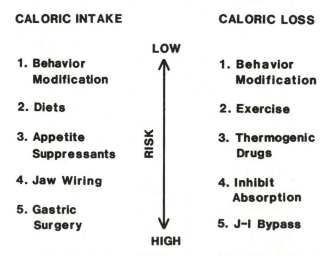

Figure 15. Treatments for obesity in relation to risk. On the left are treatments that affect energy intake and on the right are treatments that affect energy expenditure or loss. They are ranked in estimated overall order for risk with lowest risk at the top and highest risk at the bottom.

tion of the heart and other organs. Thus, simply staying in bed and engaging in no physical activity reduces energy expenditure to ~0.8 kcal/min (1150 kcal/d) for a normal-weight adult. High levels of physical activity can increase this by two- to fourfold over 24 h. Thus, for initial weight loss, decreasing food intake has the most to recommend it, whereas increasing energy expenditure through physical activity appears to have a particular attractiveness in efforts at long-term maintenance of a lower body weight.

References

1. G.A. Bray, ed. (1989) Obesity: a clinical and metabolic approach. *Med. Clin.* 73:1–269.

2. K.D. Brownell and J.P. Foreyt, eds. (1986) *Handbook of Eating Disorders. Physiology, Psychology, and Treatment of Obesity, Anorexia, and Bulimia,* Basic Books, New York.

3. J.S. Garrow (1981) *Treat Obesity Seriously,* Churchill Livingston, London.

4. W.P.T. James (1984) Obesity. *Clin. Endocrinol. Metab.* 13:435–663.

5. R.J. Wurtman and J.J. Wurtman (1987) Human obesity. *Ann. N.Y. Acad. Sci.* 499:1–349.

6. G.A. Bray (1976) *The Obese Patient. Major Problems in Internal Medicine,* W.B. Saunders, Philadelphia.

7. A. Keys, F. Fidanza, M.J. Karvonen, N. Kimuro, and H.L. Taylor (1972) Indices of relative weight and obesity. *J. Chronic Dis.* 25:329–343.

8. G.A. Bray (1987) Overweight is risking fate. Definition, classification, prevalence and risks. *Ann. N.Y. Acad. Sci.* 249:14–28.

9. S. Abraham, M.D. Carroll, M.F. Najjar, and F. Robinson (1983) *Obese and Overweight Adults in the United States.* USDHHS Publication No. (PHS) 83-1680, Vital Health and Statistics Series 11, No. 230, National Center for Health Statistics, Hyattsville, MD.

10. H.C. Lukaski (1987) Methods for the assessment of human body composition: traditional and new. *Am. J. Clin. Nutr.* 46:537–556.

11. H.C. Lukaski, P.E. Johnson, W.W. Bolonchuk, et al (1985) Assessment of fat-free mass using bioelectrical impedance measurement of the human body. *Am. J. Clin. Nutr.* 41:810–817.

12. K.R. Segal, M. Van Loan, P.I. Fitzgerald, J.A. Hodgdon, and T.B. Van Itallie (1988) Lean body mass estimation by bioelectrical impedance analysis: a four-site cross-validation study. *Am. J. Clin. Nutr.* 47:7–14.

13. L. Sjostrom, H. Kvist, A. Cederblad, and U. Tylen (1986) Determination of total adipose tissue and body fat in women by computed tomography, ^{40}K, and tritium. *Am. J. Physiol.* 250:E736–E745.

14. R.J. Kuczmarski, M.T. Fanelli, and G.G. Koch (1987) Ultrasonic assessment of body composition in obese adults: overcoming limitations of the skinfold caliper. *Am. J. Clin. Nutr.* 45:717–724.

15. S.H. Cohn, D. Vartsky, S. Yasumura, et al. (1980) Compartmental body composition based on total-body nitrogen, potassium and calcium. *Am. J. Physiol.* 239:524–530.

16. T.B. Van Itallie (1985) Health implications of overweight and obesity in the United States. *Ann. Intern. Med.* 103:983–988.

17. J.H. Wilmore (1983) Body composition in sports and exercise directions for future research. *Med. Sci. Sports Exerc.* 15:21–31.

18. P.B. Goldblatt, M.E. Moore, and A.J. Stunkard (1965) Social factors in obesity. *JAMA* 192:1039–1044.

19. D. Kromhout (1983) Changes in energy and macronutrients in 871 middle-aged men during 10 years of follow-up (the Zutphen study). *Am. J. Clin. Nutr.* 37:287–294.

20. R. Beaudoin and J. Mayer (1953) Food intakes of obese and non-obese women. *J. Am. Diet. Assoc.* 29:29–33.

21. J.E. Lincoln (1972) Calorie intake, obesity, and physical activity. *Am. J. Clin. Nutr.* 25:390–394.

22. J.A. Baecke, W.A. van Staveren, and J. Burema (1983) Food consumption, habitual physical activity, and body fatness in young Dutch adults. *Am. J. Clin. Nutr.* 37:278–286.

23. D. Kromhout (1983) Changes in energy and macronutrients in 871 middle-aged men during 10 years of follow-up (the Zutphen study). *Am. J. Clin. Nutr.* 37:287–294.

24. L.E. Braitman, E.V. Adlin, and J.L. Stanton, Jr. (1985) Obesity and caloric intake: the National Health and Nutrition Examination Survey of 1971–1975 (NHANES I). *J. Chronic Dis.* 38:727–732.

25. I. Romieu, W.C. Willett, M.J. Stampfer, et al. (1988) Energy intake and other determinants of relative weight. *Am. J. Clin. Nutr.* 47:406–412.

26. I. Romieu, W.C. Willett, M.J. Stampfer, et al. (1988) Energy intake and other determinants of relative weight. *Am. J. Clin. Nutr.* 47:406–412.

27. A.J. Stunkard and D. Kaplan (1977) Eating in public places: a review of reports of the direct observation of eating behavior. *Int. J. Obesity* 1:89–101.

28. J. Garrow (1978) *Energy Balance and Obesity,* Elsevier/North Holland, New York.

29. G.A. Bray, B. Zachary, W.T. Dahms, R.A.L. Atkinson, and T.M. Oddie (1978) Eating patterns of the massively obese individual. *J. Am. Diet. Assoc.* 72:24–27.

30. G.A. Rose and R.T. Williams (1961) Metabolic studies on large and small eaters. *Br. J. Nutr.* 15:1–9.

31. O.E. Owen, J.L. Holup, D.A. D'Alessio, et al. (1987) A reappraisal of the caloric requirements of men. *Am. J. Clin. Nutr.* 46:847–885.

32. E. Jequier and Y. Schutz (1983) Long-term measurements of energy expenditure in humans using a respiration chamber. *Am. J. Clin. Nutr.* 38:989–998.

33. J.O. De Boer, A.J.H. Van Es, J.M.A. Van Raaij, and J.G.A.J. Hautvast (1987) Energy requirements and energy expenditure of lean and overweight women, measured by indirect calorimetry. *Am. J. Clin. Nutr.* 46:13–21.

34. C. Bogardus, S. Lillioja, E. Ravussin, et al. (1986) Familial dependence of resting metabolic rates. *N. Engl. J. Med.* 315:96–100.

35. E. Ravussin, S. Lillioja, W.C. Knowler, et al. (1988) Reduced rate of energy expenditure as a risk factor for body weight gain. *N. Engl. J. Med.* 318:467–472.

36. G.A. Bray (1983) The energetics of obesity. *Med. Sci. Sports Exerc.* 15:32–40.

37. M. Waxman and A.J. Stunkard (1980) Caloric intake and expenditure of obese boys. *J. Pediatr.* 96:187–193.

38. R. Woo, R. Daniels-Kush, and E.S. Horton (1985) Regulation of energy balance. *Annu. Rev. Nutr.* 5:411–433.

39. Z. Glick, R.J. Teague, and G.A. Bray (1981) Brown adipose tissue: thermic response increased by a single low protein, high carbohydrate meal. *Science* 213:1125–1127.

40. A. Astrup, J. Bulow, J. Madsen, et al. (1985) Contribution of BAT and skeletal muscle to thermogenesis induced by ephedrine in man. *Am. J. Physiol.* 248:E507–E515.

41. K.R. Segal, B. Gutin, J. Albu, and F.X. Pi-Sunyer (1987) Thermic effects of food and exercise in lean and obese men of similar lean body mass. *Am. J. Physiol.* 252:E110–E117.

42. J. Leblanc and L. Brondel (1985) Role of palatability on meal induced thermogenesis in human subjects. *Am. J. Physiol.* 248:E333–E336.

43. A. Golay, Y. Schutz, H.V. Meyer, et al. (1982) Glucose-induced thermogenesis in nondiabetic and diabetic obese subjects. *Diabetes* 31:1023–1028.

44. P. Bjorntorp and J. Ostman (1971) Human adipose tissue. Dynamics and regulation. *Adv. Metab. Dis.* 5:277–327.

45. J.L. Knittle, K. Timmers, F. Ginsberg-Fellner, R.E. Brown, and D.P. Katz (1979) The growth of adipose tissue in children and adolescents. Cross-sectional and longitudinal studies on adipose cell number and size. *J. Clin. Invest.* 63:239–246.

46. L. Sjostrom and T. William-Olsson (1981) Prospective studies on adipose tissue development in man. *Int. J. Obesity* 5:597–604.

47. M.L. Krotkiewski, P. Sjostrom, P. Bjorntorp, G. Carlgren, G. Garellick, and U. Smith (1977) Adipose tissue cellularity in relation to prognosis for weight reduction. *Int. J. Obesity* 1:395–416.

48. J.S. Flier, K.S. Cook, P. Usher, and B.M. Spiegelman (1987) Severely impaired adipsin expression in genetic and acquired obesity. *Science* 237:405–408.

49. Society of Actuaries (1980) *Build Study of 1979.* Society of Actuaries and Association of Life Insurance Medical Directors of America, Chicago.

50. E.A. Lew and L. Garfinkel (1979) Variation in mortality by weight among 750,000 men and women. *J. Chronic Dis.* 32:563–576.

51. H.T. Waaler (1983) Height, weight and mortality: the Norwegian experience. *Acta Med. Scand.* 679(suppl):1–55.

52. J.E. Manson, M.J. Stampfer, C.H. Hennekens, and W.C. Willett (1987) Body weight and longevity. A reassessment. *JAMA* 257:353–358.

53. S.M. Garn, V.M. Hawthorne, J.J. Pilkington, and S.D. Pesick (1983) Fatness and mortality in the west of Scotland. *Am. J. Clin. Nutr.* 38:313–319.

54. J. Vague (1956) The degree of masculine differentiation of obesities: a fact for determining predisposition to diabetes, atherosclerosis, gout and uric calculus disease. *Am. J. Clin. Nutr.* 4:20–34.

55. L. Lapidus, C. Bengtsson, B. Larsson, K. Pennert, E. Rybo, and L. Sjostrom (1984) Distribution of adipose tissue and risk of cardiovascular disease and death: a 12-year follow-up of participants in the population study of women in Gothenburg, Sweden. *Br. Med. J.* 289:1257–1261.

56. B. Larsson, K. Svardsudd, L. Welin, L. Wilhelmsen, P. Bjorntorp, and G. Tibblin (1984) Abdominal adipose tissue distribution, obesity, and risk of cardiovascular disease and death: 13-year follow-up of participants in the study of men born in 1913. *Br. Med. J.* 288:1401–1404.

57. J. Stokes III, R.J. Garrison, and W.B. Kannel (1985) The independent contribution of various indices of obesity to the 22 year incidence of coronary heart disease. In: *Metabolic Complications of Obesity.* (J. Vague, P. Bjorntorp, and P. Vague, eds.), pp. 49–57, Elsevier Science Publishers, Amsterdam.

58. P. Ducimietre, J. Richard, and F. Cambien (1986) The pattern of subcutaneous fat distribution in middle-aged men and the risk of coronary heart disease: the Paris prospective study. *Int. J. Obesity* 10:229–240.

59. R.P. Donahue, R.D. Abbott, E. Bloom, D.M. Reed, and K. Yano (1987) Central obesity and coronary heart disease in men. *Lancet* 1:821–824.

60. M. Krotkiewski, P. Bjorntorp, L. Sjostrom, and U. Smith (1983) Impact of obesity on metabolism in men and women: importance of regional adipose tissue distribution. *J. Clin. Invest.* 72:1150–1162.

61. A.H. Kissebah, N. Vydelingum, and R. Murray (1982) Relation of body fat distribution to metabolic complications of obesity. *J. Clin. Endocrinol. Metab.* 54:254–256.

62. S. Fujioka, Y. Matsuzawa, K. Tokunaga, and S. Tarui (1987) Contribution of intra-abdominal fat accumulation to the impairment of glucose and lipid metabolism in human obesity. *Metabolism* 36:54–59.

63. M.H. Maxwell, A.J. Waks, P. Schroth, M. Karam, and L.P. Dornfeld (1983) Error in blood pressure measurement due to incorrect cuff size in obese patients. *Lancet* 1:33–35.

64. D. Blair, J.P. Habicht, E.A.H. Sims, D. Sylvester, and S. Abraham (1984) Evidence for an increased risk for hypertension with centrally located body fat and the effect of race and sex on this risk. *Am. J. Epidemiol.* 119:526–540.

65. A.J. Hartz, D.C. Rupley, and A.A. Rimm (1984) The association of girth measurement with disease in 32,856 women. *J. Epidemiol.* 119:71–80.

66. S.W. MacMahon, D.E.L. Wilcken, and G.J. Macdonald (1986) The effect of weight reduction on left ventricular mass: a randomized controlled trial in young, overweight hypertensive patients. *N. Engl. J. Med.* 314:334–379.

67. E.J. Drenick (1979) Definition and health consequences of morbid obesity. *Surg. Clin. North Am.* 59:963–976.

68. M. Toeller, F.A. Gries, and K. Dannehl (1982) Natural history of glucose intolerance in obesity. A ten year observation. *Int. J. Obesity* 6:145–149.

69. R.R. Henry, A. Wiest-Kent, L. Scheaffer, O. Kolterman, and J.M. Olefsky (1986) Metabolic consequences of very-low-calorie diet therapy in obese non-insulin-dependent diabetic and non-diabetic subjects. *Diabetes* 35:155–164.

70. J.T. Sharp, M. Barrocas, and C. Chokrovertys (1980) The cardiorespiratory effects of obesity. *Clin. Chest Med.* 1:103–118.

71. C.S. Ray, D.Y. Sue, G.A. Bray, J.E. Hansen, and K.R. Wasserman (1983) Effects of obesity on respiratory function. *Am. Rev. Respir. Dis.* 128:501–506.

72. M.T. Meistas, G.V. Foster, S. Margolis, and A.A. Kowarski (1982) Integrated concentrations of growth hormone, insulin, c-peptide and prolactin in human obesity. *Metabolism* 31:1224–1228.

73. A.R. Glass (1989) Endocrine aspects of obesity. *Med. Clin. North Am.* 73:139–160.

74. E. Danforth, E.S. Horton, M. O'Connell, et al. (1969) Dietary-induced alterations in thyroid hormone metabolism during overnutrition. *J. Clin. Invest.* 64:1336–1342.

75. H.K. Kley, H.G. Solbach, J.C. McKinnan, and H.L. Kruskemper (1979) Testosterone decrease and estrogen increase in male patients with obesity. *Acta Endocrinol.* 91:553–563.

76. A.J. Hartz, P.N. Barboriak, A. Wong, K.P. Katayama, and A.A. Rimm (1979) The association of obesity with infertility and related menstrual abnormalities in women. *Int. J. Obesity* 3:57–73.

77. F.W. Ashley Jr. and W.B. Kannel (1974) Relation of weight change to changes in atherogenic traits: the Framingham study. *J. Chronic Dis.* 27:103–114.

78. G.A. Bray, W.T. Dahms, R.S. Swerdloff, R.H. Fiser, R.L. Atkinson, and R.E. Carrel (1983) The Prader-Willi syndrome: a study of 40 patients and a review of the literature. *Medicine* 62:59–80.

79. A.J. Stunkard, T.I.A. Sorensen, C. Harris, et al. (1986) Adoption study of human obesity. *N. Engl. J. Med.* 314:193–198.

80. G.A. Bray (1981) The inheritance of corpulence. In: *The Body Weight Regulatory System: Normal and Disturbed Mechanisms* (L.A. Cioffi, W.P.T. James, and T.B. Van Itallie, eds.), pp. 185–195, Raven Press, New York.

81. A.J. Stunkard, T.T. Foch, and Z. Hrubec (1986) A twin study of human obesity. *JAMA* 256:51–54.

82. C. Bouchard, L. Perusse, C. Leblanc, A. Tremblay, and G. Thierault (in press) Inheritance of the amount and distribution of human body fat. *Int. J. Obesity.*

83. G.A. Bray (1984) Syndromes of hypothalamic obesity in man. *Pediatr. Ann.* 13:525–536.

84. K.D. Brownell, G.A. Marlatt, E. Lichtenstein, and G.T. Wilson (1986) Understanding and preventing relapses. *Am. Psychol.* 41:765–782.

85. G.A. Bray and D.S. Gray (1988) Obesity: I: Pathogenesis. *West. J. Med.* 149:429–441.

86. G.A. Bray (1985) Complications of obesity. *Ann. Intern. Med.* 103:1052–1062.

Chapter 5

Michael C. Latham

Protein-energy Malnutrition

Protein-energy malnutrition (PEM) in young children currently is the most important nutritional problem in the nonindustrialized countries. No accurate numbers on the world prevalence of PEM exist, and even good estimates are difficult to obtain. To some extent prevalence estimates depend on definitions, as is the case with other forms of ill health. Relatively minor changes in anthropometric cutoff points can change by millions the estimated numbers of children with PEM. The World Health Organization (WHO) has suggested that at least 500 million children in the world suffer from PEM, and this number is probably an underestimate.[1]

PEM is a relatively new term and is used to describe a broad array of clinical conditions ranging from very serious to mild. At one end of the range are kwashiorkor and nutritional marasmus, which have high fatality rates, and at the other is mild PEM in which the main detectable manifestation in children is poor growth. PEM is not confined to children but is much more prevalent during early childhood, and most descriptions of the condition concentrate on this age group. Kwashiorkor, or a kwashiorkor-like condition, and marasmus may be seen in adults during famines or in adults who suffer from certain forms of malabsorption. This condition is at first similar to mild or moderate PEM but later manifests itself as adult nutritional marasmus. However, the latter terminology is seldom used. This condition eventually can be fatal.

In the United States and in other industrialized countries as well as in developing countries cases of adult PEM can be found in hospital wards where the condition may be secondary to a wide variety of diseases including infections, such as AIDS and tuberculosis; malabsorption syndromes; renal and hepatic diseases; carcinoma and other malignancies; and anorexia nervosa.

Historical Background

That starvation or inadequate intakes of food lead to weight loss and wasting in adults and poor growth in children has been known for centuries. In the literature from previous centuries there are many descriptions of starvation accompanied by body wasting, severe emaciation, and eventually death. Although most physicians in the 19th century and early part of this century certainly recognized that low food intakes resulted in poor growth of children, nevertheless this form of undernutrition was not often described as a disease syndrome except when it led to severe wasting. There are old medical records of famines and outbreaks of measles that include descriptions of the development of debilitating edema.

It was not until the early 1930s that Dr. Cicely Williams, who was working in Ghana, gave detailed descriptions of the condition that she termed kwashiorkor,[2] using the local Ga word, which means "the disease of the displaced child." It was over a decade later before the medical world began to accept kwashiorkor as a medical syndrome and a deficiency disease. In the 1950s kwashiorkor began to excite those working in developing countries; it was thought to be mainly due to protein deficiency and for some years concentrated efforts were made to reduce the incidence of kwashiorkor,[3] which was often described as the most important form of malnutrition. The solution to the problem of malnutrition was viewed mainly as finding a means to make protein-rich foods available for children. This stress on protein led to a relative neglect of nutritional marasmus, of growth failure, and of adequate energy and total food intakes for children and adults living in poverty.

There followed a good deal of scientific interest and medical evidence of the relationship between infections and malnutrition.[4] It was recognized that common childhood infections contributed to malnutrition, adversely affected growth of children, and in other ways were associated with or acted synergistically with nutrition. In 1959 the term protein-calorie malnutrition was introduced to include both kwashiorkor and marasmus as well as intermediate forms of these syndromes.[5] The terminology was later changed to PEM.

In the mid 1970s the literature increasingly moved to the current view that most PEM is due to an inadequate intake of food and is not simply due to a lack of dietary protein. It was also recognized that nutritional marasmus is at least as prevalent and, in many localities, more prevalent than kwashiorkor[6] and that these two serious clinical forms of PEM constitute the small tip of an iceberg. In most populations studied in poor countries, the point prevalence rates for kwashiorkor and nutritional marasmus combined is 1–5% whereas 30–70% of children 0–5 y of age exhibit other manifestations of what are now termed mild or moderate PEM. These conditions are diagnosed mainly on the basis of anthropometric measurements.

Consequently, the stress on protein and protein-rich foods was replaced with efforts to improve total food intakes, to provide more frequent meals to young children, to concentrate on energy-dense foods, and more importantly to deal with the underlying causes of PEM, which include poverty and infections.

Etiology and Epidemiology

Unlike the other important nutritional deficiency diseases, PEM is a macronutrient deficiency, not a micronutrient deficiency. Although termed PEM, it is now generally accepted that in most cases PEM is due to insufficient food intake and that energy deficiency is more important and more frequent than protein deficiency. It is very often associated with infections and with micronutrient deficiencies.

However, it is naive to consider the etiology of PEM (and to some extent some other deficiency diseases prevalent in developing countries) simply in terms of inadequate intake of nutrients. Food and the nutrients they contain must be available in adequate quantity to the family; the correct balance of foods and nutrients must be fed at the right intervals; the individual must have an appetite to consume the food; there must be proper digestion and absorption of the nutrients in the food; the metabolism of the person must be reasonably normal; and conditions should not exist that prevent body cells from utilizing the nutrients nor that result in abnormal losses of nutrients. Factors that adversely influence any of these conditions can be causes of malnutrition, particularly PEM.[7] The etiology, therefore, can be complex. Certain factors that contribute to PEM, particularly in the young child, are related to the host, the

agent (the diet), and the environment. Some examples of such factors include:

- the young child's relatively higher needs for both energy and protein per kilogram than those of older family members
- staple diets that are often of low energy density (not infrequently bulky and unappetizing), low in their protein content, and not fed frequently enough to children
- inadequate availability of food for the family because of poverty, inequity, lack of sufficient arable land, and problems related to intrafamily food distribution
- infections (viral, bacterial, and parasitic) that may cause anorexia, reduce food intake and nutrient absorption and utilization, or result in nutrient losses
- famine resulting from droughts, natural disasters, wars, civil disturbances, etc.
- inappropriate weaning practices; inappropriate use of infant formula in place of breast-feeding for very young infants in poor families.

It is appropriate that we now see much less emphasis than seen previously on amino acid fortification of cereals, on single-cell or fish protein concentrate, on high-protein weaning foods, and on nutrition education efforts to ensure a much greater consumption of meat, fish, and eggs. Rather, current efforts are based on promoting breast-feeding and sound weaning, increasing consumption by young children of cereals, legumes, and other locally produced weaning foods, preventing and controlling infections and parasitic diseases, and, where appropriate, encouraging higher consumption of oil, fat, and other food items that reduce bulk and increase the energy density of foods fed to children at risk. These measures are likely to have greater impact if accompanied by growth monitoring, immunizations, oral rehydration therapy for diarrhea,[8] early treatment of diseases, deworming,[9] and attention to the underlying causes of PEM, such as poverty and inequity.[10] Many of these measures can be implemented as part of primary health care.

Nutritional Marasmus. Nutritional marasmus is common in most developing countries and is especially prevalent in children under 18 mo of age. All of the causes discussed above may be contributory factors. There is no doubt that the major cause is inadequate food intake, particularly insufficient energy to meet the requirements for both metabolism and normal growth. For infants in the first few months of life, prematurity or low birth weight may be a predisposing cause. Failure of breast-feeding because of death of the mother, separation from the mother, or lack of or insufficient breast milk may be causes in poor societies where successful breast-feeding is often the only feasible way for mothers to feed their young babies adequately.[11] Therefore, erosion of breast-feeding because of promotion of formula feeding of infants and insufficient support of breast-feeding by the medical profession and health services may be a factor in the etiology of marasmus. These causes of nutritional marasmus relate mainly to poor, uneducated mothers living in unsanitary environments with contaminated water supplies and poor kitchen facilities. Low incomes also lead mothers to overdilute formula, which may be a potent cause of nutritional marasmus. Prolonged exclusive breast-feeding without the introduction of other foods at age 4–6 mo may also contribute to growth faltering, PEM, and eventually nutritional marasmus.

Kwashiorkor. The previously held view that nutritional marasmus was due to energy deficiency and kwashiorkor was due to protein deficiency provides an oversimplified explanation of the complex etiology of these two conditions.[12] The child with kwashiorkor, with only a few exceptions, is usually consuming a diet providing too little protein and energy. However, infections often play an important part. It is likely that both endogenous and exogenous causes influence whether a child develops nutritional marasmus, with its very severe wasting; kwashiorkor, which is characterized by the presence of edema; or the intermediate form known as marasmic kwashiorkor. In a child consuming much less food than is needed to meet energy needs, energy is mobilized from body fat and from muscle, and gluconeogenesis in the liver is enhanced. As a result there is loss of subcutaneous fat and wasting of muscles. Some claim that under these circumstances especially when protein intake is very low (perhaps aggravated by nitrogen losses from infections) in relation to carbohydrates, then a series of metabolic changes take place that contribute to the development of edema. More sodium and water are retained, and much of this water collects outside the cardiovascular system in the tissues, resulting in pitting edema. The role played by infections has not been adequately explained, but certain infections cause major increases in urinary nitrogen, which comes from amino acids in muscle tissue.

There is still no agreement on the actual cause of the edema that is the definitive feature of kwashiorkor.[13] Most workers agree that relative potassium deficiency and sodium retention are important in the pathogenesis of edema. Many workers now disagree with the theory that a dietary deficiency of protein contributes to a low concentration of serum albumin that, in turn, results in edema. Arguments against

this are many but most often are based on two findings. First, there is not a good inverse correlation in the individual child with kwashiorkor between amount of edema and concentration of serum albumin. Second, limited data (not entirely convincing) suggest that previous diets consumed by children who develop edematous kwashiorkor have not been lower in protein content than diets of children who develop nutritional marasmus.[12] Certainly the metabolic state varies with different children and plays some role in the development of edema. Some suggest that kwashiorkor is a dysadaptation to protein deficiency or of hormonal origin.

A rather comprehensive review of the pathogenesis of edema in kwashiorkor concludes that "although the evidence in support of the classical theory may be incomplete and inconclusive, we cannot ignore the possibility that oedematous malnutrition is a sign of inadequate protein intake."[14] Among many arguments to support this view is the fact that edema, fatty liver, and a kwashiorkor-like condition can be induced in pigs and baboons on protein-deficient diets; there is epidemiological evidence that higher rates of kwashiorkor occur in areas such as Uganda where the staple diet is plantain, which is very low in protein.

Two new theories to explain the cause of kwashiorkor were postulated. The first is that kwashiorkor is due to aflatoxin poisoning.[15] The second is that free radicals are important in the pathogenesis of kwashiorkor and that most of the clinical features of kwashiorkor could be caused by an excess of free radical stress.[16] This hypothesis suggests that various noxae produce free-radical-mediated lipid peroxides and toxic carbonyls. Under normal metabolic and nutritional circumstances, the radicals are scavenged and dissipated. However, children subsisting on poor diets may have a deficiency of several micronutrients and, consequently, a reduction in protective mechanisms. The free radicals then cause damage that results in edema, fatty liver, and other signs of kwashiorkor. Among the important noxae in this hypothesis are various infections.[17] This new, relatively untested theory also suggests that kwashiorkor, even if produced by free radicals, is likely to occur only in children with inadequate food intakes and who are subjected to infections. Therefore, even if this theory were to be proved correct, it explains a mechanism for the pathogenesis of kwashiorkor but does not change the fact that improving diets and reducing infections will significantly reduce severe PEM and both kwashiorkor and nutritional marasmus.

Neither the aflatoxin nor the free radical theories have been proved experimentally, and there is not convincing research to uphold the view of individual dysadaptation. Surprisingly, there also are no conclusive studies either to prove similarities or differences between the dietary consumption of children developing kwashiorkor with edema and those who show clinical signs of nutritional marasmus without any edema.

In all cases of severe PEM, there is biochemical evidence and often clinical evidence of micronutrient deficiencies. It is not surprising that a child or adult consuming a grossly inadequate diet has evidence of multiple mineral and vitamin deficiencies.[17] In both nutritional marasmus and kwashiorkor (but also in moderate PEM) it is often clear from clinical examinations or biochemical tests that the sufferer has evidence of, for example, vitamin A deficiency, nutritional anemia, and/or zinc deficiency. However, there is little evidence that any one micronutrient deficiency is the cause of PEM or is by itself responsible for the edema of kwashiorkor.

Clinical Features of PEM in Children

The two extreme forms of PEM, namely kwashiorkor and nutritional marasmus, have very different appearances and clinical features. Marasmic kwashiorkor is the term used for the patient who is marasmic but also has edema. Mild and moderate forms of PEM are diagnosed mainly on the basis of anthropometric measurements. The proper use of weight-for-age, height-for-age, and weight-for-height permits the diagnosis of the relative acuteness or chronicity of the PEM.

The so-called Wellcome classification (Table 1) of severe forms of PEM has been used widely.[18] It has the advantage of simplicity because it is based on only two measures, namely the percent weight-for-age and the presence or absence of edema. It is useful for comparisons over time or between countries but is not adequate for actual clinical diagnosis.

Nutritional Marasmus in the Young Child. Nutritional marasmus may occur at any age from early infancy until old age. Most severe cases in children occur in children <2 y of age. The infant or child with advanced nutritional marasmus presents an unmistakable picture. The patient is appallingly thin, but in contrast to the rest of the body, the belly is sometimes relatively protuberant. The severe wasting and loss of subcutaneous tissue makes the ribs prominent; the face is simian in appearance; and the skin, particularly over the buttocks, hangs in wrinkles.

The main clinical features include growth failure—weight <60% of that expected for a child of that age, low length-for-age or height-for-age, little or no remaining subcutaneous fat (as judged by picking up

Table 1. Wellcome classification of severe forms of PEM

Weight (% of standard)	Edema	
	Present	Absent
60–80%	Kwashiorkor	Undernourished
<60%	Marasmic kwashiorkor	Nutritional marasmus

a skinfold between thumb and forefinger or as measured with skinfold calipers); wasting—severe and obvious muscle wasting, thin limbs, and reduced major muscle mass; infections—evidence of current or past infection including diarrhea, respiratory infection, chronic inflammation, tuberculosis, or parasitic infections including intestinal helminths (conditions that may, in fact, be secondary to a serious infection); and signs of other nutrient deficiencies—clinical and/or biochemical evidence of concomitant micronutrient deficiencies, for example, evidence of xerophthalmia, vitamin B deficiencies, nutritional anemia, and others.

Some other signs that are important in kwashiorkor are either absent or less prominent in nutritional marasmus. There is no edema nor is there fatty infiltration of the liver leading to hepatomegaly. The hair may show some changes; the child's mood and mental state may be anxious rather than apathetic and miserable; appetite may be good but anorexia is not unknown; stools are often loose and there may be severe diarrhea; and except in the case of children with febrile infections, body temperature may be low.

Kwashiorkor in the Young Child. Kwashiorkor is most commonly seen in children 1–3 y of age but can occur at younger and older ages, including in adults. There is often a history of having been weaned from the breast in the previous months, sometimes because the mother became pregnant or had a new infant. The patient is frequently a "displaced child."[2] Edema is the cardinal feature.[14]

Partly because of the edema, which may cause severe generalized swelling, but also because wasting is less marked than in nutritional marasmus, the child with kwashiorkor may not have the obvious appearance of severe undernutrition, and so the parents and untrained observers may not easily appreciate that this is severe PEM.

The main clinical features of kwashiorkor[7] are

- growth failure as judged by anthropometry but with the percent weight-for-age >60% of that expected on the basis of the Wellcome classification
- wasting of muscles and loss of subcutaneous fat that is less extreme than in nutritional marasmus

- pitting edema (In the ambulant child this usually appears in the feet and lower legs but may affect almost the whole body including legs, arms, trunk, and face.)
- hepatomegaly caused by fatty infiltration of the liver
- mental changes—almost invariably present (The child is apathetic, miserable, irritable when disturbed, and unsmiling.)
- hair alterations—common but not invariable (There are changes in texture, color, strength, and ease of pluckability. The tight curl of African hair is lost, the hair becomes straighter, the attractive dark sheen is lost, the color may become brownish, and the hair is silkier; color changes are usually generalized but occasionally may be localized leading to the "flag sign.")
- skin changes—not always seen but if present are characteristic (Initially, there may be depigmentation but eventually a dermatosis develops especially in areas of friction such as in the groin and behind the knees. Darkly pigmented patches occur that may desquamate like old peeling paint, which has given rise to the term "flaky paint dermatosis.")
- anorexia (Poor appetite is an almost constant feature of kwashiorkor [and is also a feature of laboratory animals consuming inadequate protein]; the child seems uninterested in food, which makes refeeding difficult and sometimes necessitates feeding through a nasogastric tube for a few days.)
- diarrhea (Stools are frequent, are loose or watery, and may contain undigested food particles. The diarrhea may be due to an infection but at least in part is due to a reduction in the production of digestive enzymes as a direct consequence of the disease and a flattening of the intestinal villi.)
- infections and other nutrient deficiencies (The child with kwashiorkor may have evidence of past or current infections and of micronutrient deficiencies similar to those described for nutritional marasmus. Anemia may be due to protein deficiency rather than iron or folate deficiency.)

Marasmic-kwashiorkor in Children. In many areas in which PEM is a problem, many children with severe PEM exhibit the features of marasmus with some degree of edema; others have many of the signs of kwashiorkor including edema, hair and skin changes, anorexia, and mental symptoms but are quite wasted and have a weight-for-age <60% of the standard for their age. Patients who combine the features of kwashiorkor and nutritional marasmus are diagnosed to have marasmic kwashiorkor. After a short period of treatment when the edema disappears, they may then be said to have only nutritional marasmus.

Mild to Moderate Protein-energy Malnutrition in Children. Children without the clinical features of nutritional marasmus or kwashiorkor but who have growth failure are usually said to have mild or moderate PEM. They often have abnormalities besides growth failure. By the Wellcome classification (*see* Table 1), these children who have no edema and a weight-for-age between 60% and 80% of the standard are classified as undernourished.

During the 1950s and 1960s weight-for-age, sometimes based on the Gomez classification,[19] was the main method used to assess nutritional status. Under the Gomez classification, children with a weight-for-age between 75% and 89% of the standard had grade I, or mild malnutrition; between 60% and 74% of the standard had grade II, or moderate; and <60% had grade III, or severe malnutrition.

In 1971 it was suggested that classification based only on weight-for-age had many disadvantages and that it was important to distinguish three different categories, or types, of malnutrition using weight and height measurements of children.[20] By using this method it was possible to separate malnourished children who had low weight-for-age into three categories: acute short-duration malnutrition; past chronic malnutrition; and acute, chronic, or current long-duration malnutrition. This proposed classification received a good deal of attention and led to a new suggested terminology for the three conditions.[21] Acute malnutrition was termed *wasting*, chronic malnutrition was termed *stunting*, and the combined acute on chronic malnutrition was labeled *wasting and stunting*. Although nutritionists have not reached complete agreement either on the terms to be adopted or on the anthropometric cutoff points, the concepts in this classification system are widely utilized, and there is a fair measurement of agreement that these distinctions are useful. The World Health Organization has been supportive of these efforts to rationalize the classification of mild and moderate PEM.[22]

A controversy has smoldered for years over whether each country or ethnic group should have a separate set of growth standards. However, in recent years there has been increasing acceptance of the U.S. National Center for Health Statistics (NCHS) growth standards as published by WHO.[23] An editorial in the *Lancet*, stimulated by a study in Kenya providing comparisons of anthropometric measurements on both privileged and underprivileged children, states, "Recent evidence suggests that the growth of privileged groups of children in developing countries does not differ importantly from these standards and that the poorer growth so commonly observed in the underprivileged is due to social factors—among which the malnutrition-infection complex is of primary importance—rather than to ethnic or geographic differences."[24]

There are still those who suggest that the low anthropometric measurements found in groups of children in developing countries may be normal and that smallness may be advantageous. This view is not supported by convincing evidence.[25] There is strong support for the view that ethnic differences are much less important than other factors as causes of growth failure in children.[26] Inadequate food intakes, infectious and parasitic diseases, and adverse environmental factors often associated with poverty combine to prevent children from realizing their full growth potential. Certainly genetic factors influence achieved body size and especially stature, but in prepubertal children, heredity is a less significant cause of below-average growth than are other factors. In adults both environmental factors in childhood and heredity affect stature. Recognition of these views has important policy implications.

Biochemical, Metabolic, and Related Features

The biochemical and metabolic abnormalities in nutritional marasmus, marasmic kwashiorkor, and kwashiorkor often are similar. However, in other cases there are marked differences between the findings in children with severe marasmus as compared with those with kwashiorkor.

The one biochemical test available in hospital laboratories in developing countries that is feasible and useful in the diagnosis of severe PEM is serum protein determinations. In kwashiorkor total serum protein concentrations are usually low, mainly because of reduced serum albumin concentrations (<20 g/L and not infrequently <10 g/L). The low serum albumin is due to inadequate hepatic synthesis. In marasmus the serum protein concentrations generally are normal or near normal. Serum concentrations of essential amino acids are usually low, whereas those of nonessential amino acids may be normal or high, especially in kwashiorkor.

Concomitant infections are common in children with all three clinical forms of PEM, and these may lead to increased concentrations of serum immunoglobulin G. Retinol-binding protein may be decreased and may contribute to the development of xerophthalmia.

In kwashiorkor there is fatty infiltration of the liver. Serum concentrations of free fatty acids are high, but concentrations of cholesterol and triglycerides are low. In all forms of PEM, low hemoglobin concentration and hematocrit are common. Concentrations

of urinary creatinine and hydroxyproline are low particularly in subjects with marked wasting. Blood glucose concentrations are not altered significantly.

Biochemical evidence of deficiencies of important vitamins, such as vitamin A, riboflavin, thiamin, niacin, and ascorbic acid, or of minerals, such as iron, zinc, or magnesium, is frequently present in children with severe PEM. All of these deficiencies are accompaniments of a grossly inadequate diet but are not usually the cause of the PEM. Similarly, there may be biochemical evidence of dehydration and electrolyte disturbance because of accompanying diarrhea.

It has been suggested that in severe PEM all the processes of the body show a reductive adaptation and that "no physiological function has so far been studied in severe undernutrition and found to be normal."[17] The whole body is affected, and most metabolic systems, including, for example, metabolic rate, sodium pump activity, intracellular sodium and potassium concentrations, cardiac and renal function, immune response, and many others, are affected.

Changes in Body Systems and Organs

A wide variety of abnormalities occur in body systems and organs of the severely malnourished person. In the gastrointestinal tract it is common that the villi are flattened and atrophic, and amounts of almost all digestive enzymes are reduced. This condition leads to poor digestion and absorption and may contribute to diarrhea. In kwashiorkor the liver becomes grossly infiltrated with fat, and hepatomegaly is a constant feature. Fat in liver initially is more marked in cells at the periphery of the hepatic lobules but later may involve almost all liver cells. Fat accumulation in liver is related to protein deficiency and can be produced in protein-deficient animals fed adequate quantities of other nutrients, including energy. Surprisingly, liver function is usually not seriously impaired and the condition is reversible with treatment.

Muscle wasting occurs in severe undernutrition and is clearly evident in large muscle masses in the limbs and trunk. However, muscle wasting is also apparent in the intestines, heart, and other organs. Myocardial changes may lead to reduced cardiac output and electrocardiographic changes. Although renal function may be abnormal, consistent kidney pathology has not been described.

In severe PEM, immune responses are impaired. The thymus gland, the tonsils, and other lymph tissue may be smaller in size than normal. There is evidence of reduced leucocytosis, lowered phagocytic activity of neutrophils, and poor antibody formation. Severe undernutrition both in children and adults has a marked negative effect on cell-mediated immunity.[27] This finding helps to explain why infections are often more prevalent and more severe in malnourished individuals.

Treatment

Some malnourished children show evidence of dehydration and electrolyte disturbance. These children need careful attention and usually can be treated by appropriate oral fluids rather than by intravenous therapy. Many serious children with PEM have infections, and sometimes these infections are either the precipitating or the underlying cause of malnutrition. Such infections need attention on an individual basis, with appropriate antibiotic or other therapy. Attention also should be given to micronutrient deficiencies in the first days of treatment.

As recovery begins, nutrient repletion becomes the principal consideration in most cases. In many hospitals in developing countries, an aqueous mixture containing dried skimmed milk, vegetable oil, casein, and sugar is used because it is inexpensive, easily available, and proven to be effective.[7] Initially a mixture providing ~120 kcal and 3–5 g protein per kilogram body weight per day should be provided. Usually this mixture is fed to the child at frequent feedings; in some cases the mixture is given by intragastric tube. Energy is usually limiting, and as the appetite improves and no signs of intolerance or complications are evident, the energy intake may be increased to 250 kcal/kg body weight. The diet may need to provide more than the recommended allowances of other nutrients, and evidence of any particular micronutrient deficiency requires appropriate additional nutrient supplements. Some evidence now suggests that zinc supplementation may be beneficial. Extra vitamin A and iron is often advisable. The child must be kept adequately warm. In tropical countries, nights may be cool, and hypothermia can occur and be life threatening.

Severe cases of kwashiorkor respond relatively quickly. Diuresis occurs with rapid reduction in edema, diarrhea, and other gastrointestinal symptoms. The mood of the child changes—a smile may be a better prognostic sign than is an increase of serum albumin concentration. In nutritional marasmus, response and cure are slower, and longer hospitalization may be necessary.

In all cases it is particularly important that the patient is not discharged from treatment only to return to the circumstances that led to the disease. Steps must be taken to ensure that there is follow-up and that an adequate diet will be provided after the child leaves the hospital. Health and nutrition education of the mother may be important to reduce the likelihood that the condition will recur.

Summary

PEM is the most important nutritional problem of children in nonindustrialized countries. PEM may occur at any age but is most prevalent in early childhood when it contributes importantly to high rates of morbidity and mortality. The main cause is a lack of adequate food intake, but infections also play an important role in the etiology of PEM. Underlying causes include poverty, inequity in food distribution, and unsanitary living conditions. UNICEF in its 1988 State of the World's Children[28] suggested that the monetary debt crisis for many poor nations is contributing to an increase of PEM in children. Kwashiorkor, marasmic kwashiorkor, and nutritional marasmus are the severe clinical manifestations of PEM but are much less prevalent than mild or moderate PEM, which in many countries may affect >50% of all children at some time in their lives. This form of PEM is assessed by anthropometric measurements, which are also useful in separating wasted from stunted children.

References

1. M.C. Latham (1984) Strategies for the control of malnutrition and the influence of the nutritional sciences. *Food Nutr.* 10:5–31.
2. C.D. Williams (1933) A nutritional disease of childhood associated with a maize diet. *Arch. Dis. Child.* 8:423–433.
3. H.C. Trowell, J.N.P. Davies, and R.F.A. Dean (1954) *Kwashiorkor,* Edward Arnold, London.
4. N.S. Scrimshaw, C.E. Taylor, and J.E. Gordon (1957) Interactions of nutrition and infection. WHO Monograph Series No. 57, pp. 1–52, WHO, Geneva.
5. D.B. Jelliffe (1959) Protein-calorie malnutrition: a review of the recent literature. *J. Pediatr.* 54:227–256.
6. D.S. McLaren (1974) The great protein fiasco. *Lancet* 2:93–96.
7. M.C. Latham (1979) *Human Nutrition in Tropical Africa,* FAO, Rome.
8. J. Grant (1985) *The State of the World's Children 1985,* UNICEF, New York and Oxford University Press, Oxford.
9. L.S. Stephenson (1987) *The Impact of Helminth Infections on Human Nutrition,* Taylor and Francis, London.
10. M.C. Latham (1988) Western development strategies and inappropriate modernization as causes of malnutrition and ill health. In: *Hunger and Society,* vol. 1 (M.C. Latham, L. Bondestam, R. Chorlton, and U. Jonsson, eds.), Cornell International Nutrition Monograph Series No. 17, pp. 75–95, Cornell University, Ithaca, NY.
11. D.B. Jelliffe and E.F.P. Jelliffe (1978) *Human Milk in the Modern World,* Oxford University Press, Oxford.
12. C. Gopalan (1968) Kwashiorkor and nutritional marasmus: evolution and distinguishing features. In: *Calorie Deficiencies and Protein Deficiencies* (R.A. McCance and E. Widdowson, eds.), pp. 49–58, Churchill, London.

13. J. Landman and A.A. Jackson (1980) The role of protein deficiency in the aetiology of kwashiorkor. *West Indian Med. J.* 29:229–238.

14. J.C. Waterlow (1984) Kwashiorkor revisited: the pathogenesis of oedema in kwashiorkor and its significance. *Trans. R. Soc. Trop. Med. Hyg.* 78:436–441.

15. R.G. Hendrickse (1984) The influence of aflatoxins on child health in the tropics with particular reference to kwashiorkor. *Trans. R. Soc. Trop. Med. Hyg.* 78:427–435.

16. H.M.N. Golden and D. Ramdath (1987) Free radicals in the pathogenesis of kwashiorkor. *Proc. Nutr. Soc.* 46:53–68.

17. H.M.N. Golden (1988) The effects of malnutrition in the metabolism of children. *Trans. R. Soc. Trop. Med. Hyg.* 82:3–6.

18. Wellcome Trust Working Party (1970) Classification of infantile malnutrition. *Lancet* 2:302–303.

19. F. Gomez, R. Ramos-Galvan, R. Frenk, J.M. Cravioto, R. Chavez, and J. Vasquez (1956) Mortality in second and third degree malnutrition. *J. Trop. Pediatr.* 2:77–85.

20. N. Seoane and M.C. Latham (1971) Nutritional anthropometry in the identification of malnutrition in childhood. *J. Trop. Pediatr.* 17:98–104.

21. J.C. Waterlow (1972) Classification and definition of protein-calorie malnutrition. *Br. Med. J.* 3:566–569.

22. W. Keller and C.M. Fillmore (1983) Prevalence of protein-energy malnutrition. *World Health Stat. Q.* 36(2):129–167.

23. World Health Organization (1983) *Measuring Changes in Nutritional Status,* WHO, Geneva.

24. Editorial (1984) A measure of agreement on growth standards. *Lancet* 1:142–143.

25. C. Gopalan (1983) Small is healthy? *Nutr. Fdn. India Bull.* 5:33–37.

26. L.S. Stephenson, M.C. Latham, and A. Jansen (1983) *A comparison of growth standards: similarities between NCHS, Harvard, Denver and privileged African children and differences with Kenyan rural children,* Cornell International Nutrition Monograph Series No. 12, pp. 1–109, Cornell University, Ithaca, New York.

27. R.K. Chandra (1983) Nutrition, immunity and infection: present knowledge and future directions. *Lancet* 1:688–691.

28. J. Grant (1988) *The State of the World's Children, 1988,* UNICEF, New York.

Chapter 6

Béla Szepesi

Carbohydrates

Carbohydrates are the most abundant and readily available source of food for human beings. Important food carbohydrates are polyols (aldoses, ketoses) with a general formula of $(CH_2O)_n$. Simple sugars is a term used to describe mono- and disaccharides. Oligosaccharides is a term usually applied to carbohydrates consisting of three or more monosaccharide units, whereas polysaccharides can have molecular weights in the millions. A good review of carbohydrate structure can usually be found in most current textbooks on biochemistry.

Carbohydrate Intake and Absorption

Type and Amount. Carbohydrate intake is determined by cultural and economic factors and ranges from 50% in Western countries to as high as 70% or more in some other areas of the world. The most abundant sources of dietary carbohydrates are starch, simple sugars, and cellulose. Cellulose is a straight-chain polymer of glucose molecules linked together by 1,4-β glycosidic bonds. Such polymers are linear and planar and form many hydrogen bonds to adjacent molecules, producing fibrous structures of great strength. Man and most monogastric animals can not digest cellulose. Starch is also a glucose polymer, but the glycosidic bonds are 1,4-α in straight-chain starch (amylose) or 1,4-α with branch points of 1,6-α bonds (amylopectin). Starch can form a left-handed α-helix and consequently is not able to form many hydrogen bonds with adjacent molecules.

In the Western diet 50% of the calories are derived from carbohydrate. Of this, one half (or 25% of the total) is from simple sugars (glucose, fructose, sucrose, lactose, some maltose, and traces of trehalose); the rest is from complex carbohydrates (hemicellulose, galactans, mannans, and, of course, starch). Complex carbohydrates other than starch are referred to as dietary fiber. Unlike cellulose, dietary fiber can be digested either partially or totally in the large intestine.

Digestion. The digestion of dietary carbohydrates is a physiologically regulated process associated with the anatomical structure of the gastrointestinal tract and important developmental changes that occur throughout life in some cases. The biological imperative of maintaining constant blood glucose is aided greatly by the structure and functions of the gastrointestinal tract. Regulation of the emptying of the stomach, the motility of the intestine, the secretion and activation of digestive enzymes, and the localization of some intestinal enzymes all serve to reduce the fluctuation in nutrient inflow.

Carbohydrate is ingested in three basic forms: (*1*) raw or processed (i.e., cooked, boiled, ground, etc.) vegetables, fruits, or grain, (*2*) purified carbohydrate added to foods, and (*3*) carbohydrate dissolved in various drinks. The first step in the digestion of carbohydrates is mastication of food by the teeth. During mastication starch granules are exposed or broken open, and surface area is increased by reducing particle size. Food in the mouth is mixed with salivary α-amylase that begins to break down starch immediately. Hydrolysis of starch slows or stops in the stomach because of the change in pH and resumes again in the duodenum, where pancreatic α-amylase is secreted. The cumulative action of the two amylases is to produce maltose and maltotriose from amylose and maltotriose, maltose, some glucose plus limit dextrin [3–5 glucose units (1,4-α) and one glucose unit (1,6-α) from amylopectin[1]]. Digestion of starch remnants is then completed by the brush border enzymes. Polysaccharides that are not digested in the small intestine may then undergo at least partial digestion by bacteria in the colon.

Progress in our knowledge of the enzymes of the small intestine has been rapid and has resulted in a complete alteration of our conception of how these enzymes work. Maltotriose, maltose, limit dextrins (molecules left after amylopectin is treated with β-amylase), and the major disaccharides (sucrose, lactose) are split to monosaccharide constituents in the small intestine. The small intestine is covered with microvilli that give a total absorptive surface many times the area of the planar intestinal surface. The extended surface may be as large as 200 m^2 in the average man.[1] The microvilli extend into the so-called unstirred water layer (UWL) phase of the intestinal lumen. The enzymes that complete the hydrolysis of starch digestion end products are anchored to the brush border membrane. If a limit dextrin, trisaccharide, or disaccharide enters the UWL, it is rapidly hydrolyzed by these enzymes. With the exception of trehalase, a minor component (MW 75,000), the other saccharidases of the small intestine share a number of common characteristics: a molecular weight between 200,000 and 300,000, a membrane-spanning hydrophobic portion that acts as an anchor in the brush border, two separate catalytic sites each on a separate domain, and heavy glycosylation; they also undergo extensive posttranslational processing by intracellular and extracellular (pancreatic) hydrolases.[1]

The sucrase-isomaltase complex is anchored to the brush border at its N terminal, and it is split into two peptides by pancreatic hydrolases.[2-4] The anchor peptide complex [isomaltase (maltase)] is held together with the terminal peptide complex [sucrase (maltase)] by noncovalent forces.[1-4] The maltase of this complex also is known as the heat-labile maltase. Isomaltase is the enzyme that splits the 1,6-α glycoside linkage.[1] The glucoamylase complex contains the heat-stable maltase and glucoamylase (1 and 2), which has two active sites. The two domains are held together covalently[5] and the glucoamylase is anchored to the brush border by its N terminal.[1] The β-glucosidase complex contains lactase and another peptide domain that is referred to as either glycosylceramidase or phlorizin hydrolase. This enzyme complex contains one peptide and is anchored in the brush border at its C terminal.[1] In the brush border of healthy rats and humans, enzyme activity is believed to be more than adequate to take care of all substrate that gets into the UWL.[1]

Regulation of Digestion. Digestion is regulated in part by the emptying of the stomach and the motility of the intestine. The combined result of this regulation is to reduce fluctuations in nutrient inflow and to minimize osmotic shock.[6] Because the half-lives of intestinal brush border enzymes are shorter than the life span of the intestinal cells, the activities of these enzymes can be regulated, and they are known to be adaptive.[1] Sucrase and lactase concentrations may be increased by feeding either sucrose or lactose.[7,8] Sucrase activity is decreased by both starvation[9] and starch intake.[10] Earlier studies indicated that changes in rates of synthesis were responsible for changes in sucrase concentration.[11] A recent article, however, indicates that at least in short-term experiments, sucrose and fructose depress the expression of the sucrase-isomaltase complex by a leupeptin-sensitive degradation process possibly through alteration in glycosylation.[12]

Diabetes produces very large changes in intestinal function.[1] Concentrations of intestinal enzymes[13-16] and intestinal transport[17] are increased. The UWL becomes less of a barrier to absorption[18] and the sodium gradient between intestinal lumen and intestinal cells increases.[19] The adaptation of intestinal function to diabetes speeds up digestion and increases the transport of carbohydrate into the blood stream.

Absorption and Transport of Carbohydrates. Carbohydrates, which are polyols and polar, cannot pass through nonpolar membranes without some type of transport system. There are four known types of carbohydrate transport: bacterial permease mediated, the dolichol system, Na$^+$-dependent active transport, and the facilitated carrier.[20]

Dolichol is used to transport oligosaccharides and monosaccharides into the endoplasmic reticulum and the Golgi membrane system for use in glycosylation. Dolichol has a long nonpolar portion that easily inserts into the membrane. Even before the carbohydrate-transporting proteins were isolated, their existence and a number of their properties were deduced and described by Crane.[21-23] Intestinal glucose transport was shown to be active (required energy expenditure), to be Na$^+$ dependent,[23] and to have stereospecificity for glucose and galactose.[22] It was deduced that the brush border enzymes not only provide transportable monosaccharides but somehow enhance their transport as well.[24] It is believed that this enhancing effect on transport is due to adjacent localization[24] and is particularly effective for disaccharides.[23]

Animal cells have two basic types of glucose carriers: one that is Na$^+$ dependent and another that is not.[1,20] The Na$^+$-dependent carriers are found in intestinal wall and in kidney.[20] The intestinal cell wall carrier and one of the kidney carriers have a stoichiometry of one Na$^+$ molecule per carrier, whereas the second kidney transporter works with two Na$^+$ molecules per carrier.[20] The rest of the glucose carriers also can be divided into two groups: Muscle and adipose tissue carriers are insulin-dependent; the others are not.[1,20]

The essential features of the Na$^+$-dependent glucose carrier have been described.[25,26] Sodium is pumped from the cell to create a sodium gradient between the intestinal lumen and the interior of the cell. The sodium pump requires ATP hydrolysis and the resultant sodium gradient drives the cotransporter so that one molecule of sodium and one molecule of glucose are cotransported.[20] The carriers that do not require sodium are thought to work like an enzyme except that no bonds are broken or formed. The driving force for this carrier is the glucose gradient and the entropy change that occurs when highly organized water is replaced on the carrier by glucose. The resultant change in electric fields (set up by the movement of electrons) then alters the local magnetic fields, which in turn move part of the carrier that has the glucose bound to it. Thus, glucose is moved across the membrane where it leaves the carrier. Much of this explanation is conjecture, but the kinetics of carrier action resembles enzyme kinetics.[26] The fructose carrier also is driven by a concentration gradient, and like the Na^+-independent glucose carrier, it requires no ATP. This type of transport is referred to as facilitated transport.[25,26]

Glucose transporters from many tissues have been isolated. The best known is the erythrocyte carrier that has 12 hydrophobic helical loops spanning the membrane and one external and one internal loop.[27] A number of transporters recently were cloned[28–31] and compared with the *Escherichia coli* Na^+/proline cotransporter.[32]

Malabsorption and Intolerance. Carbohydrate malabsorption and carbohydrate intolerance are not the same. Carbohydrate malabsorption is the failure to absorb carbohydrate in an appropriate manner at the appropriate site. Intolerance is the collection of abdominal symptoms that accompany malabsorption.[1]

Malabsorption may be due to a genetically determined enzyme deficiency (primary deficiency) or a deficiency induced by some disease (secondary deficiency).[1,20,25,26] It is detected by the administration of a large oral dose of a test carbohydrate; a very small rise in blood carbohydrate or elevation of hydrogen in the breath is confirming evidence of malabsorption. Disaccharidase deficiency refers to a congenital deficiency of sucrase and/or isomaltase. Primary, adult-type hypolactasia is seen in many populations of other than European origin.[1] In non-Europeans, lactase declines postweaning so that although young children can consume milk, the intake of milk in adults can cause abdominal distress. Symptoms of intolerance differ in severity, and the amount of lactose that can be tolerated varies greatly. In some areas of the world most milk is consumed as fermented products in which the amount of lactose is reduced or completely eliminated by fermentation.

Malabsorption is influenced by many factors: the quantity of the ingested sugar, the rate of gastric emptying, osmolarity of the fecal mass, fluid balance in the colon, colonic bacteria and the state of the colon, and the type and amount of carbohydrate that reaches the colon.

Concepts of Carbohydrate Utilization

Intermediary Metabolism. Carbohydrates have many roles. One very important role is to serve as metabolic fuel for all tissues, especially the brain and the nervous tissues, which use glucose almost exclusively. The absorbed monosaccharide is subjected to a complex set of controls to maintain a constant concentration of blood glucose. After intestinal transport, monosaccharides are absorbed into the portal vein and are transferred to the liver. The liver is the major organ for regulating glucose homeostasis.[33] In times of excess glucose, the liver stores glucose as glycogen or fat. In times of glucose shortage, the liver will manufacture glucose: first from liver glycogen and when that is depleted, from amino acids.[33]

Whereas the liver (and to some extent the kidney) is a net exporter of glucose, the rest of the organs are net users. Most organs convert glucose to pyruvate (gaining two high-energy phosphates in the process) and oxidize part of the pyruvate to CO_2 and NADH via the TCA cycle. Through the electron-transport system, NADH and $FADH_2$ produced in the TCA cycle are oxidized to H_2O and the bulk of the energy stored in glucose is chemically captured as high-energy phosphates in ATP.[33] Lactate produced in peripheral tissues, however, is not oxidized to CO_2 but is returned to the liver, where most of it is resynthesized to glucose and returned to the blood. The cycle of glucose to pyruvate to glucose (liver to muscle to liver) is referred to as the Cori cycle.[33] The breakdown of glucose to pyruvate is called glycolysis; the production of glucose is called gluconeogenesis.

The disposition of glucose is subject to interorgan controls and also intracellular controls. The process of reciprocal control of gluconeogenesis and lipogenesis is well understood; conditions that increase one decrease the other.[34] The intracellular controls rely on endocrine hormones. These hormones have organ and target-tissue specificity and activate only tissues where there are receptors for the hormones. Insulin, glucagon, glucocoticoids, thyroid hormone, and growth hormone are the major hormones that regulate carbohydrate metabolism, i.e., the direction of flow of carbohydrates into various pathways. (The release of insulin and the regulation of its receptor is beyond the scope of this work.) The outcome of this regulation is that there exists a complex relationship between dietary fat, dietary carbohydrate, insulin concentration, and insulin receptor.[35] Similar complexity exists with glucagon.[36] The maintenance of proper blood glucose concentration is extremely important. If blood glucose falls too low (hypoglycemia), the organism cannot function properly; fatigue, mental disorientation, and even fainting or coma may result. Elevated blood glucose (hyperglycemia) can give rise to other pathological conditions.

The glycolytic pathway (glucose to pyruvate) is the major highway of metabolism. Other monosaccharides can be converted to glucose, and glucose can be used to make other monosaccharides. The pentose phosphate shunt produces ribose (a major component of nucleic acids) and other pentoses. Glucuronic acid is used to conjugate a number of substances in the liver before they are excreted in the urine as waste products (drugs, for example). Galactose, fucose, xylose, mannose, sialic acid, and the amino derivatives of glucose, galactose, and mannose are used in the posttranslational modification of proteins and lipids.[33]

Glycolysis and gluconeogenesis take place in the same cell compartment using the same enzymes except at four control points. Each control point is a pair of enzymes, one unidirectionally gluconeogenic and the other unidirectionally glycolytic.[33] Operation of both enzymes simultaneously results in ATP hydrolysis and the net release of energy as heat. Such an event has been termed a futile cycle.[37]

Effects of Molecular Size. It has been known for many years that glucose taken by mouth elicits a greater insulin response than does glucose given intravenously.[38] The reason for this response is now known: glucose releases peptide hormones from the intestine that facilitate the release of insulin. Therefore, the idea that the intestine is capable of generating chemical regulators that affect other organs is now accepted.

Indications that there might be some special phenomena associated with the ingestion of disaccharides were found during the first decade of this century.[39] Early work indicated that consumption of sucrose or maltose initiates a faster rise in blood glucose, expired CO_2, or heat production than that initiated by the consumption of the monosaccharide equivalent. The effects referred to above were observed within 30–60 min after the ingestion of a disaccharide. After the work of Crane,[21-23] which suggested the existence of a special carrier for disaccharides, it was assumed that this special effect of disaccharides was due to a more rapid influx of monosaccharides into the blood when disaccharides were ingested. Later work on enzyme induction in livers from starved-refed rats cast doubt on this explanation.[40] In a 2-d refeeding experiment the transitory effect of sucrose feeding becomes irrelevant, because the enzyme overshoot is produced during the second day of refeeding.[39] The hypothesis was advanced that the disaccharide effect was generated by the presence of the disaccharide in the gut.[39] This hypothesis was partially validated by showing that physically sequestering glucose in the food with xanthan gum produces an enzyme response in the liver as if the carbohydrate fed were starch and by showing that if maltose is infused in a lower portion of the small intestine, it produces a smaller response of liver enzymes than if it is infused in the upper portion of the small intestine.[39]

The molecular-size hypothesis was then formulated.[39,41] According to this hypothesis the upper small intestine contains areas that are activated by the presence of disaccharides and monosaccharides. This hypothesis implies a receptor-ligand interaction that is a different mechanism from that postulated to involve an increase in insulin release because (1) the magnitude is disaccharide > monosaccharide > polysaccharide, (2) the disaccharide effect (increased lipogenic enzyme concentrations in the liver) is accompanied by increased gluconeogenic enzyme concentrations, and (3) the molecular-size effect is seen in gluconeogenic rates in liver cells from animals adapted to starch, maltose, or glucose in the diet.[42] If the effect of maltose were mediated by simply increasing glucose transport and elevating insulin concentration either directly or indirectly (via gut hormones), this effect would be expected to reduce gluconeogenesis. Because the opposite is true, we are left with a conjecture that the interaction of the simple sugar with the upper part of the small intestine produces a response that increases both gluconeogenesis and lipogenesis. Thus, simple sugars produce a partial derangement of the normal (reciprocal) control of lipogenesis and gluconeogenesis; in this action the simple sugar mimics the effects of dietary fructose,[34] obesity,[43] and diabetes.[43] A number of studies indicate the existence of an effect that is due to the molecular size of the ingested carbohydrate.[39] One of the best-characterized cases has to do with taste. Different taste receptors for glucose, maltose, and the octaglucose oligosaccharide were postulated.[44] The precise mechanism of the molecular-size effect and its importance in health is not understood.

The Glycemic Index of Food Carbohydrates. The concept of glycemic index is a measure of the ability of a carbohydrate to contribute to the concentration of blood glucose.[45] High glycemic index means that the dietary carbohydrate elevates blood glucose faster and to a higher level than a carbohydrate of lower glycemic index. Recently, the concept was challenged on the basis that the rise in blood glucose is not a precisely predictable phenomenon and is subject to variables that cannot be controlled.[46] It appears clear now that the original enthusiasm for the use of the glycemic index was somewhat exaggerated. Nevertheless, it is true that there are more categories of carbohydrates than complex and simple and that each category (or group) has a different ability to elevate blood glucose. The fact that this ability to raise blood glucose is interactive with other factors (such as state of health, meal size, amount of dietary fat, etc.) does not invalidate the concept. It merely emphasizes that the concept is not as simple and precise as originally believed.

The concept of glycemic index may be inadequate to describe the effect of starch on blood glucose. Amylose produces a slow and comparatively small rise in blood glucose and insulin; amylopectin produces a large increase in blood glucose, insulin, and glucagon.[47] The simultaneous rise in insulin and glucagon is not what would be expected from conventional knowledge. That is, we expect glucagon to decrease with increasing influx of glucose and the rise of blood insulin. The rapid inflow of glucose (from amylopectin) promotes two normally opposed responses, which may indicate that a crucial link is missing from our understanding of what takes place in the small intestine.

Carbohydrate Sensitivity. The term carbohydrate sensitivity originally was used to describe the Bureau of Home Economics (BHE) rat.[48] This rat, particularly when young, can maintain normal blood glucose concentration only by elevated blood insulin concentration. Later the concept was refined and applied to humans.[49] The test for carbohydrate sensitivity involves scoring a glucose-tolerance test (preferably by feeding sucrose). Points are given for attaining certain concentrations of insulin at certain times after carbohydrate ingestion; the scores are added and if a threshold value is exceeded, the subject is classified as carbohydrate sensitive. The difference between impaired glucose tolerance and carbohydrate sensitivity is that the former emphasizes blood glucose concentration, whereas the latter places more emphasis on the amount of blood insulin. Blood triglyceride and uric acid are positively correlated with insulin.[49]

Carbohydrate-sensitive human subjects develop elevated blood constituents (believed to be risk factors for arterial and heart disease) in response to being fed sucrose[50] or fructose.[51] Some scientists believe that the insulin overresponse to blood glucose is the beginning of a process that can develop first into pancreatic hypertrophy and with middle and advancing age into cumulative pancreatic failure (type II diabetes). This proposition, however, is far from being universally accepted.

Intracellular Carbohydrate Utilization

Glycolysis. The disposition of glucose via glycolysis is carefully regulated. The primary regulatory sites are phosphofructokinase 1 (PKF1) and a bifunctional polypeptide (MW 53,000) that has two components, phosphofructokinase 2 (PFK2) and fructose 2,6-biphosphatase (FBPase 2). PFK1 is an allosteric protein. Its activity is controlled by the need for energy (related to AMP, ADP, and ATP concentrations), the amount of free glucose, and endocrine status.[33] Another mechanism that regulates the activity of PFK1 is called feed-forward stimulation; it is controlled by the accumulation of fructose-2,6-biphosphate. The polypeptide has two functions: production of fructose-2,6-biphosphate by the action of PFK2 and removal of FBPase 2. The two activities are reciprocally controlled: Phosphorylation increases FBPase 2 and inhibits PFK2. The fructose-1,6-biphosphate accelerates the conversion of fructose-6-phosphate to fructose-1,6-biphosphate and, thus, stimulates glycolysis.

Disposition of Fructose. Fructose is metabolized primarily by the liver and then by a pathway that bypasses phosphofructokinase.[51] Fructose is phosphorylated in the 1 position and then split to the trioses by a special aldolase. This pathway is very fast so that fructose does not reach very high concentrations in the blood but is converted quickly to pyruvate, glucose, and fat in the liver. There are several consequences that arise from this event. First, suggestions that fructose is the sugar of preference for diabetics (because its transport into the muscle is independent of insulin) is based on a faulty premise, because fructose does not accumulate in the blood. Second, the side-effects of feeding fructose can be harmful, especially to the diabetic. It was noted before that fructose promotes both lipogenesis and gluconeogenesis;[34] therefore, this carbohydrate adds to the very abnormality that is present in diabetes. In addition, fructose increases lipogenesis, blood lipids, uric acid, blood insulin, and glucose and can further impair glucose tolerance in the carbohydrate-sensitive individual.[51] Fructose is reported to enhance the symptoms of some mineral deficiencies, particularly copper deficiency.[51]

Industrial production of high-fructose corn syrup from cornstarch made it possible to replace sucrose with fructose. In view of the effects of fructose cited above, the fructose level of the diet was suggested to be a concern to some scientists.[51] Critical evidence, however, is lacking.

Intracellular Glycosylation and Its Biological Role. Many proteins that are exported from the cytosol acquire carbohydrate sequences during post-translational modification.[33] Such proteins have a leader sequence that inserts into the endoplasmic reticulum and draws the protein into a membranous structure that later matures into Golgi bodies.[33] During the maturation of the Golgi bodies, carbohydrate is added either on the hydroxyl group of an amino acid such as serine or on the amino group of asparagine.[33] This process (glycosylation) is complex, but it may be summarized as follows. After a protein enters the endoplasmic reticulum a carbohydrate sequence is added either at an O or an N site. Such a carbohydrate sequence may be graphically represented as a tuning fork; attachment to the protein is via the end of the handle. Carbohydrate sequences enter the membranes by their dolichol attachment.[33] In the endoplasmic reticulum attachment of the carbohydrate sequence depends on the structure of the protein, the specific glycosyl transferases present, and the specific carbohydrate structures available for glycosylation.[52] As the membrane structure matures, one or both sides of the tuning fork structure may be shortened, added to, or both. These processes are highly specific, but the basis of specificity is just beginning to be understood.[52] The final carbohydrate sequences may be as short as a disaccharide on the glomerular basement membrane[53] or may constitute the major part of some proteins, such as keratins.[33] Recent work indicates that not only plasma and cytoplasmic proteins but some nucleoproteins, chromatin, and the cytoskeleton also are glycosylated.[54]

Once the glycosylation process is completed, the carbohydrate moieties impart diverse capabilities to the protein.[33] The first role of the carbohydrate attachments is that they serve as "postal codes" that set the destination of proteins.[33] The carbohydrate moieties act as recognition sites enabling a protein to be anchored to the membrane.[54] Carbohydrates act as recognition sites on receptors and antigens and play a crucial role in cellular adhesion.[33] The terminal sialic acid may protect some serum proteins from degradation[55] and may serve to keep albumin in the glomerulus.[56] Proteins that are used in the body as lubricants are highly glycosylated and are hydrophilic.[33]

Because most of this work has been done by molecular biologists, little is known about the effect of dietary carbohydrate on glycosylation. The possible effect of fructose on the glycosylation of intestinal disaccharidases was already mentioned.[12]

Nonenzymic Glycosylation (Glycation) and Its Consequences. Nonenzymic glycosylation means the addition of glucose, fructose, their phosphate derivatives, or triose phosphates to proteins. The process is officially designated as glycation, and this term will be used throughout.

The diverse effects of insulin-dependent diabetes mellitus (IDDM or type I) led some researchers to speculate that there was one underlying cause of all the pathology that accompanies IDDM. This one cause is now suspected to be the nonenzymic addition of glucose to protein and the subsequent crosslinking of such proteins.[57] According to the glycation hypothesis, lysine and hydroxylysine of long-lived proteins can react with glucose to produce a Schiff base.[57] The Schiff base then undergoes an Amadori re-

arrangement (shifting of the double bond to the second carbon) and a subsequent cyclization. Such structures can crosslink proteins; one particular structure of three glucose remnants crosslinking two proteins via the ϵ amino group of lysine was isolated.[57]

Glycation occurs throughout life even in individuals without diabetes.[58] A biological process is present to remove and repair damaged protein.[59] According to this hypothesis, a great deal of what we conceive as the symptoms of aging is related to the failure of the repair process to remove damaged material. The rate of damage is greatly accelerated in IDDM. Certain structures, such as the glomerular basement membrane, are especially susceptible to damage.[57] The glomerular basement membrane is not really a membrane but a complex protein network studded with heteropolysaccharides, disaccharides (glucose-galactose), and sporadic crosslinks.[57] Similar structures are found in the eye lens capsule[60] and arteries.[61] These structures become glycated and crosslinked during the course of IDDM, resulting in eventual impairment of organ function. Some of the same pathology can be observed in non-insulin-dependent diabetes mellitus (NIDDM), but in NIDDM the pathology produced by hyperlipidemia (i.e., heart attacks) is more likely to cause death than end-stage renal failure.

Reports indicate that glucose causes a relatively low rate of glycation and that fructose, phosphorylated fructose and glucose derivatives, and aldehydic phosphates of trioses may cause a glycation rate 10 or more times higher than that of glucose.[62] This finding argues against diabetics increasing fructose intake.

Glycation may be retarded by added aminoguanidine.[63] Arginine, the body's guanidine compound, is reported to be lowered in obesity[64] and, therefore, may be inadequate to prevent damage. It was proposed that the kidney is a major source of circulating arginine.[65] Hyperglycemia in IDDM or NIDDM and reduced arginine concentration may be related to the special vulnerability of kidney to damage in diabetics as well as to the link between obesity and diabetes.

Health Issues and Carbohydrate Nutrition

Enzyme Deficiencies and Toxicity. In the normal individual there is no short-term requirement for carbohydrate intake nor is there toxicity from excess carbohydrate. This does not mean that such diets are healthy in the long run. Carbohydrate intake must be controlled when some enzyme deficiencies occur. One such condition is galactosemia, in which the concentration of galactose-1-phosphate uridyl transferase is very low and results in the accumulation of toxic galactose metabolites.[33] If the intake of galactose is not restricted, mental retardation results.[66] Glycogen storage disease can be due to one of several enzyme deficiencies.[66] Individuals with this type of mutation have a very poor ability to mobilize liver glycogen, resulting in abnormally high amounts of liver glycogen and periodic episodes of hypoglycemia.[66] Exclusion of all simple sugars from the diet and the intake of small meals relatively low in carbohydrate (mostly amylose starch) is the only therapy currently available.

Simple Sugars and Health. During the 1960s and 1970s the possible role of simple sugars (sucrose, fructose) in the etiology of diabetes, obesity,[67,68] and arterial disease[68] was highly publicized. Numerous laboratories showed that feeding elevated amounts of fructose[51] or sucrose[69] elevated blood lipids, glucose, insulin, and uric acid, i.e., alterations that are believed to be risk factors in diabetes, arterial disease, and heart disease. On the basis of these reports, the Senate Select Committee on Nutrition[70] recommended that individuals limit or reduce the intake of simple sugars. However, a 1986 report of the Food and Drug Administration concluded that there was no proven health risk at current amounts of sugar consumption.[71] This conclusion was supported by a recent report of the NAS.[72] This controversy has been halted but may not yet be settled.

Special Aspects of Carbohydrate Nutrition. Several aspects of carbohydrate nutrition set it apart from other areas of nutrition: (*1*) There is no short-term requirement for carbohydrate in the diet nor is there a toxicity (in pharmacological terms) due to excess intake. (*2*) Effects of carbohydrate are relatively small, are cumulative, and are interactive with other dietary factors and genetic predisposition. (*3*) Some effects of carbohydrate (primarily those of the simple sugars) may be deleterious to some individuals (i.e., carbohydrate-sensitive individuals).

The basic nature of the human biological response to the consumption of sucrose is a particularly controversial subject. The source of the controversy is the experimental protocol used and the interpretation of the data. The effect of dietary sucrose in a human study using randomly selected people is relatively small ranging from 0% to 30% or 35%.[50] To show conclusively that such effects are statistically significant, a large number of subjects must be used.[39] Such studies are not feasible for financial and logistical reasons. This problem led some investigators to use a technique called telescoping, which means to increase the magnitude of the response and reduce the time it takes to develop the response by selecting subjects sensitive to sucrose feeding (i.e., carbohydrate-sensitive subjects) and by increasing the amount of dietary sucrose to two or three times nor-

mal. Such experiments were performed,[50] and it was found that sucrose but not starch feeding increased the risk factors associated with heart disease and NIDDM. Because of the use of telescoping, the implication that sucrose is an independent risk factor for heart disease and NIDDM is not generally accepted. Rather, it is suspected that a sucrose effect is a synergistic action between diet and genetic background.

Other Aspects of Carbohydrate Nutrition. Sucrose has been suggested as a causative agent for a number of conditions ranging from hyperactivity to juvenile delinquency. Most of these suggestions will not be addressed here, not because the ideas are outlandish, but because a systematic cause-and-effect relationship is either difficult to establish or impossible to test. However, there are indications that carbohydrates may affect mood changes,[73] and a recent report suggests that carbohydrate affects concentrations of enkephalins and endorphins.[74]

Altered Carbohydrates. The food industry has been introducing chemically altered starch for a number of years.[75] The purpose of such alterations is to change the properties of regular starch so as to produce better rheological properties, longer shelf-life, and better response to reheating or cooling. Some of these products are used in sauces, pies, and frozen ready-to-eat dinners, for example.

An interesting product is sucrose polyester, which consists of fatty acids bound to sucrose.[75] Sucrose polyester is not absorbed and is in fact a nonmetabolizable fat (even though it contains sucrose).

A number of commercially produced small carbohydrates such as sorbitol and xylitol are added to food as sweeteners. Others such as the L-sugars are being developed.

References

1. G.S. Semanza and S. Auricchio (1989) Small intestinal disaccharidases. In: *The Metabolic Basis of Inherited Disease*, 6th ed. (C.R. Scriver, A.L. Beaudet, W.S. Sly, and D. Valle, eds.), pp. 2975–2997, McGraw-Hill, New York.

2. K.A. Conklin, K.M. Vamashiro, and G.M. Gray (1975) Human intestinal sucrase-isomaltase: identification of free sucrase and isomaltase and cleavage of the hybrid into active distinct subunits. *J. Biol. Chem.* 250:5735–5741.

3. J.E. Riby and N. Kretchmer (1985) Participation of pancreatic enzymes in the degradation of intestinal sucrase-isomaltase. *J. Pediatr. Gastroenterol. Nutr.* 4:971–979.

4. H.P. Hauri, A. Quaroni, and K.J. Isselbacher (1979) Biogenesis of intestinal plasma membrane. Post-translational route and cleavage of sucrase-isomaltase. *Proc. Natl. Acad. Sci. USA* 76:5183–5186.

5. H.Y. Naim, E.E. Sterchi, and M.J. Lentze (1988) Structure, biosynthesis, and glycosylation of human small intestinal maltase-glucoamylase. *J. Biol. Chem.* 263:19709–19717.

6. T.F. Burks, J.J. Galligan, F. Porreca, and W.D. Barber (1985) Regulation of gastric emptying. *Fed. Proc.* 44:2897–2901.

7. T. Goda, S. Bustamente, and O. Koldovsky (1985) Dietary regu-

lation of intestinal lactase and sucrase in adult rats: quantitative comparison of effect of lactose and sucrose. *J. Pediatr. Gastroenterol. Nutr.* 4:998–1008.

8. J.S. Morrill, L.K. Kwong, P. Sunshine, G.M. Briggs, R.O. Castillo, and K.K. Tsuboi (1989) Dietary CHO and stimulation of carbohydrates along villus column of fasted rat jejunum. *Am. J. Physiol.* 256:G158–G165.

9. K. Yamada, T. Goda, S. Bustamente, and O. Koldovsky (1983) Different effect of starvation on activity of sucrase and lactase in rat jejunoileum. *Am. J. Physiol.* 244:G449–G455.

10. T. Goda, K. Yamada, S. Bustamente, and O. Koldovsky (1983) Dietary-induced rapid decrease in microvillar carbohydrase activity in rat jejunoileum. *Am. J. Physiol.* 245:G418–G423.

11. J.E. Riby and N. Kretchmer (1984) Effect of dietary sucrose on synthesis and degradation of intestinal sucrase. *Am. J. Physiol.* 246:G757–G763.

12. E.M. Danielsen (1989) Post-translational suppression of expression of intestinal brush border enzymes by fructose. *J. Biol. Chem.* 264:13726–13729.

13. Y. Nakabou, Y. Ishikawa, A. Misake, and H. Hagihira (1980) Effect of food intake on intestinal absorption and mucosal hydrolases in alloxan diabetic rats. *Metabolism* 29:181–185.

14. H.P. Schedl, A.S. Al-Jurf, and H.D. Wilson (1983) Elevated intestinal disaccharidase activity in the streptozotocin-diabetic rat is independent of enteral feeding. *Diabetes* 32:265–270.

15. G.R. Gourley, H.A. Korsmo, and W.A. Olsen (1983) Intestinal mucosa in diabetic rats: studies of microvillus membrane composition and microviscosity. *Metabolism* 30:1053–1058.

16. D. Wen, S.J. Henning, and R.L. Hazelwood (1988) Effect of diabetes on development of small intestinal enzymes of infant rats. *Proc. Soc. Exp. Biol. Med.* 187:51–57.

17. A.P. Morton and P.J. Hanson (1984) Monosaccharide transport by the small intestine of lean and genetically obese (ob/ob) mice. *Q. J. Exp. Physiol.* 69:117–126.

18. A.B.R. Thomson (1983) Experimental diabetes and intestinal barriers to absorption. *Am. J. Physiol.* 244:G151–G159.

19. E.S. Debnam, W.H. Karasov, and C.S. Thompson (1988) Nutrient uptake by rat enterocytes during diabetes mellitus; evidence for an increased sodium electrochemical gradient. *J. Physiol.* 397:503–512.

20. D.L. Baly and R. Horuk (1988) The biology and chemistry of the glucose transporter. *Biochim. Biophys. Acta* 947:571–590.

21. R.K. Crane (1960) Intestinal absorption of sugars. *Physiol. Rev.* 40:789–825.

22. R.K. Crane (1962) Hypothesis for mechanism of intestinal active transport of sugars. *Fed. Proc.* 21:891–895.

23. R.K. Crane (1968) Absorption of sugars. In: *Handbook of Physiology,* section 6, vol. 3 (C.F. Code and W. Heidel, eds.), pp. 1323–1351, Waverly Press, Baltimore.

24. G.M. Gray (1975) Carbohydrate digestion and absorption. Role of the small intestine. *Physiol. Med.* 292:1225–1230.

25. G.M. Gray (1981) Carbohydrate absorption and malabsorption. In: *Physiology of the Gastrointestinal Tract* (L.R. Johnson, ed.), pp. 1063–1072, Raven Press, New York.

26. E. Brot-Laroche and F. Alvarado (1983) Mechanism of sugar transport across the intestinal brush border membrane. In: *Intestinal Transport* (M. Gilles-Baillien and R. Gilles, eds.), pp. 147–169, Springer-Verlag, Berlin.

27. A.R. Walmsley (1988) The Dynamics of the glucose transporter. *Trends Biochem. Sci.* 13:226–231.

28. R.N. Fedorak, E.B. Chang, J.L. Madara, and M. Field (1987) Intestinal adaptation to diabetes. Altered Na-dependent nutrient absorption in streptozotocin-treated chronically diabetic rats. *J. Clin. Invest.* 79:1571–1578.

29. M.A. Hediger, M.J. Coady, T.S. Ikeda, and E.M. Wright (1987) Expression cloning and cDNA sequencing of the Na+/glucose cotransporter. *Nature* 330:379–381.

30. B. Thorens, H.K. Sarkar, H.R. Kaback, and H.F. Lodish (1988) Cloning and functional expression in bacteria of a novel glucose transporter present in liver, intestine, kidney and β-pancreatic islet cells. *Cell* 55:281–290.

31. H. Fukumoto, T. Kayano, J.B. Buse, et al. (1989) Cloning and characterization of the major insulin-responsive glucose transporter expressed in human skeletal muscle and other insulin-responsive tissue. *J. Biol. Chem.* 264:7776–7779.

32. M.A. Hedigar, E. Turk, and E.M. Wright (1989) Homology of the human intestinal Na+/glucose and *Escherichia coli* Na+/proline cotransporters. *Proc. Natl. Acad. Sci. USA* 86:5748–5752.

33. G. Zubay (1988) *Biochemistry,* 2nd ed, Macmillan, New York.

34. J. Tepperman and H.M. Tepperman (1970) Gluconeogenesis, lipogenesis and the Sherringtonean metaphor. *Fed. Proc.* 29:1284–1293.

35. S.J. Bhathena (1987) Insulin receptor. In: *Peptide Hormone Receptors* (M.Y. Kalimi and J.R. Hubbard, eds.), pp. 179–285, Walter de Gruyter, Berlin.

36. R.T. Premont and I. Iyengar (1987) Glucagon receptor: structure and function. In: *Peptide Hormone Receptors* (M.Y. Kalimi and J.R. Hubbard, eds.), pp. 129–177, Walter de Gruyter, Berlin.

37. M.L. Scrutton and M.F. Utter (1968) The regulation of glycolysis and gluconeogenesis in animal tissues. *Ann. Rev. Biochem.* 37:249–302.

38. N. McIntyre, C.D. Holdsworth, and D.S. Turner (1965) Intestinal factors in the control of insulin secretion. *J. Clin. Endocrinol.* 25:1317–1324.

39. B. Szepesi and O.E. Michaelis, IV (1986) 'Disaccharide effect.' Comparison of metabolic effects of the intake of disaccharides and their monosaccharide equivalents. In: *Metabolic Effects of Dietary Carbohydrates* (I. MacDonald, and A. Vrana, eds.), pp. 192–219, S. Karger, Basel, Switzerland.

40. O.E. Michaelis, IV, C.S. Nace, and B. Szepesi (1975) Demonstration of a specific metabolic effect of disaccharides in the rat. *J. Nutr.* 105:1186–1191.

41. O.E. Michaelis, IV, and B. Szepesi (1977) Specificity of the disaccharide effect in the rat. *Nutr. Metab.* 21:329–340.

42. J.H.Y. Park, C.D. Berdanier, O.E. Deaver, Jr., and B. Szepesi (1986) Effects of dietary carbohydrate on hepatic gluconeogenesis in BHE rats. *J. Nutr.* 116:1193–1203.

43. J.-S. Pan, C.D. Berdanier, and D. Hantle (in press) Glucose metabolism in obese and lean SHR and LA strains of rats. 6th Annual Meeting of NAASO, Washington, DC. *Int. J. Obes.*

44. A. Sclafani and S. Mann (1987) Carbohydrate taste preferences in rats. Glucose, sucrose, maltose, fructose and polyose compared. *Physiol. Behav.* 40:563–568.

45. D.J.A. Jenkins, T.M.S. Wolever, R.H. Taylor, et al. (1981) Glycemic index of foods: a physiological basis for carbohydrate exchange. *Am. J. Clin. Nutr.* 34:362–366.

46. C.B. Hollenbeck, A.M. Coulston, and G.M. Reaven (1988) Comparison of plasma glucose and insulin responses to mixed meals of high-, intermediate-, and low-glycemic potential. *Diabetes Care* 11:323–329.

47. K.M. Behall, D.I. Scholfield, I. Yuhaniak, and J. Canary (1989) Diets containing high amylose vs amylopectin starch: effects of metabolic variables in human subjects. *Am. J. Clin. Nutr.* 49:337–344.

48. C.D. Berdanier (1976) The BHE strain of rat: an example of the role of inheritance in determining metabolic controls. *Fed. Proc.* 35:2295–2299.

49. S. Reiser, M.C. Bickard, J. Hallfrisch, O.E. Michaelis, IV, and E.S. Prather (1981) Blood lipids and their distribution in lipoproteins in hyperinsulinemic subjects fed three different levels of sucrose. *J. Nutr.* 111:1045–1057.

50. S. Reiser (1982) Metabolic risk factors associated with heart disease and diabetes in carabohydrate-sensitive humans when consuming sucrose as compared to starch. In: *Metabolic Effects of*

Utilizable Dietary Carbohydrates (S. Reiser, ed.), pp. 239–260, Marcel Dekker, New York.

51. S. Reiser, and J. Hallfrisch (1987) *Metabolic Effects of Dietary Fructose,* CRC Press, Boca Raton, FL.

52. J.C. Paulson and K.J. Colley (1989) Glycosyltransferases. *J. Biol. Chem.* 264:17615–17618.

53. R.G. Spiro (1967) The structure of the disaccharide unit of the renal glomerular basement membrane. *J. Biol. Chem.* 242:4813–4823.

54. G.W. Hart, G.W. Holt, and R.S. Haltiwanger (1988) Nuclear and cytoplasmic glycosylation: novel saccharide linkages in unexpected places. *Trends Biochem. Sci.* 13:380–384.

55. N. Sharon and H. Lis (1981) Glycoproteins: research booming on long-ignored, ubiquitous compounds. *Chem. Eng. News* 59:21–24.

56. D.M. Brown, G.A. Andres, T.H. Hostetter, S.M. Mauer, and R. Price (1982) Kidney complications. *Diabetes* 31(suppl. 1):71–81.

57. M. Brownlee, H. Vlassara, and A. Cerami (1984) Nonenzymic glycosylation and the pathogenesis of diabetic complications. *Ann. of Intern. Med.* 101:527–537.

58. H. Vlassara, J. Valinsky, M. Brownlee, C. Cerami, S. Nishimoto, and A. Cerami (1987) Advanced glycosylation endproducts on erythrocyte cell surface induce receptor-mediated phagocytosis by macrophages. A model for turnover of aging cells. *J. Exp. Med.* 166:539–549.

59. H. Vlassara, M. Brownlee, K. Monogue, et al. (1988) Cachetin/TNF and IL-1 induced by glucose-modified proteins: role in normal tissue remodeling. *Science* 240:1546–1548.

60. S. Fukushi and R.G. Spiro (1969) The lens capsule. Sugar and amino acid composition. *J. Biol. Chem.* 244:2041–2048.

61. M. Brownlee, A. Cerami, and H. Vlassara (1988) Advanced products of nonenzymatic glycosylation and the pathogenesis of diabetic vascular disease. *Diabetes Metab. Rev.* 4:437–451.

62. J.D. McPhearson, B.H. Shilton, and D.J. Walton (1988) Role of fructose in glycosylation and cross-linking of proteins. *Biochemistry* 27:1901–1907.

63. M. Brownlee, H. Vlassara, A. Kooney, P. Ulrich, and A. Cerami (1986) Aminoguanidine prevents diabetes-induced arterial wall protein cross-linking. *Science* 232:1629–1632.

64. S. Yamini, R. Staples, and B. Szepesi (1989) Effect of obesity and dietary carbohydrate on liver and kidney urea cycle enzyme activities and plasma amino acids in the rat. *FASEB J.* 3(3, part I): A352 (abstr.).

65. W.R. Featherston, Q.R. Rogers, and R.A. Freedland (1973) Relative importance of kidney and liver in synthesis of arginine by the rat. *Am. J. Physiol.* 224:127–129.

66. F. Dickens, P.J. Randle, and W.J. Whelan, eds. (1968) *Carbohydrate Metabolism and Its Disorders,* vol. 2, Academic Press, New York.

67. A.M. Cohen, A. Teitelbaum, S. Briller, L. Yanko, E. Rosenmann, and E. Shafrir (1974) Experimental models of diabetes. In: *Sugars in Nutrition* (H.L. Sipple and K.W. McNutt, eds.); pp. 483–511, Academic Press, New York.

68. J. Yudkin (1968) Dietary intake of carbohydrate in relation to diabetes and atherosclerosis. In: *Carbohydrate Metabolism and Its Disorders,* vol. 2. (F. Dickens, P.J. Randle, and W.J. Whelan, eds.), pp. 169–183, Academic Press, London.

69. S. Reiser. Simple and complex carbohydrates (in press) In: *Nutritional Status Assessment of the Individual* (G.E. Livingston, ed.), Food and Nutrition Press, Westport, CT.

70. Senate Select Committee on Nutrition and Human Needs (1977) *Dietary Goals for the United States,* 2nd ed., U.S. Government Printing Office, Washington, DC.

71. Sugars Task Force, Health and Human Services, Food and Drug Administration (1986) *Evaluation of Health Aspects of Sugars Contained in Carbohydrate Sweeteners,* U.S. Government Printing Office, Washington, DC.

72. Committee on Diet and Health, Food and Nutrition Board, National Research Council (1989) *Implications for Reducing Chronic Disease Risk,* National Academy Press, Washington, DC.

73. R.J. Wurtman, and J.J. Wurtman (1989) Carbohydrates and Depression. *Sci. Am.* 260:68–75.

74. S.J. Bhathena, S. Reiser, B.W. Kennedy, A.S. Powell, P.M. Smith, and G. Rockwood (1988) Effect of dietary carbohydrate on plasma opiates in carbohydrate sensitive subjects. *FASEB J.* 2(5):A1202 (abstr.).

75. O.B. Wurzburg, ed. (1986) *Modified Starches: Properties and Uses,* CRC Press, Boca Raton, FL.

Chapter 7

Jacqueline Dupont

Lipids

Lipids, or fats, are generally defined as substances that are insoluble in water but soluble in organic solvents. Fat in food occurs in greatest proportion as triacylglycerol (triglyceride). Other lipids in food are sterols, fat-soluble vitamins (A, E, D, and K), phosphoglycerides (phospholipids) and sphingolipids, and some waxes and other minor complex lipidic components. Lipid metabolism includes lipid digestion, absorption, transport, synthesis, storage, utilization for energy, and structural or other functional properties. Storage and energy metabolism are described in other chapters and will be discussed here only as adjuncts to the other topics.

Physical Properties and Nomenclature

Lipids. The water insolubility of lipids is of major importance. The most hydrophobic lipids are triacylglycerols and cholesterol and its esters (Figure 1). They require special modifications or agglomerations to be transported in the aqueous medium of the blood. Sophisticated metabolic systems exist to enable lipids in the intestine to be solubilized for absorption. The insolubility of neutral lipids contributes to their function for storage as energy and for participation in membrane structures.

Any modification of a saturated hydrocarbon lipid to a more ionic form results in great effects on metabolism. Dehydration to double-bond structure (i.e., polyunsaturated fatty acids), hydroxylation (i.e., cholic acid), hydrolysis to acidic form (i.e., free fatty acids), and conjugation with other molecules (i.e., glycocholic acid) may cause neutral lipids to become more hydrophilic and even amphipathic.

Fatty Acids. Table 1 describes the nomenclature used for fatty acids of particular importance in food and nutrition. The double bonds in all of the naturally occurring fatty acids are in *cis* configuration and are three carbons apart (Figure 2). Monounsaturated, diunsaturated, and triunsaturated fatty acids are me-

tabolized by different mechanisms. Short- (4–6C), medium- (8–12C), long- (14–20C), and very-long- ($\geq$22C) chain fatty acids are metabolized by different pathways. *Trans* fatty acids occur in products derived from ruminant animals and in those that are chemically hydrogenated during processing.[5] They have physical characteristics similar to saturated fatty acids of the same length (Figure 2).

Fatty acids convey their individual physical characteristics to the lipids in which they are incorporated. Hydrolysis of the neutral lipids results in free fatty acids (FFA), that is, nonesterified fatty acids that are water soluble in acidic solution and that form acyl salts (soaps) in basic solution, hence the term saponifiable material.

Long-chain fatty acid triacylglycerols have heats of combustion of ~9.5 kcal/g.[6] With a digestibility of 95% the fuel value is 9.0 kcal/g (37.66 kJ/g). Protein and carbohydrate yield only 4.0 kcal/g (16.74 kJ/g); therefore, it is necessary to specify whether the proportion of fat in a food or diet is based on mass (weight percent, wt %) or energy value (energy percent, en %).

Sterols. Because of their hydrocarbon ring structure, sterols are extremely hydrophobic and rigid in structure (Figure 1). This characteristic accounts for their functions in nerve tissues and membranes. Steryl esters are unable to cross membranes, whereas free sterols (nonsaponifiable material) freely cross membranes by passive diffusion. Neutral sterols are hydroxylated to dialcohols and trialcohols and converted to cholanoic acids that are conjugated with glycine or taurine (i.e., the bile salts). These compounds are amphipathic and have functions directly related to their detergent effects.

Digestion and Absorption

The digestion of fat begins in the mouth, where chewing releases fat from other food components,

TRIGLYCERIDE MODELS

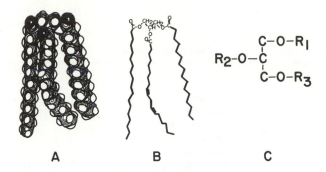

A   B   C

$$C-O-R_1$$
$$R_2-O-C$$
$$C-O-R_3$$

CHOLESTEROL MODELS

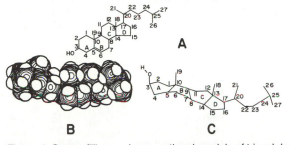

A

B   C

Figure 1. Space-filling and conventional models of triacylglycerol and cholesterol. The uncharged state of the molecules makes them hydrophobic. Triacylglycerol models: A. space-filling; B. conformational; C. stereospecific numbering (sn) of glycerides. If the R_3 substituent of an acylglycerol is PO_4, the compound is phosphatidic acid. If it is phosphoryl-choline, -ethanolamine, -inositol, etc. it is a phosphoglyceride.[1] Cholesterol models: A. conventional; B. space-filling; C. conformational. Adapted from reference 1 with permission.

and lingual lipase begins hydrolysis of triacylglycerols.[7] The average Western diet contains ~150 g triacylglycerol, 4–8 g phospholipid,[8] and 400–500 mg cholesterol.[9] In the stomach the activity of lingual lipase continues at pH 2–6 and hydrolyzes triacylglycerols to diacylglycerols and FFA. Lingual lipase has specificity for medium- and short-chain fatty acids, and these fatty acids may be absorbed from the stomach.

In the duodenum the fat from food is mixed with secretions of the bile duct that include bile salts and 7–22 g/d of lecithin (phosphatidylcholine). Fat droplets are formed and the pH is increased to 5.5–6.5. Pancreatic lipase is secreted and is activated at that pH. Bile salts and phospholipids adhere to the surface of the lipid droplets and prevent access by lipase (Figure 3). Lipolysis can occur because procolipase is secreted along with lipase by the pancreas. Procolipase is activated to colipase by pancreatic trypsin, and the colipase complexes with lipase and also binds to the lipid droplets permitting lipase to have access to triacylglycerols (Figure 3). Hydrolysis

of long-chain as well as other fatty acids occurs, yielding FFA and sn2-monoacylglycerols.

Bile micelles made of bile acids and phospholipids are formed when the proportions of the two reach a critical micellar concentration (CMC). Micellar aggregates engulf free fatty acids and monoacylglycerols, and the expanded micelle is water soluble. The process is very rapid and leads to diffusion of the micelle through the aqueous interface between the micelle and the cell membrane, an unstirred water layer (Figure 3). Passage of the micelle through the unstirred water layer is the rate-limiting step for lipid absorption.[8] The FFA and monoacylglycerols come into contact with the cell membrane and diffuse freely through the membrane. Within the mucosal cell the fatty acids and monoacylglycerols are reesterified to triacylglycerols that do not passively diffuse in the reverse direction.

Saturated fatty acids with carbon chain length of 18 are poorly absorbed in the free state but are well absorbed as sn2-monoacylglycerols. Absorption rates of very-long-chain fatty acids decrease with increasing melting points.

Medium-chain-length fatty acids occur in triacylglycerols (MCT) of milk fat and of coconut and palm kernel oils. The MCT are much more water soluble than are the long- and very-long-chain triacylglycerols. They are hydrolyzed and enter the mucosal cells similarly to other fatty acids, but they are not reesterified within the cell. They are transported via the portal circulation at a much faster rate than the longer-chain fatty acids are transported via the lymph.

Phospholipids are hydrolyzed by pancreatic phospholipase A2, which cleaves the fatty acid at the sn2 position. The resulting lysophospholipid (i.e., lysophosphatidylcholine) diffuses into the mucosal cell where the fatty acid at the A1 position is cleaved. The products are acylated to reform phospholipids by using two lysophospholipid molecules to generate a phospholipid and a glycerophosphorylcholine (or ethanolamine, etc.) molecule.[10]

Cholesterol in the gut is derived from the diet and from bile secretion, the latter normally being about the same amount as the former. Biliary cholesterol, which is in the free form, enters the gut in a micellar form, whereas dietary cholesterol must be dispersed from fat droplets to micelles. Dietary cholesterol is hydrolyzed by a pancreatic cholesteryl esterase in the gut to the free form. Estimates for absorption vary depending upon the methods used to determine absorption. Endogenous cholesterol is estimated to be absorbed at ~60–80% efficiency; dietary cholesterol is less well absorbed.[9] Passage through the unstirred water layer and subsequent passive diffusion across the mucosal membrane are analogous to the

Table 1. Some fatty acids in food fats and oils and human plasma*

Symbol	Systematic name	Common name	Typical fat source	Percentage in whole plasma Mean	SD
Saturated fatty acids					
4:0	Butanoic	Butyric	Butterfat		
6:0	Hexanoic	Caproic	Butterfat		
8:0	Octanoic	Caprylic	Coconut oil		
10:0	Decanoic	Capric	Coconut oil		
12:0	Dodecanoic	Lauric	Coconut oil		
14:0	Tetradecanoic	Myristic	Butterfat, coconut oil	0.71	0.39
15:0	Pentadecanoic	Pentadecylic		0.22	0.07
16:0	Hexadecanoic	Palmitic	Most fats and oils	19.17	1.38
18:0	Octadecanoic	Stearic	Most fats and oils	6.83	0.61
20:0	Eicosanoic	Arachidic	Lard, peanut oil	0.13	0.03
22:0	Docosanoic	Behenic	Peanut oil	0.33	0.07
24:0	Tetracosenoic	Lignoceric		0.32	0.07
Unsaturated fatty acids					
10:1n−1	9-Decenoic	Caproleic	Butterfat		
12:1n−3	9-dodecenoic	Lauroleic	Butterfat		
14:1n−5	9-tetradecanoic	Myristoleic	Butterfat		
16:1n−7	9-hexadecenoic	Palmitoleic	Fish oils	1.42	0.46
16:1n−7	Transhexadecenoic	Palmitelaidic	HVO†	0.30	0.06
18:1n−9	9-Octadecenoic	Oleic	Most fats and oils	16.65	2.54
18:1n−9	9-Octadecenoic	Elaidic	Butterfat, beef fat, HVO		
18:1n−7	11-Octadenoic	Vaccenic	Butterfat, beef fat	1.56	0.25
18:2n−6	9,12-Octadecadienoic	Linoleic	Most vegetable oils	36.00	4.16
18:3n−6	6,9,12-Octadecatrienoic	γ-linoleic		0.40	0.13
18:3n−3	9,12,15-Octadecatrienoic	α-Linolenic	Soybean, canola oils	0.44	0.13
20:1n−11	9-Eicosanoic	Gadoleic	Fish oils		
20:1n−9	11-Eicosanoic	Gondoic	Rapeseed oil	0.12	0.03
20:3n−9	5,8,11-Eicosatrienoic	Mead	EFA-deficient animals‡	0.06	0.02
20:2n−6	11,14-Eicosadienoic			0.20	0.06
20:3n−6	11,14-Eicosadienoic	Dihomogammalinolenic		1.45	0.25
20:4n−6	5,8,11,14-Eicosatetraenoic	Arachidonic	Lard	7.52	1.56
20:4n−3	8,11,14,17-Eicosatetraenoic			0.05	0.06
20:5n−3	5,8,11,14,17-Eicosapentaenoic	EPA, timnodonic	Fish oils	0.58	0.37
22:1n−9	13-Docosenoic	Erucic	Rapeseed oil	0.03	0.03
22:4n−6	7,10,13,16-Docosatetraenoic			0.26	0.08
22:5n−6	4,7,10,13,16-Docosapentaenoic			0.17	0.06
22:5n−3	7,10,13,16,19-Docosapentaenoic			0.52	0.13
22:6n−3	4,7,10,13,16,19-Docosahexaenoic	DHA, cervonic	Fish oils	2.51	0.86
24:1	15-Tetracoseanoic	Nervonic		0.36	0.09

* Adapted from references 2 (foods) and 3 (human plasma). Used with permission.
† HVO, hydrogenated vegetable oil.
‡ EFA, essential fatty acids.

processes for fatty acids. Free cholesterol is reesterified within the mucosal cell by action of acyl-coenzyme A (CoA)-cholesterol acyltransferase (ACAT).

Transport

Lipoproteins. Absorbed lipids are made water soluble for transport in blood plasma by their incorporation into lipoproteins. Triacylglycerols and cholesterol are incorporated into chylomicrons in the intestinal mucosa. The processes are similar to those for other secretory proteins. The chylomicron contains ~84% triacylglycerol encased in a hydrophilic film of phospholipid and protein. Some very-low-density lipoprotein (VLDL) is also secreted by the intestinal mucosa. The apoprotein characteristic of these particles is apo-B48.[7]

The liver secretes a particle called high-density lipoprotein (HDL) that contains a number of apoproteins and little lipid. It is secreted in a discoidal form

FATTY ACID MODELS

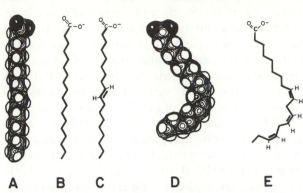

Figure 2. Space-filling and conventional models of fatty acids: A. stearic acid (18:0), space-filling; B. stearic acid, conformational; C. elaidic acid (18:1n—9t) trans, conformational; D. α-linolenic acid (18:3n—3), space-filling; E. α-linolenic acid, all cis, conformational.[3] Adapted from reference 3 with permission.

and is distributed throughout the circulation and lymph. After chylomicrons and VLDL are secreted into the lymph, the particles interact with HDL and thus acquire apoproteins E and CII (Figure 4). Apo-CII activates lipoprotein lipase at the luminal surface of the endothelium and in fat cells. Repeated actions of the lipase as the blood circulates remove most of the triglyceride of the chylomicron (Figure 4), and the resulting particle is called the remnant. Excess apo-CII is returned to HDL, and the remnant is rich in apo-E, which activates receptors in the liver. The remnant particles enter liver cells by endocytosis and are then hydrolyzed to FFA, cholesterol, and amino acids by lysosomes.[11]

Fat in the liver is present from chylomicrons, from biosynthesis from dietary carbohydrate and protein, and from fatty acids mobilized from adipose tissue. The hydrolysis products of HDL, chylomicron remnants, and low-density lipoprotein (LDL) also are available for resecretion. The lipid is secreted by incorporation into VLDL analogous to the formation of chylomicrons in the intestine; however, the apoprotein is apo-B100.[7] Secreted VLDL receives apo-CII and apo-E from HDL and is acted upon by lipoprotein lipase in the same way as are chylomicrons (Figure 4). The requirements for the enzyme, lipoprotein lipase, and a low-molecular-weight protein, apo-CII, are analogous to requirements for hydrolysis in the intestine by lipase and colipase. Both VLDL and HDL contain bile acids (VLDL 160 and HDL 320 μg/L).[12] The resulting particle is called LDL. Most of the cholesterol transported in the body is found in LDL. Adipose tissue, muscle, and liver have receptors for apo-B100, and the LDL particles are taken up by endocytosis and hydrolyzed in the lysosomes.[13]

Lipoproteins have many regulatory functions in metabolism beyond those of lipid transport. Under-

standing of the genetic basis for dyslipoproteinemias is quite advanced, and the relationships of the lipoproteins to cardiovascular disease are under intensive investigation. For more complete information on the status of this knowledge, see Steinberg.[14]

Fatty Acids. The FFA released by hydrolysis of triacylglycerols by the action of lipoprotein lipase enter cells by passive diffusion and are rapidly reesterified. They are incorporated into phospholipids for function in membranes and as precursors of icosanoids, into triacylglycerols for storage for energy, and into cholesteryl esters. FFA also may be used for energy, especially by heart, muscle, kidney, and platelets.

Some of the fatty acids released by lipoprotein lipase enter the blood stream. Most of the circulating fatty acids, however, come from lipolysis of triacylglycerols in adipose tissue during fasting. They are transported in the form of complexes with albumin. Albumin has two active binding sites that form firm but rapidly reversible complexes. In humans the liver takes up 40–50% of the fatty acids leaving plasma.

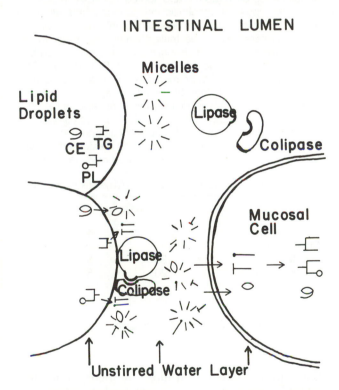

Figure 3. Processes of digestion and absorption of dietary fat. Bile micelles prevent access of pancreatic lipase to lipid droplets by adhering to their surface; colipase has a high affinity for the lipid droplets and complexes with lipase to allow hydrolysis of triacylglycerols; hydrolyzed fatty acids and monoacylglycerols are made water soluble by incorporation into micelles and thereby cross the unstirred water layer where the fatty acids enter the mucosal cells by passive diffusion. Fatty acids are then reesterified to triacylglycerols, phospholipids, and cholesteryl esters.[4] Adapted from reference 4 with permission.

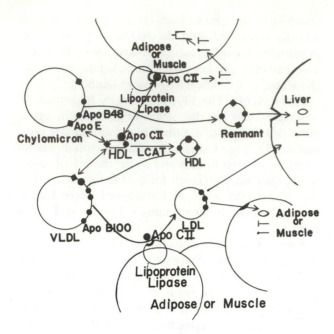

Figure 4. Lipoprotein metabolism. Chylomicrons from the intestinal lymph and very-low-density lipoprotein (VLDL) from the liver interact with discoidal high-density lipoprotein (HDL) to acquire apoprotein (apo) E and apo-CII. Apo-CII interacts with lipoprotein lipase at endothelial cell surfaces, and fatty acids and monoacylglycerols are released to enter cells by passive diffusion where they are reesterified to triglycerides for storage. The remaining fraction of chylomicrons is the remnant particle; that of VLDL is low-density lipoprotein (LDL). The apo-CII is returned to HDL, and the remnant apo-E acts as a signal for uptake by liver receptors. LDL contains apo-B100, which is recognized by receptors in liver and peripheral tissues. The particles enter the cell by endocytosis and are hydrolyzed by lysosomes. HDL interacts with circulating lipoproteins and cell surfaces to pick up free cholesterol, which is esterified by action of the HDL enzyme lecithin-cholesterol-acyltransferase (LCAT).[4]

Compound	VLDL	LDL	Chylomicron	HDL
			% of total	
Triglycerides	50	8	84	4
Cholesteryl				
Esters	15	35	5	17
Phospholipids	8	20	8	48
Cholesterol	6	7	2	3
Protein	10	25	2	48

Adapted from reference 4 with permission.

Some may be stored but most are incorporated into VLDL and secreted again into the plasma.[7]

Cholesterol Metabolism

Cholesterol is required for membrane structure, nervous tissue, bile-acid synthesis, and steroid-hormone synthesis. If it is not available to cells it must be synthesized. All mammalian cells examined have the capacity to synthesize cholesterol. The necessary precursor is acetyl-CoA. Acetyl-CoA is generated within the mitochondria and converted into citrate, which diffuses into the cytosol. Citrate is hydrolyzed by citrate lyase to yield acetyl-CoA and oxaloacetate. In the cytosol three molecules of acetyl-CoA are converted to β-hydroxy-β-methyl glutaryl (HMG)-CoA (Figure 5). The major regulatory site for cholesterol synthesis is the action of HMG-CoA reductase upon HMG-CoA to yield mevalonic acid. This enzyme is the site for feedback regulation of cholesterol synthesis by cholesterol in cells. The 5-carbon mevalonate is phosphorylated, three units are combined into the 15-carbon molecule, farnesyl-pyrophosphate, and two of those molecules are converted to squalene. Squalene is oxidized and cyclized to a steroid ring, lanosterol, in a reaction that is not reversible in the mammalian system. All steroid-ring products must be excreted from the body as steroids. Lanosterol is converted to cholesterol by the loss of three methyl groups, saturation of the side chain, and a shift of the double bond from the 8 to the 5 position (Figure 5).

Most cholesterol synthesis occurs in the liver. Exogenous cholesterol may inhibit synthesis; therefore, absorption and feedback regulation of synthesis are two major forms of regulation of cholesterol concentration in plasma and tissues. Because all of the steroid nucleus must be excreted, the third mechanism for control of total body cholesterol is excretion of neutral sterol via the bile and conversion of cholesterol to bile acids that are subsequently excreted. Whereas reabsorption of cholesterol amounts to about one-half of that secreted in the bile, bile acids are reabsorbed at ~95% efficiency.[7] The net loss of bile acids from the body accounts for 30–60% of the total sterol lost. Bile contains a large part of the total pool of bile acids, and the bile acids may be recycled many times per day.

The formation of bile acids from cholesterol is another of the irreversible metabolic steps that contribute to regulation of total body cholesterol. Cholesterol 7-α-hydroxylase places a hydroxyl group at the 7 carbon of cholesterol, and a subsequent hydroxylation at the 12-α-position is followed by inversion of the 3-β-hydroxyl to the 3-α-position. Removal of the terminal 3-carbon group is followed by conjugation with glycine or taurine, another irreversible step. These reactions result in formation of the primary bile acids, taurocholic and glycocholic acids (3-α,7-α,12-α-hydroxyl), and tauro- and glycochenodeoxycholic acids (3-α,7α-hydroxyl). Bile acids are synthesized, for the most part, in the liver, but other types of cells also have the capacity to make these compounds.[11] After the primary bile acids reach the lower intestine, they come into contact with gut microorganisms that can deconjugate and dehydroxyl-

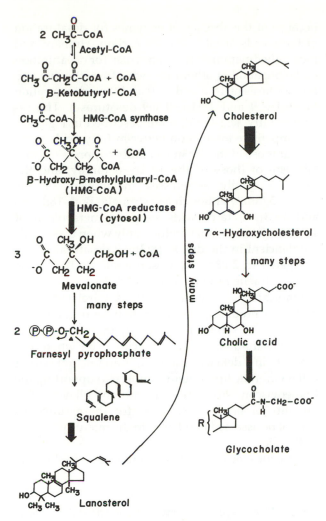

Figure 5. Formation of cholesterol and bile salts. Three molecules of acetyl-CoA form HMG-CoA which is reduced to mevalonate in an irreversible step; three mevalonate molecules condense to form farnesyl pyrophosphate, and two of those condense to form squalene. Squalene is cyclized by an oxidative reaction to form lanosterol. Many reactions remove three methyl groups and transfer the double bond from the 8–9 to the 5–6 position. By an irreversible reaction a mixed-function oxidase forms 7-α-hydroxycholesterol. Removal of the 25–27 carbons by β-oxidation leads to formation of a bile acid, and conjugation with glycine forms a bile salt.[2] Adapted from reference 2 with permission.

ate them. The products of these reactions are absorbed in the enterohepatic circulation and taken up by the liver from the portal blood. Small amounts of these secondary bile acids are found in the peripheral blood. The liver rehydroxylates and reconjugates the free bile acids, which continue to be recycled.

Cholesterol synthesis in peripheral tissues is minimal under most conditions, because ample cholesterol is provided by circulating lipoproteins. The receptor-mediated uptake of LDL is regulated by the number of receptors. The possible number of receptors is controlled genetically,[13] and their functional number is regulated by plasma LDL concentration. After the LDL enters the cell and is hydrolyzed, the free cholesterol thus released is available as a feedback inhibitor of HMG-CoA reductase and as a substrate for ACAT. Free cholesterol may pass back out of the cell by passive diffusion through the membrane where it is available for incorporation into HDL by action of LCAT. Otherwise, the cholesterol is reacylated, preferentially with oleate, to be stored. The resulting cholesteryl ester cannot exit the cell until it is hydrolyzed. This intracellular regulation of cholesterol egress from the cell is not understood. Cholesterol released by the lysosomes acts to inhibit HMG-CoA reductase, activate ACAT, and reduce recycling and synthesis of LDL receptors.

Defects in regulation of any aspect of cholesterol metabolism lead to pathological conditions. A fundamental need in nutrition science is to identify the genetic aspects of the regulation of cholesterol metabolism that are amenable to dietary intervention. Many aspects of the diet affect cholesterol metabolism: amount and composition of protein, carbohydrate, and fat; availability of all the nutrients that are necessary for enzyme activity; and total food consumption and meal patterns. Indirectly, dietary factors that impinge on other risk factors for hypercholesterolemia, i.e., diabetes, hypertension, and obesity, must be considered. Dietary factors generally implicated in hypercholesterolemia are excess total fat and saturated fatty acids and to a lesser extent excess cholesterol.[15]

Essential Fatty Acids

The first indication of the essentiality of a fatty acid was presented by Burr and Burr in 1929 (for historical primary references see Aaes-Jorgensen[16] and Mead[17]). The symptoms in rats were dry, scaly skin, excessive consumption of water, reduced growth, and male and female infertility. Later many organ abnormalities were added to the list. The first quantitative biochemical manifestation to be reported was an increase in the triene-tetraene ratio. This increase was the result of appearance of eicosatrienoic acid (20:3n−9) in tissues of rats fed fat-free diets when the fatty acids were analyzed by alkaline isomerization. In normal fat-fed rats the 20:3 was absent or barely detectable, and its ratio to arachidonic acid (20:4n−6) increased with increasing time of consumption of a fat-free diet. A ratio of ≤0.4, which was attainable with a dietary content of 1 wt % (2 en %) of linoleate, was considered to be adequate to prevent the observed symptoms. Later use of methods such as gas-liquid chromatography[16] revised the value indicating deficiency to a ratio of <0.2 in humans. The use of such a ratio to describe a very

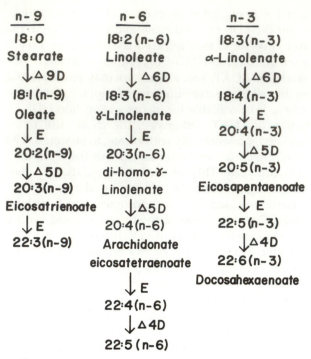

Figure 6. Families of fatty acids formed from C$_{18}$ precursors by desaturation (D) and elongation (E). The n−9 pathway is exhibited in mammals only when there is insufficient n−6 present in the diet.

complex physiological system and the conclusion that 1 wt % of the diet was sufficient was deemed to be of questionable value, even for the rat.[17] The reasons for questioning are related to the multiple functions of polyunsaturated fatty acids and the absence of evidence to explain the mechanisms for the symptoms.

Linoleate is an essential dietary factor for mammals

because of the absence of enzymes for desaturation of fatty acids distal to the δ-9 carbon. Humans and most other mammals have enzymes for desaturation and elongation of other fatty acids from the diet and for synthesis of 16:0 and 18:0 and their desaturation to 16:1n−9 and 18:1n−9 (δ9-desaturase). The resulting fatty acid families are described in Figure 6. A competitive interaction between fatty acids exists so that those of the 18:3n−3 family suppress the metabolism of those of the 18:2n−6 family, and the 18:2n−6 family suppresses metabolism of the 18:3n−3 family although less strongly. Both 18:2n−6 and 18:3n−3 fatty acids suppress metabolism of 18:1n−9 fatty acids. Therefore, only when these acids are deficient in the diet is 18:3n−9 desaturated and elongated to 20:3n−9 (eicosatrienoic acid) and the triene-tetraene ratio is increased.[18]

Linoleate has several functions unrelated to its metabolic products. It is an efficient source of energy because it is oxidized more rapidly than saturated or monounsaturated 18-C fatty acids even when animals are in a deficient state.[19] It is an integral part of cell membrane lipoprotein complexes supporting the homeoviscous structure of membrane bilayers. The quantity of linoleate required for these functions cannot be assessed in relation to the quantity needed in the diet.

A major specific function of linoleate is in skin cer-

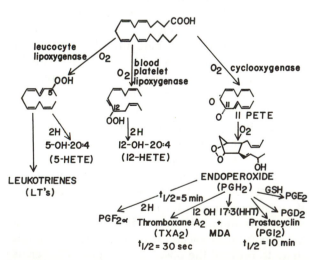

Figure 7. Icosanoid synthesis from arachidonate. HETE (hydroxyeicosatetraenoic acid), PETE (peroxyeicosatetraenoic acid), PG (prostaglandin), GSH (glutathione), and MDA (malondialdehyde).[6] Adapted from reference 6 with permission.

Table 2. Physiological functions of icosanoids and conditions of increased icosanoid formation*

System	PG involved
Physiological functions	
Cardiovascular	
Platelet aggregation	TX$_{A2}$, PGI$_2$
Blood flow	PGI$_2$, PG$_{E2}$
Closure of ductus arteriosus	PGI$_2$, PG$_{E2}$
Renal	
Renin release	PGI$_2$
Water excretion (vasopressin)	PG$_{E2}$
Blood flow	PG$_{E2}$, PGI$_2$
Gastrointestinal	
Cytoprotective effect	PG$_{E2}$
Blood flow	PG$_{E2}$
Reproductive	
Uterus contraction	PG$_{F2\alpha}$
Conditions	
Inflammation	PG$_{E2}$, LTs
Allergic reactions	PGs, TX$_{A2}$, LT$_3$
Mastocytosis	PG$_{D2}$
Hypercalcemia of cancer	PG$_{E2}$
Bartters syndrome	PGI$_2$
Patent ductus arteriosus	PG$_{E2}$, PGI$_2$
Dysmenorrhea	PG$_{F2\alpha}$

* PGI, prostacyclin; TX, thromboxane; PG, prostaglandin; LT, leukotriene.

Table 3. Recommended diet modifications to lower blood cholesterol*

	The Step-One Diet	
	Choose	Decrease
Fish, chicken, turkey, and lean meats	Fish, poultry without skin, lean cuts of beef, lamb, pork or veal, shellfish	Fatty cuts of beef, lamb, pork; spare-ribs, organ meats, regular cold cuts, sausage, hot dogs, bacon, sardines, roe
Skim and low-fat milk, cheese, yogurt, and dairy substitutes	Skim or 1% fat milk (liquid, powdered, evaporated), buttermilk	Whole milk (4% fat): regular, evaporated, condensed; cream, half and half, 2% milk, imitation milk products, most nondairy creamers, whipped toppings
	Nonfat (0% fat) or low-fat yogurt	Whole-milk yogurt
	Low-fat cottage cheese (1% or 2% fat)	Whole-milk cottage cheese (4% fat)
	Low-fat cheeses, farmer or pot cheeses (all of these should be labeled no more than 2–6 g of fat per ounce)	All natural cheeses (eg, blue, roquefort, camembert, cheddar, Swiss), low-fat or "light" cream cheese, low-fat or "light" sour cream, cream cheeses, sour cream
	Sherbet, sorbet	Ice cream
Eggs	Egg whites (two whites equal 1 whole egg in recipes), cholesterol-free egg substitutes	Egg yolks
Fruits and vegetables	Fresh, frozen, canned, or dried fruits and vegetables	Vegetables prepared in butter, cream, or other sauces
Breads and cereals	Homemade baked goods using unsaturated oils sparingly, angel food cake, low-fat crackers, low-fat cookies	Commercial baked goods: pies, cakes, doughnuts, croissants, pastries, muffins, biscuits, high-fat crackers, high-fat cookies
	Rice, pasta	Egg noodles
	Whole-grain breads and cereals (oatmeal, whole wheat, rye, bran, multigrain, etc)	Breads in which eggs are a major ingredient
Fats and oils	Baking cocoa	Chocolate
	Unsaturated vegetable oils: corn, olive, rapeseed (canola oil), safflower, sesame, soybean, sunflower	Butter, coconut oil, palm oil, palm kernel oil, lard, bacon fat
	Margarine or shortenings made from one of the unsaturated oils listed above, diet margarine	
	Mayonnaise, salad dressings made with unsaturated oils listed above, low-fat dressings	Dressings made with egg yolk
	Seeds and nuts	Coconut

* From reference 15. Used with permission.

amides.[20] The increased water consumption of rats fed linoleate-deficient diets was shown to be caused by excess transepidermal water loss. The defect can be corrected by supplementation of the diet of rats with ~0.5 en % of linoleate. Neither oleate nor α-linolenate can be substituted for linoleate, but arachidonate and the rare fatty acid columbinate [18:3(5t,9c,12c)] are effective. The linoleate is incorporated into acylglucosylceramides and acylceramides. Linoleate is the only fatty acid substantially incorporated into these sphingolipids, so it is postulated that arachidonate spares the linoleate requirement for its own synthesis and is retroconverted to linoleate.[20]

A requirement for linoleate that may account for many of the functional defects of deficiency is its use as a precursor for dihomogammalinolenic and arachidonic acids, which are the parent compounds for the one and two series icosanoids (Figure 7). The fatty acid precursors of the icosanoids are stored in phospholipids, preferentially in the sn2-position. They are released upon appropriate physiological stimulation by action of phospholipase A2. The enzymes cyclooxygenase and lipoxygenase convert them to physiologically potent end products. They act as paracrine and autocrine modulators of cellular reactions in extremely small concentrations (picograms and nanograms). Whereas linoleate is the precursor for both cyclooxygenase and lipoxygenase products, much more is known about dietary effects upon cyclooxygenase products (prostaglandins, thromboxanes, prostacyclin), and those effects will be emphasized.

It is impossible to discuss all of the possible manifestations of dietary fat effects upon icosanoid functions (partially described in Table 2) in one short chapter. Reviews are available of both general dietary[21-23] and specific organ or clinical implications.[24]

Evaluation of diet effects upon icosanoid metabolism is hampered by the difficulties of measuring icosanoid production and of interpreting results obtained in relation to in vivo conditions. Keys to evaluation of available data include the following: (1) Tissue fatty acid composition must be analyzed and not inferred from dietary fat. For example, arachidonate tissue concentration is not proportional to dietary linoleate. (2) Availability of free arachidonate is not the sole regulator of icosanoid synthesis, so providing exogenous arachidonate in the reaction medium is not appropriate. Nutrition-related conclusions should be based upon tissue endogenous fatty acid composition. (3) The act of taking a tissue sample will cause the production of unphysiological quantities of icosanoids, from 100 to 10,000 times that of in vivo production.[23]

Measurement of icosanoid metabolites in the urine seems to be the most reliable indicator of whole-body metabolism. The major disadvantages of this procedure are inability to infer the tissue of origin and contamination with icosanoids of seminal vesicle or menstrual origin.[25] Under these constraints it seems clear that deficiency of linoleate (0–1 en % in the diet for a prolonged time) depresses icosanoid synthesis.[23] Because such consumption of linoleate also causes other severe manifestations of deficiency, one may conclude that this condition of depressed icosanoid synthesis is undesirable. Analysis of results of several different kinds of experiments using graded concentrations of linoleate in the diets of rats and humans and in media for cultured cells suggested that icosanoid synthesis is enhanced by increasing dietary linoleate from 0 to 2–3 en % with a maximum value reached of twice the minimum. With dietary linoleate > 2–3 en %, synthesis of icosanoids was reduced, and a value close to the minimum was found when dietary linoleate was 5–10 en %. Consumption of linoleate > 12–15 en % of the diet resulted in a linear increase in icosanoid synthesis.[23] The ratio of dietary linoleate to saturated fatty acids seemed to have no effect when the concentrations of the two types of fat were <5 en % each. Above that amount an increase in saturated fatty acids with no change in concentration of linoleate caused increased icosanoid synthesis that was prevented by a simultaneous increase in linoleate. Consumption of >10–12 en %

linoleate causes increasing synthesis of icosanoids in some tissues.[23] Because of the ill effects associated with excessive synthesis of icosanoids (Table 2), the upper limit of consumption of linoleate suggested by the expert panel[15] seems to be prudent.

Effects of dietary fatty acids upon icosanoid metabolism are mediated by other dietary factors. Most important are the antioxidants vitamin E[26] and selenium-dependent glutathione peroxidase.[27] The conversion of arachidonate to icosanoids is a peroxidative process, and the presence of appropriate antioxidant systems at the site of synthesis is a necessary control mechanism.

In recent years it has become clear that fatty acids of the n−3 family are essential components of the diet. Linolenate (18:3n−3) is not required for growth or reproduction. Its desaturation and elongation products are not normal substrates for icosanoids. However, a large portion of the polyunsaturated fatty acids in the brain and retina are elongation and desaturation products of 18:3n−3, eicosapentaenoic, and docosahexaenoic acids. Prolonged deprivation of these fatty acids resulted in reduced visual acuity in infant monkeys and defective electroretinographic responses in monkeys and rats.[28] A few case studies in humans suggested linolenic acid deficiency. For these reasons n−3 fatty acids now are regarded as essential nutrients.[29]

Fish oils contain predominantly very-long-chain n−3 fatty acids. When marine fish, fish oils, or purified preparations of fish-oil fatty acids are consumed they are stored in tissues, replacing part of the n−6 very-long-chain fatty acids, arachidonic and docosapentaenoic. Contrary to the disposition of linoleate, α-linolenic acid is not accumulated in tissues. Eicosapentaenoic acid is converted to thromboxane A_3 when it is concentrated in tissues, and it inhibits the desaturation of linoleate. Menhaden oil consumption exacerbates the skin symptoms developed by feeding a fat-free diet to rabbits.[30]

FAO/WHO[31] recommends consumption of 3 en % of the diet as linoleate on the basis of growth of human infants. The recommendation for pregnancy and lactation is 4.5–5.7 en %. No official body has made a quantitative recommendation for linolenate. On the basis of human milk composition, Neuringer et al.[28] recommend 0.7–1.3 en % with a ratio of n−6 to n−3 fatty acids of 4:1 to 10:1.

Fat Consumption and Balance of Fatty Acids in the Diet

There is great popular interest in nutrition in relation to dietary fat because of implications for obesity, heart disease, and, lately, cancer. These concerns are accompanied by interest in the more complex aspects of cardiovascular disease, hypertension, immune system, aging, and cancer by health professionals. Current knowledge is reaching a state of better understanding of all these conditions and a consensus toward recommendations for dietary fat consumption.

The National Cholesterol Education Program Expert Panel[15] reported comprehensively on the status of hypercholesterolemia in the population, the value of changing the status, and dietary recommendations for achieving change. More than half of the population of the United States over 20 y old have cholesterol concentrations that put them at risk for atherosclerosis (>5.17 mmol/L) and half of those are at high risk (>6.20 mmol/L). It is reasonable to accept the guidelines for dietary fat recommended for those at-risk people as suitable for the population. The recommendations are to consume <30 en % of total fat in the diet, <10 en % saturated fatty acids, ≤10 en % polyunsaturated fatty acids, and 10–15 en % as monounsaturated fatty acids. The available evidence suggests that saturated fatty acids (specifically lauric, myristic, and palmitic acids)[32] are the major factor that cause an increase in plasma cholesterol, particularly LDL cholesterol.[33] Carbohydrate and monounsaturated fatty acids lower plasma cholesterol when they replace saturated fatty acids. Polyunsaturated fatty acids of 18-C chain length have a greater cholesterol-lowering effect than can be accounted for by replacement of saturated fatty acids.[32] The mechanisms of the fatty acid effects upon lipoprotein cholesterol are not understood but possibly include changing morphology of the lipoproteins, influencing LDL-receptor activity, and altering bile acid synthesis and excretion.

In addition to lowering the risk of heart disease by lowering cholesterol, increasing the proportion of polyunsaturated fatty acids in the diet (P-S ratio) changes the P-S ratio of membrane fatty acids in the same direction. Increasing linoleate in the diet increases linoleate in the platelets and decreases thromboxane synthesis and aggregability, thus lowering the propensity for thrombosis.[24] Fish oils cause a decrease in hypertriglyceridemia but do not affect cholesterol concentration. Both linoleate and fish oils may decrease hypertension.[34] Medium-chain fatty acids do not affect blood lipids, perhaps because they are rapidly oxidized by peroxisomal enzymes.

Recommendations for reduction of total dietary fat from the present 37 en % average[35] to 30 en % are consistent with the effort to decrease the incidence of obesity, heart disease, and cancer.[36] The average diet consumed in the United States in 1985 provided ~6–7 en % linoleate.[35] That amount is considered sufficient in the Surgeon General's report[36] but has been questioned in relation to cancer risk. Current knowledge suggests that tumor development requires a minimum of linoleate for cell proliferation, and the minimum depends upon the animal species and organ (Charles Elson, personal communication). Greater than the minimum requirement for linoleate does not contribute to additional tumor growth. Human epidemiological studies suggest that increasing dietary fat may elevate the risk of some cancers (breast and colon), but the type of fat is not a factor (M.N. Woods and S.L. Gorbach, personal communication).

As knowledge grows, empirical recommendations for amount and type of fat to be consumed are becoming supported by scientific information. There is not enough known to specify an ideal fatty acid mixture. The standard dietary advice to consume a variety of foods should be followed with regard to fats. Recommendations for appropriate food choices were made by an expert panel (Table 3).[15] Extremes should be avoided, and pure fatty acids should be considered to be unapproved pharmaceuticals.

References

1. G.R. Jacobson and D.E. Vance (1988) Lipids. In: *Biochemistry* (G. Zubay, ed.), pp. 154–175, Macmillan, New York.

2. J. Dupont, R.W. White, K.M. Johnston, A.A. Heggtveit, B.E. McDonald, and S.M. Grundy (in press) Food safety and health effects of canola oil. *J. Am. Coll. Nutr.*

3. E.N. Siguel and E.J. Schaefer (1988) Aging and nutritional requirements of essential fatty acids. In: *Dietary Fat Requirements in Health and Development* (J. Beare-Rogers, ed.) pp. 163–189, American Oil Chemists' Society, Champaign, IL.

4. D.E. Vance (1988) Cholesterol and related derivatives. *Biochemistry* (G. Zubay, ed.), pp. 725–748, Macmillan, New York.

5. E.A. Emken (1984) Nutrition and biochemistry of trans and positional isomers in hydrogenated oils. *Annu. Rev. Nutr.* 4:339–376.

6. A.L. Merrill and B.K. Watt (1955) *Energy Value of Foods. Basis and Derivation.* U.S. Department of Agriculture Handbook no. 74, U.S. Government Printing Office, Washington, DC.

7. W.G. Linscheer and A.J. Vergroesen (1988) Lipids. In: *Modern Nutrition in Health and Disease* (M.E. Shils and V.R. Young, eds.), pp. 72–107, Lea and Febiger, Philadelphia.

8. M.C. Carey, D.M. Small, and C.M. Bliss (1983) Lipid digestion and absorption. *Annu. Rev. Physiol.* 45:651–678.

9. S.M. Grundy (1983) Absorption and metabolism of dietary cholesterol. *Annu. Rev. Nutr.* 3:71–96.

10. S.H. Zeisel (1988) Vitamin-like molecules (A) choline. In: *Modern Nutrition in Health and Disease* (M.E. Shils and V.R. Young, eds.), pp. 440–452, Lea and Febiger, Philadelphia.

11. R.W. Mahley, D.H. Hui, T.I. Innerarity, and U. Beisiegel (1989) Chylomicron remnant metabolism. Role of hepatic lipoprotein receptors in mediating uptake. *Arteriosclerosis* 9(suppl. I):14–18.

12. J. Dupont, P.A. Garcia, B. Hennig, et al. (1988) Bile acids in extrahepatic tissues. In: *The Bile Acids*, vol. 4 (K.D.R. Setchell, D. Kritchevsky, and P.P. Nair, eds.), pp. 341–372, Plenum, New York.

13. M.S. Brown and J.L. Goldstein (1986) A receptor-mediated pathway for cholesterol homeostasis. *Science* 232:34–47.

14. S. Steinberg, S. Parthasarathy, T.E. Carew, J.C. Khoo, and J.L. Witztum (1989) Beyond cholesterol: modifications of low density lipoprotein that increase its atherogenicity. *N. Engl. J. Med.* 320: 915–924.

15. National Cholesterol Education Program Expert Panel (1988) Report on detection, evaluation, and treatment of high blood cholesterol in adults. *Arch. Intern. Med.* 148:36–69.

16. E. Aaes-Jorgensen (1982) EFA-essentiality-1980. *Prog. Lipid Res.* 20:123–128.

17. J.F. Mead (1982) The essential fatty acids: past, present, and future. *Prog. Lipid Res.* 20:1–6.

18. H. Sprecher, A.C. Voss, M. Careaga, and C. Hadjiagapiou (1987) Interrelationships between polyunsaturated fatty acid and membrane lipid synthesis. In: *Polyunsaturated Fatty Acids and Eicosanoids* (W.E.M. Lands, ed.), pp. 154–168, American Oil Chemists Society, Champaign, IL.

19. J. Dupont (1988) Fat effects on fatty acid and cholesterol metabolism in animal experiments. In: *Fat Requirements for Development and Health* (J. Beare-Rogers, ed.), pp. 87–100, American Oil Chemists Society, Champaign, IL.

20. H.S. Hansen and B. Jensen (1985) Essential function of linoleic acid esterified in acylglucosylceramide and acylceramide in maintaining the epidermal water permeability barrier. Evidence from feeding studies with oleate, linoleate, arachidonate, columbinate and a-linolenate. *Biochem. Biophys. Acta* 834:357–363.

21. H.S. Hansen (1986) Dietary essential fatty acids and prostaglandin formation in vivo. In: *Proceedings of the XIII International Congress of Nutrition* (T.G. Taylor and N.K. Jenkins, eds.), pp. 353–357, John Libbey, London.

22. J. Dupont (1987) Essential fatty acids and prostaglandins. *Prev. Med.* 16:485–492.

23. M.M. Mathias and J. Dupont (1989) Effects of dietary fat on eicosanoid production in normal tissues. In: *Carcinogenesis and Dietary Fat* (S. Abraham, ed.), pp. 29–52, Kluwer Academic, Boston.

24. J.A. Oates, G.A. FitzGerald, R.A. Branch, E.K. Jackson, H.R. Knapp, and L.J. Roberts, II (1988) Clinical implications of prostaglandin and thromboxane A2 formation. *N. Engl. J. Med.* 319:761–767.

25. A. Ferretti, J.P. Church, and V.P. Flanagan (1982) Changes in urinary PGE_2 and PGF_{2a} daily excretion rates in man during a period of 4–5 months. *Prog. Lipid Res.* 20:195–198.

26. M.P. Carpenter (1982) Antioxidants and prostaglandin synthesis. In vivo and in vitro effects. *Prog. Lipid Res.* 20:143–149.

27. R.W. Bryant and M. Bailey (1982) Role of selenium-dependent glutathione peroxidase in platelet lipoxygenase metabolism. *Prog. Lipid Res.* 20:189–194.

28. M. Neuringer, G.J. Anderson, and W.E. Connor (1988) The essentiality of n-3 fatty acids for the development and function of the retina and brain. *Annu. Rev. Nutr.* 8:517–541.

29. G.J. Anderson and W.E. Connor (1989) On the demonstration of ω-3 essential-fatty acid deficiency in humans. *Am. J. Clin. Nutr.* 49:585–587.

30. V.A. Ziboh and R.S. Chapkin (1988) Metabolism and function of skin lipids. *Prog. Lipid Res.* 27:81–105.

31. Food and Agricultural Organization—U.N. and World Health Organization (1980) *Dietary Fats and Oils in Human Nutrition,* FAO Food and Nutrition Series, Food and Agriculture Organization of the United Nations, Rome.

32. A. Keys, J.T. Anderson, and F. Grande (1965) Serum cholesterol response to changes in the diet. IV. Particular saturated fatty acids in the diet. *Metabolism* 14:776–787.

33. J. Shepherd, C.J. Packard, S.M. Grundy, D. Yeshurum, A.M. Gotto, Jr., and O.D. Taunton (1980) Effects of saturated and polyunsaturated fat diets on the chemical composition and metabolism of low density lipoproteins in man. *J. Lipid Res.* 21:91–99.

34. H.P. Knapp and G.A. FitzGerald (1989) The antihypertensive effects of fish oil: a controlled study of polyunsaturated fatty acid supplements in essential hypertension. *N. Engl. J. Med.* 320:1037–1043.

35. Human Nutrition Information Service, Nutrition Monitoring Division (1987) *Nationwide Food Consumption Survey 1985,* NFCS, CSFII, Report no. 85-3, U.S. Government Printing Office, Washington, DC.

36. U.S. Department of Health and Human Services (1988) *Surgeon General's Report on Nutrition and Health,* Summary and Recommendations, DHHS Publication no. (PHS) 88-50211, U.S. Government Printing Office, Washington, DC.

Chapter **8**   Robert D. Steele and Alfred E. Harper

Proteins and Amino Acids

The intent of this chapter is to emphasize some of the trends in research that are advancing knowledge of protein and amino acid nutrition and metabolism in new directions and to review briefly progress on some topics that usually receive only passing attention in general nutrition courses. The information presented is intended only to complement, not be a substitute for, the more complete treatments of the subject included in general textbooks on nutrition. Our approach has been to start with a summary of recent reassessments of estimates of protein requirements, then review some of the advances in basic knowledge of protein and amino acid metabolism that are expanding our understanding of protein utilization and needs, and conclude by discussing efforts to use a metabolic approach to reassess the validity of currently accepted values for amino acid requirements and the bearing of the results of these studies on evaluation of protein quality and practical nutritional problems.

Protein Requirements and Allowances

Protein requirements and allowances have been discussed and debated continuously throughout this century. No other nutrient requirement has been subjected to comparable scrutiny. The most recent comprehensive evaluation of information on this subject is provided in a 1985 report *Energy and Protein Requirements* prepared by an international committee convened by the Food and Agriculture and World Health Organizations and the United Nations University (FAO/WHO/UNU).[1] The recommendations of the FAO/WHO/UNU committee, nonetheless, have not stilled the debate on appropriate values for the protein requirements of infants[2,3] or the amino acid requirements of adults.[4,5]

The continuing debate over the validity of estimates of protein requirements of humans is difficult to resolve for several reasons. First, functional changes indicative of protein inadequacy cannot be detected in adults until protein depletion is severe. Second, the accuracy of estimates of protein requirements by the nitrogen-balance procedure is limited because of the difficulty in recovering all of the nitrogen lost from the body. Third, nitrogen retention is influenced by relatively small changes in energy intake. Fourth, human subjects can adapt to a range of protein intakes and achieve nitrogen balance with small changes in body protein content that do not appear to represent significant depletion or accumulation of body protein.

In 1965 a FAO/WHO committee[6] adopted what has been called the factorial method for estimating protein requirements, which is based on the assumption that measurement of total body nitrogen losses by subjects consuming a protein-free diet should provide an estimate of the requirement. The factorial method does not take into account Liebig's law of the minimum or the law of diminishing returns, as it is commonly called, i.e., if the intake of a nutrient is increased by equal increments, the response per increment declines owing to the gradual fall in efficiency of utilization of the nutrient as the requirement is approached.[7] It was for this reason that the results of nitrogen-balance studies were used in estimating protein requirements[8] and allowances[9] by committees of the National Research Council (NRC) in the United States.

In 1973 another FAO/WHO committee[10] modified the factorial method by including an additional component to take into account the inefficiency of utilization that occurs with even the highest quality proteins as intake approaches the requirement level. The factor needed for this correction was estimated from differences observed between values for requirements based on the factorial method and those derived from nitrogen-balance studies. In essence, the additional factor adjusted the factorial values so that it equalled the value obtained by the nitrogen-balance method. The latest FAO/WHO/UNU committee,[1] therefore, adopted as its starting point for estimating protein requirements and allowances, results obtained using the traditional methodology, i.e., "direct measurement of the nitrogen needed for zero-balance in short-term or long-term studies."

From a detailed assessment of both the older and more recent estimates of adult requirements for protein obtained with the nitrogen-balance method, the committee concluded that the average adult requirement had been underestimated previously and proposed that it be increased by ~20% to 0.6 g high-quality protein·kg body weight^{-1}·d^{-1}. The true coefficient of variation (CV) of this value was calculated to be 12.5%. The lower end of the safe range of protein intakes, taken as the average plus twice the CV, was estimated to be 0.75 g protein·kg body weight^{-1}·d^{-1}. The committee concluded also that for adults consuming usual mixed diets there was no need to adjust this value for protein quality. The FAO/WHO/UNU safe intake can be compared with the Recommended Dietary Allowance (RDA) in the United States of 0.8 g·kg body weight^{-1}·d^{-1}, which was also estimated (but by using somewhat different assumptions) from the results of nitrogen-balance studies.[9,11]

The FAO/WHO/UNU committee[1] also reevaluated protein requirements in infancy and for growth. Because of the paucity of direct measurements of requirements over the age range from 1 to 18 y, it is necessary to interpolate between the reasonably well-established values for infants and for young adults using the factorial type of approach. Maintenance nitrogen requirements were estimated from the results of several studies on older infants and young children. To these were added increments for growth based on knowledge of body composition and growth rates. The estimated increments needed for growth were increased by 50% because this increase brought the calculated values for the young infant close to the average intake of breast-fed infants. Efficiency of utilization of the nitrogen was assumed to be 70%.

The requirement values obtained in this way were further increased by two standard deviations (SDs) to allow for individual variability (CV = 12.5–15%). The safe intake of protein for the 1-y-old child was estimated to be 1.5 g·kg body weight^{-1}·d^{-1} and to fall to 1 g·kg^{-1}·d^{-1} by 6 y of age, essentially the same as the values proposed by the previous committee.[10] The RDA values in the United States for these groups are somewhat higher, 1.75 and 1.2 g·kg^{-1}·d^{-1}, respectively. For children between ages 6 and 18 y, the FAO/WHO/UNU safe intake declines from 1 to 0.8 and 0.85 g·kg^{-1}·d^{-1} for females and males, respectively. These values are above the 1973 FAO/WHO values but are below the RDA in the United States for children 7–14 y of age.

In another assessment of protein requirements of infants, Fomon[12] compared values obtained by using a modified factorial method with those obtained from information about breast-milk intakes and composition. The average requirement of the 3–4-mo-old infant for protein was estimated to be 1.2 g·kg^{-1}·d^{-1} by the factorial method and was not significantly different on the basis of breast-milk intakes after correcting for the proportion of breast-milk nitrogen (17%) that is considered to be unutilizable for protein synthesis. An epidemiological approach was used by Beaton and Chery[2] to assess the validity of the conclusion of the WHO/FAO/UNU committee[1] that the average protein requirement of the 3–4-mo-old infant is 1.47 g·kg^{-1}·d^{-1}. They used a probability model based on the distributions of protein intakes and protein requirements and calculated the incidence of inadequate intakes that would be predicted with any given protein intake. When the average protein requirement of the 3–4-mo-old infant was taken as 1.47 g·kg^{-1}·d^{-1}, the model predicted the incidence of inadequate intakes of breast-fed infants to be between 30% and 35%, an unacceptably high value. Only when the requirement value was reduced to 1.1 g·kg^{-1}·d^{-1} did the predicted incidence of inadequate intakes fall to a more probable value of between 3% and 7%. Their analysis of these results led Beaton and Chery[2] to conclude that the method used to estimate infant requirements, unlike that for estimation of adult requirements, actually provides an estimate not of the requirement per kilogram of body weight, but of the protein-to-energy ratio needed in infant foods to prevent the occurrence of deficiency in all infants. Assuming a CV of their estimated requirement of 15%, the safe intake, an amount that would essentially preclude the occurrence of deficiency, would be ~1.5 g·kg^{-1}·d^{-1}, not far from the estimate for average intakes of protein by this age group from human milk at which inadequate intakes are considered to be negligible.

Despite the immense amount of attention given to estimating protein requirements, all of the answers obviously are not yet in.[3,13] These reevaluations suggest that average protein requirements of the very young have been overestimated considerably whereas protein requirements of older children and adults have been underestimated somewhat.

Protein Digestion and Absorption

Digestion of dietary protein begins in the stomach with the action of the protease pepsin, which is secreted as an inactive proenzyme (zymogen). Activation occurs autocatalytically with the release of a small peptide fragment from the inactive precursor. The contribution of the gastric phase to overall protein digestion is mainly cleavage of dietary proteins to smaller polypeptides and accounts for <10% of total protein digestion in humans.[14] The major site of protein digestion is the small intestine. Here proteins of dietary origin (exogenous) as well as those of endogenous origin are cleaved to small peptides and free amino acids. Endogenous proteins are secretions of the oral cavity (saliva), stomach, intestine, liver (bile), and pancreas. They include hydrolytic enzymes and proteins of cells desquamated during the normal turnover of intestinal mucosa. Endogenous protein may account for up to 50% of the total protein digested.[14] The proportion will depend upon dietary protein intake.

The intestinal proteases are also secreted as proenzymes from the pancreas. A brush border enzyme, enterokinase, which is released from the intestinal mucosa by the action of bile acids, activates trypsinogen to trypsin by cleaving a hexapeptide. Trypsin in turn activates the other pancreatic proenzymes producing an array of activated proteases including endopeptidases, such as trypsin and chymotrypsin, and exopeptidases, such as the carboxypeptidases.[14] The end result of the action of these enzymes coupled with that of aminopeptidases from the brush border is a mixture of free amino acids and short peptides, mainly dipeptides and tripeptides, which are readily taken up by the enterocyte.

A number of transport systems exist for ensuring efficient absorption of the products of protein digestion. Well-defined carriers for the transport of acidic, basic, and neutral amino acids have been identified; however, the number of distinct carriers operative at the brush border membrane is still not known. There would appear to be at least nine.[15] Dependency upon sodium for transport is an accepted feature of most amino acid transport systems, and like intestinal glucose transport, sodium-dependent amino acid transport is electrogenic. On the basis of cross-inhibition studies, transport systems of the brush border membrane appear to be similar to but not identical with the well-defined transporters in nonepithelial cells.[16] The characteristic substrate specificity and cross reactivity of the intestinal transporters recently was summarized.[15] Sodium-independent amino acid transport, similar to the L system, for phenylalanine and leucine across the brush border membrane also was observed, but it appears to represent a minor route of transport.[15,17] That a number of specific amino acid transporters exist at the brush border membrane is evident from the occurrence of a variety of genetic defects of amino acid absorption in which failure to absorb either several amino acids (e.g., Hartnup's disease) or a specific amino acid (such as methionine) was observed.[14,18]

It is now clear that small peptides, primarily dipeptides and tripeptides, are transported intact across the brush border membrane by carriers distinct from any amino acid transporter.[19] The number of carrier proteins involved is not known as there are theoretically hundreds of possibilities for dipeptide transport and thousands for tripeptide transport. Available evidence, however, indicates that dipeptide transport is distinct from tripeptide transport and that both processes are electrogenic. Originally it was thought that the transport process required sodium, but more recent reports indicate that the transport mechanism involves peptide-H^+ cotransport.[19] Although such systems are relatively common in microorganisms, this finding, if confirmed, will represent the first example of proton cotransport in a mammalian system. It has been difficult to determine in vivo the quantitative significance of peptide absorption relative to free amino acid absorption because peptides, once absorbed, are rapidly hydrolyzed in the mucosal cell. However, there is general agreement, particularly in view of the satisfactory nutritional status of patients with Hartnup's disease, that the fraction is substantial.

There is unequivocal evidence that intact proteins are taken up into the intestinal mucosal cells in very small quantities, particularly in young animals.[20] This process has long been known to be important in many mammalian species as the means whereby passive immunity may be transmitted to young animals by the transport of significant amounts of maternal immunoglobulins, particularly IgG, via recognition by intestinal IgG receptors. After closure, intestinal IgG receptors disappear. In humans, uptake by this process does not appear to be significant because closure occurs at birth or very soon after. Hence, passive immunity is acquired by placental transport.[20] Uptake of other proteins appears to be primarily by transcellular endocytosis with some uptake taking place by paracellular routes at the junctions between cells. Whereas transport of intact proteins by these processes is not of nutritional significance with respect to overall nitrogen absorption, this transport process may be important in the development of food allergies and other diseases; however, knowledge of this subject remains limited.

Once inside the mucosal cell, transport of amino acids out of the cell at the basolateral membrane occurs primarily by the sodium-independent L system showing broad specificity for neutral amino acids.[15] A sodium-independent system similar to the ASC system also was identified. Sodium-dependent systems at the basolateral membrane similar to the A and ASC systems appear to occur mainly to ensure an adequate supply of amino acids to enterocytes when availability of amino acids from the lumen is limited.[15]

Intestinal Metabolism of Amino Acids

The principal fate of the absorbed products of protein digestion is release of free amino acids into the portal vein for subsequent utilization by other tissues. However, it is increasingly apparent that a considerable amount of amino acid metabolism occurs in the mucosal cells. Proteins of the intestinal mucosa represent the most rapidly turning over proteins in the body, with an estimated fractional renewal rate for protein of 136%/d.[21] This turnover is both rapid and complex because it involves synthesis of proteins for secretion, turnover of intracellular proteins, and turnover of the entire cell. Considerable evidence indicates that a luminal supply of amino acids is necessary for normal mucosal cell function and turnover;[15] for example, in animals fed parenterally the mucosa atrophies. Of all the amino acids, glutamine is likely the most extensively metabolized by the intestine, with about one-fourth of the total plasma glutamine being metabolized during each pass through the mucosal tissue bed.[22] In perfused jejunal segments from animals in the postabsorptive state, most of the glutamine carbon was oxidized to carbon dioxide, which accounted for ~35% of the total carbon dioxide produced; in contrast, glucose provided <10% of the total. The nitrogen from glutamine metabolism appears in portal blood primarily as alanine, proline, and citrulline as well as in free ammonia. Glutamine and glutamate are, therefore, major energy sources for the nutrition of intestinal cells, and the intestine is an important site of metabolism of these amino acids obtained from the diet or from other tissues, such as muscle.

The amino acid pattern in portal blood plasma, then, is similar to the dietary protein amino acid pattern except for a substantial increase in the molar fraction of alanine in the portal blood and a corresponding decrease in the fractions of aspartate, glutamate, and glutamine;[22,23] the degree of change over time, however, may be influenced by the nature of the protein fed.[24] Remesy et al.[23] found that when they raised the amount of dietary casein fed to rats from 13% to 50%, the proportion of glutamate and glutamine recovered in portal blood increased, probably because the metabolic capacity of the intestine for oxidizing these amino acids was exceeded.

Role of the Liver

The liver plays a primary role in controlling the quantities and proportions of amino acids from the portal blood that are distributed to the rest of the body. Much of the incoming load of amino acids from the portal vein is extracted by the liver and degraded. Only about one-fourth of the entering amino acids were observed by Elwyn[25] to exit the liver as such; a smaller amount was secreted in the form of plasma proteins. However, not all amino acids are removed from the circulation to the same extent,[23,25] and the proportion removed depends upon the protein content of the diet. About 25% of the portal alanine is removed by the liver in rats fed a diet containing a modest amount of protein (13%) and ~50% is removed in rats fed high-protein diets. Other amino acids, such as glycine, serine, tyrosine, phenylalanine, and threonine, show similar patterns whereas only a small proportion of the branched-chain amino acids are removed by liver. Therefore, although increases in dietary protein may result in substantial increases in portal blood amino acid concentrations, the response in the peripheral circulation is much less dramatic.

That the liver should play such a major role in extraction of circulating amino acids was shown many years ago in the classic studies by Miller,[26] who compared the extent of oxidation of amino acids by perfused rat liver and eviscerated rat carcass. Miller found that of the indispensible amino acids only the branched-chain amino acids, leucine, isoleucine, and valine, were degraded primarily by extrahepatic tissues. Subsequent studies showed that the enzymes for degradation of this group of amino acids are widely distributed.[27] When the inflow of amino acids to the liver is high, such as after the ingestion of a high-protein meal, part of the excess of amino acids is removed through increased protein synthesis and part by increased degradation to urea and glucogenic or ketogenic substrates depending upon the particular amino acid and its oxidative pathway.

Control of Amino Acid Metabolism. The degradation of amino acids in liver and other tissues is controlled by a number of factors. First, because the enzymes degrading amino acids are of relatively low affinity and high capacity [i.e., high K_m relative to liver amino acid (substrate) concentration], rates of amino acid degradation are influenced to a great extent by tissue concentrations.[28] Hence, an increase in the amount of amino acids entering the liver from the portal blood will result in a corresponding increase in oxidation thus providing an efficient short-term mechanism that contributes to maintenance of stable blood and tissue amino acid concentrations during times of variable amino acid supply, such as after a meal.

A longer-term mechanism for maintaining stable amino acid concentrations in tissues is by induction or repression of the activities of amino acid–degrading enzymes by diet or hormones. In general, activities of amino acid–degrading enzymes are low when dietary protein intake is low and may rise manyfold when the intake of protein is increased for a number of days.[29] Unlike the rapid substrate-induced changes in the rate of oxidation, dietary and hormonally induced responses of enzyme activity generally reach the maximum after hours to days, and the activity remains altered as long as the stimulus is present. These responses thus can result in long-term changes in the metabolic capacity to oxidize amino acids. For example, after adaptation of rats to high-protein feeding, plasma concentrations of most indispensable amino acids remain in the normal range even though protein consumption by the animal may have increased fivefold. Exceptions, however, are the plasma concentrations of the branched-chain amino acids, which increase steadily in animals as protein intake increases and remain elevated even in animals adapted to a high-protein diet.[27]

Recent research documented that the diet-induced alterations in the activities of several of these enzymes are the result of increases in the total amount of enzyme owing to stimulus-induced increases in the amount of translatable mRNA for the enzyme protein.[30] The availability of molecular probes for a number of these enzymes will lead to an understanding at the molecular level of the mechanism for these effects. Other studies conducted over the past few years documented that the activities of some amino acid–degrading enzymes may be regulated mainly by covalent modification and allosteric interactions. Research on regulation of the branched-chain α-keto acid dehydrogenase (BCKAD) complex and the enzymes phenylalanine hydroxylase and glycine methyltransferase illustrates these effects.

BCKAD (EC 1.2.4.4) is a multienzyme complex located in the mitochondria that catalyzes the oxidative decarboxylation of α-ketoisocaproate, α-keto-β-methylvalerate, and α-ketoisovalerate, the transamination products of leucine, isoleucine, and valine, respectively.[27] Unlike the activity of the transaminating enzyme, the activity of this complex is highly regulated in a manner resembling that of other mitochondrial dehydrogenases, such as the pyruvate dehydrogenase complex.[31] Regulation is accomplished through reversible phosphorylation (deactivation) and dephosphorylation (activation) by a tightly bound kinase and loosely bound phosphatase, respectively. Phosphorylation, occurring on the E1 subunit (dehydrogenase), causes inactivation of the complex and a reduction in the Vmax of the enzyme. Recent studies show the phosphorylation to occur exclusively at two sites on the α-subunit of E1. The phosphatase also recently was purified and characterized.[31] The kinase as well as the phosphatase of the BCKAD complex appear to be specific and do not interact with other dehydrogenase complexes. Inhibition of the kinase by the branched-chain α-keto acids themselves may represent an important mechanism for acute regulation of activity of the complex. Thus, when α-keto acid concentrations are relatively high, such as during high-protein feeding, the complex will remain active because of the inhibition of the kinase. Miller et al.[32] recently showed that liver BCKAD was 25% active in rats fed 6% casein diets and increased to 82% active and 100%

active in rats consuming 20% and 50% casein diets, respectively. In contrast, muscle BCKAD was 10%, 13%, and 22% active. By use of antibodies directed toward the E2 subunit and E1α subunit, the total amount of enzyme-protein complex was found to be unchanged as dietary protein was increased. The recent availability of cDNAs for some of the BCKAD subunits[31] will aid in furthering our understanding of this complex control process.

A second example of complex control of amino acid–degrading enzyme activity is that of phenylalanine hydroxylase. This enzyme (EC 1.14.16.1) catalyzes the irreversible conversion of phenylalanine to tyrosine[33–35] and is the initial step in the only pathway available for the complete oxidative degradation of phenylalanine. Like the BCKAD complex, phenylalanine hydroxylase may be activated by its substrate and also is controlled by reversible phosphorylation and dephosphorylation. It appears, then, that there are two phenylalanine-binding sites on the enzyme, a regulator site and a catalytic site. Kaufman's laboratory recently showed that the regulator site only becomes active when two dimers interact to form a tetramer.[34]

Unlike the BCKAD complex, phenylalanine hydroxylase is activated by phosphorylation that occurs by the action of a cAMP-dependent protein kinase. It appears that the purified hydroxylase from rat liver is partially phosphorylated and that 1 mol of phosphate is incorporated per subunit. Activation of the hydroxylase by phenylalanine and by phosphorylation appears not to be independent but rather synergistic, such that phosphorylation is stimulated by phenylalanine and phenylalanine facilitates the phosphorylation of the hydroxylase. The net effect of the responsiveness of the hydroxylase to phenylalanine would be to ensure that when phenylalanine intake is high, tissue phenylalanine concentrations do not remain elevated and produce adverse effects such as have been so well characterized in patients with classical phenylketonuria.[36]

A third example of sophisticated metabolic control of amino acid–degrading enzymes is glycine N-methyltransferase (GMT; EC 2.1.1.20). This enzyme catalyzes the methylation of glycine by S-adenosylmethionine (AdoMet) to form sarcosine and S-adenosylhomocysteine (AdoHyc). It is an abundant enzyme accounting for ~1% of soluble rat liver protein. The function of this enzyme is to remove excess methyl groups and, thus, it serves as a means of regulating the ratio of AdoMet to AdoHyc, a proposed important regulator of cellular methylation reactions.[37] Hence, GMT seems to play a critical role in the overall metabolism of the methyl group of the indispensable sulfur-containing amino acid, methionine. Wagner's laboratory[38] showed that GMT is bound by 5-methyltetrahydropteroylpentaglutamate

(5-methyl THF), which is a potent inhibitor of its activity. The activity of this methylation-controlling enzyme is then intricately linked to the folic acid–dependent remethylation of homocysteine, which forms methionine, and thereby provides an important means of generating methyl groups de novo.[39] More recently, Wagner et al.[40] found that GMT is activated by a protein kinase–dependent phosphorylation reaction, illustrating, once again, the exquisite control processes operative for many amino acid–metabolizing enzymes.

Control of Urea Synthesis. Along with catabolism of the carbon skeleton of amino acids, an efficient means of disposal of the nitrogen from amino groups is necessary to prevent the buildup of toxic levels of ammonia.[41] Stoichiometric amounts of ammonia (as carbamyl phosphate) and aspartate are necessary for synthesis of urea in the liver.[42] The small intestine is a major supplier of ammonia and of alanine, an ammonia precursor. Liver glutamate is a major ammonia precursor as well because of the action of glutamate dehydrogenase. Nitrogen flux to urea is large, amounting to 9.4 mmol urea nitrogen/d in starved 350-g rats;[22] >30% of the utilized nitrogen comes from glutamine metabolism in the small intestine.

Acini, the functioning units of the liver, extend along the liver sinusoids from the terminal venule of the portal vein to the terminal venule of the hepatic vein. Hepatocytes from different acinar locations differ in metabolic function, hence the term metabolic zonation.[43] Studies showed that detoxification of ammonia occurs through two systems: ureagenesis, located primarily in periportal regions of the acini,[44] with high capacity but relatively low affinity for ammonium ions, and glutamine synthesis by glutamine synthetase, located primarily in perivenous regions of acini, with low capacity but high affinity for ammonium ions. Having two systems connected in series for ammonium-ion removal insures against buildup of toxic nitrogenous waste during catabolism of carbon skeletons.[45]

Urea-cycle enzymes also exhibit adaptive responses to changes in dietary protein intake and to hormones such as glucagon and glucocorticoids.[46] These long-term changes in enzyme activity are the result of changes in enzyme mass, and a major goal of recent research has been to identify the regulated metabolic steps by which these changes occur. The recent availability of cloned cDNAs for all five urea-cycle enzymes has made it possible to assess whether mRNA amounts for these enzymes respond in parallel to changes in dietary protein intake.[47] Changes in abundance of mRNA for all five urea-cycle enzymes in rats fed high-protein diets were comparable with changes in enzyme activity, indicating that a pretranslational level of control was operative. However, variable responses of mRNA amounts were

found after injection of rats with dexamethasone and dibutyrl cAMP. Transcription run-on assays showed that transcription of carbamoylphosphate synthetase I and argininosuccinate synthetase was stimulated nearly fivefold within 30 min. Morris et al.[47] concluded that the variable responses of the urea-cycle enzymes to hormone treatment indicate that regulatory mechanisms for controlling amounts of the individual enzymes in this cycle may be different. The availability of molecular probes for each of these enzymes and for the corresponding DNA and mRNA sequences will be of great use for future studies on control of this metabolic pathway.

Protein Turnover

Quantitatively by far the greatest need for amino acids is for protein synthesis. It appears that the needs for aminoacyl t-RNAs for protein synthesis are assured, regardless of amino acid supply, owing to the very low K_ms and thus high affinities of the amino acid–activating enzymes relative to those of other amino acid–metabolizing enzymes. However, growth and maintenance of cells and tissues depend upon regulation of many of the individual reactions involved in both protein synthesis and protein degradation.

Considerable advances in our understanding of the biochemical steps and regulation of protein synthesis were made over the past decade and a number of comprehensive reviews appeared.[48–50] Synthesis of protein involves both an initiation phase and an elongation phase. Initiation of the formation of peptide linkages involves a series of reactions utilizing ribosomal subunits, initiator tRNA, a number of initiation factors, and energy. Elongation involves recognition and binding of an appropriate aminoacyl-tRNA by the ribosome, formation of the peptide bond by peptidyl transferase, translocation of the growing peptide chain, release of a free tRNA, and regeneration of the binding site for binding the next aminoacyl-tRNA. The free tRNA released is reacylated and may be used for further elongation. As with initiation, elongation also requires expenditure of energy. Greater rates of protein synthesis, then, may occur from stimulation of initiation or elongation or from an increase in the absolute amounts of the pathway constituents such as ribosomes or mRNA.

Degradation of cellular protein is an ongoing process and serves to provide tissues with a supply of amino acids during periods of nutrient deprivation. Cellular proteins are considered to consist of a short-lived class having half-lives of ≤10 min and accounting for <1% of total protein and long-lived proteins having half-lives hundreds of times greater and accounting for 99% of cellular protein.[51] Degradation of short-lived proteins is not thought to be under physiological control and occurs at a location other than the lysosome. Degradation of the more slowly turning over proteins is under strict control and occurs primarily in the lysosomal compartment. Lysosomal protein sequestration involves macroautophagy and microautophagy.[51,52] Macroautophagy is induced by insulin or by amino acid deprivation. Other hormones, such as glucagon, cAMP, and β-agonists, also stimulate macroautophagy in liver cells but not in myocytes. Microautophagy differs in that the "cytosolic bite"[51,52] is less, and the uptake process does not appear to be regulated as in macroautophagy. A select group of amino acids (leucine, tyrosine-phenylalanine, glutamine, proline, methionine, tryptophan, and histidine) exert inhibitory control of macroautophagy when present at 0.5 or at 4 times the normal concentration but not at normal concentration unless alanine or insulin is present. On the other hand, glucagon blocks inhibition at half normal amino acid concentration and results in maximal rates of protein degradation at normal amino acid concentrations. This rapidly evolving area of investigation is beginning to produce a more complete picture of the physiological mechanisms of protein degradation at the molecular level. A number of recent comprehensive reviews of protein degradation have appeared.[51–54]

The effects of dietary amino acids on protein synthesis appear, for the most part, to be due to their effect on secretion of hormones, principally insulin, growth hormone, glucocorticoids, thyroid hormone, and insulin-like growth factors (e.g., IGF-1). Much of this work was reviewed recently by Millward and Rivers[55] and others.[56,57]

Very small differences between the rates of these two complex processes determine whether net accumulation or loss of protein occurs. Because of the rapid rate of turnover of protein, small changes in synthesis or degradation may lead to large changes in tissue protein content. Protein synthesis rates vary considerably among tissues (Table 1). The differences are attributed primarily to differences in the RNA content of the cells;[56] however, the rate of peptide synthesis per unit ribosome, nevertheless, may change within a few hours of a change in meal composition with no change in tissue RNA content. Therefore, short-term and long-term control mechanisms of protein synthesis may be different.

Numerous isotopic methods exist for measuring protein synthesis; however, for protein breakdown adequate methods exist only for liver, where the problem of isotope reutilization has been eliminated.[21] A suitable method for measuring the rate of breakdown of whole tissue over a short time period is not yet available. Currently the best approach to obtaining a longer-term estimate of breakdown is by the indirect method of subtracting the amount of

Table 1. Protein synthesis in young rats*

Tissue	Fed	48-hr starved	Protein-free diet
	%	% change	% change
Jejeunal mucosa	123	−25	−23
Liver	86	−16	−16
Heart	20	−40	−50
Gastrocnemius muscle	17	−65	−76

* Values for the fed state are percent of the protein pool synthesized per day and for the starved and protein-free state are percent change from the fed state. Adapted from Reeds and James.[56]

protein deposited during growth from the amount synthesized as measured by isotope incorporation. Muscle protein degradation has been estimated from urinary excretion of 3-methyl histidine, a muscle constituent that is not metabolized, although the reliability of this method has been debated owing to the possible contribution to the urinary 3-methyl histidine pool from rapidly turning over tissues, such as intestine.[56,58,59]

It is now clear that each tissue has its own rate of turnover and that individual proteins within these tissues turn over at different rates. In one tissue, for example in liver, the rate of protein degradation may be the more important control point, whereas in another tissue, such as in muscle, the rate of synthesis may be more important. Nonetheless, the contribution of each process can be assessed only by in vivo studies. The mechanisms regulating these two processes and their interactions with each other as well as with other factors such as hormones are an active area of study.

Regulation of Plasma Amino Acid Concentrations

As described earlier, plasma amino acid concentrations after a meal generally reflect protein intake, but in the postabsorptive state, concentrations remain stable and are characteristic of the species. Many of the processes already discussed, such as protein synthesis and regulation of amino acid catabolic enzymes, contribute in a major way to this regulation, but other means, such as control of gastric emptying after a meal and efficient reabsorption of amino acids in the kidney, should not be overlooked. Plasma amino acid concentrations for a number of species are given in Table 2. In addition Scriver et al.[61] published values for normal plasma amino acid concentrations in humans and their variability due to physiological state and to intersubject and intrasubject variability.

Table 2. Plasma concentrations of amino acids for various species

Amino acid	Rat	Human	Dog	Chick
			$\mu mol/L$	
Alanine	342	326	442	170
Arginine	65	88	90	150
Aspartate	30	2	11	74
Cystine	14	33		116
Glutamate	109	72	26	277
Glutamine	286	241	452	
Glycine	344	270	158	353
Histidine	59	84	80	118
Isoleucine	56	59	179*	324
Leucine	132	107	—	446
Lysine	260	157	208	823
Methionine	26	18	32	
Phenylalanine	56	52	34	98
Proline	171	178	113	214
Serine	149	124	154	344
Taurine	83	79	22	
Threonine	143	143	191	78
Tyrosine	35	47	26	78
Valine	136	228	168	528

* Value is for isoleucine and leucine combined. Adapted from Silbernagl.[60]

Urinary excretion of amino acids is very small relative to the load that is filtered. As may be calculated from Table 2, the total plasma concentration of amino acids ranges from about 2 to 4 mmol/L. Assuming a glomerular filtration rate of 120 mL/min in humans, the filtered load amounts to >400 mmol/d with only ~1% of the load being excreted.[60] This amount is ≪1% of a usual protein intake of 100 g/d. The renal handling of amino acids and oligopeptides was reviewed recently by Silbernagl.[60]

The plasma amino acid profile may have an impact on the entry of amino acids into other tissues because of the presence of a relatively few transport carriers with broad specificity.[16] Of particular importance is the effect of plasma amino acid profile on the uptake of amino acids into brain, which depends upon the blood-brain barrier transport carriers for neutral, acidic, and basic amino acids.[62] Normal plasma amino acid concentrations are at or below the K_m for blood-brain barrier transport.[63] Changes in the concentration of an individual amino acid as well as the degree of change relative to those of other amino acids sharing the same transporter, as is the case for all of the large neutral amino acids, will markedly influence the uptake of the particular amino acid into the brain and, hence, will affect brain amino acid profiles and the synthesis of nonprotein substances formed from amino acids, such as neurotransmitters.[64] Therefore, under normal physiological conditions, regulation of the plasma amino acid pool assures a certain degree of stability of other amino acid pools as well, partic-

ularly in brain. If the amino acid profile of the plasma pool becomes unbalanced, a depression in voluntary food intake occurs that will reduce the effect of the imbalance.[65] With transport K_ms being high in other tissues relative to circulating amino acid concentrations, it is unlikely that competitive effects will alter the plasma amino acid profile except when deviations are severe.[66]

Metabolic activity in tissues other than brain also has an impact on plasma amino acid pools. In the postabsorptive state net release of amino acids from muscle to plasma occurs, but in kidney amino acids are taken up as substrates for gluconeogenesis and renal ammoniagenesis, in intestine as energy substrates, and in liver for gluconeogenesis and detoxification of nitrogen to urea. Release of amino acids from muscle is not reflective of the muscle amino acid profile. Glutamine and alanine account for about two-thirds of the total amino acids released but are present in much lower amounts in muscle protein and free amino acid pools, indicating substantial de novo synthesis of glutamine and alanine in muscle.[67] The interaction of branched-chain amino acids, alanine, and glutamine on interorgan aspects of amino acid metabolism was reviewed by Abumrad et al.[67]

The availability in recent years of amino acids labeled with high enrichments of the stable isotope of carbon in addition to nitrogen has led to an increase in studies to assess the dynamics of whole-body protein and amino acid metabolism in humans.[68,69] Although this tracer kinetic approach differs little in principle from earlier work conducted primarily with animals by using radioactive isotopes, it led to the beginning of an understanding of the complex nature of protein and amino acid metabolism in humans. Examples of the use of this approach in humans include the determination of the flux of phenylalanine to tyrosine in vivo,[70] the dynamics of branched-chain amino acid metabolism in humans with respect to leucine transamination to α-ketoisocaproate and subsequent oxidation or reamination back to leucine,[71] the use of plasma α-ketoisocaproate specific activities (reciprocal pool specific activities) as a more accurate means of assessing intracellular specific activities of leucine,[72] and the use of simultaneous infusions of nitrogen and carbon-labeled lysine to develop a comprehensive model of lysine metabolism in humans.[73] An extensive discussion of the application of the tracer kinetic approach in modeling protein and amino acid metabolism in humans, including its limitations, was provided recently by Bier.[69]

Protein Quality: Amino Acid Requirements

The human requirement for protein is a composite of requirements for nine amino acids that cannot be synthesized in the body and requirements for additional nitrogen. The latter can be met largely from nonspecific sources but is ordinarily obtained from the dispensable amino acids in dietary proteins. Classification of amino acids according to their nutritional essentiality and the concept of protein quality were required to deal with this complexity of the protein requirement. Both the nutritional classification of amino acids[74,75] and the concept of protein quality[76,77] have undergone transitions over the years as knowledge of metabolic relationships among amino acids expanded and as information about quantitative requirements for amino acids accumulated and were reassessed.

Nutritional Classification of Amino Acids. The distinction between dispensable (nonessential) and indispensable (essential) amino acids is strictly nutritional.[74,75] Dispensable amino acids can be synthesized in the body; indispensable amino acids must be provided in the diet. After amino acids are consumed, however, metabolic interactions occur between pairs and among groups of amino acids independently of their nutritional essentiality.

The dispensable amino acids are essential for an immense number of metabolic reactions. Serine, for example, is essential for the metabolism of methionine; proline is an essential component of collagen; in fact, dispensable amino acids are required in adequate amounts for the synthesis of all proteins. Alanine is an important, nontoxic carrier of nitrogen released during the degradation of amino acids in peripheral tissues to the liver for disposal as urea.[29] Glutamine is essential for maintenance of acid-base balance in the kidney, and both glutamate and glutamine, as mentioned, are major energy sources for the intestine.[22] Nutritional distinctions, based on dietary need, should not be allowed to obscure the importance of the dispensable amino acids for the nutrition of cells and their essentiality for normal cell and organ function.

Amino acids such as tyrosine and cystine that ordinarily are synthesized in adequate amounts in the body from their precursors, phenylalanine and tyrosine, respectively, are often referred to as semiindispensable, a self-contradictory term. The term conditionally indispensable (essential) recently was proposed by Chipponi et al.[78] for substances that are ordinarily nutritionally dispensable but that because of either metabolic impairment or the physiological state of the organism may not be synthesized in large enough amounts to meet the body's needs. Adoption of this term would contribute to clarity in discussions of nutritional needs for amino acids and for nutrients generally. It would apply to cystine and tyrosine for premature infants,[79] probably to taurine,[80,81] and possibly to carnitine.[82] Arginine and glycine might be included in any one of the three categories depending upon the species or the specific conditions under study.[74,75,83] For human infants consuming a formula containing a low amount of high-quality protein[84] or for young animals consuming diets containing mainly indispensable amino acids,[74] a nonspecific source of nitrogen for the synthesis of dispensable amino acids may be conditionally indispensable. In proposals for modification of the nutritional classification of amino acids, Jackson[83] and Laidlaw and Kopple[85] accepted the concept of conditional indispensability. Their proposals for further subdividing the current categories on the basis of metabolic distinctions among amino acids, however, seem to represent an unnecessary complication of the present simple scheme.

Histidine is often omitted from the list of amino acids required by adult humans even though its essentiality for human infants was demonstrated years ago. Studies on effects of deleting histidine from the diets of adults were reviewed by Visek[75] and by Laidlaw and Kopple.[85] Under these conditions, plasma histidine concentration and urinary histidine excretion both fell sharply; the concentration of the histidine-rich protein, hemoglobin, tended to decline; and nitrogen balance fell to zero or below. Both Cho et al.[86] and Kopple and Swendseid[87] concluded that histidine was uniquely well conserved by adults but that a dietary source was nonetheless required. Both Visek[75] and the FAO/WHO/UNU committee[1] concurred with this conclusion.

Protein Quality. The nutritional quality of a protein, i.e., the quantity needed to meet requirements for indispensable amino acids relative to that of one that is highly digestible and provides amino acids in the proportions in which they are required, depends upon its amino acid composition, digestibility, and any unique unavailability of specific amino acids. In general, the nutritional quality of proteins is still estimated indirectly from the results of growth or nitrogen-retention studies with young rats. Such methods provide only crude estimates of the value of proteins in meeting human amino acid needs and do not permit calculation of the quality of mixtures of proteins in diets.[76,77]

The chemical score procedure[88] provided a method for predicting efficiency of utilization of food proteins from comparisons of their amino acid compositions with that of a high-quality standard, whole-egg proteins. This procedure was adapted by a FAO/WHO committee[89] that substituted the amino acid score based on amino acid requirements of adult males for the whole-egg amino acid composition used as the standard for comparison in the chemical score procedure. When estimates of the amino acid requirements of women and infants became available, other committees[8,10] reassessed all of the information on amino acid requirements of humans and proposed modifications of the standard amino acid scoring pattern. In the recent FAO/WHO/UNU report,[1] the values given for amino acid requirements are essentially those proposed earlier[8,10] but changes in the estimates of protein requirements necessitated some changes in amino acid scoring patterns. The committee proposed different scoring patterns for infants, children, and adults but concluded that there was no need to adjust protein allowances of adults for protein quality. The report noted, however, that allowances should be adjusted for protein digestibility. This adjustment always should be done when protein quality is estimated from the amino acid scoring pattern.[77]

Although it is important to know how amino acid requirements change with increasing age, it is difficult to understand the rationale for proposing three different scoring patterns. Protein quality measurements are needed to assess the adequacy of diets for nations, large populations, and families. A single pattern based on the needs of the most vulnerable group, young children, as a general standard of adequacy would seem preferable. The conclusion of the FAO/WHO/UNU committee[1] that adjustment of the protein allowance for adults for protein quality is not necessary was based on calculations showing that amino acid intakes from a variety of national diets were adequate. It should be recognized in relation to this conclusion that the generally accepted amino acid requirements of adults are extremely low and that adults do require more of unbalanced proteins such as those of wheat flour than of milk or egg proteins to achieve nitrogen balance when these foods are the sole source of protein in the diet.[8]

Amino Acid Requirements of Adults. Recently, Young, Bier, and Pellett[4] concluded on the basis of results of metabolic studies that the generally accepted adult requirements for amino acids are too low. Using a stable-isotope technique, they estimated obligatory amino acid losses from measurement of the amounts of labeled carbon dioxide exhaled by adult human subjects consuming amino acid diets containing graded increments of one indispensable amino acid. From the values obtained for the amounts of each of five indispensable amino acids oxidized as the amounts consumed were increased from inadequate to more than adequate, they estimated how much of each would have to be ingested to maintain amino acid balance. They concluded, with some reservations, that requirements of adults for leucine, lysine, threonine, and tryptophan had been underestimated by two- to threefold. Millward and Rivers[5] questioned the reliability and accuracy of the oxidation procedure and the validity of the conclusion that adult amino acid requirements have been seriously underestimated.

Diets used in studies of amino acid requirements, which provide all but one of the indispensable amino acids in excess, should ensure that the limiting amino acid will be used highly efficiently for protein synthesis. Efficiency of utilization of proteins with balanced patterns of amino acids consumed at the requirement amount is only 65–70%;[8,10] therefore, if surpluses of the other amino acids improve efficiency of utilization of the one that is limiting, underestimation of amino acid requirements by ~30% would not be surprising. Nonetheless, values for amino acid requirements of infants fed amino acid diets low in a single amino acid have not been lower than requirements estimated from intakes of amino acids by infants consuming human milk or milk-based formulas in amounts just sufficient to meet the total protein requirement.[8]

It is difficult to reconcile the suggestion that amino acid requirements of adults determined with the nitrogen-balance procedure have been so seriously underestimated, because (1) nitrogen-balance studies have provided reasonable estimates of nitrogen requirements for maintenance,[1] (2) lysine intakes of adults maintained in nitrogen balance while consuming only wheat flour, which is severely limiting in lysine, are not >30% above the requirement estimated from balance studies with amino acid diets,[8] and (3) amino acid requirements of young rats estimated from growth responses agree quite well with those based on oxidation studies in which the animals were fed amino acid diets with a single limiting amino acid.[90] Millward and Rivers[5] suggested that obligatory losses of amino acids by human subjects may be overestimated by the oxidation procedure. Young et al.[4] suggested, on the other hand, on the basis of observations on nitrogen repletion of subjects who had been consuming diets low in a single amino acid, that body protein depletion that is not evident may occur during experiments in which amino acid requirements are determined using the nitrogen-balance procedure.

A saturation-kinetics model based on Michaelis-Menton analysis of growth responses of rats having a wide range of intakes of a nutrient was used by Mercer et al.[91] to estimate amino acid requirements. This model has the considerable merit of providing a method for identifying in a consistent way the amount of nutrient required for maximum response. It would provide another approach to estimating amino acid requirements of humans but would require many more values at intakes above the estimated requirement intake than are usually obtained. The latter is a distinct shortcoming of most studies of requirements for nutrients of humans.

Implications for Protein Quality. The questions that have arisen about the discrepancies between estimates of amino acid requirements of adults obtained by the balance and oxidation procedures require answers. The answers are important for an understanding of the metabolic basis of requirements for maintenance; they are also important for establishing accurate and reliable estimates of amino acid utilization for different functions in vivo. Hopefully, the controversy on this subject will stimulate research to evaluate critically methods for estimating amino acid requirements. In the meantime, use of protein-quality measurements based on the amino acid scoring pattern for young children in dealing with practical nutrition problems is not invalidated by uncertainty about the values for amino acid requirements of adults.

It should be more widely acknowledged that estimates of the protein quality of individual foods by the classical animal-growth and nitrogen-retention methods provide only crude, qualitative information of limited value in human nutrition.[76,77] Only with the amino acid scoring pattern can the nutritive value of mixtures of proteins or the complementary value of proteins for human nutrition be predicted. In assessments of the amount of protein needed by populations consuming different diets, adjustments for protein quality based on meeting the amino acid requirements of the most vulnerable group, young children, will ensure that the needs of older age groups will be met. The FAO/WHO 1973 amino acid scoring pattern based on the amino acid requirements of young children was tested for its ability to predict the amount of protein from milk and from a highly digestible vegetable mixture needed for normal growth of 2–3-y-old children.[92] The predictions were amazingly accurate, indicating that both the amino acid scoring pattern and the estimates of protein requirements for this age group were highly satisfactory.

Adoption of the procedure based on the amino acid scoring pattern for evaluating the nutritional quality of food proteins with correction of the estimated requirement for incomplete digestibility of the proteins in the available foods would represent a long overdue advance in procedures for estimating protein needs.[76,77,93] Because human diets are unlikely to be limiting in amino acids other than lysine, methionine, tryptophan, and threonine,[1,77] it seems reasonable to propose that RDA for these four amino acids be established and included as part of the RDA standard. Allowances for these amino acids for adults might be controversial at present, but values for children would be at least as accurate and probably more accurate than RDA for many vitamins and minerals.

Summary

Knowledge of interorgan relationships in amino acid metabolism, metabolism of individual amino acids by individual organs and tissues, the processes of protein synthesis and degradation, and the molecular basis for regulation of amino acid–degrading enzymes has been greatly expanded during the past decade. Steady progress also has been made in quantifying body fluxes of amino acids and changes in protein turnover in relation to changes in nutritional state and in assessing effects of dietary modifications on transport of amino acids especially into brain. These advances have improved our understanding of tissue utilization of amino acids and metabolic control of plasma and tissue amino acid concentrations, and they hold out the promise of providing a metabolic basis for establishing protein and amino acid requirements.

A detailed reassessment of information on protein requirements by an international committee has led to the conclusion that recommended intakes of protein for children > 8 y of age and for adults have been underestimated. An epidemiological assessment of protein requirements of infants suggests that requirements of infants have been overestimated. Amino acid requirements of adults, based on metabolic studies, are reported to be much higher than generally accepted values. This report has raised questions and controversy about the validity of estimates based on nitrogen-balance studies. Underestimation of amino acid requirements for adults may also raise questions about the validity of the assumption that protein quality is of little significance for adults. Controversy over requirements of adults for amino acids does not have implications for practical applications of protein-quality measurements, because the quality of dietary proteins for population groups is assessed routinely with the amino acid scoring pattern that is based on the requirements of young children.

References

1. Food and Agriculture Organization, World Health Organization, and United Nations University (1985) *Energy and Protein Requirements.* World Health Organization Technical Report Series 724, World Health Organization, Geneva.

2. G.H. Beaton and A. Chery (1988) Protein requirements of infants: a reexamination of concepts and approaches. *Am. J. Clin. Nutr.* 48:1403–1412.

3. D.J. Millward and J.P.W. Rivers (1986) Protein and amino acid requirements in the adult human. *J. Nutr.* 116:2559–2561.

4. V.R. Young, D.M. Bier, and P.L. Pellett (1989) A theoretical basis for increasing current estimates of the amino acid requirements in adult man, with experimental support. *Am. J. Clin. Nutr.* 50:80–92.

5. D.J. Millward and J.P.W. Rivers (1988) The nutritional role of indispensable amino acids and the metabolic basis for their requirements. *Eur. J. Clin. Nutr.* 42:367–393.

6. Food and Agriculture Organization and World Health Organization (1965) *Protein Requirements.* World Health Organization Technical Report Series 301, World Health Organization, Geneva.

7. S. Brody (1945) *Bioenergetics and Growth,* Reinhold Publishing Co., New York.

8. Committee on Amino Acids, Food and Nutrition Board, National

Research Council (1974) *Improvement of Protein Nutriture,* National Academy of Sciences, Washington, DC.

9. Committee on Dietary Allowances, Food and Nutrition Board, National Research Council (1974) *Recommended Dietary Allowances,* National Academy of Sciences, Washington, DC.

10. Food and Agriculture Organization and World Health Organization (1973) *Energy and Protein Requirements.* World Health Organization Technical Report Series 522, World Health Organization, Geneva.

11. National Research Council (1989) *Recommended Dietary Allowances,* 10th ed., National Academy of Sciences, Washington, DC.

12. S.J. Fomon (1986) Protein requirements of term infants. In: *Energy and Protein Needs During Infancy* (S.J. Fomon and W.C. Heird, eds.), pp. 55–68, Academic Press, Orlando, FL.

13. D.J. Millward (1989) Protein requirements of infants. *Am. J. Clin. Nutr.* 50:406–407.

14. D.H. Alpers (1987) Digestion and absorption of carbohydrates and proteins. In: *Physiology of the Gastrointestinal Tract,* 2nd ed., vol. 2 (L.R. Johnson, ed.), pp. 1469–1487, Raven Press, New York.

15. U. Hopfer (1987) Membrane transport mechanisms for hexoses and amino acids in the small intestine. In: *Physiology of the Gastrointestinal Tract,* 2nd ed. vol. 2 (L.R. Johnson, ed.), pp. 1499–1526, Raven Press, New York.

16. E.J. Collarini and D.L. Oxender (1987) Mechanisms of transport of amino acids across membranes. *Annu. Rev. Nutr.* 7:75–90.

17. B.R. Stevens, J.D. Kaunitz, and E.M. Wright (1984) Intestinal transport of amino acids and sugars: advances using membrane vesicles. *Annu. Rev. Physiol.* 46:417–433.

18. D. Wellner and A. Meister (1981) A survey of inborn errors of amino acid metabolism and transport in man. *Annu. Rev. Biochem.* 50:911–968.

19. S.A. Adibi, W. Fekl, P. Furst, and M. Oehnke, eds. (1987) *Dipeptides as New Substrates in Nutrition Therapy,* Karger, Basel.

20. M.L.G. Gardner (1988) Gastrointestinal absorption of intact proteins. *Annu. Rev. Nutr.* 8:329–350.

21. P.J. Garlick (1980) Protein turnover in the whole animal and specific tissues. In: *Comprehensive Biochemistry: Protein Metabolism,* vol. 19B, part I (M. Florkin, A. Neuberger, and L.L.M. Van Deenen, eds.), pp. 77–152, Elsevier, Amsterdam.

22. H.G. Windmueller (1982) Glutamine utilization by the small intestine. *Adv. Enzymol.* 53:201–237.

23. C. Remesy, C. Demigne, and J. Aufrere (1978) Inter-organ relationships between glucose, lactate and amino acids in rats fed on high-carbohydrate or high-protein diets. *Biochem. J.* 170:321–329.

24. I. Galibois, G. Parent, and L. Savoie (1987) Effect of dietary proteins on time-dependent changes in plasma amino acid levels and on liver protein synthesis in rats. *J. Nutr.* 117:2027–2035.

25. D.H. Elwyn (1970) The role of the liver in regulation of amino acid and protein metabolism. In: *Mammalian Protein Metabolism,* vol. IV (H.N. Munro, ed.), pp. 523–557, Academic Press, New York.

26. L.L. Miller (1962) The role of the liver and the non-hepatic tissues in the regulation of free amino acid levels in the blood. In: *Amino Acid Pools* (J.T. Holden, ed.), pp. 708–721, Elsevier, New York.

27. A.E. Harper, R.H. Miller, and K.P. Block (1984) Branched-chain amino acid metabolism. *Annu. Rev. Nutr.* 4:409–454.

28. H.A. Krebs (1972) Some aspects of the regulation of fuel supply in omnivorous animals. *Adv. Enzyme Regul.* 10:397–420.

29. A.E. Harper (1986) Enzymatic basis for adaptive changes in amino acid metabolism. In: *Proceedings of the XII International Congress of Nutrition* (T.G. Taylor and N.K. Jenkins, eds.), pp. 409–414, John Libby & Co., London.

30. M.M. Mueckler, M.J. Merrill, and H.C. Pitot (1983) Translational and pretranslational control of ornithine aminotransferase in rat liver. *J. Biol. Chem.* 258:6109–6114.

31. S.J. Yeaman (1989) The 2-oxo acid dehydrogenase complexes: recent advances. *Biochem. J.* 257:625–632.

32. R.H. Miller, R.S. Eisenstein, and A.E. Harper (1988) Effects of dietary protein intake on branched-chain keto acid dehydrogenase activity of the rat. *J. Biol. Chem.* 263:3454–3461.

33. S. Kaufman (1986) Regulation of the activity of hepatic phenylalanine hydroxylase. *Adv. Enzyme Regul.* 25:37–64.

34. S. Kaufman (1987) The enzymology of the aromatic amino acid hydroxylases. In: *Amino Acids in Health and Disease: New Perspectives* (S. Kaufman, ed.), pp. 205–232, A.R. Liss, New York.

35. A.E. Harper (1984) Phenylalanine metabolism. In: *Aspartame: Physiology and Biochemistry* (L.D. Stegink and L.J. Filer, eds.), pp. 77–109, Marcel Dekker, New York.

36. A. Tourian and J.B. Sidbury (1983) Phenylketonuria and hyperphenylalaninemia. In: *The Metabolic Basis of Inherited Disease,* 5th ed. (J.B. Stanbury, J.B. Wyngaarden, D.S. Fredrickson, J.L. Goldstein, and M.S. Brown, eds.), pp. 271–286, McGraw-Hill, New York.

37. G.L. Cantoni (1985) The role of S-adenosylhomocysteine in the biological utilization of S-adenosylmethionine. In: *Biochemistry and Biology of DNA Methylation* (G.L. Cantoni and A. Razin, eds.), pp. 47–65, A.R. Liss, Inc., New York.

38. R.J. Cook and C. Wagner (1984) Glycine N-methyltransferase is a folate binding protein of rat liver cytosol. *Proc. Natl. Acad. Sci. USA* 81:3631–3634.

39. B. Shane and E.L.R. Stokstad (1985) Vitamin B_{12}-folate interrelationships. *Annu. Rev. Nutr.* 5:115–141.

40. C. Wagner, W. Decha-Umphai, and J. Corbin (1989) Phosphorylation modulates the activity of glycine N-methyltransferase, a folate binding protein. *J. Biol. Chem.* 264:9638–9642.

41. A.J.L. Cooper and F. Plum (1987) Biochemistry and physiology of brain ammonia. *Physiol. Rev.* 67:440–519.

42. M.J. Jackson, A.L. Beaudet, and W.E. O'Brien (1986) Mammalian urea cycle enzymes. *Annu. Rev. Genet.* 20:431–464.

43. R.G. Thurman, F.C. Kauffman, and K. Jungermann, eds. (1986) *Regulation of Hepatic Metabolism: Intra- and Intercellular Compartmentation,* Plenum Press, New York.

44. A.R. Poso, K.E. Penttila, E.-M. Suolinna, and K.O. Lindros (1986) Urea synthesis in freshly isolated and in cultured periportal and perivenous hepatocytes. *Biochem. J.* 239:263–267.

45. D. Haussinger (1986) Regulation of hepatic ammonia metabolism: the intercellular glutamine cycle. *Adv. Enzyme Regul.* 25:159–180.

46. W.J. Visek (1979) Ammonia metabolism, urea cycle capacity and their biochemical assessment. *Nutr. Rev.* 37:273–282.

47. S.M. Morris, C.L. Moncman, K.D. Rand, G.J. Dizikes, S.D. Cederbaum, and W.E. O'Brien (1987) Regulation of mRNA levels for five urea cycle enzymes in rat liver by diet, cyclic AMP, and glucocorticoids. *Arch. Biochem. Biophys.* 256:343–353.

48. K. Moldave (1985) Eukaryotic protein synthesis. *Annu. Rev. Biochem.* 54:1109–1149.

49. V.M. Pain and M.J. Clemens (1980) Protein synthesis in mammalian systems. In: *Comprehensive Biochemistry: Protein Metabolism,* vol. 19B, part I (M. Florkin, A. Neuberger, and L.L.M. Van Deenen, eds.), pp. 1–76, Elsevier, Amsterdam.

50. L.A. Russo and H.E. Morgan (1989) Control of protein synthesis and ribosome formation in rat heart. *Diabetes Metab. Rev.* 5:31–47.

51. G.E. Mortimore and A.R. Poso (1987) Intracellular protein catabolism and its control during nutrient deprivation and supply. *Annu. Rev. Nutr.* 7:539–564.

52. G.E. Mortimore, A.R. Poso, and B.R. Lardeux (1989) Mechanism and regulation of protein degradation in liver. *Diabetes Metab. Rev.* 5:49–70.

53. R.J. Benyon and J.S. Bond (1986) Catabolism of intracellular protein: molecular aspects. *Am. J. Physiol.* 251:C141–C152.

54. J.S. Bond and P.E. Butler (1987) Intracellular proteases. *Annu. Rev. Biochem.* 56:333–364.

55. D.J. Millward and J.P.W. Rivers (1989) The need for indispensable amino acids: the concept of the anabolic drive. *Diabetes Metab. Rev.* 5:191–211.

56. P.J. Reeds and W.P.T. James (1983) Protein turnover. *Lancet* 1: 571–574.

57. M.A. McNurlan and P.J. Garlick (1989) Influence of nutrient intake on protein turnover. *Diabetes Metab. Rev.* 5:165–189.

58. F.J. Ballard and F.M. Tomas (1983) 3-Methylhistidine as a measure of skeletal muscle protein breakdown in human subjects: the case for its continued use. *Clin. Sci.* 65:209–215.

59. M.J. Rennie and D.J. Millward (1983) 3-Methylhistidine excretion and the urinary 3-methylhistidine/creatinine ratio are poor indicators of skeletal muscle protein breakdown. *Clin. Sci.* 65:217–225.

60. S. Silbernagl (1987) The renal handling of amino acids and oligopeptides. *Physiol. Rev.* 68:911–1007.

61. C.R. Scriver, D.M. Gregory, D. Sovetts, and G. Tissenbaum (1985) Normal plasma free amino acid values in adults: the influence of some common physiological variables. *Metabolism* 34:868–873.

62. W.M. Pardridge (1983) Brain metabolism: a perspective from the blood-brain barrier. *Physiol. Rev.* 63:1481–1535.

63. Q.R. Smith, S. Momma, M. Aoyagi, and S.A. Rapoport (1987) Kinetics of neutral amino acid transport across the blood-brain barrier. *J. Neurochem.* 49:1651–1658.

64. G. Huether, ed. (1988) *Amino Acid Availability and Brain Function in Health and Disease,* Springer-Verlag, Berlin.

65. P.M.B. Leung and Q.R. Rogers (1987) The effect of amino acids and protein on dietary choice. In: *Umami: A Basic Taste* (Y. Kawamura and M.R. Kare, eds.), pp. 565–610, Marcel Dekker, New York.

66. W.M. Pardridge (1977) Regulation of amino acid availability to the brain. In: *Nutrition and the Brain,* vol. 1 (R.J. Wurtman and J.J. Wurtman, eds.), pp. 141–204, Raven Press, New York.

67. N.N. Abumrad, P. Williams, M. Frexes-Steed, et al. (1989) Inter-organ metabolism of amino acids in vivo. *Diabetes Metab. Rev.* 5:213–226.

68. J.C. Waterlow and J.M.L. Stephen, eds. (1981) *Nitrogen Metabolism in Man,* Applied Science Publishers, London.

69. D.M. Bier (1989) Intrinsically difficult problems: the kinetics of body proteins and amino acids in man. *Diabetes Metab. Rev.* 5:111–132.

70. J.T.R. Clarke and D.M. Bier (1982) The conversion of phenylalanine to tyrosine in man. Direct measurement of continuous intravenous infusions of L-[*ring*-^{2}H$_5$]phenylalanine and L-[1-^{13}C]tyrosine in the postabsorptive state. *Metabolism* 31:999–1005.

71. D.E. Matthews, D.M. Bier, M.J. Rennie, et al. (1981) Regulation of leucine metabolism in man: a stable isotope study. *Science* 214:1129–1131.

72. W.F. Shwenk, B. Beaufrere, and M.W. Haymond (1985) Use of reciprocal pool specific activities to model leucine metabolism in humans. *Am. J. Physiol.* 249:E121–E130.

73. C.S. Irving, M.R. Thomas, E.W. Malphus, et al. (1986) Lysine and protein metabolism in young women: subdivision based on the novel use of multiple stable isotopic labels. *J. Clin. Invest.* 77: 1321–1331.

74. A.E. Harper (1983) Dispensable and indispensable amino acid interrelationships. In: *Amino Acids: Metabolism and Medical Applications* (G.L. Blackburn, J.P. Grant, and V.R. Young, eds.), pp. 105–121, John Wright PSG, Inc., Boston.

75. W.J. Visek (1984) An update of concepts of essential amino acids. *Annu. Rev. Nutr.* 4:137–155.

76. A.E. Harper (1981) McCollum and directions in the evaluation of protein quality. *J. Agric. Food Chem.* 29:429–435.

77. C.E. Bobwell, J.S. Adkins, and D.T. Hopkins, eds. (1981) *Protein Quality in Humans: Assessment and In Vitro Estimation,* Avi Publishing Co., Westport, CN.

78. J.X. Chipponi, J.C. Bleier, M.T. Santi, and D. Rudman (1982) Deficiencies of essential and conditionally essential nutrients. *Am. J. Clin. Nutr.* 35:1112–1116.

79. S.E. Snyderman (1984) Human amino acid nutrition. In: *Genetic Factors in Nutrition* (A. Velazquez and H. Bourges, eds.), pp. 269–278, Academic Press, New York.

80. K.C. Hayes and J.A. Sturman (1981) Taurine in metabolism. *Annu. Rev. Nutr.* 1:401–425.

81. C.E. Wright, H.H. Tallan, Y.Y. Lin, and G.E. Gaull (1986) Taurine: biological update. *Annu. Rev. Biochem.* 55:427–453.

82. C.R. Rebouche and D.J. Paulson (1986) Carnitine metabolism and function in humans. *Annu. Rev. Nutr.* 6:41–66.

83. A.A. Jackson (1983) Amino acids: essential and non-essential? *Lancet* 1:1034–1037.

84. S.E. Snyderman, L.E. Holt, J. Dancis, E. Roitman, A. Boyer, and M.E. Balis (1962) ''Unessential'' nitrogen: a limiting factor for human growth. *J. Nutr.* 78:57–72.

85. S.A. Laidlaw and J.D. Kopple (1987) Newer concepts of the indispensable amino acids. *Am. J. Clin. Nutr.* 46:593–605.

86. E.S. Cho, H.L. Anderson, R.L. Wixom, K.C. Hanson, and G.F. Krause (1984) Long-term effects of low histidine intake on men. *J. Nutr.* 114:369–384.

87. J.D. Kopple and M.E. Swendseid (1981) Effect of histidine intake on plasma and urine levels, nitrogen balance and N-methylhistidine excretion in normal and chronically uremic men. *J. Nutr.* 111:931–942.

88. R.J. Block and H.H. Mitchell (1946–47) The correlation of the amino acid composition of proteins with their nutritive value. *Nutr. Abstr. Rev.* 16:249–278.

89. Food and Agriculture Organization (1957) *Protein Requirements,* Food and Agriculture Organization Nutritional Studies no. 16, Food and Agriculture Organization, Rome.

90. Y.A. Kang-Lee and A.E. Harper (1977) Effect of histidine intake and hepatic histidase activity on the metabolism of histidine in vivo. *J. Nutr.* 107:1427–1443.

91. L.P. Mercer, S.J. Dodds, and D.L. Smith (1987) New method for formulation of amino acid concentrations and ratios in diets of rats. *J. Nutr.* 117:1936–1944.

92. G. Arroyave (1974) Amino acid requirements by age and sex. In: *Nutrients in Processed Foods: Proteins* (P.L. White and D.C. Fletcher, eds.), pp. 15–28, Publishing Sciences Group, Inc., Acton, MA.

93. V.R. Young and P.L. Pellett (1984) Amino acid composition in relation to protein nutritional quality of meat and poultry products. *Am. J. Clin. Nutr.* 40:737–742.

Chapter 9

Barbara O. Schneeman and Daniel D. Gallaher

Dietary Fiber

Introduction and Definition of Dietary Fiber

Dietary fiber includes the components of plant material that are not digested by the enzymes of the mammalian digestive system. This definition of fiber, which includes nonstarch structural polysaccharides, nonstarch nonstructural polysaccharides, and lignin, was presented originally by Burkitt and Trowell[1] when they proposed that a lack of fiber-rich foods in the diet may be associated with the incidence of certain chronic disorders. Although this definition has been fairly widely accepted, in recent years controversy has arisen about whether nonpolysaccharide components, such as lignin, phenolic compounds, digestive enzyme inhibitors, phytic acid, other inorganic constituents, or starch that is resistant to digestion should be included in the definition of dietary fiber. Although these fractions are minor components of most foods consumed by humans, they have physiological activities that are associated with the metabolic responses to diets rich in fiber-containing foods. This controversy clearly illustrates that it is often difficult to disassociate the responses to fiber per se from the response to consuming a diet rich in fiber-containing foods. This difficulty is especially acute when one examines the association between the risk of chronic diseases and dietary fiber. The definition given by Burkitt and Trowell is based on a physiological definition of the nondigestible fraction of foods. Perhaps fiber can be defined more accurately by the analytical methods utilized to determine the fiber content of food—if the methods allow a clear definition of the fraction in food that is estimated.

The major components of dietary fiber are the nonstarch polysaccharides that include cellulose, β-glucans, hemicelluloses, pectins, and gums.[2] Each of these fractions is characterized by sugar residues and the linkages among them. Cellulose and β-glucans are glucose polymers with β 1–4 linkages; in the glucans these linkages are interspersed with β 1–3 bonds.

Cellulose is found in all plant cell walls, and oats and barley are particularly rich sources of β-glucans. The hemicelluloses are a diverse group of polysaccharides with varying degrees of branching. These compounds may be classified according to the monosaccharide in the backbone (e.g., xylans, galactans, and mannans) and in the side chains (e.g., arabinose, galactose). The major backbone sugar for pectins is galacturonic acid, and side chains typically include galactose and arabinose. The degree of methoxylation on the uronic acid residues varies. The structural features of gums vary according to the source. Typically the gums are a minor polysaccharide constituent in most foods. However, certain gums have been fed in an isolated form in clinical trials (e.g., guar gum and locust bean gum, which are classified as galactomannans). The noncarbohydrate constituent that is included in most definitions of fiber is lignin, which has a highly complex three-dimensional structure and contains phenylpropane units. Lignin is usually not an important component of human foods, because it is generally associated with tough or woody tissue. The one exception is foods that contain intact seeds consumed with the food.

The current interest in fiber as an important component of the diet stems from the epidemiological association of a high fiber intake with a lower incidence of certain chronic disorders, such as cardiovascular disease and large bowel cancer. The epidemiological data linking a reduced risk of cancer with a high fiber intake are complex and difficult to evaluate. Greenwald et al.[3] reviewed the epidemiological evidence supporting a link between colon cancer risk and diets low in fiber and report that although an association clearly exists, the impact of total diet and the interaction of fiber with other dietary factors are important to the relationship. An example of the complexity of the interaction is pointed out by Klurfeld.[4] In Japan, where the diet is lower in fat but similar in fiber content to the U.S. diet, the incidence of colon cancer is lower; however, the incidence of gastric cancer is higher in Japan than in the United States. Recent evidence suggests that total energy intake and the fiber intake with respect to energy intake may also have an important role in determining colon cancer risk in a population. Clearly, the association between disease risk and dietary factors is multifactorial, and our present state of knowledge indicates that fiber cannot be isolated as a single factor affecting risk but must be evaluated in the context of the total dietary pattern.

Methods of Analysis

Methods of dietary fiber analysis fall into one of two categories—gravimetric or component analysis. Gravimetric methods are simpler and faster but are limited to estimates of total fiber or soluble and insoluble fiber. Component analysis yields the quantity of individual neutral sugars and the total quantity of acidic sugars (i.e., uronic acids). The total fiber content is then calculated as the sum of the individual sugars. When desired, lignin can be estimated separately and added to the sum of the individual sugars. Component analysis, however, is more involved in terms of both expertise and equipment and, consequently, is less suitable for routine dietary fiber analysis.

Gravimetric Procedures. The oldest and first official method of dietary fiber analysis was crude fiber analysis. This method measures the weight of the undigestible residue after extraction with organic solvents and digestion with dilute acid and alkali with a correction for ash. Although an official Association of Official Analytical Chemists (AOAC) method since 1955, the method does not accurately measure dietary fiber. All soluble fiber is lost along with variable amounts of insoluble fiber, thus underestimating the true fiber content of the food. Because the losses are variable, extrapolation of crude fiber values to dietary fiber is not possible.

Highly reproducible values for insoluble fiber are obtained by the neutral detergent method (NDF).[5] Food samples are boiled with a detergent (sodium dodecyl sulfate) at neutral pH, and the residue is collected by filtration. The enzymatic NDF method includes a modification to reduce starch interference by inclusion of a treatment with α-amylase and is an official method of the American Association of Cereal Chemists.[6] However, because soluble fibers are lost in the NDF procedures the fiber content of many foods, particularly fruits and vegetables, is underestimated.

The growing awareness of the potential importance of soluble fiber and the desire for a simple and reliable measure of dietary fiber led to the development of the present official AOAC method (first action) commonly referred to as Total Dietary Fiber (TDF).[7] Duplicate samples are digested with a heat-stable α-amylase at 100 °C to remove starch, followed by successive treatments with protease and amyloglucosidase to digest protein and residual starch. Fiber is precipitated with ethanol, and the precipitate is collected on a filter, dried, and weighed. The residue from one set of duplicates is incinerated to correct for ash, and the other is analyzed for nitrogen to correct for protein contamination. It is imperative that a sample blank be run with all samples because the values for the blank can be significant. Recently, a modification of the TDF procedure was suggested to reduce the high coefficient of variation of the procedure (V. Hicks, personal communication). The substitution of a buffer with no chelating ability for the phosphate buffer currently used reduces the formation of calcium phosphate precipitates, which form in variable amounts at the concentration of ethanol used to precipitate the fiber.

Gravimetric procedures that measure total fiber can be modified to give estimates of soluble and insoluble fiber.[8] This is accomplished by filtering the fiber digest before precipitation with ethanol; the filter residue contains the insoluble fraction whereas the filtrate contains the soluble fraction. The soluble fraction is then precipitated with ethanol, collected by filtration, dried, and weighed.

Component Analysis Procedures. The primary difference between component analysis and the gravimetric methods is in the manner of quantitating the fiber residue obtained after digestion and collection of the fiber residue. Component analysis involves hydrolyzing the residue with strong acids, usually sulfuric acid, and quantitation of the monomeric sugars. Neutral sugars are determined colorimetrically by refractive index after separation by high-performance liquid chromatography or, more commonly, by gas chromatography after derivitization. Acidic sugars are quantitated by decarboxylation and measurement of the carbon dioxide released or colorimetrically by the use of any of several compounds that produce chromophores with uronic acids in the presence of hot sulfuric acid. Summation of the monomeric sugars then yields a value for total dietary fiber. Minor modifications allow estimates of cellulose, soluble and insoluble fiber, and noncellulosic polysaccharides (essentially hemicellulose).

The newer methods of component analysis, such as those of Englyst et al.[9] or Theander and Westerlund,[10] correlate well with the AOAC TDF procedure but are generally lower.[11,12] The difference appears to be largely due to lignin, which is not measured in the method of Englyst et al.,[9,13] and to residual starch in some food samples that are retained by the TDF procedure.

In contrast to the advances made in measuring the carbohydrate component of dietary fiber, almost no improvement has been made in the measurement of lignin. Uncertainty about the chemical structure, differences in the solubility of lignins in acid, and reactions of lignins with proteins and other food components complicate the analysis. Hydrolysis with 72% sulfuric acid and correction for ash yielding Klason lignin is the classical procedure for lignin determination. However, cutin and certain Maillard reaction products resist this hydrolysis and, thus, interfere. Similarly, the permanganate oxidation[14] and acetyl bromide[15] methods have shortcomings. Although the lignin content of most foods is quite low, lignin is not degraded in the colon by bacteria and may have greater influence on colonic events than its minor presence suggests.

The demonstration that some starch in foods, particularly thermally processed foods, escapes digestion within the small intestine led to the concept of resistant starch.[16] Resistant starch is formed during retrogradation of amylose and consequently is formed in large amounts in high-amylose foods such as potatoes.[17] By its resistance to the action of amylolytic enzymes, resistant starch is not removed in enzymatic-gravimetric procedures such as the TDF and consequently is measured as dietary fiber in these procedures. Currently, there is disagreement as to whether resistant starch should be considered as dietary fiber or as a separate entity.[18,19] Resistant starch may be measured by the method of Englyst et al.[9,10] as the additional glucose present in a fiber sample dispersed in buffer instead of dimethylsulfoxide.

Physical Properties of Dietary Fiber

The chemical composition of dietary fibers has provided little insight into their physiological effects. Progress in understanding the action of different types of dietary fiber in the intestinal tract has come primarily from the characterization of their physical properties. Therefore, determining such characteristics as the water-holding capacity, viscosity, bile acid–binding capacity, and cation-exchange capacity is more likely to be useful than is the detailed chemical composition provided by component analysis.

The water-holding capacity (WHC) of a fiber source refers to its ability to retain water within its matrix. Interest in the WHC of fiber preparations stems from the suggestion that fibers with a large WHC will increase stool weight.[20] WHC can be measured by saturating the fiber with water and then removing unretained water by centrifugation, filtration,[21] or osmotic suction.[22] Water can be bound to

a fiber or merely entrapped by it. Filtration and centrifugation appear to measure both entrapped and bound water, whereas the osmotic suction technique measures only bound water. Therefore, values obtained by osmotic suction are much lower. Soluble fibers such as pectin and the gums have a much higher WHC than do insoluble fibers such as cellulose and wheat bran. Vegetable fibers have intermediate values. Unfortunately, the WHC determined in vitro does not predict the fecal bulking ability of a fiber source that is due to fermentation of the fiber and increase in microbial mass in the colon.[23] The potential WHC (PWHC) of a fiber source is a measure developed to account for these factors.[24] The PWHC, which is determined by osmotic suction, is essentially the WHC of the fiber-source residue and microbial mass after in vitro fermentation. When fiber sources with a broad range of WHC and fermentability were used, the PWHC ranked the fibers in the same order as their fecal-bulking ability. Although the PWHC is more difficult to determine than the WHC, it appears to be a physiologically meaningful measure.

Certain groups of dietary fiber can form highly viscous solutions. These groups include pectins, various gums, O-glucans, and algal polysaccharides, such as agar and carrageenan. Within a group the viscosity is highly dependent upon the chemical structure of the compound. For example, the viscosity of pectin is dependent upon both the molecular weight and methyl ester content; a reduction in either will reduce its viscosity. Soluble fibers exhibit pseudoplastic (shear thinning) behavior, i.e., as the shear rate increases, the apparent viscosity decreases. Because the shear rate within the small intestine is unknown, the viscosity of the contents within the small intestinal lumen after consumption of a viscous fiber cannot be determined exactly. Guar gum consumption, however, clearly increases intestinal contents viscosity[25] (D.D. Gallaher, unpublished observations).

Dietary fiber is capable of binding bile acids both in vitro[26,27] and in vivo.[28] In general, cellulose binds very little, wheat bran and alfalfa somewhat more, pectin and guar gum moderate amounts, and lignin a great deal. Caution should be exercised in regard to lignin binding, however, because lignin preparations most often used in these studies are isolated from wood by using harsh procedures and, therefore, may bear little resemblance to lignins in food. Bile acid binding is greatest at acid pH and declines as the pH increases.[29,30] The nature of the binding first was proposed to be a hydrophobic attraction of bile acids to the lignin component of the fiber sources on the basis of the decrease in binding after delignification.[30] Binding due to the presence of saponins also was proposed,[31] although this finding could not be confirmed.[32] On the other hand, Selvendran et al.[2] reported that, in cell wall material from runner bean pods, bile acid binding was reduced in depectinated material and in material in the hydrogenated form. Their results suggest that bile acid binding is hydrophilic in nature and that pectin is the responsible component. The reason for these disparate results is not apparent, although the two types of binding are not mutually exclusive. Differences in the conditions used for measuring binding and in the fiber preparation may account for the lack of agreement.

Many fiber sources have a demonstrable cation exchange capacity (CEC) and, thus, may bind minerals within the gastrointestinal tract. The functional group primarily responsible for binding cations is the carboxyl group of uronic acids. However, the pectin content of a food is not a reliable indicator of the CEC because the majority of the uronic acids are esterified in most foods and, therefore, are unavailable for cation exchange.

Physiological Response to Sources of Dietary Fiber

Several physiological responses, such as lowering of plasma cholesterol levels, modification in the glycemic response, improving large bowel function, and lowering nutrient availability, have been associated with isolated fiber fractions or diets rich in fiber-containing foods. From mediation of these responses, it is clear that the physical properties of dietary fibers affect the functioning of the gastrointestinal tract and influence the rate and site of nutrient absorption. Hence, discussing our current understanding of these physiological responses will be done in the context of dietary fiber's effects on gastrointestinal function.

The effect of fiber on the rate of gastric emptying has been associated with its ability to blunt the glycemic response to a glucose load and to slow nutrient absorption. Viscous polysaccharides but not insoluble fiber sources such as cellulose were reported to delay gastric emptying.[33,34] Because viscous polysaccharides can form a gel matrix, they are likely to trap nutrients in the matrix and delay their emptying from the stomach. The glucose-flattening ability of various fiber supplements is correlated with their viscosities.[35-37]

Within the small intestine the digestible components of the diet are broken down by hydrolysis, and nutrients are absorbed through the mucosal cells. In vitro data indicate that various fiber sources can inhibit the activity of pancreatic enzymes that digest carbohydrates, lipids, and proteins.[38] The mechanisms for inhibiting digestive enzyme activity are not clearly established, but in some nonpurified fiber sources, specific enzyme inhibitors may exist.[39] It is difficult to assess the physiological importance of this inhibition, because an excess of digestive enzyme activity occurs in response to a meal. However, several lines of evidence indicate that specific fibers may reduce the availability of the enzyme for hydrolyzing triacylglycerides, starch, and proteins within the intestinal contents. Gallaher and Schneeman[40] reported that a diet high in cellulose (20% by weight) delayed the disappearance of labeled triolein but not labeled cholesterol from the small intestine. The high-cellulose content of the diet interfered with triolein breakdown but not with overall lipid absorption. Lairon et al.[41,42] reported that an inhibitor of pancreatic lipase is present in wheat bran and wheat germ. The characteristics of this inhibitor suggest that it may be active in the small intestine and capable of slowing the digestion of triacylglycerides. Legumes were reported to contain amylase inhibitors that could slow the hydrolysis of starch in the small intestine.[39] Inhibition of amylase in human pancreatic or duodenal fluid by wheat bran, xylan, cellulose, guar gum, and psyllium was reported.[38] Many cereals and legumes contain pancreatic protease inhibitors that can decrease protein digestibility. These inhibitors often are inactivated by heat treatment; however, some inhibitor activity potentially can survive normal processing conditions and remain active in the gut. Carageenan, a highly sulfated polysaccharide, inhibits trypsin activity both in vivo and in vitro (D.D. Gallaher, unpublished observation). In patients with pancreatic insufficiency the activity of amylase, trypsin, chymotrypsin, and lipase available from pancreatic replacement treatment was significantly reduced when the patients were given a meal containing pectin or wheat bran. This finding suggests that it is possible for these fiber sources to reduce digestive enzyme capacity in the small intestine.[43] In addition to direct inhibition of digestive enzyme activity, the presence of plant cell wall matrix in a food can provide a physical barrier to digestion.[44-46] An intact cell wall may slow the penetration of digestive enzymes into plant foods. Consequently, grinding of the fiber source to a very fine particle size may disrupt the cell wall structure sufficiently to make digestible nutrients more available for hydrolysis.

The physical characteristics of the intestinal contents are changed by the physical properties of the fiber sources in the diet. The bulk or amount of material in the small intestine will increase because the fiber is not digestible, and hence this material remains during the transit of digesta through the small intestine.[47] The volume of the intestinal contents can increase because of the WHC of the fiber source. Sandberg et al.[48,49] reported that addition of wheat bran or pectin to a low-fiber meal increased the volume of ileostomy fluid by ~20–30%. In addition, animal data indicate that a greater dry and wet weight of intestinal contents is associated with the addition of a fiber supplement to experimental diets.[47] The presence of certain viscous polysaccharides in the fiber source will increase the viscosity of the contents and in particular of the aqueous phase of the intestinal contents from which nutrients are absorbed.[25,50,51] An increase in the bulk, volume, or viscosity of the intestinal contents is likely to slow diffusion of enzymes, substrates, and nutrients to the absorptive surface, all of which can lead to a slower appearance of nutrients in the plasma after a meal.

The bile acid– and phospholipid-binding capacities of various fibers are likely to affect micelle formation in the small intestine and consequently the rate and site of lipid absorption. Vahouny et al.[52,53] demonstrated that addition of soluble fiber supplements to rat diets can slow the appearance of fatty acids and cholesterol in the lymph. The ability of this form of fiber to slow fatty acid absorption and to interfere with cholesterol absorption undoubtedly contributes to the effect of these fiber sources on plasma lipid levels. Studies in human subjects indicate that diets supplemented with oat bran, pectin, or guar gum but not wheat bran or cellulose lower plasma cholesterol levels by 5–18%.[54]

The experimental evidence suggests that through a variety of mechanisms certain fiber sources, especially those containing viscous polysaccharides, can slow the process of digestion and absorption, although total nutrient absorption is not necessarily reduced. Because of the effect of fiber on the rate of absorption, a greater proportion of nutrients from a diet high in fiber will undoubtedly be absorbed from the lower half of the small intestine. This pattern of nutrient absorption is likely to contribute to the physiological responses to various fiber sources. For example, the rate of nutrient absorption will affect the pattern of hormone release in response to diet and the rate of nutrient delivery to the tissues.[36] Evidence also exists that the presence of nutrients in the ileum can influence food intake, gastric emptying, and the composition and size of chylomicrons.[55,56] The presence of fiber in the gut has an important function in maintaining the gastrointestinal system by regulating the rate and site of nutrient absorption. Sigleo et al.[57] demonstrated that chronic feeding of fiber supplements will alter the morphology of the small intestine. Both the distribution of nutrient absorption in the small intestine as well as the influence of bulk in the small intestine on intestinal cell renewal likely contribute to this response.[58]

Our current state of understanding has indicated that the physical-chemical properties of dietary fiber, such as viscosity and bile acid binding, exert effects within the small intestine and stomach that are important in understanding the mechanisms by which fiber sources lower plasma cholesterol, blunt the glycemic response, and slow nutrient absorption. In addition to these effects in the upper gut, the metabolism of dietary fiber sources within the large intestine is important to understanding the overall physiological response to sources of fiber.

The presence of fiber in the diet can influence large bowel function by reducing transit time, increasing stool weight and frequency, and diluting large intestinal contents because of fermentation by the microflora normally present in the large intestine. All these factors are influenced by the source of fiber in the diet as well as by other dietary and nondietary factors. According to the summary in the LSRO report,[54] transit time in 14 studies was shown to decrease because of the addition of wheat bran and fruits and vegetables to the diet. In two studies cellulose was reported to decrease transit time and in two other studies to have no effect.[54] Pectin, on the basis of three studies, does not affect transit time.[54] Transit time is related to stool weight but not, however, in a simple linear manner. By examining population data from healthy subjects, Spiller[59] reported that a low stool weight is associated with delayed transit time. As stool weight increases, transit time tends to decrease. However, once a transit time of 20–30 h is achieved, further increases in stool weight do not shorten transit time significantly.

Stool weight can be increased by sources of fiber. Cummings[60] summarized a number of studies by estimating the increase in fecal weight relative to the weight of fiber fed. Fiber sources that contain insoluble fiber components, such as wheat bran, tend to have the greatest effect on stool weight, whereas soluble fiber sources, such as gums or pectin, increase stool weight only moderately. An increase in stool weight typically is associated with an increase in the microbial cell mass, the undigested fecal residue, and/or the noncellular matrix in the feces. Hence, the fecal-bulking ability of a fiber source is related to a change in one or all of these phases. For example, wheat bran is more effective in increasing the amount of undigested residue, whereas the fiber in fruits and vegetables and soluble polysaccharides can be fermented extensively and are more likely to increase the microbial cell mass of the feces. Changes in the physical characteristics of a fiber source, such as reducing particle size or altering WHC, are likely to result in a different effect of the fiber source on stool weight.

The effects of fiber on stool weight and transit time, although inherently variable, are physiological responses important for maintenance of large-bowel function, for which there is a consensus of opinion that dietary fiber has an important role.[54] Other metabolic consequences of fiber in the large intestine are more poorly understood and, thus, are more difficult to define in terms of physiological significance. For example, during the fermentation of the polysaccharides associated with dietary fiber, the microflora produce short-chain fatty acids (SCFA). The SCFA can be utilized by large intestinal cells as an energy source. The presence of highly fermentable polysaccharides can stimulate large intestinal cell growth that in turn can promote tumor formation when an initiator is administered in an animal model.[61] In contrast, other investigators speculated that production of certain SCFA may be protective against colon cancer. In addition, it was proposed that because the highly fermentable fibers are more likely to lower the glycemic response and blood cholesterol levels, perhaps absorption of SCFA into the portal blood influences glucose or cholesterol metabolism in the liver.[62] The production of SCFA in the large intestine is obviously an important consequence of consuming fiber sources that contain soluble polysaccharides; however, we still have a poor understanding of the availability of the SCFA and the metabolic consequences of their production.[63]

Adequacy of Fiber Intake

Recently several groups proposed recommendations for fiber intake. The challenge to nutritionists in making these recommendations has been to evaluate the adequacy of fiber intake given our current knowledge about the physiological responses to different sources of fiber in the diet. To assess the adequacy of intake, two approaches are possible. One is to determine an optimal intake of dietary fiber based on studying the intake of different population groups that vary in the risk of chronic disorders. The second approach is to use a physiological index to assess adequacy. Both approaches have limitations.

Bingham[64] pointed out two systematic biases inherent in comparing the fiber intake of different populations. These are differences in the methods of estimating food consumption and in the methods for estimating dietary fiber content of foods. Additionally, dietary factors other than fiber intake may influence disease risk. For example, the intake of nonstarch polysaccharides is similar in Japan and the United Kingdom, yet Japan is a population at low risk for colon cancer and diverticular disease compared with the United Kingdom.[4,64] Differences in the consumption of meat and fat, variations in the dietary fiber sources, as well as nonnutritional factors all could contribute to the differences in disease risk between these populations. Population data can provide guidance for the range of fiber intakes that

is likely to be safe but are inadequate to determine the fiber intake that is nutritionally adequate.

In this chapter we have reviewed the effects of dietary fiber in the gastrointestinal tract with respect to lowering of plasma cholesterol, blunting the glycemic response, decreasing nutrient bioavailability, and having an impact on large-bowel function. Use of the first two responses as criteria to assess nutritional adequacy of fiber intake is limited, because fasting plasma cholesterol levels or plasma glucose and insulin levels may not change in healthy subjects. Consequently, a wide range in fiber intakes will be associated with similar responses. These indices may be more useful in monitoring improvement due to dietary intervention as a means of therapeutic management of hyperlipidemia or hyperglycemia. Evaluating mineral status relative to nutrient bioavailability is likely to be useful in setting the maximum amount of fiber or fiber-rich foods to be consumed, because excessive fiber intake could compromise mineral status. These three physiological responses are all limited relative to assessment in that the criteria tend to be directed at a disease state rather than normal physiological function.

Dietary fiber clearly has an important physiological role in normal large-bowel functioning by providing bulk and substrates for fermentation. Recommendations were made that stool weight and transit time, as indicators of large-bowel function, are useful in assessing the adequacy of dietary fiber intake.[54,59] In this context the adequacy of fiber intake could be assessed using normal physiological function as the criterion. Currently the greatest limitation in using these indices is that we do not have enough information on the dose-response relationship between fiber intake (using a variety of fiber sources) and transit time or stool weight. We do know that there is a high degree of individual variability in these indices, suggesting that a wide range of fiber intakes is likely to be adequate. One possible approach toward assessment, given our current knowledge, would be to evaluate the diet as a whole with respect to fiber-containing foods. Food selection could be evaluated with respect to meeting the recommendations from USDA and HHS for consumption of fruits, vegetables, cereals, grains, and legumes.[65,66] Meeting these recommendations and selecting items higher in fiber (e.g., fruit vs. fruit juice, whole-grain vs. milled grains) would encourage the use of fiber-containing foods in the diet.

This work was supported in part by NIH grant DK20446. Parts of this text have been reproduced with permission from the Proceedings for the Third Washington, D.C., Conference on Dietary Fiber and the American Health Foundation Symposium on Assessment of Nutrition Status.

References

1. D.P. Burkitt and H. Trowell (1975) *Refined Carbohydrate Foods and Disease,* Academic Press, New York.

2. R.R. Selvendran, B.J.H. Stevens, and M.S. Du Pont (1987) Dietary fiber: chemistry, analysis and properties. *Adv. Food Res.* 31:117–209.

3. P. Greenwald, E. Lanza, and G.A. Eddy (1987) Dietary fiber in the reduction of colon cancer risk. *J. Am. Diet. Assoc.* 87:1178–1188.

4. D.M. Klurfeld (1987) The role of dietary fiber in gastrointestinal disease. *J. Am. Diet. Assoc.* 87:1172–1177.

5. H.K. Goering and P.J. Van Soest (1970) *Forage Fiber Analyses.* Handbook no. 379, p. 1, U.S. Department of Agriculture, U.S. Government Printing Office, Washington, DC.

6. J.B. Robertson and P.J. Van Soest (1977) Dietary fiber estimation in concentrate feed stuffs. *J. Anim. Sci.* 45(suppl. 1):254–255.

7. L. Prosky, N.-G. Asp, I. Furda, J.W. Devries, T.F. Schweizer, and B.F. Harland (1985) Determination of total dietary fiber in foods and food products: collaborative study. *J. Assoc. Off. Anal. Chem.* 68:677–679.

8. L. Prosky, N.-G. Asp, T. Schweizer, J.W. Devries, and I. Furda (1988) Determination of insoluble, soluble and total dietary fiber in foods and food products: interlaboratory study. *J. Assoc. Off. Anal. Chem.* 71:1017–1023.

9. H. Englyst, H.S. Wiggins, and J.H. Cummings (1982) Determination of the non-starch polysaccharides in plant foods by gas-liquid chromatography of constituent sugars as alditol acetates. *Analyst* 107:307–318.

10. O. Theander and E.A. Westerlund (1986) Studies on dietary fiber. 3. Improved procedures for analysis of dietary fiber. *J. Agric. Food Chem.* 34:330–336.

11. R. Mongeau and R. Brassard (1986) A rapid method for the determination of soluble and insoluble dietary fiber: comparison with AOAC total dietary fiber procedure and Englyst's method. *J. Food Sci.* 51:1333–1336.

12. J.A. Marlett and D. Navis (1988) Comparison of gravimetric and chemical analyses of total dietary fiber in human foods. *J. Agric. Food Chem.* 36:311–315.

13. H. Englyst and J.H. Cummings (1984) Simplified method for the measurement of total non-starch polysaccharides by gas-liquid chromatography of constituent sugars as alditol acetates. *Analyst* 109:937–942.

14. P.J. Van Soest and R.H. Wine (1968) Determination of lignin and cellulose in acid-detergent fiber with permanganate. *J. Assoc. Off. Anal. Chem.* 51:780–785.

15. I.M. Morrison (1972) Improvements in the acetyl bromide technique to determine lignin and digestibility and its application to legumes. *J. Sci. Food Agric.* 23:1463–1469.

16. H.N. Englyst and J.H. Cummings (1987) Digestion of polysaccharides of potato in the small intestine of man. *Am. J. Clin. Nutr.* 45:423–431.

17. C.S. Berry (1986) Resistant starch: formation and measurement of starch that survives exhaustive digestion with amylolytic enzymes during the determination of dietary fibre. *J. Cereal Sci.* 4:301–314.

18. H.N. Englyst, H. Trowell, D.A.T. Southgate, and J.H. Cummings (1987) Dietary fiber and resistant starch. *Am. J. Clin. Nutr.* 46:873–874.

19. N.-G. Asp, I. Furda, T.F. Schweizer, and L. Prosky (1988) Dietary fiber definition and analysis. *Am. J. Clin. Nutr.* 48:688–690.

20. A.A. McConnell, M.A. Eastwood, and W.D. Mitchell (1974) Physical characteristics of vegetable foodstuffs that could influence bowel function. *J. Sci. Food Agric.* 25:1457–1464.

21. J.A. Robertson, M.A. Eastwood, and M.M. Yeoman (1980) An investigation into the physical properties of fibre prepared from several carrot varieties at different stages of development. *J. Sci. Food Agric.* 31:633–638.

22. J.A. Robertson and M.A. Eastwood (1981) A method to measure the water-holding properties of dietary fibre using suction pressure. *Br. J. Nutr.* 46:247–255.

23. A.M. Stephen and J.H. Cummings (1979) Water-holding by dietary fibre in vitro and its relationship to faecal output in man. *Gut* 20:722–729.

24. M.I. McBurney, P.J. Horvath, J.L. Jeraci, and P.J. Van Soest (1985) Effect of in vitro fermentation using human faecal inoculum on the water-holding capacity of dietary fibre. *Br. J. Nutr.* 53:17–24.

25. N.A. Blackburn and I.T. Johnson (1981) The effect of guar gum on the viscosity of the gastrointestinal contents and on glucose uptake from the perfused jejunum in the rat. *Br. J. Nutr.* 46:239–246.

26. D. Kritchevsky and J. Story (1974) Binding of bile salts in vitro by nonnutritive fiber. *J. Nutr.* 104:458–462.

27. G.V. Vahouny, R. Tombes, M.M. Cassidy, D. Kritchevsky, and L.L. Gallo (1980) Dietary fibers: V. Binding of bile salts, phospholipids and cholesterol from mixed micelles by bile acid sequestrants and dietary fibers. *Lipids* 15:1012–1018.

28. D. Gallaher and B.O. Schneeman (1986) Intestinal interaction of bile acids, phospholipids, dietary fibers and cholestyramine. *Am. J. Physiol.* 250:G420–G426.

29. M.A. Eastwood and D. Hamilton (1968) Studies on the adsorption of bile salts to non-absorbed components of diet. *Biochim. Biophys. Acta* 152:165–173.

30. M.A. Eastwood and L. Mowbray (1976) The binding of the components of mixed micelle to dietary fiber. *Am. J. Clin. Nutr.* 29:1461–1467.

31. D.G. Oakenfull and D.E. Fenwick (1978) Adsorption of bile salts from aqueous solution by plant fibre and cholestyramine. *Br. J. Nutr.* 40:299–309.

32. G.D. Calvert and R.A. Yeates (1982) Adsorption of bile salts by soya-bean flour, wheat bran, lucerne (*Medicago sativa*), sawdust and lignin; the effect of saponins and other plant constituents. *Br. J. Nutr.* 47:45–52.

33. S.E. Schwartz, R.A. Levine, A. Singh, J.R. Scheidecker, and N.S. Track (1982) Sustained pectin ingestion delays gastric emptying, *Gastroenterology* 83:812–817.

34. A.R. Leeds, N.R. Bolster, R. Andrews, A.S. Truswell (1979) Meal viscosity, gastric emptying and glucose absorption in the rat. *Proc. Nutr. Soc.* 38:44A.

35. K. Ebihara, R. Masuhara, S. Kiriyama, and M. Manabe (1981) Correlation between viscosity and plasma glucose- and insulin-flattening activities of pectins from vegetables and fruits in rats. *Nutr. Rep. Int.* 23:985–992.

36. D.J.A. Jenkins (1978) Action of dietary fiber in lowering fasting serum cholesterol and reducing postprandial glycemia: gastrointestinal mechanisms. In: *International Conference on Atherosclerosis* (L.A. Carlson, ed.), pp. 173–182, Raven Press, New York.

37. D.J.A. Jenkins, T.M.S. Wolever, A.R. Leeds, et al. (1978) Dietary fibres, fibre analogues and glucose tolerance: importance of viscosity, *Br. Med. J.* 1:1392–1394.

38. B.O. Schneeman and D. Gallaher (1986) Effects of dietary fiber on digestive enzymes. In: *Handbook of Dietary Fiber in Human Nutrition* (G.A. Spiller, ed.), pp. 305–312, CRC Press, Boca Raton, FL.

39. D. Gallaher and B.O. Schneeman (1986) Nutritional and metabolic response to plant inhibitors of digestive enzymes. In: *Advances in Experimental Medicine and Biology, vol. 199: Nutritional and Toxicological Significance of Enzyme Inhibitors in Foods* (M. Friedman, ed.), pp. 167–184, Plenum Press, New York.

40. D. Gallaher and B.O. Schneeman (1985) Effect of dietary cellulose on site of lipid absorption. *Am. J. Physiol.* 249:G184–G191.

41. D. Lairon, D. Lafont, J.L. Vigne, G. Nalbone, J. Leonardi, and J.C. Hauton (1985) Effects of dietary fibers and cholestyramine on the activity of pancreatic lipase in vitro. *Am. J. Clin. Nutr.* 42:629–638.

42. D. Lairon, P. Borel, E. Termine, R. Grataroli, C. Chabert, and J.C. Hauton (1985) Evidence for a proteinic inhibitor of pancreatic lipase in cereals, wheat bran and wheat germ, *Nutr. Rep. Int.* 32:1107–1113.

43. G. Isaksson, I. Lundquist, B. Akesson, and I. Ihse (1984) Effects of pectin and wheat bran on intraluminal pancreatic enzyme activities and on fat absorption as examined with the triolein breath test in patients with pancreatic insufficiency. *Scand. J. Gastroenterol.* 19:467–472.

44. G. Collier and K. O'Dea (1982) Effect of physical form of carbohydrate on the postprandial glucose, insulin and gastric inhibitory polypeptide responses in type 2 diabetes. *Am. J. Clin. Nutr.* 36:10–14.

45. P. Snow and K. O'Dea (1981) Factors affecting the rate of hydrolysis of starch in food. *Am. J. Clin. Nutr.* 34:2721–2727.

46. S. Wong and K. O'Dea (1983) Importance of physical form rather than viscosity in determining the rate of starch hydrolysis in legumes. *Am. J. Clin. Nutr.* 37:66–70.

47. B.O. Schneeman (1982) Pancreatic and digestive function. In: *Dietary Fiber in Health and Disease* (G.V. Vahouny and D. Kritchevsky, eds.), pp. 73–83, Plenum Press, New York.

48. A.S. Sandberg, A. Ahderinne, H. Andersson, B. Hallgren, and L. Hulten (1983) The effect of citrus pectin on the absorption of nutrients in the small intestine. *Hum. Nutr. Clin. Nutr.* 37C:171–183.

49. A.S. Sandberg, H. Andersson, B. Hallgren, K. Hasselblad, B. Isaksson, and L. Hulten (1981) Experimental model for in vivo determination of dietary fibre and its effect on the absorption of nutrients in the small intestine. *Br. J. Nutr.* 45:283–294.

50. B. Elsenhans, U. Sufke, R. Blume, and W.F. Caspary (1980) The influence of carbohydrate gelling agents on rat intestinal transport of monosaccharides and neutral amino acids in vitro. *Clin. Sci.* 59:373–380.

51. I.T. Johnson and J.M. Gee (1981) Effect of gel-forming gums on the intestinal unstirred layer and sugar transport in vitro. *Gut* 22:398–403.

52. G.V. Vahouny, S. Satchitanandam, I. Chen, et al. (1988) Dietary fiber and intestinal adaptation: effect on lipid absorption and lymphatic transport in the rat. *Am. J. Clin. Nutr.* 47:201–206.

53. G.V. Vahouny (1982) Dietary fibers and intestinal absorption of lipids. In: *Dietary Fiber in Health and Disease* (G.V. Vahouny and D. Kritchevsky, eds.), pp. 203–227, Plenum Press, New York.

54. LSRO (Life Sciences Research Office) (1987) *Physiological Effects and Health Consequences of Dietary Fiber* (S.M. Piltch, ed.), Federation of American Societies for Experimental Biology, Bethesda, MD.

55. A.L. Wu, S.B. Clark, and P.R. Holt (1980) Composition of lymph chylomicrons from proximal or distal rat small intestine. *Am. J. Clin. Nutr.* 33:582–589.

56. R.C. Spiller, I.F. Trotman, T.E. Adrian, S.R. Bloom, J.J. Misiewicz, and D.B.A. Silk (1988) Further characterization of the 'ileal brake' reflex in man: effect of ileal infusion of partial digests of fat, protein and starch on jejunal motility and release of neurotension, enteroglucagon and peptide YY. *Gut* 29:1042–1051.

57. S. Sigleo, M.J. Jackson, and G.V. Vahouny (1984) Effects of dietary fiber constituents on intestinal morphology and nutrient transport. *Am. J. Physiol.* 246:G34–G39.

58. L.R. Johnson (1988) Regulation of gastrointestinal mucosal growth. *Physiol. Rev.* 68:456–502.

59. G.A. Spiller (1986) Suggestions for a basis on which to determine a desirable intake of dietary fiber. In: *CRC Handbook of Dietary Fiber in Human Nutrition* (G.A. Spiller, ed.), pp. 281–283, CRC Press, Inc., Boca Raton, FL.

60. J.H. Cummings (1986) The effect of dietary fiber on fecal weight and composition. In: *CRC Handbook of Dietary Fiber in Human Nutrition* (G.A. Spiller, ed.), pp. 211–280, CRC Press, Inc. Boca Raton.

61. L.R. Jacobs and J.R. Lupton (1984) Effect of dietary fibers on rat large bowel mucosal growth and cell proliferation. *Am. J. Physiol.* 246:G378–385.

62. W.-J.L. Chen and J.W. Anderson (1984) Propionate may mediate the hypocholesterolemic effects of certain soluble plant fibers in cholesterol-fed rats. *Proc. Soc. Exp. Biol. Med.* 175:215–218.

63. J.H. Cummings and H.N. Englyst (1987) Fermentation in the human large intestine and the available substrate. *Am. J. Clin. Nutr.* 45:1243–1255.

64. S. Bingham (1987) Definitions and intakes of dietary fiber. *Am. J. Clin. Nutr.* 45:1226–1231.

65. U.S. Department of Agriculture (1979) *Food.* Home and Garden Bulletin no. 228, U.S. Government Printing Office, Washington, DC.

66. U.S. Departments of Agriculture and Health and Human Services (1985) *Nutrition and Your Health. Dietary Guidelines for Americans,* 2nd ed. Home and Garden Bulletin no. 232, U.S. Government Printing Office, Washington, DC.

Chapter 10

Herbert F. Janssen

Water

Introduction

In spite of its abundance on this planet, water is one of the most closely regulated compounds in most living organisms. The phylogenetic roots of the animal kingdom are deeply embedded in water. Perhaps this link is the key to the dependence upon water that is seen in most advanced animals. All mammals spend part of their life cycles in an aquatic environment. In man and most other terrestrial mammals a substantial portion of the homeostatic regulatory mechanisms are designed to maintain body fluid balance. Failure to maintain this balance can result in severe physiological abnormalities that can shorten or end life. This chapter will explore the physicochemical properties of water, the function of water in biological systems, water intake, water loss, pathological alterations that affect water balance, and the use of diuretics.

Physicochemical Properties of Water

The two hydrogen atoms and one oxygen atom that constitute water are arranged so that the molecule is an electric dipole. The two hydrogen atoms are separated at an angle of 105° and are covalently bound to the oxygen atom. This unique structural arrangement enables water to dissolve a wide variety of solutes and serve as the biological solvent.[1] In addition to its role as a solvent, water possesses several other characteristics beneficial to life on earth. The density of water is greatest at ~4 °C and decreases as temperature changes in either direction. As temperature decreases and ice forms, hydrogen bonding occurs between adjacent water molecules. This bonding produces an unusual lattice-like structure in ice and results in ice having a density less than water.[1] As a result, ice floats, thus allowing life to exist under the polar caps and in lakes covered by ice.

The rate of water evaporation at planetary temperatures is critical. The evaporation of water from our skin surface provides a cooling mechanism that allows us to survive at high ambient temperatures. From a meteorological standpoint, the evaporation of water from oceans provides the rains to replenish fresh-water lakes and supply moisture for croplands and forests.

The Function of Water in Biological Systems

The Role of Water in Human Physiology. Water comprises 60–70% of body weight in humans. The ratio is higher in adult males and lower in females. The percentage is also lower in obese individuals and decreases in normal individuals with advancing age.[2] Approximately two-thirds of the total body water is found in the intracellular compartment whereas the remaining one-third is found in the extracellular space. The extracellular space is composed of plasma, interstitial fluid, and a small transcellular fluid volume (Figure 1).

The concentration of solutes in body fluid varies substantially among the various compartments. For example, the concentration of protein is high in the intracellular compartment, lower in the plasma, and further reduced in the interstitial space. The extracellular compartment has a high concentration of sodium and a low concentration of potassium. The intracellular concentration of these ions is reversed. Active transport is required to maintain this difference in sodium and potassium concentration across the cell membrane. Failure of this active-transport system results in the movement of sodium into the cell, which produces an osmotic gradient that will attract water causing the cell to swell.

In addition to the effect of active transport on ion balance, the Donnan effect also influences the distribution of ions across a semipermeable membrane (Figure 2). This effect occurs if a nondiffusible

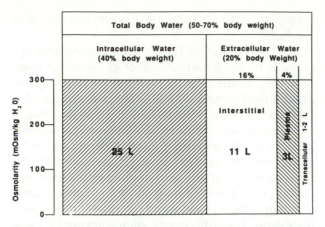

Figure 1. Distribution of water in a normal human. Approximately 60% of body weight results from total body water. Intracellular water volume is equal to ~40% of body weight whereas extracellular water is ~20% of body weight.

charged particle is trapped in one of the two compartments separated by a semipermeable membrane. The elevated protein concentration of the plasma in the interstitial space creates such a situation. The negative charge of the nondiffusible protein attracts positively charged diffusible ions. This attraction of the positively charged ions to the protein-rich compartment produces a further elevation in the number of effective osmotic particles in this space. The combined osmotic effect of the protein molecules and the diffusible ions displaced by the Donnan effect is referred to as oncotic pressure.[3]

If the osmolality and number of dissociable particles per molecule of the solution are known, osmotic pressure can be expressed in mm Hg using van't Hoff's equation.[1]

$$\Pi = n\mathrm{CRT} \qquad (1)$$

where Π is osmotic pressure, n is the number of dissociable particles per molecule, C is mol $\times$ kg H_2O^{-1}, R is gas constant (0.082 L ATM $\cdot$ °C^{-1} $\cdot$ mol^{-1}), and T is degrees Kelvin. A practical limitation of this procedure arises because protein concentration and protein molecular weight are frequently unknown. Fortunately, the effective oncotic pressure can be estimated experimentally in the laboratory.

The osmotic pressure exerted by a 1 mol/kg H_2O solution at body temperature is equal to the pressure achieved when 1 mol of an ideal gas is compressed to a volume of 1 L and the temperature is adjusted to body temperature [i.e., (22.4 L/mol) $\times$ 760 mm Hg $\times$ (310 °K/273 °K)]. From this calculation it can be seen that a nondissociated compound in solution at a concentration of 1 mmol/L H_2O will exert a pressure of 19.3 mm Hg. If the compound dissociates in solution, the increase in particle number also must

be considered, because this increase will produce an increase in the osmotic pressure proportional to the number of particles formed by the dissociation.

Movement of Water Across Membranes in Biological Systems. The active transport of water across biological membranes has been discounted by most investigators; however, a few contend that it has not been disproven in all invertebrate species.[4] In mammals it is widely accepted that water movement occurs across membranes as the result of osmotic gradients and/or differences in hydraulic pressures. (In this chapter blood pressure will be referred to as hydraulic instead of hydrostatic. Hydrostatic indicates that blood is static or not moving, which is an obvious misnomer.) An important step in proving this relationship was provided by Starling[5] at the turn of the century. He demonstrated the existence of a colloid osmotic force in plasma that attracts water from surrounding spaces. This outstanding work led to the development of the Starling equilibrium equation.

$$Q = K_f[(P_c - P_t) - (\Pi_c - \Pi_t)] \qquad (2)$$

where Q is fluid exchange across the capillary, K_f is the permeability coefficient, P_c is hydraulic pressure in the capillary, P_t is hydraulic pressure in the tissue, Π_c is oncotic pressure in the capillary, and Π_t is oncotic pressure in the tissue. This equation describes fluid flux across capillaries as a balance in hydraulic and oncotic forces.

Although investigators disagree as to the actual values for hydraulic and oncotic pressure at the capillary level, it is agreed that fluid movement from the arterial end of the capillary into the interstitial space occurs primarily because hydraulic pressure from the heart exceeds plasma oncotic pressure. As the blood flows through the capillary, its hydraulic pressure decreases as a result of resistance to flow in the capillary. On the venous end of the capillary, plasma oncotic pressure exceeds hydraulic pressure and, thus, most of the filtered water is reabsorbed into the circulation.[3] The lymphatic system removes the small volume of water (and protein) that remains behind in the interstitial space and helps to maintain the balance in interstitial fluid volume and concentration. Figure 3 illustrates the movement of fluid across a capillary.

The values listed for each of the forces are only estimates and should not be considered to represent actual values. Alterations in the movement of fluid across the capillary can occur because of a number of factors. Tissue edema will occur if the volume of fluid that remains in the interstitial space exceeds the amount that can be removed by the lymphatic system. This can occur as a result of increased capillary permeability, increased capillary hydraulic pressure, decreased plasma oncotic pressure, or a malfunction

Donnan's Equilibrium

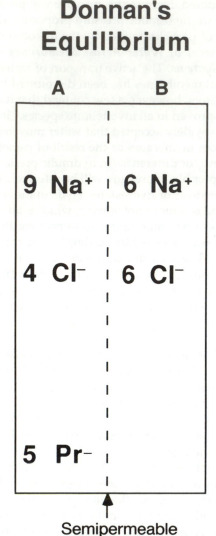

Figure 2. Distribution of diffusible sodium and chloride ions in two compartments separated by a semipermeable membrane. One of the two compartments contains a negatively charged nondiffusible protein. The number of positive and negative charges in compartment A are equal, the number of positive and negative charges in compartment B are equal, and the number of diffusible ions in the compartment containing the nondiffusible protein (A) is greater than in the opposite compartment (B).

in the lymphatic drainage system.[6] All edematous conditions can be explained by an inappropriate shift in the Starling equation.

Water Intake

Regulation of Thirst. In the normal human, water intake is usually controlled by thirst. Thirst is defined as a conscious awareness of the desire for water. Although this mechanism can be overridden by social influences, thirst remains the primary mechanism of supplying water that is not consumed with food products.

The main stimulant for the drinking response appears to be the hypertonicity of extracellular fluid. In healthy adults an increase of only 2–3% in extracellular fluid osmolarity will produce a strong desire for water.[7] The osmoreceptors that detect this change in plasma osmolarity are located in the hypothalamus and can be stimulated by either dehydration or by the infusion of hypertonic saline. Interestingly, the infusion of hypertonic urea or glucose does not produce a similar thirst stimulation. In addition to plasma osmolarity, hypovolemia and hypotension also stimulate thirst. These dipsogenic stimuli are not as strong as those produced by plasma osmolarity.[7] However, they may play a significant physiological role in the appropriate setting. The mechanisms through which hypovolemia and hypotension produce their response are not clearly understood; however, they appear to parallel those required for the release of vasopressin (antidiuretic hormone—ADH).

Thirst can be stimulated experimentally by the introduction of ADH into the circulation or into the cerebral spinal fluid. This is interesting from an experimental standpoint but may be insignificant as a normal physiological control mechanism because animals incapable of producing ADH continue to exhibit a normal dipsogenic response.[7]

Water from Food Metabolism. Metabolic water refers to water gained from the metabolism of food. The volume of water gained in this fashion varies with the type of food being metabolized. The metabolism of 1 g protein yields 0.39 g water; of 1 g starch, 0.56 g water; and of 1 g fat, 1.07 g water. In spite of the larger volume produced by fat metabolism, starch often supplies a larger amount of metabolic water because of the abundance of starch in most diets.[8] In humans, metabolic water is usually of little consequence and constitutes only a minimal amount of our daily water needs. However, some desert rodents are capable of surviving totally on metabolic water. Obviously, survival is possible only if the animal possesses a very effective renal concentrating mechanism.

Water Loss

Extrarenal Water Loss in Humans. Loss of water can occur through several mechanisms. Insensible water loss refers to the volume of water that is lost with expiration and from evaporation of skin surface water. In an inactive person at room temperature, this water loss may be <1 mL/min. As the person's activity and the ambient temperature increase, the insensible water loss will increase greatly and under extreme conditions can reach 20–25 L/d.[7] Such con-

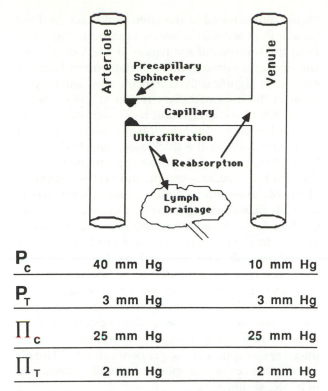

P_c	40 mm Hg	10 mm Hg
P_T	3 mm Hg	3 mm Hg
Π_c	25 mm Hg	25 mm Hg
Π_T	2 mm Hg	2 mm Hg

Figure 3. Movement of water in a typical capillary. The movement of water across the capillary membrane can be determined on the basis of the Starling equilibrium equation. On the arterial side of the capillary, hydraulic pressure (P_C) is great enough to cause the movement of fluid out of the capillary into the interstitial space. On the venous side of the capillary, P_C has decreased and water is reabsorbed into the capillary because of the force exerted by the capillary oncotic pressure (Π_C).

ditions can be tolerated only for short periods and only if adequate water replacement can be achieved.

Water lost through the gastrointestinal tract is normally low; however, vomiting and diarrhea can increase water loss immensely. In addition to severe dehydration, vomiting can produce substantial electrolyte and acid-base abnormalities by removing stomach secretions from the system.[9] Diarrhea has been reported to produce fluid loss as high as 1 L/h. It can also result in significant potassium and bicarbonate ion depletion. Hypernatremia or hyponatremia can occur depending upon the stimulus that produced the diarrhea.[9] Failure to correct these situations can be life threatening.

● *Renal Excretion of Water.* With the exception of the kidney in birds and the Malpighian tubule in insects, mammals have the only kidney capable of excreting a hypertonic urine.[4] The mammalian kidney serves as the main regulatory organ for the balance of body water. This unique kidney has enabled mammals to inhabit fresh- and salt-water environments as well as extremely arid regions of the earth. Life in extreme environmental conditions can fre-

quently be correlated with structural differences in the kidney. For example, the beaver, which spends most of its life in a fresh-water environment, can excrete copious amounts of dilute urine but has not retained the ability to produce a highly concentrated urine of low volume.[10] In contrast, the arid-adapted kangaroo rat and Australian hopping mouse can produce urine with a concentration exceeding plasma osmolarity 10-fold and 26-fold, respectively.[11] The mechanisms used by marine mammals to maintain water balance are not fully understood. In marine mammals that have been studied, it appears that plasma osmolarity is maintained at ~300 mmol, which is 700 mmol less than the surrounding ocean water. Marine mammals such as seals apparently do not drink ocean water but gain needed water from the fish in their diets.[8]

Salt water teleosts maintain plasma osmolarity in the range of 350–450 mmol. These animals apparently drink large volumes of seawater to replace the body fluid lost to the hypertonic environment. Removal of the unwanted salt ingested with the sea water is accomplished through renal mechanisms and active transport of the salt from the blood into the surrounding water by the gills. Extrarenal salt transport mechanisms also have been identified in the nasal glands of several species of marine birds.[8]

In the mammalian kidney water enters the renal tubules as an ultrafiltrate of plasma in the glomerulus. The same forces responsible for the filtration of water in a peripheral capillary produce the ultrafiltrate of plasma in the kidney; however, the value of each force is substantially different from that occurring in the peripheral capillary (Figure 4).

The glomerular capillary allows the free passage of small-molecular-weight compounds while almost totally restricting the movement of plasma proteins. Because of this low permeability to protein and the rapid removal of water from plasma in the glomerulus, the oncotic pressure of the plasma increases substantially as plasma passes through the glomerular capillary. Although unproven in the human, the increase in plasma oncotic pressure may reach a balance with the hydraulic forces near the end of the glomerular capillary (Figure 5). The site in the capillary where this theoretical balance occurs is referred to as the site of filtration equilibrium.[12] If the renal vein is ligated, the entire glomerular capillary will reach a state of filtration equilibrium, and the formation of an ultrafiltrate in the glomerulus will cease.[13]

The rate at which the ultrafiltrate of plasma enters Bowman's space is referred to as the glomerular filtration rate (GFR). In a normal human, GFR is ~100–120 mL/min or 180 L/d. This rate of glomerular filtration is closely maintained over the normal range

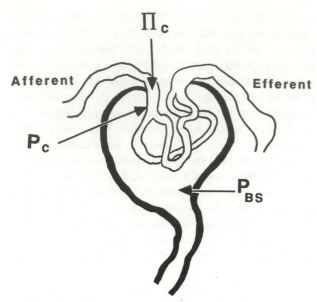

Π_C

Afferent   Efferent

P_C

P_{BS}

Figure 4. A glomerulus. The formation of an ultrafiltrate of plasma in the glomerulus is favored by the hydraulic pressure in the glomerulus (P_C) and opposed by the oncotic pressure in the capillary (Π_C) and by the hydraulic pressure in Bowman's space (P_{BS}). Unlike the situation in a typical capillary bed (Figure 3) P_C does not decrease along the length of the capillary and Π_C increases.

of blood pressure by a yet uncharacterized method of autoregulation.[14] Compensatory dilation or constriction of the afferent and/or efferent arteriole is accomplished to maintain renal blood flow and GFR at a constant value between the blood pressures of 80 and 160 mL/mm Hg.

Approximately two-thirds of the water filtered in the glomerulus is reabsorbed as the fluid passes through the proximal tubule. This water reabsorption is closely linked to the reabsorption of sodium but is also influenced by the peritubular capillary oncotic pressure and the hydraulic pressure existing in the interstitial space surrounding the proximal tubule. In the proximal tubule water reabsorption is said to be isosmotic, because the osmolality of the tubular fluid does not change appreciably. This lack of change occurs because proportionately equal amounts of water and solute are reabsorbed from the tubule into the peritubular capillary.[15]

Water leaving the proximal tubule and entering the descending limb of the loop of Henle is apparently isosmotic with plasma. As fluid moves down the loop, water is removed from the tubule as a result of osmotic forces existing in the intramedullary region of the kidney. This hyperosmotic interstitium is developed by the active transport of sodium chloride from the thick ascending limb of the loop. The ascending limb has a low water permeability, and water does not follow the sodium that is reabsorbed in this section of the tubule. As a result sodium becomes

highly concentrated in the interstitial space, and the tubular fluid becomes dilute as it returns to the cortex from the intramedullary region of the kidney. The countercurrent arrangement of the loop of Henle is capable of significantly enhancing the osmotic gradient in the intramedullary region of the kidney.[15] The ability to accomplish this task is dependent upon (1) the length of the loop, (2) the maintenance of active transport in the thick ascending limb of the loop, (3) the maintenance of an appropriate flow rate through the tubular segment, and (4) the impermeability of the ascending limb to water. Approximately 25% of all sodium reabsorption occurs in the ascending limb. In addition, significant amounts of several divalent cations are reabsorbed in the thick ascending limb. The driving force for the divalent ion reabsorption is provided by the positive charge that develops in the lumen as a result of passive potassium backflow. A decrease in the active transport mechanism in the thick ascending limb will lead to diuresis, reduced reabsorption of sodium, and reduced reabsorption of the divalent cations.[15] The effect of diuretics on this mechanism will be discussed in a later section.

In the distal portion of the nephron, water reabsorption is almost totally dependent upon the presence of ADH. In the presence of ADH, the cortical regions of the distal nephron become permeable to water whereas the intramedullary regions of the collecting duct become permeable to both water and urea.[16] Water reabsorption from the collecting duct into the interstitial space occurs as a result of the osmotic concentration developed by the loop of Henle mechanisms described earlier. The reabsorption of water from the cortical collecting duct into the interstitial space produces an increased concentration of urea in the tubular fluid. As this tubular fluid moves into the intramedullary regions of the kidney, the increased permeability of the tubular lumen to urea coupled with the elevated urea concentration of the tubular fluid enhances the reabsorption of urea into the interstitial space. In states of antidiuresis (abundant ADH present) urea contributes 40–50% of the intramedullary osmotic gradient.[15] This elevated osmotic gradient continues to contribute to the movement of water from the collecting duct, and in humans the final urine osmolarity can reach 1200–1400 mmol.

Water reabsorbed from the thin descending limb of the loop of Henle and from the collecting duct is returned to the renal circulation by the vasa recta. The vasa recta is an extension of the peritubular capillary network that reaches into the intramedullary region of the kidney along with the loop of Henle. Unlike the loop, the vasa recta does not exhibit the ability to reabsorb or secrete solutes by active trans-

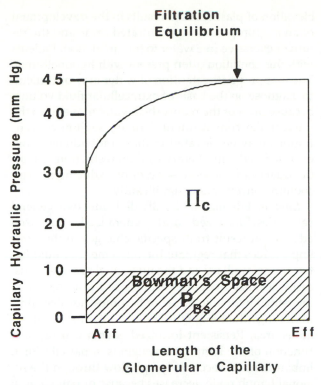

Filtration Equilibrium

Figure 5. Oncotic and hydraulic pressures that influence the movement of water across the glomerular capillary. The capillary hydrostatic pressure (Π_C) entering the glomerulus is thought to be ~45 mm Hg and does not decrease along the length of the glomerular capillary because of the relatively large cross-sectional area. P_{Bs} is the hydraulic pressure in Bowman's space and is considered to be 10 mm Hg. Because the glomerular capillary rapidly filters water while retaining virtually all plasma proteins, the oncotic pressure of the plasma increases as it moves along the length of the glomerular capillary. If enough water is removed from the plasma in the glomerulus, the oncotic pressure of the plasma will increase to a level sufficient to restrict additional water movement (known as filtration equilibrium).

port. Although attempts have been made to explain mechanisms of water reabsorption in the vasa recta, only a limited amount of experimental data is available. Several mathematical models were proposed to explain the function of the vasa recta; however, none has been universally accepted.[17]

Free-water Excretion. Free-water excretion refers to the volume of water that must be added to or removed from the excreted urine to make it isosmotic with plasma. Free-water clearance is calculated using equation 3.

$$C_{H_2O} = V - \frac{U_{Osm}V}{P_{Osm}} \qquad (3)$$

where C_{H_2O} is free-water clearance, V is urine flow per minute, U_{Osm} is urine osmolality, and P_{Osm} is plasma osmolality.

A negative free-water clearance indicates that a concentrated urine is being formed, and if other factors are constant, plasma osmolarity should decrease. A positive value indicates a dilute urine and increasing plasma osmolality. The free-water clearance value is expressed in mL/min and is indicative of the rate at which the plasma osmolarity will change. Physicians can use this value to determine the rate at which intravenous fluids should be given to a patient.

Regulation of Water Excretion in the Kidney. The regulation of water excretion in the kidney is controlled primarily by hormones. In the glomerulus autoregulation of glomerular filtration rate apparently is controlled by an interaction of prostaglandins and angiotensin II. Experimental evidence indicated an involvement of both hormones in the control of vascular resistance in the afferent and efferent arterioles. The release of these hormones can be stimulated by changes in renal perfusion pressure as well as through alterations in the fluid moving through the region of the distal tubule containing the macula densa cells. The kidney uses the latter mechanism to closely control renal blood flow and glomerular filtration rate. Although all investigators do not agree on the exact mechanism, the macula densa cells apparently detect changes in the distal tubular flow of sodium or sodium chloride or shifts in tubular fluid osmolarity. In response, the macula densa cells trigger the release of renin from the juxtaglomerular cells, which in turn produces the desired changes in renal blood flow and glomerular filtration rate.[18] Quite likely, prostaglandins play a role in the autoregulatory process either directly or by modulating the effect of angiotensin II.

The reabsorption of water in the distal nephron is controlled hormonally by ADH. An increase in extracellular fluid osmolality is the primary stimulus for the release of ADH. Secondary stimuli for ADH release are hypovolemia, hypotension, and circulating angiotensin II. Individually or in combination, these stimuli provoke a release of ADH from the posterior pituitary into the circulation.[7] The hormone is then carried through the circulation to the distal nephron, where it acts through cyclic AMP to increase water permeability in both the cortical and medullary collecting ducts and urea permeability in the medullary collecting duct. This increase in permeability allows the reabsorption of water from the collecting duct into the interstitial space, where it can be returned to the circulation via the vasa recta.

Aldosterone is released from the adrenal cortex in response to angiotensin II and alterations in plasma potassium levels and, to a lesser degree, in response to plasma sodium concentration and ACTH. In the distal nephron aldosterone has been reported to increase the luminal membrane permeability to both sodium and potassium, increase the production of

ATP, and stimulate sodium-potassium ATPase.[15] These effects increase potassium secretion and sodium reabsorption. Unless ADH is specifically blocked, water will follow the reabsorption of sodium, thus allowing aldosterone to increase total body content of both sodium and water. Although this hormone can lower plasma potassium concentration, it will not alter plasma sodium concentration under normal conditions. The increase in total body sodium that occurs as a result of aldosterone is prevented from elevating plasma sodium concentration by the influx of water that dilutes the reabsorbed sodium. An effect of aldosterone on plasma sodium concentration can occur only if ADH is inhibited and water cannot follow the reabsorbed sodium.

Pathological Alterations That Affect Water Balance

Suppressed ADH Secretion or Action. Neurogenic or nephrogenic diabetes insipidus can increase urinary volume by altering the control ADH normally maintains over water homostasis. Neurogenic diabetes insipidus results from a deficiency in ADH secretion. The problem can result from surgical or accidental trauma, tumors, infection, or other pathological conditions that destroy the production, transport, or storage of ADH. Additionally, damage to the receptor area of the hypothalamus also will result in a decreased release of ADH. A congenital defect in ADH release has been reported; this condition is transmitted on an autosomal dominant gene.[7]

Nephrogenic diabetes insipidus occurs when the kidney cannot respond to circulating ADH. The exact mechanism responsible for this insensitivity to ADH is uncertain. Anatomical and histological alterations that occur in these kidneys may be the result rather than the cause of diabetes insipidus. In addition to induced nephrogenic diabetes insipidus, the condition also can be transmitted genetically as an X-linked recessive trait.[7]

Patients with diabetes insipidus demonstrate a notable increase in urine volume and a decrease in urine osmolality. Plasma osmolality often rises in these patients as a result of increased urinary free water. This increase in plasma osmolality results in an increase in the thirst mechanism and induces polydipsia. The increased water intake restores balance between intake and output, but plasma osmolality usually stays elevated at a level that closely approximates the osmotic stimulus for thirst.[7]

Syndrome of Inappropriate ADH Secretion (SIADH). Clinical disorders associated with SIADH occur when ADH is released in excessive amounts independent of an appropriate stimulus. Continued elevation of plasma ADH results in the development of an inappropriately concentrated urine and the return of excessive free water to the circulation. Patients with this condition often present with hyponatremia. The inappropriate retention of water may be difficult to diagnose on the basis of extracellular fluid volume because most of the reabsorbed water moves into the intracellular compartment. Urinary sodium concentrations may be elevated in these individuals; however, if faced with dietary sodium restriction, the individuals can conserve sodium by reducing urinary sodium concentration significantly.[7]

Edema. Edema can be divided into two general categories, localized and generalized. Localized edema can result from specific changes in the Starling's forces that regulate the movement of fluid between the capillary and the interstitial space. In most cases, localized edema becomes self-limiting when interstitial hydraulic pressure becomes elevated, thus inhibiting additional fluid movement into the edematous area. Persistent localized edema can result if function of the lymphatic system is impaired.[6] Such impairment can occur if lymph flow through the regional lymph node decreases because of pathological reasons or if the lymph node is removed surgically to prevent the spread of cancer cells.

Generalized edema can result from a number of pathological conditions. Failure of the kidneys, liver, or heart are some of the most common. In elderly individuals congestive heart failure is an important cause of body fluid retention and can result in edema, which is most frequently observed in the dependent limbs. Clinical treatment of this condition is accomplished by cardiac stimulants and diuretic compounds.[19] Unfortunately, renal and liver failure are usually not so easily treated and may require more heroic measures.

Diuretics

Physicians frequently use diuretics to increase the urinary excretion of water. The mechanism and site of action for the various diuretics vary substantially. With the exception of osmotic diuretics, there are four sites where the diuretic effect of the compound can be expressed. These sites include (*1*) the proximal tubule, (2) the thick ascending limb of the loop of Henle, (3) the distal tubule, and (4) the collecting duct.[19]

Osmotic diuretic compounds produce their effect along the length of the nephron at any site where water reabsorption can occur. Compounds that enter the renal tubule and are not reabsorbed will produce an osmotic diuretic effect. Examples of such compounds include glucose excreted in the urine and mannitol. As the osmotic diuretic is excreted, it carries with it an obligatory volume of water, thus reducing the water that can be reabsorbed.

Diuretics that inhibit carbonic anhydrase produce their effect in the proximal tubule by decreasing the reabsorption of sodium and the obligatory water that normally follows. These diuretics receive limited use because they can produce metabolic acidosis as a result of excessive bicarbonate loss in the urine.

The most potent diuresis can be produced by compounds that decrease active sodium chloride reabsorption in the thick ascending limb of the loop of Henle. Blockade of this active-transport mechanism leads to a reduction in the intramedullary osmotic gradient. This reduced intramedullary osmotic gradient in turn decreases water reabsorption from the thin descending limb of the loop of Henle and from the collecting duct. When the diuretic effect is fully expressed, the final urine osmolality will approach that of plasma, and water reabsorption occurs only as a result of obligatory water movement in response to solute reabsorption.

Thiazide diuretics interfere with active sodium reabsorption in the distal tubule, thereby reducing the obligatory water reabsorption that normally follows sodium reabsorbed in this section of the nephron. The relative potency of these diuretics is less than loop diuretics because only 5–10% of filtered sodium is normally reabsorbed in the distal tubule.

Potassium-sparing diuretics alter the transport of sodium and potassium in the cortical collecting duct. One group of these diuretics blocks the effect of aldosterone by competitive inhibition. Other potassium-sparing diuretics decrease sodium reabsorption by reducing the luminal entry of sodium into the tubular cell or by altering sodium reabsorption through other means. The potassium-sparing characteristics of these compounds are produced by directly altering the membrane permeability to potassium or by preventing the development of a negative electrical potential in the tubular lumen.[19]

With the exception of potassium-sparing diuretics, most diuretics increase the urinary excretion of potassium and can severely deplete body potassium if used for an extended period. The increased potassium excretion occurs because of increased sodium delivery to the distal nephron and increased flow rate of fluid through this section of the nephron. In the distal nephron potassium is normally secreted into the tubular lumen to replace the positively charged sodium that is reabsorbed. The increased distal delivery of sodium increases sodium reabsorption at this site and thus stimulates potassium secretion. The increased tubular flow rate speeds the removal of the potassium excreted into the distal nephron, which increases the gradient for additional potassium secretion. When

used separately or in combination with other diuretics, potassium-sparing diuretics help to prevent potassium depletion by blocking the sodium-potassium exchange. Patients receiving this combined drug therapy or dietary potassium supplements must be managed properly to insure that the severe side effects of potassium imbalance are prevented.

References

1. C.L. Prosser, ed. (1973) *Comparative Animal Physiology*, W.B. Saunders, Philadelphia.
2. D.D. Fanestil (1987) Compartmentation of body water. In: *Clinical Disorders of Fluid and Electrolyte Metabolism* (M.H. Maxwell, C.R. Kleeman, and R.G. Narins, eds.), pp. 5–10, McGraw-Hill, New York.
3. H. Valtin (1983) *Renal Function; Mechanisms Preserving Fluid and Solute Balance in Health*, Little, Brown and Co., Boston.
4. R. Eckert, D. Randall, and G. Augustine (1988) *Animal Physiology: Mechanisms and Adaptations*, 3rd ed., W.H. Freeman & Co., New York.
5. E.H. Starling (1899) The glomerular functions of the kidney. *J. Physiol. (Lond.)* 24:317–330.
6. A.C. Guyton (1986) *Textbook of Medical Physiology*, W.B. Saunders, Philadelphia.
7. G.L. Robertson and T. Berl (1986) Water Metabolism. In: *The Kidney*, vol. I (B.M. Brenner and F.C. Rector, Jr., eds.), pp. 385–432, W.B. Saunders, Philadelphia.
8. K. Schmidt-Nielsen (1983) *Animal Physiology: Adaptation and Environment*, 3rd ed., Cambridge University Press, Cambridge.
9. J.M. Weinberg (1986) Fluid and electrolyte disorders and gastrointestinal diseases. In: *Fluids and Electrolytes* (J.P. Kokko and R.L. Tannen, eds.), pp. 742–759, W.B. Saunders, Philadelphia.
10. B. Schmidt-Nielsen and R. O'Dell (1961) Structure and concentrating mechanism in the mammalian kidney. *Am. J. Physiol.* 200: 1119–1124.
11. R.E. MacMillian and A.K. Lee (1967) Australian desert mice: independence of exogenous water. *Science* 158:383–385.
12. L.D. Dworkin and B.M. Brenner (1985) Biophysical basis of glomerular filtration. In: *The Kidney: Physiology and Pathophysiology*, vol. 1 (D.W. Seldin and G. Giebisch, eds.), pp. 397–426, Raven Press, New York.
13. A.N. Richards (1920–21) Kidney function. *Harvey Lect.* 16:163–187.
14. F.S. Wright (1981) Feedback control of glomerular filtration rate: a symposium. *Fed. Proc.* 40:77–115.
15. M.B. Burg (1986) Renal handling of sodium, chloride, water, amino acids and glucose. In: *The Kidney*, 3rd ed., vol. I (B.M. Brenner and F.C. Rector, Jr., eds.), pp. 145–175, W.B. Saunders, Philadelphia.
16. J.P. Kokko and F.C. Rector, Jr. (1972) Countercurrent multiplication system without active transport in inner medulla. *Kidney Int.* 2: 214–223.
17. D.R. Roy and R.L. Jamison (1985) Countercurrent system and its regulation. In: *The Kidney: Physiology and Pathophysiology*, vol. I (D.W. Seldin and G. Giebisch, eds.), pp. 903–932, Raven Press, New York.
18. J. Schnermann and J. Biggs (1985) Function of the juxtaglomerular apparatus: local control of glomerular hemodynamics. In: *The Kidney: Physiology and Pathophysiology*, vol. I (D.W. Seldin and G. Giebisch, eds.), pp. 669–698, Raven Press, New York.
19. B.E. Berger and D.G. Warnock (1986) Clinical uses and mechanisms of action of diuretic agents. In: *The Kidney*, 3rd ed., vol. I (B.M. Brenner and F.C. Rector, Jr., eds.), pp. 433–455, W.B. Saunders, Philadelphia.

11   James A. Olson

··

Vitamin A

Night blindness and some eye disorders, which were well recognized in ancient Egypt, were treated by the topical application of juice squeezed from cooked liver or by prescribing liver in the diet. This medical lore was lost over the centuries, and night blindness, called "this curious and obscure disease" by R.J. Hicks, a surgeon serving with the Confederate army in the American Civil War, plagued armies throughout the world in the nineteenth century.[1] The active principle of liver in treating eye disease was vitamin A, which was identified as a necessary fat-soluble factor for rat growth in 1914 and was structurally elucidated in 1930. The biological conversion of β-carotene into vitamin A was shown the same year. These early studies on vitamin A are well reviewed in Moore's fine treatise.[2]

Chemistry and Nomenclature

The parent compound in the vitamin A group is called all-*trans* retinol (Figure 1A).[3] Its aldehyde and acid forms are retinal (Figure 1B) and retinoic acid (Figure 1C). The active form of vitamin A in vision is 11-*cis* retinal (Figure 1D), and a therapeutically useful form (accutane, isotretinoin) is 13-*cis* retinoic acid (Figure 1E). Retinyl palmitate (Figure 1F) is a major storage form, and retinoyl β-glucuronide is a biologically active, water-soluble metabolite (Figure 1G). A synthetic aromatic analog (etretin), which has therapeutic usefulness, is depicted in Figure 1H. Finally, β-carotene, a major provitamin A carotenoid is shown in Figure 1I.

In a nutritional sense the vitamin A family includes all naturally occurring compounds with the biological activity of retinol. Because provitamin A carotenoids are nutritionally active, they are included in the vitamin A family. Only 50 of approximately 600 carotenoids found in nature, however, are converted into vitamin A. On the other hand, most carotenoids,

including those with provitamin A activity, also can serve as singlet oxygen quenchers and as antioxidants under certain conditions. These characteristics are not possessed by retinol. Thus, in considering the biological actions of carotenoids, it is important to differentiate between provitamin A activity and other possible effects.

Retinoids are a class of chemical substances possessing many of the structural features of vitamin A and, in particular, the extensive system of conjugated double bonds in vitamin A. Approximately 2500 retinoids have been synthesized chemically, and many have been tested for their therapeutic efficacy against neoplasms and skin disorders. Etretin (Figure 1H) is a member of this class of substances. The vitamin A family, excluding provitamin A carotenoids, are a chemical subclass of the retinoids. Although the term *retinoid* was coined in the framework of therapeutic utility, retinoid now is used generally as a generic term in both biological and clinical contexts, e.g., retinoid-binding proteins, retinoid toxicity. Because vitamin A is important in small amounts in nutrition and retinoids are useful in large doses in treating certain clinical conditions, care must also be taken in differentiating between their nutritional and pharmacological effects.

Methods of Analysis

Because of its conjugated system of double bonds, vitamin A absorbs blue light very well. Thus, the maximal absorption wavelengths and molecular extinction coefficients in ethanol are 325 nm (ϵ 52,480) for all-*trans* retinol, 381 nm (ϵ 43,400) for all-*trans* retinal, and 350 nm (ϵ 45,200) for all-*trans* retinoic acid.[4] *Cis* isomers absorb less strongly at somewhat lower wavelengths. Carotenoids tend to show triple maxima, e.g., all-*trans* β-carotene shows maximal absorption in ethanol at 453 nm (ϵ 140,700) with a

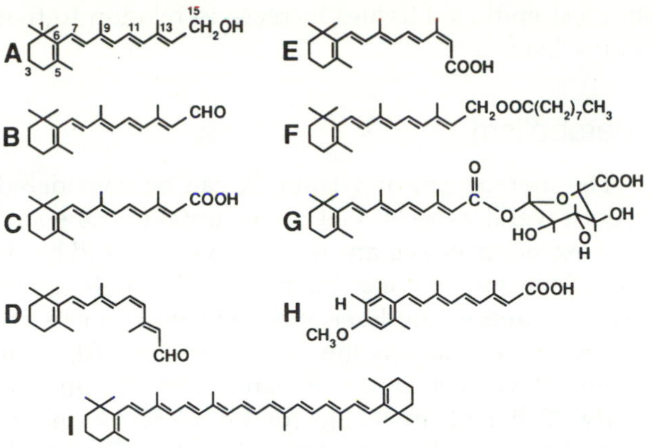

Figure 1. Formulas of major retinoids and of β-carotene. A, all-trans retinol; B, all-trans retinal; C, all-trans retinoic acid; D, 11-cis retinal; E, 13-cis retinoic acid; F, all-trans retinyl palmitate; G, all-trans retinoyl β-glucuronide; H, the trimethyl methoxyphenol analog of all-trans retinoic acid (etretin, acitretin); I, all-trans β-carotene.

shoulder at 427 nm and a secondary peak at 477 nm.[5] These spectroscopic properties primarily are used in quantitating vitamin A and carotenoids in tissues and in pharmaceutical preparations. Although many chromatographic systems are available for separating vitamin A and carotenoids, the most commonly used procedure is high-pressure liquid chromatography (HPLC). Straight-phase, reverse-phase, isocratic, and gradient HPLC systems are used for specific needs.[6–11] A very rapid procedure exists for measuring holo-RBP in blood.[12] Mass spectrometry is used both for the characterization and for the quantitation of retinoids.[13,14] Many other analytical procedures, including fluorescence and colorimetric assays, also are employed.[15]

To assess a marginal status of vitamin A nutriture, the relative dose response (RDR),[16] the modified relative dose response (MRDR),[17] and the conjunctival impression cytology (CIC) assay[18] have proven to be useful. For assessing clinical deficiency various stages of xerophthalmia, night blindness, and low serum retinol values (<0.35 μmol/L) are used effectively.[19] The concentration of vitamin A in tears, which is low in vitamin A–depleted children, increases significantly in response to a dose of vitamin A.[20] In the future, tear analysis also may prove to be of help in assessing vitamin A status.

Absorption, Transport, and Storage

Preformed vitamin A in foods is present largely as retinyl ester. During proteolytic digestion in the stomach, retinyl ester and provitamin A carotenoids are released from foods and aggregate together with other lipids. In the small intestine, because of the combined action of bile and pancreatic esterases, esters of retinol and carotenols (xanthophylls) are hydrolyzed. Together with hydrocarbon carotenoids, retinol and carotenols are transported in micellar form across the plasmalemma of the absorptive epithelial cells of the intestinal villus.[21,22]

The absorption efficiency of dietary vitamin A in healthy persons who ingest significant amounts of fat (>10 g/d) is >80%. Dietary carotenoids (in the range of 1–3 mg) are absorbed approximately half as well as vitamin A. As the amount of carotenoids in the diet increases, however, the absorption efficiency decreases.[23] The intestinal absorption of carotenoids is much more critically dependent on the presence of bile salts than is that of vitamin A.[21,22]

The major pathway for the conversion of β-carotene and other provitamin A carotenoids into vitamin A is by oxidative cleavage of the central 15,15' double bond.[24] In some plants and microorganisms, excentric cleavage of carotenoids also occurs to yield β-apo carotenoids, which in turn can be converted into vitamin A.[24] Whether excentric cleavage also occurs to some extent in mammals is still unclear.

Within the intestinal epithelia the retinal produced by carotenoid cleavage presumably is bound to a cellular retinoid binding protein, CRBP Type II.[25] Bound retinal then is reduced to bound retinol, which is then esterified both by transacylation from the α-position of lecithin[26] and from acyl-coenzyme A.[21] The resultant retinyl ester, together with a small amount of unesterified retinol, hydrocarbon carotenoids, and xanthophylls, then is incorporated into chylomicra that are released into the lymph. The triacylglycerols of chylomicra are hydrolyzed rapidly by plasma lipoprotein lipase, leaving chylomicron remnants with associated carotenoids and vitamin A. These remnants are taken up mainly by parenchymal cells of the liver and, presumably, to some degree by other tissues.

In the fasting state both vitamin A and carotenoids circulate in the plasma. The major form of circulating vitamin A is holo-retinol-binding protein (holo-RBP), which consists of a 1:1 complex of all-trans retinol with RBP (molecular weight 21,000). The plasma concentration of holo-RBP, which is synthesized and released from parenchymal cells, is homeostatically controlled by mechanisms that are not well defined. Only when liver reserves of vitamin A are nearly depleted do plasma concentrations of retinol decrease significantly.[27] Other endogenous compounds of vitamin A that circulate in the plasma, albeit at much lower concentrations, are retinyl ester, retinoic acid, retinyl β-glucuronide, and retinoyl β-glucuronide.[28,29] Little is known about the regulation of these components in plasma or about their modes of uptake by cells.

Major plasma carotenoids include lutein, lycopene, canthaxanthin, α-carotene, and β-carotene as well as traces of other species.[30] The hydrocarbon carotenoids are associated primarily with low-density lipoproteins (LDL), whereas the xanthophylls are distributed more evenly among LDL and high-density lipoproteins (HDL).[30] Of total plasma carotenoids, β-carotene usually comprises 15–30%. Unlike the plasma concentration of holo-RBP, both the total carotenoid concentration in plasma and the relative amounts of individual components are dependent on the ingested diet.

Vitamin A is very well stored in the body, with >90% of the total being found in the liver of well-nourished individuals. Two major cell types are involved in storage: the parenchymal cells and the stellate cells. The parenchymal cells, which are the predominant cell type of liver, contain very small amounts of retinol and significant amounts of retinyl ester. These cells take up and process chylomicron remnants as well as synthesize and release plasma RBP.[31] Stellate cells, also termed fat-storing cells, lipocytes, and Ito cells, are distinct, relatively small, nonphagocytic cells of the liver that line the Space of Disse.[32] Stellate cells comprise 5–15% of total liver cells. In well-nourished humans and animals, >80% of the total vitamin A of the liver is stored in special vitamin A–containing globules in these cells. Stellate cells can take up either free retinol or holo-RBP from the serum but do not seem to contain either mRNA for RBP or RBP in appreciable amounts.[33] Ingested vitamin A is taken up first by the parenchymal cells of the liver and then is transferred to the stellate cells.[34] Although retinol clearly is the chemical form that is transferred, the mode of transfer is uncertain. RBP was suggested for this role on the basis of antibody-blocking studies.[34] The way in which retinol is released from liver stellate cells into the plasma also is uncertain. One pathway would involve its initial transfer to parenchymal cells, where it would combine with apo-RBP and be secreted into the plasma.[31,33] Retinyl ester is found in most tissues, at least in small amounts. Stellate cells also are involved in retinyl ester storage in many tissues other than liver.[32]

As liver reserves are depleted, the ratio of vitamin A in stellate cells relative to parenchymal cells markedly decreases.[35] Thus, the concentration of vitamin A in parenchymal cells of the liver is much less affected by total body reserves of vitamin A than is that in stellate cells. In a vitamin A–depleted state, the relative amounts of vitamin A in the kidney and in most epithelial tissues increase in relation to that in the liver.

Metabolism

The metabolism of vitamin A can be considered from several aspects: kinetics of uptake, transport, and excretion; enzymatic transformations; and binding to specific proteins. Vitamin A, although extensively stored in the liver and depleted from its reserves at the relatively low net rate of 0.5%/d,[36,37] is nonetheless in a highly dynamic state within the body. The half-life value for holo-RBP bound to transthyretin in human plasma is ~11 h,[31] and administered vitamin A equilibrates with total body reserves largely within 2 wk and completely within 26 d. The rapid and extensive recycling of retinol from the liver to holo-RBP in the plasma and then from peripheral tissues back to the liver was quantitated by sophisticated in vivo kinetic studies.[38] Because mRNA for RBP is present in the kidney and in some other tissues, retinol may well be transported back to the liver, at least in part, as holo-RBP.[39] Lipoprotein-bound retinyl ester, however, may also play a role in recycling. Retinoid β-glucuronides, which are released as endogenous components of bile, are reabsorbed from the intestine and also recirculated back to the liver.[21,22] The leakage of holo-RBP into the urine during the passage of blood through the kidney is extremely small under normal conditions.[31] Thus, a variety of conservation mechanisms exist to minimize the loss of vitamin A from the body. These mechanisms may well have developed to foster survival during evolution because of the crucial functional roles that vitamin A plays in mammalian physiology.

Vitamin A undergoes many enzymatic transformations in mammals. As already indicated, retinyl esters in food are hydrolyzed to retinol by pancreatic esterase in the intestinal lumen and provitamin A carotenoids are oxidatively cleaved to retinal in the intestinal mucosa. Retinal is reversibly reduced to retinol and irreversibly converted to retinoic acid in many tissues.[40] β-Carotene and presumably other provitamin A carotenoids also are cleaved in many tissues, the major end products being retinol and retinoic acid.[41] Retinol also is conjugated in several ways; namely, to form retinyl esters by trans-acylation both from phospholipid[26,42] and from acyl-coenzyme A,[43] to form retinyl β-glucuronide by interaction with UDP-glucuronic acid,[21] and to form, albeit in small amounts, retinyl phosphate by phosphate transfer from ATP.[44] Retinyl phosphate can react with GDP-mannose to yield retinyl phosphomannose.[44] Retinol can form Schiff bases with ϵ-

amino groups of proteins, the most specific and important interaction being between 11-*cis* retinal and opsin in the eye. Retinoic acid can form retinoyl β-glucuronide by reaction with UDP-glucuronic acid[21,22] and probably retinoyl coenzyme A via a conventional ATP and coenzyme A activation reaction.[45] Both retinoyl β-glucuronide and retinoyl coenzyme A might transfer the retinoyl moiety to form esters with hydroxyl, amino, and sulfhydryl groups. Possible functional implications of these transfer reactions are discussed later. Conjugated forms of vitamin A, of course, can also be hydrolyzed back to the parent compounds.

Some, if not all, of the biological activity of vitamin A is retained during the above transformations. In contrast, vitamin A is inactivated by hydroxylation, epoxidation, dehydration, and carbon-carbon bond cleavage.[46] The major hydroxylation reaction occurs at the 4 position of the cyclohexene ring, and further oxidation yields the 4-oxo derivative.[46] Other sites of hydroxylation are the five methyl groups in the molecule. The primary site of epoxidation is the 5-6 double bond. The resultant 5-6 epoxy derivative is <10% as active as vitamin A in several biological tests.[47] Some tumor cells enzymatically dehydrate vitamin A to the inactive product anhydroretinol. Finally, the conjugated side chain of vitamin A can be oxidatively shortened to yield a wide variety of products, the best characterized of which is retinotaurine.[48] Major metabolic transformations are summarized in Figure 2.

In addition, both biological and chemical isomerization of carotenoids and vitamin A occur. The most significant biological isomerization reaction is the conversion of all-*trans* to 11-*cis* retinol in the eye.[49] The biological interconversion of all-*trans* and 13-*cis* forms of vitamin A is of considerable interest relative to therapeutic, toxic, and teratogenic actions. Interestingly, *cis*-isomers of retinyl esters are hydrolyzed by retinyl ester hydrolases more rapidly than the all-*trans* forms.[50]

Retinol, retinal, and retinoic acid are primarily bound to specific retinoid-binding proteins within the plasma, intercellular spaces, and cells. Retinol is bound in plasma by RBP and in cells by the cellular binding proteins CRBP and CRBP Type II (in the intestine). Retinol is bound in the eye by cellular retinal-binding protein (CRALBP) as well as by CRBP Type II. Retinoic acid is bound by cellular retinoic acid–binding protein (CRABP) in many tissues and in some tissues of the newborn by CRABP Type II. In the interphotoreceptor space of the eye, retinol is bound by an interphotoreceptor (interstitial)-binding protein (IRBP).[51,52] The three-dimensional structure and ligand-binding site of several of these retinoid-

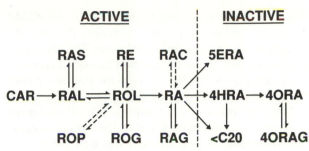

Figure 2. Major metabolic transformations of vitamin A. CAR, provitamin A carotenoids; RAL, retinal; RAS, Schiff base of retinal; ROL, retinol; RE, retinyl ester; ROP, retinyl phosphate; ROG, retinyl β-glucuronide; RA, retinoic acid; RAC, retinoyl coenzyme A; RAG, retinoyl β-glucuronide; 4HRA, 4-hydroxyretinoic acid; 5ERA, 5,6-epoxyretinoic acid; 4ORA, 4-oxoretinoic acid; 4ORAG, 4-oxoretinoyl β-glucuronide; <C20, oxidized metabolites with fewer than 20 carbon atoms. Single arrows denote irreversible reactions; double arrows, interconvertible compounds; dotted arrows, minor or not fully established in vivo reactions.

binding proteins were determined, and nearly all were cloned and sequenced. Several other retinoid-binding proteins were partially characterized from specific tissues and selected species. The retinoid-binding proteins are involved in the transport of vitamin A in the body, in the biological transformation of vitamin A and its protection from oxidation and nonspecific enzymic reactions, and in the protection of membranes and other lipid structures of cells from the amphiphilic surface-active properties of vitamin A.

Functions

The best defined function of vitamin A is in vision. The pathway for the delivery of vitamin A to the eye involves the following steps: (*1*) interaction of plasma holo-RBP with specific cell-surface receptors on retinal pigment epithelial (RPE) cells, (*2*) uptake of retinol by RPE cells and its enzymatic isomerization to 11-*cis* retinol, (*3*) transport by IRBP to the rod outer segment, (*4*) enzymatic oxidation to 11-*cis* retinol, and (*5*) nonenzymatic association of the latter with a specific lysine group in the membrane-bound protein opsin.[53] The 11-*cis* retinal in the resultant rhodopsin when exposed to light isomerizes to a transoid intermediate, which, in turn, triggers a series of conformational changes in the protein. An intermediate form, metarhodopsin II, interacts with a complex G protein, termed transducin, which causes the α unit of the latter to replace bound GDP with GTP.[54] The GTP–α unit complex of transducin activates phosphodiesterase, which in turn hydrolyzes cGMP to GMP. cGMP is involved in keeping the sodium channels of the rod outer segment open. As cGMP decreases, sodium ion entry decreases thereby hyperpolarizing the rod cell membrane. The change in membrane potential is transmitted through a complex set of synapses to the brain where the pulses received at a given time are integrated.[54]

Activated processes of temporal importance must be returned to the basal state. In the visual cascade, metarhodopsin II is converted through other conformational states to opsin and all-*trans* retinal, neither of which activates transducin. Phosphorylation of opsin also prevents its ultimate activation of transducin. Transducin possesses a GTPase activity that ultimately converts the active GTP complex to an inactive GDP-binding form. Thus, phosphodiesterase activity decreases, cGMP again increases, and the sodium channel opens. The all-*trans* retinal produced from metarhodopsin is reduced to all-*trans* retinol, transported to the RPE, and isomerized to 11-*cis* retinol. Both 11-*cis* and all-*trans* forms of retinol can be esterified and stored as retinyl esters in lipid globules of the RPE. Events occurring in the rod outer segment are summarized in Figure 3. A similar metabolic sequence seems to occur in the color-sensing cone cells of the retina.

A second major function of vitamin A is in cellular differentiation. The recent discovery of four retinoic acid receptors, termed RAR-α through RAR-γ, in the nucleus of cells has clarified, at least in part, the molecular mode of action of vitamin A.[55,56] A major hypothesis, initially defined by Chytil and Ong[57] and modified to include the RAR, is depicted in Figure 4. Retinoic acid, transported to the nucleus on CRABP, interacts with one or more of the RAR. The RAR, like other members of a superfamily of steroid, thyroid, and retinoic acid receptors, has six domains: an amino-terminal activation domain (A/B), a highly conserved DNA-binding domain (C), a hinge region (D), a ligand-binding domain (E), and a carboxy-terminal tail of less certain function.[55,56] Not all receptors are in all cells, but at least one RAR seems to be present in cells that respond to retinoic acid. The RAR, activated by binding retinoic acid, interacts with the hormone response element of appropriate genes. In embryonic development, homeobox genes are unquestionably activated (L. Gudas, personal communication, 1989), whereas in macrophages and keratinocytes, the transglutaminase gene is transcribed early.[58] Although many genes are ultimately transcribed in response to retinoic acid, the initial steps and the precise sequence are poorly defined. The discovery of the RAR, however, greatly stimulated interest and progress in understanding the mode of action of vitamin A. Although retinol and retinoic acid induce somewhat different patterns of differentiation in some cell types, a nuclear receptor for retinol has not been identified. Interestingly, the retinoid β-glucuronides seem to stimulate cellular differentiation without being hydrolyzed.[59]

In addition to vision, vitamin A has been implicated in many physiological processes, including spermatogenesis, fetal development, immune response, taste, hearing, appetite, and growth. Most of these processes depend directly or indirectly on cellular differentiation. The actions of vitamin A, including its deficiency, on these specific processes have been reviewed.[21,22,60,61]

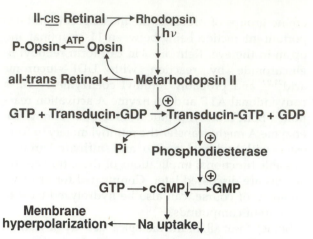

Figure 3. Visual pathway for transducing light energy into an enhanced membrane potential in the rod outer segment. + denotes stimulated reactions or enzymes.

Deficiency

Vitamin A deficiency is a major public health problem in many areas of the less-industrialized world. It was estimated that 500,000 preschool-age children become blind each year because of vitamin

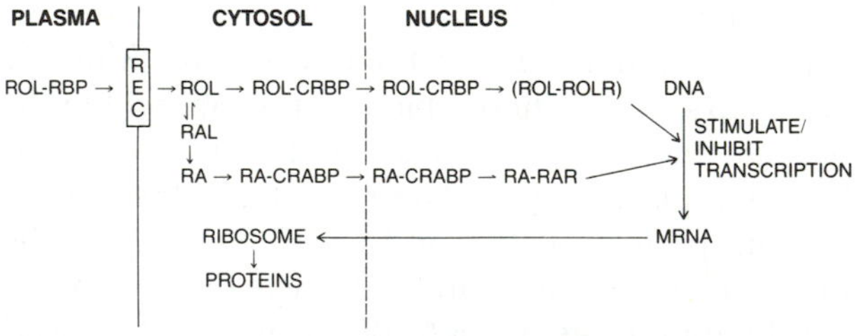

Figure 4. The modified Chytil-Ong hypothesis for the molecular action of vitamin A in cellular differentiation. ROL, retinol; RAL, retinal; RA, retinoic acid; RBP, plasma retinol-binding protein; CRBP, cellular retinol-binding protein; CRABP, cellular retinoic acid-binding protein; REC, cell-surface receptor for ROL-RBP; RAR, nuclear retinoic acid receptor; (ROLR), putative nuclear retinol receptor. (Reprinted from reference 22 by courtesy of Marcel Dekker, Inc.)

Table 1. Indicators of vitamin A status in preschool children*

Indicator	Deficient	Marginal	Satisfactory	Excessive	Toxic
Liver vitamin A (μmol/g)	<0.017	0.017–0.07	0.07–0.70	0.70–1.05	>1.05
Night blindness	+	±	0	0	0
Xerophthalmia	+	0	0	0	0
Conjunctival impression cytology (CIC)	+	±	0	0	0
Plasma vitamin A (μmol/L)	<0.35	0.35–0.70	0.70–1.75	1.75–3.5	>3.5†
Relative dose response (%)	>50	50–20	<20	<20	<20
Diet (RE/d)	<60	60–200	200–2000	2000–5000	>5000
Breast-milk vitamin A (μmol/L)‡	<0.35	0.35–1.05	1.05–3.5	—	—

* For subjective indicators (night blindness, xerophthalmia, and CIC), + signs denote clear abnormalities, ± denotes milder signs or positive reactions in only part of the range, and 0 is normal. RE is retinol equivalents.

† In excessive and toxic states, an increasing portion is present as retinyl ester (>20%).

‡ For nursing infants only.

A deficiency.[62] Many blind children do not survive.[62] Thus, the lack of a common, inexpensive dietary ingredient causes untold suffering and death. The clinical signs of vitamin A deficiency are primarily night blindness and various stages of xerophthalmia.[19,62,63] Follicular hyperkeratosis appears in some cases. The most useful clinical indicator of vitamin A deficiency in young children is Bitot's spots. Bitot's spots are foamy white accumulations of sloughed cells that usually appear on the temporal quadrant of the conjunctiva. They usually disappear in young children but disappear to a lesser extent in older children after dosing with vitamin A.[60,62] Bitot's spots are a gross manifestation of squamous metaplasia of the conjunctival epithelia in which keratinized cells replace goblet cells and normal epithelial cells.

As already noted, a new assay technique, called conjunctival impression cytology (CIC), provides an early measure of the histological changes in the eye.[18,64] The CIC assay procedure recently was simplified.[65] Although night blindness is difficult to measure quantitatively in small children, an alternative procedure that has proven useful, where specific terms for night blindness exist in the local language, is an interview with the mother.[62] Low concentrations (<0.35 mmol/L) of serum retinol also are closely associated with clinical signs of deficiency.[19] Liver concentrations of vitamin A are usually <0.02 μmol/g liver when signs of deficiency appear. The RDR and MRDR already were mentioned in relation to marginal vitamin A status.[16,17] Vitamin A deficiency is commonly associated with protein-calorie malnutrition, a low intake of fat, malabsorption syndromes, and respiratory disease.[21,22,60,62]

Requirements and Recommended Intakes

Vitamin A status can be classified in five categories: deficient, marginal, satisfactory, excessive, and toxic.

The deficient state is characterized by clinical signs as discussed earlier. In a marginal state an individual does not show clinical signs of deficiency but has an inadequate total body reserve and is at an unacceptable risk of developing a deficiency. An increased risk of morbidity (i.e., infections) and mortality also is associated with the marginal state.[64] Nutritional interactions are evident under these conditions; for example, vitamin A administered to children in a marginal state may well show improved iron status and enhanced growth.[64] The satisfactory state implies the absence of clinical signs, full physiological functions that are dependent either directly or indirectly on vitamin A, and an adequate total body reserve to meet stresses of various kinds and/or a given period of low dietary intake.

The most general indicator of vitamin A status is the total body reserve of the vitamin. Mean total body contents of vitamin A that fulfill all functions of the vitamin and provide a 3-mo reserve on a low vitamin A intake for a 76-kg male and for a 62-kg female are 0.18 mmol and 0.14 mmol, respectively. These values are derived from a satisfactory liver vitamin A concentration of 0.07 μmol vitamin A/g in both sexes.[37,66,67] The reasons for selecting this value recently were discussed in detail.[37,66–68] The RDR assay,[16] the MRDR assay,[17] and the isotope-dilution assay[69] all provide useful indicators of marginal and, by given normal values, satisfactory states of nutriture. The relation of various indicators to various states of vitamin A nutriture is summarized in Table 1. It must be stressed that the values given are reasonable estimates for an average healthy individual. Because of the heterogeneity in human populations and the influence of various factors, including nutrient interactions and disease, the values given should not be considered as individual cutoff points.

Genetic defects in vitamin A metabolism, storage, and transport are rare, probably because a homozygous defect in the regulation of this essential nutrient is not consistent with survival. Recently, however, a heterozygotic reduction of plasma RBP was reported.[70] Possible cases of vitamin A intolerance, in which toxic signs appear in some individuals who ingest only moderate amounts of vitamin A, also may have a genetic basis.[71]

The average daily amount of vitamin A that should be ingested by healthy individuals varies with age, body mass, metabolic activity, and special conditions, e.g., pregnancy and lactation. The operational endpoint also must be defined: namely, whether the objective is just to prevent deficiency or to provide as well for a suitable body reserve.[72] Finally, the heterogeneity of the population must be considered if the recommended intake is intended to meet the needs of a specified portion of the population group. In general, recommended dietary intakes for population groups tended to decrease as more information became available.

Three sets of recommended dietary intakes (RDI) for vitamin A are presented in Table 2: the new recommendations from the Food and Agriculture Organization and the World Health Organization (FAO/WHO),[67] the RDI that were suggested by an expert committee on nutrient recommendations in the United States,[37,66] and the 1989 recommendations, termed RDAs, of the Food and Nutrition Board, U.S. National Academy of Sciences.[73] Of particular interest is the use of a two-tier system in the FAO/WHO recommendations in which their basal amount corresponds to an intake that prevents signs of deficiency and their safe amount corresponds to that with an appropriate (0.07 μmol/g) liver reserve, i.e., to the suggested RDI in the United States.[37,67,72] The different recommended amounts for adults in the RDI of the FAO/WHO[67] and for the United States[37] refer solely to the different weights of reference persons, 65 kg and 55 kg for men and women in the FAO/WHO report and 76 kg and 62 kg, respectively, in the U.S. report.[37] Mean and median dietary intakes of vitamin A for adults in the United States are ~1000 and ~624 μg retinol equivalents (RE), respectively.[37] Thus, with the inevitable exception of some individuals with bizarre diets and of individuals with chronic lipid malabsorption syndromes, liver abnormalities, or genetic disease, the American people are adequately nourished in vitamin A.

In addition to dietary sources, commercial supplements of vitamin A are used extensively by the American people.[74] In most cases the supplemental intake is <5000 IU, or 1.5 times the RDA of preformed vitamin A. On the other hand, vitamin A supplements containing 10,000, 25,000, and occasionally 50,000 IU per pill are available in health

Table 2. Recommended dietary intakes of vitamin A in retinol equivalents*

Group	FAO/WHO (1989)†		Shils/Young (1988)‡	NRC-US (1989)§
	Basal	Safe		
Infants				
0–0.5 y	180	350	375	375
0.5–1 y	180	350	375	375
Children				
1–2 y	200	400	375	400‖
2–6 y	200	400	400	500¶
6–10 y	250	400	500	700**
Males				
10–12 y	300	500	600	1000††
12–70+ y	300‡‡	600	700	1000
Females				
10–70+ y	270‡‡	500	600	800
Pregnancy				
0–3 mo	+100	+100	+0	+0
3–6 mo	+100	+100	+0	+0
6–9 mo	+100	+100	+200	+0
Lactation				
0–6 mo	+180	+350	+400	+500
>6 mo	+180	+350	+320	+400

* A retinol equivalent is defined as 2 μg retinol, which is considered equal to 6 μg β-carotene or 12 μg of mixed provitamin A carotenoids.
† Reference 67.
‡ Reference 66.
§ Reference 73.
‖ 1–3 y.
¶ 4–6 y.
** 7–10 y.
†† 11–14 y.
‡‡ 18–70+ y only.

food stores. Thus, some individuals are almost certainly ingesting very large, unneeded, and possibly toxic supplements of vitamin A.

Food Sources

Common dietary sources of preformed vitamin A in the United States are liver; various dairy products, such as milk, cheese, butter, and ice cream; and fish, such as herring, sardines, and tuna. The richest sources of preformed vitamin A, although rarely ingested now in the United States, are liver oils of the shark; of marine fish, such as cod and halibut; and of marine mammals, such as the polar bear.

Common dietary sources of provitamin A carotenoids are carrots, yellow squash, dark-green leafy vegetables, corn, tomatoes, papaya, and oranges. The color of fruits and vegetables is not necessarily an indicator of its concentration of provitamin A; tomatoes, for example, are particularly rich in lycopene, which is nutritionally inactive, and the green color of leafy vegetables is due to chlorophyll, which masks the yellow color of the carotenoids.

In the United States ~75% of the RE in ingested foods are derived from preformed vitamin A and 25% from provitamin A carotenoids.[37] In terms of international units (IU), the ratio of preformed vitamin A to provitamin A carotenoids is ~1. The expression of dietary vitamin A intakes in two different units, RE and IU, has created untold confusion. The contribution of provitamin A carotenoids to the total vitamin A intake is much less when RE are used than when IU are used. Although RDI throughout the world are given largely in RE, values in food composition tables are given mainly in IU. However, the recent revised edition of Handbook 8, the major food composition table in the United States, expresses values both as RE and as IU.[75]

The problem originated because the provitamin A activity for humans of carotenoids in foods was found to be much lower than originally thought on the basis of animal studies with β-carotene in oil. In essence, the IU for provitamin A carotenoids was devalued threefold in 1967 by the FAO/WHO expert committee on the RDI for vitamin A,[76] and most national committees since have accepted the suggested conversion ratio of 1 μg retinol equals 6 μg β-carotene. To clarify this relation, the IU of vitamin A was denoted IU_a and that of β-carotene, IU_c. Currently, 1 IU_a equals 3 IU_c.[37]

The confusion about IU includes expression of the RDA for adult males in the United States in IU. In older versions the RDA of vitamin A was 5000 IU, which consisted of 50% preformed vitamin A and 50% provitamin A carotenoids in the diet. By appropriate calculation, 5000 IU is equal to 1000 RE. If only supplements of preformed vitamin A are considered, however, the RDA is 3333 IU, not 5000 IU. Suitable ways for interconverting these units were summarized.[37]

Toxicity

When ingested in large doses, vitamin A can be toxic.[77-79] There are three categories of toxicity: acute, chronic, and teratogenic. Acute toxicity is produced by one or several closely spaced very large doses of vitamin A, usually ≥100 times the recommended intake (RDI or RDA), in both adults and children. Early signs of acute toxicity include nausea, vomiting, headache, vertigo, blurred vision, muscular incoordination, and, in infants, bulging of the fontanelle. These signs are usually transient and disappear within a few days.[77-79] When the dose is very large, a second phase, characterized by drowsiness, malaise, inappetence, physical inactivity, itching, skin exfol-iation, and recurrent vomiting, follows during the next week.[80] When lethal doses are given to monkeys, the terminal phase includes coma, convulsions, respiratory abnormalities, and then death by respiratory failure or convulsions within 1–16 d.[80] For young monkeys the LD_{50} value, i.e., the single intramuscular dose that killed half of the treated animals, was 168 mg retinol (560,000 IU)/kg body weight.[80] All monkeys that received 100 mg (333,000 IU)/kg survived.[80] Rodents are much more resistant than young monkeys to acute hypervitaminosis A. In humans the only comparable case is that of a 1-mo-old male infant weighing 2.25 kg who died after receiving 1,000,000 IU of vitamin A during a 11-d period, or a total dose of ~440,000 IU/kg.[81] Infants receiving single doses of ~100,000 IU/kg body weight suffered from toxicity but did not die.[77] It, therefore, seems that children are more susceptible than are young monkeys to single lethal doses of vitamin A. Acute toxicity was reported in young children with single doses of 100,000–900,000 IU (20,000–100,000 IU/kg) and in adults with doses >1,000,000 IU/d (>14,000 IU·kg^{-1}·d^{-1}) for several days.[77] Recovery is usually complete within weeks after the termination of dosing.

Chronic toxicity, which is much more common than acute toxicity, is induced by the recurrent ingestion over a period of weeks to years of excessive doses of vitamin A that are usually ≥10 times the recommended intake (RDI or RDA). Toxic signs commonly include headache, alopecia, cracking of the lips, dry and itchy skin, hepatomegaly, bone and joint pain, as well as many other complaints.[77,78] Most cases of chronic hypervitaminosis were reported in children with daily intakes of 12,000–600,000 IU (2,000–60,000 IU·kg^{-1}·d^{-1}) and in adults with daily intakes of 50,000–1,000,000 IU (700–15,000 IU·kg^{-1}·d^{-1}).

In a few cases signs of chronic toxicity were noted in children and adults who are presumably ingesting much lower amounts of vitamin A daily, i.e., 6000–53,000 IU, or 200–800 IU·kg^{-1}·d^{-1}.[71] Some of these cases of vitamin A intolerance clearly have a genetic basis, whereas others are associated with apparently exacerbating clinical conditions.[71,79] After terminating dosing, most patients recover fully from toxicity. Permanent damage to liver, bone, and vision as well as chronic muscular and skeletal pain, however, results in some cases.

Fetal resorption, abortion, birth defects, and permanent learning disabilities in the progeny are the most serious teratogenic effects of vitamin A. Permanent learning disabilities in animals occur at significantly lower doses than those that cause gross abnormalities.[82] Generally, the drugs accutane (13-cis retinoic acid) and etretinate, an aromatic analog of the ethyl ester of all-*trans* retinoic acid, were most implicated in producing human terata.[83] In comparison with all-*trans* retinoic acid, both all-*trans* retinol and 13-*cis* retinoic acid are less toxic in several pregnant animal models.[84] Fetal development in various species differs greatly in sensitivity to retinoids. Humans are considered to be one of the most sensitive.[84] Because of these large differences in sensitivity between species and in all likelihood among individuals, the extrapolation of dose amounts from available animal models to humans is not warranted. Interestingly, high doses of all-*trans* retinoyl β-glucuronide and of some retinoylamides are not teratogenic in rodent models.[84,85]

The quantitative effects of retinoids, including vitamin A, on fetal development in humans can be considered to be in three categories: effects of the drugs 13-*cis* retinoic acid and etretinate; effects of ingested large doses of vitamin A, usually as retinyl ester; and associations between vitamin A intake early in pregnancy and abnormal outcomes. Doses of 13-*cis* retinoic acid of 0.5–1.5 $mg \cdot kg^{-1} \cdot d^{-1}$, or ~30–90 mg/d, taken early in pregnancy induce a high incidence (relative risk of 25.6) of abortions and a characteristic set of birth defects.[83] Etretinate, which is well stored in the body, produces similar effects even after therapy has been discontinued for several months.[86] Although high doses of retinol and its esters are known to produce similar birth defects in animals, quantitative data on humans are derived from only a few cases.[79,86] Birth defects noted after the mother consumed one or more doses of 100,000–500,000 IU (33–167 mg) of vitamin A early in pregnancy are in all likelihood caused by excessive vitamin A intake. Lower doses (18,000–60,000 IU/d, or 6–20 mg/d) also were associated with birth defects, although causative relations are less clear in these cases. Because the integrated area under the maternal plasma concentration curve of a teratogen seems to be closely related to the risk of fetal defects in experimental animals, the total dose taken during the first 2 mo of pregnancy may well be a better predictor of abnormal outcome than the daily dose alone.

The key issue is that the no-observed-effect level (NOEL) for vitamin A ingestion in early pregnancy is not known. Inasmuch as early pregnancy imposes no additional requirements for vitamin A, the RDI for vitamin A is the same during the first two trimesters of pregnancy as in the nonpregnant woman.[37] Because of concern about birth defects that might be caused by excessive intakes of vitamin A, the International Vitamin A Consultative Group (IVACG)[87] recommends average daily intakes of 650 RE for pregnant women. IVACG approves the use of daily supplements of 10,000 IU for pregnant women to prevent deficiency-induced fetal abnormalities only in regions of the world where vitamin A deficiency is common. The Teratology Society[88] recommends that women of child-bearing age limit their total daily intake of preformed vitamin A, including food and supplements, to ≤8000 IU and that supplements, if taken, be in the form of provitamin A carotenoids. The Council for Responsible Nutrition,[89] a trade association of the nutritional-supplement industry, advises pregnant women to limit their daily intake of supplements to 10,000 IU. Thus, several groups with different orientations suggest maximal daily intakes of ≤10,000 IU of preformed vitamin A during pregnancy.

Supplements are not needed by healthy persons ingesting a balanced diet. In this regard, the American Institute of Nutrition, the American Society for Clinical Nutrition, and the American Dietetic Association[90] issued a formal joint statement that supplements of vitamins and minerals were not needed by well-nourished, healthy individuals, including pregnant women, except for some specific exceptions.

Carotenoids in foods are not known to be toxic even when ingested in large amounts. Hypercarotenosis, a benign condition characterized by a jaundice-like yellowing of the skin and high plasma carotenoid concentrations, however, can result when large amounts of carotene-rich foods, i.e., tomato juice, carrot juice, or daily β-carotene supplements (>30 mg), are ingested.[91] The only known toxic manifestation of carotenoid intake is canthaxanthin retinopathy, which may occur in patients treated therapeutically with large daily doses (50–100 mg) of this 4,4'-diketo derivative of β-carotene for long periods.[92] As an action independent from their conversion into vitamin A, both nutritionally active and nutritionally inactive carotenoids, e.g., lutein and lycopene, may have protective effects in reducing oxidative stress and some forms of chronic disease.[93] The extent to which carotenoid ingestion affects the onset of chronic disease in humans, however, is unclear.

Summary

Vitamin A, ingested either as preformed vitamin A or as provitamin A carotenoids, is required in small amounts for vision and cellular differentiation. A deficient or marginal vitamin A status is a common condition among preschool children in the less-industrialized world. Several new methods for diagnosing marginal vitamin A status have been developed. The digestion and absorption of vitamin A is closely associated with lipid absorption. Vitamin A normally is stored in ester form in the liver and is chaperoned in the plasma, across intercellular spaces, and within cells by several specific retinoid-binding proteins. Biologically active, water-soluble retinoid β-glucuronides are formed in several tissues, and retinoic acid receptors in the nucleus serve as transcription regulatory proteins. FAO/WHO developed an appropriate, operationally defined, two-tier system of recommended dietary intakes that countries might well emulate. Foods containing vitamin A and provitamin A carotenoids, although widespread, inexpensive, and available, are not eaten by preschool children in many societies primarily because of cultural patterns and food aversions. Excessive ingestion of vitamin A, but not of most carotenoids, can cause several forms of toxicity, the most serious of which are birth defects. The dose of vitamin A, as distinct from the retinoid drugs, that can cause abortion or birth defects, although probably quite high, is not well defined. In the absence of a clear need for vitamin A supplements, women of child-bearing age should exercise prudence in the use of such supplements.

This work was supported in part by grants from NIH (EY03677, DK-32793, DK-39733, CA-46406), USDA (CRGO-SEA-87-CRCR-1-2320), the Thrasher Research Fund (2800-8), the World Food Institute of Iowa State University (0124), the Allen Whitfield Memorial Cancer Fund, the Wilfred S. Martin Fund, and the Iowa Agriculture and Home Economics Experiment Station, Ames, IA (Project 2534).

References

1. R.J. Hicks (1867) Night blindness in the Confederate army. *Richmond Med. J.* 3:34–38.
2. T. Moore (1957) *Vitamin A.* Elsevier, Amsterdam.
3. American Institute of Nutrition (1987) Nomenclature policy: generic descriptors and trivial names for vitamins and related compounds. *J. Nutr.* 117:7–14.
4. M. Kofler and S.H. Rubin (1960) Physicochemical assay of vitamin A and related compounds. *Vitam. Horm.* 18:315–339.
5. O. Isler (1971) *Carotenoids.* Birkhauser Verlag, Basel.
6. H.C. Furr, O. Amedee-Manesme, and J.A. Olson (1984) Gradient reversed-phase high pressure liquid chromatographic separation of naturally occurring retinoids. *J. Chromatogr.* 309:299–307.
7. H.C. Furr, D.A. Cooper, and J.A. Olson (1986) Separation of retinyl esters by non-aqueous reversed-phase high-pressure liquid chromatography. *Chromatography* 378:45–53.
8. G.M. Landers and J.A. Olson (1988) Rapid simultaneous determination of isomers of retinaldehyde, retinal oxime and retinol by high-performance liquid chromatography. *J. Chromatogr.* 438:383–392.
9. F. Khachik and G.R. Beecher (1988) Separation and identification of carotenoids and carotenol fatty esters in some squash products by liquid chromatography 1. *J. Agric. Food Chem.* 36:929–937.
10. A.P. DeLeenheer, H.J. Nelis, W.E. Lambert, and R.M. Bauwens (1988) Chromatography of fat-soluble vitamins in clinical chemistry. *J. Chromatogr.* 429:3–58.
11. P.V. Bhat and P.R. Sundaresan (1988) High-performance liquid chromatography of vitamin A compounds. *CRC Crit. Rev. Anal. Chem.* 20:197–218.
12. H.C. Furr and J.A. Olson (1988) A direct microassay for serum retinol (vitamin A alcohol) by using size-exclusion high-pressure liquid chromatography with fluorescence detection. *Anal. Biochem.* 171:360–365.
13. V.M. Papa, J. Hupert, H. Friedman, P.S. Ng, E.F. Robbins, and S. Mobarhan (1988) Analysis of retinoids by direct exposure probe mass spectrometry. *Biomed. Environ. Mass Spectrom.* 16:323–325.
14. A.J. Clifford, A.D. Jones, Y. Tondeur, H.C. Furr, and J.A. Olson (1986) Assessment of vitamin A status of humans by isotope dilution. *Proc. Conf. Mass. Spectrom. Allied Topics* 34:327–328.
15. C.A. Frolik and J.A. Olson (1984) Extraction, separation and chemical analysis of retinoids. In: *The Retinoids*, Vol. 1 (M.B. Sporn, A.B. Roberts, and D.S. Goodman, eds.), pp. 181–233, Academic Press, Orlando, FL.
16. H. Flores, F. Campos, C.R.C. Araujo, and B.A. Underwood (1984) Assessment of marginal vitamin A deficiency in Brazilian children using the relative dose response. *Am. J. Clin. Nutr.* 40:1281–1289.
17. S.A. Tanumihardjo, P.G. Koellner, and J.A. Olson (1989) The modified relative dose response (MRDR) using 3,4-didehydroretinol and its application to a population of well-nourished children. *FASEB J.* 3:A465 (abstr.).
18. O. Amedee-Manesme, R. Luzeau, J.R. Wittpen, A. Hanck, and A. Sommer (1988) Impression cytology detects subclinical vitamin A deficiency. *Am. J. Clin. Nutr.* 47:875–878.
19. World Health Organization (1982) *Control of Vitamin A Deficiency and Xerophthalmia.* Technical Report Series 672. WHO, Geneva.
20. E.J. van Agtmaal, M.W. Bloem, A.J. Speck, S. Saowakontha, W.H.P. Schreurs, and N.J. Van Haeringen (1988) The effect of vitamin A supplementation on tear fluid retinol levels of marginally nourished preschool children. *Curr. Eye Res.* 7:43–48.
21. J.A. Olson (1988) Vitamin A, retinoids and carotenoids. In: *Modern Nutrition in Health and Disease*, 7th ed. (M.E. Shils and V.R. Young, eds.), pp. 293–312, Lea & Febiger, Philadelphia.
22. J.A. Olson (in press) Vitamin A. In: *Handbook of Vitamins*, 2nd ed. (L.J. Machlin, ed.), Dekker, New York.
23. G. Brubacher and H. Weiser (1985) The vitamin A activity of beta-carotene. *Int. J. Vitam. Nutr. Res.* 55:5–15.
24. J.A. Olson (1989) The provitamin A function of carotenoids. *J. Nutr.* 119:105–108.
25. B.P. Kakkad and D.E. Ong (1988) Reduction of retinaldehyde bound to cellular retinol-binding protein (type II) by microsomes from rat small intestine. *J. Biol. Chem.* 263:12916–12919.
26. P.N. MacDonald and D.E. Ong (1988) Evidence for a lecithin-retinol acyltransferase activity in the rat small intestine. *J. Biol. Chem.* 263:12478–12482.
27. J.A. Olson (1984) Serum levels of vitamin A and carotenoids as reflectors of nutritional status. *JNCI* 73:1439–1444.
28. M.G. DeRuyter, W.E. Lambert, and A.P. DeLeenheer (1979) Retinoic acid: an endogenous compound of human blood. *Anal. Biochem.* 98:402–409.
29. A.B. Barua, R.O. Batres, and J.A. Olson (1989) Characterization of retinyl β-glucuronide in human blood. *Am. J. Clin. Nutr.* 50:370–374.
30. R.S. Parker (1989) Carotenoids in human blood and tissues. *J. Nutr.* 119:101–104.
31. D.S. Goodman (1984) Plasma retinol-binding protein. In: *The Retinoids*, vol. 2 (M.B. Sporn, A.B. Roberts, and D.S. Goodman, eds.), pp. 41–88, Academic Press, Orlando.
32. K. Wake (1980) Perisinusoidal stellate cells (fat-storing cells, interstitial cells, lipocytes), their related structure in and around the

liver sinusoids, and vitamin A-storing cells in extrahepatic organs. *Int. Rev. Cytol.* 66:303–353.

33. M. Yamada, W.S. Blaner, D.R. Soprano, J.L. Dixon, H.M. Kjeldbye, and D.S. Goodman (1987) Biochemical characteristics of isolated rat liver stellate cells. *Hepatology* 7:1224–1229.

34. R. Blomhoff, T. Berg, and K.R. Norum (1988) Transfer of retinol from parenchymal to stellate cells in liver is mediated by retinol-binding protein. *Proc. Natl. Acad. Sci. (USA)* 85:3455–3458.

35. R.O. Batres and J.A. Olson (1987) A marginal vitamin A status alters the distribution of vitamin A among parenchymal and stellate cells in rat liver. *J. Nutr.* 117:874–879.

36. H.E. Sauberlich, R.E. Hodges, D.L. Wallace, et al. (1974) Vitamin A metabolism and requirements in the human studied with the use of labelled retinol. *Vitam. Horm.* 32:251–275.

37. J.A. Olson (1987) Recommended dietary intakes (RDI) of vitamin A in humans. *Am. J. Clin. Nutr.* 45:704–716.

38. M.H. Green, L. Uhl, and J.B. Green (1985) A multi-compartmental model of vitamin A kinetics in rats with marginal liver vitamin A stores. *J. Lipid Res.* 26:806–818.

39. D.R. Soprano, K.J. Soprano, and D.S. Goodman (1986) Retinol-binding protein messenger-RNA levels in the liver and in extra-hepatic tissues of the rat. *J. Lipid Res.* 27:166–171.

40. P.V. Bhat, L. Poissant, P. Falardeau, and A. LaCroix (1988) Enzymatic oxidation of all-*trans* retinal to retinoic acid in rat tissues. *Biochem. Cell Biol.* 66:735–740.

41. J.L. Napoli and K.R. Race (1988) Biogenesis of retinoic acid from beta-carotene: differences between the metabolism of β-carotene and retinal. *J. Biol. Chem.* 263:17372–17377.

42. J.C. Saari and D.L. Bredberg (1988) CoA- and non-CoA-dependent retinol esterification in retinal pigment epithelium. *J. Biol. Chem.* 263:8084–8090.

43. M.D. Ball (in press) Acyl-CoA-dependent retinol esterification. *Methods Enzymol.*

44. L.M. De Luca, C.S. Silverman-Jones, D. Rimoldi, and K.E. Creek (1987) Retinoids and glycosylation. *Chem. Scripta* 27:193–198.

45. D.A. Miller and H.F. De Luca (1985) Activation of retinoic acid by coenzyme A for the formation of ethyl retinoate. *Proc. Natl. Acad. Sci. (USA)* 82:6419–6422.

46. C.A. Frolik (1984) Metabolism of retinoids. In: *The Retinoids,* vol. 1 (M.B. Sporn, A.B. Roberts, and D.S. Goodman, eds.), pp. 177–208, Academic Press, Orlando, FL.

47. W.K. Sietsema and H.F. De Luca (1982) A new vaginal smear for vitamin A in rats. *J. Nutr.* 112:1481–1489.

48. K.L. Skare, H.K. Schnoes, and H.F. De Luca (1982) Biliary metabolites of all-*trans* retinoic acid: isolation and identification of a novel polar metabolite. *Biochem.* 21:3308–3317.

49. P.S. Bernstein, W.C. Law, and R.R. Rando (1987) Isomerization of all-*trans* retinoids to 11-*cis* retinoids in vitro. *Proc. Natl. Acad. Sci. (USA)* 84:1849–1853.

50. D.A. Cooper and J.A. Olson (1988) Hydrolysis of *cis* and *trans* isomers of retinyl palmitate by retinyl ester hydrolase of pig liver. *Arch. Biochem. Biophys.* 260:705–711.

51. S.-L. Fong, G.I. Liou, R.A. Landers, et al. (1984) The characterization, localization and biosyntheses of an interstitial retinol-binding protein in the human eye. *J. Neurochem.* 42:1667–1676.

52. B. Wiggert, C.L. Kapoor, L. Lee, R.L. Somers, and G.L. Chader (1988) Phosphorylation of interphotoreceptor retinoid-binding protein (IRBP). *Neurochem. Int.* 13:81–87.

53. C.D.B. Bridges (1984) Retinoids in photosensitive systems. In: *The Retinoids,* vol. 2 (M.B. Sporn, A.B. Roberts, and D.S. Goodman, eds.), pp. 125–176, Academic Press, Orlando, FL.

54. L. Stryer (1988) *Textbook of Biochemistry,* 3rd ed., pp. 1027–1038, W.H. Freeman, New York.

55. M. Petkovich, N.J. Brand, A. Krust, and P. Chambon (1987) A human retinoic acid receptor which belongs to the family of nuclear receptors. *Nature* 330:444–450.

56. V. Giguere, E.S. Ong, P. Segui, and R.M. Evans (1987) Identification of a receptor for the morphogen retinoic acid. *Nature* 330:624–629.

57. F. Chytil and D.E. Ong (1987) Intracellular vitamin A-binding proteins. *Annu. Rev. Nutr.* 7:321–335.

58. P.J.A. Davies, J.P. Basilion, E.A. Chiocca, J. Johnson, S. Poddar, and J.P. Stein (1988) Retinoids as generalized regulators of cellular growth and differentiation. *Am. J. Med. Sci.* 31:164–170.

59. J.M. Gallup, A.B. Barua, H.C. Furr, and J.A. Olson (1987) Effects of retinoid β-glucuronides and *N*-retinoyl amines on the differentiation of HL-60 cells in vitro. *Proc. Soc. Exp. Biol. Med.* 186:269–274.

60. B.A. Underwood (1984) Vitamin A in animal and human nutrition. In: *The Retinoids,* vol. 1 (M.B. Sporn, A.B. Roberts, and D.S. Goodman, eds.), pp. 281–392, Academic Press, Orlando, FL.

61. G. Dennert (1984) Retinoids and the immune system: immunostimulation by vitamin A. In: *The Retinoids,* vol. 2 (M.B. Sporn, A.B. Roberts, and D.S. Goodman, eds.), pp. 373–390, Academic Press, Orlando, FL.

62. A. Sommer (1982) *Nutritional Blindness,* Oxford University Press, Oxford.

63. J.C. Bauernfeind, ed. (1987) *Vitamin A Deficiency and Its Control.* Academic Press, Orlando, FL.

64. A. Sommer (1989) New imperatives for an old vitamin (A). *J. Nutr.* 119:96–100.

65. O. Amedee-Manesme, R. Luzeau, C. Carlier, and A. Ellrodt (1987) Simple impression cytology method for detecting vitamin A deficiency. *Lancet* 1:1263.

66. M.E. Shils and V.R. Young, eds. (1988) *Modern Nutrition in Health and Disease,* 7th ed. 7, Lea & Febiger, Philadelphia.

67. Food and Agriculture Organization/World Health Organization (1989) *Requirements of Vitamin A, Iron, Folate, and Vitamin B$_{12}$.* Report of a joint FAO/WHO Expert Committee. FAO Food and Nutrition Series 23, FAO, Rome.

68. J.A. Olson (1987) The storage and metabolism of vitamin A. *Chem. Scripta* 27:179–183.

69. H.C. Furr, O. Amedee-Manesme, A.J. Clifford, H.R. Bergen III, A.D. Jones, and J.A. Olson (1989) Relationship between liver vitamin A concentrations determined by isotope dilution assay with tetradeuterated vitamin A and by biopsy in generally healthy adult humans. *Am. J. Clin. Nutr.* 49:713–716.

70. T. Matsuo, N. Matsuo, F. Shiraga, and N. Koide (1988) Keratomalacia in a child with familial hypo-retinol-binding proteinemia. *Jpn. J. Ophthalmol.* 32:249–254.

71. J.A. Olson (1989) Upper limits of vitamin A in infant formulas, with some comments on vitamin K. *Am. J. Clin. Nutr.* 119:1820–1824.

72. G.H. Beaton (1986) Towards harmonization of dietary, biochemical, and clinical assessments: the meanings of nutritional status and requirements. *Nutr. Rev.* 44:349–358.

73. National Research Council (1989) *Recommended Dietary Allowances,* 10th ed., National Academy Press, Washington, DC.

74. M.L. Stewart, J.L. McDonald, A.S. Levy, R.E. Schucker, and D.R. Henderson (1985) Vitamin/mineral supplement use: a telephone survey of adults in the United States. *J. Am. Diet. Assoc.* 85:1585–1590.

75. U.S. Dept. of Agriculture, Consumer and Food Economics Institute (1976–84) *Composition of Foods: Agriculture Handbook No. 8-1 to 8-12,* U.S. Government Printing Office, Washington, DC.

76. Food and Agriculture Organization/World Health Organization (1967) *Requirements of Vitamin A, Thiamine, Riboflavin, and Niacin.* FAO Series no. 8, WHO Technical Report Series no. 362, FAO, Rome and WHO, Geneva.

77. J.C. Bauernfeind (1980) *The safe use of vitamin A.* International vitamin A consultative group, Nutrition Foundation, Washington, DC.

78. J.A. Olson (1983) Adverse effects of large doses of vitamin A and retinoids. *Semin. Oncol.* 10:290–293.

79. A. Bendich and L. Langseth (1989) Safety of vitamin A. *Am. J. Clin. Nutr.* 49:358–371.

80. M.P. Macapinlac and J.A. Olson (1981) A lethal hypervitaminosis A syndrome in young monkeys following a single intramuscular dose of a water-miscible preparation containing vitamins A, D_2 and E. *Int. J. Vitam. Nutr. Res.* 51:331–341.

81. M.E. Bush and B.B. Dahms (1984) Fatal hypervitaminosis in a neonate. *Arch. Pathol. Lab. Med.* 108:838–842.

82. G.A. Nolan (1986) The effects of prenatal retinoic acid on the viability and behavior of the offspring. *Neurobehav. Toxicol. Teratol.* 8:643–654.

83. E.J. Lammer, D.T. Chen, R.M. Hoar, et al. (1985) Retinoic acid embryopathy. *N. Engl. J. Med.* 313:837–841.

84. W.B. Howard and C.C. Willhite (1986) Toxicity of retinoids in humans and animals. *J. Toxicol. Toxin Rev.* 5:55–94.

85. D.B. Gunning, A.B. Barua, and J.A. Olson (1989) Retinoyl β-glucuronide is not teratogenic in rats. *FASEB J.* 3:A467(abstr.).

86. F.W. Rosa, A.L. Wilk, and F.O. Kelsey (1986) Teratogen update: vitamin A congeners. *Teratology* 33:355–364.

87. B.A. Underwood (1986) *The Safe Use of Vitamin A by Women During the Reproductive Years,* International Vitamin A Consultative Group, ILSI-Nutrition Foundation, Washington, DC.

88. Teratology Society Position Paper (1987) Recommendations for vitamin A use during pregnancy. *Teratology* 35:269–275.

89. Council for Responsible Nutrition (1986) *Safety of Vitamins and Minerals: A Summary of Findings of Key Reviews,* Council for Responsible Nutrition, Washington, DC.

90. American Institute of Nutrition, American Society of Clinical Nutrition, and American Dietetic Association (1987) Joint statement on vitamin and mineral supplements. *J. Nutr.* 117:1649.

91. M.S. Micozzi, E.D. Brown, P.R. Taylor, and E. Wolfe (1988) Carotenodermia in men with elevated carotenoid intake from foods and β-carotene supplements. *Am. J. Clin. Nutr.* 48:1061–1064.

92. B. Daicker, K. Schiedt, J.J. Adnet, and P. Bermend (1987) Canthaxanthin retinopathy: an investigation by light and electron microscopy and physicochemical analysis. *Graefes Arch. Clin. Exp. Ophthalmol.* 225:189–197.

93. A. Bendich and J.A. Olson (1989) Biological actions of carotenoids. *FASEB J.* 3:1927–1932.

Vitamin D

Vitamin D is essential for life in higher animals. It is one of the most important biological regulators of calcium metabolism. Along with the two peptide hormones parathyroid hormone and calcitonin, vitamin D has long been known to be responsible for the minute-by-minute as well as the day-to-day maintenance of calcium-mineral homeostasis. It is now agreed that these important biological effects are achieved as a consequence of the metabolism of vitamin D into a family of daughter metabolites. One of these metabolites, 1,25-dihydroxycholecalciferol [$1,25(OH)_2D_3$], produces the bulk of the biological responses attributed to the parent vitamin D through its acting in the fashion of a steroid hormone. Thus, the existence of a vitamin D endocrine system is now understood and accepted.

It has become increasingly apparent in the 1980s that vitamin D also plays an important multidisciplinary role in tissues not primarily related to mineral metabolism, e.g., the hematopoietic system, effects on cell differentiation and proliferation including interaction with cancer cells, and participation in the process of insulin secretion. The purpose, then, of this chapter is to provide a succinct overview of our current understanding of the important nutritional substance vitamin D and the mechanisms by which it mediates biological responses. The interested reader is referred to a plethora of other reviews in the recent scientific literature that provide differing coverages and perspectives.[1-9]

Historical Background

Man is reported to have been aware since early antiquity of the substance we now know as vitamin D.[10] The first scientific description of a vitamin D deficiency, namely rickets, was provided in the 17th century by both Dr. Daniel Whistler (1645) and Professor Francis Glisson (1650).[1] The major breakthrough in understanding the causative factors of rickets was the development of nutrition as an experimental science and the appreciation of the existence of vitamins. Considering the fact that now we accept that the biologically active form of vitamin D is a hormone, it is somewhat ironic that vitamin D, through a historical accident, became classified as a vitamin. It was in 1919–1920 that Sir Edward Mellanby[11] working with dogs raised exclusively indoors (in the absence of sunlight or ultraviolet light) devised a diet that allowed him to establish unequivocally that rickets was caused by a deficiency of a trace component present in the diet. In 1921 he wrote, "The action of fats in rickets is due to a vitamin or accessory food factor which they contain, probably identical with the fat-soluble vitamin." Moreover, he established that cod-liver oil was an excellent antirachitic agent. Shortly thereafter, McCollum et al.[12] by bubbling oxygen through a preparation of the "fat soluble vitamin" were able to distinguish between vitamin A, which was inactivated, and vitamin D, which retained activity. In 1923 Goldblatt and Soames[13] published data that clearly showed that when skin was irradiated with sunlight or ultraviolet light, a substance equivalent to the fat-soluble vitamin was produced. Hess and Weinstock[14] confirmed the dictum that light equals vitamin D. They excised a small portion of skin, irradiated it with ultraviolet light, and then fed it to groups of rachitic rats. The skin that had been irradiated provided protection against rickets, whereas the unirradiated skin provided no protection whatsoever. Clearly, these animals possessed endogenous body mechanisms to produce adequate quantities of "the fat-soluble vitamin," suggesting that it was not an essential dietary trace constituent. Because of the rapid rise of the science of nutrition—and the discovery of the family of water-soluble and fat-soluble vitamins—it rapidly became firmly established that the antirachitic factor was a vitamin.

The chemical structures of the vitamins D were

determined in the 1930s in the laboratory of Professor A. Windaus at the University of Gottingen. Vitamin D, which could be produced by ultraviolet irradiation of ergosterol, was chemically characterized in 1932.[15] Cholecalciferol (vitamin D_3) was not chemically characterized until 1936,[16] when it was shown to result from the ultraviolet irradiation of 7-dehydrocholesterol. Virtually simultaneously, the elusive antirachitic component of cod-liver oil was shown to be identical to the newly characterized vitamin D_3.[17] These results clearly established that the antirachitic substance vitamin D was chemically a steroid, more specifically a secosteroid.

Chemistry of Vitamin D

The structures of ergocalciferol (vitamin D_2) and vitamin D_3 and their provitamins are presented in Figure 1. Vitamin D is a generic term and indicates a molecule of the general structure shown for rings A, B, C, and D with differing side-chain structures. Technically the steroid vitamin D is a secosteroid. Secosteroids are those in which one of the rings has undergone fission; in vitamin D, this ring is ring B, and it is indicated by the inclusion of "9,10-seco" in the nomenclature.

Vitamin D (synonym calciferol) is named according to the new revised rules of the International Union of Pure and Applied Chemists (IUPAC). Because vitamin D is derived from a steroid, the structure retains its numbering from the parent compound. Asymmetric centers are named using R,S notation; the configurations of the double bonds are notated E for *trans* and Z for *cis*. Thus the official name of vitamin D_3 is 9,10-seco(5Z,7E)-5,7,10(19)-cholestatriene-3β-ol. The official name of vitamin D_2 is 9,10-seco(5Z,7E)-5,7,10(19),22-ergostatetraene-3β-ol.

Vitamin D_3 can be produced photochemically by the action of sunlight or ultraviolet light from a precursor sterol 7-dehydrocholesterol, which is present in the epidermis or skin of most higher animals.[18] The chief structural prerequisite of a provitamin D is that it be a sterol with a $\delta 5$–7 diene double-bond system in ring B (*see* Figure 1). The conjugated double-bond system in this specific location of the molecule allows the absorption of light quanta at certain wavelengths in the ultraviolet range thus initiating a complex series of transformations (not summarized in Figure 1) that ultimately result in the appearance of vitamin D. It is important to appreciate that vitamin D_3 can be endogenously produced and that as long as an animal has access on a regular basis to sunlight there is no dietary requirement for the vitamin.

Vitamin D_2 is a synthetic form of vitamin D that is produced by irradiation of the plant steroid ergosterol. The general structural similarity of the vitamin

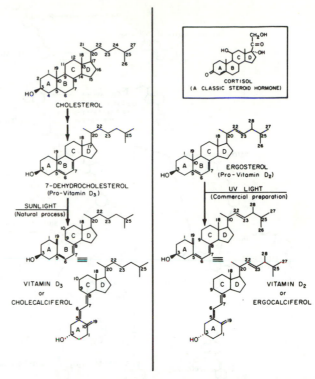

Figure 1. Structural representations of vitamin D_3 (left panel) and vitamin D_2 (right panel) and the relationship to their respective precursors, namely 7-dehydrocholesterol and ergosterol. The inset panel shows the structure of a typical steroid hormone, cortisol.

D secosteroids to that of classical steroids is illustrated in Figure 1 by comparison with the structure of cortisol; all steroids are derived from the cyclopentanoperhydrophenanthrene ring system.

Vitamin D Endocrine System

A detailed study of the mode of action of vitamin D was not possible until the availability in the 1960s of preparations of radioactive vitamin D.[19] As a consequence of efforts in many laboratories, a new model emerged to describe the biological mechanism of action of vitamin D. This model is based on the concept that, in terms of its structure and mode of action, vitamin D is similar to the classic steroid hormones, e.g., aldosterone, testosterone, estrogen, cortisol, and ecdysterone.[20] The current concept of the mechanism of action of steroid hormones is that a biochemical description of their mode of action must be sought in terms of their interaction with genetic information.[21]

Vitamin D_3 is, in reality, a prohormone leading by metabolism to a number of daughter metabolites. Two of these metabolites, $1,25(OH)_2D_3$ and $24R,25(OH)_2D_3$ (both of which are produced by the kidney), are viewed as being the mediators of the

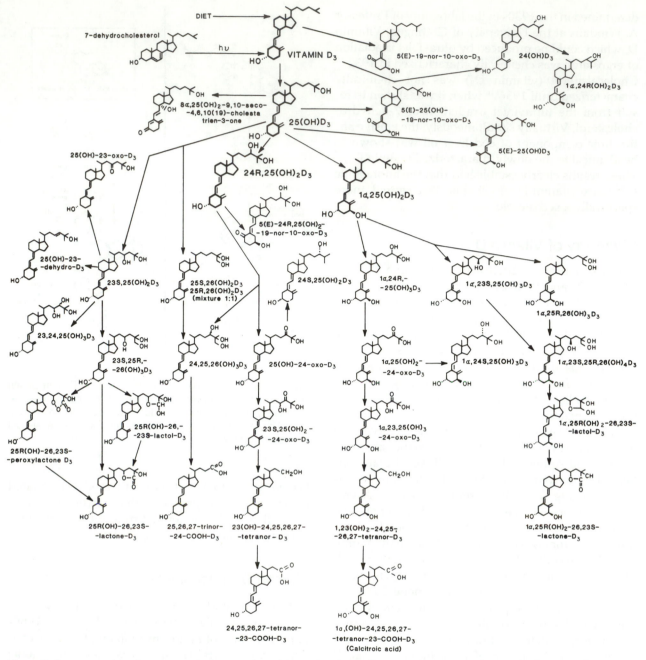

Figure 2. Summary of the known metabolites produced from vitamin D_3. The principal metabolites are 25(OH)D_3, 1,25(OH)$_2D_3$, and 24R,25(OH)$_2D_3$; the other metabolites are believed to represent catabolites of the main metabolites. (For a detailed discussion see reference 22).

spectrum of biological responses attributable to the parent vitamin D. These effects are generated in the classic target organs of vitamin D action: the intestine, the skeletal system, and the kidney. However, many new target tissues for 1,25(OH)$_2D_3$ recently have been identified, leading to the appreciation that the vitamin D endocrine system extends far beyond the original sites of action.

The elements of the vitamin D endocrine system are identified as follows: (1) photoconversion of 7-

dehydrocholesterol to vitamin D or dietary intake of vitamin D_3; (2) metabolism of vitamin D_3 by the liver to 25(OH)D_3, which is an entry steroid for further metabolism into an extensive family of daughter metabolites (Figure 2); (3) conversion of 25(OH)D_3 by the kidney (functioning as an endocrine gland to produce biologically active steroid hormones) into the two principal dihydroxylated metabolites, namely 1,25(OH)$_2D_3$ and 24R,25(OH)$_2D_3$; (4) systemic transport of the two dihydroxylated metabolites to distal target organs; (5) binding of the dihydroxylated metabolites, particularly $1,25(OH)_2D_3$, to a receptor at the target organs; and (6) interaction of the $1,25(OH)_2D_3$ steroid-receptor complex on selected genes to produce selected biological responses.

Metabolism of Vitamin D

In the liver vitamin D_3 undergoes its initial transformation, which involves the addition of a hydroxyl group to C_{25}. The enzyme catalyzing this transformation is vitamin D-25-hydroxylase, a cytochrome P_{450}–like enzyme present in the microsomes and mitochondria.[23] The metabolite thus formed is $25(OH)D_3$, which is the major circulating form of vitamin D. Like other steroids that circulate in the plasma, vitamins D_2 and D_3 are bound to their specific transport protein, the vitamin D–binding protein (DBP).[24]

From the liver, $25(OH)D_3$ is returned to the circulatory system where it is transported to the kidney by the plasma DBP. In the kidney, which functions as an endocrine gland to produce a steroid hormone in physiologically regulated amounts, a second hydroxyl group is added to C_1 of the substrate $25(OH)D_3$ yielding the product $1,25(OH)_2D_3$; this metabolite was chemically characterized simultaneously in 1971 by three laboratories.[25–27] The enzyme responsible for the 1-α-hydroxylation of $25(OH)D_3$ is 25-OH-vitamin D-1-hydroxylase. The 1-hydroxylase, also a cytochrome P_{450}–containing enzyme, is located in mitochondria of the proximal tubules of the kidney.[28] The enzyme belongs to a class of enzymes known as mitochondrial mixed-function oxidases. Mixed-function oxidases use molecular oxygen as the oxygen source instead of water. The 1-hydroxylase is composed of three proteins that are integral components of the mitochondrial membrane; they are renal ferredoxin reductase, renal ferredoxin, and cytochrome P_{450}.[29]

The most important point of regulation of the vitamin D endocrine system occurs through the stringent control of the activity of the renal-1-hydroxylase. In this way the production of the hormone $1,25(OH)_2D_3$ can be modulated according to the calcium needs of the organism. The chief regulatory factors are $1,25(OH)_2D_3$ itself, parathyroid hormone (PTH), and the serum concentrations of calcium[29,30] and phosphate.[31] Probably the most important determinant of 1-hydroxylase activity is the vitamin D status of the animal. When circulating concentrations of $1,25(OH)_2D_3$ are low, production of $1,25(OH)_2D_3$ by the kidney is high, and when circulating concentrations of $1,25(OH)_2D_3$ are high, synthesis of $1,25(OH)_2D_3$ by the kidney is low.

A second dihydroxylated metabolite of vitamin D, $24R,25(OH)_2D_3$, is produced by the kidney. The enzyme responsible for the production of $24R,25(OH)_2D_3$ is the 25-OH-vitamin D-24-hydroxylase, which is also associated with the mitochondria of the proximal tubule. The activity of this enzyme is regulated so that when $1,25(OH)_2D_3$ concentrations are low, the activity of 24-hydroxylase is also low, but when $1,25(OH)_2D_3$ concentrations are high, the activity of 24-hydroxylase is high. Under normal physiological conditions both $1,25(OH)_2D_3$ and $24R,25(OH)_2D_3$ are secreted from the kidney and circulated in the plasma of all classes of vertebrates. A discussion of the biological role of $24,25(OH)D_3$ is complex and controversial: the interested reader is referred to other publications.[5,32–34]

Figure 2 summarizes current understanding of the metabolism of vitamin D_3. In addition to the three key vitamin D_3 metabolites, $25(OH)D_3$, $1,25(OH)_2D_3$, and $24R,25(OH)_2D_3$, some 35 other vitamin D_3 metabolites were isolated and chemically characterized[22] and the existence of others appears likely. Most of the known metabolites appear to be intermediates in degradation pathways of $1,25(OH)_2D_3$. None of these other metabolites have been shown to have biological activity except for the $1,25(OH)_2D_3$-26,23-lactone, which may have selective actions on bone.[35] The activation of vitamin D_2 occurs via the same metabolic pathway as does the activation of vitamin D_3, but to date only some nine metabolites of vitamin D_2 have been characterized.[36]

Other evidence supports the existence of a paracrine system for the metabolism of $25(OH)D_3$ into $1,25(OH)_2D_3$ or $24R,25(OH)_2D_3$ by hematopoietic cells, particularly activated macrophages (see lower left box of Figure 3).[37,38] A detailed discussion of this aspect of vitamin D metabolism and its role in biology is beyond the scope of this review. The interested reader is referred elsewhere.[39,40]

Biochemical Mode of Action

The availability of high-specific-activity tritiated $1,25(OH)_2D_3$ facilitated study of the mode of action of this hormonally active form of vitamin D in a variety of its target tissues. In fact it was in the target intestine that $1,25(OH)_2D_3$ was first discovered.[41] In the steroid-hormone model of action, target tissues are defined by the presence in selected cells of specific, high-affinity receptors for the hormone in question. A model for the steroid hormone action of $1,25(OH)_2D_3$ is shown in Figure 4. In a target tissue, the $1,25(OH)_2D_3$ enters the cell (probably passively) and binds to the unoccupied form of the receptor, which is partitioned between the nucleus and the cytosol of the cell. After the steroid-receptor complex, RS, is formed, it becomes tightly associated with the

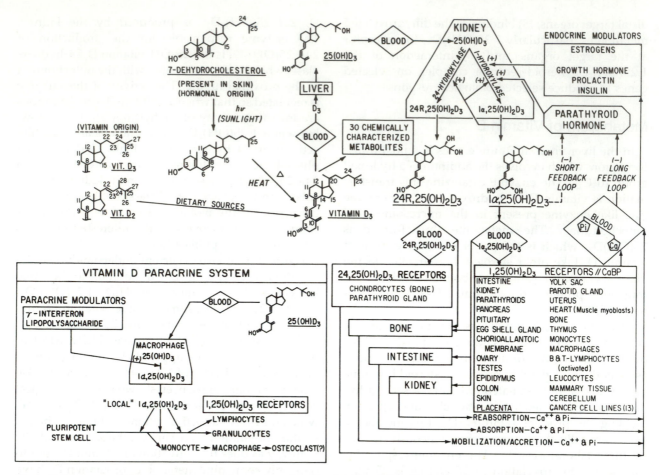

Figure 3. Summary of the vitamin D endocrine system. hν, ultraviolet irradiation; P$_i$, inorganic phosphate.

chromatin and more specifically with recognition elements for the 1,25(OH)$_2$D$_3$-receptor that are specifically present in the promoter region of genes that are regulated by 1,25(OH)$_2$D$_3$. Then modulation of

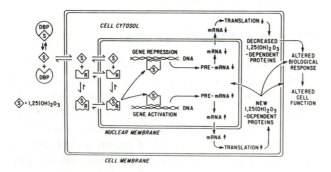

Figure 4. Proposed model to describe the actions of 1,25(OH)$_2$D$_3$ in regulating gene expression. Target organs and cells for 1,25(OH)$_2$D$_3$ by definition contain receptors for this secosteroid which converge upon them the ability to modulate genomic events. The interaction of 1,25(OH)$_2$D$_3$ with genomic material is thought to be analogous to the mode of action of other classic steroid hormones. S, steroid hormone; R, receptor protein; DBP, vitamin D serum binding protein; P, RNA polymerase.

specific gene transcription results in either induction or repression of specific mRNAs, ultimately resulting in changes in protein synthesis needed to produce the required biological responses.

The receptor for 1,25(OH)$_2$D$_3$ is the key to understanding the details of the secosteroid's mode of action as well as appreciating the breadth of the vitamin D endocrine system. Receptors for 1,25(OH)$_2$D$_3$ were detected in an astonishing array of tissues (see box, lower right corner of Figure 3). Although it was not surprising to find receptors for 1,25(OH)$_2$D$_3$ in intestine, bone, and kidney, all known sites of action of the parent vitamin D, it was exciting to learn that the biological sphere of influence of vitamin D also extended to the pancreas (β cell and insulin secretion)[42-44] and parathyroid (regulation of PTH secretion).[45] It is now generally accepted that the presence of a 1,25(OH)$_2$D$_3$ receptor in a cell is reflective of the ability of this secosteroid to mediate specific biological effects within that cell. The full spectrum of the vitamin D endocrine system and the sphere of action of 1,25(OH)$_2$D$_3$ are summarized in Figure 3.

The 1,25(OH)$_2$D$_3$ receptor was first discovered in chick intestine in 1969;[46,47] since that time it has been studied extensively by a large number of laboratories.[5,6] The $1,25(OH)_2D_3$ receptor is a protein with a molecular weight of $\sim$60,000–67,000. It has a high affinity for $1,25(OH)_2D_3$ with a K_d in the range of 1–50×10^{-11}. The receptor binds vitamin D metabolites and analogs with a specificity that parallels the biological activity of these compounds. Recently the cDNA for the human $1,25(OH)_2D_3$ receptor was cloned;[48] the amino acid and nucleotide sequence data indicate that the $1,25(OH)_2D_3$ receptor is structurally homologous to the other classical steroid hormone receptors as well as to the thyroid hormone receptor and the retinoic acid receptor (*see* figure 3 of reference 2), all of which have been postulated to belong to a super-gene family.[49]

One of the major positive gene transcriptional effects of $1,25(OH)_2D_3$ in many of its target tissues is the induction of a calcium-binding protein named calbindin-D. In the mammalian kidney and brain and in the chick, a larger form of the protein is expressed, calbindin-D_{28k}, whereas in the mammalian intestine and placenta a smaller form is expressed, calbindin-D_{9k}. Early experiments showed that actinomycin D and α-amanitin, which are transcriptional inhibitors, could block the induction of calbindin-D_{28k} by $1,25(OH)_2D_3$.[50] Later experiments showed that $1,25(OH)_2D_3$ stimulated total RNA synthesis in chick intestine[51] in addition to specifically inducing the mRNA for calbindin-D_{28k}.[52] Nuclear transcription assays showed that transcription of calbindin-D_{28k} mRNA is directly induced by $1,25(OH)_2D_3$ in chick intestine and is correlated to the number of occupied $1,25(OH)_2D_3$ receptors.[53] Recently the entire chick gene for calbindin-D_{28k} was sequenced;[54] it is currently under intensive study to identify the specific sites of interaction of the $1,25(OH)_2D_3$ receptor. $1,25(OH)_2D_3$ and its receptor also were shown to regulate the following genes; preproPTH, calcitonin, type I collagen, fibronectin, bone matrix GLA protein, interferon-γ, c-myc, c-fos, c-fms, and prolactin.[2]

Nutritional Requirements

The World Health Organization (WHO) has responsibility for defining the International Unit of vitamin D_3. Their most recent definition, provided in 1950, stated that "the International Unit of vitamin D recommended for adoption is the vitamin D activity of 0.025 μg of the international standard preparation of crystalline vitamin D_3."[55] Thus 1.0 IU vitamin D_3 is 0.025 μg, which is equivalent to 65.0 pmol. With the discovery of the metabolism of vitamin D_3 to other active secosteroids, particularly $1,25(OH)_2D_3$, Norman[56] proposed that 1.0 IU $1,25(OH)_2D_3$ be set equivalent in molar terms to that of the parent vitamin D_3. Thus 1.0 IU of $1,25(OH)_2D_3$ is equivalent to 65 pmol.

The vitamin D requirement for healthy adults has never been precisely defined. Because vitamin D_3 is produced in the skin after exposure to sunlight, the human does not have a requirement for vitamin D when sufficient sunlight is available. However, vitamin D becomes an important nutritional factor in the absence of sunlight. In addition to geographical and seasonal factors, ultraviolet light from the sun may be blocked by many means; air pollution blocks ultraviolet rays, for example. Man's tendency to wear clothes, to live in cities where tall buildings block adequate sunlight from reaching the ground, to live indoors, to use synthetic sunscreens that block ultraviolet rays, and to live in geographical regions of the world that do not receive adequate sunlight all contribute to the inability of the skin to biosynthesize sufficient amounts of vitamin D. Under these conditions vitamin D becomes a true vitamin in that it must be supplied in the diet on a regular basis.

Because vitamin D_3 can be produced by the body and because it is retained for long periods of time by vertebrate tissue, it is difficult to determine with precision the minimum daily requirements for this secosteroid. The requirement for vitamin D also is known to be dependent on the concentration of calcium and phosphorus in the diet, the physiological stage of development, age, sex, degree of exposure to the sun, and the amount of pigmentation in the skin.[57]

The current allowance of vitamin D recommended by the National Research Council is 5 μg (200 IU)/d for adults,[58] but it should be appreciated that this is an arbitrary figure and may represent the upper limit of vitamin D required. In 1970 the Expert Committee of the FAO/WHO[59] reviewed data that showed that, in full-term infants, greater absorption of calcium and faster growth rates occur in those children given 400 IU vitamin D_3/d than in those given 100 IU/d, although 100 IU/d is known to be enough to prevent rickets.

Hypervitaminosis D

Excessive amounts of vitamin D are not available from normal dietary sources. However, vitamin D intoxication can be a concern in patients being treated with vitamin D or vitamin D analogs for hypoparathyroidism, vitamin D–resistant rickets, renal osteodystrophy, osteoporosis, psoriasis, or some cancers or in individuals who take excessive amounts of supplemental vitamins. Symptoms of intoxication include hypercalcemia, hypercalciuria, anorexia, nausea, vomiting, thirst, polyuria, muscular weakness, joint pains, diffuse demineralization of bones, and

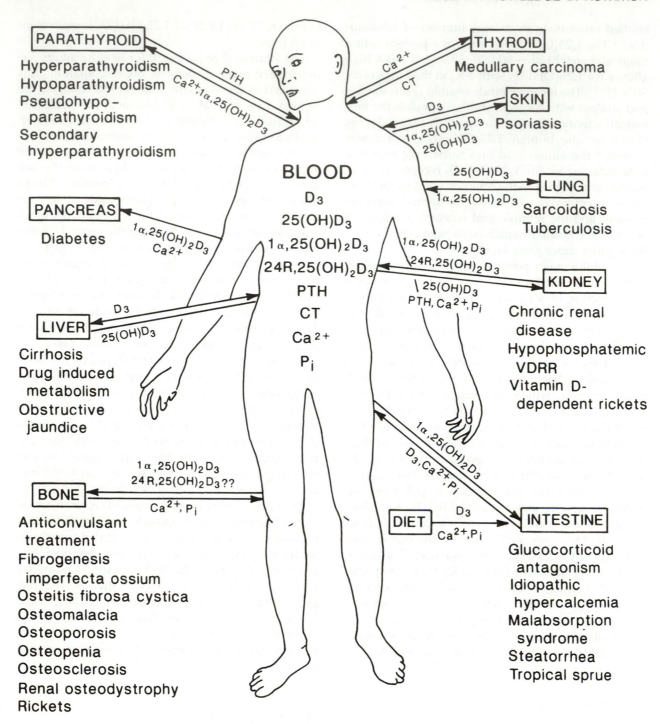

PARATHYROID
Hyperparathyroidism
Hypoparathyroidism
Pseudohypo-
  parathyroidism
Secondary
  hyperparathyroidism

THYROID
Medullary carcinoma

SKIN
Psoriasis

BLOOD
D_3
$25(OH)D_3$
$1\alpha,25(OH)_2D_3$
$24R,25(OH)_2D_3$
PTH
CT
Ca^{2+}
P_i

LUNG
Sarcoidosis
Tuberculosis

PANCREAS
Diabetes

KIDNEY
Chronic renal
  disease
Hypophosphatemic
  VDRR
Vitamin D-
  dependent rickets

LIVER
Cirrhosis
Drug induced
  metabolism
Obstructive
  jaundice

BONE
Anticonvulsant
  treatment
Fibrogenesis
  imperfecta ossium
Osteitis fibrosa cystica
Osteomalacia
Osteoporosis
Osteopenia
Osteosclerosis
Renal osteodystrophy
Rickets

DIET

INTESTINE
Glucocorticoid
  antagonism
Idiopathic
  hypercalcemia
Malabsorption
  syndrome
Steatorrhea
Tropical sprue

Figure 5. Disease states in man that have been shown to have some association with vitamin D.

general disorientation. If vitamin D intoxication is allowed to go unchecked, death will eventually occur.

Vitamin D intoxication is thought to occur as a result of high plasma concentrations of 25(OH)D rather than high plasma concentrations of 1,25-$(OH)_2D$.[60] Patients suffering from hypervitaminosis D were shown to exhibit a 15-fold increase in plasma 25(OH)D concentration as compared with normal individuals; however, $1,25(OH)_2D$ concentrations are

not substantially altered.[60] It also was shown that large concentrations of $25(OH)D_3$ can mimic the actions of $1,25(OH)_2D_3$ at the level of the receptor.[61]

Disease States in Man Related to Vitamin D

Figure 5 presents a schematic diagram of the metabolic processing of vitamin D via its endocrine system. Listed under each of the substeps of the various metabolic or regulatory steps are disease states that are known to be clinically focused at that particular locus. Conceptually, human clinical disorders related to vitamin D can be considered as those arising because of (1) altered availability of vitamin D; (2) altered conversion of vitamin D_3 to $25(OH)D_3$; (3) altered conversion of $25(OH)D_3$ to $1,25(OH)_2D_3$ and/or $24R,25(OH)_2D_3$; (4) variations in end organ responsiveness to $1,25(OH)_2D_3$ or possibly $24R,25(OH)_2D_3$; and (5) other conditions of uncertain relation to vitamin D. Thus, the clinician-nutritionist-biochemist is faced with a problem in a diagnostic sense, of identifying indices of hypersensitivity, antagonism, or resistance (including genetic aberrations) to vitamin D or one of the other of its metabolites as well as identifying perturbations of metabolism that result in problems in production and/or delivery of the hormonally active form, $1,25(OH)_2D_3$. A detailed consideration of this area is beyond the scope of this presentation; the interested reader should consult other publications.[3,62]

Summary

Current evidence supports the concept that the classical biological actions of the nutritionally important fat-soluble vitamin D in mediating calcium homeostasis are supported by the combined presence of two daughter dihydroxylated metabolites, namely $1,25(OH)_2D_3$ and $24R,25(OH)_2D_3$. A complex endocrine system coordinates the metabolism of vitamin D_3 into these hormonally active forms (Figure 3). It is now clear that the vitamin D endocrine system embraces many more target tissues than simply the intestine, bone, and kidney. Notable additions to this list include pancreas, pituitary, breast, placenta, hematopoietic cells, skin, and cancer cells of various origins. Key advances in understanding the diversity of the vitamin D endocrine system, particularly with respect to the interaction of $1,25(OH)_2D_3$, were made through study of the tissue distribution of specific receptors for this ligand as well as study of the tissue distribution and subcellular localization of the gene products induced by this steroid hormone.

References

1. A.W. Norman (1979) *Vitamin D: The Calcium Homeostatic Steroid Hormone,* Academic Press, New York.
2. P.P. Minghetti and A.W. Norman (1988) $1,25(OH)_2$-vitamin D_3 receptors: gene regulation and genetic circuitry. *FASEB J.* 2:3043–3053.
3. H. Reichel, H.P. Koeffler, and A.W. Norman (in press) The role of the vitamin D endocrine system in health and disease. *N. Engl. J. Med.*
4. I. Nemere and A.W. Norman (1982) Vitamin D and cell membranes. *Biochim. Biophys. Acta* 694:307–327.
5. A.W. Norman, J. Roth, and J. Orci (1982). The vitamin D endocrine system: steroid metabolism, hormone receptors and biological response (calcium binding proteins). *Endocr. Rev.* 3:331–366.
6. M.R. Haussler (1986) Vitamin D receptors: nature and function. *Annu. Rev. Nutr.* 6:527–562.
7. A.W. Norman, K. Schaefer, H.G. Grigoleit, and D.v. Herrath, eds. (1988) *Vitamin D: Molecular, Cellular and Clinical Endocrinology,* Walter de Gruyter, Berlin.
8. D.R. Fraser (1980) Regulation of the metabolism of vitamin D. *Physiol. Rev.* 60:551–613.
9. D.E.M. Lawson, ed. (1978) *Vitamin D,* Academic Press, New York.
10. R.S. Soleki (1971) *Shanidar: The Humanity of Neanderthal Man,* Knopf, New York.
11. E. Mellanby (1921) Experimental rickets. *Med. Res. Counc. Spec. Rep. Ser.* (Lond.) 61:68.
12. E.V. McCollum, N. Simmonds, J.E. Becker, and P.G. Shipley (1922) Studies on experimental rickets XXI. An experimental demonstration of the existence of the vitamin which promotes calcium deposition. *J. Biol. Chem.* 53:293–312.
13. H. Goldblatt and K.N. Soames (1923) A study of rats on a normal diet irradiated daily by the mercury vapor quartz lamp or kept in darkness. *Biochem. J.* 17:247–294.
14. A.F. Hess and M. Weinstock (1925) The antirachitic activity of irradiated cholesterol and physterol II. Further evidence of a change in biological activity. *J. Biol. Chem.* 64:181–191.
15. A. Windaus, O. Linsert, A. Luttringhaus, and G. Weidlich (1932) About crystalized vitamin D. *Justus Liebigs Ann. Chem.* 492:226–241.
16. A. Windaus, F. Schenck, and F. von Werder (1936) About the antirachitic irradiation product of 7-dehydrocholesterol. *Hoppe-Seyler's Z. Physiol. Chem.* 241:100–103.
17. H. Brockmann (1937) The isolation of the antirachitic vitamin from halibut liver oil. *Hoppe-Seyler's Z. Physiol. Chem.* 245:96–102.
18. M.F. Holick, J.A. MacLaughlin, M.B. Clark, et al. (1980) Photosynthesis of previtamin D_3 in human skin and the physiologic consequences. *Science* 210:203–205.
19. A.W. Norman and H.F. DeLuca (1963) The preparation of H^3-vitamins D_2 and D_3 and their localization in the rat. *Biochemistry* 2:1160–1168.
20. A.W. Norman (1968) The mode of action of vitamin D. *Biol. Rev.* 43:97–137.
21. A.W. Norman and G. Litwack (1987) *Hormones,* Academic Press, Orlando, FL.
22. H.L. Henry and A.W. Norman (1985) Interactions between aluminum and the actions and metabolism of vitamin D_3 in the chick. *Calcif. Tissue Int.* 37:484–490.
23. I. Bjorkhem and I. Holmberg (1978) Assay and properties of a mitochondrial 25-hydroxylase active on vitamin D_3. *J. Biol. Chem.* 253:842–849.
24. H. van Baelen and R. Bouillon (1986) Purification of the serum vitamin D-binding protein (DBP) from different species. *Binding Proteins of Steroid Hormones,* vol. 149 (M.G. Forest and M. Pugeat, eds.), pp. 69–83, John Libbey, London.
25. D.E.M. Lawson, D.R. Fraser, E. Kodicek, H.R. Morris, and D.H. Williams (1971) Identification of 1,25-dihydroxycholecalciferol, a new kidney hormone controlling calcium metabolism. *Nature* 230:228–230.
26. M.F. Holick, H.K. Schnoes, H.F. DeLuca, T. Suda, and R.J. Cousins (1971) Isolation and identification of 1,25-dihydroxycholecalciferol: a metabolite of vitamin D active in intestine. *Biochemistry* 10:2799–2804.
27. A.W. Norman, J.F. Myrtle, R.J. Midgett, H.G. Nowicki, V. Williams, and G. Popjak (1971) 1,25-Dihydroxycholecalciferol: identification of the proposed active form of vitamin D_3 in the intestine. *Science* 173:51–54.
28. H.L. Henry, R.J. Midgett, and A.W. Norman (1974) Studies on

calciferol metabolism IX. Characteristics of the renal 25-hydroxy-vitamin D3-1-hydroxylase. *J. Biol. Chem.* 249:7529–7535.

29. H.L. Henry and A.W. Norman (1984) Vitamin D: metabolism and biological actions. *Annu. Rev. Nutr.* 4:493–520.

30. H.L. Henry, R.J. Midgett, and A.W. Norman (1974) Studies on calciferol metabolism X. Regulation of 25-hydroxyvitamin D_3-1-hydroxylase, in vivo. *J. Biol. Chem.* 249:7584–7592.

31. L.A. Baxter and H.F. DeLuca (1976) Stimulation of 25-hydroxyvitamin D_3-1-hydroxylase by phosphate depletion. *J. Biol. Chem.* 251:3158–3161.

32. H.L. Henry and A.W. Norman (1978) Vitamin D: two dihydroxylated metabolites are required for normal chicken egg hatchability. *Science* 201:835–837.

33. A.W. Norman, V.L. Leathers, and J.E. Bishop (1983) Studies on the mode of action of calciferol XVIII. Normal egg hatchability requires the simultaneous administration to the hen of $1\alpha,25$-dihydroxyvitamin D_3 and 24R,25-dihydroxyvitamin D_3. *J. Nutr.* 113: 2505–2515.

34. Y. Tanaka, H.F. DeLuca, Y. Kobayashi, T. Taguchi, N. Ikekawa, and M. Morisaki (1979) Biological activity of 24,25-difluoro-25-hydroxyvitamin D_3: effect of blocking of 24-hydroxylation on the functions of vitamin D. *J. Biol. Chem.* 254:7163–7167.

35. S. Ishizuka, M. Kiyoka, N. Kurihara, et al. (1988) Effects of diastereoisomers of 1,25-hydroxyvitamin D_3-26-23-lactone on alkaline phosphatase and collagen synthesis in osteoblastic cells. *Mol. Cell. Endocrinol.* 55:77–86.

36. A.W. Norman (in press) AIN/ASCN Symposium on Nutritional Adaption. *Am. J. Clin. Nutr.*

37. H. Reichel, H.P. Koeffler, and A.W. Norman (1987) Synthesis in vitro of 1,25-dihydroxyvitamin D_3 and 24,25-dihydroxyvitamin D_3 by interferon-γ-stimulated normal human bone marrow and alveolar macrophages. *J. Biol. Chem.* 262:10931–10937.

38. H. Reichel, H.P. Koeffler, R. Barbers, and A.W. Norman (1987) Regulation of the 1,25-dihydroxyvitamin D_3 production by cultured alveolar macrophages from normal human donors and from patients with pulmonary sarcoidosis. *J. Clin. Endocrinol. Metab.* 65: 1201–1209.

39. W.F.C. Rigby (1988) The immunobiology of vitamin D. *Immunol. Today* 9:54–58.

40. H. Reichel and A.W. Norman (1989) Systemic effects of vitamin D. *Ann. Rev. Med.* 40:71–78.

41. M.R. Haussler, J.F. Myrtle, and A.W. Norman (1968) The association of a metabolite of vitamin D_3 with intestinal mucosa chromatin in vivo. *J. Biol. Chem.* 243:4055–4064.

42. S. Christakos and A.W. Norman (1981) Studies on the mode of action of calciferol XXIX. Biochemical characterization of 1,25-dihydroxyvitamin D_3 receptors in chick pancreas and kidney cytosol. *Endocrinology* 108:140–149.

43. A.W. Norman, B.J. Frankel, A.M. Heldt, and G.M. Grodsky. Vitamin D deficiency inhibits pancreatic secretion of insulin. *Science* 209: 823–825.

44. S. Kadowaki and A.W. Norman (1985) Demonstration that the vitamin D metabolite 1,25(OH)$_2$-vitamin D_3 and not 24R,25(OH)$_2$-vitamin D_3 is essential for normal insulin secretion in the perfused rat pancreas. *Diabetes* 34:314–320.

45. W.R. Wecksler, H.L. Henry, and A.W. Norman (1977) Studies on

the mode of action of calciferol. Subcellular localization of 1,25-dihydroxyvitamin D_3 in chicken parathyroid glands. *Arch. Biochem. Biophys.* 183:168–175.

46. M.R. Haussler and A.W. Norman (1969) Chromosomal receptor for a vitamin D metabolite. *Proc. Natl. Acad. Sci. USA* 62:155–162.

47. H.C. Tsai and A.W. Norman (1973) Studies on calciferol metabolism VIII. Evidence for a cytoplasmic receptor for 1,25-dihydroxyvitamin D_3 in the intestinal mucosa. *J. Biol. Chem.* 248:5967–5975.

48. A.R. Baker, D.P. McDonnell, M. Hughes, et al. (1988) Cloning and expression of full-length cDNA encoding human D receptor. *Proc. Natl. Acad. Sci. USA* 85:3294–3298.

49. S. Green and P. Chambon (1986) A superfamily of potentially oncogenic hormone receptors. *Nature* 307:745–747.

50. R.A. Corradino and R.H. Wasserman (1968) Actinomycin inhibition of vitamin D_3-induced calcium-binding protein (CaBP) formation in chick duodenal mucosa. *Arch. Biochem. Biophys.* 219:286–296.

51. H.C. Tsai, R.J. Midgett, and A.W. Norman (1973) Studies on calciferol metabolism VII. The effects of actinomycin D and cycloheximide on the metabolism, tissue and subcellular localization, and action of vitamin D_3. *Arch. Biochem. Biophys.* 157:339–347.

52. G. Theofan and A.W. Norman (1986) Effects of α-amanitin and cycloheximide on 1,25-dihydroxyvitamin D_3-mediated induction in the chick intestine of a 28K calcium binding protein and its mRNA. *J. Biol. Chem.* 261:7311–7315.

53. G. Theofan, A.P. Nguyen, and A.W. Norman (1986) Regulation of calbindin-D$_{28K}$ gene expression by 1,25-dihydroxyvitamin D_3 is correlated to receptor occupancy. *J. Biol. Chem.* 261:16943–16947.

54. P.P. Minghetti, L. Cancela, Y. Fujisawa, G. Theofan, and A.W. Norman (1988) Molecular structure of the chicken vitamin D-induced calbindin-D$_{28K}$ gene reveals eleven exons, six Ca^{2+}-binding domains, and numerous promoter regulatory elements. *Mol. Endocrinol.* 2:355–367.

55. World Health Organization Expert Committee on Biological Standardization (1950) Report of the subcommittee on fat-soluble vitamins. Technical Report Series 3:7, WHO, Geneva.

56. A.W. Norman (1972) Problems relating to the definition of an international unit for vitamin D and its metabolites. *J. Nutr.* 102: 1243–1245.

57. E.R. Yendt (1970) Vitamin D: Part II. XIII. Pharmacological activities of vitamin D. *Int. Encycl. Pharmacol.* 1;Sect 51:139–195.

58. National Research Council (1989) Recommended Dietary Allowances, 10 ed., National Academy Press, Washington, DC.

59. FAO/WHO (1970) Requirement of ascorbic acid, vitamin D, vitamin B-12, folate and iron. Technical Report Series no. 452, World Health Organization, Geneva.

60. M.R. Hughes, D.J. Baylink, P.G. Jones, and M.R. Haussler (1976) Radioligand receptor assay for 25-hydroxyvitamin D_2/D_3 and 1 alpha, 25-dihydroxyvitamin D_2/D_3. *J. Clin. Invest.* 58:61–70.

61. P.F. Brumbaugh and M.R. Haussler (1973) 1 Alpha, 25-dihydroxyvitamin D_3 receptor: competitive binding of vitamin D analogs. *Life Sci.* 13:1737–1746.

62. M.R. Haussler and T.A. McCain (1977) Basic and clinical concepts related to vitamin D metabolism and action. *N. Engl. J. Med.* 297: 974–983, 1041–1050.

Vitamin E

History

Vitamin E was discovered in 1922 by Evans and Bishop, who observed that rats did not reproduce when fed a purified diet in which lard was the source of fat. They found that a component in lipid extracts of various grains would correct the infertility, and this unknown substance was termed the antisterility factor. A few years later it was designated vitamin E.[1] In all vitamin E–deficient experimental animals, reproductive difficulties were shown to be due to abnormalities in both the male and female. In the male, degeneration of the seminiferous tubules of the testes occurred; in the female an inability to maintain the fetus resulted in fetal death and resorption.

In addition to reproductive tissue effects, muscle in many animal species was observed to become dystrophic. Eventually death ensued.

In vitamin E–deficient chicks, changes in capillary function led to vascular leakage. Deficient animals also showed an abnormal dark pigmentation in adipose and other tissues, leading investigators to propose a general protective action of vitamin E on unsaturated fatty acids throughout the body.

In spite of many years of intensive research on vitamin E in animals, it was more than 30 y after its discovery that clear evidence became available showing that humans did, indeed, also require the vitamin.

Chemistry

Structures. In the early isolation of vitamin E from plant oils, chemists obtained four compounds with very similar structures. Evans proposed the name *tocopherol* for vitamin E, and when four components were found they were designated by the first four letters of the Greek alphabet: α, β, γ, and δ. Their structures (Figure 1) have two primary parts, a complex ring (chroman) and a long saturated side chain.

The four tocopherols differ only in the number and position of the methyl groups on the ring. In addition to these four compounds, another related series of compounds, *tocotrienols*, has three double bonds in the side chain. These compounds are less widely distributed in nature, generally have lower biological activity than the tocopherols, and are of lesser nutritional importance.

Because tocopherols contain three asymmetric carbon atoms, there are eight possible diastereoisomers. Only one of these configurations is found in nature and is termed *RRR*. Thus, the most commonly occurring and also the most active tocopherol, α, is designated *RRR*-α-tocopherol (formerly *d*-α-tocopherol). When this vitamin is synthesized, a mixture of the eight isomers is obtained, and the product is designated all-*rac*-α-tocopherol (formerly *dl*-α-tocopherol).[2]

Chemical Properties. Tocopherols are readily oxidized by air, especially in the presence of iron and other metals. When oxidized, the hydroxyl group on the ring is changed to an oxy group, the ring opens, and a quinone is formed. This compound, tocopheryl quinone, has no biological activity. To prevent this oxidation, most nutritional supplements of α-tocopherol are esterified with acetic acid to yield α-tocopherol acetate. This form of the vitamin is resistant to oxidation but has no biological activity until hydrolyzed. In the gastrointestinal tract, enzymes hydrolyze the ester and the free tocopherol is absorbed.

In addition to tocopheryl quinone, a large number of other oxidation products were produced in the laboratory with a variety of oxidizing agents. None of the oxidation products has significant biological activity.

Methods of Analysis. Early methods of tocopherol analysis were based on its ability to be oxidized. A variety of purification steps were necessary, and for some materials the procedure was long and difficult

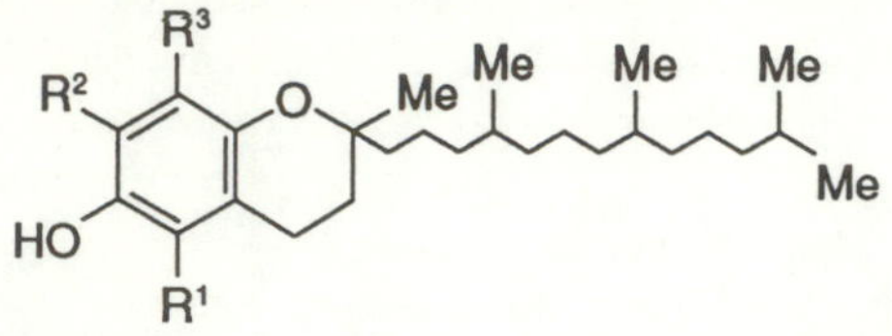

Figure 1. Structure and biological equivalence of naturally occurring tocopherols.

Compound	R^1	R^2	R^3
α-Tocopherol	Me	Me	Me
β-Tocopherol	Me	H	Me
γ-Tocopherol	H	Me	Me
δ-Tocopherol	H	H	Me

because of possible oxidation losses. An excellent review of the variety of such methods is available.[3] These earlier methods, however, are largely obsolete, and the current method of choice is high-performance liquid chromatography (HPLC). This technique permits very rapid analysis of plasma. As little as ≤0.1 mL can be analyzed for α- and γ-tocopherols as well as for retinol (vitamin A) in 7 min.[4] The method also has been applied to platelets, and the sensitivity has been increased by use of a fluorescent detector.[5] A variation of this procedure permits the analysis of tocopherols in homogenates of animal tissues and in subcellular fractions.[6]

HPLC is also the method of choice for determining the numerous tocopherols and tocotrienols in food. The vitamin E components in fruits and vegetables[7] and fats and oils[8] of Finnish foods were reported. As more such data become available, the accuracy of calculating the vitamin E content of diets will improve greatly.

Absorption and Transport

The absorption of vitamin E is associated with fat absorption. If for any reason an individual does not digest dietary fat (triglyceride) and absorb fatty acids, there will be a marked decrease in tocopherol absorption. A primary requirement is normal bile secretion to facilitate emulsification for hydrolysis by pancreatic lipase. Additionally, if pancreatic function is not normal, fat digestion and tocopherol absorption will be impaired.

Esterified α-tocopherol is completely hydrolyzed, and only free tocopherol appears in chylomicrons in the lymph. Efficiency of absorption of tocopherol is relatively low compared with triglyceride absorption. Studies in humans show a wide range, from 20–80%, with an average of ∼50% at normal intakes of 5–15 mg/d.[9,10] As the intake increases, the percentage of

tocopherol absorbed decreases, suggesting a saturation process.

Tocopherol in lymph passes into the circulation where it first appears in chylomicrons but rapidly equilibrates with other lipoproteins as the chylomicrons are cleared. In the postabsorptive state most tocopherol is carried by the low-density lipoproteins (LDL) in males whereas in females the high-density lipoproteins (HDL) carry more than the LDL. The percentage distributions for males and females, respectively, are 59 and 42 for LDL, 33 and 59 for HDL, and 8 and 12 for very-low-density lipoproteins (VLDL).[11] There is a high correlation between plasma tocopherol concentration and plasma total lipids; there is a slightly lower correlation with total cholesterol. For practical purposes the ratio of tocopherol to cholesterol plus triglycerides is as useful as the ratio to total lipids for evaluating tocopherol status.[12] In the author's experience, the relationship between plasma tocopherol and plasma lipids is much weaker for normolipemic subjects than it is for subjects with low or high lipid values.

In normal adults, plasma total tocopherols range from 11.6 to 26.9 μmol/L; values for α-tocopherol only are 10–20% lower (the difference is primarily γ-tocopherol). Children have slightly lower values than adults and, thus, different norms should be used in evaluating plasma values.[13,14]

Tissues slowly accumulate tocopherol by transfer from plasma lipoproteins. The process is not understood clearly.[15] Liver and adipose tissue have the highest concentrations, but muscle also accounts for much of body tocopherol. In order to double plasma concentration, approximately a 10-fold intake of tocopherol is required.

Biochemical Function

Very shortly after the tocopherols had been isolated, it was discovered that they were effective antioxidants for protecting unsaturated lipids from autooxidation. Observations in experimental animals led to the hypothesis that vitamin E also functioned in this manner in tissues to prevent oxidative damage to lipids, particularly the polyunsaturated fatty acids in membranes. It has become clear in recent years that numerous enzyme systems produce a variety of potentially damaging oxidative products and that the body has a complex system of defense against them.[16] Primary in this defense system is vitamin E, which, being lipid soluble, is a component of cellular membranes and thus is intimately associated with phospholipids.[17] Other nutrients also participate in regulating tissue-damaging oxidations, primarily the trace element selenium (as a functional part of the enzyme glutathione peroxidase) and vitamin C (ascorbic acid). Whether vitamin E has other functions apart from its scavenging of free radicals and reacting with active forms of oxygen has not been established.

Physiological Effects

A well-established function of vitamin E in animals, related to its antioxidant action, is its ability to protect against a variety of toxicants. These include heavy metals such as lead and mercury; hepatotoxic compounds such as carbon tetrachloride, benzene, and cresol; and a variety of drugs.[18,19] In most of these toxicities, the compound is thought to initiate free radicals. Model systems in animals[20] and cell cultures[21] also have shown that vitamin E protects against environmental pollutants such as ozone and nitrous oxide. Supplements of vitamin E given to normal adults provided suggestive evidence of increased protection from ozone exposure.[22] However, there is no direct evidence that tocopherol supplements are beneficial to populations exposed to abnormal levels of atmospheric pollutants, probably because normal adults in the U.S. population have relatively high tissue concentrations of vitamin E,[23] and additional intakes may have no effect.

Animal experiments have shown interesting effects of vitamin E on several other physiological processes. Some of these effects can be shown only in deficient animals, but some occur after normal animals are dosed with tocopherol. Several aspects of the immune function in chicks, mice, and rats are altered by large intakes of α-tocopherol.[24,25] Similar effects in humans, however, have not been shown.

An area of recent interest and research activity is the possible relationship of vitamin E to cancer. Prospective studies of blood vitamin E concentrations in cancer patients and matched, noncancerous control subjects suggested a relationship of lower plasma α-tocopherol with certain cancer sites, especially lung and breast cancer.[26–28] Other nutrients, vitamin A, β-carotene, and selenium are confounding variables in these relationships so that it is not clear how significant these epidemiological observations may be. With regard to vitamin E, certain experimental cancers in animals can be prevented or altered by oral or topical administration of α-tocopherol, e.g., rat mammary tumors[29] and hamster buccal (oral) cancer.[30] As in the prospective human studies, selenium often is a confounding factor in animal experiments. Current studies hopefully will clarify the possible relationship between specific nutrients and cancer.

Deficiency

Malabsorption Disorders. Individuals with a variety of intestinal disorders associated with fat malabsorption have low plasma tocopherol levels.[31,32] Among such disorders are celiac disease, pancreatitis, sprue, and biliary cirrhosis. When malabsorption occurs in adults, it may take several years for the blood vitamin E concentration to decrease to <9.3 μmol/L. For a long time it was thought that this relatively tocopherol-deficient state in adults was a benign condition. It has become clear, however, that after 5–10 y neurological abnormalities, often very subtle, may appear.[33–35]

In children born with certain genetic diseases in which fat absorption may be impaired, such as cystic fibrosis, or with congenital abnormalities, such as biliary atresia, a vitamin E–deficient condition can develop relatively rapidly with serious consequences, primarily neurological, if the vitamin E deficiency is not corrected.[36,37] If vitamin E treatment is not initiated early in the lives of these children or if rigorous means are not taken to ensure that blood tocopherol concentrations are increased, the developing neuropathy is only partially reversible.[38] Neuropathologic changes in these patients include neuroaxonal dystrophy affecting the gracile nucleus; the lesions are similar to those observed in animals with vitamin E deficiency.[39]

Premature Infants. It has been known for many years that newborn infants have low plasma tocopherol values compared with children aged ≥6 mo. Premature infants are even more precarious with respect to vitamin E status, and a number of the medical complications that these very small babies exhibit have been suggested to be related to their low blood tocopherol concentrations. Considerable interest has focused on the hemolytic anemia in low-birth-weight neonates and the efficacy of vitamin E therapy.[39] Although it is generally agreed that formulas for the premature infant should have an adequate α-tocopherol content in relation to polyunsaturated fatty acids, recent studies indicate that larger supplements of vitamin E do not confer any extra benefit for the hematological picture.[40]

Other medical problems of premature infants in which vitamin E has been tried include hyperbilirubinemia, respiratory-distress syndrome, periventricular hemorrhage, and retrolental fibroplasia. In the latter two conditions, tocopherol therapy appeared to be beneficial in some but not all cases.[39,41] It is not clear what critical blood concentrations of tocopherol need to be achieved to provide greater protection against these conditions.

Hematologic Disorders. Several hereditary diseases are characterized by episodes of excessive red cell hemolysis or abnormal red cell structure. The more common of these diseases are thalassemia, sickle cell anemia, and glucose-6-phosphate dehydrogenase (G-6-PD) deficiency in red cells. A number of studies showed some patients with these diseases have low plasma α-tocopherol concentrations but others have plasma and red cell α-tocopherol concentrations that are normal.[39,42,43] The explanation for the low plasma values is not obvious unless one assumes a chronic low degree of red cell breakdown, the products of which could destroy plasma tocopherol. Evidence for this hypothesis, however, is not available. Treatment of patients with these diseases with oral supplements of vitamin E yielded promising results. However, in the case of G-6-PD deficiency, not all patients show improvement with vitamin E treatment.

Kidney patients undergoing hemodialysis have been noted to have lower-than-normal plasma or red cell α-tocopherol concentrations, with accompanying anemia. Supplements of vitamin E to these patients are reported to decrease red cell fragility and partially correct the anemia.[44,45]

The number of medical conditions in which vitamin E is claimed to have a beneficial effect continues to grow, and the reader is referred to a review of this subject.[39] Most of the claims made for vitamin E in a variety of diseases have not stood the test of time. Many interesting observations made in in vitro studies or in experimental animals cannot be shown to hold for humans.

Allowances and Intakes

The Food and Nutrition Board of the U.S. National Academy of Sciences[46] recommended a daily allowance of 8 mg of α-tocopherol equivalents for women and 10 mg for men, with proportionately lesser amounts for children. These intakes of vitamin E daily throughout life establish the normal blood concentrations of the vitamin and also give rise to appropriate tissue concentrations. The allowances, however, will not be adequate in individuals who for a variety of reasons do not absorb fat efficiently or who may have medical conditions that for unknown reasons appear to produce an abnormal vitamin E status in the blood and tissues.

Animal experiments showed that the requirement for vitamin E increases when the intake of polyunsaturated fatty acids (PUFA) is increased. In human diets the PUFA content is primarily linoleic acid. This increased tocopherol requirement, however, appears to be significant only at relatively high PUFA intakes.[47]

The vitamin E content of U.S. diets varies widely, depending primarily on the amount of vegetable oils present.[32] Several studies of composite diets of 2000–3000 kcal found daily intakes in the U.S. ranging from 7 to 10 mg α-tocopherol equivalents. Information from other countries indicates similar or lower

intakes.[32] When diets contain considerable amounts of corn and soybean oils, as in the United States, the γ-tocopherol often exceeds the α-tocopherol. Because γ-tocopherol has ~10% of the biological activity of α-tocopherol, one-tenth of the amount of γ-tocopherol should be calculated to provide the total α-tocopherol equivalents in the diet.[46]

Toxicity

Reports of adverse symptoms from large doses of vitamin E are largely subjective and based on limited observations. The most commonly occurring complaint is gastrointestinal upset of short duration. Animal studies have shown that large intakes of vitamin E can interfere with the absorption of vitamins A and K. This relationship may have occurred in a male subject who consumed 1200 mg tocopherol equivalents while on anticoagulation therapy for a heart condition.[48] The subject experienced excessive hemorrhages that disappeared when vitamin E supplementation was discontinued. Examination of a large number of blood tests in a normal population taking vitamin E supplements did not reveal any abnormalities.[49,50] Most of the evidence indicates that a daily intake in the range of 200–600 mg is innocuous for most adults. In infants, however, large oral doses of tocopherol have been associated with a significantly higher incidence of necrotizing enterocolitis than is seen in control infants.[51] This effect may have been partially due to the high osmolarity of the aqueous vitamin E preparation used. In 1983, toxicity and death occurred in premature infants given an intravenous vitamin E solution.[52] Whether this was caused by the tocopherol or by the surface-active agent in the vehicle was not determined.

References

1. H.M. Evans (1963) The pioneer history of vitamin E. *Vitam. Horm.* 20:379–387.
2. S. Kasparek (1980) Chemistry of tocopherols and tocotrienols. In: *Vitamin E, a Comprehensive Treatise* (L.J. Machlin, ed.), pp. 7–66, Marcel Dekker, Inc., New York.
3. I.D. Desai (1980) Assay methods. In: *Vitamin E, a Comprehensive Treatise* (L.J. Machlin, ed.), pp. 67–98, Marcel Dekker, Inc., New York.
4. J.G. Bieri, T.J. Tolliver, and G.L. Catignani (1979) Simultaneous determination of alpha-tocopherol and retinol in plasma or red cells by high pressure liquid chromatography. *Am. J. Clin. Nutr.* 32:2143–2149.
5. J. Lehmann and H.L. Martin (1982) Improved direct determination of alpha- and gamma-tocopherols in plasma and platelets by liquid chromatography with fluorescence detection. *Clin. Chem.* 28:1784–1787.
6. J.K. Lang, K. Gohil, and L. Packer (1986) Simultaneous determination of tocopherols, ubiquinols, and ubiquinones in blood, plasma, tissue homogenates, and subcellular fractions. *Anal. Biochem.* 157:106–116.

7. V. Piironen, E.L. Syvaoja, P. Varo, K. Salminen, and P. Koivistoinen (1986) Tocopherols and tocotrienols in Finnish foods: vegetables, fruits and berries. *J. Agric. Food Chem.* 34:742–746.

8. E.L. Syvaoja, V. Piironen, P. Varo, P. Koivistoinen, and K. Salminen (1986) Tocopherols and tocotrienols in Finnish foods: oils and fats. *J. Am. Oil Chem. Soc.* 63:328–329.

9. R. Blomstrand and L. Forsgren (1968) Labelled tocopherols in man. *Int. Z. Vitaminforsch.* 38:328–344.

10. M.T. MacMahan and G. Neale (1970) The absorption of alpha-tocopherol in control subjects and in patients with intestinal malabsorption. *Clin. Sci.* 38:197–210.

11. W.A. Behrens, J.N. Thompson, and R. Madere (1982) Distribution of alpha-tocopherol in human plasma lipoproteins. *Am. J. Clin. Nutr.* 35:691–696.

12. D.I. Thurnham, J.A. Davies, B.J. Crump, R.D. Situnayake, and M. Davis (1986) The use of different lipids to express serum tocopherol: lipid ratios for the measurement of vitamin E status. *Ann. Clin. Biochem.* 23:514–520.

13. S.L. Levine, A.J. Adams, M.D. Murphy, and P.M. Farrell (1976) Survey of vitamin E status in children. *Pediatr. Res.* 10:356–358.

14. K. Mino, M. Kitagawa, and S. Nakagawa (1985) Red blood cell tocopherol concentrations in a normal population of Japanese children and premature infants in relation to assessment of vitamin E status. *Am. J. Clin. Nutr.* 41:631–638.

15. C.A. Thellman and R.B. Shireman (1985) In vitro uptake of (^{3}H)-alpha-tocopherol from low density lipoproteins by cultured human fibroblasts. *J. Nutr.* 115:1673–1679.

16. H.J. Forman and A.B. Fisher (1981) Antioxidant defenses. In: *Oxygen and Living Processes; an Interdisciplinary Approach* (D.L. Gilbert, ed.), pp. 235–249, Springer-Verlag, New York.

17. G.W. Burton and K.U. Ingold (1986) Vitamin E application of the principles of physical organic chemistry to the exploration of its structure and function. *Accounts Chem. Res.* 19:194–201.

18. J. Ono, T. Mimaki, and H. Yabuuchi (1986) Effects of phenobarbital on lipid peroxidation in vitamin E-deficient rats. *Pediatr. Pharmacol.* 5:223–227.

19. G.A. Pascoe and D.J. Reed (1987) Vitamin E protection against chemical-induced cell injury. II. Evidence for a threshold effect of cellular alpha-tocopherol in prevention of adriamycin toxicity. *Arch. Biochem. Biophys.* 256:159–166.

20. D.B. Menzel (1980) Protection against environmental toxicants. In: *Vitamin E, a Comprehensive Treatise* (L.J. Machlin, ed.), pp. 474–494, Marcel Dekker, New York.

21. A.W.T. Konings (1986) Mechanism of ozone toxicity in cultured cells. 1. Reduced clonogenic ability of polyunsaturated fatty acid-supplemented fibroblasts. Effect of vitamin E. *J. Toxicol. Environ. Health* 18:491–497.

22. E.J. Calabrese, J. Victor, and M.A. Stoddard (1985) Influence of dietary vitamin E on susceptibility to ozone exposure. *Bull. Environ. Contam. Toxicol.* 34:417–422.

23. J.G. Bieri and R.P. Evarts (1975) Tocopherols and polyunsaturated fatty acids in human tissues. *Am. J. Clin. Nutr.* 28:717–720.

24. R.P. Tengerdy (1980) Effect of vitamin E on immune responses. In: *Vitamin E, a Comprehensive Treatise* (L.J. Machlin, ed.), pp. 429–444, Marcel Dekker, New York.

25. A. Bendich, E. Gabriel, and L.J. Machlin (1986) Dietary vitamin E requirement for optimum immune response in the rat. *J. Nutr.* 116:675–681.

26. J.T. Salonen, R. Salonen, R. Lappetelainen, P.H. Maenpaa, G. Alfthan, and P. Puska (1985) Risk of cancer in relation to serum concentrations of selenium and vitamins A and E: matched case-control analysis of prospective data. *Br. Med. J.* 290:417–420.

27. M.S. Menkes, G.W. Comstock, J.P. Vuilleumier, K.J. Helsing, A.A. Rider, and R. Brookmeyer (1986) Serum beta-carotene, vitamins A and E, selenium and the risk of lung cancer. *N. Engl. J. Med.* 315:1250–1254.

28. N.J. Wold, J. Boreham, J.L. Hayward, and R.D. Bulbrook (1984) Plasma retinol, beta-carotene and vitamin E levels in relation to the future risk of breast cancer. *Br. J. Cancer* 49:321–324.

29. C. Ip (1985) Attenuation of the anticarcinogenic action of selenium by vitamin E deficiency. *Cancer Lett.* 25:325–331.

30. D. Trickler and G. Shklar (1987) Prevention by vitamin E of experimental oral carcinogenesis. *JNCI* 78:165–169.

31. P.M. Farrell (1980) Deficiency states, pharmacological effects, and nutrient requirements. In: *Vitamin E, a Comprehensive Treatise* (L.J. Machlin, ed.), pp. 520–620, Marcel Dekker, New York.

32. J.G. Bieri (1987) Dietary role of vitamin E. In: *Lipids in Modern Nutrition* (M. Horisberger and U. Bracco, eds.), pp. 123–132, Raven Press, New York.

33. R.J. Sokol (1984) Vitamin E deficiency in adults. *Ann. Intern. Med.* 100:769.

34. S. Satya-Murti, L. Howard, G. Krohel, and B. Wolf (1986) The spectrum of neurological disorder from vitamin E deficiency. *Neurology* 36:917–921.

35. G.P. Jeffrey, D.P.R. Muller, A.K. Burroughs, et al. (1987) Vitamin E deficiency and its clinical significance in adults with primary biliary cirrhosis and other forms of liver disease. *J. Hepatol.* 4: 307–317.

36. E. Elias, D.P.R. Muller, and J. Scott (1981) Association of spino-cerebellar disorders with cystic fibrosis or chronic childhood cholestasis and very low serum vitamin E. *Lancet* 2:1319–1321.

37. M.A. Guggenheim, S.P. Ringel, A. Silverman, B.E. Grabert, and H.E. Neville (1982) Progressive neuromuscular disease in children with chronic cholestasis and vitamin E deficiency: clinical and muscle biopsy findings and treatment with alpha-tocopherol. *Ann. N.Y. Acad. Sci.* 393:84–93.

38. D.P.R. Muller (1986) Vitamin E—its role in neurological function. *Postgrad. Med. J.* 62:107–112.

39. J.G. Bieri, L. Corash, and V.S. Hubbard (1983) Medical uses of vitamin E. *N. Engl. J. Med.* 308:1063–1071.

40. Anonymous (1988) Vitamin E supplementation of premature infants. *Nutr. Rev.* 46:122–123.

41. S. Sinha, N. Toner, J. Davies, S. Bogle, and M. Chiswick (1987) Vitamin E supplementation reduces frequency of periventricular hemorrhage in very preterm babies. *Lancet* 1:466–470.

42. C. Natta and L.J. Machlin (1979) Plasma levels of tocopherol in sickle cell anemia subjects. *Am. J. Clin. Nutr.* 32:1359–1362.

43. E.A. Rachmilewitz, A. Shifter, and I. Kakane (1979) Vitamin E deficiency in beta-thalassemia major: changes in hematological and biochemical parameters after a therapeutic trial with alpha-tocopherol. *Am. J. Clin. Nutr.* 32:1850–1858.

44. K. Ono (1985) Effects of large dose vitamin E supplements on anemia in hemodialysis patients. *Nephron* 40:440–445.

45. R. Lubrano, M.T. Galluci, V. Mazzarella, et al. (1986) Relationship between red blood cell lipid peroxidation, plasma hemoglobin, and red blood cell osmotic resistance before and after vitamin E supplementation in hemodialysis patients. *Artif. Organs* 10:245–250.

46. National Research Council (1989) *Recommended Dietary Allowances*, 10th ed., National Academy Press, Washington, DC.

47. F.C. Jager (1972) Linoleic acid intakes and vitamin E requirements in rats and chicks. *Ann. N.Y. Acad. Sci.* 203:199–211.

48. J.J. Corrigan, Jr. (1979) Coagulation problems relating to vitamin E. *Am. J. Pediatr. Hematol. Oncol.* 1:169–173.

49. P.M. Farrell and J.G. Bieri (1975) Megavitamin E supplementation in man. *Am. J. Clin. Nutr.* 28:1381–1386.

50. A. Bendich and L.J. Machlin (1988) Safety of oral intake of vitamin E. *Am. J. Clin. Nutr.* 48:612–619.

51. N.N. Finer, K.L. Peters, Z. Hayek, and C.L. Merkel (1984) Vitamin E and necrotizing enterocolitis. *Pediatrics* 73:387–393.

52. S.L. Alade, R.E. Brown, and A. Paquet, Jr. (1986) Polysorbate 80 and E-Ferol toxicity. *Pediatrics* 77:593–597.

Chapter 14

John W. Suttie

Vitamin K

History

Vitamin K was discovered in the early 1930s when Dam noted a hemorrhagic syndrome in chicks fed a lipid-free diet. This condition could be cured by the addition of alfalfa meal to the diet or by the administration of a lipid extract of green plants. By 1939 a series of investigations led by Dam in Denmark, Almquist at Berkeley, and Doisy at St. Louis University established that the form of the vitamin in alfalfa, now called vitamin K_1 or phylloquinone, was 2-methyl-3-phytyl-1,4-naphthoquinone. Bacterial forms of the vitamin, a series of multiprenyl menaquinones with an unsaturated side chain that were originally called vitamin K_2, were subsequently characterized. The hemorrhagic condition that resulted from the dietary lack of vitamin K originally was thought to be due solely to a lowered concentration of plasma prothrombin (factor II), but it was shown later that the synthesis of clotting factors VII, IX, and X also was depressed in the deficient state. This early history of vitamin K research has been adequately reviewed.[1,2]

Knowledge of the biochemical events involved in the production of the plasma protein prothrombin by the liver and the regulation of these metabolic events developed largely during the last 20 years. By the early 1940s the 4-hydroxy-coumarins were identified as indirect anticoagulants that functioned by antagonizing the action of vitamin K. It was, therefore, possible to regulate the production of prothrombin in an attempt to understand its synthesis. However, the lack of a general understanding of the mechanism of protein biosynthesis prevented serious experimental approaches to the cellular and molecular mechanisms involved until the mid 1960s. By the early 1970s it was possible to demonstrate that the vitamin was a cosubstrate for a liver enzyme involved in the conversion of inactive precursors of the vitamin K-dependent proteins to the biologically active plasma forms.

Chemistry

Natural compounds with vitamin K activity are 2-methyl-1,4-naphthoquinones that contain a hydrophobic substituent at the 3 position (Figure 1). Phylloquinone, vitamin K_1, the form isolated from green plants, has a phytyl group, whereas bacterially synthesized forms of the vitamin (menaquinones) have an unsaturated multiprenyl group at this position. Although a wide range of menaquinones are synthesized by bacteria, menaquinones with 6–10 isoprenoid groups in the side chain (MK-6 to MK-10) are the most common.[3,4] The synthetic compound, menadione (2-methyl-1,4-naphthoquinone), is commonly used as a source of the vitamin in animal feeds and is known to be alkylated to MK-4 by mammalian liver.[5]

Vitamin K is extracted from plant and animal tissues with nonpolar solvents, and the small amount of vitamin present in the crude complex-lipid extract made quantitation of the vitamin difficult. Advances in high-performance liquid chromatography (HPLC) separations and development of new methods of detection in column effluents corrected this problem,[6] and what appear to be reproducible values for the plasma concentration of phylloquinone in the human now are available. These concentrations are low, and most individuals have postabsorption values of ≤ 2 nmol/L.[7,8] A few measurements of human liver vitamin K concentrations now are also available, and values reported are in the range of 4–40 nmol phylloquinone/g liver.[7,9] A spectrum of menaquinones also are found in liver, and the total menaquinone concentration appears to be about 10-fold higher than that of phylloquinone. Studies of the influence of dietary vitamin K on the concentration of circu-

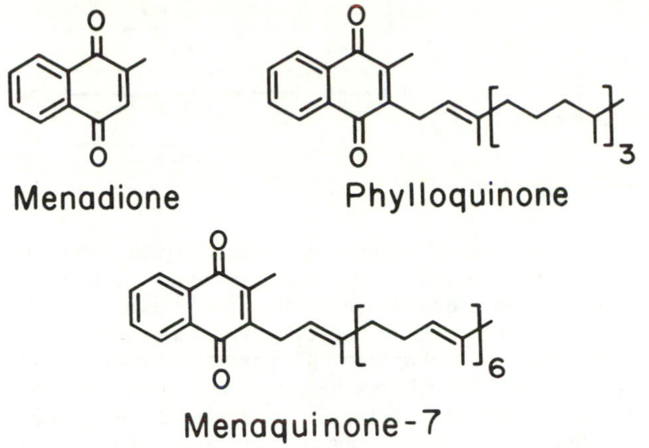

Figure 1. Structures of the biologically active forms of vitamin K.

lating and stored vitamin K are just beginning, and rapid progress in this area should be made in the next few years.

Absorption, Transport, and Metabolism

Absorption of phylloquinone from the gut is via the lymphatic system, and conditions that result in a general impairment of lipid absorption also adversely influence vitamin K absorption.[10] The vitamin is rapidly concentrated in liver, but in contrast to the other fat-soluble vitamins, it has a very rapid turnover in this organ. Excretion of phylloquinone occurs predominantly in feces via the bile, but significant amounts are excreted in the urine. Very little dietary phylloquinone is excreted unmetabolized, and the major metabolites appear to represent the stepwise oxidation of the side chain at the 3 position to various degrees, followed by glucuronide conjugation.[11] The metabolic role of the vitamin as a substrate for the liver microsomal γ-glutamyl-carboxylase results in the production of the 2,3-epoxide of the vitamin, and this metabolite appears to be subject to the same oxidative degradation as the parent vitamin.[12]

Early studies with germ-free animals indicated that they had an increased vitamin K requirement,[13] and prevention of coprophagy is commonly used to produce a vitamin K deficiency in the rat. The human gut also contains large quantities of bacterially produced menaquinones; the nutritional significance of this potential source of the vitamin is not yet clear. The extent of absorption of these menaquinones from the lower bowel is not clearly established, although it was demonstrated that liver contains a significant quantity of menaquinone. The relative turnover rate of the menaquinone liver pool compared with that of the liver phylloquinone pool is not established,

nor has it been determined if one form of the vitamin is preferentially used by the hepatic vitamin K–dependent enzymes. The principal homologue in plasma is phylloquinone; menaquinones are not detectable in plasma unless hyperlipemia exists. The limited information available suggests that the pathway of degradative metabolism of menaquinones is similar to that of phylloquinone.

Biochemical Function

From the time of their discovery until the early 1970s, it was assumed that the classical vitamin K–dependent clotting factors were the only proteins requiring the vitamin for their synthesis, and studies directed toward an understanding of this role concentrated on an understanding of the biosynthesis of prothrombin. A number of indirect studies in the mid-1960s strongly suggested that vitamin K was involved in converting an inactive precursor to active prothrombin. This hypothesis was strengthened by the observation of immunochemically similar but biologically inactive prothrombin molecules that increased in the plasma of anticoagulant-treated patients.[14] Characterization of this abnormal bovine prothrombin revealed that its amino acid composition, amino- and carboxyl-terminal amino acids, and molecular weight appeared to be identical to those of prothrombin.[15,16] The abnormal prothrombin could be electrophoretically separated from prothrombin in the presence but not the absence of calcium ions, and, in contrast to normal prothrombin, it was not adsorbed by barium salts. Calcium ions are required to bind prothrombin to a phospholipid surface during its activation to thrombin, and the abnormal prothrombin lacked the specific calcium-binding sites present in normal prothrombin[17,18] and did not demonstrate a calcium-dependent association with phospholipid surfaces.[19] The isolation and characterization of this abnormal plasma prothrombin suggested that it might be similar to the postulated liver prothrombin precursor, and the existence of this precursor was demonstrated in the livers of vitamin K–deficient or anticoagulant-treated rats.[20]

The lack of calcium-binding ability of the plasma abnormal prothrombin suggested that the function of vitamin K was to attach a calcium-binding prosthetic group to a liver precursor of this plasma protein. A low-molecular-weight, calcium-binding peptide could be isolated from enzymatic digests of normal but not abnormal prothrombin.[21] Acidic peptides of this type were subsequently shown to contain γ-carboxyglutamic acid (Gla), a previously unrecognized acidic amino acid.[22,23] Further investigation of the chemistry of prothrombin revealed that all 10 of the glutamic acid residues in the first 42 residues of bovine prothrombin have been modified in this fashion (Figure 2).[24] These residues, which are effective calcium-binding groups, are formed by a post-translational vitamin K–dependent modification of a liver precursor protein.

Plasma clotting factors VII, IX, and X also depend on vitamin K for their synthesis and contain Gla residues. The amino-terminal regions of these proteins are very homologous,[25] and the Gla residues are in essentially the same position in all of these clotting factors. Two more homologous Gla-containing plasma proteins, protein C[26] and protein S,[27] play an anticoagulant rather than a procoagulant role in normal hemostasis. Another Gla-containing bovine plasma protein (protein Z) was described, but its function is not yet known.[28]

The demonstration that a Gla-containing protein, subsequently called osteocalcin or bone Gla protein, could be isolated from bone[29,30] raised the possibility that vitamin K–dependent proteins might serve important physiological functions in a number of tissues. There is no apparent structural homology between this protein and the vitamin K–dependent plasma proteins and its function is not known, but it is most likely involved in some aspect of the control of tissue mineralization.[31,32] The demonstration that the concentration of this protein in plasma varies in some metabolic bone diseases suggested possible clinical implications[33] as has the demonstration that the synthesis of this protein is to some extent regulated by vitamin D.[34] A second structurally related protein originally isolated from bone and called matrix Gla protein is known to be present in other tissues,[35] but its physiological role is also unclear. It is, however, clear that the vitamin K–dependent reaction is present in most tissues and that a reasonably large number of proteins are subjected to this post-translational modification. The physiological role of these proteins has not yet been established.

Vitamin K–dependent Metabolic Reactions

The reactions shown in Figure 3 summarize the known major metabolic transformation of vitamin K in rat liver microsomes and indicate that, at least in in vitro incubations, three forms of vitamin K (the quinone, the hydroquinone, and the 2,3-epoxide) can feed into this liver vitamin K cycle. The quinone and hydroquinone of the vitamin are interconverted by a number of NAD(P)H-linked reductases, including one that appears to be a microsomal-bound form of the extensively studied liver DT-diaphorase activity,[36,37] and also by a dithiol-dependent reductase.[38] Vitamin KH_2, the reduced form of the vitamin, can

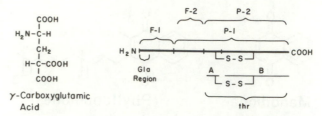

Figure 2. Structure of γ-carboxyglutamic acid (Gla) and a representation of the prothrombin molecule. Specific proteolysis of prothrombin by thrombin and factor Xa will cleave prothrombin into the specific large peptides shown: fragment-1 (F-1), fragment-2 (F-2), prethrombin-1 (P-1), prethrombin-2 (P-2), and thrombin (thr). The Gla residues in bovine prothrombin are located at residues 7, 8, 15, 17, 20, 21, 26, 27, 30, and 33, and they occupy homologous positions in the other vitamin K–dependent plasma proteins.

serve as a substrate for a microsomal internal monooxygenase that converts the vitamin to its 2,3-epoxide.[39] This epoxide, discovered in the early 1970s as the major liver metabolite of the vitamin,[40] is the substrate for another microsomal enzyme, the 2,3-epoxide reductase. The enzyme utilizes a sulfhydryl compound as a reductant and appears to be the enzyme that is the site of the physiological action of the 4-hydroxycoumarins as anticoagulants.[41,42] In in vitro systems dithiothreitol will also reduce vitamin K to vitamin KH_2 in a 4-hydroxycoumarin–sensitive reaction, and there are data to suggest that this step might be of physiological importance in the action

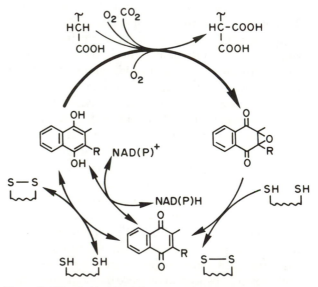

Figure 3. Vitamin K–dependent reactions catalyzed by crude liver microsomes. Current evidence suggests that the carboxylation and epoxidation activities are catalyzed by the same enzyme. The dithiol-dependent reductions of the epoxide and of vitamin K quinone are extremely sensitive to the action of coumarin anticoagulants such as warfarin.

of these anticoagulants.[43] Whether this reduction is catalyzed by the same enzyme that reduces the epoxide is not yet known, but current evidence suggests that the quinone is the initial product of the reduction of vitamin K-2,3-epoxide and that this product is then further reduced. Recent evidence suggests that the physiological reductant for the enzyme(s) that catalyzes the reduction of vitamin K epoxide to vitamin KH_2 may be thioredoxin.[44,45]

The discovery of Gla residues in prothrombin led to the demonstration that crude rat liver microsomal preparations contain an enzymatic activity that promotes a vitamin K–dependent incorporation of $H^{14}CO_3^-$ into microsomal precursors of these vitamin K–dependent proteins to form Gla residues.[46] The enzyme activity was soon shown to be active in a number of detergent-solubilized systems, and it was demonstrated that the pentapeptide Phe-Leu-Glu-Glu-Val would be a substrate for this enzyme.[47] Most subsequent studies utilized this or similar peptide substrates rather than the endogenous substrates to study enzyme activity.

Early studies of the requirements of this enzymatic system were reviewed.[48] The initial report of the vitamin K–dependent carboxylation reaction utilized a postmitochondrial supernatant preparation with no added reductant. Studies with washed microsomes demonstrated a requirement for NAD(P)H and/or a reduced pyridine nucleotide–generating system, and it was demonstrated subsequently that vitamin KH_2 could substitute for these cytoplasmic factors. Early studies also demonstrated that the carboxylation reactions did not require ATP, and the available data are consistent with the view that the energy to drive this carboxylation reaction is derived from the reoxidation of vitamin KH_2. This unique carboxylase requires O_2, and a number of studies appear to have ruled out the involvement of biotin in the system. These findings and a direct study of this requirement would suggest that CO_2 rather than HCO_3^- is the active species in the reaction.

A number of substances are known to inhibit this carboxylase. The vitamin K antagonist 2-chloro-3-phytyl-1,4-naphthoquinone is an effective inhibitor of the carboxylase, and the reduced form of this analog was shown to be competitive vs. the reduced vitamin site.[49] Substitution of a trifluoromethyl group at the 2 position also results in an inhibitory compound.[50] Sulfhydryl poisons, spin trapping agents, chelating agents, and CN^- were reported to inhibit the reaction, whereas pyridoxyl phosphate and Mn^{2+} stimulate the reaction.[48] The significance of these observations in the crude systems that often were used is difficult to assess at this time.

The activities of various homologs and analogs of vitamin K as substrates for the enzyme were determined. Review of these studies suggests that the only important structural features of this substrate in a detergent-solubilized system are a 2-methyl-1,4-naphthoquinone substituted at the 3 position with a rather hydrophobic group.[48] Methyl substitution of the benzenoid ring has little effect or decreases binding.[49] Synthesis and assay of a large number of low-molecular-weight peptide substrates of the enzyme failed to reveal any unique sequence needed as a signal for carboxylation.[51] In general, peptides with Glu-Glu sequences are better substrates than those with single Glu residues. Gln, D-Glu, or Homo-Glu residues were demonstrated to be noncarboxylated residues, whereas Asp residues are poorly carboxylated.[52,53] Why only the first of the two adjacent Glu residues is carboxylated by the enzyme is not yet apparent. Some larger peptides were reported to be excellent substrates,[54] and consensus sequences within the Gla region that may be important for efficient carboxylation were identified.[55] Details of the current understanding of the specificity of the various substrates for the carboxylase are available in a recent review.[56]

The rough microsomal fraction of liver is highly enriched in carboxylase activity, and lower but significant amounts are found in smooth microsomes. Mitochondria, nuclei, and cytosol have negligible activities.[57] The addition of 0.2% Triton X-100 to intact microsomes results in a 10–20-fold stimulation of carboxylation of peptide substrates, suggesting that the enzyme system may be accessible only from the lumen of the microsomal membrane. This finding is supported by the inaccessibility of any strongly rate-limiting component of the carboxylase to trypsin in the absence of detergents. The data obtained are consistent with the hypothesis that the carboxylation event occurs on the lumen side of the rough endoplasmic reticulum.

Mechanism of Carboxylation. Early studies of the mechanism of this apparently unique carboxylation reaction considered two possibilities: that the vitamin was a cofactor utilized to abstract the hydrogen on the γ-position of the glutamyl residue to allow for attack of CO_2 at this position or that it was involved as a CO_2 carrier. Little evidence to support the latter hypothesis was ever obtained. Use of the substrate Phe-Leu-Glu-Glu-Leu, tritiated at the γ-carbon of each Glu residue, demonstrated that the enzyme catalyzed a vitamin $K H_2$-dependent and O_2-dependent but CO_2-independent release of tritium from this substrate.[58] These data established that the role of the vitamin was to remove the γ-hydrogen of the Glu substrate. Present understanding of the mechanism of the carboxylation reaction stresses its relationship to a microsomal vitamin K epoxidase activity that converts vitamin K hydroquinone to the 2,3-epoxide of the vitamin. Early studies demonstrated that this activity was closely associated with the vitamin K–dependent carboxylase activity, and epoxide formation was subsequently shown to be stimulated by the presence of a Glu site substrate of the carboxylase.[59] At saturating concentrations of CO_2 there is an apparent equivalent stoichiometry between epoxide formation and Gla formation,[60] but at lower CO_2 concentrations a large excess of vitamin K epoxide is produced. The degree to which these two reactions are coupled in routine incubations is, therefore, strongly dependent on incubation conditions.

How epoxide formation is coupled to γ-hydrogen abstraction has not yet been established, but one possibility would be through the action of an oxygenated intermediate, such as a hydroperoxide, that would be a logical intermediate on the pathway to epoxide formation. Such an intermediate has not been demonstrated, and the evidence for its presence is indirect. Any detailed mechanism of how an oxygenated form of vitamin K could be used to drive the carboxylation reaction is speculative, and direct abstraction of a proton to leave a formal carbanion on the glutamyl residue and a radical-mediated sequence of events both have been considered. Hydrogen abstraction is known to be stereospecific, and it is the pro-S hydrogen at the γ-position that is removed.[61] The enzyme will catalyze a vitamin KH_2 and oxygen-dependent exchange of ^3H from ^3H_2O into the γ-position of a Glu residue in the substrate Boc-Glu-Glu-Leu-OMe.[62] Exchange of ^3H with the γ-carbon hydrogen is decreased as the concentration of HCO_3^- in the media is increased. It was also demonstrated that the fate of the activated Glu residue in the absence of CO_2 is to protonate rather than form an adduct with some other component of the incubation that would result in an altered Glu residue.[63] More recent studies utilizing γ-^3H–labeled Glu substrates demonstrated a close association between epoxide formation, Gla formation, and γ-C-H bond cleavage.[64] The efficiency of the carboxylation reaction, Gla formed/γ-C-H bond cleaved, was found to be independent of Glu substrate concentration, and the data suggest that this ratio approaches unity at high CO_2 concentrations. The available data place severe constraints on a radical mechanism and are consistent with the model shown in Figure 4, which indicates that the role of vitamin K is to abstract the γ-hydrogen to leave a carbanion. The data do not rule out the possibility that a radical is formed initially and carbanion formation is a subsequent event. Proof of either hy-

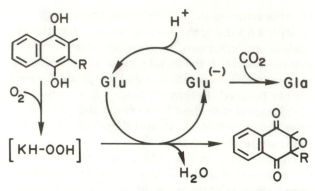

Figure 4. Proposed mechanism for the vitamin K–dependent carboxylase-epoxidase system. The available data strongly support the vitamin K–dependent formation of a carbanion at the γ-carbon of the Glu residue followed by carboxylation in a step not involving the vitamin. Neither the chemical nature of the proposed oxygenated vitamin K intermediate nor the mechanism by which hydrogen abstraction is linked to epoxide formation can be determined from the available data.

pothesis will, however, depend on a clearer understanding of the mechanism by which hydrogen abstraction is coupled to epoxide formation and will probably require progress in purifying this membrane-bound enzyme system.

Involvement of the "Propeptide" in Carboxylation. The specific γ-carboxylation of vitamin K–dependent proteins raises a number of questions relative to the control and targeting of this posttranslational event. Knowledge of the intracellular intermediates involved in the carboxylation is becoming available. The major prothrombin species that accumulates in the hepatic microsomes of intact rats treated with warfarin[65] or in cultured human liver cells[66] and that appears to be the substrate for the vitamin K–dependent carboxylase is a high mannose form. Comparison of the aglyco forms of plasma prothrombin and its intracellular precursors indicated that the intracellular form is $\sim$1500 daltons larger and is more basic. Structural information obtained through cDNA sequencing revealed that the primary gene product of the vitamin K–dependent proteins contains a basic amino acid–rich "propeptide" between the signal peptide region and the amino-terminal end of the plasma form of the protein.[67] An amino-terminal extension homologous to this region also was observed in the precursor form of the vitamin K–dependent bone Gla protein.[68] This protein shows little other sequence homology to the plasma vitamin K–dependent proteins, again suggesting that this amino-terminal extension might be an important recognition site for the carboxylation system.

Isolated plasma abnormal (des-γ-carboxy) prothrombin was found to be a poor substrate for the vitamin K–dependent carboxylase;[54] isolated rat liver microsomal prothrombin precursor preparations are a much better substrate.[69,70] Because the major difference in these two preparations is the presence or absence of the propeptide, these data support the hypothesis that this region may be important in the interaction of the enzyme with its macromolecular substrate. Utilization of plasmids encoding constructs of protein C, which contain or lack a partial propeptide region, also were used to assess this relationship.[71] When these proteins were expressed in E. coli, only those proteins containing a partial propeptide region were substrates for an in vitro carboxylase assay. The physiological importance of these observations was confirmed by the demonstration that effective carboxylation of constructs of factor IX[72] or protein C[73] expressed in mammalian cell lines is dependent on the presence of a native propeptide region. The covalent attachment of a synthetic propeptide region to a low-molecular-weight peptide substrate also was shown to result in an excellent carboxylase substrate.[74] A 20-residue peptide containing the octadeca propeptide of human factor X was shown to strongly stimulate the activity of the vitamin K–dependent carboxylase toward a noncovalently attached low-molecular-weight peptide substrate.[75] This stimulation is seen at less than micromole-per-liter propeptide concentrations and is accompanied by a decrease in K_m of the Glu site substrate. These data raise the possibility that this region of the normal carboxylase substrates has both an enzyme recognition role and a regulatory role.

Vitamin K Deficiency in Man

Primary vitamin K deficiency is uncommon in the healthy human population. There is a widespread distribution of phylloquinone in plants, and the microbiological flora of the normal gut synthesize menaquinones in amounts that may supply a portion of the daily requirement for vitamin K. The causes of acquired deficiencies in the vitamin K–dependent coagulation factors in the adult are largely secondary to disease or drug therapy.

The hemorrhagic disease of the newborn is a long recognized syndrome that is in part responsive to vitamin K.[76] Vitamin K stores are low at birth because of poor placental transfer, and the sterile gut of the newborn precludes any possible synthesis of menaquinones during early life. The condition is complicated by a general hypoprothrombinemia in infants caused by the inability of immature liver to synthesize normal amounts of clotting factors.[77] The low vitamin K content of breast milk[78] and low milk intake[79,80] are contributing factors to vitamin K deficiency in the newborn. Formulas are now routinely supplemented with vitamin K, and the American Academy of Pediatrics[81] recommends intramuscular administration of phylloquinone at birth as routine prophylaxis.

It is now clear that the most common condition known to result in a vitamin K–responsive hemorrhagic event occurs in patients who have a low dietary intake of vitamin K and are also receiving antibiotics.[82,83] These cases are numerous and were reviewed by Savage and Lindenbaum.[84] The prevalence of this condition suggests that patients with restricted food intake or on total parenteral nutrition who are also receiving antibiotics should be closely observed for signs of vitamin K deficiency. Historically, these episodes were attributed to an interference with the synthesis of menaquinones in the gut, but evidence to substantiate the effect is lacking. The second- and third-generation cephalosporins were implicated in a large number of hypoprothrombinemic episodes, and, although it was suggested that these drugs have a direct effect on the vitamin K–dependent carboxylase,[85] it is more likely that they are exerting a weak coumarin-like response in patients with low vitamin K status.[86]

Vitamin K deficiency was reported in patients subjected to long-term total parenteral nutrition,[87] and supplementation of the vitamin is advised under these circumstances. Supplementation in the case of biliary obstruction is also advisable, because the impairment of lipid absorption resulting from the lack of bile salts also will adversely affect vitamin K absorption. Depression of the vitamin K–dependent coagulation factors frequently has been found in malabsorption syndromes[84] and in other gastrointestinal disorders (for example, cystic fibrosis, sprue, celiac disease, ulcerative colitis, regional ileitis, ascaris infection, and short-bowel syndrome) and has usually been observed to respond to vitamin K administration.

The low requirement and the relatively large amounts of vitamin K found in most diets prevented an accurate assessment of the requirement until recent years. In starved, intravenously fed, debilitated patients given antibiotics to decrease intestinal vitamin K synthesis, it was found that 0.1 μg phylloquinone$\cdot$kg$^{-1}\cdot$d^{-1} was not sufficient to maintain normal prothrombin concentrations and that 1.5 μg$\cdot$kg$^{-1}\cdot$d^{-1} was sufficient to prevent any decreases in clotting factor synthesis.[88] These data indicate that the requirement was of the order of 1 μg$\cdot$kg$^{-1}\cdot$d^{-1}. Prothrombin concentrations were depleted to <50% in 20 wk in two normal subjects fed a chemically defined diet providing <10 μg vitamin K/d.[89] Mineral oil and antibiotics were administered during a portion of this period in an attempt to decrease vitamin absorption and synthesis. Administration of $\sim$0.5 μg vitamin $K \cdot kg^{-1} \cdot d^{-1}$ rapidly restored clotting activity to normal in these subjects. It was concluded from this study that $\sim$1 μg vitamin $K \cdot kg^{-1} \cdot d^{-1}$ was sufficient to maintain normal clotting factor synthesis in the normal adult human. Four normal volunteers were maintained on a diet containing $\sim$25 μg vitamin K/d and administered antibiotics to decrease intestinal menaquinone synthesis.[90] Prothrombin activity was maintained in a normal range of from 70% to 100% of normal during a 5-wk period; lower values were observed near the end of the study. These data suggest that prothrombin concentrations can be maintained near the low end of the normal range on a diet containing $\sim$0.5 μg vitamin $K \cdot kg^{-1} \cdot d^{-1}$. The limited studies available, therefore, suggest that the vitamin requirement of the human is in the range of 0.5–1.0 μg vitamin $K \cdot kg^{-1} \cdot d^{-1}$. A recent study modifying the vitamin K intake of young adults by restriction of foods with a high phylloquinone content resulted in mild deficiency symptoms and alterations of circulating phylloquinone concentrations.[91] These responses were reversed by additional dietary vitamin, and the data obtained are consistent with a requirement in the range previously suggested.

Recent advances in methodology have made it possible to routinely measure circulating concentrations of phylloquinone,[6] and it appears that normal postadsorptive plasma concentrations are in the range of $\leq$2 nmol/L. The factors influencing these concentrations and their relationship to dietary intake are not yet clarified, but alteration of plasma phylloquinone by dietary restriction of the vitamin was reported in studies of limited scope[91,92] and was shown to be low in debilitated patient populations.[86,93] Assessment of adequacy by use of the rather insensitive one-stage prothrombin time (clinical Pro Time) meant that a rather large decrease in vitamin K–dependent clotting factor synthesis was needed to produce an apparent deficiency. More sensitive clotting assays[91] and the ability to immunochemically detect circulating des-γ-carboxy prothrombin[94] provide an opportunity to monitor much milder forms of vitamin K deficiency. These advances in technology will make it possible to establish the relationship between dietary vitamin K and circulating concentrations of the vitamin and to reexamine current estimates of requirement. The question of menaquinone utilization by the human also is unsolved and will depend on the utilization of newer methods of analysis and adequacy assessment.

Sources of Vitamin K

Comprehensive tables of the vitamin K content of foods are not currently available. The few available analyses are summarized in standard nutrition texts[95] and reviews.[1] Many of the values used to develop the available tables were obtained from chick biological assays of vitamin content of foods before a suitable standard was available and should be used with a great deal of caution. In general, green vegetables are the major source of phylloquinone in the diet, and such foods as spinach, broccoli, brussels sprouts, kale, and turnip greens are excellent sources of the vitamin. These foods contain a few hundred micrograms of phylloquinone per 100 g fresh weight, whereas the more commonly consumed green vegetables such as peas, green beans, cabbage, and lettuce furnish between 10 and 100 μg/100 g fresh weight. Methods for the analysis of the phylloquinone content of foods by HPLC were developed, and more values should soon be added to the existing database. The usual intake of the vitamin in the human diet has been assumed to be 300–500 μg/d,[95] but at least one recent study showed that this range of intake is a rather high estimate and that the intake of young adults was only $\sim$100 μg/d.[91] Liver is known to provide a significant dietary intake of menaquinones, but, except for some fermented food products consumed by the oriental population, the major source of vitamin in the diet is phylloquinone of plant origin.

Toxicity

There is no known toxicity associated with the administration of high doses of phylloquinone, a natural form of the vitamin.[96] Administration of menadione to infants was shown to be associated with hemolytic anemia and liver toxicity, and phylloquinone is now prescribed to prevent hemorrhagic disease of the newborn. The toxicity of dietary menadione is, however, relatively low, and animals have been fed as much as 1000 times the daily requirement with no adverse effect.

References

1. J.W. Suttie (1984) Vitamin K. In: *Handbook of Vitamins: Nutritional, Biochemical, and Clinical Aspects* (L.J. Machlin, ed.), pp. 147–198, Marcel Dekker, New York.
2. R.E. Olson and J.W. Suttie (1978) Vitamin K and γ-carboxyglutamate biosynthesis. *Vitam. Horm.* 35:59–108.
3. K. Ramotar, J.M. Conly, H. Chubb, and T.J. Louie (1984) Production of menaquinones by intestinal anaerobes. *J. Infect. Dis.* 150:213–218.
4. F. Fernandez and M.D. Collins (1987) Vitamin K composition of anaerobic gut bacteria. *FEMS Microbiol. Lett.* 41:175–180.
5. W.V. Taggart and J.T. Matschiner (1969) Metabolism of menadione-6,7-³H in the rat. *Biochemistry* 8:1141–1146.
6. M.J. Shearer (1983) High-performance liquid chromatography of K vitamins and their antagonists. In: *Advances in Chromatography*.

(J.C. Giddings, E. Grushka, J. Cazes, and P.R. Brown, eds.), pp. 243–301, Marcel Dekker, New York.

7. M.J. Shearer, P.T. McCarthy, O.E. Crampton, and M.B. Mattock (1988) The assessment of human vitamin K status from tissue measurements. In: *Current Advances in Vitamin K Research* (J.W. Suttie, ed.), pp. 437–452, Elsevier Science Publishers, New York.

8. J.A. Sadowski, D.S. Bacon, S. Hood, et al. (1988) The application of methods used for the evaluation of vitamin K nutritional status in human and animal studies. In: *Current Advances in Vitamin K Research* (J.W. Suttie, ed.), pp. 453–463, Elsevier Science Publishers, New York.

9. K. Uchida and T. Komeno (1988) Relationships between dietary and intestinal vitamin K and urinary Gla. In: *Current Advances in Vitamin K Research* (J.W. Suttie, ed.), pp. 477–492, Elsevier Science Publishers, New York.

10. J.W. Suttie (1985) Vitamin K. In: *The Fat-soluble Vitamins* (A.T. Diplock, ed.), pp. 225–311, William Heinemann, Ltd., London.

11. M.J. Shearer, A. McBurney, and P. Barkhan (1974) Studies on the absorption and metabolism of phylloquinone (vitamin K_1) in man. *Vitam. Horm.* 32:513–542.

12. M.J. Shearer, A. McBurney, A.M. Breckenridge, and P. Barkhan (1977) Effect of warfarin on the metabolism of phylloquinone (vitamin K_1): dose-response relationships in man. *Clin. Sci. Mol. Med.* 52:621–630.

13. B.E. Gustafson (1959) Vitamin K deficiency in germfree rats. *Ann. NY Acad. Sci.* 78:166–174.

14. P.O. Ganrot and J.E. Nilehn (1968) Plasma prothrombin during treatment with dicumarol II. Demonstration of an abnormal prothrombin fraction. *Scand. J. Clin. Lab. Invest.* 22:23–28.

15. J. Stenflo (1972) Vitamin K and the biosynthesis of prothrombin. II. Structural comparison of normal and dicumarol-induced bovine prothrombin. *J. Biol. Chem.* 247:8167–8175.

16. G.L. Nelsestuen and J.W. Suttie (1972) The purification and properties of an abnormal prothrombin protein produced by dicumarol-treated cows. A comparison of normal prothrombin. *J. Biol. Chem.* 247:8176–8182.

17. G.L. Nelsestuen and J.W. Suttie (1972) Mode of action of vitamin K. Calcium binding properties of bovine prothrombin. *Biochemistry* 11:4961–4964.

18. J. Stenflo and P.O. Ganrot (1973) Binding of Ca^{2+} to normal and dicumarol-induced prothrombin. *Biochem. Biophys. Res. Commun.* 50:98–104.

19. C.T. Esmon, J.W. Suttie, and C.M. Jackson (1975) The functional significance of vitamin K action. Differences in phospholipid binding between normal and abnormal prothrombin. *J. Biol. Chem.* 250: 4095–4099.

20. J.W. Suttie (1973) Mechanism of action of vitamin K. Demonstration of a liver precursor of prothrombin. *Science* 179:192–194.

21. G.L. Nelsestuen and J.W. Suttie (1973) The mode of action of vitamin K. Isolation of a peptide containing the vitamin K-dependent portion of prothrombin. *Proc. Natl. Acad. Sci. USA* 70:3366–3370.

22. G.L. Nelsestuen, T.H. Zytkovicz, and J.B. Howard (1974) The mode of action of vitamin K identification of γ-carboxyglutamic acid as a component of prothrombin. *J. Biol. Chem.* 249:6347–6350.

23. J. Stenflo, P. Fernlund, W. Egan, and P. Roepstorff (1974) Vitamin K dependent modifications of glutamic acid residues in prothrombin. *Proc. Natl. Acad. Sci. USA* 71:2730–2733.

24. S. Magnusson, L. Sottrup-Jensen, T.E. Petersen, H.R. Morris, and A. Dell (1974) Primary structure of the vitamin K-dependent part of prothrombin. *FEBS Lett.* 44:189–193.

25. D.A. Walz, D. Hewett-Emmett, and M.-C. Guillin (1986) Amino acid sequences and molecular homology of the vitamin K-dependent clotting factors. In: *Prothrombin and Other Vitamin K Proteins* (W.H. Seegers and D.A. Walz, ed.), pp. 125–160, CRC Press, Boca Raton, FL.

26. J. Stenflo (1976) A new vitamin K-dependent protein. Purification from bovine plasma and preliminary characterization. *J. Biol. Chem.* 251:355–363.

27. R.G. DiScipio, M.A. Hermodson, S.G. Yates, and E.W. Davie (1977) A comparison of human prothrombin, factor IX (Christmas factor), factor X (Stuart factor), and protein S. *Biochemistry* 16:698–706.

28. C.V. Prowse and M.P. Esnouf (1977) The isolation of a new warfarin-sensitive protein from bovine plasma. *Biochem. Soc. Trans.* 5:255–256.

29. P.V. Hauschka, J.B. Lian, and P.M. Gallop (1975) Direct identification of the calcium-binding amino acid γ-carboxyglutamate in mineralized tissue. *Proc. Natl. Acad. Sci. USA* 72:3925–3929.

30. P.A. Price, A.S. Otsuka, J.W. Poser, J. Kristaponis, and N. Raman (1976) Characterization of a γ-carboxyglutamic acid-containing protein from bone. *Proc. Natl. Acad. Sci. USA* 73:1447–1451.

31. P.A. Price, M.K. Williamson, T. Haba, R.B. Dell, and W.S.S. Jee (1982) Excessive mineralization with growth plate closure in rats on chronic warfarin treatment. *Proc. Natl. Acad. Sci. USA* 79: 7734–7738.

32. J.B. Lian (1988) Osteocalcin: functional studies and postulated role in bone resorption. *Current Advances in Vitamin K Research* (J.W. Suttie, ed.), pp. 245–257, Elsevier Science Publishers, New York.

33. C.M. Gundberg (1988) The concentration of osteocalcin in serum is a clinically useful marker for bone disease. In: *Current Advances in Vitamin K Research* (J.W. Suttie, ed.), pp. 275–280, Elsevier Science Publishers, New York.

34. P.A. Price and S.A. Baukol (1980) 1,25-Dihydroxyvitamin D_3 increases synthesis of the vitamin K-dependent bone protein by osteosarcoma cells. *J. Biol. Chem.* 255:11660–11663.

35. J.D. Fraser and P.A. Price (1988) Lung, heart, and kidney express high levels of mRNA for the vitamin K-dependent matrix Gla protein. Implications for the possible functions of matrix Gla protein and for the tissue distribution of the γ-carboxylase. *J. Biol. Chem.* 263: 11033–11036.

36. R. Wallin, O. Gebhardt, and H. Prydz (1978) NAD(P)H dehydrogenase and its role in the vitamin K (2-methyl-3-phytyl-1,4-naphthoquinone)-dependent carboxylation reaction. *Biochem. J.* 169:95–101.

37. M.J. Fasco and L.M. Principe (1982) Vitamin K_1 hydroquinone formation catalyzed by DT-diaphorase. *Biochem. Biophys. Res. Commun.* 104:187–192.

38. M.J. Fasco and L.M. Principe (1980) Vitamin K_1 hydroquinone formation catalyzed by a microsomal reductase system. *Biochem. Biophys. Res. Commun.* 97:1487–1492.

39. J.A. Sadowski, H.K. Schnoes, and J.W. Suttie (1977) Vitamin K epoxidase: properties and relationship to prothrombin synthesis. *Biochemistry* 16:3856–3863.

40. J.T. Matschiner, R.G. Bell, J.M. Amelotti, and T.E. Knauer (1970) Isolation and characterization of a new metabolite of phylloquinone in the rat. *Biochim. Biophys. Acta* 201:309–315.

41. D.S. Whitlon, J.A. Sadowski, and J.W. Suttie (1978) Mechanism of coumarin action: significance of vitamin K epoxide reductase inhibition. *Biochemistry* 17:1371–1377.

42. E.F. Hildebrandt and J.W. Suttie (1982) Mechanism of coumarin action: sensitivity of vitamin K metabolizing enzymes of normal and warfarin-resistant rat liver. *Biochemistry* 21:2406–2411.

43. M.J. Fasco, E.F. Hildebrandt, and J.W. Suttie (1982) Evidence that warfarin anticoagulant action involves two distinct reductase activities. *J. Biol. Chem.* 257:11210–11212.

44. L.J.M. van Haarlem, B.A.M. Soute, and C. Vermeer (1987) Vitamin K-dependent carboxylase. Possible role for thioredoxin in the reduction of vitamin K metabolites in liver. *FEBS Lett.* 222:353–357.

45. R.B. Silverman and D.L. Nandi (1988) Reduced thioredoxin: a possible physiological cofactor for vitamin K epoxide reductase.

Further support for an active site disulfide. *Biochem. Biophys. Res. Commun.* 155:1248–1254.

46. C.T. Esmon, J.A. Sadowski, and J.W. Suttie (1975) A new carboxylation reaction. The Vitamin K-dependent incorporation of $H^{14}CO_3^-$ into prothrombin. *J. Biol. Chem.* 250:4744–4748.

47. J.W. Suttie, J.M. Hageman, S.R. Lehrman, and D.H. Rich (1976) vitamin K-dependent carboxylase: development of a peptide substrate. *J. Biol. Chem.* 251:5827–5830.

48. J.W. Suttie (1985) Vitamin K-dependent carboxylase. *Ann. Rev. Biochem.* 54:459–477.

49. A.Y. Cheung, G.M. Wood, S. Funakawa, C.P. Grossman, and J.W. Suttie (1988) Vitamin K-dependent carboxylase: substrates, products, and inhibitors. In: *Current Advances in Vitamin K Research* (J.W. Suttie, ed.), pp. 3–16, Elsevier Science Publishers, New York.

50. C.P. Grossman, J.W. Suttie, T. Taguchi, Y. Suda, and Y. Kobayashi (1988) Synthesis of trifluoromethyl analogs of vitamin K as substrates for the liver microsomal vitamin K-dependent carboxylase. *BioFactors* 1:255–259.

51. D.H. Rich, S.R. Lehrman, M. Kawai, H.L. Goodman, and J.W. Suttie (1981) Synthesis of peptide analogues of prothrombin precursor sequence 5–9. Substrate specificity of vitamin K dependent carboxylase. *J. Med. Chem.* 24:706–711.

52. S.E. Hamilton, D. Tesch, and B. Zerner (1982) Vitamin K$_1$ dependent carboxylase: β-carboxylation of t-butyloxycarbonylaspartic acid α-benzyl ester. *Biochem. Biophys. Res. Commun.* 107:246–249.

53. J.J. McTigue, M.K. Dhaon, D.H. Rich, and J.W. Suttie (1984) Vitamin K-dependent carboxylase: carboxylation of aspartyl residues to β-carboxyaspartyl residues in synthetic substrates. *J. Biol. Chem.* 259:4272–4278.

54. B.A.M. Soute, C. Vermeer, M. De Metz, H.C. Hemker, and H.R. Lijnen (1981) In vitro prothrombin synthesis from a purified precursor protein. III. Preparation of an acid-soluble substrate for vitamin K-dependent carboxylase by limited proteolysis of bovine descarboxyprothrombin. *Biochim. Biophys. Acta* 676:101–107.

55. P.A. Price, J.D. Fraser, and G. Metz-Virca (1987) Molecular cloning of matrix Gla protein: implications for substrate recognition by the vitamin K-dependent γ-carboxylase. *Proc. Natl. Acad. Sci. USA* 84:8335–8339.

56. J.W. Suttie (1988) Vitamin K-dependent carboxylation of glutamyl residues in proteins. *BioFactors* 1:55–60.

57. T.L. Carlisle and J.W. Suttie (1980) Vitamin K-dependent carboxylase: subcellular location of the carboxylase and enzymes involved in vitamin K metabolism in rat liver. *Biochemistry* 19:1161–1167.

58. P.A. Friedman, M.A. Shia, P.M. Gallop, and A.E. Griep (1979) Vitamin K-dependent γ-carbon-hydrogen bond cleavage and the non-mandatory concurrent carboxylation of peptide bound glutamic acid residues. *Proc. Natl. Acad. Sci. USA* 76:3126–3129.

59. J.W. Suttie, L.O. Geweke, S.L. Martin, and A.K. Willingham (1980) Vitamin K epoxidase: dependence of epoxidase activity on substrates of the vitamin K-dependent carboxylation reaction. *FEBS Lett.* 109:267–270.

60. A.E. Larson, P.A. Friedman, and J.W. Suttie (1981) Vitamin K-dependent carboxylase: stoichiometry of carboxylation and vitamin K 2,3-epoxide formation. *J. Biol. Chem.* 256:11032–11035.

61. R. Azerad, P. Decottignies-Le Marechal, C. Ducrocq, et al. The vitamin K-dependent carboxylation of peptidic substrates: stereochemical features and mechanistic studies with substrate analogues. In: *Current Advances in Vitamin K Research* (J.W. Suttie, ed.), pp. 17–23, Elsevier Science Publishers, New York.

62. J.J. McTigue and J.W. Suttie (1983) Vitamin K-dependent carboxylase: demonstration of a vitamin K- and O_2-dependent exchange of ^3H from ^3H_2O into glutamic acid residues. *J. Biol. Chem.* 258:12129–12131.

63. D.L. Anton and P.A. Friedman (1983) Fate of the activated γ-carbon-hydrogen bond in the uncoupled vitamin K-dependent γ-glutamyl carboxylation reaction. *J. Biol. Chem.* 258:14084–14087.

64. G.M. Wood and J.W. Suttie (1988) Vitamin K-dependent carboxylase. Stoichiometry of vitamin K epoxide formation, γ-carboxyglutamyl formation, and γ-glutamyl-^3H cleavage. *J. Biol. Chem.* 263:3234–3239.

65. J.C. Swanson and J.W. Suttie (1985) Prothrombin biosynthesis: characterization of processing events in rat liver microsomes. *Biochemistry* 24:3890–3897.

66. S. Karpatkin, T.H. Finlay, A.L. Ballesteros, and M. Karpatkin (1987) Effect of warfarin on prothrombin synthesis and secretion in human HEP G2 cells. *Blood* 70:773–778.

67. E.W. Davie (1987) The blood coagulation factors: their cDNAs, genes, and expression. In: *Hemostasis and Thrombosis: Basic Principles and Clinical Practice* (R.W. Colman, J. Hirsh, V.J. Mardar, and E.W. Salzman, eds.), pp. 242–267, Lippincott, Philadelphia.

68. L.C. Pan and P.A. Price (1985) The propeptide of rat bone γ-carboxyglutamic acid protein shares homology with other vitamin K-dependent protein precursors. *Proc. Natl. Acad. Sci. USA* 82:6109–6113.

69. D.V. Shah, J.C. Swanson, and J.W. Suttie (1983) Vitamin K-dependent carboxylase: effect of detergent concentrations, vitamin K status, and added protein precursors on activity. *Arch. Biochem. Biophys.* 222:216–221.

70. M.R. Evans, M.W.P. Sung, and M.P. Esnouf (1984) The early stages in the biosynthesis of prothrombin. *Biochem. Soc. Trans.* 12:1051–1052.

71. J.W. Suttie, J.A. Hoskins, J. Engelke, et al. (1987) Vitamin K dependent carboxylase: possible role of the "propeptide" as an intracellular recognition site (γ-carboxyglutamic acid protein C). *Proc. Natl. Acad. Sci. USA* 84:634–637.

72. M.J. Jorgensen, A.B. Cantor, B.C. Furie, C.L. Brown, C.B. Shoemaker, and B. Furie (1987) Recognition site directing vitamin K-dependent γ-carboxylation residues on the propeptide of factor IX. *Cell* 48:185–191.

73. D.C. Foster, M.S. Rudinski, B.G. Schach, et al. (1987) Propeptide of human protein C is necessary for gamma-carboxylation. *Biochemistry* 26:7003–7011.

74. M.M.W. Ulrich, B. Furie, M.R. Jacobs, C. Vermeer, and B.C. Furie (1988) Vitamin K-dependent carboxylation. A synthetic peptide based upon the γ-carboxylation recognition site sequence of the prothrombin propeptide is an active substrate for the carboxylase in vitro. *J. Biol. Chem.* 263:9697–9702.

75. J.E. Knobloch and J.W. Suttie (1987) Vitamin K-dependent carboxylase. Control of enzyme activity by the "propeptide" region of factor X. *J. Biol. Chem.* 262:15334–15337.

76. P.A. Lane and W.E. Hathaway (1985) Vitamin K in infancy. *J. Pediatr.* 106:351–359.

77. M. Andrew, B. Paes, R. Milner, et al. (1987) Development of the human coagulation system in the full-term infant. *Blood* 70:165–172.

78. J.M. Sutherland, H.I. Glueck, and G. Gleser (1967) Hemorrhagic disease of the newborn. *Am. J. Dis. Child.* 113:524–533.

79. R.v. Kries, M.J. Shearer, M. Haug, G. Harzer, and U. Gobel (1988) Vitamin K deficiency and vitamin K intake in infants. In: *Current Advances in Vitamin K Research* (J.W. Suttie, ed.), pp. 515–523, Elsevier Science Publishers, New York.

80. K. Motohara, M. Matsukura, I. Matsuda, et al. (1984) Severe vitamin K deficiency in breast-fed infants. *J. Pediatr.* 105:943–945.

81. American Academy of Pediatrics, Committee on Nutrition (1971) Vitamin K supplementation for infants receiving milk substitute infant formulas and for those with fat malabsorption. *Pediatrics* 48:483–487.

82. J.E. Ansell, R. Kumar, and D. Deykin (1977) The spectrum of vitamin K deficiency. *JAMA* 238:40–42.

83. J.B. Alperin (1987) Coagulopathy caused by vitamin K deficiency in critically ill, hospitalized patients. *JAMA* 258:1916–1919.

84. D. Savage and J. Lindenbaum (1983) Clinical and experimental human vitamin K deficiency. In: *Nutrition in Hematology* (J. Lindenbaum, ed.), pp. 271–320, Churchill Livingstone, New York.

85. J.J. Lipsky (1988) Antibiotic-associated hypoprothrombinaemia. *J. Antimicrob. Chemother.* 21:281–300.

86. M.J. Shearer, H. Bechtold, K. Andrassy, et al. (1988) Mechanism of cephalosporin-induced hypoprothrombinemia: relation to cephalosporin side chain, vitamin K metabolism, and vitamin K status. *J. Clin. Pharmacol.* 28:88–95.

87. S.J. Dudrick, D.W. Wilmore, H.M. Vars, and J.E. Rhoads (1968) Long-term total parenteral nutrition with growth, development and positive nitrogen balance. *Surgery* 64:134–142.

88. P.G. Frick, G. Riedler, and H. Brogli (1967) Dose response and minimal daily requirement for vitamin K in man. *J. Appl. Physiol.* 23:387–389.

89. E.A. Doisy (1971) In: *Symposium Proceedings on the Biochemistry, Assay and Nutritional Value of Vitamin K and Related Compounds,* pp. 79–92, Association of Vitamin Chemists, Chicago.

90. R.A. O'Reilly (1971) Vitamin K in hereditary resistance to oral anticoagulant drugs. *Am. J. Physiol.* 221:1327–1330.

91. J.W. Suttie, L.L. Mummah-Schendel, D.V. Shah, B.J. Lyle, and J.L. Greger (1988) Vitamin K deficiency from dietary vitamin K restriction in humans. *Am. J. Clin. Nutr.* 47:475–480.

92. P.M. Allison, L.L. Mummah-Schendel, C.G. Kindberg, C.S. Harms, N.U. Bang, and J.W. Suttie (1987) Effects of a vitamin K-deficient diet and antibiotics in normal human volunteers. *J. Lab. Clin. Med.* 110:180–188.

93. H. Cohen, S.D. Scott, I.J. Mackie, et al. (1988) The development of hypoprothrombinaemia following antibiotic therapy in malnourished patients with low serum vitamin K_1 levels. *Br. J. Haematol.* 68:63–66.

94. R.A. Blanchard, B.C. Furie, M. Jorgensen, S.F. Kruger, and B. Furie (1981) Acquired vitamin K-dependent carboxylation deficiency in liver disease. *N. Engl. J. Med.* 305:242–248.

95. R.E. Olson (1988) Vitamin K. In: *Modern Nutrition in Health and Disease* (M.E. Shils and V.R. Young, eds.), pp. 328–339, Lea & Febiger, Philadelphia.

96. National Research Council (1987) *Vitamin Tolerance of Animals,* National Academy Press, Washington, DC.

Ascorbic Acid

Brief History of Vitamin C

Scurvy, now known to be the consequence of a deficiency in vitamin C, was described by ancient Greeks, Egyptians, and Romans. Scurvy was historically a scourge of armies, navies, and explorers. Armies on long marches, including the crusaders, suffered from the consequences of scurvy. Wars, including the U.S. Civil War, were menaced by scurvy. Sea voyagers were ravaged by scurvy. As examples, the majority of the crews were lost to scurvy during the long voyages of Vasco da Gama (in 1498), of Magellan (in 1519), and of Jacques Cartier (in Newfoundland in 1535). During the voyage of Admiral George Anson in 1740–1744, over a thousand sailors of an initial crew of 1955 were lost, mainly to scurvy. The British naval surgeon James Lind investigated extensively the problem of scurvy in the British navy. His experiences were recorded in 1753 in his *Treatise of the Scurvy*.[1] During the California gold rush, thousands of prospectors succumbed to scurvy. Not until 1907, with the discovery by Holst and Fröhlich that a scorbutic condition could be produced in the guinea pig, was it fully accepted that scurvy was the result of a dietary deficiency.[2,3]

Subsequently, during the period of 1928–1931, Szent-Györgyi extracted a substance from cabbage, oranges, paprika, and adrenal glands, which he named hexuronic acid.[4–7] Shortly thereafter, Waugh and King[8,9] reported that hexuronic acid was the same as the vitamin C that they had isolated from oranges and lemons. Svirbely and Szent-Györgyi[10,11] also demonstrated that the isolated hexuronic acid had antiscorbutic activity. The structural formula was determined and the compound was synthesized in 1933.[6,12] L-Ascorbic acid is now synthesized in considerable tonnage for human nutrition, pharmaceutical uses, animal feeds, and industrial applications.

Those interested in the history of scurvy should read the extensive, fascinating, and well-documented book of K.J. Carpenter.[13] Several other recent publications provide additional related information.[14–17]

Chemistry, Structure, and Chemical Properties

Vitamin C, a six-carbon compound, is closely related to glucose. The white crystalline material has a molecular weight of 176.1, melts at 190–192 °C, has a sharp acidic taste, and is highly soluble in water. Water solutions are unstable. Ascorbic acid rapidly oxidizes in the presence of oxygen, a reaction that is accelerated by copper, iron, or an alkaline pH. Normally, most of the vitamin exists as ascorbic acid, which can be reversibly oxidized to dehydroascorbic acid (Figure 1). Further oxidation results in irreversible formation of diketogulonic acid and other products that possess no antiscorbutic activity.

The stereoisomer of L-ascorbic acid, known as erythrobic acid or D-isoascorbic acid, has little if any antiscorbutic activity for humans or guinea pigs.[18–26] However, when given in a sufficiently high dose, erythorbic acid was reported to replace ascorbic acid in guinea pigs.[18,24,25] Other studies with guinea pigs suggest that erythorbic acid may have an antagonistic effect that may reduce the amount of ascorbate present in tissues by inhibiting the tissue uptake or storage of ascorbic acid.[27]

Both ascorbic acid and erythorbic acid are used extensively in the United States as antioxidants in the food industry. Items such as frankfurters, beef bologna, bacon, and ham may contain 0.15–0.58 mg erythorbic acid/g (H.E. Sauberlich, unpublished observations, 1988).[28] Nonchromatographic methods for measuring ascorbate levels in foods are unable to distinguish between the erythorbic acid and ascorbic acid. Consequently, reported vitamin C contents of some food items may be erroneously high.

Methods of Analysis

Numerous methods are available for determining vitamin C in animal tissue extracts, fluids, and

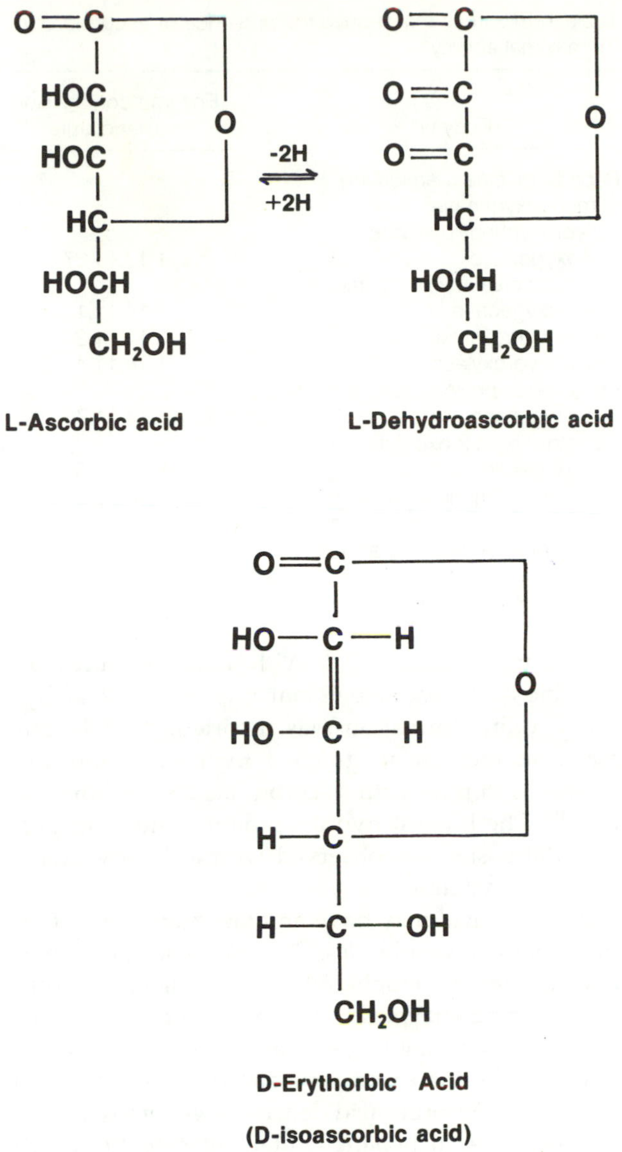

L-Ascorbic acid

L-Dehydroascorbic acid

D-Erythorbic Acid

(D-isoascorbic acid)

Figure 1. Vitamin C.

foods.[29–31] The procedures usually either measure the reduced form of ascorbic acid or determine total ascorbic acid based upon the oxidation of ascorbic acid followed by the formation of a hydrazone or fluorophor.[29,32,33] Colorimetric methods for the determination of ascorbic acid usually are based on the reduction of 2,6-dichlorophenolindophenol or the formation of a colored dinitrophenylhydrazine derivative of the vitamin.[32–35] The dinitrophenylhydrazine method measures both dehydroascorbic acid and total ascorbic acid. The 2,6-dichlorophenolindophenol method measures only reduced ascorbic acid. Automated procedures were described for both methods.[29,36] Metaphosphoric acid, perchloric acid, or trichloracetic acid is generally used for the extraction and stabilization of ascorbic acid in assay samples. Other colorimetric methods used to measure ascorbic acid include the ferrozine method and the iodometric method adopted by the United States Pharmacopeia.[37,38] An enzyme method for ascorbic acid analysis using ascorbic acid oxidase was described, but the procedure has received only limited application.[39] The α,α'-dipyridyl complex procedure is a fast and simple procedure that has been used frequently.[32,33,40] The fluorometric method of Deutsch and Weeks[41] is a highly specific and sensitive method for the determination of ascorbic acid. The method is based on the oxidation of ascorbic acid to dehydroascorbic acid and the condensation of dehydroascorbic acid with O-phenylenediamine to form the fluorophor quinoxaline.

More recently high-performance liquid chromatography (HPLC) procedures have become the methods of choice for the measurement of ascorbic acid in biological materials and foods.[27,29,42–49] Procedures vary in the type of column, mobile phase, detection system, and stabilization of extracts. The HPLC methods are rapid, specific, and sensitive. When applied to serum or plasma specimens, the ferrozine, dinitrophenylhydrazine, O-phenylenediamine, and HPLC methods provide comparable results. Somewhat higher values are obtained with the α,α'-dipyridyl and 2,6-dichlorophenolindophenol methods.[25] Unlike other methods, the HPLC procedures are capable of distinguishing between ascorbic acid and erythorbic acid.[25,27,28,42–47,50–52] With the use of an electrochemical detector, subnanogram quantities of the isomers may be measured.[44]

Absorption and Transport

The relatively high amounts of ascorbic acid that are present in fresh, frozen, and canned strawberries, tomatoes, citrus fruits, and other vegetables and fruits are considered readily available and efficiently absorbed.[53] For the human, intakes up to 100 mg ascorbic acid/d are 80–90% absorbed.[54–56] The efficiency of absorption falls with higher intakes.[57,58] In the human and other vitamin C–dependent animals, the majority of the ascorbic acid is absorbed in the distal region of the small intestine where a sodium-dependent active-transport system (K_m of ~1 mmol/L) is present.[26,58–67] Ascorbic acid absorption occurs also at a low rate by simple diffusion.[59,61,66–68] In rats ascorbic acid is absorbed from the intestine in a passive process.[69]

The upper level of ascorbic acid in the blood is limited by kidney clearance with a Tm of 85 μmol/L. Ascorbic acid appears to be transferred into the central nervous system and other tissues by a facilitated saturable process.[70] Thus, human leukocytes may accumulate ascorbic acid in the cytosol in concentrations that may exceed the plasma concentration by over 80-fold.[70,71] Dehydroascorbic acid, the oxidative product of ascorbic acid, appears to be transported by diffusion. Dehydroascorbic acid is the preferred form of vitamin C for uptake by erythrocytes, lymphocytes, and neutrophils.[72] Within the erythrocyte, dehydroascorbic acid is reduced to ascorbic acid by a glutathione-dependent, dehydroascorbic-acid-reducing enzyme.[63] Diabetic subjects were reported to have elevated serum levels of dehydroascorbic acid.[73] Dehydroascorbic acid also was observed to have an inhibitory effect on insulin secretion from mouse pancreatic islets.[74]

The accumulation of ascorbic acid at the concentrations observed in tissues such as the adrenals and the pituitary gland requires the transportation of the vitamin against a concentration gradient. A stereospecific, active transport mechanism is thought to exist.[70]

High intakes of iron, copper, zinc, and pectin were observed to have an adverse effect on vitamin C metabolism. It is uncertain whether these effects reflect a direct influence on the absorption of ascorbic acid or represent changes in the amount of the vitamin oxidized before absorption. Vitamin C is highly labile to oxidation, which may be enhanced by the presence of iron, zinc, and copper.

Biochemical Functions

The biochemical functions of ascorbic acid were reviewed by England and Seifter[75] and Hornig et al.[64,76] Chiefly, vitamin C serves as a reducing agent in a number of important hydroxylation reactions in the body.[77,78] Table 1 indicates some of the enzymes that are influenced by the presence of ascorbic acid.[75] However, vitamin C appears to have additional metabolic roles.[79]

Vitamin C participates in the hydroxylation of proline to hydroxyproline and lysine to hydroxylysine.[80–82] Consequently, a deficiency in ascorbic acid results in an impairment of collagen synthesis.[83] The defect in collagen synthesis is reflected in failure of wounds to heal, defects in tooth formation, and rupture of capillaries. Ascorbic acid is required for normal function of fibroblasts and osteoblasts. The vitamin participates in the hydroxylation of trimethyllysine and α-butyrobetaine in carnitine synthesis.[75] Vitamin C participates in the synthesis of adrenal hormones and vasoactive amines, microsomal drug metabolism, leukocyte functions, tyrosine metabolism, wound healing, and folate metabolism.[84–96] The functions of ascorbic acid in endocrine systems were the subject of an extensive review.[97] However, despite extensive investigations the molecular function of ascorbic acid in vivo remains uncertain.[75]

Several studies indicate a role for ascorbic acid in

Table 1. Enzymes that require the presence of ascorbic acid for maximal activity*

Enzyme	Enzyme commission nomenclature
Peptidyl glycine α-amidating monooxygenase	—
4-Hydroxyphenylpyruvate dioxygenase	1.13.11.27
γ-Butyrobetaine, 2-oxoglutarate 4-dioxygenase	1.14.11.1
Proline hydroxylase	1.14.11.2
Lysine hydroxylase	1.14.11.4
Procollagen-proline 2-oxoglutarate dioxygenase	1.14.11.7
Trimethyllysine-2-oxoglutarate dioxygenase	1.14.11.8
Dopamine β-monooxygenase	1.14.17.1

* From references 19 and 22.

periodontal disease.[98–101] With tissue cultures an ascorbic acid dose-dependent improvement of hydroxyproline formation was reported.[102–104] In humans an increase in gingival hydroxyproline and proline occurred with ascorbic acid supplementation.[105] The highest hydroxyproline content in periodontal tissue was observed with a dietary intake of 100 mg vitamin C.

Ascorbic acid may have an ameliorative effect on the toxicity of xenobiotics.[106–111] Xenobiotics, such as polychlorinated biophenyls, induce hepatic drug-metabolizing enzymes.[106,107] To attain maximum induction of the enzymes, the requirement for ascorbic acid may be increased severalfold in experimental animals.[106] Ascorbic acid deficiency generally results in a decrease in hepatic content of cytochrome P-450 and a decrease in hepatic activity of drug-metabolizing enzymes.[84,112] In guinea pigs ascorbic acid deficiency does not interfere with the synthesis of the heme essential for cytochrome P-450 formation.

Ascorbic acid has been considered as a nitrosation inhibitor with potential importance as an in vivo nitrite scavenger.[113] Vitamin C also has been considered a nutrient with cancer-prevention properties.[114–117] Epidemiologic studies suggest that the consumption of vitamin C–rich foods is associated with a lower risk of stomach and esophageal cancers.[118]

Although numerous studies have been conducted on the effects of ascorbic acid on cholesterol and triglyceride metabolism, the significance of the results is difficult to assess.[65,119] Hypercholesterolemia and hypertriglyceridemia occur in guinea pigs fed a vitamin C–deficient diet.[120,121] Elevated intakes of ascorbic acid may lower blood concentrations of cholesterol and triglycerides in guinea pigs, monkeys, rats, and other laboratory animals.[65,121–124] Other studies indicate that high concentrations of ascorbic acid intakes may make copper unavailable for regulating cholesterol metabolism.[65,125]

Metabolites

Ascorbic acid is widely distributed throughout the tissues of the human body. Concentrations range considerably among tissues; highest concentrations are in the pituitary gland, adrenals, and leukocytes (Table 2).[32,43,70,71,73] However, the major portion of the ascorbate pool in the body resides in the skeletal muscle, brain, and liver.

Absorbed vitamin C equilibrates readily with the body pool of the vitamin. The average adult man has a body pool of vitamin C of 1.2–2.0 g, which is utilized at a rate of 3–4%/d.[127–131] A body pool of ~1.5 g may be provided with a daily intake of ~75 mg of ascorbic acid.[129,131,132] Saturation of the total-body ascorbate pool in young adult males would require an estimated daily intake of 138 mg.[133]

Ascorbic acid is metabolized to 2,3-diketogulonic acid and oxalate and is excreted in the urine.[26,67] However, excess intakes of vitamin C are largely excreted unchanged. The renal threshold for ascorbic acid is ~85 μmol/L of plasma. Vitamin C intakes >200 mg/d result in the formation of carbon dioxide from ascorbic acid.[57]

In humans, guinea pigs, and monkeys, ascorbic acid metabolites identified in the urine include dehydroascorbic acid, diketogulonic acid, ascorbate-2-sulfate, oxalate, 2-O-methyl ascorbate, and 2-ketoascorbitol.[65,67] Ascorbate-2-sulfate is found in high concentrations in brine shrimp cysts. An important metabolic role for ascorbate-2-sulfate appears unlikely because the compound is not antiscorbutic for the guinea pig or monkey.[26,122,134] Ascorbate-2-sulfate can, however, replace ascorbic acid in fish.[135,136]

Deficiency

In humans deficiency in vitamin C results in scurvy, a long-recognized disease. Experimentally, scurvy is characterized by petechiae, bleeding gums, follicular hyperkeratosis, perifollicular hemorrhage, arthralgia and joint effusions, fatigue, depression, and hypochondriasis.[63,127–131,137] Neuropathy and components of the sicca syndrome may occur. Resistance to infections is compromised.[67] In developed countries the rare occurrence of scurvy is usually associated with alcoholism, nutritional ignorance, and poverty.[137]

In neonates a vitamin C deficiency may result in scurvy or in a transient tyrosinemia.[89–92,138] Although neonatal scurvy is extremely rare, it is manifested by tenderness of the lower extremities, hemorrhage of

Table 2. Ascorbic acid concentrations in human tissues*

Tissue	Concentration	
	mg/100 g wet tissue	mmol/kg wet tissue
Pituitary gland	40–50	2.3–2.8
Adrenals	30–40	1.7–2.3
Liver	10–16	0.6–0.9
Spleen	10–15	0.6–0.9
Lungs	7	0.4
Kidneys	5–15	0.3–0.9
Heart muscle	5–15	0.3–0.9
Brain	13–15	0.8–0.9
Pancreas	10–15	0.6–0.9
Aqueous humor	18.6	1.06
Eye lens	25–31	1.4–1.8
Testes	3	0.2
Thyroid	2	0.1
Skeletal muscle	3–4	0.2–0.3
Saliva	0.07–0.09	0.004–0.005
Plasma	0.3–1.0	0.017–0.057
Erythrocytes	0.3–1.0	0.017–0.057
Granulocytes	21	1.2
Monocytes	65	3.7
Platelets	30	1.7

* See references 22, 47, 70, 71, 78, 128.

the costochondral cartilages, fever, and irritability. A transient tyrosinemia may occur in up to 30% of premature infants and 10% of full-term infants. The tyrosinemia results from a partial deficiency of the p-hydroxyphenylpyruvic acid oxidase enzyme. The activity of this enzyme is increased with the administration of ascorbic acid. Although the tyrosinemia is generally considered harmless, mild impairment of mental development during late childhood was reported.[90,91] To protect against possible adverse effects of transient tyrosinemia, an intake of 100 mg ascorbic acid/d during the first week of life is recommended.[91]

Evaluation of Vitamin C Status

The measurement of plasma or serum concentrations of ascorbic acid is the most commonly used and practical procedure for evaluation of vitamin C nutritional status.[25,30,33,139,140] Plasma vitamin C concentrations of 11–17 μmol/L are considered indicative of low or inadequate intakes of the vitamin. Plasma ascorbate concentrations of 34–43 μmol/L are usually maintained in normal adults with daily intakes of 60–75 mg (340–426 μmol) of ascorbic acid. Whole blood, erythrocyte, and leukocyte ascorbate concentrations also were used to assess vitamin status.[25,30,33,47,99,141–143] The measurement of leukocyte vitamin C concentrations is somewhat more tedious to perform and more prone to analytical errors. Leukocyte vitamin C concentrations have been thought to provide information concerning body stores of ascorbic acid.[33,144]

Requirements

A wide variety of plant and animal species synthesize ascorbic acid from carbohydrate precursors. However, humans, other primates, guinea pigs, certain insects, invertebrates, fish, bats, and birds cannot synthesize ascorbic acid.[63,73,145–153] The absence of the microsomal enzyme L-gulonolactone oxidase (EC 1.1.3.8) results in an inability to synthesize the vitamin.[154–157] Although rats normally have the ability to synthesize ascorbic acid, a strain of rat was observed to lack the L-gulonolactone oxidase enzyme (EC 1.1.3.8) and, hence, has a dietary requirement for vitamin C.[158,159] The willow ptarmigan also appears unique in that it can synthesize some ascorbic acid but requires an additional dietary source to meet its need to survive.[160]

Human requirements for vitamin C have been guided by the 1989 Recommended Dietary Allowances.[92] These allowances were derived from the amount of ascorbic acid that will cure or prevent scurvy, the amount that is metabolized in the body, and the amount necessary to maintain adequate body reserves.

Recent studies demonstrated that the vitamin C requirement for adult nonpregnant women would be marginally met by an intake of 60 mg (340 μmol) ascorbic acid/d.[25]

Vitamin C requirements of cigarette smokers are higher than those of nonsmokers by as much as 40%.[54,161,162] Smokers have lower plasma ascorbate levels and an increased metabolic turnover of the vitamin.[54,161–167] In addition to smoking, a number of other factors may influence the needs for ascorbic acid. Acute emotional or environmental stress, such as exposure to elevated temperatures, was reported to increase the amount of vitamin C required to maintain normal plasma ascorbate concentrations.[91,168–171] Drugs, including aspirin and oral contraceptives, were reported to affect vitamin C requirement, although the significance of these data is not certain.[172–176]

Studies showed that elderly men have significantly lower plasma ascorbic acid concentrations than do elderly women at similar intakes of the vitamin.[139,177,178] Over half of the healthy elderly men examined had plasma concentrations of ascorbic acid of <17 μmol/L. The results suggested that elderly men and women have an increased requirement for vitamin C. Daily intakes of ascorbic acid of 125 mg and 75 mg were recommended for healthy elderly

men and women, respectively.[139,178] However, another report concluded that there was little evidence that the RDA for vitamin C should be altered for elderly people.[179]

The absorption of nonheme iron from the diet can be enhanced fourfold or more by the simultaneous ingestion of 25–75 mg vitamin C.[180–182] To be effective vitamin C and iron must be consumed in the same meal.[183] The inhibition of iron absorption by phytates in the diet also can be significantly counteracted by ascorbic acid.[184] Aspirin treatment of rheumatoid-arthritis patients can reduce ascorbic acid concentrations in platelets and plasma; the reduction can be prevented by vitamin C supplements.[185]

Food Sources

Relatively high amounts of vitamin C are present in strawberries, citrus fruits, tomatoes, and various vegetables, including cabbage, cauliflower, broccoli, and greens (Table 3). However, the ascorbic acid content in foods may be influenced by numerous factors.[186] Postharvest storage will affect the vitamin C content of raw fruits and vegetables commensurate with the time and temperature of storage, extent of cellular tissue damage, and the presence of ascorbic acid oxidase. Tomatoes and other seed-containing tissues show striking changes in the concentration of vitamin C during maturation. Extremely variable distribution of ascorbic acid may be observed within an individual fruit or vegetable. Because of its lability to destruction by oxidation, prolonged cooking, particularly in the presence of iron and copper, may result in appreciable losses of the vitamin.

Toxicity

Megadoses of ascorbic acid have been reported to have beneficial effects on resistance to the common cold and various diseases.[13,79,187,188] These claims, however, have not been well documented or accepted. For most individuals ascorbic acid has a low toxicity and, hence, excessive intakes are tolerated. Adverse effects of high ascorbate supplements have been reported on occasion, such as hypoglycemia, induced uricosuria,[189] dependency or rebound effect,[142] and hemolysis in patients with erythrocyte glucose-6-phosphate dehydrogenase deficiency.[187,190]

With excessive intake the absorbed ascorbic acid is largely excreted into the urine. Only a small amount is metabolized to oxalate regardless of the level of intake.[25,33] However, studies indicate that individuals who form kidney stones should avoid the intake of high doses of vitamin C.[191] This also is true for patients with renal impairment or who are on chronic hemodialysis.[192]

Table 3. Vitamin C content of selected foods*

Food item	Vitamin C content	Food item	Vitamin C content
	mg/100 g		*mg/100 g*
Willow leaves	415	Arctic dwarf raspberry	38
Green pepper, raw	128	Collard greens, cooked	30
Scurvy grass (stems and seed pods)	111	Spinach, cooked	28
Broccoli, cooked	90	Rutabaga, cooked	26
Brussels sprouts, cooked	86	Tomato, fresh	23
Turnip greens, cooked	69	Tomato juice	16
Watercress, raw	68	Potato, baked in skin	20
Kale, cooked	62	Potato, boiled	16
Strawberries, fresh	59	Vegetable juice	9
Cauliflower, cooked	55	Pineapple juice	9
Cereals, fortified	52	Grape juice	Trace
Oranges, fresh	49	Fruits (peach, pear, apricot, banana, plum, apple, grape)	≤10
Orange juice	49		
Mustard greens, cooked	49	Carrot, celery, and lettuce	≤10
Cabbage, raw, green	46	Milk, 2% fat	1
Kohlrabi, cooked	42	Fried chicken	0
Cranberry juice	40	Roast beef	0
Grapefruit juice	38	Eggs, fresh or cooked	0
Cheese, various	0	Hamburger, regular, plain	0

* From references 150 and 186. The vitamin C content of additional items may be obtained from the U.S. Department of Agriculture Handbooks on composition of foods.

References

1. J. Lind (1753) *A Treatise of the Scurvy*. Edinburgh.
2. A. Holst and T. Frölich (1907) Experimental studies relating to ship-beri-beri and scurvy. II. On the etiology of scurvy. *J. Hyg. (Lond)* 7:634–671.
3. B.C. Johnson (1954) Axel Holst. *J. Nutr.* 53:3–16.
4. A. Szent-Györgyi (1928) Observations on the function of the peroxidase systems and the chemistry of the adrenal cortex. Description of a new carbohydrate derivative. *Biochem. J.* 22:1387–1409.
5. A. Szent-Györgyi (1931) The function of hexuronic acid in the respiration of the cabbage leaf. *Biochem. J.* 90:385–393.
6. R.G. Ault, D.K. Baird, H.C. Carrington, et al. (1933) Synthesis of d- and l-ascorbic acid and of analogous substances. *J. Chem. Soc.* 1419–1423.
7. C.G. King (1953) The discovery and chemistry of vitamin C. *Proc. Nutr. Soc.* 12:219–227.
8. C.G. King and W.A. Waugh (1932) The chemical nature of vitamin C. *Science* 75:357–358.
9. W.A. Waugh and C.G. King (1932) Isolation and identification of vitamin C. *J. Biol. Chem.* 97:325–331.
10. J.L. Svirbely and A. Szent-Györgyi (1932) The chemical nature of vitamin C. *Biochem. J.* 26:865–870.
11. J.L. Svirbely and A. Szent-Györgyi (1933) Chemical nature of vitamin C. *Biochem. J.* 27:279–285.
12. T. Reichstein, A. Gruessner, and R. Oppenauer (1933) Synthesis of d- and l-ascorbic acid (vitamin C). *Helv. Chim. Acta* 16:1019–1033.
13. K.J. Carpenter (1986) *The History of Scurvy and Vitamin C.* Cambridge University Press, New York.
14. F.J. Stare and I.M. Star (1988). Charles Glen King, 1896–1988. *J. Nutr.* 118:1272–1277.
15. T.H. Jukes (1988) The identification of vitamin C, an historical summary. *J. Nutr.* 118:1290–1293.
16. R.W. Moss (1987) *Free Radical: Albert Szent-Györgyi and the Battle over Vitamin C.* Paragon House, New York.
17. K.J. Carpenter (1988) *Free Radical: Albert Szent-Gyorgyi and the Battle over Vitamin C.* R.W. Moss, ed. Book review. *J. Nutr.* 118:1422–1423.
18. J. Fabianek and A. Heys (1969) Antiscorbutic activity of D-araboascorbic acid. *Proc. Soc. Exp. Biol. Med.* 125:462–465.
19. M.M. Wang, K.H. Fisher, and M.L. Dodds (1962) Comparative metabolic response to erythorbic acid and ascorbic acid by the human. *J. Nutr.* 77:443–447.
20. J.M. Rivers, E.D. Huang, and M.L. Dodds (1963) Human metabolism of L-ascorbic acid and erythorbic acid. *J. Nutr.* 81:163–168.
21. J.S. Reiff and A.H. Free (1959) Nutritional studies with isoascorbic acid in the guinea pig. *J. Agric. Food Chem.* 7:55–56.
22. R.E. Hughes and R.J. Hurley (1969) The uptake of D-araboascorbic acid (D-isoascorbic acid) by guinea-pig tissues. *Br. J. Nutr.* 23:211–216.
23. O. Pelletier and C. Godin (1969) Vitamin C activity of D-isoascorbic acid for the guinea pig. *Can. J. Physiol. Pharmacol.* 47:985–991.
24. H.M. Goldman, B.S. Gould, and H.N. Munro (1981) The antiscorbutic action of L-ascorbic acid and D-isoascorbic acid (erythorbic acid) in the guinea pig. *Am. J. Clin. Nutr.* 34:24–33.
25. H.E. Sauberlich, M.J. Kretsch, P.C. Taylor, H.L. Johnson, and J.H. Skala (1989) Ascorbic acid and erythorbic metabolism in nonpregnant women. *Am. J. Clin. Nutr.* 50:1039–1049.
26. D. Hornig (1975) Metabolism of ascorbic acid. *World Rev. Nutr. Diet.* 23:225–258.
27. N. Arakawa, E. Suzuki, T. Kurata, M. Otsuka, and C. Inagaki (1986) Effect of erythorbic acid administration on ascorbic acid content in guinea pig tissues. *J. Nutr. Sci. Vitaminol. (Tokyo)* 32:171–181.
28. M.A. Kutnink and S.T. Omaye (1987) Determination of ascorbic acid, erythorbic acid, and uric acid in cured meats by high performance liquid chromatography. *J. Food Sci.* 52:53–56.
29. H.E. Sauberlich, M.D. Green, and S.T. Omaye (1982) Determination of ascorbic acid and dehydroascorbic acid. In: *Ascorbic Acid: Chemistry, Metabolism and Uses* (P.A. Seib and B.M.

Tolbert, eds.), Advances In Chemistry Series, no. 200, pp. 200–221, American Chemical Society, Washington, DC.

30. H.E. Sauberlich (1975) Vitamin C status: methods and findings. *Ann. N.Y. Acad. Sci.* 258:438–450.

31. O. Pelletier (1985) Vitamin C (L-ascorbic and dehydro-L-ascorbic acids). In: *Methods of Vitamin Assay,* 4th ed., pp. 303–347, Wiley-Interscience, New York.

32. S.T. Omaye, J.D. Turnbull, and H.E. Sauberlich (1979) Selected methods for the determination of ascorbic acid in animal cells, tissues and fluids. *Methods Enzymol.* 62:3–11.

33. H.E. Sauberlich (1981) Ascorbic acid (vitamin C). *Clin. Lab. Med.* 1:673–684.

34. J.H. Roe and C.H. Kuether (1943) The determination of ascorbic acid in whole blood and urine through the 2,4-dinitrophenylhydrazine derivative of dehydroascorbic acid. *J. Biol. Chem.* 147:399–407.

35. R.R. Schaffert and G.R. Kingsley (1955) A rapid, simple method for the determination of reduced, dehydro-, and total ascorbic acid in biological materials. *J. Biol. Chem.* 212:59–69.

36. H.E. Sauberlich, W.C. Goad, J.H. Skala, and P.P. Waring (1976) Procedure for mechanized (continuous-flow) measurement of serum ascorbic acid (vitamin C). *Clin. Chem.* 22:105–110.

37. E.L. McGown, M.G. Rusnak, C.M. Lewis, and J.A. Tillotson (1982) Tissue ascorbic acid analysis using ferrozine compared with the dinitrophenylhydrazine method. *Anal. Biochem.* 119:55–61.

38. P. Finholt, R.B. Paulssen, and T. Higuchi (1963) Rate of anaerobic degradation of ascorbic acid in aqueous solution. *J. Pharm. Sci.* 52:948–954.

39. T.Z. Liu, N. Chin, M.D. Kiser, and W.N. Bigler (1982) Specific spectrophotometry of ascorbic acid in serum and plasma by use of ascorbate oxidase. *Clin. Chem.* 28:2225–2228.

40. V. Zannoni, M. Lynch, S. Goldstein, and P. Sato (1974) A rapid method for the determination of ascorbic acid in plasma and tissues. *Biochem. Med.* 11:41–48.

41. M.J. Deutsch and C.E. Weeks (1965) Microfluorometric assay for vitamin C. *J. Assoc. Off. Anal. Chem.* 48:1248–1256.

42. C.S. Tsao and S.L. Salimi (1982) Differential determination of L-ascorbic acid and D-isoascorbic acid by reversed-phase high-performance liquid chromatography with electrochemical detection. *J. Chromatogr.* 245:355–358.

43. J.M. Coustard and G. Sudraud (1981) Separation des acides ascorbique et isoascorbique par chromatographie des paires d'ions sur phase inverse. *J. Chromatogr.* 219:338–342.

44. M.A. Kutnink, J.H. Skala, H.E. Sauberlich, and S.T. Omaye (1985) Simultaneous determination of ascorbic acid, isoascorbic acid (erythorbic acid) and uric acid in human plasma by high-performance liquid chromatography with amperometric detection. *J. Liquid Chromatogr.* 8:31–46.

45. L.W. Donar and K.B. Kicks (1981) High-performance liquid chromatographic separation of ascorbic acid, erythorbic acid, dehydroascorbic acid, dehydroerythorbic acid, diketogulonic acid, and diketogluconic acid. *Anal. Biochem.* 115:225–230.

46. N. Narakawa, M. Otsuka, T. Kurata, and C. Inagaki (1981) Separative determination of ascorbic acid and erythorbic acid by high-performance liquid chromatography. *J. Nutr. Sci. Vitaminol. (Tokyo)* 27:1–7.

47. S.T. Omaye, E.E. Schaus, M.A. Kutnink, and W.C. Hawkes (1987) Measurement of vitamin C in blood components by high-performance liquid chromatography. *Ann. N.Y. Acad. Sci.* 498:389–401.

48. E.E. Schaus, M.A. Kutnink, D.K. O'Connor, and S.T. Omaye (1986) A comparison of leukocyte ascorbate levels measured by the 2,4-dinitrophenylhydrazine method with high-performance liquid chromatography using electrochemical detection. *Biochem. Med. Metab. Biol.* 36:369–376.

49. A. Lopez-Anaya and M. Mayersohn (1987) Ascorbic and dehydroascorbic acids simultaneously quantified in biological fluids by liquid chromatography with fluorenscence detection, and comparison with a colorimetric assay. *Clin. Chem.* 33:1874–1878.

50. M.H. Bui-Nguyen (1980) Application of high-performance liquid chromatography to the separation of ascorbic acid and isoascorbic acid. *J. Chromatogr.* 196:163–165.

51. J. Geigert, D.S. Hirano, and S.L. Neidleman (1981) High-performance liquid chromatographic method for the determination of L-ascorbic acid and D-isoascorbic acid. *J. Chromatogr.* 206:396–399.

52. J.W. Finley and E. Duang (1981) Resolution of ascorbic, dehydroascorbic, and diketogulonic acids by paired-ion reversed-phase chromatography. *J. Chromatogr.* 207:449–452.

53. H.E. Sauberlich (1985) Bioavailability of vitamins. *Prog. Food Nutr. Sci.* 9:1–33.

54. A. Kallner (1987) Requirement for vitamin C based on metabolic studies. *Ann. NY. Acad. Sci.* 498:418–423.

55. A. Kallner, D. Hartman, and D. Hornig (1977) On the absorption of ascorbic acid in man. *Int. J. Vitam. Nutr. Res.* 47:383–388.

56. A. Kallner, D. Hornig, and D. Hartman (1982) Kinetics of ascorbic acid in humans. In: *Ascorbic Acid: Chemistry, Metabolism and Uses* (P.A. Seib and B.M. Tolbert, eds.), Advances In Chemistry Series, no. 200, pp. 335–348, American Chemical Society, Washington, DC.

57. A. Kallner, D. Hornig, and R. Pellikka (1985) Formation of carbon dioxide from ascorbate in man. *Am. J. Clin. Nutr.* 41:609–613.

58. M. Mayersohn (1972) Ascorbic acid absorption in man—pharmacokinetic implications. *Eur. J. Pharmacol.* 19:140–142.

59. R.C. Rose (1985) Intestinal transport of vitamins. *J. Inherited Metab. Dis.* 8:13–16.

60. R.C. Rose, A.M. Hoyumpa, Jr., R.H. Allen, H.M. Middleton, III, L.M. Henderson, and I.H. Rosenberg (1984) Transport and metabolism of water-soluble vitamins in intestine and kidney. *Fed. Proc.* 43:2423–2429.

61. A. Mellors, D. Nahrwold, and R. Rose (1977) Ascorbic acid flux across mucosal border of guinea pig and human ileum. *Am. J. Physiol.* 233:E374–E379.

62. N.R. Stevenson (1974) Active transport of L-ascorbic acid in human ileum. *Gastroenterology.* 67:952–956.

63. N.R. Stevenson and M.K. Brush (1969) Existence and characteristics of Na$^+$-dependent active transport of ascorbic acid in guinea pig. *Am. J. Clin. Nutr.* 23:318–326.

64. D. Hornig (1975) Metabolism of ascorbic acid. *World Rev. Nutr. Diet.* 23:225–258.

65. S.T. Omaye, J.A. Tillotson, and H.E. Sauberlich (1982) Metabolism of L-ascorbic acid in the monkey. In: *Ascorbic Acid: Chemistry, Metabolism and Uses* (P.A. Seib and B.M. Tolbert, eds.), Advances In Chemistry Series, no. 200, pp. 317–334, American Chemical Society, Washington, DC.

66. R.C. Rose (1988) Transport of ascorbic acid and other water-soluble vitamins. *Biochim. Biophys. Acta.* 979:335–366.

67. R.C. Rose (1981) Transport and metabolism of water-soluble vitamins in intestine. *Am. J. Physiol.* 240:G67–G101.

68. R. Rose (1980) Water-soluble vitamin absorption in intestine. *Annu. Rev. Physiol.* 42:157–171.

69. R.P. Spencer, S. Purdy, R. Hoeldtke, T.M. Bow, and M.A. Marksulis (1963) Studies on intestinal absorption of L-ascorbic acid. *Gastroenterology* 44:768–773.

70. U. Moser (1987) Uptake of ascorbic acid by leukocytes. *Ann. N.Y. Acad. Sci.* 498:200–215.

71. D. Hornig (1975) Distribution of ascorbic acid, metabolites and analogues in man and animals. *Ann. N.Y. Acad. Sci.* 258:103–118.

72. R.H. Bigley and L. Stankova (1974) Uptake and reduction of oxidized and reduced ascorbate by human leukocytes. *J. Exp. Med.* 139:1084–1092.

73. C.R. Chaudhuri and I.B. Chatterjee (1969) L-ascorbic acid synthesis in birds: phylogenetic trends. *Science* 164:435–436.

74. L.A. Pence and J.H. Mennear (1979) The inhibitory effect of dehydroascorbic acid on insulin secretion from mouse pancreatic islets. *Toxicol. Appl. Pharmacol.* 50:57–65.

75. S. England and S. Seifter (1986) The biochemical functions of ascorbic acid. *Annu. Rev. Nutr.* 6:365–406.

76. D.H. Hornig, U. Moser, and B.E. Glatthaar (1988) Ascorbic acid. In: *Modern Nutrition In Health and Disease* (M.E. Shils and V.R. Young, eds.), 7th ed., pp. 417–435, Lea & Febiger, Philadelphia.

77. M. Levine (1986) New concepts in the biology and biochemistry of ascorbic acid. *N. Engl. J. Med.* 314:892–902.

78. M. Levine and W. Hartzell (1987) Ascorbic acid: the concept of optimum requirements. *Ann. N.Y. Acad. Sci.* 498:424–444.

79. C.J. Schorah (1981) The level of vitamin C reserves required in man: towards a solution to the controversy. *Proc. Nutr. Soc.* 40:147–154.

80. R. Myllyla, E.-R. Kuitti-Savolainen, and K.I. Kivirikko (1978) The role of ascorbate in the prolyl hydroxylase reaction. *Biochem. Biophys. Res. Commun.* 83:441–448.

81. R.I. Schwarz, P. Kleinman, and N. Owens (1987) Ascorbate can act as an inducer of the collagen pathway because most steps are tightly coupled. *Ann. N.Y. Acad. Sci.* 498:172–185.

82. R.A. Berg and D.J. Prockop (1973) Affinity column purification of protocollagen proline hydroxylase from chick embryos and further characterization of the enzyme. *J. Biol. Chem.* 248:1175–1182.

83. S.R. Pinnell, S. Murad, and D. Darr (1987) Induction of collagen synthesis by ascorbic acid. *Arch. Dermatol.* 123:1684–1686.

84. V.G. Zannoni, E.J. Holsztynska, and S.S. Lau (1982) Biochemical functions of ascorbic acid in drug metabolism. In: *Ascorbic Acid: Advances In Chemistry, Metabolism and Uses* (P.A. Seib and B.M. Tolbert, eds.), Advances in Chemistry Series, no. 200, pp. 349–368, American Chemical Society, Washington, DC.

85. V.G. Zannoni and P.H. Sato (1975) Effects of ascorbic acid on microsomal drug metabolism. *Ann. N.Y. Acad. Sci.* 258:119–131.

86. P.G. Shilotri (1977) Glycolytic, hexose monophosphate shunt and bactericidal activities of leukocytes in ascorbic acid deficient guinea pigs. *J. Nutr.* 107:1507–1512.

87. P.G. Shilortri (1977) Phagocytosis and leukocyte enzymes in ascorbic acid deficient guinea pigs. *J. Nutr.* 107:1513–1516.

88. M.C. Goldschmidt, W.J. Masin, L.R. Brown, and P.R. Wyde (1988) The effect of ascorbic acid on leukocyte phagocytosis and killing of *Actinomyces viscosus*. *Int. J. Vitam. Nutr. Res.* 58:326–334.

89. I.J. Light, H.K. Berry, and J.M. Sutherland (1956) Aminoacidemia of prematurity. Its response to ascorbic acid. *Am. J. Dis. Child.* 112:229–236.

90. M.E. Avery, C.L. Clow, J.H. Menkes, et al. (1967) Transient tyrosinemia of the newborn: dietary and clinical aspects. *Pediatrics* 39:378–384.

91. M.I. Irvin and B.K. Hutchins (1976) A conspectus of research on vitamin C requirements of man. *J. Nutr.* 106:823–879.

92. National Research Council (1989) *Recommended Dietary Allowances,* 10th ed., National Academy of Sciences, Washington, DC.

93. P.L. Schwartz (1970) Ascorbic acid in wound healing—a review. *J. Am. Diet. Assoc.* 56:497–503.

94. P.L. Stokes, V. Melikian, R.L. Leeming, H. Portman-Graham, J.A. Blair, and W.T. Cooke (1975) Folate metabolism in scurvy. *Am. J. Clin. Nutr.* 28:126–129.

95. K.R. Thien, J.A. Blair, R.J. Leeming, W.T. Cooke, and V. Melikian (1977) Serum folates in man. *J. Clin. Pathol.* 30:438–448.

96. C.M. Lewis, E.L. McGown, M.G. Rusnak, and H.E. Sauberlich (1982) Interactions between folate and ascorbic acid in the guinea pig. *J. Nutr.* 112:673–680.

97. M. Levine and K. Morita (1985) The function of ascorbic acid in endocrine systems. *Vitam. Horm.* 42:1–64.

98. P.J. Leggott, P.B. Robertson, D.C. Rothman, P.A. Murray, and R.A. Jacob (1986) The effect of controlled ascorbic acid depletion and supplementation on periodontal health. *J. Periodontal.* 57:480–485.

99. R.A. Jacob, S.T. Omaye, J.H. Skala, P.J. Leggott, D.L. Rothman, and P.A. Murray (1987) Experimental vitamin C depletion and supplementation in young men. *Ann. N.Y. Acad. Sci.* 498:333–346.

100. S.N. Woolfe, E.B. Kenney, W.R. Hume, and F.A. Carranza, Jr. (1984) Relationship of ascorbic acid levels of blood and gingival tissue with response to periodontal therapy. *J. Clin. Periodontol.* 11:159–165.

101. S.L. Melnick, J.O. Alvarez, J.M. Navia, R.B. Cogen, and J.M. Roseman (1988) A case-control study of plasma ascorbate and acute necrotizing ulcerative gingivitis. *J. Dent. Res.* 67:855–860.

102. R.A. Berg, B. Steinmann, S.I. Rennard, and R.G. Crystal (1983) Ascorbate deficiency results in decreased collagen production: underhydroxylation of proline leads to increased intracellular degradation. *Arch. Biochem. Biophys.* 226:681–686.

103. J. Sodek, J. Feng, E.H.K. Yen, and A.H. Melcher (1982) Effect of ascorbic acid on protein synthesis and collagen hydroxylation in continuous flow organ cultures of adult mouse peridontal tissues. *Calcif. Tissue Int.* 34:408–415.

104. S. Tajima and S.R. Pinnell (1982) Regulation of collagen synthesis by ascorbic acid. Ascorbic acid increases type I procollagen mRNA. *Biochem. Biophys. Res. Commun.* 106:632–637.

105. R. Buzina, J. Aurer-Kozelj, K. Srdak-Jorgic, E. Buhler, and K.F. Gey (1986) Increase in gingival hydroxyproline and proline by improvement of ascorbic acid status in man. *Int. J. Vitam. Nutr. Res.* 56:367–372.

106. F. Horio, K. Ozaki, M. Kohmura, A. Yoshida, S. Makino, and Y. Hayashi (1986) Ascorbic acid requirement for the induction of microsomal drug-metabolizing enzymes in a rat mutant unable to synthesize ascorbic acid. *J. Nutr.* 116:2278–2289.

107. F. Horio and A. Yoshida (1982) Effects of some xenobiotics on ascorbic acid metabolism in rats. *J. Nutr.* 112:416–425.

108. F. Horio, M. Kimura, and A. Yoshida (1983) Effect of several xenobiotics on the activities of enzymes affecting ascorbic acid synthesis in rats. *J. Nutr. Sci. Vitaminol. (Tokyo)* 29:233–247.

109. K. Chatterjee, S.K. Banerjee, R. Tiwari, K. Mazumdar, A. Bhattacharya, and G.C. Chatterjee (1981) Studies on the protective effects of L-ascorbic acid in chronic chlordane toxicity. *Int. J. Vitam. Nutr. Res.* 51:254–265.

110. R.K. Tiwari, S.K. Bandyopadhyay, K. Chatterjee, A. Mitra, A. Banerjee, and G.C. Chatterjee (1982) Effects of high dose application of lindane to rats and influence of L-ascorbic acid supplementation. *Int. J. Vitam. Nutr. Res.* 52:448–455.

111. V.G. Zannoni, J.I. Brodfuehrer, R.C. Smart, and R.L. Susick, Jr. (1987) Ascorbic acid, alcohol, and environmental chemicals. *Ann. N.Y. Acad. Sci.* 498:364–388.

112. J.D. Turnbull and S.T. Omaye (1980) Synthesis of cytochrome P-450 heme in ascorbic acid-deficient guinea pigs. *Biochem. Pharmacol.* 29:1255–1260.

113. S.R. Tannenbaum and J.S. Wishnok (1987) Inhibition of nitrosamine formation by ascorbic acid. *Ann. N.Y. Acad. Sci.* 498:364–388.

114. R.R. Watson and T.K. Leonard (1986) Selenium and vitamins A, E, and C: nutrients with cancer prevention properties. *J. Am. Diet. Assoc.* 86:505–510.

115. S.L. Romney, J. Basu, S. Vermund, P.R. Palan, and C. Duttogupta (1987) Plasma reduced and total ascorbic acid in human uterine cervix dysplasias and cancer. *Ann. N.Y. Acad. Sci.* 498:132–143.

116. A.B. Hanck (1987) Vitamin C and cancer. *Prog. Clin. Biol. Res.* 259:307–320.

117. D. Hornig, B. Glatthaar, and U. Moser (1984) General aspects of ascorbic acid function and metabolism. In: *Proceedings of Workshop on Ascorbic Acid in Domestic Animals* (I. Wegger,

F.J. Tagwerker, and J. Moustgaared, eds.), Royal Danish Agricultural Society, Copenhagen.

118. B.E. Glatthaar, D.H. Hornig, and U. Moser (1986) The role of ascorbic acid in carcinogenesis. *Adv. Exp. Med. Biol.* 206:357–377.

119. P.F. Jacques, S.C. Hartz, R.B. McGandy, R.A. Jacob, and R.M. Russell (1987) Vitamin C and blood lipoproteins in an elderly population. *Ann. N.Y. Acad. Sci.* 498:100–109.

120. D. Hornig and H. Weiser (1976) Ascorbic acid and cholesterol: effect of graded oral intakes on cholesterol conversion to bile acids in guinea-pigs. *Experientia* 32:687–689.

121. E. Ginter (1979) Chronic marginal vitamin C deficiency: biochemistry and pathophysiology. *World Rev. Nutr. Diet.* 33:104–141.

122. L.J. Machlin, F. Garcia, W. Kuenzig, C.B. Richter, H.E. Spiegel, and M. Brin (1976) Lack of antiscorbutic activity of ascorbate 2-sulfate in the rhesus monkey. *Am. J. Clin. Nutr.* 29:825–831.

123. J.P. Kotze, I.V. Menne, J.H. Spies, and W.A. deKlerk (1975) Effect of ascorbic acid on serum lipid levels and depot cholesterol of the baboon (*Papio ursinus*). *S. Afr. Med. J.* 49:906–909.

124. B. Nambisan and P.A. Kurup (1975) Ascorbic acid and glycosaminoglycan and lipid metabolism in guinea pigs fed normal and atherogenic diets. *Atherosclerosis* 22:447–461.

125. D.B. Milne and S.T. Omaye (1980) Effect of vitamin C on copper and iron metabolism in the guinea pig. *Int. J. Vitam. Nutr. Res.* 50:301–308.

126. G.R. Reiss, P.G. Werness, P.E. Zollman, and R.F. Brubaker (1986) Ascorbic acid levels in the aqueous humor of nocturnal and diurnal mammals. *Arch. Ophthalmol.* 104:753–755.

127. E.M. Baker, R.E. Hodges, J. Hood, H.E. Sauberlich, and S.C. March (1969) Metabolism of ascorbic-1-^{14}C acid in experimental human scurvy. *Am. J. Clin. Nutr.* 22:549–558.

128. E.M. Baker, H.E. Sauberlich, S.C. March, and R.E. Hodges (1968) Experimental scurvy in man. Army Science Conference Proceedings. I:1–14, Office, Chief of Research and Development, U.S. Department of the Army, Washington, DC.

129. E.M. Baker, R.E. Hodges, J. Hood, H.E. Sauberlich, S.C. March, and J.E. Canham (1971) Metabolism of [14]C- and ^{3}H-labeled L-ascorbic acid in human scurvy. *Am. J. Clin. Nutr.* 24:444–454.

130. R.E. Hodges, E.M. Baker, J. Hood, H.E. Sauberlich, and S.C. March (1969) Experimental scurvy in man. *Am. J. Clin. Nutr.* 22:535–548.

131. R.E. Hodges, J. Hood, J.E. Canham, H.E. Sauberlich, and E.M. Baker (1971) Clinical manifestations of ascorbic acid deficiency in man. *Am. J. Clin. Nutr.* 24:432–443.

132. A. Kallner, D. Hartman, and D. Hornig (1979) Steady-state turnover and body pool of ascorbic acid in man. *Am. J. Clin. Nutr.* 32:530–539.

133. R.A. Jacob, J.H. Skala, and S.T. Omaye (1987) Biochemical indicies of human vitamin C status. *Am. J. Clin. Nutr.* 46:818–826.

134. W. Kuenzig, R. Avenia, and J. Kamm (1974) Studies on the antiscorbutic activity of ascorbate 2-sulfate in the guinea pig. *J. Nutr.* 104:952–956.

135. J.E. Halver, R.R. Smith, B.M. Tolbert, and E.M. Baker (1975) Utilization of ascorbic acid in fish. *Ann. N.Y. Acad. Sci.* 258:81–102.

136. D. Hornig (1975) Distribution of ascorbic acid, metabolites and analogues in man and animals. *Ann. N.Y. Acad. Sci.* 258:103–118.

137. J.B. Reuler, V.C. Broudy, and T.G. Cooney (1985) Adult scurvy. *JAMA* 253:805–807.

138. G.R. Pereira and A.H. Zucker (1986) Nutritional deficiencies in the neonate. *Clin. Perinatol.* 13:175–189.

139. P.J. Garry, D.J. Vanderjagt, and W.C. Hunt (1987) Ascorbic acid intakes and plasma levels in healthy elderly. *Ann. N.Y. Acad. Sci.* 498:90–99.

140. H.E. Sauberlich, R.P. Dowdy, and J.H. Skala (1974) *Laboratory Tests for the Assessment of Nutritional Status,* CRC Press, Boca Raton, FL.

141. E. Ginter, P. Bobek, and M. Jurcovicova (1982) Role of L-ascorbic acid in lipid metabolism. In: *Ascorbic Acid: Advances In Chemistry, Metabolism, and Uses* (P.A. Seib and B.M. Tolbert, eds.), Advances In Chemistry Series, no. 200, pp. 381–393, American Chemical Society, Washington, DC.

142. S.T. Omaye, J.H. Skala, and R.A. Jacob (1986) Plasma ascorbic acid in adult males: effect of depletion and supplementation. *Am. J. Clin. Nutr.* 44:257–264.

143. W. Lee, K.A. Davis, R. Rettmer, and R.F. Labbe (1988) Ascorbic acid status: biochemical and clinical considerations. *Am. J. Clin. Nutr.* 48:286–290.

144. J.D. Turnbull, J.H. Sudduth, H.E. Sauberlich, and S.T. Omaye (1981) Depletion and repletion of ascorbic acid in the rhesus monkey: relationship between ascorbic acid concentration in blood components with total body pool and liver concentration of ascorbic acid. *Int. J. Vitam. Nutr. Res.* 51:47–53.

145. I.B. Chatterjee, A.K. Majumder, B.K. Nandi, and N. Subramanian (1975) Synthesis and some function of vitamin C. *Ann. N.Y. Acad. Sci.* 258:24–47.

146. I.B. Chatterjee (1978) Ascorbic acid metabolism. *World Rev. Nutr. Diet.* 30:69–87.

147. F.A. Loewus, G. Wagner, and J.C. Yang (1975) Biosynthesis and metabolism of ascorbic acid in plants. *Ann. N.Y. Acad. Sci.* 258:7–23.

148. F.A. Loewus and J.P. Helsper (1982) Metabolism of L-ascorbic acid in plants. In: *Ascorbic Acid: Chemistry, Metabolism and Uses* (P.A. Seib and B.M. Tolbert, eds.), Advances In Chemistry Series, no. 200, pp. 249–261, American Chemical Society, Washington, DC.

149. E.C. Birney, R. Jenness, and K.M. Ayaz (1976) Inability of bats to synthesize L-ascorbic acid. *Nature* 260:626–628.

150. J.C. Bauernfeind (1982) Ascorbic acid technology in agricultural, pharmaceutical, food, and industrial applications. In: *Ascorbic Acid: Chemistry, Metabolism and Uses* (P.A. Seib and B.M. Tolbert, eds.), Advances In Chemistry Series, no. 200, pp. 395–497, American Chemical Society, Washington, DC.

151. T. Murai, J.W. Andrews, and J.C. Bauernfeind (1978) Use of L-ascorbic acid, ethocel coated ascorbic acid and ascorbate-2-sulfate in diets for channel catfish, *Ictalurus punctatus. J. Nutr.* 108:1761–1766.

152. K.J. Kramer and P.A. Seib (1982) Ascorbic acid and the growth and development of insects. In: *Ascorbic Acid: Chemistry, Metabolism and Uses* (P.A. Seib and B.M. Tolbert, eds.), Advances In Chemistry Series, no. 200, pp. 275–291, American Chemical Society, Washington, DC.

153. T.M. John, J.C. George, J.W. Hilton, and S.J. Slinger (1979) Influence of dietary ascorbic acid on plasma lipids levels in the rainbow trout. *Int. J. Vitam. Nutr. Res.* 49:400–405.

154. P. Sato, M. Nishikimi, and S. Udenfriend (1976) Is L-gulonolactone oxidase the only enzyme missing in animals subject to scurvy? *Biochem. Biophys. Res. Commun.* 71:293–299.

155. M. Nishikimi and S. Udenfriend (1976) Immunologic evidence that the gene for L-gulono-γ-lactone oxidase is not expressed in animals subject to scurvy. *Proc. Natl. Acad. Sci. USA* 73:2066–2068.

156. P. Sato and S. Udenfriend (1978) Scurvy-prone animals, including man, monkey, and guinea pig, do not express the gene for gulonolactone oxidase. *Arch. Biochem. Biophys.* 187:158–162.

157. P.H. Sato, L.A. Roth, and D.M. Walton (1986) Treatment of a metabolic disease, scurvy, by administration of the missing enzyme. *Biochem. Med. Metab. Biol.* 35:59–64.

158. Y. Mizushima, T. Harauchi, and S. Makino (1984) A rat mutant unable to synthesize vitamin C. *Experientia* 40:359–361.

159. F. Horio, K. Ozaki, A. Yoshida, S. Makino, and Y. Hayashi (1985)

Ascorbic acid requirement in a rat mutant unable to synthesize ascorbic acid. *J. Nutr.* 115:1630–1640.

160. I. Hanssen, H.J. Grav, J.B. Steen, and H. Lysnes (1979) Vitamin C deficiency in growing willow ptarmigan. *J. Nutr.* 109:2260–2278.

161. J.L. Smith and R.E. Hodges (1987) Serum levels of vitamin C in relation to dietary and supplemental intake of vitamin C in smokers and nonsmokers. *Ann. N.Y. Acad. Sci.* 498:144–152.

162. A.B. Kallner, D. Hartmann, and D.H. Hornig (1981) On the requirements of ascorbic acid in man: steady-state turnover and body pool in smokers. *Am. J. Clin. Nutr.* 34:1347–1355.

163. J.H. Calder, R.C. Curtis, and H. Fore (1963) Comparison of vitamin C in plasma and leukocytes of smokers and nonsmokers. *Lancet* 1:556.

164. M. Brook and J.J. Grimshaw (1968) Vitamin C concentration of plasma and leukocytes as related to smoking habit, age, and sex of humans. *Am. J. Clin. Nutr.* 21:1259–1267.

165. O. Pelletier (1968) Smoking and vitamin C levels in humans. *Am. J. Clin. Nutr.* 21:1259–1267.

166. O. Pelletier (1970) Vitamin C status of cigarette smokers and nonsmokers. *Am. J. Clin. Nutr.* 23:520–524.

167. E.P. Norkus, H. Hsu, and M.R. Cehelsky (1987) Effect of cigarette smoking on the vitamin C status of pregnant women and their offspring. *Ann. N.Y. Acad. Sci.* 498:500–501.

168. H.E. Sauberlich and E.M. Baker (1967) Studies in human nutrition. In: *Annual Research Progress Report,* 30 June 1967, pp. 180–187, U.S. Army Medical Research and Nutrition Laboratory, San Francisco, CA.

169. M.E. Visagie, J.P. DuPlessis, G. Groothof, A. Alberts, and N.F. Laubacher (1974) Change in vitamin A and C levels in black mine-workers. *S. Afr. Med. J.* 48:2502–2506.

170. M.E. Visagie, J.P. DuPlessis, and N.F. Laubacher (1975) Effect of vitamin C supplementation on black mine-workers. *S. Afr. Med. J.* 49:889–892.

171. G.I. Bondarev, K.K. Glikov, and K.A. Laricheva (1975) Vitamin C allowance for sailors against the background of qualitatively differing nutrition. *Vopr. Pitan.* 1:11–13.

172. M. Brook and J.J. Grimshaw (1968) Vitamin C concentration of plasma and leukocytes as related to smoking habit, age, and sex of humans. *Am. J. Clin. Nutr.* 21:1254–1258.

173. H.S. Loh and C.W.M. Wilson (1971) Relationship of human ascorbic acid metabolism to ovulation. *Lancet* 1:110–112.

174. M. Briggs and M. Briggs (1972) Vitamin C requirements and oral contraceptives. *Nature* 238:277.

175. V.J. McLeroy and H.E. Schendel (1973) Influence of oral contraceptives on ascorbic acid concentration in healthy, sexually mature women. *Am. J. Clin. Nutr.* 26:191–196.

176. J.M. Rivers and M.M. Devine (1975) Relationships of ascorbic acid to pregnancy and oral contraceptive steroids. *Ann. N.Y. Acad. Sci.* 258:465–482.

177. P.J. Garry, J.S. Goodwin, W.C. Hunt, and B.A. Gilbert (1982) Nutritional status in a healthy elderly population: vitamin C. *Am. J. Clin. Nutr.* 36:332–339.

178. D.J. VanderJagt, P.J. Garry, and H.N. Bhagavan (1987) Ascorbic acid intake and plasma levels in healthy elderly people. *Am. J. Clin. Nutr.* 46:290–294.

179. P.M. Suter and R.M. Russell (1987) Vitamin requirements of the elderly. *Am. J. Clin. Nutr.* 45:501–512.

180. L. Hallberg, M. Brune, and L. Rossander-Hulthen (1987) Is there a physiological role of vitamin C in iron absorption? *Ann. N.Y. Acad. Sci.* 498:324–332.

181. E.R. Monsen, L. Hallberg, M. Layrisse, D.M. Hegsted, J.D. Cook, W. Mertz, and C.A. Finch (1978) Estimation of available iron. *Am. J. Clin. Nutr.* 31:134–141.

182. D.P. Derman, D. Ballot, T.H. Bothwell, et al. (1987) Factors influencing the absorption of iron from soy-bean protein products. *Br. J. Nutr.* 57:345–353.

183. L. Halberg, M. Brune, and L. Rossander (1986) Effect of ascorbic acid on iron absorption from different types of meals. *Hum. Nutr. Appl. Nutr.* 40A:97–113.

184. L. Hallberg, M. Brune, and L. Rossander (1989) Iron absorption in man: ascorbic acid and dose-dependent inhibition by phytate. *Am. J. Clin. Nutr.* 40:140–144.

185. M.A. Sahud and R.J. Cohen (1971) Effect of aspirin ingestion on ascorbic acid levels in rheumatoid arthritis. *Lancet* 1:937–938.

186. J.W. Erdman, Jr. and B.P. Klein (1982) Harvesting, processing, and cooking influences on vitamin C in foods. In: *Ascorbic Acid: Chemistry, Metabolism and Uses* (P.A. Seib and B.M. Tolbert, eds.), Advances In Chemistry Series, no. 200, pp. 499–532, American Chemical Society, Washington, DC.

187. J.M. Rivers (1987) Safety of high-level vitamin C ingestion. *Ann. N.Y. Acad. Sci.* 498:445–454.

188. F. Erden, S. Gulenc, M. Torun, Z. Kocer, B. Simsek, and S. Nebioglu (1985) Ascorbic acid effect on some lipid fractions in human beings. *Acta Vitaminol. Enzymol.* 7:131–138.

189. H.G. Stein, A. Hasan, and I.H. Fox (1976) Ascorbic acid-induced uricosuria. A consequence of megavitamin therapy. *Ann. Intern. Med.* 84:385–388.

190. A. Hanck (1982) Tolerance and effects of high doses of ascorbic acid. *Int. J. Vitam. Nutr. Res.* 23(suppl):221–238.

191. A.H. Chalmers, D.M. Cowley, and J.M. Brown (1986) A possible etiological role for ascorbate in calculi formation. *Clin. Chem.* 32:333–336.

192. P. Balchke, P. Schmidt, J. Zazgornik, H. Kopsa, and A. Haubenstock (1984) Ascorbic acid aggravates secondary hyperoxalemia in patients on chronic hemodialysis. *Ann. Intern. Med.* 101:344–345.

Chapter 16

Thiamin

Beriberi, a thiamin-deficiency disease that causes extensive damage to the nervous and cardiovascular systems, was known long before the vitamin was discovered.[1-3] Takaki, a surgeon in the Japanese navy during the late 19th century, demonstrated that addition of meat and whole grains to the usual ship's rations resulted in a decrease in the incidence of what was then called shipboard beriberi. Apparently this finding provided the first substantive evidence that beriberi was caused by a dietary deficiency. Fifteen or so years thereafter, Eijkmann, a physician in the Dutch East Indies, reported a beriberi-type neurological syndrome in birds that were fed a diet of highly polished rice. No such disease occurred in birds fed rice bran. Some years later Grijns, another physician, suggested that the disease was caused by lack of a dietary constituent in polished rice that was present in the whole grain. The unknown constituent, vitamin B-1, now known as thiamin, was isolated in 1926 by Jansen and Donath and was synthesized 10 years later by Williams and Cline.[4]

Chemistry

Thiamin is a relatively simple compound. It comprises a pyrimidine ring and a thiazole ring linked by a methylene bridge (Figure 1). Commercially, the vitamin is available in the hydrochloride and mononitrate forms. Thiamin hydrochloride is stable in dry form and in acid solution. It is unstable in alkaline solution, and decomposition accelerates as temperature increases. Thiamin mononitrate is more stable to heat than is the hydrochloride.

Thiamin is extremely sensitive to sulfite, which splits the molecule into the pyrimidine and thiazole moieties thus destroying vitamin activity.

Absorption and Transport

Thiamin absorption occurs by at least two mechanisms.[5-7] At low concentrations (>1 μmol/L) thiamin is absorbed by an active-transport system, is carrier-mediated, and requires Na^+. At high concentrations absorption is primarily by passive diffusion and apparently is inefficient. Absorption takes place primarily in the jejunum. The ileum is not involved to any great extent.

The vitamin is phosphorylated to form the pyrophosphate (Figure 2) in the jejunal mucosa. Phosphorylated thiamin is transported in blood cells; free thiamin is primarily in plasma.

Total body thiamin content in the adult human is estimated to be ~30 mg. Highest concentrations appear to be in liver, kidney, and heart and are two to three times greater than the concentration in brain.[8] Free thiamin comprises <5% of body thiamin. The remainder is primarily pyrophosphate.[9]

Biochemical Function

Thiamin pyrophosphate (TPP) is the major coenzyme form of thiamin (Figure 2). Phosphorylation requires ATP. TPP is involved in two major kinds of reactions: (1) the oxidative decarboxylation of α-keto acids to carboxylic acids (i.e., pyruvate $\rightarrow$ acetyl CoA and α-ketoglutarate $\rightarrow$ succinyl CoA) catalyzed by dehydrogenase complexes and (2) the transketolase reaction of the pentose phosphate pathway.

Oxidative decarboxylation takes place in the mitochondria and is pivotal to formation of acetyl CoA from pyruvate and for the production of succinyl CoA in the citric acid cycle. In addition, acetyl CoA is necessary for synthesis of lipids and other essential compounds such as acetylcholine.

The transketolase reaction of the pentose phosphate shunt takes place in the cytosol and involves the transfer of an α-keto group from xylulose-5-phosphate to ribose-5-phosphate to form sedoheptulose-7-phosphate and glyceraldehyde-3-phosphate. The reactions of the pentose phosphate shunt are not directly in the main glycolytic pathway for

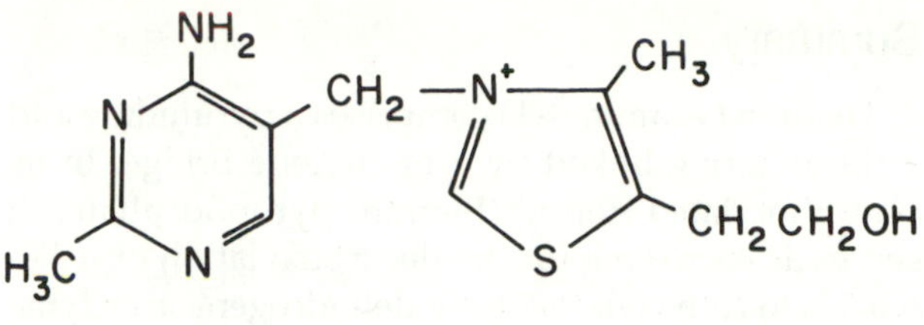

Figure 1. Thiamin.

carbohydrate metabolism. This pathway, however, is the major source of pentoses for nucleic acid synthesis and NADPH for fatty acid and other syntheses. The stimulation of erythrocyte transketolase by in vitro addition of TPP is the basis for the currently preferred method for measuring thiamin nutritional status.[10,11] Activity of transketolase is lowered early in thiamin deficiency. In young rats, for example, reduced transketolase activity can be detected in red blood cells before growth rate is affected.[10]

Although all enzymes of the pentose phosphate shunt are present in brain, this pathway is of minor importance in brain of adult animals. In young developing animals, however, the pentose phosphate shunt may metabolize as much as half of all glucose present.[7] This high activity likely is related to the role of NADPH in numerous synthetic processes and of ribose phosphate for nucleic acid synthesis.

Although TPP is the principal and possibly the only active thiamin coenzyme, the monophosphate (TMP) and the triphosphate (TTP) are present in small amounts in most tissues. In brain, for example, the percentages of thiamin and its phosphates were reported to be 4% for free thiamin, 11% for TMP, 79% for TPP, and 5% for TTP.[7] Similar ratios were found in heart, liver, and kidney.

Thiamin Antagonists

Although several thiamin antagonists are known, only two, oxythiamin and pyrithiamin, have been studied extensively.[12,13] Oxythiamin has an hydroxyl group instead of an amino group in the pyrimidine moiety. Pyrithiamin contains a pyridine ring instead of the thiazole ring of thiamin. Oxythiamin can be converted to the pyrophosphate and competes in the thiamin pyrophosphate enzyme systems. Pyrithiamin

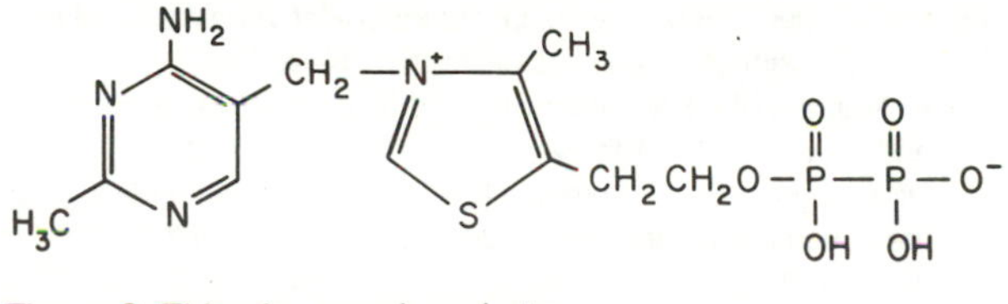

Figure 2. Thiamin pyrophosphate.

affects the activity of thiamin kinase, the enzyme that catalyzes thiamin phosphorylation, and thus prevents the formation of thiamin pyrophosphate.

Amprolium, a 2-n-propyl pyrimidine used in the treatment of coccidiosis in chickens, also has anti-thiamin activity.[13]

Thiaminases

Naturally occurring thiamin antagonists, thiaminases, occur in some foods.[14,15] Two types of thiaminases are known. Thiaminase I catalyzes cleavage of the vitamin so that the methylene group of the pyrimidine group is displaced and the vitamin becomes inactive. Thiaminase II catalyzes cleavage of the molecule into the pyrimidine and thiazole moieties. Thiaminases are found in certain raw fish as well as plant sources such as tea, coffee, betel nuts, blueberries, and red cabbage. In cultures in which large amounts of such foods are consumed, thiaminases may contribute to thiamin deficiency.[16]

Analysis

The classic method for thiamin analysis involves conversion of the vitamin by potassium ferricyanide in alkaline solution to thiochrome, a fluorescent compound.[17] Initially thiamin phosphates were converted to thiamin by action of a suitable enzyme, such as takadiastase, followed by removal of interfering substances by use of an ion-exchange resin. More recently high-performance liquid chromatography permitted analysis of thiamin and its phosphate esters.[11,18,19]

Metabolites

A number of thiamin metabolites were identified in mammalian urine.[20] Apparently the thiamin molecule initially is split to the pyrimidine and thiazole moieties. In a study of thiamin excretion in subjects on a low-thiamin diet, both pyrimidine and thiazole were excreted, and urinary concentrations remained high even after thiamin excretion ceased. Further degradation also occurs, splitting the thiazole ring so that carbon-2 is released as carbon dioxide.[20] Thiamin labeled with ^{14}C in both the pyrimidine and thiazole rings indicated at least 22 breakdown products from pyrimidine and 29 products from thiazole.[21]

Deficiency

Beriberi causes extensive damage to the nervous and cardiovascular systems. Dry beriberi is accompanied by severe muscle wasting whereas wet beriberi is accompanied by edema. The disease may also be manifested in mental confusion, muscular weakness, loss of ankle and knee jerks, painful calf muscles, or peripheral paralysis. Beriberi is particularly devastating in infants. Symptoms include cyanosis, dyspnea, tachycardia, and aphonia (soundless crying). Death often occurs suddenly from cardiac failure.

Haas[8] discussed in detail changes in the neurotransmitter systems and nerve conduction in simple thiamin deficiency and in deficiency produced by oxythiamin and pyrithiamin in animals. Many of the symptoms and defects are similar to those seen in the Wernicke-Korsakoff syndrome. This syndrome is characterized by mental confusion, memory disturbances, ataxia, opthalmoplegia, and nystagmus. The syndrome is most commonly seen in malnourished alcoholic individuals and can be alleviated by treatment with thiamin. Tomasulo et al.[22] presented evidence that thiamin absorption is decreased by alcohol. A more recent study suggested that neither alcoholism nor acute exposure to alcohol significantly limits intestinal uptake of thiamin.[23] However, in that study there was wide variation among subjects, and severely malnourished subjects were not included in the study for ethical reasons.

Recent studies in patients with Alzheimer's disease indicated structural abnormalities of red cell transketolase[24] as well as reduced activities of the 2-ketoglutarate dehydrogenase and transketolase of brain tissue from patients dying from the disease.[25] The latter observations did not appear to be accounted for by postmortem changes. How these changes are effected is unknown.

Requirements and Allowances

The Recommended Dietary Allowance of 0.5 mg/1000 kcal for thiamin is nearly four times the amount at which signs of deficiency were observed and is well within the range observed to be consistent with good health.[26] Data in older persons (age >60 y) suggest the 0.5 mg/1000 kcal is sufficient for this age group. A minimum intake of 1 mg/d was recommended for individuals consuming <2000 kcal/d.

Sources

Unrefined and enriched cereals, organ meats, legumes, and nuts are good sources of thiamin. Of the meats and meat products, pork muscle is an exceptionally good source. Thiamin is widely distributed in foods and, therefore, intake of a variety of foods including whole grains or enriched grains can insure an adequate intake.

Summary

Thiamin (vitamin B-1) comprises a pyrimidine and a thiazole ring linked by a methylene bridge. In its phosphorylated form, thiamin pyrophosphate, it serves as coenzyme for the decarboxylation of α-ketoacids to carboxylic acids by dehydrogenase enzyme complexes and in the formation of ketoses by the transketolase enzyme in the pentose phosphate pathway. The latter reaction currently is the basis for what is considered to be the most sensitive measure of thiamin nutrition status.

Severe deficiency of the vitamin results in the disease beriberi, which is characterized by extensive damage to the nervous and cardiovascular systems. Beriberi occurs most commonly among populations in which highly refined grains are a major component of the diet. In the United States thiamin deficiency is rare except among malnourished alcoholic individuals. The symptoms most often encountered are classified as Wernicke-Korsakoff syndrome, which responds to administration of thiamin.

References

1. R.R. Williams (1961) *Toward the Conquest of Beriberi*, Harvard University Press, Cambridge, MA.
2. H.M. Wuest (1982) The history of thiamine. *Ann. N.Y. Acad. Sci.* 378:576–601.
3. R.A. Peters (1969) The biochemical lesion and its historical development. *Br. Med. Bull.* 25:223–226.
4. R.R. Williams and J.K. Cline (1936) Synthesis of vitamin B₁. *J. Am. Chem. Soc.* 58:1504–1505.
5. G. Rindi and V. Ventura (1972) Thiamin intestinal transport. *Physiol. Rev.* 52:821–827.
6. A. Hoyumpa, R. Strickland, J.J. Sheehan, et al. (1982) Dual system of intestinal thiamine transport in humans. *J. Lab. Clin. Med.* 90:701–708.
7. B.B. Bowman, D.B. McCormick, and I.H. Rosenberg (1989) Epithelial transport of water-soluble vitamins. *Annu. Rev. Nutr.* 9:187–189.
8. R.H. Haas (1988) Thiamin and the brain. *Annu. Rev. Nutr.* 8:483–515.
9. G. Rindi and L. deGiuseppi (1961) A new chromatographic method for the determination of thiamine and its mono-, di- and tri-phosphates in animal tissues. *Biochem. J.* 78:602–606.
10. M. Brin, M. Tai, A.S. Ostashever, et al. (1960) Effect of thiamine deficiency on activity of erythrocyte hemolysate transketolase. *J. Nutr.* 71:273–280.
11. H.E. Sauberlich (1984) Newer laboratory methods for assessing nutriture of selected B-complex vitamins. *Annu. Rev. Nutr.* 4:377–407.
12. E.F. Rogers (1970) Thiamine antagonists. In: *Methods in Enzymology*, vol. 18, part A (D.B. McCormick and L.D. Wright, eds.), pp. 245–258, Academic Press, New York.
13. C.J. Gubler (1984) Thiamin. In: *Handbook of Vitamins* (L. Machlin ed.), pp. 245–297, Marcel Dekker, Inc., New York.
14. K. Murata (1982) Actions of two types of thiaminase on thiamin and its analogues. *Ann. N.Y. Acad. Sci.* 378:146–156.
15. D.M. Hilker and J.C. Somogyi (1982) Antithiamins of plant origin: their chemical nature and mode of action. *Ann. N.Y. Acad. Sci.* 378:137–145.
16. S. Vimokesant, S. Kunjara, K. Rungruangask, et al. (1982) Beriberi

caused by antithiamin factors in food and its prevention. *Ann. N.Y. Acad. Sci.* 378:123–136.

17. Association of Official Analytical Chemists (1980) *Official Methods of Analysis,* AOAC, Arlington, VA.

18. M. Kimura and Y. Itokawa (1985) Determination of thiamine and its phosphate esters in human and rat blood by high-performance liquid chromatography with post-column derivatization. *J. Chromatogr.* 332:181–188.

19. J.R. Cooper and T. Matsuda (1986) Separation and determination of thiamin and its phosphate esters by SP-Sephadex chromatography. *Methods Enzymol.* 122:20–24.

20. Z.Z. Ziporin, W.T. Nunes, R.C. Powell, et al. (1965) Excretion of thiamine and its metabolites in the urine of young adult males receiving restricted intakes of the vitamin. *J. Nutr.* 85:287–296.

21. R.A. Neal (1970) Isolation and identification of thiamin catabolites in mammalian urine; isolation and identification of some products of bacterial catabolism of thiamin. In: *Methods in Enzymology,* vol. 18, part A (D.B. McCormick and A.D. Wright, eds.), pp. 133–140, Academic Press, New York.

22. P.A. Tomasulo, R.M.H. Kater, and F.L. Iber (1968) Impairment of thiamin absorption in alcoholism. *Am. J. Clin. Nutr.* 21:1341–1344.

23. K.J. Breen, R. Buttigieg, S. Iossifidis, et al. (1985) Jejunal uptake of thiamin hydrochloride in man: influence of alcoholism and alcohol. *Am. J. Clin. Nutr.* 42:121–126.

24. G.E. Gibson, K.-F.R. Shew, J.P. Bloss, et al. (1988) Reduced activities of thiamine-dependent enzymes in the brains and peripheral tissues of patients with Alzheimer's disease. *Arch. Neurol.* 45:836–840.

25. K.-F.R. Shew, D.D. Clarke, Y.-T. Kim, et al. (1988) Studies of transketolase abnormality in Alzheimer's disease. *Arch. Neurol.* 45:841–845.

26. National Research Council (1989) *Recommended Dietary Allowances,* National Academy Press, Washington, DC.

Riboflavin

Riboflavin (vitamin B_2) and related natural flavins participate in numerous and diverse reactions, perhaps more than for any other vitamin-coenzyme group. The ongoing discovery of new forms of flavins and the proteins with which they associate is periodically updated in volumes resulting from symposia held every 3 y on flavins and flavoproteins; the most recent (ninth) of such proceedings was published in 1987.[1] Briefer coverage of riboflavin can be found in chapters of texts emphasizing clinical and nutritional aspects.[2,3]

Natural Flavins

All flavins are isoalloxazines, which are 10-substituted derivatives of alloxazine, the parent tricyclic ring system, with nitrogens in positions 1, 3, and 5. The variations in structures of naturally occurring flavins, with a dashed line between atoms in positions 1 and 5 to allow for oxidized (quinoid), half-reduced (semiquinoid or radical), and fully reduced (hydroquinoid) forms, are summarized in Figure 1. Approximately 30 different flavoquinones have been isolated from natural sources.

Riboflavin [7,8-dimethyl-10-(1'-D-ribityl)isoalloxazine] is a yellow fluorescent compound that is widely distributed throughout the plant and animal kingdoms. Studies with bacteria and fungi, particularly *Ashbya gossypii* and *Eremothecium ashbyii*, that can biosynthesize rather large quantities of riboflavin have revealed a pathway from GTP through 6,7-dimethyl-8-D-ribityllumazine to yield the vitamin.[4] Though most flavins derive from further actions upon riboflavin, at least two, namely roseoflavin with an 8-dimethylamino function produced by *Streptomyces davawensis* and coenzyme F_{420} with a 5-carba-5-deaza nucleus formed in *Methanobacterium* sp., must arise in variations of the usual biosynthetic pathway. Structures of these native flavins, with substituents noted in respect to Figure 1, are summarized in Table

1. Higher organisms, notably the human and other mammals, cannot biosynthesize the isoalloxazine system; therefore, riboflavin is a water-soluble vitamin (i.e., required nutrient) for such species.

Flavocoenzymes

The coenzyme forms of riboflavin that function as the prosthetic groups of numerous holoenzymes that catalyze diverse and often essential one- and two-electron oxidation-reduction reactions are flavin mononucleotide (FMN) and the more frequently encountered flavin adenine dinucleotide (FAD). Moreover, a small but significant fraction of both coenzymes occurs in some organelles and organisms as forms altered at positions 6, 8, or 8α. Structures of the coenzyme-level flavins with substituents noted in respect to Figure 1 are summarized in Table 2.

Sources for the coenzyme-level flavins were summarized in a previous review.[5] Briefly, however, it can be noted that the 6-hydroxy derivatives of both FMN and FAD may arise from oxidative turnover of the predominate natural coenzymes during function. So far the 6-S-cysteinyl-FMN, 8-hydroxy flavins, and 8α-O-tyrosyl-FAD have been found only in certain bacterial systems, but the 8α-S-cysteinyl- and both 8α-N^1- and N^3-histidyl-FAD forms are found in several lower and higher organisms. The covalent attachment of FAD via an 8α-linkage to a cysteinyl residue in mitochondrial monoamine oxidase (both A and B types) and such linkage to the N^3 of an imidazole of histidyl residues in mitochondrial succinate and sarcosine dehydrogenases are important examples in our bodies. The N^1 linkage occurs, among other places, in L-gulonolactone oxidase that allows certain animals, e.g., rats, to biosynthesize L-ascorbic acid.

Absorption, Transport, and Uptake

After ingestion of diverse natural flavins, most of which occur as coenzymes, riboflavin and traces of

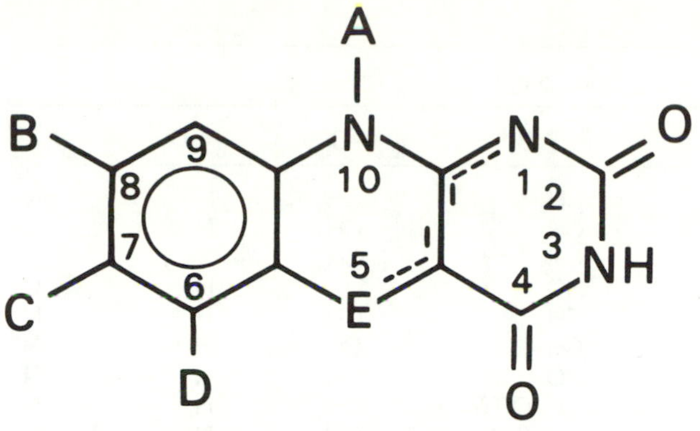

Figure 1. Generalized structure for flavins and derivatives that occur naturally. Particular substituents are given in the text and tables that refer to diverse types.

flavinyl peptides are released by nonspecific hydrolytic activities in the gastrointestinal tract. Earlier investigations on general aspects of absorption in humans were updated by studies with sections of gut[6] and isolated cells[7] from other mammals. Enterocytes in the upper small bowel absorb riboflavin by initial rapid uptake that is Na^+ dependent and inhibited by ouabain, reflecting an ATPase-involved active cotransport system. Metabolic trapping by conversion to FMN and FAD occurs before release of the vitamin to circulation by nonspecific pyrophosphatase and phosphatase.[8,9] Some consideration has been given to developmental aspects of riboflavin transport in the intestine associated with maturation and aging.[10,11] Antacid effects on absorption,[12] an effect of fiber on pharmacologic doses of the vitamin,[13] and impaired absorption in experimental uremia[14] were noted.

Transport of flavin by blood plasma is known to involve both loose association with albumin and tight associations with some globulins. Among the latter, immunoglobulins were identified as the major binding proteins for riboflavin in serum from normal humans[15,16] and from patients with certain types of cancer.[17] By use of flavinyl-affinity chromatography, different immunoglobulin subclasses, viz., IgG, IgM, and IgA, were isolated and shown to have both κ and λ light chains.[18] Papain cleavage of the immunoglobulins yields Fab fragments that still bound riboflavin. Hence, at least a portion of the antigenic binding site may be involved. In this connection, it is interesting to note that antiflavin antibodies were elicited in response to haptenic challenges.[19]

Some riboflavin-binding proteins are pregnancy specific, including the classic case of the estrogen-induced egg white protein. This subject was reviewed in recent years[20,21] and ongoing work is extending knowledge of those interesting cases in mammals. Examples include binding proteins from pregnant

cows,[22] rats,[23] bonnet monkeys,[24] and humans.[25,26] These proteins appear similar to the avian riboflavin-binding protein because their epitopes are recognized by monoclonal antibodies to the chicken riboflavin-binding protein.[27] They are essential for fetal development because immunization of animals with the avian protein or injection of antibodies against the avian protein terminates pregnancy in rats,[28] mice,[29] and the bonnet monkey.[30] Fetal degeneration accompanies lowering of FAD levels in the fetus.[31,32] The exact cause of the effect on level of flavocoenzyme is not known, but an interaction between chick liver flavokinase and riboflavin-binding protein was shown.[33] Placental transfer of riboflavin seems to involve binding proteins that help vector the vitamin and enhance supply to the fetus. In perfused human placenta, differential rates of uptake were noted at maternal and fetal surfaces.[34,35] There are differences in riboflavin concentration in maternal and cord blood in the human,[36] carrier proteins were isolated from both,[26] and a flavin-containing placental protein was isolated.[37]

Uptake processes for flavins by mammalian cells have some characteristics in common, but there are both qualitative and quantitative differences among different cell types. Hepatocytes exhibit an initial rapid uptake followed by slower passive diffusion of the vitamin, which becomes metabolically trapped by flavokinase-catalyzed phosphorylation.[38] The uptake process is relatively insensitive to both Na^+ and ouabain and probably reflects a facilitated, carrier-mediated system. With proximal tubular epithelial cells from rat kidney, the faster facilitated phase of flavin uptake exhibits Na^+ dependence (like small intestine but unlike liver) but is insensitive to ouabain (like liver but unlike small intestine).[39] An ATP requirement reflects, as for other cells, the trapping of riboflavin by phosphorylation, a process that can be impeded by other flavin substrates or inhibitors of flavokinase.

Coenzyme Formation and Interconversion

Current knowledge on the way in which flavins are interconverted to coenzymic forms is summarized in Figure 2. As noted in an update on this subject,[40]

Table 1. Native flavins formed by microorganisms

Name	Substituent				
	A	B	C	D	E
Riboflavin	1'-D-ribityl	CH_3	CH_3	H	N
Roseoflavin	1'-D-ribityl	$(CH_3)_2N$	CH_3	H	N
5-Deazaflavin	1'-D-ribityl	HO	H	H	CH

Table 2. Flavocoenzymes found with flavoenzymes

Name	Substituent				
	A	B	C	D	E
FMN	1'-D-ribityl-5'-phosphate	CH$_3$	CH$_3$	H	N
6-Hydroxy-FMN	1'-D-ribityl-5'-phosphate	CH$_3$	CH$_3$	HO	N
6-S-Cysteinyl-FMN	1'-D-ribityl-5'-phosphate	CH$_3$	CH$_3$	S-Cys	N
Coenzyme F$_{420}$	1'-D-ribityl-5'-phospholactyldiglutamate	HO	H	H	CH
FAD	1'-D-ribityl-5'-ADP	CH$_3$	CH$_3$	H	N
6-Hydroxy-FAD	1'-D-ribityl-5'-ADP	CH$_3$	CH$_3$	HO	N
8-Hydroxy-FAD	1'-D-ribityl-5'-ADP	HO	CH$_3$	H	N
8α-O-Tyrosyl-FAD	1'-D-ribityl-5'-ADP	CH$_2$-O-Tyr	CH$_3$	H	N
8α-S-Cysteinyl-FAD	1'-D-ribityl-5'-ADP	CH$_2$-S-Cys	CH$_3$	H	N
8α-N^1-Histidyl-FAD	1'-D-ribityl-5'-ADP	CH$_2$-N^1-His	CH$_3$	H	N
8α-N^3-Histidyl-FAD	1'-D-ribityl-5'-ADP	CH$_2$-N^3-His	CH$_3$	H	N

it was only within the last decade that relatively homogeneous preparations of flavokinase were obtained, first from rat liver,[41] then from mung beans,[42] and most recently from a bacterium.[43] Though not identical in molecular properties, the mammalian (28,000 M.W.) and plant (30,000–35,000 M.W.) kinases cannot further catalyze formation of FAD from FMN, whereas the bacterial enzyme (38,000 M.W.) is both a flavokinase and an FAD synthetase. The synthetase from liver is a larger enzyme (100,000 M.W. dimer) but cannot function as a flavokinase.[44] In all cases, Zn^{2+} is preferred for kinase activity and Mg^{2+} for synthetase activity. The phylogenic differences among flavokinases and FAD synthetases located in the cytosol are interesting and may have bearing on the controls that can modulate levels of flavocoenzyme formed in higher organisms with separate but probably interactive enzymes. As reviewed in the preceding edition of this volume,[45] there is significant endocrine control of flavocoenzyme level, most especially as involves thyroid hormone-induced increase in biosynthesis. One of the more important recent additions to this knowledge is that increase in triiodothyronine in rats leads to an increase in a more active form of liver flavokinase and a concomitant decrease in a less active form.[46]

The nonspecific hydrolytic enzymes that break down FMN and FAD have been observed in extracts from numerous sources.[47] Mammalian phosphatases that can hydrolyze FMN to riboflavin and inorganic phosphate not only include those with somewhat acidic pH optima,[48] such as those located in lysosomes, but also include those with alkaline optima,[8,9] such as in plasma membranes and the intestinal brush border. FAD pyrophosphatases from both liver[49] and intestine[8,9] are optimal at alkaline pH. Though there are age-related decreases in the hydrolytic activities for both FMN and FAD in rat liver,[50] the pyrophosphate is elevated in liver carcinoma induced by p-dimethylaminoazobenzene[51] and in serum from some patients with liver disease.[52]

The means by which subsequent modifications of flavocoenzymes occur is not yet completely understood. However, it is certain that FMN and more commonly FAD are preformed before fractions of these coenzymes are covalently attached to specific apoenzymes. Studies on incorporation of ^{14}C-riboflavin into the covalently bound FAD of enzymes from rat liver mitochondria also suggested that formation of FAD preceded attachment.[53–55] The fact that certain synthetic 8α-substituted riboflavins (e.g., S-cysteinyl or N^3-histidyl derivatives) were not converted by flavokinase to the corresponding FMN analog[41,56] and that synthetic 8α-imidazole FMN is not a substrate for the FAD synthetase[57] would also argue against covalent linkage to such systems as are in monoamine oxidase or succinate dehydrogenase until after FAD is formed.

Work with cell-free synthesis of 6-hydroxy-D-nicotine oxidase obtained from *Arthrobacter oxidans*, an enzyme with an 8α-N^3-histidyl FAD, has established that intact FAD is incorporated into nascent polypeptide chains during ribosomal translation.[58,59] This has been extended to the similarly linked FAD within bacterial succinate and fumarate dehydrogenases.[60,61] The apoenzyme of the hydroxynicotine oxidase could be transformed into holoenzyme in the presence of FAD, ATP, phosphoenolpyruvate, and pyruvate kinase.[62] This finding indicates flavinylation is enzyme

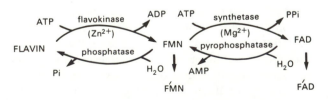

Figure 2. Interconversions of flavin and flavocoenzymes.

catalyzed and may proceed through a phosphointermediate.

Catabolism and Excretion

Though certain bacteria of the *Pseudomonas* genus can extensively degrade both the ring system[63] and side chains[64,65] of flavins, mammals are more limited in their abilities to catabolize the vitamin.[1,40,47,66] The diversity of flavin-derived products in mammalian urine, however, reflects metabolic events that occur in gastrointestinal microbes as well as in the somatic cells and additionally is augmented by photochemical events that occur at the dermal level. The present and fairly extensive knowledge of these events is summarized in Figure 3.

Cleavage of the side chain at position 10 seems mainly if not entirely attributable to intestinal microflora and light. Action of the former on riboflavin was shown to lead to partial fragmentation to form the 10-formylmethylflavin found in urine from ruminants,[67] which can interconvert this product with the 10-hydroxyethylflavin formed as a result of pyridine-nucleotide-dependent dehydrogenase in tissue.[68] The 10-hydroxyethylflavin is also found in urine from rats[69] and humans.[70] Lumichrome-level compounds not only can result from complete removal of the side chain by microflora, such as can be decreased by antibiotic administration,[69,71] but also accompany lumiflavin as a photoproduct from action of light on flavin within the dermal tissue.[69-71] A significant fraction of fecal radioactivity obtained from

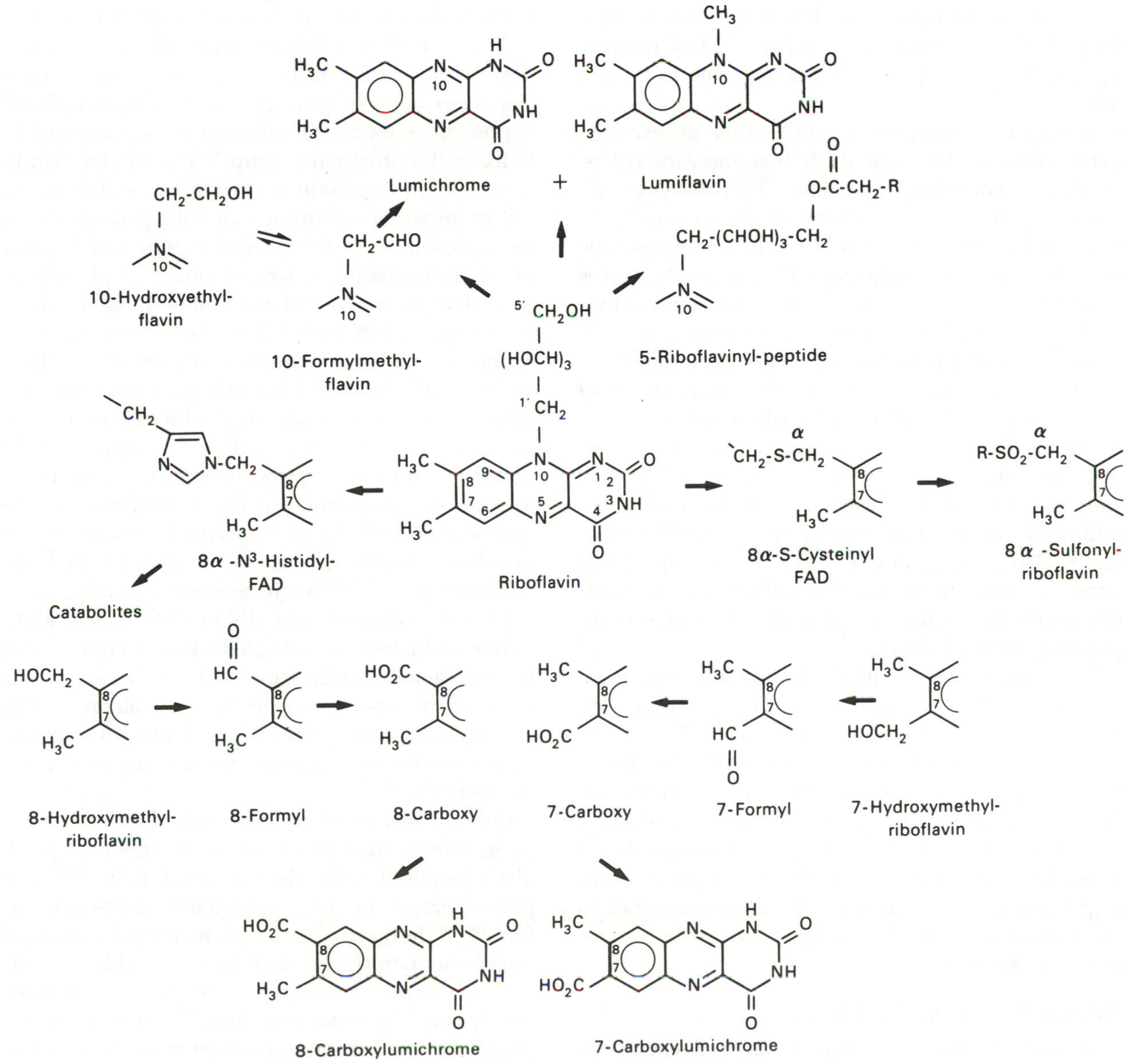

Figure 3. Catabolism and photodegradation of riboflavin reflected by urinary products from mammals.

rats administered $[2-^{14}C]$riboflavin was also found to be chloroform soluble and at the level of lumichrome.[71] A portion of the formylmethylflavin can also be oxidized by alimentary bacteria of the ruminant and human to form the 10-carboxymethylflavin.[72]

No enzymatic activity able to lead to such chain-shortened products has been identified within tissues.[73] Rather those catabolites of riboflavin that primarily derive from oxidations within tissue are the 7- and 8-hydroxymethylriboflavins (7α- and 8α-hydroxyriboflavins) found especially in human urine[70,74] and the 7- and 8-carboxylumichromes that occur in considerable amounts in rat urine.[69,75] These methyl-oxidized products reflect microsomal mixed-function oxidase activity.[76] Other flavin catabolites include those from 8α-(amino acid)riboflavins released from covalently bonded FAD.[77] An 8α-sulfonylriboflavin found in human urine may derive from the 8α-cysteinyl-FAD of monoamine oxidase.[70] Most recently a peptide ester of riboflavin was reported in human urine.[78]

We can now account for >95% of flavins excreted in human urine. For normal adults eating varied diets, riboflavin comprises 60–70%; 7-hydroxymethylriboflavin, 10–15%; 8α-sulfonylriboflavin, 5–10%; 8-hydroxymethylriboflavin, 4–7%; riboflavinyl peptide ester, 5%; and 10-hydroxyethylflavin, 1–3%. Traces of lumiflavin and varyingly the 10-formylmethyl- and carboxymethylflavins may be present.

Secretion of flavin into milk was reexamined on the basis of newer techniques for separation and identification.[40] In addition to riboflavin as a predominant flavin, lesser amounts of FMN, FAD, and a flavin with retention time suggestive of the 8α-sulfonylriboflavin are present in fresh (raw) milk from both cow and human. Some 7-hydroxymethylriboflavin also appears in cow milk. Processing of this latter substance to yield the typical commercial product results in breakdown of most of the FAD and putative sulfonyl flavin.

There are yet other metabolic derivatives of flavin known to occur naturally. Among these are glycosides[79] and a cyclic phosphodiester[80] of the ribityl side chain and even schizoflavins[81] that derive from oxidations at the 5′-hydroxymethyl terminus. A riboflavinyl 5′-malonate has been obtained from *Avena* coleoptiles.[82] However, these compounds are generally associated with bacterial, fungal, or plant organisms and are not normally of consequence to the human. The riboflavinyl α-D-glucoside was reported in rat urine.[83]

Newer Aspects of Deficiency

Human riboflavin requirements and metabolic consequences of deficiency in man and animals were covered in recent reviews.[84,85] Appropriate overviews of the nature and causes for deficiency of riboflavin, particularly as concerns the human, have been adequately covered in current texts on clinical[2] and medical nutrition,[3] in texts on medicine per se,[86] and in the previous edition of this volume.[45] Although riboflavin has a wide distribution in foodstuffs, especially eggs, lean meats, milk, broccoli, and enriched breads and cereals, many people live for long periods on low intakes. Consequently, biochemical reflections of suboptimal intake and even minor signs of deficiency are common in many parts of the world. More recent reports include infants in New Guinea[87] and children and pregnant women in Gambia[88–91] and Nigeria.[92–94] Deficiency is encountered almost invariably in combination with deficits of other water-soluble vitamins. In fact classically described deficiency symptoms such as glossitis and dermatitis may have resulted from other complicating deficiencies.

Severe riboflavin deficiency can affect the conversion of vitamin B-6 to its coenzyme.[95] Isolation and characterization of pure pyridoxine (pyridoxamine) 5′-phosphate oxidase confirmed its requirement for FMN as the prosthetic group.[96] The similar skin lesions seen in riboflavin and vitamin B-6 deficiencies reflect impaired maturation of collagen, which has been attributed to the need for pyridoxal 5′-phosphate, the formation of which from the 5′-phosphates of pyridoxine and pyridoxamine requires riboflavin operating as FMN with this oxidase.[97] A putative response of the carpal tunnel syndrome to riboflavin and to riboflavin combined with pyridoxine has been rationalized as also reflecting the important function of the FMN-dependent oxidase.[98] A low FMN-dependent pyridoxine 5′-phosphate oxidase activity due to a red-cell deficiency of FMN, confirmed by response to oral riboflavin, was reported in the majority of subjects with D-glucose 6-phosphate dehydrogenase deficiency.[99,100] Such cases seem to have an accelerated conversion of FMN to FAD so that glutathione reductase is saturated. This contrasts with heterozygous β-thalassemia, where there is an inherited slow red-cell conversion of riboflavin to FMN, a decrease in subsequent FAD, and a high stimulation of the erythrocyte glutathione reductase by extraneous FAD.[100,101]

Other diseases also affect riboflavin status.[3,102] Some effects arise as a result of treatment, e.g., dialysis required with chronic renal failure[103,104] or phototherapy in the potentially kernicteric infant.[105–107] In these cases supplements are warranted. Supplementation also may be reasonable with the use of certain drugs. Some affect riboflavin absorption[108] or renal excretion;[109] others seemingly impair flavocoenzyme formation or utilization, e.g., chlorpromazine[110,111] and antimalarials, some of which are flavin analogs.[112,113] In this latter connection, it is interesting that a relative riboflavin deficiency confers some protection against plasmodia infection as has been observed in rats[114] and humans.[115]

There has been an expansion in our knowledge of those inborn errors of metabolism that are the result of genetic defects in formation of functional flavoproteins.[116–118] Some involve enzymes of mitochondrial general electron transfer, whereas others are associated with β-oxidation of fatty acyl-CoA. In most cases, therapeutic levels of riboflavin have a beneficial effect.

Summary

Although riboflavin is the precursor for the predominant flavocoenzymes, FMN and FAD, there are other natural flavins that arise from divergences in the biosynthetic pathway for the vitamin, and a fraction of the coenzyme forms are covalently attached to the enzymes with which they function.

Circulatory transport after Na^+-dependent absorption from the upper small intestine is by tight complexing with immunoglobulins as well some loose association with albumin, and additional pregnancy-specific proteins enhance the transfer process in many animals including the human. The means by which the vitamin is taken in by different cells within the body differs somewhat, though rapid metabolic trapping that involves flavokinase-catalyzed phosphorylation is a common feature.

Much of the control on riboflavin utilization is at the level of flavocoenzyme formation, especially with flavokinase, which is subject to the thyroid-hormone–induced conversion from a less active to a more active form. Action by FAD synthetase is required to complete the major coenzyme before the larger fraction is noncovalently and a smaller fraction covalently bound to preformed apoenzymes.

The diverse degradative products from flavin that are excreted largely in the urine reflect turnover of coenzymes by hydrolytic and oxidative processes followed by tissue mixed-function oxidation of methyl groups of the free flavin and by ribityl side-chain cleavage that is largely the result of microfloral activity in the gut and exposure of skin to light.

Uncomplicated riboflavin deficiency is uncommon, but dietary lack of the vitamin can lead to deficit not only in flavocoenzyme functions but also in conversion of vitamin B-6 to pyridoxal phosphate that is required for other functions. Certain diseases and their treatment as well as infrequent genetic defects in flavoprotein function require supplementation, but normal individuals receive ample vitamin by eating a variety of foods.

References

1. D.E. Edmondson and D.B. McCormick, eds. (1987) *Flavins and Flavoproteins,* Ninth international symposium, de Gruyter, Berlin.
2. D.B. McCormick (1986) Riboflavin. In: *Textbook of Clinical Chemistry* (N.W. Tietz, ed.), pp. 927–964, W.B. Saunders, Philadelphia.
3. D.B. McCormick (1988) Riboflavin. In: *Modern Nutrition in Health and Disease* (M.E. Shils and V.R. Young, eds.), 7th ed., pp. 362–369, Lea and Febiger, Philadelphia.
4. D.W. Young (1986) The biosynthesis of the vitamins thiamin, riboflavin, and folic acid. *Nat. Prod. Rep.* 3:395–419.
5. A.H. Merrill, Jr., J.D. Lambeth, D.E. Edmondson, and D.B. McCormick (1981) Formation and mode of action of flavoproteins. *Annu. Rev. Nutr.* 1:281–317.
6. H. Daniel, U. Wille, and G. Rehner (1983) In vitro kinetics of the intestinal transport of riboflavin in rats. *J. Nutr.* 113:636–643.
7. E. Hegazy and M. Schwenk (1983) Riboflavin uptake by isolated enterocytes of guinea pigs. *J. Nutr.* 113:1702–1707.
8. T. Akiyama, J. Selhub, and I.H. Rosenberg (1982) FMN phosphatase and FAD pyrophosphatase in rat intestinal brush borders: role in intestinal absorption of dietary riboflavin. *J. Nutr.* 112:263–268.
9. H. Daniel, U. Wille, and G. Rehner (1983) Hydrolysis of FMN and FAD by alkaline phosphatase of the intestinal brush-border membrane. *Int. J. Vitam. Nutr. Res.* 53:109–114.
10. H.M. Said and D. Hollander (1985) Does aging affect the intestinal transport of riboflavin? *Life Sci.* 36:69–73.
11. H.M. Said, F.K. Ghishan, H.L. Greene, and D. Hollander (1985) Development maturation of riboflavin intestinal transport in the rat. *Pediatr. Res.* 19:1175–1178.
12. S. Feldman and W. Hedrick (1983) Antacid effects on the gastrointestinal absorption of riboflavin. *J. Pharm. Sci.* 72:121–123.
13. D.A. Roe, H. Kalkwarf, and J. Stevens (1988) Effect of fiber supplements on the apparent absorption of pharmacological doses of riboflavin. *J. Am. Diet. Assoc.* 88:211–213.
14. N.D. Vaziri, H.M. Said, D. Hollander, et al. (1985) Impaired intestinal absorption of riboflavin in experimental uremia. *Nephron* 41:26–29.
15. A.H. Merrill, Jr., J.A. Froehlich, and D.B. McCormick (1981) Isolation and identification of alternative riboflavin-binding proteins from human plasma. *Biochem. Med.* 25:198–206.
16. W.S.A. Innis, D.B. McCormick, and A.H. Merrill, Jr. (1985) Variations in riboflavin binding by human plasma: identification of immunoglobulins as the major proteins responsible. *Biochem. Med.* 34:151–165.
17. W.S. Innis, D.W. Nixon, D.R. Murray, D.B. McCormick, and A.H. Merrill, Jr. (1986) Immunoglobulins associated with elevated riboflavin binding by plasma from cancer patients. *Proc. Soc. Exp. Biol. Med.* 181:237–241.
18. A.H. Merrill, Jr., W.S.A. Innis-Whitehouse, and D.B. McCormick (1987) In: Characterization of human riboflavin-binding immunoglobulins. *Flavins and Flavoproteins* (D.E. Edmondson and D.B. McCormick, ed.), pp. 445–448, de Gruyter, Berlin.
19. M.J. Barber, D.C. Eichler, L.P. Solomonson, and B.A. Achrell (1987) Anti-flavin antibodies. *Biochem. J.* 242:89–95.
20. A. Kozik (1985) Riboflavin-binding proteins. *Postepy Biochem.* 31:263–281.
21. H.B. White, III and A.H. Merrill, Jr. (1988) Riboflavin-binding Proteins. *Annu. Rev. Nutr.* 8:279–299.
22. A.H. Merrill, Jr., J.A. Froehlich, and D.B. McCormick (1979) Purification of riboflavin-binding proteins from bovine plasma and discovery of a pregnancy-specific riboflavin-binding protein. *J. Biol. Chem.* 254:9362–9364.
23. K. Muniyappa and P.R. Adiga (1980) Isolation and characterization of riboflavin-binding protein from pregnant-rat serum. *Biochem. J.* 186:537–540.

24. S.S. Visweswariah and P.R. Adiga (1987) Purification of a circulatory riboflavin carrier protein from pregnant bonnet monkey (*M. radiata*): comparison with chicken egg vitamin carrier. *Biochim. Biophys. Acta* 915:141–148.

25. C.V.R. Murthy and P.R. Adiga (1982) Isolation and characterization of a riboflavin-carrier protein from human pregnancy serum. *Biochem. Int.* 5:289–296.

26. S.S. Visweswariah and P.R. Adiga (1987) Isolation of riboflavin carrier proteins from pregnant human and umbilical cord serum: similarities with chicken egg riboflavin carrier protein. *Biosci. Rep.* 7:563–571.

27. S.S. Visweswariah, A.A. Karande, and P.R. Adiga (1987) Immunological characterization of riboflavin carrier proteins using monoclonal antibodies. *Mol. Immunol.* 24:969–974.

28. K. Muniyappa and P.R. Adiga (1980) Occurrence and functional importance of a riboflavin-carrier protein in the pregnant rat. *FEBS Lett.* 110:209–212.

29. U. Natraj, A.R. Kumar, and P. Kadam (1987) Termination of pregnancy in mice with antiserum to chicken riboflavin-carrier protein. *Biol. Reprod.* 36:677–685.

30. P.B. Seshagiri and P.R. Adiga (1988) Pregnancy suppression in the bonnet monkey by active immunisation with chicken riboflavin carrier protein. *J. Reprod. Immunol.* 12:93–107.

31. K. Krishnamurthy, N. Surolia, and P.R. Adiga (1984) Mechanism of foetal wastage following immunoneutralization of riboflavin carrier protein in the pregnant rat: disturbances in flavin coenzyme levels. *FEBS Lett.* 178:87–91.

32. N. Surolia, K. Krishnamurthy, and P.R. Adiga (1985) Enzymic basis of deranged foetal flavin-nucleotide consequent on immunoneutralization of maternal riboflavin carrier protein in the pregnant rat. *Biochem. J.* 230:363–367.

33. M. Slomczynska and Z. Zak (1987) The effect of riboflavin binding protein (RBP) on flavokinase catalytic activity. *Comp. Biochem. Physiol.* 37B:681–685.

34. J. Dancis, J. Lehanka, and M. Levitz (1985) Transfer of riboflavin by the perfused human placenta. *Pediatr. Res.* 19:1143–1146.

35. J. Dancis, J. Lehanka, and M. Levitz (1988) Placental transport of riboflavin: differential rates of uptake at the maternal and fetal surfaces of the perfused human placenta. *Am. J. Obstet. Gynecol.* 158:204–210.

36. N.W. Kirshenbaum, J. Dancis, M. Levitz, J. Lehanka, and B.K. Young (1987) Riboflavin concentration in maternal and cord blood in human pregnancy. *Am. J. Obstet. Gynecol.* 157:748–752.

37. H. Bohn and W. Winckler (1987) Isolation and characterization of a flavin-containing placental protein (PP3). *Arch. Gynecol.* 240:201–206.

38. T.Y. Aw, D.P. Jones, and D.B. McCormick (1983) Uptake of riboflavin by isolated rat liver cells. *J. Nutr.* 113:1249–1254.

39. D.M. Bowers-Komro and D.B. McCormick (1987) Riboflavin uptake by isolated rat kidney cells. In: *Flavins and Flavoproteins* (D.E. Edmondson and D.B. McCormick, eds.), pp. 449–453, de Gruyter, Berlin.

40. D.B. McCormick, W.S.A. Innis, A.H. Merrill, Jr., D.M. Bowers-Komro, M. Oka, and J.L. Chastain (1987) An update on flavin metabolism in rats and humans. In: *Flavins and Flavoproteins* (D.E. Edmondson and D.B. McCormick, eds.), pp. 459–471, de Gruyter, Berlin.

41. A.H. Merrill, Jr. and D.B. McCormick (1980) Affinity chromatographic purification and properties of flavokinase (ATP:riboflavin 5'-phosphotransferase) from rat liver. *J. Biol. Chem.* 255:1335–1338.

42. J. Sobhanaditya and N. Appaji Rao (1981) Plant flavokinase. Affinity-chromatographic procedure for the purification of the enzyme from mung-bean (*Phaseolus aureus*) seeds and conformational changes in its interaction with orthophosphate. *Biochem. J.* 197:227–232.

43. D.J. Manstein and E.F. Pai (1986) Purification and characterization of FAD synthetase from *Brevebacterium ammoniagenes*. *J. Biol. Chem.* 261:16169–16173.

44. M. Oka and D.B. McCormick (1987) Complete purification and general characterization of FAD synthetase from rat liver. *J. Biol. Chem.* 262:7418–7422.

45. R.S. Rivlin (1984) Riboflavin. In: *Present Knowledge in Nutrition* (R.E. Olson, H.P. Broquist, C.D. Chichester, W.J. Darby, A.C. Kolbye, Jr., and R.M. Stalvey, eds.), 5th ed, pp. 285–302, The Nutrition Foundation, Inc., Washington, DC.

46. S.-S. Lee and D.B. McCormick (1985) Thyroid hormone regulation of flavocoenzyme biosynthesis. *Arch. Biochem. Biophys.* 237:197–201.

47. D.B. McCormick (1975) Metabolism of riboflavin. In: *Riboflavin* (R.S. Rivlin, ed.), pp. 153–198, Plenum Press, New York.

48. D.B. McCormick and M. Russell (1962) Hydrolysis of flavin mononucleotide by acid phosphatases from animal tissues. *Comp. Biochem. Physiol.* 5:113–121.

49. N. Krishnan (1971) Metabolism of water soluble vitamins: studies on enzymes from sheep liver and from livers of fresh water fishes (*Wallag attu*) that hydrolyze nucleotides. Ph.D. thesis, Department of Biochemistry, Indian Institute of Science, Bangalore 12, India.

50. S.-S. Lee and D.B. McCormick (1983) Effect of riboflavin status on hepatic activities of flavin-metabolizing enzymes in rats. *J. Nutr.* 113:2274–2279.

51. W.-K. Yang and J.-L. Sung (1966) Riboflavin metabolism in liver diseases. IV. Enzymic splitting and synthesis of flavine adenine dinucleotide in the *p*-dimethylaminoazobenzene-induced rat liver carcinoma tissue. *Taiwan I Hsueh Hui Tsa Chih* 65:299.

52. W.-K. Yang and J.-L. Sung (1966) Riboflavin metabolism in liver diseases. V. Clinical studies on the enzymic splitting of flavine adenine dinucleotide in serum. *Taiwan I Hsueh Hui Tsa Chih* 65:306.

53. K. Yagi, Y. Nakagawa, O. Suzuki, and N. Ohishi (1976) Incorporation of riboflavin into covalently-bound flavins in rat liver. *J. Biochem.* 79:841–843.

54. R. Addison and D.B. McCormick (1978) Biogenesis of flavoprotein and cytochrome components in hepatic mitochondria from riboflavin-deficient rats. *Biochem. Biophys. Res. Commun.* 81:133–138.

55. M. Sato, N. Ohishi, and K. Yagi (1984) Localization and identification of covalently bound flavoproteins in rat liver mitochondria by prelabeling of their flavin moiety. *J. Biochem.* 96:553–562.

56. A.H. Merrill, Jr. and D.B. McCormick (1979) Preparation and properties of immobilized flavokinase. *Biotech. Bioeng.* 21:1629–1638.

57. D.B. Bowers-Komro, Y. Yamada, and D.B. McCormick (1988) Substrate and affinity-matrix specificity of mammalian FAD synthetase. *Fed. Proc.* 2:no. 4 (abstr. no. 349).

58. H.-H. Hamm and K. Decker (1978) FAD is covalently attached to peptidyl-tRNA during cell-free synthesis of 6-hydroxy-D-nicotine oxidase. *Eur. J. Biochem.* 92:449–454.

59. H.-H. Hamm and K. Decker (1980) Cell-free synthesis of a flavoprotein containing the 8α-(N³-histidyl)-riboflavin linkage. *Eur. J. Biochem.* 104:391–395.

60. R. Brandsch and V. Bichler (1985) In vivo and in vitro expression of the 6-hydroxy-D-nicotine oxidase gene of *Arthrobacter oxidans*, cloned into *Escherichia coli*, as an enzymatically active, covalently flavinylated polypeptide. *FEBS Lett.* 192:204–208.

61. R. Brandsch and V. Bichler (1986) Studies in vitro on the flavinylation of 6-hydroxy-D-nicotine oxidase. *Eur. J. Biochem.* 160:285–289.

62. R. Brandsch and V. Bichler (1987) Covalent flavinylation of 6-hydroxy-D-nicotine oxidase involves an energy-requiring process. *FEBS Lett.* 224:121–124.

63. L. Tsai and E.R. Stadtman (1971) In: Riboflavin degradation. *Vitamins and Coenzymes, Methods in Enzymology*, vol. 18B (D.B.

McCormick and L.D. Wright, eds.), pp. 557–571, Academic Press, New York.

64. T. Yanagita and J.W. Forster (1956) A bacterial riboflavin hydrolase. *J. Biol. Chem.* 221:593–607.

65. C.S. Yang and D.B. McCormick (1967) Substrate specificity of a riboflavin hydrolase from *Pseudomonas riboflavina. Biochim. Biophys. Acta* 132:511–513.

66. D.B. McCormick, W.S.A. Innis, A.H. Merrill, Jr., and S.-S. Lee (1984) Mammalian metabolism of flavins. In: *Flavins and Flavoproteins* (R.C. Bray, P.C. Engel, and S.G. Mayhew, eds.), pp. 833–846, de Gruyter, Berlin.

67. E.C. Owen and D.W. West (1971) Isolation and identification of 7,8-dimethyl-10-formylmethylisoalloxazine as a product of the bacterial degradation of riboflavin. In: *Vitamins and Coenzymes, Methods in Enzymology,* vol. 18B (D.B. McCormick and L.D. Wright, eds.), pp. 579–581, Academic Press, New York.

68. E.C. Owen and D.W. West (1971) Isolation and identification of 7,8-dimethyl-10-(α^1-hydroxyethyl)isoalloxazine from natural sources. In: *Vitamins and Coenzymes, Methods in Enzymology,* vol. 18B (D.B. McCormick and L.D. Wright, eds.), pp. 574–579, Academic Press, New York.

69. J.L. Chastain and D.B. McCormick (1987) Clarification and quantitation of primary (tissue) and secondary (microbial) catabolites of riboflavin that are excreted in mammalian (rat) urine. *J. Nutr.* 117:468–475.

70. J.L. Chastain and D.B. McCormick (1987) Flavin catabolites: identification and quantitation in human urine. *Am. J. Clin. Nutr.* 46:830–834.

71. C.S. Yang and D.B. McCormick (1978) Degradation and excretion of riboflavin in the rat. *J. Nutr.* 93:445–453.

72. D.W. West and E.C. Owen (1973) Degradation of riboflavin by alimentary bacteria of the ruminant and man: production of 7,8-dimethyl-10-carboxymethylisoalloxazine. *Br. J. Nutr.* 29:33–41.

73. M. Oka and D.B. McCormick (1985) Urinary lumichrome-level catabolites of riboflavin are due to microbial and photochemical events and not tissue enzymic cleavage of the ribityl chain. *J. Nutr.* 115:496–499.

74. H. Ohkawa, N. Ohishi, and K. Yagi (1983) New metabolites of riboflavin appear in human urine. *J. Biol. Chem.* 258:5623–5628.

75. H. Ohkawa, N. Ohishi, and K. Yagi (1983) New metabolites of riboflavin appeared in rat urine. *Biochem. Int.* 6:239–247.

76. H. Ohkawa, N. Ohishi, and K. Yagi (1983) Hydroxylation of the 7- and 8-methyl groups of riboflavin by the microsomal electron transfer system of rat liver. *J. Biol. Chem.* 258:5629–5633.

77. C.P. Chia, R. Addison, and D.B. McCormick (1978) Absorption, metabolism, and excretion of 8α-(amino acid)riboflavins in the rat. *J. Nutr.* 108:373–381.

78. J.L. Chastain and D.B. McCormick (1988) Characterization of a new flavin metabolite from human urine. *Biochim. Biophys. Acta* 967:131–134.

79. L.G. Whitby (1971) Glycosides of riboflavin. In: *Vitamins and Coenzymes, Methods in Enzymology,* vol. 18B (D.B. McCormick and L.D. Wright, eds.), pp. 404–413, Academic Press, New York.

80. S. Tachibana (1967) The formation of new flavin phosphates by molds. *J. Vitaminol. (Kyoto)* 13:70–79.

81. S. Tachibana and T. Murakami (1980) Isolation and identification of schizoflavins. In: *Vitamins and Coenzymes, Methods in Enzymology,* vol. 66 (D.B. McCormick and L.D. Wright, eds.), pp. 333–338, Academic Press, New York.

82. S. Ghisla, R. Mack, G. Blankenhorn, P. Hemmerich, E. Krienitz, and T. Kuster (1984) Structure of a novel flavin chromophore from avena coleoptiles, the possible "blue light" photoreceptor. *Eur. J. Biochem.* 138:339–344.

83. H. Ohkawa, N. Ohishi, and K. Yagi (1983) Occurrence of riboflavinyl glucoside in rat urine. *J. Nutr. Sci. Vitaminol. (Tokyo)* 29:515–522.

84. H.E. Sauberlich (1984) Implications of nutritional status on human biochemistry, physiology, and health. *Clin. Biochem.* 17:132–142.

85. C.J. Bates (1987) Human riboflavin requirements, and metabolic consequences of deficiency in man and animals. *World Rev. Nutr. Diet* 50:215–265.

86. J.D. Wilson (1982) Riboflavin. In: *Harrison's Principles of Internal Medicine,* 10th ed. (R.G. Petersdorf, R.D. Adams, E. Braunwald, K.J. Isselbacher, J.B. Martin, and J.D. Wilson, eds.), p. 466, McGraw-Hill, New York.

87. S.J. Oppenheimer, R. Bull, and D.J. Thurnham (1983) Riboflavin deficiency in Madang infants. *Papua New Guinea Med. J.* 26:17–20.

88. H.J. Powers, C.J. Bates, A.M. Prentice, W.H. Lamb, M. Jepson, and H. Bowman (1983) The relative effectiveness of iron and iron with riboflavin in correcting a microcytic anaemia in men and children in rural Gambia. *Hum. Nutr. Clin. Nutr.* 37:413–425.

89. C.J. Bates, A. Flewitt, A.M. Prentice, W.H. Lamb, and R.G. Whitehead (1983) Efficacy of a riboflavin supplement given at fortnightly intervals to pregnant and lactating women in rural Gambia. *Hum. Nutr. Clin. Nutr.* 37:427–432.

90. C.J. Bates, A.M. Prentice, M. Watkinson, et al. (1984) Efficacy of a food supplement in correcting riboflavin deficiency in pregnant Gambian women. *Hum. Nutr. Clin. Nutr.* 38:363–374.

91. H.J. Powers, C.J. Bates, and W.H. Lamb (1985) Haematological response to supplements of iron and riboflavin to pregnant and lactating women in rural Gambia. *Hum. Nutr. Clin. Nutr.* 39:117–129.

92. O.A. Ajayi (1984) Biochemical ariboflavinosis among Nigerian rural school children. *Hum. Nutr. Clin. Nutr.* 38:383–389.

93. O.A. Ajayi and O.A. James (1984) Effect of riboflavin supplementation on riboflavin nutriture of a secondary school population in Nigeria. *Am. J. Clin. Nutr.* 39:787–791.

94. O.A. Ajaji (1985) Incidence of biochemical riboflavin deficiency in Nigerian pregnant women. *Hum. Nutr. Clin. Nutr.* 39:149–153.

95. Anonymous (1981) Genetic determination of coenzyme synthesis in red cells. *Nutr. Rev.* 39:331–334.

96. M.N. Kazarinoff and D.B. McCormick (1975) Rabbit liver pyridoxamine (pyridoxine) 5'-phosphate oxidase. Purification and properties. *J. Biol. Chem.* 250:3436–3442.

97. R. Prasad, A.V. Lakshmi, and M.S. Bamji (1983) Impaired collagen maturity in vitamins B_2 and B_6 deficiency—probable molecular basis of skin lesions. *Biochem. Med.* 30:333–341.

98. K. Folkers, A. Wolaniuk, and S. Vadhanavikit (1984) Enzymology of the response of the carpal tunnel syndrome to riboflavin and to combined riboflavin and pyridoxine. *Proc. Natl. Acad. Sci. U.S.A.* 81:7076–7078.

99. H.J. Powers and C.J. Bates (1985) A simple fluorimetric assay for pyridoxamine phosphate oxidase in erythrocyte haemolysates: effects of riboflavin supplementation and of glucose 6-phosphate dehydrogenase deficiency. *Hum. Nutr. Clin. Nutr.* 39:107–115.

100. B.B. Anderson, J.E. Clements, G.M. Perry, C. Studds, C. Vullo, and G. Salsini (1987) Glutathione reductase activity in G6PD deficiency. *Eur. J. Haematol.* 38:12–20.

101. B.B. Anderson, G.M. Perry, and J.E. Clements (1984) Red cell enzyme activities in thalassaemia. *Br. J. Haematol.* 57:711–714.

102. G.E. Nicholalds (1981) Riboflavin. *Clin. Lab. Med.* 1:685–698.

103. G. Stein, H. Sperschneider, and S. Koppe (1985) Vitamin levels in chronic renal failure and need for supplementation. *Blood Purif.* 3:52–62.

104. F. Marumo, K. Kamata, and M. Okubo (1986) Deranged concentrations of water-soluble vitamins in the blood of undialyzed and dialyzed patients with chronic renal failure. *Int. J. Artif. Organs* 9:17–24.

105. R. Hodr, E. Knobloch, E. Proch'azkov'a, J. Skutilov'a, and V. Houdkov'a (1986) Riboflavin hypovitaminosis in phototherapy of neonatal hyperbilirubinemia. *Cesk. Pediatr.* 41:206–207.

106. R. Hodr, E. Knobloch, E. Proch'azkov'a, J. Skutilov'a, and V. Houdkov'a (1986) Prevention of riboflavin hypovitaminosis and a favorable therapeutic effect during phototherapy and neonatal hyperbilirubinemia. *Cesk. Pediatr.* 41:271–274.

107. T.R. Sisson (1987) Photodegradation of riboflavin in neonates. *Fed. Proc.* 46:1883–1885.

108. D.A. Roe (1983) Drugs and nutrient absorption. *Curr. Concepts Nutr.* 12:129–138.

109. J.T. Pinto and R.S. Rivlin (1987) Drugs that promote renal excretion of riboflavin. *Drug. Nutr. Interact.* 5:143–151.

110. N. Pelliccione, J. Pinto, Y.P. Huang, and R.S. Rivlin (1983) Accelerated development of riboflavin deficiency by treatment with chlorpromazine. *Biochem. Pharmacol.* 32:2949–2953.

111. J. Pinto, Y.P. Huang, and R.S. Rivlin (1985) Inhibition by chlorpromazine of thyroxine modulation of flavin metabolism in liver, cerebrum and cerebellum. *Biochem. Pharmacol.* 34:93–95.

112. W.B. Cowden, G.A. Butcher, N.H. Hunt, I.A. Clark, and F. Yoneda (1987) Antimalarial activity of a riboflavin analog against *Plasmodium vinckei* in vivo and *Plasmodium falciparum* in vitro. *Am. J. Trop. Med. Hyg.* 37:495–500.

113. W.B. Cowden, I.A. Clark, and N.H. Hunt (1988) Flavins as potential antimalarials. 1. 10-(Halophenyl)-3-methylflavins. *J. Med. Chem.* 31:799–801.

114. P. Kaikai and D.I. Thurnham (1983) The influence of *Plasmodium gerghei* infection in rats. *Trans. R. Soc. Trop. Med. Hyg.* 77:680–686.

115. D.I. Thurnham, S.J. Oppenheimer, and R. Bull (1983) Riboflavin status and malaria in infants in Papua New Guinea. *Trans. R. Soc. Trop. Med. Hyg.* 77:423–424.

116. K. Bartlett (1983) Vitamin-responsive inborn errors of metabolism. *Adv. Clin. Chem.* 23:141–198.

117. N. Gregersen (1985) Riboflavin-responsive defects of beta-oxidation. *J. Inherited Metab. Dis.* (suppl. 8) 1:65–69.

118. C. Vianey-Liaud, P. Divry, N. Gregersen, and M. Mathieu (1987) The inborn errors of mitochondrial fatty acid oxidation. *J. Inherited Metab. Dis.* (suppl. 10) 1:159–200.

Chapter **18**   Alfred H. Merrill, Jr., and Faith S. Burnham

Vitamin B-6

The vitamin B-6 group is composed of three natural compounds—pyridoxine (pyridoxol, PN), pyridoxamine (PM), and pyridoxal (PL). The history of vitamin B-6 was summarized recently beginning with the discovery of an agent that prevented dermatitis in rats by Gyorgy in 1934 to identification of the coenzymatically active form of vitamin B-6 as pyridoxal 5'-phosphate (PLP) by Snell, Gunsalus, and others.[1] The importance and diversity of the biochemical pathways that utilize these compounds have engendered numerous investigations covered in recent reviews and symposia.[2-9] This chapter gives an overview of basic knowledge about vitamin B-6 and updates earlier treatments in this series[2] with topics such as bioavailability and toxicity.

Chemistry

Structure. The three vitamers are 2-methyl-3-hydroxy-5-hydroxymethyl pyridines with a hydroxymethyl (PN), aminomethyl (PM), or formyl (PL) group at position 4 (Figure 1). The major degradation form (pyridoxic acid, 4-PA) has a carboxyl group at position 4. All three vitamers exist primarily as the 5'-phosphates in tissues. Plant foods contain variable portions of the 5'-glucosides of pyridoxine, which affects the bioavailability.[10] During food processing N4'-pyridoxyl-lysine is sometimes formed from PLP,[11] and 6-hydroxy-PN can be formed in ascorbate-rich foods.[12]

Chemical Properties. Pyridoxine is sold commercially as the hydrochloride salt for use in dietary supplementation. The salts of PN, PL, and PM and the 5'-phosphates of these compounds are water soluble. In neutral solution the ring is zwitterionic with ionized phenolate and pyridinium groups. PL exists partially as the hemiacetal of the aldehyde and 5'-hydroxyl group; 4-PA exists largely as the stable lactone. Solutions of PL and PLP that also contain compounds with free amino groups (e.g., amino acids, Tris buffer, etc.) will spontaneously form the (yellow) Schiff bases; cysteine forms a stable thiazolidine derivative that has been useful in dissociating the coenzyme from PLP-dependent enzymes to yield the apoforms.

Vitamin B-6 compounds absorb light in the ultraviolet (and for most Schiff bases, the visible) region and are somewhat fluorescent. (4-PA is highly fluorescent.) They are light sensitive especially at alkaline pH. The spectroscopic properties of these compounds have been valuable in elucidating their mechanism of action and in the development of sensitive assays.[6,13]

Methods of Analysis. The methods for determination of vitamin B-6 in foods and other biological materials were reviewed recently by Gregory.[10] They range from microbiological assays to high-performance liquid chromatography.[14,15] The advantage of the latter is that it allows analysis of all seven major forms of the B-6 compounds in a single run. Many laboratories analyze PLP by mixing the sample with an apoPLP-dependent enzyme (such as apotyrosine decarboxylase) and measuring the reconstituted activity by sensitive methods.[16]

Absorption and Transport

The overall scheme of vitamin B-6 transport and metabolism is shown in Figure 2.

Intestinal Uptake. Pyridoxine is encountered in foods in the free form and as the glycoside, which is readily taken up by the intestine directly or after hydrolysis by lumenal enzymes and/or microflora.[17] PL and PM are present in foods primarily as the 5'-phosphates and require hydrolysis by the nonspecific phosphatases of the gastrointestinal tract.[18] The bioavailability of vitamin B-6 varies with the type of food and method of processing.[19]

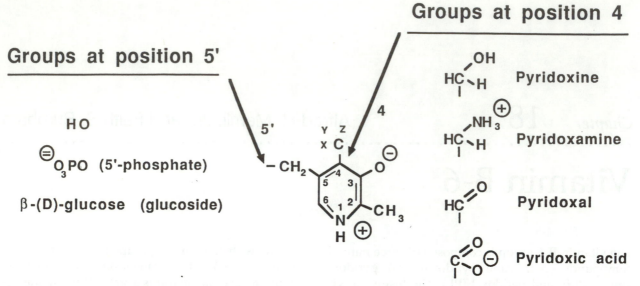

Figure 1. Major naturally occurring forms of vitamin B-6 and metabolites. Shown are the three vitamers (pyridoxine, pyridoxamine, and pyridoxal) that vary in the x, y, and z substitutions on the carbon at position 4 of the pyridinium ring (shown in the dianionic form present at neutral pH) and the dead-end catabolite (pyridoxic acid). The vitamers have a hydroxyl on the 5'-carbon and are metabolized to the 5'-phosphates. Pyridoxine is also encountered in plants as the β-glucoside.

The three forms are absorbed in the jejunum by a nonsaturable process followed by metabolic trapping by phosphorylation.[20,21] In the rat the uptake has been shown to decrease from the proximal to distal small intestine,[21] and PLP utilization was affected by pH, which might indicate that agents that raise the gastric pH could affect the utilization of vitamin B-6.[18] The B-6 vitamers exit the intestinal cells via the basolateral membrane in mainly the nonphosphorylated forms.[20]

Transport via Circulation. In blood, PL and PLP are tightly bound by albumin.[22] PN and PL are also rapidly accumulated by erythrocytes because of metabolism and trapping of the PL by binding to hemoglobin.[23]

Metabolism. Most of the absorbed vitamin B-6 is taken up by liver, where the phosphorylated forms are hydrolyzed by the plasma membrane alkaline phosphatase, and enters the hepatocytes by a facilitated process and diffusion followed by metabolic trapping.[24,25] The various aspects of vitamin B-6 metabolism were reviewed in depth[26-28] with emphasis on human metabolism.[27] The three vitamers are converted to pyridoxine 5'-phosphate (PNP), pyridoxamine 5'-phosphate (PMP), and PLP by a single kinase;[29] then PNP and PMP are oxidized to PLP by a flavin-dependent oxidase.[30] PLP is bound by apoenzymes or released into plasma as PLP, PL, or 4-PA (after hydrolysis and oxidation).[31] Analyses of the relative activities of these enzymes in human liver indicate that the kinase and phosphatase have similar activities at physiological pH, which accounts for the

rapid accumulation of the vitamers as the 5'-phosphates but also allows dephosphorylation of PLP that is not protein bound to facilitate its release from the hepatocytes as PL or degradation to 4-PA.[32] Another site of regulation of vitamin B-6 metabolism is the conversion of PNP and PMP to PLP, which is highly sensitive to product inhibition so that excess PLP limits the flux through this step.[33,34]

Other Aspects. Because essentially all tissues contain PL kinase, but few have significant levels of PNP(PMP) oxidase, it is thought that liver is responsible for converting dietary PN and PM to PL (via PLP) and that other tissues only make PLP from the PL taken up from circulation. This may not be the whole story because aminotransferases interconvert PMP and PLP; however, this route has not been evaluated quantitatively. In addition to interorgan metabolism and transport, PLP is required by several enzymes in the mitochondria, necessitating intracellular transport systems. The uptake of PLP into isolated rat-liver mitochondria is energy independent and is most consistent with passive diffusion facilitated by protein binding.[35]

Catabolism and Excretion. The liver is the major source of plasma PLP,[36] although muscle has been suggested to be an additional source during conditions of muscle turnover.[27] The PLP is primarily carried to tissues where it is utilized if needed, and the remainder is oxidized to 4-PA. Because PLP is tightly bound to albumin while in circulation, the hydrolysis by alkaline phosphatase is central to its availability for both tissue uptake and catabolism. The marked

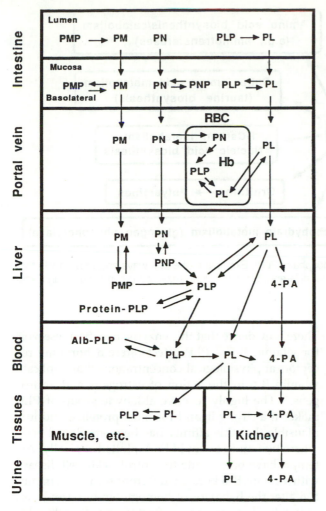

Figure 2. Overview of vitamin B-6 transport and metabolism. The involvement of different organs in the uptake, transport, metabolism, and excretion of vitamin B-6 are summarized. The enzymes involved in these interconversions are pyridoxal (PL) kinase for the phosphorylation of pyridoxine (PN), pyridoxamine (PM), and PL; PNP(PMP) oxidase for pyridoxal 5'-phosphate (PLP) synthesis from pyridoxine 5'-phosphate (PNP) and pyridoxamine 5'-phosphate (PMP) (there is also interconversion of PLP and PMP by aminotransferases, not shown); alkaline phosphatase to remove the 5'-phosphates; and PL oxidase and, possibly, PL dehydrogenase to form pyridoxic acid (4-PA). The PL and PLP can be bound by albumin (Alb) and hemoglobin (Hb) in red blood cells (RBC).

increase in circulating PLP in patients with hypophosphatasia, an inborn error characterized by deficient activity of this enzyme, underscores the role of alkaline phosphatase in PLP clearance.[37]

Because 4-PA is a dead-end catabolite, the balance between PL uptake by cells vs. catabolism is important to the efficient utilization of this micronutrient. It appears that the PL released in circulation has access to peripheral tissues first; then the excess is taken up by liver, which is thought to be the major site of

4-PA formation.[38] Because the hepatic kinase and PL oxidase have comparable activities in liver,[32] they compete about equally well for PL, and a substantial portion is rapidly converted to 4-PA.[39] The kidney also takes up PL and PN and probably contributes to the catabolism and elimination of vitamin B-6[40]; however, the role of this organ has not yet been characterized fully. The two major forms of vitamin B-6 found in urine are PL and 4-PA.

Biochemical Functions

Pyridoxal 5'-phosphate is utilized by over 60 enzymes. Except where noted, only mammalian enzymes will be discussed here; for recent reviews, see references 6 and 7. They typically bind the coenzyme tightly in a Schiff base linkage with the ϵ-amino group of an active-site lysine, and for most of the enzymes, the incoming substrate displaces the lysine to form a new Schiff base. This action results in a strong electron sink adjacent to several of the bonds on the substrate and facilitates a variety of chemical reactions, as illustrated by the following examples and the summary in Figure 3.

Aminotransferase Reactions. The interconversions of amino acids and their respective α-ketoacids by aminotransferases (e.g., alanine aminotransferase, aspartate aminotransferase, etc.) are central to the biosynthesis and catabolism of essential and nonessential amino acids. In many instances they provide a simple link between the amino acid and intermediates of glycolysis (e.g., alanine and pyruvate) and the tricarboxylic acid cycle (e.g., aspartate and oxaloacetate, glutamate and α-ketoglutarate). Not all aminotransferases act on the α-amino group, however, as illustrated in the conversion of ornithine to pyrroline-5-carboxylate by ornithine-δ-aminotransferase.

Decarboxylation Reactions. The synthesis of polyamines, serotonin, tyramine, histamine, and γ-amino butyric acid (GABA) (for examples) involves the decarboxylation of precursor amino acids. The de novo formation of phosphatidylethanolamine (which is also an intermediate in the synthesis of choline and phosphatidylcholine) by decarboxylation of phosphatidylserine is thought to utilize a PLP-dependent enzyme.

Decarboxylation with Carbon-carbon Bond Formation. The initial and regulatory enzymes of heme (δ-amino levulinate synthetase) and sphingolipid (serine palmitoyltransferase) biosynthesis condense glycine with succinyl-CoA and serine and palmitoyl-CoA, respectively.

Side-chain Cleavage Reactions. The key step in initiation of one-carbon metabolism is the transfer

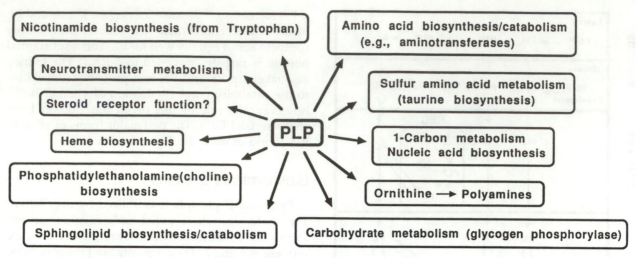

Figure 3. Overview of metabolic pathways utilizing pyridoxal 5'-phosphate (PLP). Example of the pathways and/or products that directly utilize PLP are shown. Each example may include several different PLP-dependent enzymes (as in sulfur amino acid metabolism).

of a hydroxymethyl group from serine to tetrahydrofolate (catalyzed by serine hydroxymethyltransferase) to form glycine and N^5,N^{10}-methylenetetrahydrofolate. Another example of a side-chain cleavage reaction is the splitting of cystathionine (by cystathionase) in cysteine biosynthesis from methionine. Vitamin B-6 has long been known to be intimately involved in sulfur amino acid metabolism at multiple sites (it is also utilized in taurine synthesis), and sulfur amino acid metabolism is adversely affected in vitamin B-6 deficiencies and in individuals with congenital defects in PLP utilization.[41] Tryptophan catabolism and its utilization in nicotinamide biosynthesis also proceed via an intermediate that is cleaved by a PLP-dependent enzyme; the accumulation of various intermediates and side products of this pathway in response to a tryptophan load has been used as a test of vitamin B-6 status.[42]

Dehydratase Reactions. Another type of side-chain modification reaction (β-elimination) is exemplified in the deamination and dehydration of serine to pyruvate, ammonia, and water by L-serine dehydratase.

Racemization Reactions. Many bacteria contain PLP-dependent enzymes that catalyze the interconversion of D- and L-amino acids, although such enzymes are not thought to be found in mammals. These enzymes permit the synthesis of optically active amino acids and have been the target of antimicrobial drugs that act as mechanism-based ("suicide") inhibitors.

Other Functions. Several other systems use PLP in a different manner from these examples. Glycogen phosphorylase requires PLP, perhaps because the phosphate is involved in the catalytic mechanism.

There is evidence that this enzyme may be a reservoir for vitamin B-6.[27] PLP affects steroid hormone receptors at physiological concentrations that implicate vitamin B-6 in the action of estrogens and androgens.[43] The highly reactive aldehyde group of PLP makes it a strong ligand for most proteins, and it is plausible that this affinity has been employed elsewhere by nature or could be exploited clinically. Attempts have been made to control sickle cell disease with vitamin B-6 because different forms of vitamin B-6 alter the behavior of hemoglobin in vitro; however, it has not yet proven effective in a clinical trial.[44]

Deficiency

Dietary Deficiencies. Deficiencies in vitamin B-6 alone are relatively uncommon in humans; instead, one usually encounters inadequate consumption of many B-complex vitamins.[3,8,9] Early biochemical signs of low vitamin B-6 are a decrease in plasma PLP and urinary PL and 4-PA, an increased excretion of xanthurenic acid (especially after a tryptophan load), an increase in the apoform of serum and red cell transaminases, and sometimes an increase in urinary cystathionine after a methionine load. The physiological indicators of vitamin B-6 deficiency are electroencephalographic abnormalities (including the possibility of convulsions in the young), dermatitis with cheilosis and glossitis, impaired humoral and cell-mediated immunity, reduced delayed-hypersensitivity responses, depletion of thoracic-duct lymphocytes and reduced lymphocyte proliferation, impaired thymic epithelial cell function, maintenance of normal T-cell function in vivo, and possibly a normocytic, microcytic, or sideroblastic anemia.[45]

Iatrogenic Deficiencies. One of the more common ways of encountering vitamin B-6 deficiency is as a side effect of drugs that form a complex with PL and PLP (e.g., isoniazid, cycloserine, penicillamine, and carbonyl reagents in general);[46] hence, the recommended therapy is to administer these drugs with a vitamin B-6 supplement. These effects are caused by the formation of adducts with the aldehyde group of PL and PLP that inhibits vitamin B-6 metabolism and coenzyme binding by apoenzymes.[47]

Genetic Defects. Pyridoxine supplementation is indicated in a number of functional vitamin B-6 deficiencies wherein a genetic defect in a PLP-dependent enzyme does not allow the enzyme to utilize its coenzyme effectively.[8,9,48] Examples of this defect are PN-responsive convulsions caused by inadequate γ-butyric acid synthesis, homocystinuria and cystathioninuria arising from cystathionine β-synthase and cystathioninase deficiencies, xanthurenic aciduria caused by kynureninase deficiency, ornithinemia (gyrate atrophy) caused by a defective ornithine aminotransferase, and primary oxalosis (type I), where PN seems to increase the removal of glyoxylic acid to glycine. As already noted, one congenital defect (hypophosphatasia) was proven to alter vitamin B-6 metabolism.[37]

Disease. Diseases also affect vitamin B-6 status, as was reviewed recently.[9,28,49] Plasma PLP is significantly lower in cirrhosis and other hepatic and biliary diseases, apparently because of increased turnover of circulating PLP. It is not clear, however, whether or not this apparent B-6 deficiency contributes to the abnormal metabolism of amino acids and other compounds. Low plasma PLP also is found in patients with chronic renal failure and in patients undergoing maintenance hemodialysis, intermittent peritoneal dialysis, or kidney transplant with or without normal or nearly normal kidney function. Carpal tunnel syndrome has been reported to respond to megadoses of pyridoxine in some instances, although this therapy remains controversial. There is no solid evidence that pyridoxine therapy is of benefit in other neurological disorders (Downs syndrome, epilepsy).

Requirements and Allowances

The current Recommended Dietary Allowance (RDA) for vitamin B-6 is ~2.0 mg/d for adult males and 1.6 mg/d for adult females.[50] The RDA for infants begins at 0.3 mg/d and increases to 0.6 mg/d for older infants consuming a mixed diet and increases from 1 to 2 mg/d from childhood through adolescence. Pregnancy and lactation add 0.6 and 0.5 mg/d, respectively, to the RDA for women.

Several methods have been suggested to assess human requirements for vitamin B-6 and to identify deficiencies of this vitamin.[3] These include measuring plasma PLP,[51] urinary 4-PA,[51,52] stimulation of various serum and erythrocyte aminotransferases by PLP,[53] and urinary metabolites of pathways sensitive to depletion of vitamin B-6.[41,42] Plasma PLP is most often studied and is a reasonable indicator of human vitamin B-6 status. However Lui et al.[51] suggest that urinary 4-PA is a better indicator of intake and that plasma PLP content reflects the body store.

Among healthy individuals these indices seem to give an adequate picture of normal vitamin B-6 status. For example, Driskell et al.[54] studied 22 healthy males (aged 20–37 y, of different races) and found that they all had plasma PLP within the normal range. Calculated values of vitamin B-6 in the foods consumed indicated intakes of 1.22–1.67 mg vitamin B-6/d; however, analysis of the foods eaten for the 4 wk gave vitamin B-6 intakes of only 0.75–0.98 mg/d. This finding indicates that consumption slightly below the RDA still provides normal vitamin B-6 status as reflected by plasma PLP levels.

Combined deficiencies of B vitamins exacerbate minor deficiencies in any single vitamin. For example, van der Beek et al.[55] reported changes in aerobic power and onset of blood lactate accumulation in a double-blind study of a combined restriction of thiamin, riboflavin, vitamin B-6, and vitamin C at 21.3–32.5% of the Dutch RDA. There are many interrelationships between these micronutrients that could account for this response, as for example the utilization of a flavin-dependent enzyme in vitamin B-6 metabolism.[56] Other factors that affect these variables include protein consumption,[57] age,[58] and degree of activity.[59]

As with other nutrients, there is ongoing reevaluation of the adequacy of the current dietary levels of vitamin B-6 in providing optimal benefit against more subtle and/or chronic disorders. There has been discussion of vitamin B-6 as a possible factor in coronary heart disease, cancer, and premenstrual syndrome. These possibilities warrant additional attention; however, there do not appear to be compelling reasons to make major changes in the current dietary recommendations for vitamin B-6 except to consider the issue of bioavailability and to emphasize the known needs for greater consumption in pregnancy and lactation and the specific disorders discussed in the previous sections.

In the meantime, more is being learned about the effects of pyridoxine supplementation and human vitamin B-6 pools.[60] A dose of ≥ 1 mg of vitamin B-6 is necessary to obtain measurable changes in metabolism,[39] and at >25 mg there is little increase in plasma PLP.[61] These findings appear to bracket the practical range of dietary manipulation except in persons with severe disorders.

Sources

Vitamin B-6 is present in most foods in variable amounts and with different bioavailabilities.[62,63] Beef (3–8 μg/g), poultry ($\leq$7 μg/g for white meat), fish (3–4 μg/g), and pork (3 μg/g) are good sources as are some fruits (bananas, 5 μg/g), nuts (peanuts, $\leq$7 μg/g), whole grains (whole wheat, 2 μg/mg, and soybean flour, 7 μg/g), and vegetables (1–3 μg/g). As already noted, losses can occur during storage and preparation. The major dietary supplement is pyridoxine hydrochloride.

Toxicity

The acute toxicity of pyridoxine is low; however, prolonged consumption of amounts considerably above the RDA results in neurotoxicity, as was first shown for man by Schaumberg et al.[64] The symptoms include peripheral neuropathy with atactic gait disorders; absence of limb reflexes; impairment of the sensations of touch, vibration, temperature, pinprick, and joint position; absence of action potentials in sensitive nerves; and in some instances bone pains and muscle weakness.[46,64–66] This syndrome has been reported with patients taking oral pyridoxine supplements from 0.1 to 6 g/d; however, no systematic study of the lower doses has been made and pyridoxine has been used at 0.1–0.5 g/d clinically with few observations of side effects.[48] In most but not all cases the patients recover normal function after they stop taking the megadoses.

A few other problems have been associated with taking large amounts of pyridoxine. Administration of pyridoxine for neonatal seizures was reported to cause acute hypotonia requiring assisted ventilation.[67] Pyridoxine was suggested to inhibit prolactin secretion and lactation, but this point was challenged.[48,68] All together, the data indicate that the possibility of side effects should be considered in individuals taking pyridoxine in amounts exceeding several hundred milligrams per day.

Summary

Vitamin B-6 occurs in foods mainly as pyridoxal and pyridoxamine (and the 5′-phosphates) and pyridoxine (and the 5′-glucoside); the bioavailability depends on the type of food and processing. After intestinal absorption most of the vitamin B-6 is transported to liver where it is converted to pyridoxal 5′-phosphate, a cofactor for over 60 enzymes. Pyri-

doxal and the 5′-phosphate are released into circulation for use by other tissues. Amounts of vitamin B-6 in excess of tissue needs are eliminated in urine as pyridoxal and pyridoxic acid. The enzymes that utilize pyridoxal 5′-phosphate span carbohydrate, amino acid, lipid, nucleic acid, polyamine, heme, nicotinamide, and neurotransmitter biosynthesis and catabolism, and a possible role in steroid receptor function has been indicated. Vitamin B-6 deficiencies arise typically because of inadequate consumption of B vitamins, but deficiencies also can occur as complications of disease and drug therapy. Several genetic diseases respond to pyridoxine supplementation. The vitamin B-6 requirement depends on age, sex, pregnancy and lactation, overall health, and amount of dietary protein. Although moderate pyridoxine supplementation above the RDA appears safe, megadoses can cause peripheral neuropathy.

References

1. E.E. Snell (1986) Pyridoxal phosphate: history and nomenclature. In: *Pyridoxal Phosphate: Chemical, Biochemical and Medical Aspects, Part A* (D. Dolphin, R. Poulson, and O. Avramovic, eds.), vol. 1A, pp. 1–12, John Wiley & Sons, New York.
2. L.M. Henderson (1984) Vitamin B$_6$. In: *Present Knowledge in Nutrition, 5th ed.* (R.E. Olson, H.P. Broquist, C.D. Chichester, W.J. Darby, A.C. Kolbye, Jr., and R.M. Stalvey, eds.), pp. 303–317, The Nutrition Foundation, Inc., Washington, D.C.
3. J.E. Leklem and R.D. Reynolds, eds. (1980) *Methods in Vitamin B-6 Nutrition, Analysis and Assessment*, Plenum Press, New York.
4. A.E. Evangelopoulos, ed. (1983) *Chemical and Biological Aspects of Vitamin B$_6$ Catalysis, Parts A & B*, International Union of Biochemists Symposium 121, Alan R. Liss, Inc., New York.
5. R.D. Reynolds and J.E. Leklem, eds. (1985) *Vitamin B-6: Its Role in Health and Disease, Current Topics in Nutrition and Disease*, vol. 13, Alan R. Liss, Inc., New York.
6. D. Dolphin, R. Poulson, and O. Avramovic, eds. (1986) *Pyridoxal Phosphate: Chemical, Biochemical and Medical Aspects, Parts A and B*, vol. 1A and 1B, John Wiley & Sons, New York.
7. T.K. Korpela and P. Christen, eds. (1987) *Biochemistry of Vitamin B$_6$, Proceedings of the 7th International Congress on Chemical and Biological Aspects of Vitamin B$_6$ Catalysis*, Birkhauser Congress Reports, Life Sciences, vol. 2, Birkhauser Verlag, Basel.
8. R.D. Reynolds and J.E. Leklem, eds. (1987) *Clinical and Physiological Applications of Vitamin B-6, Current Topics in Nutrition and Disease*, vol. 19, Alan R. Liss, Inc., New York.
9. D.B. McCormick (1988) Vitamin B$_6$. In: *Modern Nutrition in Health and Disease* (M.E. Shils and V.N. Young, eds.), pp. 376–382, Lea and Febiger, Philadelphia.
10. J.F. Gregory (1988) Methods for determination of vitamin B$_6$ in foods and other biological materials: a critical review. *J. Food Comp. Anal.* 1:105–123.
11. J.F. Gregory and J.R. Kirk (1978) Vitamin B$_6$ activity for rats of ϵ-pyridoxyllysine bound to dietary protein. *J. Nutr.* 108:1192–1199.
12. K. Tadera, M. Arima, S. Yoshino, and F. Yagi (1986) Conversion of pyridoxine to 6-hydroxypyridoxine by food components, especially ascorbic acid. *J. Nutr. Sci. Vitaminol. (Tokyo)* 32:267–277.
13. B.I-Y. Yang and D.E. Metzger (1979) Pyridoxal 5′-phosphate and analogs as probes of coenzyme-protein interaction. *Methods Enzymol.* 62:528–551.

14. S.P. Coburn and J.D. Mahuren (1986) Cation-exchange high-performance liquid chromatographic analysis of vitamin B$_6$. *Methods Enzymol.* 122:102–110.

15. B. Hollins and J.M. Henderson (1986) Analysis of B$_6$ vitamers in plasma by reversed-phase column liquid chromatography. *J. Chromatogr.* 16:157–168.

16. L. Lumeng, A. Lui, and T.-K. Li (1981) Microassay of pyridoxal phosphate using tyrosine apodecarboxylase. In: *Methods in Vitamin B-6 Nutrition, Analysis and Assessment* (J.E. Leklem and R.D. Reynolds, eds.), pp. 57–78, Plenum Press, New York.

17. P.R. Trumbo and J.F. Gregory (1988) Metabolic utilization of pyridoxine β-glucoside in rats: influence of vitamin B-6 status and route of administration. *J. Nutr.* 118:1336–1342.

18. H.M. Middleton (1986) Intestinal hydrolysis of pyridoxal 5'-phosphate in vitro and in vivo in the rat. Effect of protein binding and pH. *Gastroenterology* 91:343–350.

19. J.F. Gregory and S.L. Ink (1985) The bioavailability of vitamin B-6. In: *Vitamin B-6: Its Role in Health and Disease, Current Topics in Nutrition and Disease* (R.D. Reynolds and J.E. Leklem, eds.), vol. 13, pp. 3–23, Alan R. Liss, Inc., New York.

20. L.M. Henderson (1985) Intestinal absorption of B-6 vitamers. In: *Vitamin B-6: Its Role in Health and Disease, Current Topics in Nutrition and Disease* (R.D. Reynolds and J.E. Leklem, eds.), vol. 13, pp. 25–33, Alan R. Liss, Inc., New York.

21. H.M. Middleton (1985) Uptake of pyridoxine by in vivo perfused segments of rat small intestine: a possible role for intracellular vitamin metabolism. *J. Nutr.* 115:1079–1088.

22. W.B. Dempsey and H.N. Christensen (1962) The specific binding of pyridoxal 5'-phosphate to bovine plasma albumin. *J. Biol. Chem.* 237:1113–1120.

23. H. Mehansho and L.M. Henderson (1980) Transport and accumulation of pyridoxine and pyridoxal by erythrocytes. *J. Biol. Chem.* 255:11901–11907.

24. H. Mehansho, D.D. Buss, M.W. Hamm, and L.M. Henderson (1980) Transport and metabolism of pyridoxine in rat liver. *Biochim. Biophys. Acta* 631:112–123.

25. A. Kozik and D.B. McCormick (1984) Mechanism of pyridoxine uptake by isolated rat liver cells. *Arch. Biochem. Biophys.* 229:187–193.

26. S.L. Ink and L.M. Henderson (1984) Vitamin B$_6$ metabolism. *Annu. Rev. Nutr.* 4:455–470.

27. J.E. Leklem (1987) Vitamin B-6 metabolism and function in humans. In: *Clinical and Physiological Applications of Vitamin B-6, Current Topics in Nutrition and Disease* (R.D. Reynolds and J.E. Leklem, eds.), vol. 19, pp. 3–28, Alan R. Liss, Inc., New York.

28. A.H. Merrill, Jr. and J.M. Henderson (1987) Diseases associated with defects in vitamin B$_6$ metabolism or utilization. *Annu. Rev. Nutr.* 7:137–156.

29. D.B. McCormick, M. Gregory, and E.E. Snell (1961) Pyridoxal phosphokinases. I. Assay, distribution, purification, and properties. *J. Biol. Chem.* 236:2076–2084.

30. M.N. Kazarinoff and D.B. McCormick (1975) Rabbit liver pyridoxamine (pyridoxine) 5'-phosphate oxidase. Purification and properties. *J. Biol. Chem.* 250:3436–3442.

31. L. Lumeng and T.-K. Li (1980) Mammalian vitamin B$_6$ metabolism: regulatory role of protein-binding and the hydrolysis of pyridoxal 5'-phosphate in storage and transport. In: *Vitamin B$_6$ Metabolism and Role in Growth* (G.P. Tryfiates, ed.), pp. 27–51, Food and Nutrition Press, Westport, CT.

32. A.H. Merrill, Jr., J.M. Henderson, E. Wang, B.W. McDonald, and W.J. Millikan (1984) Metabolism of vitamin B-6 by human liver. *J. Nutr.* 114:1664–1674.

33. H. Wada and E.E. Snell (1961) The enzymatic oxidation of pyridoxine and pyridoxamine phosphate. *J. Biol. Chem.* 236:2089–2095.

34. A.H. Merrill, Jr., K. Horiike, and D.B. McCormick (1979) Evidence for the regulation of pyridoxal 5'-phosphate formation in liver by pyridoxamine (pyridoxine) 5'-phosphate oxidase. *Biochem. Biophys. Res. Commun.* 83:984–990.

35. A. Lui, L. Lumeng, and T.-K. Li (1982) Transport of pyridoxine and pyridoxal 5'-phosphate in isolated rat liver mitochondria. *J. Biol. Chem.* 257:14903–14906.

36. L. Lumeng, R.E. Brashear, and T.-K. Li (1974) Pyridoxal 5'-phosphate in plasma: source, protein-binding and cellular transport. *J. Lab. Clin. Med.* 84:334–343.

37. M.P. Whyte, J.D. Mahuren, L.A. Vrabel, and S.P. Coburn (1985) Markedly increased circulating pyridoxal 5'-phosphate levels in hypophosphatasia. *J. Clin. Invest.* 76:752–756.

38. L. Lumeng, S. Schenker, T.-K. Li, R.E. Brashear, and M.C. Compton (1984) Clearance and metabolism of plasma pyridoxal 5'-phosphate in the dog. *J. Lab. Clin. Med.* 103:59–69.

39. J.R. Wozenski, J.E. Leklem, and L.T. Miller (1980) The metabolism of small doses of vitamin B-6 in men. *J. Nutr.* 110:275–285.

40. M.W. Hamm, H. Mehansho, and L.M. Henderson (1980) Management of pyridoxine and pyridoxal in the isolated kidney of the rat. *J. Nutr.* 110:1597–1609.

41. J.A. Sturman (1986) Vitamin B$_6$ and sulfur amino acid metabolism, inborn errors, brain function, and megavitamin therapy. In: *Pyridoxal Phosphate: Chemical, Biochemical and Medical Aspects, Part B* (D. Dolphin, R. Poulson, and O. Avramovic, eds.), vol. 1B, pp. 507–572, John Wiley & Sons, New York.

42. E.A. Donald (1986) Nutritional aspects of vitamin B$_6$. In: *Pyridoxal Phosphate: Chemical, Biochemical and Medical Aspects, Part B* (D. Dolphin, R. Poulson and O. Avramovic, eds.), vol. 1B, pp. 477–505, John Wiley & Sons, New York.

43. D.A. Bender (1988) Oestrogens and vitamin B6—actions and interactions. *World Rev. Nutr. Diet.* 51:140–188.

44. J.D. Reed, R. Redding-Lallinger, and E.P. Orringer (1987) Nutrition and sickle cell disease. *Am. J. Hematol.* 24:441–455.

45. C. Ha, L.T. Miller, and N.I. Kerkvliet (1984) The effect of vitamin B$_6$ deficiency on cytotoxic immune responses of T cells, antibodies, and natural killer cells, and phagocytosis by macrophages. *Cell. Immunol.* 85:318–329.

46. R.C. Young and J.P. Blass (1982) Iatrogenic nutritional deficiencies. *Annu. Rev. Nutr.* 2:201–227.

47. D.B. McCormick, B.M. Guirard, and E.E. Snell (1960) Comparative inhibition of pyridoxal kinase and glutamic acid decarboxylase by carbonyl reagents. *Proc. Soc. Exp. Biol. Med.* 104:554–557.

48. K.H. Bassler (1988) Megavitamin therapy with pyridoxine. *Int. J. Vitam. Nutr. Res.* 58:105–118.

49. A. Lui and L. Lumeng (1986) Pharmacology and therapeutic usage of vitamin B$_6$. In: *Pyridoxal Phosphate: Chemical, Biochemical and Medical Aspects, Part B* (D. Dolphin, R. Poulson, and O. Avramovic, eds.), vol. 1B, pp. 601–674, John Wiley & Sons, New York.

50. National Research Council (1989) *Recommended Dietary Allowances*, 10th ed. National Academy Press, Washington, DC.

51. A. Lui, L. Lumeng, G.R. Aronoff, and T.-K. Li (1985) Relationship between body store of vitamin B$_6$ and plasma pyridoxal-P clearance: metabolic balance studies in humans. *J. Lab. Clin. Med.* 106:491–497.

52. K. Schuster, L.B. Bailey, J.J. Cerda, and J.F. Gregory (1984) Urinary 4-pyridoxic acid excretion in 24-hour versus random urine samples as a measurement of vitamin B$_6$ status in humans. *Am. J. Clin. Nutr.* 39:466–470.

53. L.W.J.J.M. Westerhuis and J.C.M. Hafkenscheid (1983) Apoenzyme content of serum aninotransferases in relation to plasma pyridoxal 5'-phosphate concentration. *Clin. Chim.* 29:789–792.

54. J.A. Driskell, B.M. Chrisley, F.W. Thye, and L.K. Reynolds (1988) Plasma pyridoxal phosphate concentrations of men fed different levels of vitamin B-6. *Am. J. Clin. Nutr.* 48:122–126.

55. E.J. van der Beek, W. van Dokkum, J. Schrijver, et al. (1988)

Thiamin, riboflavin, and vitamins B-6 and C: impact of combined restricted intake on functional performance in man. *Am. J. Clin. Nutr.* 48:1451–1462.

56. K.M. Rasmussen, P.M. Barsa, D.B. McCormick, and D.A. Roe (1980) Effect of strain, sex and dietary riboflavin on pyridoxamine (pyridoxine) 5′-phosphate oxidase activity in rat tissues. *J. Nutr.* 110:1940–1946.

57. L.T. Miller, J.E. Leklem, and T.D. Schultz (1985) The effect of dietary protein on the metabolism of vitamin B_6 in humans. *J. Nutr.* 115:1663–1672.

58. A.K. Kant, P.B. Moser-Veillon, and R.D. Reynolds (1988) Effect of age on changes in plasma, erythrocyte, and urinary B-6 vitamers after an oral vitamin B-6 load. *Am. J. Clin. Nutr.* 48:1284–1290.

59. D.M. Dreon and G.E. Butterfield (1986) Vitamin B-6 utilization in active and inactive young men. *Am. J. Clin. Nutr.* 43:816–824.

60. S.P. Coburn, D.L.N. Lewis, W.J. Fink, J.D. Mahuren, W.E. Schaltenbrand, and D.L. Costill (1988) Human vitamin B-6 pools estimated through muscle biopsies. *Am. J. Clin. Nutr.* 48:291–294.

61. J.B. Ubbink, W.J. Serfontein, P.J. Becker, and L.S. de Villiers (1987) Effect of different levels of oral pyridoxine supplementation on plasma pyridoxal 5′-phosphate and pyridoxal levels and urinary vitamin B-6 excretion. *Am. J. Clin. Nutr.* 46:78–85.

62. D.H. Alpers, R.E. Clouse, and W.F. Stenson (1983) In: *Manual of Nutritional Therapeutics,* pp. 11–15, Little, Brown and Co., Boston.

63. H.E. Sauberlich and J.E. Canham (1973) Vitamin B_6. In: *Modern Nutrition in Health and Disease* (R.R. Goodhard and M.E. Shils, eds.), 5th ed., pp. 210–220, Lea and Febiger, Philadelphia.

64. H. Schaumberg, J. Kaplan, A. Windebank, et al. (1983) Sensory neuropathy from pyridoxine abuse: a new megavitamin syndrome. *N. Engl. J. Med.* 309:445–447.

65. G.J. Parry and D.E. Bredesen (1985) Sensory neuropathy with low-dose pyridoxine. *Neurology* 35:1466–1468.

66. K. Dalton and M.J.T. Dalton (1987) Characteristics of pyridoxine overdose neuropathy syndrome. *Acta Neurol. Scand.* 76: 8–11.

67. J.S. Kroll (1985) Pyridoxine for neonatal seizures: an unexpected danger. *Dev. Med. Child. Neurol.* 27:377–379.

68. M.B. Andon, M.P. Howard, P.B. Moser, and R.D. Reynolds (1985) Nutritionally relevant supplementation of vitamin B_6 in lactating women: effect on plasma prolactin. *Pediatrics* 76: 769–773.

Chapter **19**

Robert A. Jacob and Marian E. Swendseid

Niacin

The term *niacin* is the generic descriptor for nicotinic acid (pyridine-3-carboxylic acid) and derivatives exhibiting qualitatively the biological activity of nicotinamide (nicotinic acid amide). Nicotinic acid (NA) was isolated as a pure chemical substance in 1867, but not until 1937 was it demonstrated to be the anti-black-tongue factor in dogs[1] and the antipellagra vitamin for humans.[2] Before this time it had been suggested that pellagra was due to a deficiency of tryptophan (Trp) in corn, but the biosynthetic pathway for the formation of a niacin derivative from Trp was not established until after both niacin and nicotinamide were shown separately to be antipellagragenic.

Chemistry and Analytical Methods

The structure of NA and nicotinamide (NAm) are shown in Figure 1. The compounds are both stable, white crystalline solids. Nicotinamide is more soluble in water, alcohol, and ether than is nicotinic acid. The acid or amide form can be determined by a chemical reaction with cyanogen bromide and organic bases, by liquid chromatographic procedures,[3] or by microbiologic methods using a variety of bacteria requiring niacin for growth.[4] The active coenzyme forms of niacin, the pyridine nucleotides NAD (NADH) and NADP (NADPH), can be determined by enzyme-cycling colorimetric[5] or high-performance liquid chromatography (HPLC)[6] methods.

The urinary metabolites of niacin, including the methylated derivatives N^1-methylnicotinamide (NMN) and N^1-methyl-2-pyridone-5-carboxamide (2-pyridone), are measured by fluorescence or HPLC techniques. Ketones react with NMN in alkaline solution to form a fluorescent product.[7] Chemical methods for determining 2-pyridone are more tedious than for NMN; however, HPLC methods have been developed for both metabolites.[8–10]

The biological activity of niacin-containing foods can be determined by the dog pellagra test (black tongue disease) or growth tests in chicks and rats.

Many niacin antagonists have been synthesized and tested on bacteria. Some that are effective as antivitamins in animals include acetylpyridine, 6-aminonicotinamide, and 2-amino,1,3,4thiazole. These compounds have teratogenic effects when administered to pregnant animals and some of them have antitumor effects.[11]

Metabolism and Biochemistry

Absorption and Transport. Nicotinic acid and nicotinamide are rapidly absorbed from the stomach or the intestine.[12] At low concentrations absorption occurs as an Na^+-dependent facilitated diffusion, but at higher concentrations passive diffusion predominates. Three to 4 g of niacin given orally can be almost completely absorbed. Nicotinamide is the major form in the bloodstream, and arises from enzymatic hydrolysis of NAD in the intestinal mucosa and liver.[13–15] The intestinal mucosa is rich in niacin conversion enzymes such as NAD glycohydrolase. Nicotinamide is released from NAD in the liver and intestines by glycohydrolases for transport to tissues that synthesize NAD as needed. Tissues apparently take up both forms of the vitamin by simple diffusion; however, evidence indicates a facilitated transport of niacin into erythrocytes.[16]

Excretion. Excess niacin is methylated in the liver to NMN, which is excreted in the urine along with the 2- and 4-pyridone oxidation products of NMN (Figure 2). The two major excretion products are NMN and 2-pyridone; minor amounts of niacin or niacin oxide and hydroxyl forms also are excreted.[17] The pattern of niacin products excreted after niacin ingestion depends somewhat on the amount and form of niacin ingested and the niacin status of the individual.

Biosynthetic Pathways and Their Regulation. Niacin is biosynthesized from quinolinate in all organisms studied. In mammals, quinolinic acid arising from dietary Trp through the kynurenine pathway

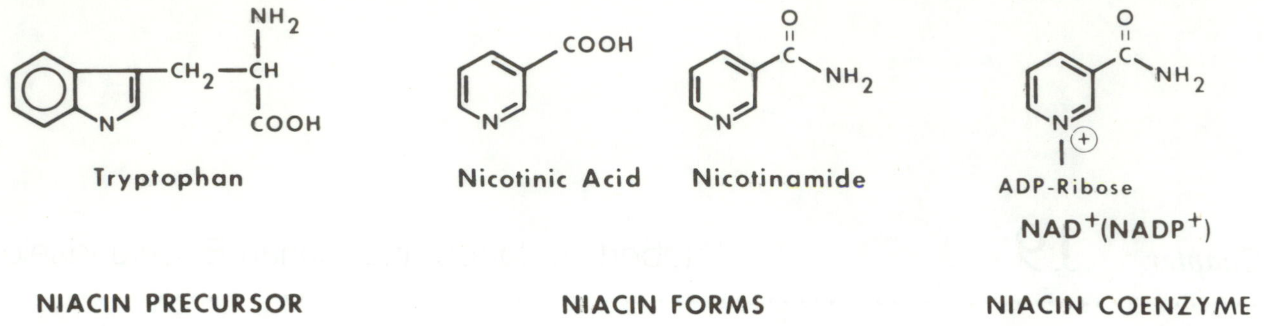

Figure 1. Niacin-related structures.

is converted to nicotinic acid ribonucleotide (Figure 2).[18] This conversion is apparently regulated by the enzyme quinolinate phosphoribosyltransferase. In humans the biosynthesis of niacin from Trp is an important route for meeting the body's niacin requirement. The efficiency of conversion of dietary Trp to niacin is affected by nutritional (protein, energy, pyridoxine, riboflavin, and niacin) and hormonal factors. Deficiencies of vitamin B-6 or riboflavin slow the conversion because these vitamins are essential cofactors for enzymes involved in the pathway. Conversion efficiency increases with restricted protein, Trp, energy, or niacin intakes, because of changes in activities of pathway enzymes including tryptophan oxygenase, quinolinate phosphoribosyltransferase, and picolinate carboxylase.[18-21] Irrespective of dietary factors, large individual differences in the conversion efficiency of Trp to niacin have been reported.[22] To estimate nutritional intake or niacin equivalents (NE) from Trp, an average conversion ratio of 60 mg Trp to 1 mg niacin was recommended by the Food and Nutrition Board of the National Research Council.[23] The 60-to-1 conversion value is based primarily on the conversion of Trp to niacin metabolites found in studies of humans.[24] A notable exception to the 60-to-1 conversion ratio is data showing a threefold increase in conversion efficiency in pregnant women during the third trimester.[25] This increase presumably is due to the stimulation by estrogen of tryptophan oxygenase, a suggested rate-limiting enzyme in the pathway.[26]

An amino acid imbalance, particularly excessive dietary leucine, was reported to antagonize the Trp-to-niacin conversion, probably by altering kynureninase activity. Other studies showed addition of 5% leucine to the diet increased the activity of hepatic NAD(P) glycohydrolase and, thus, decreased the NAD. It was observed in isolated rat liver cells that 2-oxoisocaproate, the 2-oxo analog of leucine, decreases NAD biosynthesis from both Trp and nicotinic acid. Whether excess dietary leucine compromises niacin status, however, remains open to question because some studies in rats[27] and humans[22,28,29] showed no effects of excess leucine on niacin metabolism or status.

The niacin coenzymes NAD and NADP are synthesized in all tissues of the body from nicotinic acid and/or nicotinamide (Figure 2).[15,30] Evidence for mitochondrial synthesis of these pyridine nucleotides from nicotinamide was reported.[31] Tissue concentrations of NAD appear to be regulated by the concentration of extracellular nicotinamide, which in turn is under hepatic control and is hormonally influenced. In the liver excess plasma nicotinamide is converted to storage NAD (i.e., NAD not bound to enzymes) and metabolites of niacin that are excreted. Trp and nicotinic acid also contribute to storage NAD, and recent studies with rats suggest that the liver synthesizes NAD(P) predominantly from Trp rather than from preformed niacin.[32,33] In the degradation of NAD, the nicotinamide formed can be reconverted to NAD via nicotinamide ribonucleotide. Human tissue cells contain little nicotinamide deamidase, but nicotinamide can be deamidated in the intestinal tract by intestinal microflora.[34] Hydrolysis of hepatic NAD allows release of nicotinamide for transport to tissues that lack the ability to synthesize the NAD(P) coenzymes from Trp.

Biochemical Functions. Niacin is essential in the form of the coenzymes NAD and NADP in which the nicotinamide moiety acts as electron acceptor or hydrogen donor in many biological redox reactions. Thus, NAD functions as an electron carrier for intracellular respiration as well as participates as a codehydrogenase with enzymes involved in the oxidation of fuel molecules such as glyceraldehyde 3-phosphate, lactate, alcohol, 3-hydroxybutyrate, pyruvate, and α-ketoglutarate dehydrogenases. NADP functions as a hydrogen donor in reductive biosyntheses such as in fatty acid and steroid syntheses and, like NAD, as a codehydrogenase such as in the oxidation of glucose 6-phosphate to ribose 5-phosphate in the pentose phosphate pathway.

Previous mention was made of glycohydrolases

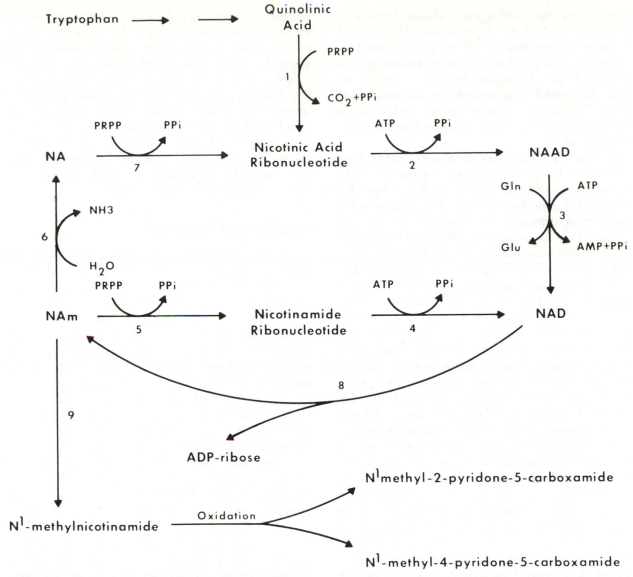

Figure 2. Pathways of niacin metabolism. NA, nicotinic acid; NAm, nicotinamide; NAAD, nicotinic acid adenine dinucleotide; PRPP, phosphoribosyl pyrophosphate. Enzymes: 1, quinolinate phosphoribosyltransferase; 2 & 4, adenyltransferases; 3, NAD synthetase; 5, nicotinamide phosphoribosyltransferase; 6, nicotinamide deamidase; 7, nicotinate phosphoribosyltransferase; 8, poly (ADP-ribose) synthetase or NAD glycohydrolase; 9, N^1-methyltransferase.

that cleave the β-N-glycoside link of NAD to provide nicotinamide and ADP ribose (ADPR) from ingested or storage NAD. Mammalian glycohydrolases also catalyze the transfer of the ADP ribose moiety to other bases and macromolecules (M) forming the basis for an important nonredox function of NAD, ADP-ribosylation:

$$ADPR-NAm^+(NAD^+) + M \rightarrow$$

$$ADPR-M + NAM + H^+$$

Examples of ADP-ribose transfer products in prokaryote cells are diphtheria toxin, which inhibits protein synthesis, and cholera toxin, which regulates adenylate cyclase activity.

The nuclei of eukaryote cells contain poly ADP-ribose polymerase that catalyzes the transfer of many ADP-ribose moieties to acceptor molecules such as the histones. The nuclear poly ADP-ribose proteins appear to be involved in DNA replication, DNA repair, and cell differentiation.[35] Parallel changes in NAD levels and ADP-ribose residues of proteins in rat liver because of differing nicotinamide intakes suggest that niacin status can play an important role in the extent of ADP ribosylation of proteins.[36]

A recent study demonstrated that quiescent human peripheral blood lymphocytes continually produce NAD and utilize it for poly-ADP ribosylation.[37] Oxidant or DNA strand-break stressors were shown to cause rapid depletion of the cellular NAD pool in lymphocytes and murine macrophages because of excessive poly-ADP-ribose synthesis.[37,38] In such situations the generation of ATP may be impaired.

Nicotinic acid was found to be part of the glucose tolerance factor, an organochromium complex isolated from yeast that potentiates the insulin response.[39] The role of the niacin moiety in the glucose tolerance factor is unknown because free niacin has no similar effect.

Biochemical Assessment of Niacin Status. Measurement of the urinary excretion of the two major methylated metabolites, NMN and 2-pyridone, has been used as a method of determining niacin status. The Interdepartmental Committee on Nutrition for National Defense published criteria for interpreting urinary NMN excretion amounts in adults and pregnant women and suggested 24-h excretions for adults of <5.8 μmol/d as representing deficient niacin status and 5.8 to <17.5 μmol/d as representing low status.[40] The use of creatinine corrections to allow for assay of random fasting urine samples rather than 24-h collections makes interpretation difficult because of differences in creatinine excretion by age.[40] The ratio of 2-pyridone to NMN was suggested as a niacin deficiency marker independent of age and creatinine excretion.[40] Shibata and Matsuo,[41,42] however, found that the urinary pyridone–NMN ratio in rats and humans was strongly dependent on the level of protein intake and that the ratio was a measure of protein adequacy rather than niacin status. A recent experimental study of niacin deficiency in adult males found the ratio to be insensitive to a marginal niacin intake of 10 niacin equivalents (NE)/d and not totally reliable for evaluating an intake of 6 NE/d.[28] In the same study urinary excretion of <8.8 μmol/d of either NMN or 2-pyridone reliably identified subjects receiving the lowest niacin intake of 6 NE/d, but the NMN was a more sensitive marker in subjects ingesting 10 NE/d.

No tests of niacin derivatives in blood have been in general used as markers of niacin status. Although Vivian et al.[43] reported a nearly 40% decrease in blood pyridine nucleotides in human subjects fed a niacin-deficient experimental diet, subsequent studies reported mixed results on the effects of pellagra or experimental niacin deficiency on concentrations of blood pyridine nucleotides.[29] In the recent experimental study of niacin deficiency cited above,[28] erythrocyte NAD levels decreased by ~70% whereas NADP levels remained unchanged when adult male subjects were fed low-niacin diets of either 6 or 10 NE/d.[29] The results suggest that the erythrocyte NAD concentration may serve as a sensitive indicator of niacin depletion and that a ratio of erythrocyte NAD to NADP < 1.0 may identify subjects at risk of developing niacin deficiency.[29]

Concentrations of niacin and niacin metabolites in plasma are normally quite low, and these tests generally have not been shown to be useful markers of niacin status. Results from a recent experimental study, however, indicated that 2-pyridone but not NMN in plasma could be a reliable marker of niacin deficiency because the 2-pyridone metabolite dropped below detection limits after a low niacin intake.[28] With an oral niacin load (20 mg NAm/70 kg body weight) postdose changes in the 2-pyridone metabolite were more responsive to niacin status than was the NMN metabolite, and these changes occurred in plasma as well as in urine.[28]

Requirement for Niacin

The Recommended Dietary Allowance (RDA) expressed as NE ranges from 13 to 19 NE/d for adults or 6.6 NE/1000 kcal.[23] This amount provides for differences in various diets consumed in terms of the bioavailability of niacin and the contribution of Trp. Recognizing that variations occur in the amount of Trp converted to niacin, the Food and Nutrition Board recommended that an average value of 60 mg Trp be considered as equivalent to 1 mg niacin. The evidence on which these allowances are based was studies in adult men and women conducted during the 1950s. There is no information on niacin requirements of children from infancy through adolescence. In infants, milk from well-nourished mothers appears adequate to meet niacin needs, and on the basis of the niacin content of human milk, the allowance for infants up to age 6 mo is 8 NE/1000 kcal. There are no direct data on niacin requirements during pregnancy and lactation. The RDA provides an increase of 2 NE/d for pregnant women on the basis of an increased energy requirement of 300 kcal/d. During lactation it is calculated that 1.5 mg niacin/850 mL milk will be lost. Added to this is an increase of energy expenditure to support lactation resulting in a recommended additional allowance of 5.0 NE/d for the lactating woman.

Food Sources

Niacin is widely distributed in plant and animal foods. Good sources are yeast, meats including liver, cereals, legumes, and seeds. Milk, green leafy vegetables, and fish as well as coffee and tea also contain this vitamin in appreciable amounts. Niacin is present in uncooked foods mainly as the pyridine nucleotides NAD and NADP, but some hydrolysis of these nucleotides to free forms may occur during food preparation. In plants niacin may be bound to macromolecules and be unavailable as food sources to mammals. In wheat there are several forms of bound niacin containing various peptides, hexoses, and pentoses (sometimes referred to as niacinogen or niacytin). In corn the bioavailability of bound niacin is increased by pretreatment with lime water, a procedure used in Central America and Mexico for preparation of tortillas. Roasting green coffee beans removes the methyl group from trigonellin (1-methylnicotinic acid), resulting in an increase in nicotinic acid. New varieties of corn such as Opaque-2 that contain more Trp and niacin than conventional sources are now available. Niacin is unique among the vitamins in that an amino acid, Trp, is a precursor that can contribute substantially to niacin needs by its conversion to a niacin derivative in mammalian liver tissue. A dietary intake of 60 mg Trp is considered in humans to be equivalent to 1 mg niacin. Because most proteins contain ~1% Trp, it is theoretically possible to maintain adequate niacin status on a diet devoid of niacin but containing >100 g protein.

Deficiency States

The classic dietary deficiency disease, pellagra, was observed in the mid-18th century in Spain and described more fully a few years later by physicians in northern Italy who used the term pellagra (raw skin) for the first time. The disease is associated with poorer social classes whose chief dietary staple often consists of some type of cereal such as maize (corn) or sorghum. The connection between maize-eating and pellagra was shown by Goldberger (1920), who conducted epidemiological studies indicating that pellagra was a deficiency disease caused by lack of a dietary factor in maize.[2] In 1937 nicotinic acid was established as this factor by its demonstrated effectiveness in curing pellagra.[2] In experimental studies with humans, clinical signs of pellagra develop in 50–60 d after the initiation of a corn diet. The most common signs of a niacin deficiency are changes in the skin; in the mucosa of the mouth, tongue, stomach, and intestinal tract; and in the nervous system. The symptoms associated with the skin are most characteristic. A pigmented rash develops symmetrically in areas exposed to sunlight and is similar to a sunburn although in chronic cases a darker color may develop. Changes in the digestive tract are associated with vomiting, constipation, or diarrhea, and the tongue becomes bright red. Neurological symptoms include depression, apathy, headache, fatigue, and loss of memory. Pellagra was common in the United States and parts of Europe in the early twentieth century, but it has now virtually disappeared from industrialized countries except for its occurrence in some alcoholics. It is still endemic in India and parts of China and Africa. An analysis of diets described in historical studies of human pellagra indicated that many had NE in excess of the RDA, but a low intake of riboflavin was common. These results suggest that the etiology of the U.S. pellagra epidemic of the early 1900s has not been explained satisfactorily.[44]

Reports of pellagra-like syndromes also were described in situations where the absence of dietary niacin deficiency was documented.[45] In each case the pellagra resulted from a reduction in the conversion of Trp to niacin. Pellagra sometimes occurred with the carcinoid syndrome, where Trp is preferentially hydrolyzed to 5-OH Trp and serotonin. Prolonged treatment with the drug Isoniazid also may lead to niacin deficiency by competition of the drug with pyridoxal phosphate, a coenzyme required in the Trp-to-niacin pathway. Patients with Hartnup's disease, an autosomal recessive disorder, develop pellagra because of a defect in the absorption process for Trp and other monocarboxylic amino acids in the intestine and kidney. Nicotinamide treatment (40–250 mg/d) resulted in marked improvement in skin and neurologic abnormalities.[46]

Niacin deficiency has been produced in dogs, pigs, monkeys, chickens, trout, and rats.[47] Pigs are particularly sensitive and exhibit a scaly dermatitis. There is generally poor growth and lack of appetite as well as inflammation of mouth and tongue mucosa (black tongue disease in dogs). Skin lesions do not always occur, as, for example, in young monkeys.

Pharmacological Effects and Toxicity

That large doses of nicotinic acid can reduce serum cholesterol concentrations in human subjects was first reported in 1955.[48] Subsequent studies revealed that triglyceride concentrations were also decreased and that these effects were not observed when nicotinamide was given. The administration of nicotinic acid in the Coronary Drug Project was associated with a reduction in recurrent myocardial infarctions and in long-term total mortality.[49] Nicotinic acid given as a drug in doses of 1.5–3 g/d decreases total and LDL-cholesterol concentrations and increases HDL-cholesterol concentrations. There are side effects including flushing of the skin, hyperuricemia, abnormalities in liver function, and occasionally hyperglycemia. These effects are reversed if the drug is reduced in amount or discontinued. The lipid-decreasing effect of nicotinic acid has been extensively investigated but the mechanism of action is not known. It does not appear related to any vitamin coenzyme function, because nicotinamide does not have a similar effect.

Experiments with rats showed that injections of nicotinamide (1 g/kg) caused phosphaturia that results from an increased NAD concentration in the renal cortex.[50] NAD is an inhibitor or modulator of the Na^+-dependent transport of phosphate through the membranes of the proximal kidney tubules. In adult rats large doses of nicotinamide were shown to induce activities of drug metabolizing enzymes including components of the hepatic microsomal mixed-function oxidase system and uridine diphosphoglucuronyl transferase in normal and tumor-bearing rats.[50] Chronic administration of large doses of nicotinamide to rats also produces increased lipid and decreased choline concentrations in liver.[51]

The LD_{50} (oral) for the rat is 3.5 g/kg for nicotinamide and 4.5–5.2 g/kg for nicotinic acid. Nicotinamide fed at concentrations of 1–2% of the diet inhibits growth.[52]

References

1. C.A. Elvehjem, R.J. Madden, F.M. Strong, and D.W. Woopley (1938) The isolation and identification of the anti-black tongue factor. *J. Biol. Chem.* 123:137–149.

2. T.D. Spies, C. Cooper, and M.A. Blankenhorn (1938) The use of nicotinic acid in the treatment of pellagra. *JAMA* 110:622–627.

3. L.M. Henderson (1983) Niacin. *Annu. Rev. Nutr.* 3:289–307.

4. H. Baker and O. Frank, eds. (1968) *Clinical Vitaminology, Methods, and Interpretation,* Interscience Publishers, New York.

5. J.S. Nisselbaum and S. Green (1969) A simple ultramicromethod for determination of pyridine nucleotides in tissues. *Anal. Biochem.* 27:212–217.

6. V. Stocchi, L. Cucchiarini, F. Canestrari, M. Piacentini, and G. Fornaini (1987) A very fast ion-pair reversed-phase HPLC method for the separation of the most significant nucleotides and their degradation products in human red blood cells. *Anal. Biochem.* 167:181–190.

7. O. Pelletier and R. Brassard (1977) Automated and manual determination of N^1-methylnicotinamide in urine. *Am. J. Clin. Nutr.* 30:2108–2116.

8. R.W. McKee, Y.A. Kang-Lee, M. Panaqua, and M.E. Swendseid (1982) Determination of nicotinamide and metabolic products in urine by high performance liquid chromatography. *J. Chromatogr.* 230:309–318.

9. K. Shibata, T. Kawada, and K. Iwai (1987) High performance liquid chromatographic determination of nicotinamide in rat tissue samples and blood after extraction with diethyl ether. *J. Chromatogr.* 422:257–262.

10. K. Shibata, T. Kawada, and K. Iwai (1988) Simultaneous microdetermination of nicotinamide and its major metabolites, N^1-methyl-2-pyridone-5-carboxamide and N^1-methyl-4-pyridone-3-carboxamide, by high performance liquid chromatography. *J. Chromatogr.* 424:23–28.

11. M. Weiner and J. Van Eys (1983) Nicotinic acid anatonists. In: *Nicotinic Acid: Nutrient-Cofactor-Drug* (M. Weiner, ed.), pp. 109–131, Marcel Dekker, Inc., New York.

12. H. Bechgaard and S. Jespersen (1977) GI absorption of niacin in humans. *J. Pharm. Sci.* 66:871–872.

13. L.M. Henderson and C.J. Gross (1979) Transport of niacin and niacinamide in perfused rat intestine. *J. Nutr.* 109:646–653.

14. L.M. Henderson and C.J. Gross (1979) Metabolism of niacin and niacinamide in perfused rat intestine. *J. Nutr.* 109:654–662.

15. J. Preiss and P. Handler (1958) Biosynthesis of diphosphopyridine nucleotide I. Identification of intermediates. *J. Biol. Chem.* 233:488–500.

16. S.J. Lan and L.M. Henderson (1968) Uptake of nicotinic acid and nicotinamide by rat erythrocytes. *J. Biol. Chem.* 243:3388–3394.

17. J.E. Mrocheck, R.L. Jolley, D.S. Young, and W.J. Turner (1976) Metabolic response of humans to ingestion of nicotinic acid and nicotinamide. *Clin. Chem.* 22:1821–1827.

18. U. Satyanarayana and B.S. Narasinga Rao (1980) Dietary tryptophan level and the enzymes of tryptophan-NAD pathway. *Br. J. Nutr.* 43:107–113.

19. I. Nakagawa, T. Takahashi, T. Suzuki, and Y. Masana (1969) Effect in man of the addition of tryptophan or niacin in the diet on the excretion of their metabolites. *J. Nutr.* 99:325–330.

20. U. Satyanarayana and B.S. Narasinga Rao (1977) Effect of dietary protein level on some key enzymes of tryptophan-NAD pathway. *Br. J. Nutr.* 38:39–45.

21. U. Satyanarayana and B.S. Narasinga Rao (1977) Effect of diet restriction on some key enzymes of tryptophan-NAD pathway in rats. *J. Nutr.* 107:2213–2218.

22. J.I. Patterson, R.R. Brown, H. Linkswiler, and A.E. Harper (1980) Excretion of tryptophan-niacin metabolites by young men: effects of tryptophan, leucine, and vitamin B_6 intakes. *Am. J. Clin. Nutr.* 33:2157–2167.

23. National Research Council (1989) *Recommended Dietary Allowances,* 10th ed., National Academy of Sciences, Washington, DC.

24. M.K. Horwitt, A.E. Harper, and L.M. Henderson (1981) Niacin-tryptophan relationships for evaluating niacin equivalents. *Am. J. Clin. Nutr.* 34:423–427.

25. A.W. Wertz, M.E. Lojkin, B.S. Bouchard, and M.B. Derby (1958) Tryptophan-niacin relationships in pregnancy. *J. Nutr.* 64:339–353.

26. D.P. Rose and I.P. Braidman (1971) Excretion of tryptophan metabolites as affected by pregnancy, contraceptive steroids, and steroid hormones. *Am. J. Clin. Nutr.* 24:673–683.

27. N.E. Cook and K.J. Carpenter (1987) Leucine excess and niacin status in rats. *J. Nutr.* 117:519–526.

28. R.A. Jacob, M.E. Swendseid, R.W. McKee, C.S. Fu, and R.A. Clemens (1989) Biochemical markers for assessment of niacin status in young men: urinary and blood levels of niacin metabolites. *J. Nutr.* 119:591–598.

29. C.S. Fu, M.E. Swendseid, R.A. Jacob, and R.W. McKee (in press) Biochemical markers for assessment of niacin status in young men: levels of erythrocyte niacin coenzymes and plasma tryptophan. *J. Nutr.*

30. L.S. Dietrich, L. Fuller, I.L. Yero, and L. Martinez (1966) Nicotinamide mononucleotide pyrophosphorylase activity in animal tissues. *J. Biol. Chem.* 241:188–191.

31. R.A. Lange and M.K. Jacobson (1977) Synthesis of pyridine nucleotides by the mitochondrial fractions of yeast. *Biochem. Biophys. Res. Commun.* 76:424–428.

32. D.A. Bender and R. Olufunwa (1988) Utilization of tryptophan, nicotinamide and nicotinic acid as precursors for nicotinamide nucleotide synthesis in isolated rat liver cells. *Br. J. Nutr.* 59:279–287.

33. G.M. McCreanor and D.A. Bender (1986) The metabolism of high intakes of tryptophan, nicotinamide, and nicotinic acid in the rat. *Br. J. Nutr.* 56:577–586.

34. C. Bernofsky (1980) Physiologic aspects of pyridine nucleotide regulation in mammals. *Mol. Cell. Biochem.* 33:135–143.

35. P.H. Pekala and B.M. Anderson (1982) Non-oxidation-reduction reactions of pyridine nucleotides. In: *The Pyridine Nucleotide Coenzymes* (J. Everse, B. Anderson, and K.S. You, eds.), pp. 326–369, Academic Press, New York.

36. R. Bredehorst, H. Lengyel, H. Hilz, D. Stark, and G. Siebert (1980) Increase of mono (ADP-ribose) protein conjugate level in rat liver induced by nicotinamide administration. *Hoppe-Seylers Z. Physiol. Chem.* 361:559–562.

37. D.A. Carson, S. Seto, and D.B. Wasson (1987) Pyridine nucleotide cycling and poly (ADP-ribose) synthesis in resting human lymphocytes. *J. Immunol.* 138:1904–1907.

38. I.U. Schraufstatter, D.B. Hinshaw, P.A. Hyslop, R.G. Spragg, and C.G. Cochrane (1986) Oxidant injury of cells: DNA strand breaks activate polyadenosine diphosphate-ribose polymerase and lead to depletion of nicotinamide adenine dinucleotide. *J. Clin. Invest.* 77:1312–1320.

39. W. Mertz (1975) Effects and metabolism of glucose tolerance factor. *Nutr. Rev.* 33:129–135.

40. H.E. Sauberlich, R.P. Dowdy, and J.H. Skala (1974) *Laboratory Tests for the Assessment of Nutritional Status,* CRC Press Inc., Boca Raton, FL.

41. K. Shibata and H. Matsuo (1988) Relationship between protein intake and the ratio of N[1]-methyl-2-pyridone-5-carboxamide and N[1]-methyl-4-pyridone-3-carboxamide to N[1]-methylnicotinamide excretion. *Agric. Biol. Chem.* 52:2747–2752.

42. K. Shibata and H. Matsuo (1989) Effect of supplementing low protein diets with the limiting amino acids on the excretion of N[1]-methylnicotinamide and its pyridones in the rat. *J. Nutr.* 119:896–901.

43. V.M. Vivian, M.M. Chaloupka, and M.S. Reynolds (1958) Some aspects of tryptophan metabolism in human subjects. I. Nitrogen balances, blood pyridine nucleotides, and urinary excretion of N-methylnicotinamide and N-methyl-2-pyridone-5-carboxamide on a low niacin diet. *J. Nutr.* 56:587–598.

44. K.J. Carpenter and W.J. Lewin (1985) A reexamination of the composition of diets associated with pellagra. *J. Nutr.* 115:543–552.

45. D.B. McCormick (1988) Niacin. In: *Modern Nutrition in Health and Disease,* 7th ed. (M.E. Shils and V.R. Young, eds.), pp. 370–375, Lea and Febiger, Philadelphia.

46. K. Halversen and S. Halversen (1963) Hartnup disease. *Pediatrics* 31:29–38.

47. H.E. Sauberlich (1987) Nutritional aspects of pyridine nucleotides. In: *Pyridine Nucleotide Coenzymes,* vol. 2B, (D. Dolphun, R. Poulson, and O. Aramovic, eds.), pp. 608–609, John Willey & Sons, Inc., New York.

48. Z. Altchul, A. Hoffer, and J.D. Stephen (1955) Influences of nicotinic acid on serum cholesterol in man. *Arch. Biochem. Biophys.* 54:558–559.

49. P.L. Canner, K.G. Berge, N.K. Wenger, et al. (1986) Fifteen-year mortality in Coronary Drug Project patients: long-term benefit with niacin. *J. Am. Coll. Cardiol.* 8:1245–1255.

50. K. Nomura, M. Shui, K. Sano, C. Umezawa, and T. Shimada (1983) Effect of nicotinamide administration to rats on the liver microsomal drug metabolizing enzymes. *Int. J. Vitam. Nutr. Res.* 53:35–43.

51. Y.A. Kang-Lee, R.W. McKee, S.M. Wright, M.E. Swendseid, D.J. Jenden, and R.S. Jope (1982) Metabolic effects of nicotinamide administration to rats. *J. Nutr.* 113:215–221.

52. W. Friedrich (1988) *Vitamins,* W. de Gruyter, New York.

Chapter 20

Victor Herbert

Vitamin B-12

A fatal anemia that was due to "some disorder of the digestive and assimilative organs" (that is, defective nutrition) was first described by Combe[1] in the 1820s. For a century this anemia was invariably fatal, hence the name, pernicious anemia. This name still is used for the disease even though the Nobel Prize–winning discovery by Minot and Murphy[2] in 1926 proved that the disease could be cured by feeding large quantities of liver, and the demonstration by Castle and Townsend[3] that the causative mechanism was "an inability to carry out some essential step in the process of gastric digestion." Castle's work was seminal in helping develop the concept that all deficiencies of vitamin B-12 (or indeed of any vitamin) could arise in one of six fundamental ways: three inadequacies (ingestion, absorption, or utilization) or three increases (requirement, excretion, or destruction).[4] Ironically, he did not share the Nobel Prize with Minot and Murphy, but the prize was rather shared with Whipple,[5] who with Robscheit-Robbins showed that beef liver enhanced hemoglobin formation in chronically bled dogs. In 1936, 2 y after the Nobel Prize in Medicine was awarded for liver therapy of pernicious anemia, it became apparent that the reason the dogs responded to liver was the iron content of the liver and not the vitamin B-12 content.[6]

The search for the active principle in liver culminated with the isolation of the vitamin in 1948 by a pharmaceutical industry research team of Merck scientists[7] working in the United States and a British team at Glaxo Laboratories in England,[8] whose publication of the identical discovery was preceded by a margin of only 3 wk. Yet another Nobel Prize (Chemistry, 1964) was awarded to Dorothy Hodgkin for her part in the elucidation of the chemical structure of vitamin B-12 by x-ray crystallography.

Nomenclature

Figure 1 indicates the nomenclature for vitamin B-12.[9-13] The four reduced pyrrole rings linked together become a macrocyclic ring designated corrin because it is the core of the vitamin B-12 molecule; the letters "co" of corrin are not derived from the fact that vitamin B-12 contains cobalt. All of the compounds containing this ring are designated corrinoids. "Cob" designates that the compound contains cobalt. As the figure indicates, the cobalamins contain the entire structure in the figure, and the permissive (semisystematic, trivial) term cobalamin (or vitamin B-12) is used to describe the vitamin B-12 molecule without the cyanide group. The term cobalamin is prefixed by the designation of the anionic R group attached to the cobalt. The permissive names are more widely used than are the systemic names, which are more cumbersome. For example, the systemic name for vitamin B-12 is α-(5,6-dimethylbenzimidazolyl)-cobamide cyanide. Cyanocobalamin is the permissive name for vitamin B-12, and the name vitamin B-12 without qualification means exclusively cyanocobalamin. In practice, the term vitamin B-12 has two meanings. To the chemist it means only cyanocobalamin. In the nutrition and pharmacology literature, it is a generic term for all the cobamides active in humans. So far, all the cobamides found to play a role in human metabolism have been cobalamins. The two cobalamins currently known to be coenzymatically active in humans are methylcobalamin and 5′-deoxyadenoxyl cobalamin (also known as coenzyme B-12 although it is only one of the two vitamin B-12 coenzymes with known activity in humans).

Sources in Food

All vitamin B-12 found in nature is made by microorganisms. Thus, the vitamin is absent in plants except when they are contaminated by microorganisms.[10,14] (For example, the root nodules of certain legumes contain small quantities of vitamin B-12 made by the microorganisms that live in those nodules.) Fruits, vegetables, grains, and grain products

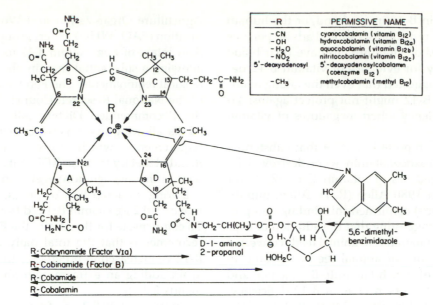

−R	PERMISSIVE NAME
− CN	cyanocobalamin (vitamin B₁₂)
− OH	hydroxcobalamin (vitamin B₁₂ₐ)
− H₂O	aquocobalamin (vitamin B₁₂ᵦ)
− NO₂	nitritocobalamin (vitamin B₁₂꜀)
5'−deoxyadenosyl	5'−deoxyadenosylcobalamin (coenzyme B₁₂)
− CH₃	methylcobalamin (methyl B₁₂)

Figure 1. The structural formula of Vitamin B-12. The numbering system for the corrin nucleus is made to correspond to that of the porphin nucleus by omitting the number 20. The corrin nucleus is in the plane of the page. The R group is above it; the rest of the molecule is below it.

are devoid of vitamin B-12 except insofar as they are unwashed and contaminated with fecal matter used as fertilizer. Feces contain a large amount of vitamin B-12 because microorganisms in the colon synthesize large amounts of the vitamin. The vitamin, however, is not absorbed from the colon. Strict vegetarians generally develop vitamin B-12 deficiency very slowly over a period of many years. Delay in development of vitamin B-12 deficiency in vegetarian children may relate in part to cleanliness. The less thoroughly they wash their hands after defecating and the more frequently they suck their fingers, the more they protect themselves against developing vitamin B-12 deficiency. Both normal people and patients with pernicious anemia excrete ~3.7 nmol/d of vitamin B-12 in the feces, although most recent work suggests a substantial portion of fecal B-12 may be analogues of the vitamin.[10,15,16] Some seaweeds containing vitamin B-12 from microbial synthesis can help vegetarians ward off vitamin B-12 deficiency, but spirulina may not.[10,15]

The usual dietary sources of vitamin B-12 are meat and meat products (including shellfish, fish, poultry, and eggs) and to a lesser extent milk and milk products. The source of vitamin B-12 in animal products is via the animal's ingestion of microorganisms containing vitamin B-12 or the vitamin B-12–producing activity of microorganisms high enough in the animal's alimentary tract for absorption and storage in the animal's tissues.

Rich sources of vitamin B-12 (>10 μg/100 g wet weight) include organ meats, such as lamb or beef liver, kidney, and heart, and bivalves, such as clams and oysters, which siphon large quantities of vitamin

B-12–synthesizing microorganisms from the sea. Moderately large amounts (3–10 μg/100 g wet weight) occur in nonfat dry milk, some seafoods (crabs, rockfish, salmon, sardines), and egg yolks. Moderate amounts (1–3 μg wet weight) occur in muscle meats, some seafoods (lobster, scallops, flounder, haddock, swordfish, tuna), and fermenting cheeses such as Camembert and Limburger. Fluid milk products, cheddar cheese, and cottage cheese contain <1 μg vitamin B-12/100 g wet weight.

When milk is pasteurized for 2–3 s, it loses 7% of its available vitamin B-12; boiling for 2–5 min destroys 30%; sterilization in a bottle for 13 min at 119–120 °C causes a loss of 77%; rapid sterilization (3–4 s) with superheated steam of 143 °C destroys only ~10% of the vitamin.[17] Overprocessed milk as a sole source of vitamin B-12 may be inadequate.[18]

Effects of Megadoses of Vitamin C on Vitamin B-12

Megadoses (500 mg) of vitamin C may adversely affect availability of vitamin B-12 from food,[19] and persons taking even greater megadoses of vitamin C (1 g/meal) may develop vitamin B-12–deficiency disease.[20] The Roche group[17] was unable to demonstrate destruction of vitamin B-12 in food by vitamin C. Other work[15] suggests that one reason for their failure was that the pharmaceutical assay for vitamin B-12 does not discriminate between the vitamin and some of its analogues, nor does a radioassay that does not use pure intrinsic factor as binder.[21] Until the question of whether megadoses of vitamin

C damage vitamin B-12 in food and/or the human body is resolved, nutritionists should advise persons taking megadoses of vitamin C to have their blood checked regularly for evidence of vitamin B-12 deficiency. It was suggested that even the taking of additional vitamin B-12 might not protect against vitamin B-12 deficiency when megadoses of vitamin C are taken.[20]

Herbert et al.[22] reported in 1979 that substantial amounts of hydroxocobalamin were destroyed by exposure to megadoses of vitamin C at 37 °C for one-half hour. In 1980 Allen (R. H. Allen, unpublished observations) confirmed this finding and presented evidence suggesting that the addition of copper, thiamin, and vitamin C to animal feeds converted a substantial amount of animal feed cobalamin to analogues, some of which had anti–B-12 action and theoretically could worsen vitamin B-12 deficiency. In 1982 Herbert et al.[23] reported that 10–30% of the vitamin B-12 in multivitamin preparations appeared to be converted to analogues by the antioxidant action of vitamin C, iron, and other antioxidant nutrients in the same preparations from Allen's laboratory. Kondo et al.[24] reported that two of the analogues in one of their preparations blocked vitamin B-12 metabolism in mammalian cells.

Nutritional Requirements

Vitamin B-12 requirements have been estimated from three different types of studies.[14,25–28] One type of study demonstrates the minimal quantity of vitamin B-12 that when injected can produce and maintain hematologic response in uncomplicated vitamin B-12 deficiency; the minimal amount was found to be in the range of 0.1 μg/d, with 0.5–1 μg producing maximal hematologic responses. Another type of study correlates concentrations of vitamin B-12 in serum and liver in deficient and healthy subjects; moderately deficient individuals were shown to have an average liver vitamin B-12 concentration of 0.12 nmol/g wet weight of liver to be associated with serum vitamin B-12 concentrations of 59–96 pmol/L and an average total body vitamin B-12 of ~185 nmol. Individuals with lesser degrees of deficiency, who had not yet developed morphological evidence of blood damage, had an average liver vitamin B-12 concentration of ~0.21 nmol/g wet weight, associated with serum levels between 96 and 148 pmol/L and an average total body vitamin B-12 concentration of ~390 nmol. The third type of study correlating body stores and turnover rates of vitamin B-12 measured with tracer doses of radioactive vitamin indicated radioactivity turnover of between 0.1% and 0.2% daily regardless of whether body vitamin B-12 stores were normal or reduced.

On the basis of such findings, the joint Food and Agriculture Organization and World Health Organization (FAO/WHO) expert group[25] recommends a daily intake of 1 μg vitamin B-12 for the normal adult, allowing a substantial margin above normal physiological requirements. The Food and Nutrition Board of the National Research Council[26] suggests 2 μg as the Recommended Dietary Allowance (RDA) for adults, allowing an even greater margin above normal requirements, which mirrors Herbert's[27] recommended dietary intakes (RDI). Vitamin B-12 is abundant in the average nonvegetarian diet.[29]

During the latter half of pregnancy, the fetus removes ~0.2 μg vitamin B-12/d from maternal stores. To compensate for this drain, the FAO/WHO group recommends that the total daily intake of vitamin B-12 be increased in pregnancy to 1.4 μg. The RDA, again adding an extra margin above need, recommends 2.2 μg.

Approximately 0.3 μg of vitamin B-12 is lost daily in the breast milk of nursing mothers.[25] To compensate for this loss, the FAO/WHO group recommends a total daily intake during lactation of 1.3 μg, and the RDA recommends 2.6 μg.

Because nutritional vitamin B-12 deficiency in infants is corrected by 0.1 μg vitamin B-12/d, the FAO/WHO group recommends 0.1 μg as the daily intake for infants on artificial feeding. Herbert[27] recommended 0.3 μg in months 0–2.9, 0.4 μg in months 3–5.9, and 0.5 μg in months 6–11.9. The RDA essentially mirrors Herbert in recommending 0.3 μg in months 0–5.9 and 0.5 μg in months 6–12. Milk from marginally vitamin B-12–deficient mothers whose serum contains vitamin B-12 concentrations above the lower limit of normal (that is, 148 pmol/L) is usually adequate.

Assessment of Vitamin B-12 Nutriture

As a general rule, a serum vitamin B-12 concentration < 1.11 pmol/L is diagnostic for negative vitamin B-12 balance.[4,20,30] Red cell vitamin B-12 concentrations in normal and deficient subjects frequently overlap.[31] The red cell vitamin B-12 tends to be low not only in vitamin B-12 deficiency but also in folate deficiency[32] and iron deficiency.[33] During pregnancy when folate deficiency frequently appears,[34] there is a gradual fall in serum vitamin B-12 concentration,[10] that rises to normal when the patient is treated with folate. Human serum contains not only cobalamins[35] but also vitamin B-12 analogs.[36] Radioassays using pure intrinsic factor (IF) as binder measure only cobalamins,[36,37] radioassays using R binder measure the total of cobalamin plus analogs, and radioassays using mixtures of IF and R measure both. Both microbiologic assays and radioassays appear similarly able to separate normal from B-12–deficient sera.[38–42]

Methylmalonate and homocysteine accumulate in serum and are excreted in the urine in increased quantities in vitamin B-12 deficiency, because vitamin B-12 is required for their normal metabolism, as indicated in Figure 2. The majority of patients with vitamin B-12 deficiency have methylmalonic aciduria but some do not, even after oral loading doses of valine and/or isoleucine.[43–46]

The deoxyuridine (dU) suppression test is of value in biochemical assessment of vitamin B-12 nutriture.[47–51] In this test, bone marrow cells,[48,49] peripheral blood lymphocytes,[50] or whole blood samples[51] from an individual are preincubated in a test tube with nonradioactive dU and then with a radioactive precursor of DNA. By the amount of radioactivity incorporated into the DNA of the cells in the absence vs. the presence of vitamin B-12 added to the test tube, vitamin B-12 deficiency and its correction by supplying vitamin B-12 can be determined. This test will detect past vitamin B-12 deficiency even after the start of treatment, because resting lymphocytes are impervious to B vitamins and so reflect the nutritional status of the patient at the time the lymphocyte was made (an average of 1–2 mo earlier).[52] This test also will recognize vitamin deficiency even when serum and red cell vitamin concentrations are normal[53] as when cobalamin metabolism is damaged by nitrous oxide anesthesia.[54,55]

Going from normality to vitamin B-12 deficiency is a slowly to rapidly (depending on individual circumstances) overlapping continuum of four stages of negative B-12 balance (Figure 3).[4,56] Reduced absorption of B-12 produces negative balance, defined as when the amount of nutrient lost each day exceeds the amount absorbed. Negative balance can be transient or progressive. The left-hand column in Figure 3

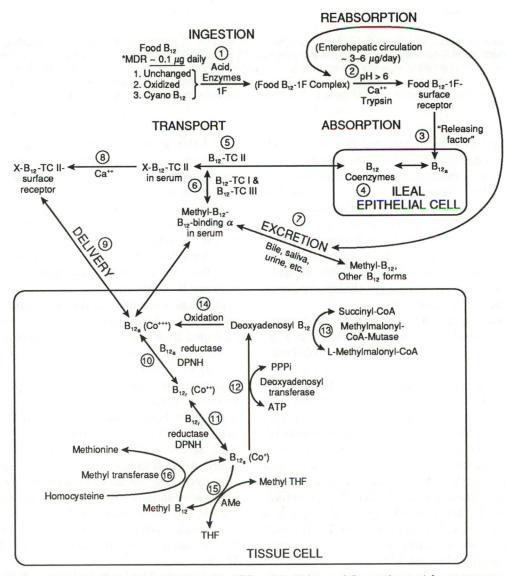

Figure 2. Flow chart of vitamin B-12 metabolism in man. MDR, adult minimum daily requirement from exogenous sources to sustain normality.

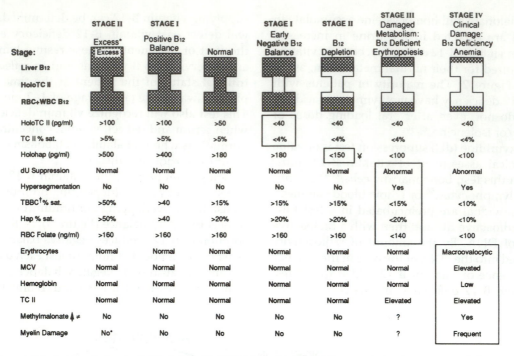

Stage:	STAGE II Excess*	STAGE I Positive B12 Balance	Normal	STAGE I Early Negative B12 Balance	STAGE II B12 Depletion	STAGE III Damaged Metabolism: B12 Deficient Erythropoiesis	STAGE IV Clinical Damage: B12 Deficiency Anemia
Liver B12							
HoloTC II							
RBC+WBC B12							
HoloTC II (pg/ml)	>100	>100	>50	<40	<40	<40	<40
TC II % sat.	>5%	>5%	>5%	<4%	<4%	<4%	<4%
Holohap (pg/ml)	>500	>400	>180	>180	<150 ↓	<100	<100
dU Suppression	Normal	Normal	Normal	Normal	Normal	Abnormal	Abnormal
Hypersegmentation	No	No	No	No	No	Yes	Yes
TBBC† % sat.	>50%	>40	>15%	>15%	>15%	<15%	<10%
Hap % sat.	>50%	>40	>20%	>20%	>20%	<20%	<10%
RBC Folate (ng/ml)	>160	>160	>160	>160	>160	<140	<100
Erythrocytes	Normal	Normal	Normal	Normal	Normal	Normal	Macroovalocytic
MCV	Normal	Normal	Normal	Normal	Normal	Normal	Elevated
Hemoglobin	Normal	Normal	Normal	Normal	Normal	Normal	Low
TC II	Normal	Normal	Normal	Normal	Normal	Elevated	Elevated
Methylmalonate ↑ ≠	No	No	No	No	No	?	Yes
Myelin Damage	No*	No	No	No	No	?	Frequent

Figure 3. Sequential stages of vitamin B-12 status. © 1990 Victor Herbert. *Cyanocobalamin excesses (injected or intranasal) produce transient rise in B-12 analogues on B-12 delivery protein (TC II); the significance of such rises is unknown. Cyanocobalamin acts as an anti–B-12 in a rare congenital defect in B-12 metabolism. #In serum and urine. †Total B-12 binding capacity. ↓Low holohaptocorrin correlates with liver cell B-12 depletion. There may be hematopoietic cell and glial cell B-12 depletion before liver cell depletion, and those cells may be in stage III or IV negative B-12 balance while liver cells are still in stage II.

lists tests used in assessment, and the box in each negative-balance column encloses those tests which, by becoming abnormal, mark the onset of the stage of negative balance represented by that column. The first two stages of negative nutrient balance are stages of depletion: stage I is serum depletion (i.e., the highway is delivering less); stage II is cell-store depletion (i.e., the storehouse is bare). The last two are stages of deficiency: stage III is biochemical deficiency (subtle inadequate function); stage IV is clinical deficiency (obvious inadequate function).

The earliest serum marker of subnormal vitamin B-12 (cobalamin) absorption and, therefore, of negative B-12 balance is low serum holotranscobalamin II (holo-TC II; B-12-TC II), which precedes a low total serum B-12 concentration by weeks to months.[57] Normally, ~20% of serum B-12 is on TC II and 80% is on haptocorrin, the circulating B-12 storage glycoprotein. The half-time for B-12 clearance from TC II is only ~6 min and the B-12 is taken up by many tissues, whereas the half-time for B-12 clearance from haptocorrin is 240 h and this B-12 is taken up largely (and possibly exclusively) by the liver.[58,59] Therefore, it would be expected that when B-12 absorption is reduced, B-12 would disappear from TC II much more rapidly than it would disappear from haptocorrin, and such is the case.[57,60,61]

Much more common in the population than generally appreciated are the three stages of negative B-12 balance that precede clinical B-12 deficiency. At any given time there are probably twice as many people in these three stages as there are with clinical nutrient deficiency manifested by anemia, which occurs only in the final stage (stage IV) of negative B-12 balance (Figure 2).[56,57] Studies in elderly people[46,62] revealed that focusing only on patients who have been in progressive negative balance so long that they are anemic will miss many patients in negative B-12 balance.

In the absence of liver damage, which artificially raises serum holohaptocorrin by releasing it from damaged liver cells,[63] liver-store depletion is measured by low serum holohaptocorrin (B-12 haptocorrin). Liver-cell surface receptors (but none on kidney, heart, or spleen cells) for holohaptocorrin were first demonstrated in 1958;[64] recent evidence suggests that serum holohaptocorrin is in equilibrium with liver B-12 stores.[63,65] Despite tissue depletion of B-12, serum B-12 may be not only normal but actually elevated in liver disease[63] and myeloproliferative disorders[66] because of the release into the serum in these situations of abnormal B-12 binders (from the liver in the former and from granulocytes and mononuclear cells in the latter), which do not deliver B-12 to tissues that have receptors only for B-12 on TC II.

As distinguished from depletion, which means that vitamin stores are low (and may be much lower in one cell line than in another), deficiency means inadequate intracellular B-12 in one or more cell lines for normal biochemical and clinical function in those lines.[10,11] Reduced absorption of B-12 reduces packaging of B-12 on TC II, the circulating B-12 transport protein[57] and, therefore, reduces delivery of B-12 to hematopoietic and other cells that depend solely on surface holo-TC II receptors to acquire needed B-12.

Early stage III negative balance is recognized by slowed DNA synthesis, demonstrable biochemically by the diagnostic dU suppression test,[4,47,53] and demonstrable morphologically by an elevated granulocytic leukocyte nuclear lobe average seen on a peripheral blood smear.[4,53] These findings precede rise in serum and urine homocysteine and methylmalonate.[46,61,67]

Figure 3 is modified by selective nutrient deficiency in one cell line but not another, with stage IV negative balance in some tissue, such as hematopoietic tissue, which has cell surface receptors only for holo-TC II and may have low B-12 stores. At the same time liver cells may be only in stage I or II negative balance, because liver cells have surface receptors for both holo-TC II and holohaptocorrin and may have high B-12 stores.[68,69] When liver is in stage I and II, nerve tissue may be in stage IV, damaged by metabolite (homocysteine, methylmalonate, B-12 analogue) changes related to B-12 deficiency.[55,70,71] Such selective deficiency is confirmed by therapeutic trial. Within 1–2 wk after a 1-mg B-12 injection, the degree of granulocyte segmentation in the hematopoietic system falls sharply, and in the neuropsychiatric system, anorexia, malaise, cognitive dysfunction, and paranoia all improve. These findings were observed in patients who had normal total serum B-12 concentrations but who had low serum holo-TC II and abnormal peripheral blood dU suppression tests that were corrected in the test tube by B-12.[61,67]

Metabolism

A flow chart of vitamin B-12 metabolism in humans is presented in Figure 2[14] and the interrelations of vitamins B-12 and folate in Figure 4.[14,72] As indicated in Figure 2, a vitamin B-12–containing enzyme removes the methyl group from methylfolate, thereby regenerating tetrahydrofolate (THF) from which is made the 5,10-methylene THF required for thymidylate synthesis. Because methylfolate is the predominant form of the vitamin in human serum and liver and because methylfolate only returns to the body's folate pool via the vitamin B-12–dependent step, vitamin B-12 deficiency results in folate being trapped as methylfolate and thus becoming metabolically useless. The folate-trap hypothesis explains the fact that the hematologic damage of vitamin B-12 deficiency is indistinguishable from that

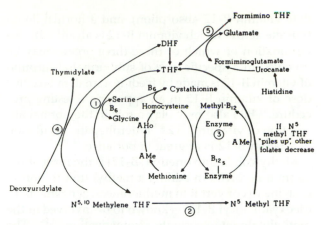

Figure 4. Interrelations in man between vitamin B-12 and folate (and vitamin B-6). Numbers represent enzymes: 1, serine hydroxymethyl-transferase; 2, methylene tetrahydrofolate (THF) reductase; 3, homocysteine transmethylase (methyltransferase); 4, thymidylate synthetase; 5, formininotransferase. AMe, S-adenosylmethionine; DHF, dihydrofolate; B-12, reduced vitamin B-12.

of folate deficiency by alleging that in both instances the defective synthesis of DNA results from the same final common pathway defect, namely an inadequate quantity of 5,10-methylene THF to participate adequately in DNA synthesis.[73,74] Although several workers attacked this hypothesis,[75] the flaws in their arguments were pointed out by others.[14,70,76] Two important facets of the folate-trap hypothesis are that vitamin B-12 is required for folate uptake by cells[72] and that the role of vitamin B-12 in folate polyglutamate synthesis is not in getting from monoglutamate (THF) to polyglutamate but rather in getting from methyl-THF to THF, which is the preferred precursor for folate polyglutamates.[76] The blockade in getting from methyl-THF to THF causes methyl-THF to leak from the vitamin B-12–deficient red cell. The folate trap is no longer hypothesis but fact[14,70,77,78] and may also control folate metabolism by regulating the supply of formate.[79] In 1968 Metz et al.[48] reported formylfolate best corrected the dU suppression test in vitamin B-12 deficiency. Some investigators claimed that they were unable to demonstrate methylfolate trapping but in the same study reported demonstrating such trapping by both a rise in liver methyl-THF polyglutamate in the "first 24 hours after nitrous oxide exposure due to cessation of methyl transfer to homocysteine" and a "rise in plasma methylfolate which persists for the duration of the nitrous oxide exposure."[79]

As indicated in Figure 2, for normal vitamin B-12 absorption one needs a normal stomach (because gastric acid and enzymes help free vitamin B-12 from its tight protein bonds in food, and the gastric parietal cells secrete intrinsic factor, a glycoprotein essential for vitamin B-12 absorption from the ileum), a normal pancreas (because trypsin[68,80] and bicarbonate facilitate vitamin B-12 absorption), and a normal ileum (the site across which vitamin B-12 is absorbed). Determination of which of these three organs may be involved in a specific case of subnormal absorption of vitamin B-12 is made by feeding a small radioactive dose of vitamin B-12 in an appropriate testing procedure.[81] Bile also may play a role in the normal absorption of vitamin B-12.[69] Enterohepatic circulation of vitamin B-12 is of great importance.[14,16,30]

Methylcobalamin (methyl–B-12) is the form of the vitamin involved in adding a methyl unit to homocysteine to convert it to methionine. Coenzyme B-12 (deoxyadenosyl B-12) is known to be involved in the methylmalonate-succinate isomerization.[10,14] The forms of vitamin B-12 involved in other metabolic functions currently are unknown.[14]

Vitamin B-12 and the Nervous System

Vitamin B-12 deficiency produces patchy, diffuse, and progressive demyelination.[45,46,67,82] The clinical picture resulting from the diffuse, uneven demyelination is one of an insidiously progressive neuropathy often beginning in the peripheral nerves and progressing centrally to involve the posterior and lateral columns of the spinal cord (producing subacute combined degeneration, also called combined system disease and posterolateral sclerosis or funicular degeneration) and the brain (megaloblastic madness).[82] Frenkel[83] described defects in the fatty acids of myelin in patients with vitamin B-12 deficiency, but whether these defects play a role in the demyelination is not yet known. Scott et al.[71] reported that nitrous oxide–induced, subacute, combined degeneration in monkeys could be prevented by dietary supplementation with methionine. Their data strongly suggest that the neurologic damage of vitamin B-12 deficiency may be due to methyl group deficiency as a result of inability to synthesize methionine and S-adenosyl methionine (SAM) or to homocysteine pileup being toxic to the brain. As they noted, cycloleucine, which inhibits activation of methionine to SAM, causes neurologic damage identical to subacute combined degeneration in rodents.[71]

Vitamin B-12 Therapy and Megatherapy

The only established therapeutic use of vitamin B-12 is in treating deficiency of the vitamin.[10] When the deficiency is due to inadequate ingestion of the vitamin as may occur in strict-vegetarian patients, an oral dose of 1 μg/d of the vitamin supplied as liquid or tablet is adequate treatment.

When the vitamin B-12 deficiency is due to inadequate absorption, 1 μg/d of the vitamin by injection is adequate therapy. A single injection of $\geq$100 μg will produce complete remission in a patient whose

vitamin B-12 deficiency is not complicated by unrelated systemic disease or other factors. The remission is sustained for life by monthly injections of 100 μg vitamin B-12.[10,14]

The only legitimate need for megatherapy with vitamin B-12 is in the very rare patient with a congenital defect in vitamin B-12 metabolism, such as vitamin B-12-responsive methylmalonic acidemia.[84] In fact, prenatal therapy of methylmalonic acidemia is possible with large amounts of vitamin B-12 administered to the mother,[85] although whether such prenatal therapy accomplishes anything is debatable.[86] Large doses of hydroxocobalamin have been used as an antidote to acute cyanide poisoning.[87]

Aside from the above indications, the use of vitamin B-12 in various neurologic disorders (with the possible and highly debatable exception of tobacco amblyopia[88]) has no known value. The red color of the vitamin along with its almost total lack of known toxicity[10] makes it an almost ideal placebo, and it is so used by many physicians. Unfortunately, it is used also by promoters who sell oral tablets, intranasal gels, or injections containing megaquantities of the vitamin for much-inflated prices for a wide range of claimed but nonexistent effects.[89,90]

Summary

Vitamin B-12 is a substituted corrin synthesized by bacteria and is present in animal foods. It is required for normal hemopoiesis by facilitating the cyclic metabolism of folic acid, which is essential for thymidine and thus DNA synthesis. Its methyl-group transfer activity is essential for a normally functioning nervous system.

The average adult requirement for vitamin B-12 is ~1 μg/d. The RDA for adults is 2 μg/d.

The circulating vitamin B-12–delivery protein, transcobalamin II, is of great importance in vitamin B-12 metabolism[58,66] as are the folate-binding proteins in folic acid metabolism.[91] Gastric intrinsic factor is necessary for vitamin B-12 absorption. Recent work suggests that salivary nonintrinsic factor cobalamin binders may play a role in the development of vitamin B-12 deficiency.[14,57,92]

References

1. J.S. Combe (1824) History of a case of anaemia. *Trans. Med. Chirurg. Soc. Edinburgh* 1:194–204.
2. G.R. Minot and W.P. Murphy (1926) Treatment of pernicious anemia by special diet. *JAMA* 87:470–476.
3. W.B. Castle and W.C. Townsend. Observations on the etiologic relationship of achylia gastrica to pernicious anemia. II. The effect of the administration to patients with pernicious anemia of beef muscle after incubation with normal human gastric juice. *Am. J. Med. Sci.* 178:764–777.
4. V. Herbert (1987) The 1986 Herman award lecture. Nutrition science

as a continually unfolding story: the folate and vitamin B-12 paradigm. *Am. J. Clin. Nutr.* 46:387–402.

5. G.H. Whipple and F.S. Robscheit-Robbins (1925) Blood regeneration in severe anemia: favorable influence of liver, heart and skeletal muscle in diet. *Am. J. Physiol.* 72:408–418.

6. G.H. Whipple and F.S. Robscheit-Robbins (1936) I. Iron and its utilization in experimental anemia. *Am. J. Med. Sci.* 191:1124–1143.

7. E.L. Rickes, N.G. Brink, F.R. Koniuszy, et al. (1948) Crystalline vitamin B-12. *Science* 107:396–397.

8. E.L. Smith and L.F.J. Parker (1948) Purification of anti-pernicious anaemia factor. *Biochem. J.* 43:vii–ix.

9. B. Zagalak and W. Friedrich, eds. (1979) *Vitamin B-12. Proceedings of the Third European Symposium on Vitamin B-12 and Intrinsic Factor,* Walter de Gruyter, New York.

10. V. Herbert (1988) Vitamin B-12: plant sources, requirements, and assay. *Am. J. Clin. Nutr.* 48:852–858.

11. B.M. Babior, ed. (1975) *Cobalamin Biochemistry and Pathophysiology,* John Wiley and Sons, New York.

12. IUPAC-IUB Commission on Biochemical Nomenclature (1974) The nomenclature of corrinoids (1973 recommendations). *Biochemistry* 13:1550–1560.

13. J.M. Pratt (1972) *Inorganic Chemistry of Vitamin B-12,* Academic Press, New York.

14. V. Herbert and N. Colman (1988). Folic acid and vitamin B-12. In: *Modern Nutrition in Health and Disease* (M.E. Shils and V.R. Young, eds.), pp. 388–416, Lea and Febiger, Philadelphia.

15. V. Herbert and G. Drivas (1982) Spirulina and vitamin B-12. *JAMA* 248:3096–3097.

16. S. Kanazawa, V. Herbert, B. Herzlich, et al. (1983) Removal of cobalamin analogue in bile by enterohepatic circulation. *Lancet* 1:707–708.

17. V. Herbert (1981) Vitamin B-12. *Am. J. Clin. Nutr.* 34:971–972.

18. V. Herbert, C. Manusselis, G. Drivas, et al. (1983) Low vitamin B-12 content of heavily processed milks may explain vitamin B-12 deficiency in young adults in Mexico. *Clin. Res.* 31:241A (abstr.).

19. V. Herbert, E. Jacob, K.-T.J. Wong, et al. (1978) Low serum vitamin B-12 levels in patients receiving ascorbic acid in megadoses: studies concerning the effect of ascorbate on radioisotope vitamin B-12 assay. *Am. J. Clin. Nutr.* 31:253–258.

20. J.D. Hines (1975) Ascorbic acid and vitamin B-12 deficiency. *JAMA* 234:24.

21. V. Herbert (1983) Folic acid and vitamin B-12. In: *Nuclear Medicine in Vitro* (B. Rothfeld, ed.), pp. 337–354, J.B. Lippincott, Philadelphia.

22. V. Herbert, L. Landau, R. Bash, et al. (1979). In: *Vitamin B-12. Proceedings of the Third European Symposium on Vitamin B-12 and Intrinsic Factor* (B. Zagalak and W. Friedrich, eds.), pp. 1069–1077, Walter de Gruyter, New York.

23. V. Herbert, G. Drivas, R. Foscaldi, et al. (1982) Multivitamin/mineral food supplements containing vitamin B-12 may also contain analogues of vitamin B-12. *N. Engl. J. Med.* 307:255–256.

24. H. Kondo, M.J. Binder, J.F. Kolhouse, et al. (1982) Presence and formation of cobalamin analogues in multivitamin-minerals pills. *J. Clin. Invest.* 70:889–898.

25. Joint FAO/WHO Expert Group (1988) *Requirements of Vitamin A, Iron, Folate, and Vitamin B-12.* FAO Food and Nutrition Series no. 23, Food and Agriculture Organization, Rome.

26. National Research Council (1989) *Recommended Dietary Allowances,* 10th ed., National Academy Press, Washington, DC.

27. V. Herbert (1987) Recommended dietary intakes (RDI) of vitamin B-12 in humans. *Am. J. Clin. Nutr.* 45:671–678.

28. L.W. Sullivan and V. Herbert (1965) Studies on the minimum daily requirements for vitamin B-12. Hematopoietic responses to 0.1 microgram of cyanocobalamin or coenzyme B-12 and comparison of their relative potency. *N. Engl. J. Med.* 272:340–346.

29. D.S. McLaren (1981) The luxus vitamins—A and B-12. *Am. J. Clin. Nutr.* 34:1611–1616.

30. V. Herbert (1983). Hematology and the anemias. In: *Nutritional Support of Medical Practice,* 2nd ed. (H.A. Schneider and C.E. Anderson, eds.), pp. 386–407, Harper and Row, Philadelphia.

31. V. Herbert (1975). The erythrocyte as a biopsy tissue in the evaluation of nutritional status. In: *Red Blood Cell,* 2nd ed. (D.M. Surgenor, ed.), pp. 386–407, Harper and Row, Philadelphia.

32. R.J. Harrison (1971) Vitamin B-12 levels in erythrocytes in anaemia due to folate deficiency. *Br. J. Haematol.* 20:623–628.

33. R.J. Harrison (1971) Vitamin B-12 levels in erythrocytes in hypochromic anaemia. *J. Clin. Pathol.* 24:698–700.

34. V. Herbert (1977). Anemias. In: *Nutritional Disorders of American Women* (M. Winick, ed.), pp. 79–90, John Wiley and Sons, New York.

35. E. Nexo and H. Olesen (1981). Quantitation of cobalamin analogues in human serum. In: *B-12,* vol. 2, *Biochemistry and Medicine* (D. Dolphin, ed.), pp. 87–104, Wiley Interscience, New York.

36. J.F. Kolhouse, H. Kondo, N.C. Allen, et al. (1978) Cobalamin analogues are present in human plasma and can mask cobalamin deficiency because current radioisotope dilution assays are not specific for true cobalamin. *N. Engl. J. Med.* 299:785–792.

37. C.W. Gottieb, F.P. Retief, and V. Herbert (1967) Blockade of vitamin B-12–binding sites in gastric juice, serum and saliva by analogues and derivatives of vitamin B-12 and by antibody to intrinsic factor. *Biochim. Biophys. Acta* 141:560–572.

38. J.M. England and J.C. Linnell (1980) Problems of the serum vitamin B-12 assay. *Lancet* 2:1072–1074.

39. D.L. Mollin, A.V. Hoffbrand, P.G. Ward, et al. (1980) Interlaboratory comparison of serum vitamin B-12 assay. *J. Clin. Pathol.* 33:243–248.

40. International Commission for Standardization in Haematology (1986) Proposed serum standard for human serum vitamin B-12 assay. *Br. J. Haematol.* 64:809–811.

41. V. Herbert and N. Colman (1981) Evidence humans may use some analogues of B-12 as cobalamins (B-12): pure intrinsic factor (IF) radioassay may "diagnose" clinical vitamin B-12 deficiency where it does not exist. *Clin. Res.* 29:571A (abstr.).

42. V. Herbert, N. Colman, D. Palat, et al. (1984) Is there a "gold standard" for human serum vitamin B-12 assay? *J. Lab. Clin. Med.* 104:828–841.

43. E.V. Cox and A.M. White (1962) Methylmalonic acid excretion: an index of vitamin B-12 deficiency. *Lancet* 2:853–856.

44. S.B. Kahn, W.J. Williams, L.A. Barness, et al. (1965) Methylmalonic acid excretion, a sensitive indicator for vitamin B-12 deficiency in man. *J. Lab. Clin. Med.* 66:75–83.

45. J. Lindenbaum, E.B. Healton, D.G. Savage, et al. (1988) Neuropsychiatric disorders caused by cobalamin deficiency in the absence of anemia or macrocytosis. *N. Engl. J. Med.* 318:1720–1728.

46. V. Herbert, E.J. Norman, T.A. Alston, et al. (1988) Cobalamin deficiency and neuropsychiatric disorders. *N. Engl. J. Med.* 319:1733–1735.

47. K.C. Das and V. Herbert (1989) *In vitro* DNA synthesis by megaloblastic bone marrow: effect of folates and cobalamins on thymidine incorporation and *de novo* thymidine synthesis. *Am. J. Hematol.* 31:11–20.

48. J. Metz, A. Kelly, V.C. Swett, et al. (1968) Deranged DNA synthesis by bone marrow from vitamin B-12–deficient humans. *Br. J. Haematol.* 14:575–592.

49. V. Herbert, G. Tisman, L.T. Go, et al. (1973) The dU suppression test using ^{125}IUdR to define biochemical megaloblastosis. *Br. J. Haematol.* 24:713–723.

50. K.C. Das and A.V. Hoffbrand (1970) Lymphocyte transformation in megaloblastic anaemia. Morphology and DNA synthesis. *Br. J. Haematol.* 19:459–468.

51. K.C. Das, C. Manusselis, and V. Herbert (1980) Simplifying lymphocyte culture and the deoxyuridine suppression test by using whole blood (0.1 ml) instead of separated lymphocytes. *Clin. Chem.* 26:72–77.

52. K.C. Das and V. Herbert (1978) The lymphocyte as a marker of past nutritional status: persistence of abnormal lymphocyte deoxyuridine (dU) suppression test and chromosomes in patients with past deficiency of folate and vitamin B-12. *Br. J. Haematol.* 38:219–233.

53. K.C. Das, V. Herbert, N. Colman, et al. (1978) Unmasking covert folate deficiency in iron-deficient subjects with neutrophil hypersegmentation: dU suppression tests on lymphocytes and bone marrow. *Br. J. Haematol.* 39:357–375.

54. H. Kondo, M.L. Osborne, J.F. Kolhouse, et al. (1981) Nitrous oxide has multiple deleterious effects on cobalamin metabolism. *J. Clin. Invest.* 67:1270–1283.

55. J. van der Westhuyzen, F. Fernandes-Costa, J. Metz, et al. (1982) Cobalamin (vitamin B-12) analogues are absent in plasma of fruit bats exposed to nitrous oxide. *Proc. Soc. Exp. Biol. Med.* 171:88–91.

56. V. Herbert (1989) Staging nutrient status from too little to too much by appropriate laboratory tests. In: *Nutritional Status Assessment of the Individual* (G.E. Livingston, ed.), pp. 147–167, Food & Nutrition Press, Trumball, CT.

57. B. Herzlich and V. Herbert (1988) Depletion of serum holotranscobalamin II: an early sign of negative vitamin B-12 balance. *Lab. Invest.* 58:332–337.

58. C. Hall (1989) The proteins of transport of the cobalamins. In: *Folates and Cobalamins* (J.A. Zittoun and B.A. Cooper, eds.), pp. 53–70, Springer-Verlag, New York.

59. R.H. Allen (1982) Cobalamin (vitamin B-12) absorption and malabsorption. *Viewpoints Dig. Dis.* 14:17–20.

60. V. Herbert, T. Stopler, O. Shevchuk, et al. (1988) Enhancing the value of serum cobalamin as the primary screening test for cobalamin (vitamin B-12) status by partitioning it into cobalamin or transcobalamin II and on haptocorrin, and determining percent saturation of transcobalamin II. *Blood* 72 (suppl. 1):43a (abstr.).

61. V. Herbert, W. Fong, T. Stopler, et al. (1989) Low serum holotranscobalamin II (B-12-TC II) diagnoses both negative B-12 balance (B-12 malabsorption) and reduced B-12 delivery to marrow in AIDS prior to high serum homocysteine (HCY). *Blood* 74 (suppl. 1):6a.

62. V. Herbert (1959) *The Megaloblastic Anemias,* Grune & Stratton, New York.

63. S. Kanazawa and V. Herbert (1985) Total corrinoid, cobalamin (vitamin B-12), and cobalamin analogue levels may be normal in serum despite cobalamin depletion in liver in patients with alcoholism. *Lab. Invest.* 53:108–110.

64. V. Herbert (1959) Studies on the role of intrinsic factor in vitamin B-12 absorption, transport, and storage. *Am. J. Clin. Nutr.* 7:433–443.

65. O. Shevchuk, T. Huebscher, and V. Herbert (1988) Evidence that vitamin B-12 regulates synthesis of proteins involved in corrinoid metabolism. *FASEB J.* 2:A1086 (abstr.).

66. E. Jacob, S.J. Baker, and V. Herbert (1980) Vitamin B-12–binding proteins. *Physiol. Rev.* 60:918–959.

67. V. Herbert, L. Cohen, T. Stopler, et al. (in press) Rediscovering selective nutrient deficiency in one cell line but not another: low serum holotranscobalamin II (Holo-TC II) may identify negative vitamin B-12 balance only in cells (ex: hematopoietic) with surface receptors solely for TC II, and not in cells (ex: liver) with receptors also for haptocorrin: In AIDS, there may be stage IV negative B-12 balance in hematopoietic and neuropsychiatric cells with liver cells only in stage I-II. *Clin. Res.*

68. S. Kanazawa and V. Herbert (1983) Mechanism of enterohepatic circulation of vitamin B-12; movement of vitamin B-12 from bile R binder to intrinsic factor due to the action of pancreatic trypsin. *Clin. Res.* 31:531A (abstr.).

69. B. Herzlich and V. Herbert (1984) The role of the pancreas in cobalamin (vitamin B-12) absorption. *Am. J. Gastroenterol.* 79:489–493.

70. J.M. Scott, J.J. Dinn, P. Wilson, et al. (1981) The methyl-folate trap and the supply of S-adenosylmethionine. *Lancet* 2:755.

71. J.M. Scott, J.J. Dinn, P. Wilson, et al. (1981) Pathogenesis of subacute combined degeneration: a result of methyl group deficiency. *Lancet* 2:334–337.

72. V. Herbert (1971) Recent developments in cobalamin metabolism. In: *The Cobalamins* (H.R.V. Arnstein and R.J. Wrighton, eds.), pp. 2–16, Churchill Livingstone, Edinburgh.

73. V. Herbert and R. Zalusky (1962) Interrelations of vitamin B-12 and folic acid metabolism: folic acid clearance studies. *J. Clin. Invest.* 41:1263–1276.

74. J.M. Noronha and M. Silverman (1962). On folic acid, vitamin B-12, methionine and formiminoglutamic acid metabolism. In: *Vitamin B-12 and Intrinsic Factor,* Second European Symposium, pp. 728–736, Enke, Stuttgart.

75. I. Chanarin (1979) *The Megaloblastic Anemias,* Blackwell, Oxford.

76. Y.L. Shin, K.U. Buhring, and E.L.R. Stokstad (1975) The relationships between vitamin B-12 and folic acid and the effect of methionine on folate metabolism. *Mol. Cell. Biochem.* 9:97–108.

77. H. Sauer and W. Willmanns (1977) Cobalamin dependent methionine synthesis and methyl-folate-trap in human vitamin B-12 deficiency. *Br. J. Haematol.* 36:189–198.

78. J. Zittoun, J. Marquet, and R. Zittoun (1978) Effect of folate and cobalamin compounds on the deoxyuridine suppression test in vitamin B-12 and folate deficiency. *Blood* 51:119–128.

79. I. Chanarin, R. Deacon, M. Lumb, et al. (1980) Vitamin B-12 regulates folate metabolism by the supply of formate. *Lancet* 2:505–507.

80. R.H. Allen, B. Seetharam, N.C. Allen, et al. (1978) Correction of cobalamin malabsorption in pancreatic insufficiency with a cobalamin analogue that binds with high affinity to R protein but not to intrinsic factor. *J. Clin. Invest.* 61:1628–1634.

81. V. Herbert (1975) Detection of malabsorption of vitamin B-12 due to gastric or intestinal dysfunction. *Semin. Nucl. Med.* 2:220–234.

82. E. Jacob and V. Herbert (1980). Vitamin B-12 and the nervous system. In: *Biochemistry of Brain* (S. Kumar, ed.), pp. 127–142, Pergamon Press, New York.

83. E.P. Frenkel (1973) Abnormal fatty acid metabolism in peripheral nerves of patients with pernicious anemia. *J. Clin. Invest.* 1237–1245.

84. W.A. Fenton and L.E. Rosenberg (1989) Inherited disorders of cobalamin transport and metabolism. In: *The Metabolic Basis of Inherited Disease* (R. Scriver, A.L. Beaudet, W.S. Sly, and D. Valle, eds.), pp. 2065–2082, McGraw-Hill, New York.

85. M.G. Ampola, M.J. Mahoney, E. Nakamura, et al. (1975) Prenatal therapy of a patient with vitamin B-12–responsive methylmalonic acidemia. *N. Engl. J. Med.* 293:313–317.

86. W.L. Nyhan (1975) Prenatal treatment of methylmalonic acidemia. *N. Engl. J. Med.* 293:353–354.

87. J.E. Cottrell, P. Casthely, J.D. Brodie, et al. (1978) Prevention of nitroprusside-induced cyanide toxicity with hydrocobalamin. *N. Engl. J. Med.* 298:809.

88. J. Wilson, J.C. Linnel and D.M. Matthews (1971) Plasma-cobalamins in neuro-ophthalmological diseases. *Lancet* 1:259–261.

89. V. Herbert (1980) *Nutrition Cultism: Facts and Fictions,* George F. Stickley Company, Philadelphia.

90. V. Herbert and S. Barrett (1981) *Vitamins and "Health" Foods: The Great American Hustle.* George F. Stickley Company, Philadelphia.

91. N. Colman and V. Herbert (1980) Folate binding proteins. *Annu. Rev. Med.* 31:433–439.

92. B. Herzlich, G. Drivas, and V. Herbert (1982) Abnormal binders with high specificity for cobalamin at pH 8 in gastric juice of patients with pernicious anemia: production by pancreatic enzymes. *Clin. Res.* 30:283A (abstr.).

Carlos L. Krumdieck

Chapter 21

Folic Acid

The history of the isolation and characterization of the vitamin folic acid was reviewed in detail.[1] A number of seemingly unrelated investigations led to the recognition that the active principle in liver and yeast extracts that cured the "pernicious anemia of pregnancy" described by Wills[2] had many properties in common with bacterial "growth factors"[3] present in liver and spinach leaves[4] and with a dietary factor required to prevent the development of anemia in chicks[5] and monkeys.[6] Because all isolation attempts had to start from large batches of crude homogenates rich in degradative enzymes and because there was no a priori reason to protect the preparations from air oxidation, folic acid, the biologically active molecule isolated in the end, was a fully oxidized, partially degraded derivative of the natural cofactors. We now know that folic acid (pteroylglutamic acid) occurs in minimal quantities, if at all, in biological materials and must, therefore, be recognized as an artifact of isolation. The two most fundamental structural modifications in going from the natural folates to folic acid are loss of the poly-γ-glutamyl chain and oxidation of the pyrazine ring from its naturally occurring dihydro or tetrahydro forms to an aromatic form. In addition, there is loss of the one-carbon substituents in positions 5 and/or 10 found in most naturally occurring forms. Two enzymes, dihydrofolate reductase (DHFR) and pteroylpolyglutamyl synthetase, acting in sequence, are required for the regeneration of 5,6,7,8-tetrahydrofolyl polyglutamates, the parent compounds from which all the folate coenzymes active in vivo are derived. Failure of either one impedes the normal utilization of the vitamin and if severe is incompatible with life.

The folates serve as coenzymes for one-carbon transfer reactions and as substrates of oxidation-reduction reactions that change the oxidation state of folate-bound one-carbon fragments. Folate-requiring one-carbon transfers are needed for the biosynthesis of purine nucleotides and of deoxythymidylic acid,

essential for RNA and DNA synthesis and hence for cell replication. They are also needed to provide de novo synthesized methyl groups to sustain a large number of S-adenosylmethionine–mediated methylation reactions under conditions of limited methionine intake. Not surprisingly the metabolism of the folates is subject to complex regulatory mechanisms that are still incompletely understood. The central role played by these cofactors in the multiplication of all living things from viruses to man makes them logical targets for the development of analogs used as drugs with a wide range of applications, including virucidal, antibacterial, and antiparasitic drugs as well as immunosuppressant and cancer chemotherapeutic agents. Nutritional folate deficiency is very common and endangers, in particular, pregnant women, premature infants, and elderly people.

The Naturally Occurring Folates: Synthesis and Analysis

Figure 1 summarizes the structures, numbering system, and nomenclature of the folates. Folic acid (pteroylglutamic acid) is named in the chemical literature as a derivative of L-glutamic acid: N-[4-[[(2-amino - 1,4 - dihydro - 4 - oxo - 6 - pteridinyl)methyl]-amino]benzoyl-L-glutamic acid.

Upon reduction to 5,6,7,8-tetrahydrofolic acid, a second asymmetric carbon is created at position 6 (the first is at the α carbon of the glutamyl residue). The absolute configuration at C-6 in the natural diastereoisomers of the tetrahydrofolates is known[7] and the designations R and S or R,S (for the racemic mixture) should be used as given in Figure 1.

Because the pirazine ring (atoms 4a,5,6,7,8, and 8a) can occur at three states of reduction with six different one-carbon substituents present at N-5 and/or N-10, and because the polyglutamyl chain may have as many as 12 glutamyl residues, the natural folates include a very large number of compounds.

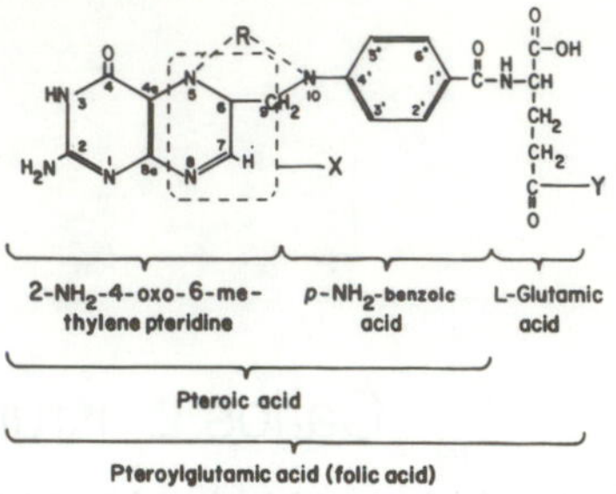

X	R	Name of Compound
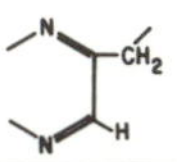	-H at N^{10}	Pteroyl glutamic acid (folic acid)
	-CHO at N^{10}	10-formyl folic acid
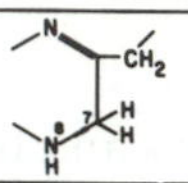	-H at N^{10}	7,8 dihydro folic acid
	$-CH_3$ at N^5	5-methyl " " "
	-CHO at N^{10}	10-formyl " " "
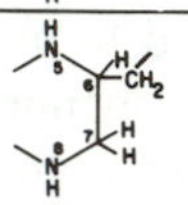	-H at N^{10}	5,6,7,8 tetrahydro folic acid [6S]*
	$-CH_3$ at N^5	5-methyl " " " [6S]
	-CHO at N^5	5-formyl " " " [6S]
	-CHNH at N^5	5-formimino " " "
	-CHO at N^{10}	10-formyl " " " [6R]
Note: asymetric C at position 6, ∴ optical isomers R,S	=CH= at N^5-N^{10}	5,10-methenyl or (methylidyne) " " " [6R]
	$-CH_2-$ at N^5-N^{10}	5,10-methylene " " " [6R]
Y	-OH	Pteroyl - mono glutamate
	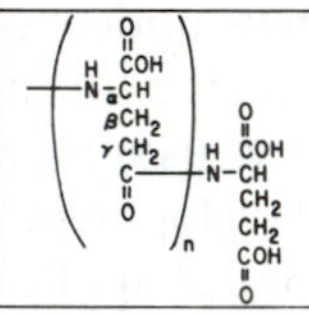	$n \geq 0$ = Pteroyl-poly-γ-glutamates $n+2$ = number of glutamic acid residues attached to pteroic acid.

Figure 1. Summary of structures, numbering system, and nomenclature of the folates. *Natural stereoisomers.

By far the majority of intracellular folates are polyglutamates. Pentaglutamates and hexaglutamates predominate in animal tissues; longer derivatives (up to 12 Glu residues) are found in bacteria. In contrast, extracellular folates (i.e., in plasma, spinal fluid, bile, and urine) are monoglutamate derivatives.[1,8]

Most natural folates are unstable and are degraded by heat, oxidation, and ultraviolet light.[9] Some tetrahydro derivatives, notably 5-formyl-tetrahydrofolic acid (5-CHO-THFA) and 5-methyl-tetrahydrofolic acid ($5\text{-}CH_3$-THFA) are relatively heat stable. The former compound is also stable to air oxidation. Tetrahydrofolic acid (THFA) and 5,10-methylenetetrahydrofolic acid ($5,10\text{-}CH_2$-THFA) are destroyed by acid, but 5,10-methenyl-tetrahydrofolic acid (5,10-CH=THFA) is stable and resistant to air oxidation in acid.

Several synthetic procedures were developed for creating fully oxidized pteroylpoly-γ-glutamates of any desired chain length.[10–12] From these procedures all reduced one-carbon–substituted derivatives (with the possible exception of the 5-formiminotetrahydrofolates) can be chemically synthesized.[1] Because of the multiplicity and lability of the natural forms and their low concentrations in biological materials, the development of analytical methods for the quantitation of all folate forms in biological samples was difficult. New procedures of extraction that minimize interconversions of one-carbon–substituted forms and prevent enzymatic degradation of the polyglutamyl chain were developed[13] and should be more universally adopted.

Most methodologies for the analysis of folylpolyglutamates resort to a simplification of the analytical problem (at the expense of loss of information) by cleaving the C9–N10 bond and resolving the resulting homologous series of *p*-aminobenzoyl polyglutamates as a function of their chain lengths.[1] An improved differential cleavage method that permits the quantitation and chain-length determination of three pools of folates was developed.[14–16] Pool one includes unsubstituted dihydro ($DHFAGlu_n$) and tetrahydro ($THFAGlu_n$) folates plus 5,10-methylenetetrahydrofolyl polyglutamates ($5,10\text{-}CH_2\text{-}THFAGlu_n$), pool two is made up solely of 5-methyl-tetrahydrofolates ($5\text{-}CH_3\text{-}THFAGlu_n$), and pool three includes all reduced folates with one-carbon substituents at the formyl oxidation level: 5,10-methenyl-tetrahydrofolyl polyglutamates ($5,10\text{-}CH{=}THFAGlu_n$), 5- and 10-formyl-tetrahydrofolyl polyglutamates (5-CHO- and $10\text{-}CHO\text{-}THFAGlu_n$), and 5-formimino-tetrahydrofolyl polyglutamates ($5\text{-}CHNH\text{-}THFAGlu_n$). An elegant analytical approach introduced by Priest et al.[17,18] is based on the use of the enzyme thymidylate synthase to selectively extract and incorporate $5,10\text{-}CH_2\text{-}THFAGlu_n$ into a stable, covalently linked, ternary complex with radiolabeled 5-fluoro-2-deoxy-[^{3}H]uridylate ([^{3}H]FdUMP). The high-molecular-weight complexes of enzyme-$5,10\text{-}CH_2THFAGlu_n$-[^{3}H]FdUMP then are resolved electrophoretically in relation to polyglutamyl chain lengths of the bound 5,10-methylene-tetrahydrofolyl polyglutamates. The quantitation and chain-length determination of other one-carbon–substituted pools are obtained by the use of enzyme-catalyzed procedures that specifically convert the desired folate pools to the $5,10\text{-}CH_2\text{-}THFAGlu_n$ to which the assay responds.[19–22] A recently proposed analytical method[23] extracts the folates by binding them to a folate milk-binder affinity column. The major purification achieved by this extraction procedure permits the application of the affinity column eluate directly to a high-performance liquid chromatography (HPLC) column. Monitoring the elution at four wavelengths allows the independent quantitation of coeluting compounds that differ in their UV spectral properties. In spite of these significant advances, it is fair to say that the complete analysis of the folates in a biological sample remains a formidable task.

Biosynthesis

De novo biosynthesis of folates occurs only in bacteria and plants. The biosynthetic pathway depicted in the fourth edition of this book remains unchallenged.[24] Note that dihydrofolic acid is the first folate product of the pathway; fully oxidized folic acid is not an intermediate. (For further details the interested reader should consult references 25 and 26.)

The ability to synthesize the ring system is sharply limited to plants and bacteria. Most recent biosynthetic studies dealt with the formation of the poly-γ-glutamyl chain, which is present in all forms of life.

The general reaction can be written as follows:

$$THFAGlu_n + ATP + \text{L-Glu} \rightarrow$$

$$THFAGlu_{n+1} + ADP + P$$

This reaction is catalyzed by a single enzyme, pteroylpoly-γ-glutamate synthetase, in nearly all systems studied. The activity in prokaryotes is much higher than in eukaryotes. The synthetases are quite specific for L-glutamate but accept various forms of folates and folate analogs as substrates.[27] Unsubstituted tetrahydrofolates are the preferred substrates, a fact that acquires special significance in vitamin B-12 deficiency when, because of decreased activity of the vitamin B-12–requiring methionine synthase, 5-methyl-tetrahydrofolates ($5\text{-}CH_3\text{-}THFAGlu_n$) accumulate and diminish the pool size of the unsubstituted $THFAGlu_n$. The biosynthesis of longer-chain polyglutamates, which are best retained intracellularly, is impaired and results in decreased tissue folate concentrations.[28,29] Folylpoly-γ-glutamyl synthetases of various sources exhibit greater affinity for polyglutamates of medium chain length; longer-chain polyglutamates (i.e., those with six or more Glu residues) are poor substrates. This property is believed to be primarily responsible for the general observation that the chain length of tissue folates increases when folate concentrations are low and decreases when they are high. However, exceptions to this rule were noted,[30] which suggests that factors other than tissue folate concentrations play a role in determining the average chain length. Because changes in chain length affect the affinity of several key folate-requiring enzymes for their folate cofactors,[30] it was postulated that such changes play a role in the regulation of one-carbon metabolism (see below).

Metabolic Functions—Regulation

For a brief, insightful review of folate metabolism the reader is directed to reference 31. Figure 2 summarizes the transfer and oxidation-reduction reactions of one-carbon fragments that require folate coenzymes. Names of the enzymes catalyzing each reaction are listed in the figure legend. Two crucial groups of reactions compete in the cell for available folates, i.e., the reactions of nucleotide biosynthesis and a large number of S-adenosylmethionine–requiring methylation reactions that are dependent on a steady supply of methionine.

The internalization of extracellular folates (reaction 19) occurs via an active-transport carrier-mediated mechanism driven by anion gradients. The same mechanism mediates the uptake of classical antifolate analogs in normal cells.[32] There is evidence, however, that in hemopoietic cells the uptake of fully oxidized folic acid occurs by a different pathway.[33] Conversion of the internalized monoglutamates to polyglutamates (reaction 3) locks the folates inside the cell at concentrations of one or two orders of magnitude greater than the extracellular concentrations. Polyglutamylation requires prior reduction of folic acid to tetrahydrofolic acid (reaction 2) or demethylation of the circulating form 5-methyl-tetrahydrofolic acid by the vitamin B-12–requiring reaction 7. The pathway of incorporation of 5-formyl-tetrahydrofolic acid (trivial names: leucovorin, folinic acid, and citrovorum factor; the latter refers to the 6S diastereoisomer) into the folylpolyglutamate pool is not well understood. It may involve prior dehydration to 5,10-methenyl-tetrahydrofolic acid (reaction 18), an irreversible ATP-dependent reaction,[34] or it may proceed directly from the 5-formyl form. There is much uncertainty regarding the biochemistry of this compound for which there is no known biosynthetic route[31] but which is found in appreciable quantities in eukaryotic cells[29,35] analyzed under conditions that preclude its formation from other folates.[36] Despite the limited information available on the metabolism of leucovorin, it is extensively utilized to reverse the toxicity of methotrexate and, more recently, to potentiate the cytotoxic effects of 5-fluorouracil.[37]

Reaction 4, going in the direction of glycine synthesis, is the main de novo generator of one-carbon fragments. Note that serine, the one-carbon donor molecule, is a nonessential amino acid biosynthesized from glucose in unlimited amounts by most cells. A notable exception to this is the lymphocyte, which apparently lacks the capacity to make serine from glucose.[38] The folate products of reaction 4, the $5,10\text{-}CH_2\text{-}THFAGlu_n$, are key intermediates for which the irreversible reactions 5 and 14 compete. The products of reaction 5, the $5\text{-}CH_3\text{-}THFAGlu_n$, are trapped in that form and can only re-enter the pool of metabolically active unsubstituted tetrahydrofolates via the vitamin B-12-requiring reaction 7. As pointed out by Huennekens et al.,[31] ". . . the role of the 5-methyl-$THFAGlu_n$ is not altogether clear. They may

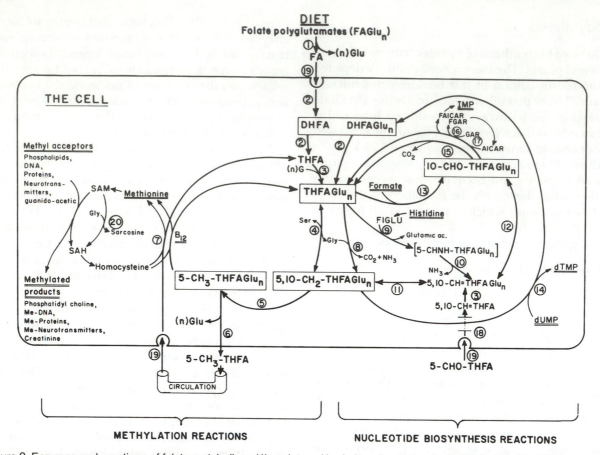

Figure 2. Enzymes and reactions of folate metabolism: (1) γ-glutamyl hydrolase (brush border ?) (EC 3.4.22.12), (2) dihydrofolate reductase (EC 1.5.1.3), (3) folyl poly-γ-glutamate synthase (EC 6.3.2.17), (4) serine hydroxymethyl transferase (EC 2.1.2.1), (5) methylene tetrahydrofolate reductase (EC 1.7.99.5), (6) γ-glutamyl hydrolase (lysosomal ?) (EC 3.4.22.12), (7) cobalamin-dependent methionine synthase (EC 2.1.1.13), (8) glycine cleavage enzyme system (EC 1.4.4.2; 2.1.2.10), (9) glutamate formiminotransferase (EC 2.1.2.5), (10) formiminotetrahydrofolate cyclodeaminase (EC 4.3.1.4), (11) methylene tetrahydrofolate dehydrogenase (EC 1.5.1.5), (12) methenyl tetrahydrofolate cyclohydrolase (EC 3.5.4.9), (13) formyl tetrahydrofolate synthetase (EC 6.3.4.3), (14) thymidylate synthase (EC 2.1.1.45), (15) formyl tetrahydrofolate dehydrogenase (EC 1.5.1.6), (16) phosphoribosyl glycinamide (GAR) formyl transferase (EC 2.1.2.2), (17) phosphoribosyl aminoimidazole carboxamide (AICAR) formyl transferase (EC 2.1.2.3), (18) 5-formyl tetrahydrofolate cycloligase (EC 6.3.3.2), (19) folate/MTX transport mechanism, and (20) glycine methyl transferase (EC 2.1.1.20).

provide: (1) a stable storage form for reduced folates which can be mobilized as needed by activation of reaction 7; (2) a mechanism for suppressing the synthesis of purines and thymidylate by sequestering reduced folates; or (3) a route for the production of methionine when the latter is unavailable from external sources." These three possible roles are not mutually exclusive; in fact all three probably occur simultaneously. This conclusion is suggested by the multiple and complex regulatory influences to which methylene tetrahydrofolate reductase (the enzyme catalyzing reaction 5) is subjected. It is inhibited by S-adenosyl methionine (SAM)[39] and by polyglutamyl derivatives of dihydrofolic acid.[40] If the former decreases, more folates are committed to the remethylation of homocysteine (reaction 7) as required by role 3; if thymidylate synthesis (reaction 14) increases, formation of the other products of that reaction, the

$DHFAGlu_n$, also increases, leading to inhibition of reaction 5 and the commitment of additional folates to the nucleotide biosynthesis pathways as required by role 2. The putative storage role presumably served also by the $5\text{-}CH_3\text{-}THFAGlu_n$ is supported by observations suggesting that the ratio of total folates made up by these forms decreases during folate deficiency. The extent of the decrease in $5\text{-}CH_3\text{-}THFAGlu_n$ will, however, be influenced by the simultaneous presence or absence of methyl group deficiency (i.e., methionine-choline deficiency). If the supply of methyl groups is satisfied from dietary sources, much of the pool of 5-methyl–substituted folates can be converted to the forms required for cell replication and would, in effect, be allowed to drop because of the sustained inhibition of methylene tetrahydrofolate reductase (reaction 5) by the normal concentrations of SAM.

Reaction 14 is the sole de novo path for thymidylate synthesis and the only folate-requiring reaction in which the cofactor serves the dual purpose of one-carbon donor and reducing agent. This reaction can only proceed if there is regeneration of $5,10\text{-}CH_2\text{-}THFAGlu_n$ by the sequential action of dihydrofolate reductase (reaction 2) and, predominantly, of serine hydroxymethyl transferase (reaction 4), although other paths for conversion of $THFAGlu_n$ to $5,10\text{-}CH_2\text{-}THFAGlu_n$ exist (see below). Inhibition of reaction 2 by methotrexate or other dihydrofolate reductase inhibitors effectively prevents thymidylate synthesis and, hence, cell replication.

The biosynthesis of purine nucleotides involves two folate-dependent reactions that insert carbon atoms C-2 (reaction 16) and C-8 (reaction 17) in the purine ring. AICAR formyltransferase, the enzyme catalyzing reaction 17, is strongly inhibited by polyglutamates of dihydrofolic acid ($DHFAGlu_n$) and by other oxidized folates that accumulate in methotrexate-treated cells.[41,42] The folate cofactors for reactions 16 and 17 are $10\text{-}CHO\text{-}THFAGlu_n$, which originate either from $5,10\text{-}CH_2\text{-}THFAGlu_n$ via reactions 11 and 12 or by the ATP-requiring reaction 13. The latter, together with reactions 9 and 10 of the degradation pathway of histidine and the glycine cleavage reaction 8, are minor contributors to the de novo synthesis of one-carbon fragments. Reactions 11, 12, and 13 are catalyzed by a single trifunctional enzyme.[43] The enzyme catalyzing reactions 9 and 10 also is a single bifunctional protein.[44] Both these multifunctional proteins use preferentially polyglutamyl substrates that do not leave the protein until acted upon by the various enzyme activities,[44] a phenomenon called channeling that is kinetically advantageous.[45,46]

The metabolic role of reaction 15 is believed to be the regeneration of $THFAGlu_n$ when $10\text{-}CHO\text{-}THFAGlu_n$ are present in excess. If so, the function of this enzyme should be solely regulatory.[47] The mechanism of egress of $5\text{-}CH_3\text{-}THFA$ to the extracellular milieu must involve prior cleavage of the polyglutamyl chain, a process indicated by reaction 6. Little is known regarding the details of this reaction, which must, however, play a significant role in the redistribution of folates from the liver to peripheral tissues and also in the enterohepatic circulation of folates.[48] In the latter process, $5\text{-}CH_3\text{-}THFA$ and $10\text{-}CHO\text{-}THFA$ monoglutamates are excreted into bile at concentrations 3–10 times higher than in plasma. The role of the enterohepatic circulation is not yet clear. We postulate that it may serve to provide a steady supply of folates to the enterocytes that apparently can satisfy their folate needs from intraluminal as opposed to circulating folates. This hypothesis is supported by the finding by Herbert[49] of normal jejunal epithelium after >17 wk of experimentally induced folate deficiency resulting from the ingestion of a diet very low in folates. At that time the plasma folate concentrations had remained <1.0 nmol/L for >12 wk, and overt megaloblastic changes in the bone marrow indicative of severe deficiency were apparent. Under these circumstances intraluminal folates derived from the very limited folate content of the diet or from folates in bile must have been the only sources of the vitamin available to the enterocytes.

Two other reactions not shown in Figure 2 give rise to $5,10\text{-}CH_2\text{-}THFAGlu_n$ from the oxidation products of choline metabolism. Choline is oxidized to betaine, which in the liver can be used to remethylate homocysteine back to methionine with the formation of dimethylglycine. The latter is further demethylated to monomethylglycine (sarcosine) and finally to glycine by the enzymes dimethylglycine dehydrogenase and sarcosine dehydrogenase, respectively. Cytosolic and mitochondrial forms of these enzymes were identified that transfer the methyl groups to $THFAGlu_n$ with the formation of $5,10\text{-}CH_2\text{-}THFAGlu_n$. The physiological significance of these reactions is not clear.[50]

The regulation of the network of one-carbon transfer and interconversion reactions is very complex. In addition to the regulatory influences exerted by changes in the concentration of effectors (i.e., substrates, products, and cofactors, such as THFA, $DHFAGlu_n$, and SAM) that instantaneously activate or inhibit certain folate-requiring reactions, a slow-response regulatory mechanism based on the covalent modification of the polyglutamyl chain length of the folates was proposed. This "two-tier" hypothesis of regulation,[30] involving fast and slow responses, is based on compelling evidence that the chain length of cellular folates varies in vivo in response to a large number of physiological or pathological stimuli that alter the steady-state equilibrium of one-carbon metabolism. Changes in chain length occur with developmental age, tissue regeneration, infection, starvation, alcohol ingestion, and methionine-choline deficiency.[30] In addition, the chain-length distribution of folylpolyglutamates differs from organ to organ within the same species. Because there can be no doubt that the requirements for one-carbon transfer reactions are different from one organ to another, this finding is in keeping with the hypothesis that changes in chain length are involved in the regulation of one-carbon metabolism. It also was shown that changes in polyglutamate chain length develop slowly and only in response to persistent stimuli. The regulatory role played by these changes therefore is thought to serve to correct long-lasting deviations rather than short-lived fluctuations of an otherwise constant steady state. The slow-response mechanism is believed to protect the concentrations of certain critical effectors, such as SAM, from long-term deviations from normal values. For example, in methyl group (choline-methionine) deficiency, the initial drop in SAM concentrations that relieves the inhibition of methylene tetrahydrofolate reductase (reaction 5) committing more folates to the remethylation of homocysteine cannot be indefinitely sustained without deleterious effects. Persistently low concentrations of SAM would inexorably lead to the malfunction of some of the many SAM-dependent methylation reactions. A mechanism that can shift the flow of one-carbon fragments in the same direction or otherwise allow SAM to regain its normal concentration is believed to exist. This role presumably is served by modifications in the length of the polyglutamyl chain of the folate cofactors. Studies based on the kinetics of pig liver methylenetetrahydrofolate reductase (reaction 5) and thymidylate synthase (reaction 14) for their common substrate, $5,10\text{-}CH_2\text{-}THFAGlu_n$, indicate that the flow of one-carbon fragments would be twice as likely to go toward reduction to $5\text{-}CH_3\text{-}THFAGlu_n$ when hexaglutamate $5,10\text{-}CH_2\text{-}THFAGlu_n$ rather than pentaglutamate are used as substrates.[51] These results further support the putative regulatory role of changes in polyglutamyl chain length.

An intriguing new mechanism of regulation also involving changes in length of the polyglutamyl chain was postulated by Wagner et al.[52] These authors showed that the SAM-dependent enzyme, glycine-N-methyl transferase (reaction 20), is inhibited by $5\text{-}CH_3\text{-}THFAGlu_n$ and that the strength of this inhibition increases with the number of glutamyl residues in the chain. This enzyme consumes SAM for the synthesis of sarcosine, a molecule for which no known metabolic function exists. It is postulated that reaction 20 serves to reduce the concentrations of SAM when this substance is present in excess. Conversely, the reaction should be inhibited when sparing of SAM is required. In keeping with this hypothesis, Cook et al.[53] demonstrated pronounced inhibition of glycine-N-methyl transferase in methionine-choline deficiency. Importantly, the activity of the enzyme decreased but the amount of enzyme was not diminished. This finding suggests an increase in the concentration of its endogenous inhibitor $5\text{-}CH_3\text{-}THFAGlu_n$ or an increase in its potency by chain elongation. Recent results showing no change in the total concentration of $5\text{-}CH_3\text{-}THFAGlu_n$ in the livers of the methyl-group–deficient animals[54] and marked chain elongation of the overall folate pool (C.L. Krumdieck, I. Eto, S. Henning, and M.E. Swenseid, unpublished observations, 1989) support the latter interpretation.

Absorption

Since 1969 it has been known that dietary folates, most of which are polyglutamyl derivatives, undergo hydrolysis to monoglutamates before appearing in the mesenteric blood.[55] The requirement for hydrolysis decreases the availability of folylpolyglutamates compared with that of folic acid.[56] Intraluminal polyglutamate hydrolysis is catalyzed by an intestinal enzyme found in the brush border. This brush border pteroylpolyglutamate hydrolase (BB-PPH) is an exopeptidase that cleaves the polyglutamyl chain one residue at a time starting from the carboxyl end. It has a pH optimum near neutrality and is activated by Zn^{2+}.[57,58] The enzyme is absent from intestinal juice. A second intracellular pteroylpolyglutamate hydrolase (IC-PPH) is found in the lysosomes of intestinal cells. It is an endopeptidase with an acidic pH optimum.[59] It is believed, although not conclusively demonstrated, that BB-PPH is involved primarily in the digestion of dietary folates. The role of IC-PPH is unknown. The rate of hydrolysis of dietary folates by BB-PPH greatly exceeds that of transport of the pteroylmonoglutamates. Halsted et al.[60] calculated that the amount of BB-PPH activity in 10 cm of human jejunum is enough to hydrolyze the adult recommended daily allowance of folates in 10 min. Inhibition of polyglutamate hydrolysis, therefore, is not a likely cause of folate malabsorption.

The effects of chronic alcohol consumption on dietary folate hydrolysis were studied recently in the pig.[61] BB-PPH activity in the alcohol-fed pigs was decreased. A similar effect in humans is likely to occur but probably is not sufficient to explain the folate malabsorption of alcoholic individuals. Enterocyte damage from folate deficiency and ethanol toxicity is considered a more important causative factor.

Recommended Dietary Intakes in Humans

The current Recommended Dietary Allowances (RDAs) for folates are set at 200 $\mu g/d$ for adult males and 180 $\mu g/d$ for adult females.[62] This represents a significant reduction from the previously recommended amount of 400 $\mu g/d$ for adult males and females. Before the publication of the tenth edition of the RDAs,[62] Herbert[63] discussed available evidence that, in his view and that of other experts, warranted reducing the RDA for nonpregnant, nonlactating adults and adolescents to 3 $\mu g \cdot kg$ body $wt^{-1} \cdot d^{-1}$. Much of the rationale for these reductions is based on the calculated folate content of diets consumed in this country (T. Tamura and E.L.R. Stokstad, unpublished observations cited in reference 63) and the mean national daily folate intakes in Canada[64] and in the United Kingdom,[65,66] which range from 180 to

$250~\mu g$ folate, determined by microbiological assays after pteroyl polyglutamate hydrolase treatment. These intakes are sufficient to maintain liver stores $>3~\mu g/g$ ($<1~\mu g/g$ is associated with overt manifestations of deficiency) and normal circulating concentrations in the majority of the population. In pregnancy and lactation, folate requirements clearly increase[67] and the RDA is now set at $400~\mu g/d$ during pregnancy and at $280~\mu g/d$ during the first 6 mo of lactation. It should be noted, however, that a study of 10 nonpregnant women followed for 92 d in a metabolic unit arrived at a higher recommended intake of $300~\mu g/d$ to meet requirements and provide an allowance for storage.[68] The recommended folate intake for healthy infants from birth to age 1 y is set at $3.6~\mu g \cdot kg^{-1} \cdot d^{-1}$.

Assessment of Nutritional Status: Homocysteinemia and Folate Deficiency

Manifestations of folate deficiency and laboratory procedures for evaluation of nutritional status were presented in previous editions of this book[24,69] and were reviewed comprehensively by Chanarin[70] and Cooper.[71] They will not be discussed here. For a lucid discussion of the use of laboratory tests for the assessment of folate status, reference 72 should be consulted.

Recently, the measurement of plasma concentration of homocysteine was shown to be a good indicator of folate and vitamin B-12 nutritional status. The folate-vitamin B-12–requiring remethylation of homocysteine to methionine (Figure 2, reaction 7) normally converts $\sim50\%$ of available homocysteine back to methionine. Its inhibition, because of vitamin B-12 deficiency[73] or inborn errors of vitamin B-12[74] or folate metabolism,[75] was shown to elevate the concentration of circulating homocysteine to values thought to represent an important risk factor for the development of occlusive vascular disease.[76,77]

The possible association of folate deficiency with homocysteinemia was investigated recently by Kang et al.[78] and later by Stabler et al.,[73] who demonstrated a striking negative correlation between serum folate concentrations and protein-bound homocysteine. Moderate to severe homocysteinemia was present in all subjects with serum folate concentrations <4.5 nmol/L and in the majority of subjects with low-normal serum concentrations (4.5–8.8 nmol/L). It must be noted that this important finding is predicated on the use of a method that measures total homocysteine. Homocysteine spontaneously binds covalently to protein and readily forms the disulfide homocystine as well as mixed disulfides with cysteine. Consequently, the concentrations of free homocysteine in plasma decline with time to very low values. Unless the procedure used cleaves the disulfides and bound forms and prevents their re-formation, the correlation between homocysteinemia and folate deficiency will not be observed. Stabler et al.,[73] using capillary gas chromatography–mass spectrometry, found elevated serum homocysteine concentrations ranging from 17 to 185 μmol/L (normal: 7–22 μmol/L) in 18 of 19 folate-deficient individuals. These findings provide a new biochemical test for the assessment of folate nutritional status. As discussed below, however, their significance seems to extend far beyond that.

In most of the subjects studied by Kang et al.,[79] folate deficiency was caused by nutritional inadequacy. In two individuals, however, a defective methylene tetrahydrofolate reductase (Figure 2 reaction 5), characterized by increased thermolability and marginally decreased activity, was detected. Both subjects had plasma homocysteine concentrations 8–15 times above normal. The homocysteinemia was corrected by oral folic acid supplements (1 mg/d) but reappeared 12 wk after the supplements were discontinued. At age 45 y one of these patients had already suffered three heart attacks and one cerebrovascular accident. In addition, he gave a positive family history of coronary heart disease. Kang et al.[80] investigated the incidence of this defect among coronary artery disease patients using the enzyme's thermolability as a marker of the trait. A surprisingly high proportion ($>20\%$) of coronary heart disease patients were found to have the thermolabile 5,10-methylene tetrahydrofolate reductase. The high prevalence of folate deficiency among bearers of this enzyme variant is as yet unexplained. The half-life of their body folates seems to be shorter than normal as indicated by the rapid reappearance of homocysteinemia after discontinuation of the folic acid supplements in patient 1 of Kang et al.[79] Assuming that correction of the homocysteinemia diminishes the risk of vascular disease and given the apparent high prevalence of the trait, a vast opportunity for prevention of coronary disease by giving these patients supplemental folic acid may exist.

Localized Folate Deficiency and Preneoplastic Lesions in Oral-contraceptive Users and in Smokers

In 1973 Whitehead et al.[81] described the presence of megaloblastic changes in cervical epithelial cells from women who used oral contraceptive agents (OCA). As many as 19% of the OCA users showed cytological abnormalities which, although not associated with systemic evidence of folate or vitamin B-

12 deficiency, were corrected by the administration of oral folic acid. The authors postulated that a localized deficiency of folates in the cervix had developed as a result of the use of contraceptive steroids. Later Butterworth et al.,[82] on the basis of morphological similarity of folate-deficient cervical epithelial cells and the cells observed in the preneoplastic lesion of cervical dysplasia, postulated that contraceptive steroids might produce localized alterations in folic acid metabolism such as to favor neoplastic transformation. A double-blind trial of OCA users diagnosed as having cervical dysplasia, half of whom received a daily supplement (10 mg) of folic acid, showed cytological improvement and significantly less-severe lesions evaluated by biopsy among the supplemented subjects.

Tobacco smoking is believed to represent a second model of localized deficiency often associated with preneoplastic changes of the affected tissues. Oxidizing components present in tobacco smoke are known to inactivate folate and vitamin B-12 cofactors in vitro[83] and are presumably responsible for the in situ destruction of these substances in the respiratory epithelia. The deficient tissues are thought to be more susceptible to neoplastic transformation by carcinogens in the smoke. A recent study showing improvement in the atypia of squamous metaplasia in smokers after a period of folic acid and vitamin B-12 supplementation supports the above hypothesis.[84] The results of the studies on OCA users and smokers await verification and must be cautiously interpreted at present. In particular the conclusion that folic acid supplements protect chronic smokers against lung cancer must be avoided.

Toxicity

A report by Milne et al.[85] described greater fecal losses of zinc during a period of oral folic acid supplementation (400 μg every other day) in four human subjects studied under metabolic-ward conditions. Zinc balance was not affected, presumably because of a concomitant decrease in urinary zinc losses. Another study on folate-zinc interactions indicated the presence of a mutually inhibitory effect of zinc and folate on intestinal transport in the rat.[86] Such an effect, however, was not observed by Keating et al. in either rats or humans.[87] In keeping with these results, Butterworth et al.[88] showed that the concentration of zinc in plasma and erythrocytes did not change significantly after folate supplements of 10 mg/d were administered for up to 4 mo to a group of 27 women. The long-held view that toxicity of oral folic acid in moderate doses is virtually nonexistent is supported by the latter studies.

References

1. C.L. Krumdieck, T. Tamura, and I. Eto (1983) Synthesis and analysis of the pteroylpolyglutamates. *Vitam. Horm.* 40:45–94.
2. L. Wills (1931) Treatment of "pernicious anaemia of pregnancy" and "tropical anaemia" with special reference to yeast extract as a curative agent. *Br. Med. J.* 1:1059–1064.
3. E.E. Snell and W.H. Peterson (1940) Growth factors for bacteria. X. Additional factors required by certain lactic acid bacteria. *J. Bacteriol.* 39:273–285.
4. H.K. Mitchell, E.E. Snell, and R.J. Williams (1941) The concentration of "folic acid." *J. Am. Chem. Soc.* 63:2284.
5. A.G. Hogan and E.M. Parrott (1940) Anemia in chicks caused by a vitamin deficiency. *J. Biol. Chem.* 132:507–517.
6. L. Wills and H.S. Bilimoria (1932) Studies in pernicious anemia of pregnancy. Part V. Production of a macrocytic anemia in monkeys by deficient feeding. *Indian J. Med. Res.* 20:391–404.
7. R.L. Blakley and S.J. Benkovic (1984) Nomenclature. In: *Folates and Pterins*, vol. 1 (R.L. Blakley and S.J. Benkovic, eds.), pp. xi–xiv, John Wiley and Sons, Inc., New York.
8. E.A. Cossins (1984) Folates in biological materials. In: *Folates and Pterins*, vol. 1 (R.L. Blakley and S.J. Benkovic, eds.), pp. 1–60, John Wiley and Sons, Inc., New York.
9. J.D. O'Broin, I.J. Temperley, J.P. Brown, and J.M. Scott (1975) Nutritional stability of various naturally occurring monoglutamate derivatives of folic acid. *Am. J. Clin. Nutr.* 28:438–444.
10. C.L. Krumdieck and C.M. Baugh (1969) The solid phase synthesis of polyglutamates of folic acid. *Biochemistry* 8:1568–1572.
11. J. Meienhofer, P.M. Jacobs, H.A. Godwin, and I.H. Rosenberg (1970) Synthesis of hepta-gamma-L-glutamic acid by conventional and solid-phase techniques. *J. Org. Chem.* 35:4137–4140.
12. A. Abraham, M.G. Nair, R.L. Kisliuk, and J. Galivan (in press) Folate analogues. 33: Synthesis of folates and antifolate poly-gamma-glutamates by Fmoc chemistry and biological evaluation of certain methotrexate polyglutamate polylysine conjugates and anhydromethotrexate as inhibitors of the growth of H35 hepatoma cells. *J. Med. Chem.*
13. S.D. Wilson and D.W. Horne (1983) Evaluation of ascorbic acid in protecting labile folic acid derivatives. *Proc. Natl. Acad. Sci. USA* 80:6500–6504.
14. I. Eto and C.L. Krumdieck (1980) Determination of three different pools of reduced one-carbon substituted folates. I. A study of the fundamental chemical reactions. *Anal. Biochem.* 109:167–184.
15. I. Eto and C.L. Krumdieck (1981) Determination of three different pools of reduced one-carbon substituted folates. II. Quantitation and chain-length determination of the pteroylpolyglutamates of rat liver. *Anal. Biochem.* 115:138–145.
16. I. Eto and C.L. Krumdieck (1982) Determination of three different pools of reduced one-carbon substituted folates. III. Reversed-phase high performance liquid chromatography of the azo dye derivatives of p-amino-benzoylpoly-gamma-glutamates and its application to the study of unlabeled endogenous pteroylpolyglutamates of rat liver. *Anal. Biochem.* 120:323–329.
17. D.G. Priest, K.K. Happel, and M.T. Doig (1980) Electrophoretic identification of poly-gamma-glutamate chain lengths of 5,10-methylenetetrahydrofolate using thymidylate synthetase complexes. *J. Biochem. Biophys. Methods* 3:201–206.
18. D.G. Priest, K.K. Happel, M. Mangum, J.M. Bednarek, M.T. Doig, and C.M. Baugh (1981) Tissue folylpolyglutamate chain length characterization by electrophoresis as thymidylate synthetase-fluorodeoxyuridylate ternary complexes. *Anal. Biochem.* 115:163–169.
19. M.T. Doig, J.R. Peters, P. Sur, M. Dang, and D.G. Priest (1985) Determination of mouse liver 5-methyltetrahydrofolate concentration and polyglutamate forms. *J. Biochem. Biophys. Methods* 10:287–294.

20. M.T. Doig, P. Sur, J.R. Peters, and D.G. Priest (1984) Enzymatic determination of tissue dihydrofolate. *Anal. Lett.* 17:2067–2073.

21. V. Kesavan, D.G. Priest, and M.T. Doig (1986) Radioenzymatic determination of subpicomole quantities of folic acid and dihydrofolate based on differential reduction by dihydrofolate reductase. *Microchem. J.* 33:326–330.

22. V. Kesavan, M.T. Doig, and D.G. Priest (1986) A radioenzymatic method for the determination of tissue 10-formyltetrahydrofolate. *J. Biochem. Biophys. Methods* 12:311–317.

23. J. Selhub and D. Fell (1988) Newer techniques for the analysis of tissue folate composition. *Fed. Proc.* A1089 (abstr.).

24. C.L. Krumdieck (1976) Folic acid. In: *Present Knowledge in Nutrition*, 4th ed., (D.M. Hegsted, C.O. Chichester, W.J. Darby, K.W. McNutt, R.M. Stalvey, and E.H. Stotz, eds.), pp. 175–190, The Nutrition Foundation, Washington, DC.

25. T. Shiota (1984) Biosynthesis of folate from pterin precursors. In: *Folates and Pterins*, vol. 1 (R.L. Blakley and S.J. Benkovic, eds.), pp. 121–134, John Wiley and Sons, Inc., New York.

26. G.M. Brown (1985) Biosynthesis of pterins. In: *Folates and Pterins*, vol. 2 (R.L. Blakley and S. Benkovic, eds.), pp. 115–154, John Wiley and Sons, Inc., New York.

27. J.J. McGuire and J.K. Coward (1984) Pteroylpolyglutamates: biosynthesis, degradation, and function. In: *Folates and Pterins*, vol. 1 (R.L. Blakley and S.J. Benkovic, eds.), pp. 135–190, John Wiley and Sons, Inc., New York.

28. Anonymous (1987) Mammalian folylpoly-γ-glutamate synthetase. *Nutr. Rev.* 45:186–188.

29. K. Fujii, T. Nagasaki, K.S. Vitols, and F.M. Huennekens (1983) Polyglutamylation as a factor in the trapping of 5-methyltetrahydrofolate by cobalamin-deficient L1210 cells. In: *Folyl and Antifolyl Polyglutamates* (I.D. Goldman, B.A. Chabner, and J.R. Bertino, eds.) pp. 375–397, Plenum Press, New York.

30. C.L. Krumdieck and I. Eto (1986) Folates in tissues and cells. Support for a "two-tier" hypothesis of regulation of one-carbon fragments. In: *Chemistry and Biology of Pteridines* (B.A. Cooper and V.M. Whitehead, eds.), pp. 447–466, Walter de Gruyter & Co., Berlin.

31. F.M. Huennekens, T.H. Duffy, and K.S. Vitols (1987) Folic acid metabolism and its disruption by pharmacologic agents. *NCI Monogr.* 5:1–8.

32. G.B. Henderson (1986) Transport of folate compounds into cells. In: *Folates and Pterins*, vol. 3 (R.L. Blakley and S.J. Benkovic, eds.), pp. 207–250, John Wiley and Sons, Inc., New York.

33. K.C. Das and A.V. Hoffbrand (1970) Studies of folate uptake by phytohaemagglutinin-stimulated lymphocytes. *Br. J. Haematol.* 19:203–221.

34. F.M. Huennekens, G.B. Henderson, K.S. Vitols, and C.E. Grimshaw (1984) Enzymatic activation of 5-formyltetrahydrofolate via conversion to 5,10-methenyltetrahydrofolate. *Adv. Enzyme Regul.* 22:3–13.

35. R.G. Moran, W.C. Werkheiser, and S.F. Zakrzewski (1976) Folate metabolism in mammalian cells in culture. I. Partial characterization of the folate derivatives present in L1210 mouse leukemia cells. *J. Biol. Chem.* 251:3569–3575.

36. C. Temple, Jr., R.D. Elliott, J.D. Rose, and J.A. Montgomery (1979) Preparation and purification of L-(±)-5-formyl-5,6,7,8-tetrahydrofolic acid. *J. Med. Chem.* 22:731–734.

37. S. Waxman and H. Bruckner (1982) The enhancement of 5-fluorouracil antimetabolic activity by leucovorin, menadione and alphatocopherol. *Eur. J. Cancer Clin. Oncol.* 18:685–692.

38. P.B. Rowe, D. Sauer, D. Fahey, G. Craig, and E. McCairns (1985) One-carbon metabolism in lectin-activated human lymphocytes. *Arch. Biochem. Biophys.* 236:277–288.

39. C. Kutzbach and E.R.L. Stokstad (1971) Mammalian methylenetetrahydrofolate reductase. Partial purification, properties, and inhibition by S-adenosylmethionine. *Biochem. Biophys. Acta* 250:459–477.

40. R.G. Matthews and C.M. Baugh (1980) Interactions of pig liver methylenetetrahydrofolate reductase with methylenetetrahydropteroylpolyglutamate substrates and with dihydropteroylpolyglutamate inhibitors. *Biochemistry* 19:2040–2045.

41. C.J. Allegra, J.C. Drake, and J. Jolivet (1985) Inhibition of phosphoribosylaminoimidazolecarboxamide transformylase by methotrexate and dihydrofolic acid polyglutamates. *Proc. Natl. Acad. Sci. USA* 82:4881–4885.

42. J.E. Baggott, W.H. Vaughn, and B.B. Hudson (1986) Inhibition of 5-aminoimidazole-4-carboxamide ribotide transformylase, adenosine deaminase and 5'-adenylate deaminase by polyglutamates of methotrexate and oxidized folates and by 5-aminoimidazole-4-carboxamide riboside and ribotide. *Biochem. J.* 236:193–200.

43. L.U.L. Tan, E.J. Drury, and R.E. MacKenzie (1977) Methylenetetrahydrofolate dehydrogenase-methenyltetrahydrofolate cyclohydrolase-formyltetrahydrofolate synthetase. A multifunctional protein from porcine liver. *J. Biol. Chem.* 252:1117–1122.

44. E.J. Drury, L.S. Bazor, and R.E. MacKenzie (1975) Formiminotransferase-cyclodeaminase from porcine liver. Purification and physical properties of the enzyme complex. *Arch. Biochem. Biophys.* 169:662–668.

45. J. Paquin, C.M. Baugh, and R.E. MacKenzie (1985) Tetrahydrofolate polyglutamates and the function of formiminotransferase-cyclodeaminase. In: *Proceedings of the Second Workshop on Folyl and Antifolyl Polyglutamates* (I.D. Goldman, ed.), pp. 105–113, Praeger, New York.

46. R.E. MacKenzie and C.M. Baugh (1983) Interaction of tetrahydropteroylpolyglutamates with two folate-dependent multifunctional enzymes. In: *Folyl and Antifolyl Polyglutamates* (I.D. Goldman, B.A. Chabner, and J.R. Bertino, eds.), pp. 19–34, Plenum Press, New York.

47. R.G. Matthews (1984) Methionine biosynthesis. In: *Folates and Pterins*, vol. 1 (R.L. Blakley and S.J. Benkovic, eds.), pp. 497–553, John Wiley and Sons, Inc., New York.

48. S.E. Steinberg, C.L. Campbell, and R.S. Hillman (1979) Kinetics of the normal folate enterohepatic cycle. *J. Clin Invest.* 64:83–88.

49. V. Herbert (1962) Experimental nutritional folate deficiency in man. *Trans. Assoc. Am. Physicians* 75:307–320.

50. R.E. MacKenzie. Biogenesis and interconversion of substituted tetrahydrofolates. In: *Folates and Pterins*, vol. 1 (R.L. Blakley and S.J. Benkovic, eds.), pp. 255–306, John Wiley and Sons, Inc., New York.

51. R.G. Matthews, Y. Lu, J.M. Green, and R.E. MacKenzie (1983) The polyglutamate specificities of four folate-dependent enzymes from pig liver. In: *Folyl and Antifolyl Polyglutamates* (I.D. Goldman, B.A. Chabner, and J.R. Bertino, eds.), pp. 35–44, Plenum Press, New York.

52. C. Wagner, W.T. Briggs, and R.J. Cook (1985) Inhibition of glycine N-methyl transferase activity by folate derivatives: implications for regulation of methyl group metabolism. *Biochem. Biophys. Res. Commun.* 127:746–752.

53. R.J. Cook, D.W. Horne, and C. Wagner (in press) Effect of dietary methyl group deficiency on one-carbon metabolism. *J. Nutr.*

54. D.W. Horne, R.J. Cook, and C. Wagner (in press) Effect of dietary methyl group deficiency on folate metabolism. *J. Nutr.*

55. C.E. Butterworth, C.M. Baugh, and C.L. Krumdieck (1969) A study of folate absorption in man utilizing carbon-14-labeled polyglutamates synthesized by the solid phase method. *J. Clin. Invest.* 48:1131–1142.

56. C.H. Halsted, A.M. Reisenauer, B. Shane, and T. Tamura (1978) Availability of monoglutamyl and polyglutamyl folates in normal subjects and in patients with celiac sprue. *Gut* 19:886–891.

57. A.M. Reisenauer, C.L. Krumdieck, and C.H. Halsted (1977) Folate conjugase: two separate activities in human jejunum. *Science* 198:196–197.

58. C.J. Chandler, T.T.Y. Wang, and C.H. Halsted (1986) Pteroylpoly-

glutamate hydrolase from human jejunal brush borders: purification and characterization. *J. Biol. Chem.* 261:928–933.

59. T.T.Y. Wang, C.J. Chandler, and C.H. Halsted (1986) Intracellular pteroylpolyglutamate hydrolase from human jejunal mucosa: isolation and characterization. *J. Biol. Chem.* 261:13551–13555.

60. C.H. Halsted, W.H. Beer, C.J. Chandler, et al. (1986) Clinical studies of intestinal folate conjugases. *J. Lab. Clin. Med.* 107:228–232.

61. C.A. Naughton, A.M. Reisenauer, C.J. Chandler, and C.H. Halsted (1988) Intestinal absorption of folates in alcoholic pigs. *FASEB J.* 2:A-1614.

62. National Research Council (1989) *Recommended Dietary Allowances,* 10th ed., National Academy Press, Washington, DC.

63. V. Herbert (1987) Recommended dietary intakes (RDI) of folate in humans. *Am. J. Clin. Nutr.* 45:661–670.

64. Bureau of Nutritional Sciences, Nutrition Canada (1983) *Food Consumption Patterns Report,* Department of National Health and Welfare, Ottawa, Canada.

65. J.A. Spring, J. Robertson, and D.H. Buss (1979) Trace nutrients. III. Magnesium, copper, zinc, vitamin B6, vitamin B12 and folic acid in the British household food supply. *Br. J. Nutr.* 41:487–493.

66. C.J. Bates, A.E. Black, D.R. Phillips, A.J.A. Wright, and D.A.T. Southgate (1982) The discrepancy between normal folate intakes and the folate RDA. *Hum. Nutr. Appl. Nutr.* 36A:422–429.

67. I. Chanarin, D. Rothman, A. Ward, and J. Perry (1968) Folate status and requirement in pregnancy. *Br. Med. J.* 2:390–394.

68. H.E. Sauberlich, M.J. Kretsch, J.H. Skala, H.L. Johnson, and P.C. Taylor (1987) Folate requirements and metabolism in nonpregnant women. *Am. J. Clin. Nutr.* 46:1016–1028.

69. C. Wagner (1984) Folic acid. In: *Present Knowledge in Nutrition,* 5th ed. (R.E. Olson, H.P. Broquist, C.O. Chichester, W.J. Darby, A.C. Kolbye, Jr., and R.M. Stalvey, eds.), pp. 332–346, The Nutrition Foundation, Inc., Washington, DC.

70. I. Chanarin (1986) Folate deficiency. In: *Folates and Pterins,* vol. 3 (R.L. Blakley and V.M. Whitehead, eds.), pp. 75–146, John Wiley and Sons, Inc., New York.

71. B.A. Cooper (1986) Folate nutrition in man and animals. In: *Folates and Pterins,* vol. 3 (R.L. Blakley and V.M. Whitehead, eds.), pp. 49–74, John Wiley and Sons, Inc., New York.

72. V. Herbert (1987) Making sense of laboratory tests of folate status: folate requirements to sustain normality. *Am. J. Hematol.* 26:199–207.

73. S.P. Stabler, P.D. Marcell, E.R. Podell, R.H. Allen, D.G. Savage, and J. Lindenbaum (1988) Elevation of total homocysteine in the serum of patients with cobalamin or folate deficiency detected by capillary gas chromatography-mass spectrometry. *J. Clin. Invest.* 81:466–474.

74. B.A. Cooper and D.S. Rosenblatt (1987) Inherited defects of vitamin B12 metabolism. *Annu. Rev. Nutr.* 7:291–320.

75. P.B. Rowe (1983) Inherited disorders of folate metabolism. In: *The Metabolic Basis of Inherited Disease,* 4th ed. (J.B. Stanbury, J.B. Wyngaarden, and D.S. Fredrickson, eds.), pp. 498–521, McGraw-Hill, New York.

76. E.R. Baumgartner, H. Wick, H. Ohnacker, et al. (1980) Vascular lesions in two patients with congenital homocystinurias due to different defects of remethylation. *J. Inherited Metab. Dis.* 3:101–103.

77. S.S. Kang, P.W.K. Wong, H.Y. Cook, M. Norusis, and J.V. Messer (1986) Protein-bound homocyst(e)ine. A possible risk factor for coronary artery disease. *J. Clin. Invest.* 77:1482–1486.

78. S.S. Kang, P.W.K. Wong, and M. Norusis (1987) Homocysteinemia due to folate deficiency. *Metabolism* 36:458–462.

79. S.S. Kang, J. Zhou, P.W.K. Wong, J. Kowalisyn, and G. Strokosch (in press) Intermediate homocysteinemia: a thermolabile variant of methylenetetrahydrofolate reductase. *Am. J. Hum. Genet.*

80. S.S. Kang, P.W.K. Wong, J. Zhou, et al. (1988) Thermolabile methylenetetrahydrofolate reductase in patients with coronary artery disease. *Metabolism* 37:611–613.

81. N. Whitehead, F. Reyer, and J. Lindenbaum (1973) Megaloblastic changes in the cervical epithelium: association with oral contraceptive therapy and reversal with folic acid. *JAMA* 226:1421–1424.

82. C.E. Butterworth, Jr., K.D. Hatch, H. Gore, H. Mueller, and C.L. Krumdieck (1982) Improvement in cervical dysplasia associated with folic acid therapy in users of oral contraceptives. *Am. J. Clin. Nutr.* 35:73–82.

83. D.C. Heimburger, C.L. Krumdieck, C.B. Alexander, R. Birch, S.R. Dill, and W.C. Bailey (1987) Localized folic acid deficiency and bronchial metaplasia in smokers: hypothesis and preliminary report. *Nutr. Int.* 3:54–60.

84. D.C. Heimburger, C.B. Alexander, R. Birch, C.E. Butterworth, Jr., W.C. Bailey, and C.L. Krumdieck (1988) Improvement of bronchial metaplasia in smokers treated with folate and vitamin B$_{12}$ (report of a preliminary randomized, double-blind intervention trial). *JAMA* 259:1525–1530.

85. D.B. Milne, W.K. Canfield, J.R. Mahalko, and H.H. Sandstead (1984) Effect of oral folic acid supplements on zinc, copper, and iron absorption and excretion. *Am. J. Clin. Nutr.* 39:535–539.

86. F.K. Ghishan, H.M. Said, P.E. Wilson, J.E. Murrell, and H.L. Greene (1987) Intestinal transport of zinc and folic acid: a mutual inhibitory effect. *Am. J. Clin. Nutr.* 45:122–125.

87. J.N. Keating, L. Wada, E.L.R. Stokstad, and J.C. King (1987) Folic acid: effect on zinc absorption in humans and in the rat. *Am. J. Clin. Nutr.* 46:835–839.

88. C.E. Butterworth, Jr., K. Hatch, P. Cole, et al. Zinc concentration in plasma and erythrocytes of subjects receiving folic acid supplementation. *Am. J. Clin. Nutr.* 47:484–486.

Chapter **22**

Donald M. Mock

Biotin

Although the water-soluble vitamin biotin was discovered more than 60 years ago, there was relatively little progress in the study of biotin nutrition in humans until the last 15 years. This lack of progress arose from several factors: (1) Overt clinical deficiency of biotin was recognized only rarely. (2) Biotin concentrations in blood and urine are typically one or two orders of magnitude less than those of other water-soluble vitamins, which makes analysis more difficult. (3) The critical role of biotin as a cofactor in mammalian carboxylases was not clearly defined until the seminal observations by Wakil and Lynen and others led to much of our current understanding of biotin enzymology in the 1960s and 1970s.[1,2]

Insight into the biochemistry of biotin provided the basis for the recent dramatic advances in understanding of inherited defects in its metabolism and also for the development of unequivocal methods of documenting biotin deficiency. Subsequent genetic and nutritional investigations acted synergistically to enhance our knowledge of the clinical and biochemical consequences of biotin deficiency and abnormalities in biotin metabolism. Several excellent reviews and symposia have appeared.[3–7]

History

Although a growth requirement for a bios fraction had been demonstrated in yeast, Boas[8] was the first to demonstrate the requirement in a mammal. In rats fed protein derived from egg white, Boas observed a syndrome of severe dermatitis, hair loss, and neuromuscular dysfunction known as egg-white injury. A factor present in liver cured the egg-white injury and was named protective factor X. It is now recognized that the critical event in egg-white injury of both the human and the rat is the highly specific and tight binding ($K_d = 10^{-15}$ mol/L) of biotin by avidin, a glycoprotein found in egg white.[9] Native avidin is resistant to intestinal proteolysis in both the free and biotin-combined forms. Thus, avidin in diets containing uncooked egg white binds and prevents the absorption of both dietary biotin and any biotin synthesized by intestinal bacteria.

Structure and Chemistry of Biotin

The structure of biotin is shown in Figure 1. Because biotin has three asymmetric carbons in its structure, eight stereoisomers exist; of these only one, designated d-(+)-biotin, is found in nature and is enzymatically active. This compound generally is referred to simply as biotin. Biotin is a bicyclic compound; the ureido ring is fused with a tetrahydrothiophene ring that has a valeric acid side chain. On the basis of studies of the binding of biotin analogs[9] and x-ray crystallography,[10] the ureido ring of the molecule is the most important region with respect to the binding of biotin to avidin and to streptavidin, a protein similar to avidin that is excreted by *Streptomyces avidinii*.[9] However, other studies suggest that the length of the side chain or the apolar nature of the -CH$_2$- moieties in the side chain also play a role in the interaction of biotin and its hydrophobic binding site on avidin.[11–15]

Methodology for Measuring Biotin

Measurement of pharmacologic amounts of biotin (e.g., 100 μmol/L) typically has been done by measuring the decrease in optical absorbance at 280 nm that occurs when biotin displaces an optical dye bound reversibly to a known quantity of avidin.[12,13] An analogous method based on displacement of a fluorescent dye recently was published;[14–16] this method offers greater sensitivity and perhaps more specificity when used in biologic fluids.

For measuring biotin at physiologic concentrations (e.g., 1 nmol/L to 1 μmol/L) in physiologic fluids, a variety of assays have been proposed, and a limited

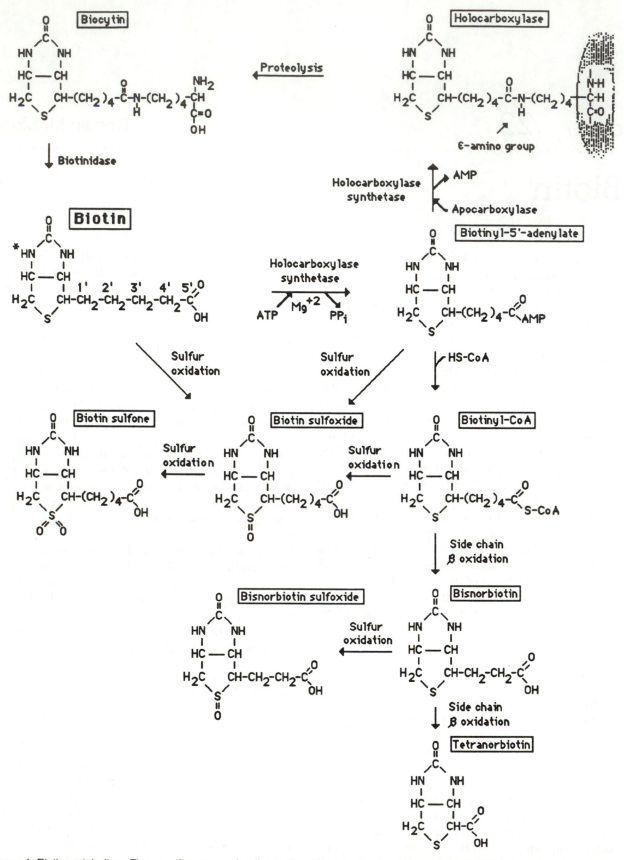

Figure 1. Biotin metabolism. The specific systems leading to the sulfoxides have not been defined. ATP, adenosine triphosphate; AMP, adenosine monophosphate; HS-CoA, coenzyme A; PP$_i$, pyrophosphate; *site of attachment of carboxyl moiety.

number have been used to study biotin nutriture. All of the published studies of biotin nutriture utilized one of three basic types of biotin assays: bioassays (most studies), avidin-binding assays (several recent studies), or a fluorescent derivative assay (one published study).

Bioassays generally have adequate sensitivity to measure physiologic concentrations of biotin.[17-21] However, as noted by Baker and Frank:[20] "None [no bacteria] have been applied satisfactorily for assaying biotin in biologic fluids." The bacterial bioassays (and perhaps the eukaryotic bioassays as well) suffer interference from unrelated substances,[2,22,23] variable growth response to biotin analogs,[24-29] and give conflicting results if biotin is bound to protein.[30] For some bioassay organisms, prior acid and/or enzymatic hydrolysis is required to release the biotin from protein.[18,20,29,31] However, for other organisms (e.g., *Kloeckera brevis*), the detectable biotin decreases with enzymatic hydrolysis.[21]

Avidin-binding assays generally measure the ability of biotin to do one of the following: (1) compete with [^{3}H]biotin, [^{125}I]biotin, or [^{14}C]biotin for binding to avidin (isotope dilution assays);[32-39] (2) bind to [^{125}I]avidin and thus prevent [^{125}I]avidin from binding to a biotinylated protein adsorbed to plastic (sequential, solid-phase assay);[40,41] (3) prevent the binding of a biotinylated enzyme to avidin and, thereby, prevent the consequent inhibition of the enzyme activity;[42,43] or (4) induce a change in fluorescence, fluorescence polarization, or chemiluminescence of native or derivatized avidin.[44-47] Avidin-binding assays have been criticized for being cumbersome, requiring highly specialized equipment or reagents, or performing poorly when applied to biological fluids.[37,39] In a manner analogous to the pioneering work of Wright et al.,[28] three groups recently coupled chromatographic separation to an avidin-binding assay of the chromatographic fractions;[39,48,49] these methods hold promise for both sensitivity and chemical specificity.

Hayakawa and Oizumi[50] recently reported measurement of biotin in plasma with high-performance liquid chromatography (HPLC) separation and fluorescence tagging. Because these investigators detected 10–100 times more biotin than is typically detected by bioassays and avidin-binding assays,[19-21,30,32-34,37,41] validity of the method remains to be proven. Biotin assays based on the conversion of biotin to a fluorescent compound[51] or upon its incorporation into pyruvate apocarboxylase in yeast cells[52] were published but have not yet been applied to biologic fluids. The stated sensitivity of the latter method should be adequate for physiologic samples.

Absorption and Transport

Digestion of Protein-bound Biotin. The content of free biotin and protein-bound biotin in foods is variable, but the majority of biotin in meats and cereals appears to be protein bound.[53-55] Wolf et al.[56] postulated that biotinidase may play a critical role in the release of biotin from covalent binding to protein as one might expect if mucosal biotinidase were involved in the release of biotin from biotinyl oligopeptides, the presumed products of intestinal proteolysis. Biotinidase in pancreatic juice releases biotin during the luminal phase of proteolysis, or biotinyl oligopeptides may be absorbed directly, either by a specific biotin transporter or by a nonspecific pathway for peptide absorption.[57] The mechanism remains to be established.

Biotinidase is present in pancreatic juice and in intestinal mucosa, but the activity is not enriched in intestinal brush border membranes.[56] In patients with biotinidase deficiency, doses of free biotin that do not greatly exceed 150 μg/d appear adequate to prevent the symptoms of biotinidase deficiency, presumably by preventing biotin deficiency.[58] These observations are consistent with a mechanism in which biotinidase deficiency contributes to biotin deficiency via impaired intestinal digestion of protein-bound biotin.

Intestinal Absorption. Understanding of the intestinal absorption of biotin evolved rapidly in the last decade. Substantial evidence suggests that, contrary to earlier conclusions, passive diffusion is neither the only nor the most important process for the intestinal absorption of biotin. Rather, a picture is emerging of a specific, regulated system.

Animal studies. The earliest studies of biotin absorption by rat intestine were performed using everted gut sacs; these studies led to the conclusion that the absorption of both biotin and biocytin (biotin linked to the ϵ-amino group of lysine) occurs by passive diffusion.[59] However, these studies were performed at high substrate concentrations (e.g., 100 μmol/L), required long incubation times, and relied upon bioassays rather than radioactive tracers. Later, Spencer and Brody[60] found that at a biotin concentration of 10 μmol/L hamster intestine transports biotin against a concentration gradient. Berger et al.[61] demonstrated that biotin transport is Na$^+$ dependent and saturable; however, the K$_m$ for the saturable transport exceeded the solubility of biotin in water. Thus, the applicability of these results to biotin transport in vivo was uncertain.

To address these deficiencies, Bowman and coworkers[62] used tracer [^{3}H]biotin in an intestinal-loop technique in vivo using [^{14}C]inulin for volume correction. They detected two distinct mechanisms for biotin uptake. One system was saturable with a K_m of 9.6 μmol/L; the other system was not saturable and was thought to represent the passive diffusion seen by earlier investigators. Using [^{3}H]biotin and everted gut sacs from rats, Said and Redha[63] confirmed the presence of the two biotin transport systems and found a similar K_m for the saturable system. In brush border membrane vesicles, these investigators demonstrated inhibition by structural analogs of biotin; energy, temperature, and Na$^+$ dependence; and electroneutrality.[64] Using [^{3}H]biotin and brush border membrane vesicles, Said and Mock[65] demonstrated that transport of biotin in both the jejunum and the ileum of the rat is appropriately up- and down-regulated by biotin deficiency and biotin supplementation, respectively. The increase in biotin transport was mediated by changes in V_{max} of the transport process, suggesting that changes in the number of transport carriers is the mechanism of regulation.

In everted gut sacs from rats, Dakshinamurti et al.[66] also identified both carrier-mediated active transport and transport by diffusion. However, the K_m for the carrier-mediated system was two orders of magnitude smaller than those determined by Bowman et al.[62] and by Said and Redha.[63]

Gore and coworkers studied biotin transport in isolated enterocytes from rats[67] and hamsters[68] and concluded that biotin uptake in the rat is the result of passive diffusion alone and that biotin transport in the hamster is the result of carrier-mediated diffusion. Thus, their conclusions conflict with the studies cited above.

In the rat, biotin transport is most active in the upper small bowel. Bowman et al.[62] found less biotin uptake in the ileum than in the jejunum. Said and Redha[63] also demonstrated a dramatic reduction in biotin transport preceding from jejunum to ileum to colon; colonic transport was ~3% of jejunal values. On the basis of additional studies in the rat, Bowman and Rosenberg[69] concluded that, although carrier-mediated transport of biotin was most active in the proximal small bowel, the absorption of biotin from the proximal colon was significant. This evidence supports the potential nutritional significance of biotin synthesized by enteric flora.

The ontogenesis of biotin transport was examined in suckling, weanling, and adult rats by Said and Redha[70] using the everted sac technique. In all age groups biotin transport was dependent on Na$^+$, energy, and temperature and was inhibited by structural analogs. Both the K_m and Vmax of the saturable system increased with age, and the site of maximal transport by the carrier-mediated system increased aborally with age, shifting from the ileum to the jejunum. In contrast, the rate of transport by the non-saturable process decreased progressively with age. In studies of aging rats using intestinal brush border membrane vesicles, Said et al.[71] demonstrated that carrier-mediated intestinal biotin transport increased from 3 mo to 24 mo of age; the increase was due to increases in the number (or activity) of carriers and was not caused by changes in the affinity of the carrier.

The putative intestinal transporter for biotin has not been definitively identified and characterized. Dakshinamurti et al.[66] subjected cytosol and solubilized brush border membrane from rat intestine to density-gradient separation and examined biotin binding to ammonium sulfate–precipitated protein. They found a close correlation between biotin-binding activity and biotinidase activity and concluded that biotinidase is the only protein in the brush border membrane that binds biotin. However, the observation that biotinidase is not enriched in the brush border membrane of the rat suggests that biotinidase may not be the protein responsible for binding and transporting biotin into the enterocyte.[56] Moreover, the observation that absorption of biotin is normal in patients with biotinidase deficiency also provides evidence against biotinidase as the protein primarily responsible for intestinal transport of biotin.[72]

Human studies. Intestinal transport of biotin in the human is similar to biotin transport in the rat. Using brush border membrane vesicles from human intestine, Said et al.[73] demonstrated the existence of a carrier-mediated process that is Na$^+$ dependent, electroneutral, and capable of accumulating biotin against a concentration gradient. Biotin transport by the carrier-mediated process decreased from duodenum to jejunum to ileum. The decrease was mediated by a decrease in the V_{max} of the transport process without a significant change in the apparent K_m and indicated that the number (or activity) of transporters decreased without changes in the transporter affinity. These investigators also demonstrated that biotin transport increases with a decrease in pH of the incubation solution from 8 to 5.5 because of an increase in transport by the diffusion-mediated process.[74] The exit of biotin from the enterocyte (i.e., transport across the basolateral membrane) also is carrier mediated but is independent of Na$^+$, is electrogenic, and cannot accumulate biotin against a concentration gradient.[75]

Clinical studies also provided evidence that biotin is absorbed from the human colon.[76,77] When biotin is instilled directly into the lumen of the colon, biotin absorption occurs as judged by increases in the plasma concentration of biotin; however, absorption is greater when the same dose of biotin is given orally.

Transport of Biotin from the Intestine to Peripheral Tissues. Little has been established concerning the transport of biotin to the liver and peripheral tissues after absorption from the intestine. Investigation of the binding of biotin to proteins in plasma and serum is proceeding along two distinct lines: investigation of the biotin-binding properties of biotinidase and empirical assessment of covalent and reversible binding of biotin to whole plasma and fractionated plasma proteins.

Wolf et al.[58] originally hypothesized that biotinidase might serve as a biotin-binding protein in plasma or perhaps even as a carrier protein for the transport of biotin into the cell. Chuahan and Dakshinamurti[78] provided evidence to support this hypothesis. Biotin binding to purified biotinidase, albumin, α- and β-globulins, and fractionated human serum was assessed both by [^{3}H]biotin binding to protein using ammonium sulfate and precipitation equilibrium dialysis. Nonspecific binding was assessed by parallel experiments using a 1000-fold excess of unlabeled biotin; only specific binding was considered. These investigators concluded that biotinidase is the only protein in human serum that specifically binds biotin. They identified two biotin-binding sites on biotinidase. One had a K_d of 3 nmol/L and a maximum binding capacity (B_{max}) of 0.065 mol biotin/mol biotinidase; the other had a K_d of 59 nmol/L and a B_{max} of 0.79 mol/mol. For comparison, the K_m of the substrate biocytin is 6.2 μmol/L. Thus, the product of the reaction (biotin) binds at least 100-fold more tightly than the substrate (biocytin); this surprising result led these investigators to speculate that the K_m for biocytin may be decreased in vivo by a modifier or that in plasma biotinidase may function primarily as a biotin carrier rather than as a hydrolytic enzyme.

Studies of biotin nutritional status, biotin transport into the central nervous system, and renal handling of biotin conducted in vivo require accurate measurements of total plasma biotin and its distribution among the pools in plasma. For example, in studies of the transport of biotin into the central nervous system using intravenous infusion of [^{3}H]biotin, knowledge of the proportion of [^{3}H]biotin that is free rather than reversibly bound is necessary for estimating the K_m for transport;[79] whether the binding is specific or nonspecific is not relevant. The typical assumption in such studies is that only the free vitamin is available to bind to the transporter. To obtain this type of information, a different experimental approach was taken; total biotin in plasma was assumed to be distributed among three compartments: in solution in plasma (free), reversibly bound to plasma protein, and covalently bound to plasma protein.

Biotin in one or more of those compartments was measured by various investigators. Using the *Ochromonas danica* bioassay, Frank et al.[80] measured the biotin bound to various plasma proteins; the biotin was released for assay by extensive enzymatic proteolysis. In relation to total biotin in whole human plasma, high amounts of biotin were detected in the α-globulin, β-globulin, and albumin fractions. Whether the biotin was bound reversibly or covalently was not determined. Using an avidin-binding assay, Suchy and Wolf[30] found a sixfold increase in detectable biotin between serum and acid-hydrolyzed serum; the increase was attributed to release of bound biotin. These investigators speculated that the discrepancy in plasma concentrations for total biotin between bioassays and avidin-binding assay might arise from incomplete detection of protein-bound biotin by bioassays. Whether the biotin released by acid hydrolysis was covalently bound or reversibly bound could not be determined from this type of experiment.

The question of reversible vs. covalent binding of biotin was addressed by Mock and coworkers.[81,82] Using tracer [^{3}H]biotin and centrifugal ultrafiltration to examine reversible binding in plasma from the rabbit[81] and human,[82] these investigators found that <10% of the total pool of free plus reversibly bound biotin is reversibly bound to plasma macromolecules (presumably protein) under physiologic conditions during relevant time intervals (minutes to days). Thus, only a small part (approximately one-twentieth) of the increase in biotin detected with acid hydrolysis of plasma can be attributed to release of reversibly bound biotin. This reversible binding of biotin to plasma protein did not saturate at biotin concentrations three orders of magnitude greater than physiologic concentrations; hence, the system appeared to be a low-affinity, high-capacity system. A similar biotin-binding system was detected in experiments with physiologic concentrations of human serum albumin.

The results of the two approaches discussed above apparently conflict; the differences may arise from differences in both the experimental approach and the definition of binding. The importance of either type of biotin binding to the transport of biotin between tissues is not yet clear. It may well be that the binding detected by Mock and coworkers represents a structurally nonspecific interaction between the hydrophobic portions of the biotin molecule and one or more of the hydrophobic binding sites on a serum protein, such as albumin. The binding may be analogous to the binding of apolar optical and fluorescent dyes to the hydrophobic binding sites on albumin and avidin.[9,13–15]

Transport of Biotin into Liver and Peripheral Tissues. The uptake of biotin by liver and peripheral tissues from mammals was the subject of several recent investigations; many of these studies used cultured cells.

Dakshinamurti and Chalifour[83,84] examined the absorption of biotin by HeLa cells in culture. The rate of uptake of free biotin was temperature dependent and linear with the external concentration of biotin, thus resembling fluid-phase pinocytosis. Uptake of biotin complexed to avidin was enhanced severalfold compared with uptake of free biotin and demonstrated saturation as the external concentration of the complex was increased; the K_d was 55 pmol/L. Transport of the biotin-avidin complex also was dependent on temperature and energy and was impaired by colchicine, cycloheximide, and trypsin. A similar system for uptake of the biotin-avidin complex was detected in human fibroblasts in culture.[85] Taken together, these observations are consistent with receptor-mediated pinocytosis, and these investigators postulated that the biotin:avidin complex was mimicking a complex of biotin and a natural biotin-binding protein that could be required for biotin transport into cells. Binding of the complex to rat liver plasma membranes also was demonstrated, although the apparent K_d of 35 nmol/L was quite different from that found with intact cells.[86]

In fully differentiated 3T3-L1 mouse fibroblasts that resemble adipocytes, Cohen and Thomas[87] demonstrated that biotin uptake was dependent on temperature and on external biotin concentration in a nonlinear fashion. The latter was consistent with transport by two distinct processes: a saturable carrier-mediated process with an apparent K_m of 22 μmol/L and a diffusion-mediated process. The terminal carboxyl group appeared to play a significant role in the uptake of the vitamin.

Using rat hepatocytes isolated by collagenase perfusion and corrected for subsequent metabolism of the [³H]biotin to bisnorbiotin, Bowers-Komro and McCormick[88] found that biotin is taken up by a saturable transport system with an apparent K_m of 0.1 μmol/L; transport was dependent on Na^+, temperature, and ATP. On the basis of inhibition by ouabain, cholate, and bilirubin, these investigators proposed that an acid-anion carrier (e.g., ligandin) is involved in biotin uptake.[89]

Transport of Biotin into the Central Nervous System. For water-soluble substances to reach the central nervous system (CNS), they must cross a hydrophobic barrier: either the blood-brain barrier or the blood-cerebrospinal fluid barrier (CSF) or both. Specific carriers evolved to promote the transport of such substances into the CNS.[90] Because the activity of biotinidase in the brain is low compared with other tissues and hence the brain may be unable to recycle biotin, the CNS may be particularly dependent on the transport of biotin across the blood-brain or blood-CSF barrier.[91]

Animal studies. Using an in situ rat brain perfusion technique and tracer [³H]biotin, Spector and Mock[81] demonstrated that biotin is transported across the blood-brain barrier by a saturable system; the apparent K_m was ~100 μmol/L (a value several orders of magnitude greater than the concentration of free biotin in plasma). Inhibition of transport by structural analogs suggested that an unesterified carboxylate group in biotin was important to transport presumably because of structural specificity of a biotin transport protein. Transfer of biotin directly into the CSF via the choroid plexus did not appear to be an important mechanism of biotin entry into the CNS. In additional studies that used either intravenous or intraventricular injection of [³H]biotin into adult rabbits,[79] these investigators found that [³H]biotin was cleared from the CSF more rapidly than mannitol was, suggesting specific transport systems for biotin uptake into the neurons after biotin crosses the blood-brain barrier. Two hours after intraventricular injection, only minimal metabolism of biotin and covalent binding to brain proteins was observed; however, after 18 h, approximately one-third of the biotin was incorporated into brain protein. This finding suggests that biotin enters the brain by a saturable transport system that does not depend upon the subsequent metabolism of biotin or its trapping by incorporation into brain proteins.

Human studies. Analysis of the data of Baker et al.[92] yields a ratio of about 0.2 for biotin concentration in CSF and blood in humans. The CSF-plasma ratios of substances that cross the blood-brain barrier by simple passive diffusion (e.g., mannitol and sucrose) are ~0.1–0.2; the CSF-blood ratio for thiamin, which enters the CNS by a specific transport system, is 0.9.[89] Thus, the data from Baker et al.[92] suggest that in humans biotin enters the CNS by passive diffusion. However, the method used for measuring biotin requires extensive proteolysis,[20] and both bound and free biotin were probably measured. Mock (unpublished observations, 1989) measured the concentrations of free biotin (i.e., total avidin-binding substances) in human CSF and ultrafiltrates of plasma; the ratio was 0.85 ± 0.5 for 11 subjects. In pooled CSF and blood, CSF-plasma ratio for biotin per se (determined by HPLC) was 0.5. These ratios are similar to the CSF-plasma ratios determined for biotin by Spector and Mock[81] in the rabbit, a species that has a specific system for biotin transport across the blood-brain barrier.[79]

Renal Handling of Biotin. Specific systems for the reabsorption of water-soluble vitamins from the glomerular filtrate may contribute importantly to conservation of water-soluble vitamins;[93] such systems were described in renal brush border membranes for ascorbic acid in the rat[94] and for nicotinic acid in the rabbit.[95] A biotin-transport system was reported by Podevin and Barbarat,[93] who studied biotin uptake by both brush border and basal lateral membrane vesicles from rabbit kidney cortex. Uptake by brush border membrane vesicles was saturable, occurred against a biotin concentration gradient, and was dependent on an inwardly directed Na^+ gradient. The K_m was 28 $\mu mol/L$ and transport exhibited structural specificity. In contrast, the uptake of biotin by basolateral membrane vesicles was not sensitive to a Na^+ gradient. Spencer and Roth[96] demonstrated that slices of rat kidney cortex transported biotin against a concentration gradient; transport was dependent on temperature. In brush border membrane vesicles, transport was dependent upon a Na^+ gradient, saturable (K_m of 0.2 $\mu mol/L$), and inhibited by equimolar concentrations of biocytin.

For the human, in vitro studies of biotin transport by renal tissue preparations have not been published. Baumgartner and coworkers[29,72,97–99] measured the renal clearance of biotin in vivo and calculated biotin-creatinine clearance ratios. In normal adults and children who are not receiving biotin supplementation, the clearance ratio is ~0.4. In patients with biotinidase deficiency, renal wasting of biotin and biocytin occurs; biotin-creatinine clearance ratios typically exceed 1, and half-lives for clearance are about half of the normal value. The mechanism for the increased renal excretion of biotin in biotinidase deficiency has not been defined, but this observation suggests that there may be a role for biotinidase in the renal handling of biotin.

Placental Transport of Biotin. Specific systems for transport of some water-soluble nutrients from the mother to the fetus are defined. However, systems for biotin transport have not been reported. Using the *O. danica* assay to measure total biotin in cord blood and maternal venous blood, Baker et al.[100] found a mean neonate-to-mother ratio of 1.5 for term infants.

Transport of Biotin into Human Milk. Little is known about the chemical form, metabolite content, compartmentalization, or bioavailability of biotin in human milk. Hood and Johnson[101] showed that dietary supplementation of nursing mothers with biotin (3000 $\mu g/d$) results in >10-fold increases in the biotin content (i.e., total avidin-binding substances) in the milk.

Biochemical Functions

Incorporation into Carboxylases. After entering the cell, biotin is converted to biotinyl 5'-adenylate (Figure 1) in the first of two serial reactions catalyzed by holocarboxylase synthetase. In the second reaction, the biotinyl moiety of biotinyl 5'-adenylate is covalently attached to the apocarboxylase, yielding the active holocarboxylase and releasing AMP (Figure 1). Attachment of biotin to the apocarboxylase is a condensation reaction that forms an amide bond between the carboxyl group of biotin and the ε-amino group of a specific lysyl residue in the apocarboxylase; these regions contain sequences of amino acids that tend to be highly conserved within and between species for the individual carboxylases.[102] Alternatively, biotinyl 5'-adenylate can be converted to biotinyl-CoA and oxidized by the mitochondrial fatty acid oxidation pathway to bisnorbiotin and tetranorbiotin (metabolites with two and four fewer carbons in the valeric acid side chain, respectively; Figure 1).

In the normal turnover of cellular proteins, holocarboxylases are degraded to biotin linked to lysine (biocytin) or biotin linked to an oligopeptide containing at most a few amino acid residues (Figure 1). Because the amide bond between biotin and lysine is not hydrolyzed by cellular proteases, biotinidase is required to release biotin for recycling.[58] Genetic deficiencies of holocarboxylase synthetase and biotinidase cause the two distinct types of multiple carboxylase deficiency that were previously designated the neonatal and juvenile forms.[5,103,104] These two diseases are discussed in several places in this chapter because studies of these patients have provided important insights into biotin nutrition and the pathogenesis of clinical findings of biotin deficiency.

Mammalian Carboxylases. In mammals biotin serves as an essential cofactor for four enzymes, each of which catalyzes a critical step in intermediary metabolism.[1–7] All four of the enzymes are carboxylases and, as such, catalyze the incorporation of bicarbonate into a substrate as a carboxyl group. In the carboxylase reactions, the carboxyl moiety is first attached to biotin at the ureido nitrogen opposite the side chain; the carboxyl group then is transferred to the substrate. Energy to drive the reaction is provided by the conversion of ATP to ADP and inorganic phosphate. Subsequent reactions in each of these four pathways release CO_2 from the product of the carboxylase reaction. Thus, these reaction sequences rearrange the substrates into more useful intermediates but do not violate the classic observation that mammalian metabolism does not result in the net fixation of CO_2.

One of the four biotin-dependent carboxylases is cytosolic; the other three are mitochondrial. The cytosolic enzyme is acetyl-CoA carboxylase (ACC). ACC catalyzes the incorporation of bicarbonate into acetyl-CoA to form malonyl-CoA (Figure 2). This three-carbon compound then serves as a substrate

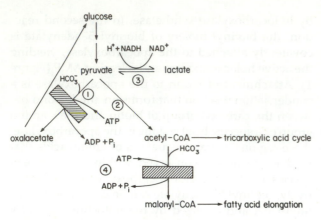

Figure 2. Lactate and pyruvate metabolism. Deficiencies of PC and ACC (striped bar) can affect the metabolic fate of intermediates related to lactic acid. Abbreviations as in Figure 1. NAD⁺ and NADH, oxidized and reduced nicotinamide adenine dinucleotide; ADP, adenosine diphosphate; P_i, inorganic phosphate. Enzymes catalyzing numbered reactions: (1) pyruvate carboxylase (PC), (2) pyruvate dehydrogenase, (3) lactate dehydrogenase, (4) acetyl-CoA carboxylase (ACC). Reprinted by permission of Raven Press from reference 105.

for the fatty acid synthetase complex; the net result is the elongation of the fatty acid substrate by two carbons and the loss of the third carbon as CO_2.

Pyruvate carboxylase (PC) catalyzes the incorporation of bicarbonate into pyruvate to form oxaloacetate, an intermediate in the tricarboxycilic acid cycle (Figure 2). In gluconeogenic tissues (i.e., liver and kidney) oxaloacetate can be converted to glucose. Deficiency of PC was proposed as the cause of the lactic acidemia, central nervous system lactic acidosis, and abnormalities in glucose regulation observed in biotin deficiency and biotinidase deficiency as discussed below.

Methylcrotonyl-CoA carboxylase (MCC) catalyzes an essential step in the degradation of the branch-chained amino acid leucine (Figure 3). Deficient activity of this enzyme (whether because of an isolated genetic deficiency,[5] multiple carboxylase deficiency,[5,103,104] or biotin deficiency per se[105,106]) leads to metabolism of its substrate 3-methylcrotonyl-CoA by an alternate pathway to 3-hydroxyisovaleric acid and/or 3-methylcrotonyl-glycine. Thus, increased urinary excretion of these abnormal metabolites reflects deficient activity of MCC and can reflect biotin depletion in genetically normal individuals.

Propionyl-CoA carboxylase (PCC) catalyzes the incorporation of bicarbonate into propionyl-CoA to form methylmalonyl-CoA, which, in turn, is isomerized to succinyl-CoA and enters the tricarboxycilic acid cycle (Figure 4). The three-carbon propionic acid moiety originates from several sources: (1) catabolism of the branch-chained amino acids isoleucine, valine, methionine, and threonine; (2) catabo-

lism of the side chain of cholesterol; (3) β oxidation of odd-numbered fatty acids; and (4) fermentation of dietary carbohydrate by intestinal flora. In a fashion analogous to MCC deficiency, deficiency of PCC leads to increased urinary excretion of 3-hydroxypropionic acid and 2-methylcitric acid.[5,103,105,106]

Other biotin-containing proteins distinct from the four carboxylases and their degradation products were identified in the mitochondria of 3T3-L1 cells by Chandler and Ballard.[107] Identities and functions of the proteins, however, are unknown.

Other Effects of Biotin. Effects of biotin on cell growth, glucose homeostasis, DNA synthesis, etc. were reported;[108–110] for these effects, a direct relationship to biotin's role as a cofactor for the four carboxylases has not been defined. It is unclear whether one or more of the effects will prove to be the indirect result of carboxylase deficiency.

Several recent studies examined the growth that biotin induces in various cell lines in culture. Vesely[111] reported that biotin concentrations as low as 1 μmol/L activate guanylate cyclase in vitro in homogenates of heart, liver, kidney, colon, and cerebellum. Spence and Koudelka[112] confirmed the activation of guanylate cyclase in cultured rat hepatocytes and provided evidence that the activation results in increased in-

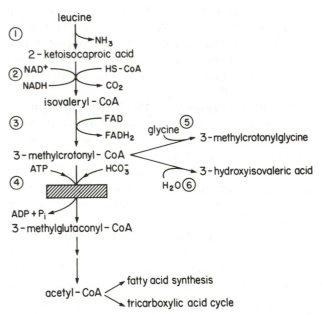

Figure 3. Leucine degradation. A deficiency (striped bar) of MCC causes increased urinary excretion of 3-methylcrotonylglycine and 3-hydroxyisovaleric acid. Abbreviations as in Figures 1 and 2. FAD and FADH₂, oxidized and reduced flavin adenine dinucleotide. Enzymes catalyzing numbered reactions: (1) leucine-isoleucine transaminase, (2) branched-chain 2-keto acid dehydrogenase, (3) isovaleryl-CoA dehydrogenase, (4) methylcrotonyl-CoA carboxylase (MCC), (5) glycine N-acylase, (6) enoyl hydratase (crotonase). Reprinted by permission of Raven Press from reference 105.

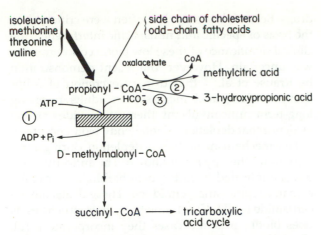

Figure 4. Propionate metabolism. Propionate is derived primarily from amino acid degradation and to a lesser extent from cholesterol and odd-chain fatty acids; a deficiency (striped bar) of PCC causes increased urinary excretion of methylcitric and 3-hydroxypropionic acids. Abbreviations as in Figures 1–3. Enzymes catalyzing numbered reactions: (1) propionyl-CoA carboxylase (PCC), (2) citrate synthetase, (3) β-oxidation or direct ω-hydroxylation. Reprinted by permission of Raven Press from reference 105.

tracellular levels of cyclic GMP, a putative mediator of the growth-promoting effects of biotin. These investigators hypothesized that this action of biotin did not represent a physiologic effect because the concentration required for activation of guanylate cyclase exceeded physiologic plasma concentrations by two orders of magnitude. However, Vesely et al.[113] recently reported isolation of a biotin receptor on the basis of binding studies conducted on plasma membranes from mouse liver. The estimated K_m of binding was 0.1–1 μmol/L. These investigators speculated that this receptor might mediate the activation of guanylate cyclase. Moreover, Singh and Dakshinamurti[114] reported that exposure of biotin-deficient HeLa cells and fibroblasts to 10 μmol biotin/L was associated with increased guanylate cyclase activity, increased cyclic GMP concentrations, and increased RNA polymerase II activity.

As early as the 1960s, biotin was linked to hyperglycemia and decreased utilization of glucose.[115–117] Recently, Coggeshall et al.[118] demonstrated that pharmacologic doses of biotin lowered fasting concentrations of blood glucose in insulin-dependent diabetic subjects during insulin withdrawal. In insulin-resistant diabetic mice, Reddi et al.[119] demonstrated improved glucose tolerance and reduced insulin resistance in response to pharmacologic amounts of biotin. The mechanism of the effects of biotin on glucose homeostasis is unknown; effects on fatty acid metabolism via ACC and pyruvate metabolism via PC were proposed.[118,119]

Metabolites

Contrary to the tacit assumption of many early attempts at biotin balance studies,[120–126] it now appears that a significant proportion of biotin undergoes metabolism before excretion and that much of the total avidin-binding substances in human urine and plasma is attributable to biotin analogs rather than to biotin per se.

In 1956, Wright and coworkers[28] published a pioneering study of the biotin metabolites in human urine. The endogenous biotin analogs in urine were separated by paper chromatography and detected by bioassay using *Neurospora crassa* (total biotin) and *Lactobacillus plantarum*; biotin metabolites were identified by comparison with retention times of the pure biotin analogs. This semiquantitative study detected significant amounts of the metabolites biocytin sulfoxide and biotin sulfoxide; however, the authors speculated that the biotin sulfoxide might have been produced artificially during the chromatographic procedure. In subsequent studies, Lee et al.[127] injected rats intraperitoneally with biotin labeled with ^{14}C in the carbonyl moiety. Radioactive metabolites in urine were fractionated using ion-exchange chromatography and were identified as biotin *l*-sulfoxide, biotin *d*-sulfoxide, bisnorbiotin, and biotin. The absence of production of $^{14}CO_2$ and [^{14}C]urea provided evidence that biotin is not immediately degraded to these simple compounds. Rather, it appears that, although the side-chain carbons and the sulfur ring undergo oxidation, the bicyclic ring is excreted largely intact. During incubation of [^{14}C]biotin with rat liver homogenates, the same four biotin metabolites were produced, although in different proportions. The bisnorbiotin was thought to result from mitochondrial β-oxidation of the side chain and the sulfoxides from oxidation of the thioether sulfur, probably by an NADPH, oxygen-dependent microsomal enzyme system. Similar results were found for the metabolites arising from the intraperitoneal injection of the [^{14}C]biotin-avidin complex.[128]

Recently, several groups initiated studies designed to more accurately and quantitatively define the content of biotin and biotin metabolites in human urine and plasma using HPLC methods for separation of biotin metabolites[49,129–132] in combination with avidin-binding assays based either on isotopic dilution[49] or a sequential, solid phase assay.[40,41] Mock et al.[48,133] reported that a substantial percentage of the total avidin-binding substances in ultrafiltrates in human plasma is attributable to biotin analogs rather than to biotin per se. On the basis of HPLC retention times, biotin, bisnorbiotin, and biotin sulfoxide were detected in mole ratios of ~3:2:1. Chan and Bartlett[39] and Sourmala et al.[49] found that patients with biotinidase deficiency excreted increased quantities of biocytin. Sourmala et al.[49] further demonstrated that treatment with pharmacologic doses of biotin produces the expected striking increases in urinary excretion of biotin, but the increases in the urinary excretion of biocytin are modest; in addition, their patients with biotinidase deficiency excreted significant amounts of other avidin-binding substances that were speculated to be bisnorbiotin and oxidation products of bisnorbiotin, biocytin, and biotin.

The relationship of the metabolite profile to biotin nutritional status has not been defined. Lee et al.[127] observed that a greater portion of [^{14}C]biotin is excreted as biotin metabolites rather than as the unchanged vitamin when a smaller amount of biotin (e.g., 0.5 vs. 1000 μg biotin/100 g body weight) is injected intraperitoneally into the rat.

Deficiency

Circumstances Leading to Deficiency. The fact that the normal human has a requirement for biotin was documented in two situations: prolonged consumption of raw egg white[106,134–137] and parenteral nutrition without biotin supplementation in patients with short-gut syndrome and other causes of malabsorption.[138–148]

Biotin deficiency also was clearly demonstrated in biotinidase deficiency,[5,103] and many clinical findings and biochemical abnormalities caused by biotinidase deficiency are similar to those of biotin deficiency. Common findings include periorificial dermatitis, conjunctivitis, alopecia, ataxia, and developmental delay.[104,149,150] These similarities support the hypothesis that the pathogenesis of biotinidase deficiency involves a secondary biotin deficiency. However, the signs and symptoms of biotin deficiency and biotinidase deficiency are not identical. Seizures, irreversible neurosensory hearing loss, and optic atrophy were observed in biotinidase deficiency[104,151] but have not been reported in human biotin deficiency. Cerebral atrophy and apparent stretching of the optic nerve were reported in one patient with biotin deficiency.[146] Moreover, Heard et al.[152] reported that biotin deficiency causes impaired auditory brainstem function in young biotin-deficient rats.[152]

Accumulating data provide evidence that long-term anticonvulsant therapy in adults can lead to biotin depletion that can be severe enough to interfere with amino acid metabolism. Krause et al.[153,154] based the diagnosis of biotin deficiency on decreased plasma concentrations of biotin as determined by the *L. plantarum* bioassay; the incidence of biotin concentrations below the normal range was ~75% in a cumulative study group of 274 adults undergoing long-term therapy with a variety of anticonvulsant drugs. Because bioassay data often were criticized on the basis of specific and nonspecific interference, the clinical significance of these low biotin concentrations was uncertain. However, the recent demonstration by Krause et al.[155] that urinary excretion of 3-hydroxyisovaleric acid increased in adults receiving long-term anticonvulsant therapy provides strong evidence that depletion of total body biotin occurred.

The mechanism of biotin depletion during anticonvulsant therapy is not known. The anticonvulsant drugs implicated include phenobarbital, phenytoin, carbamazepine, and primidone. These drugs have a carbamide (–NH–CO–) moiety in their structures as does biotin; in some cases they incorporate a full ureido group (–NH–CO–NH–). Said et al.[156] found that physiologic concentrations of primidone and carbamazepine specifically and directly inhibit biotin uptake by brush border membrane vesicles from human intestine and suggested that impaired intestinal absorption is one, but perhaps not the only, mechanism leading to biotin deficiency. Chuahan and Dakshinamurti[78] also found that phenobarbital, phenytoin, and carbamazepine displace biotin from biotinidase and thus conceivably could have an effect on plasma transport of biotin, renal handling of biotin, or cellular uptake of biotin.

Biotin deficiency was reported or inferred in several other circumstances. Leiner's disease is a severe form of seborrheic dermatitis that occurs in infancy. Although a number of studies reported prompt resolution of the rash with biotin therapy,[157–159] biotin was ineffective in the only double-blind therapeutic trial.[160] Moreover, few studies reported biotin concentrations in plasma, and no study examined organic acid excretion. Thus, the role of biotin in Leiner's disease remains unclear.[2,5,161] Biotin deficiency in the chick produces a fatal hypoglycemic disease called fatty liver-kidney syndrome. Impaired gluconeogenesis because of deficient activity of PC is the cause of the hypoglycemia.[162–165] Hood, Johnson, and Heard[166,167] proposed that biotin deficiency may cause sudden infant death syndrome (SIDS) by an analogous mechanism[166,167] and supported their hypothesis by demonstrating that hepatic biotin is significantly lower at autopsy in SIDS infants than in infants dying from other causes. Additional studies (e.g., concentrations of hepatic PC, urinary organic acids, and blood glucose) are needed to confirm or refute this hypothesis.

Concerns about the teratogenic effects of biotin deficiency led to studies of biotin status during human gestation. Low plasma concentrations of biotin were detected in some[168,169] but not all studies.[170]

Patients undergoing chronic hemodialysis[171] as well as those with chronic liver, gastric, and intestinal diseases[2,172] were reported to have low plasma concentrations of biotin. Yatzidis et al.[173] reported nine patients on chronic hemodialysis who developed either encephalopathy or peripheral neuropathy. All responded to biotin therapy; however, biotin and lactate concentrations, and organic acid excretion were not reported, and the general applicability of these results remains to be determined.

Findings of Frank Deficiency. Whether caused by egg-white feeding or omission of biotin from parenteral nutrition, the clinical findings of frank biotin deficiency in adults and older children are similar to those reported by Sydenstricker[134] in his pioneering study of egg white feeding.[139,140,143,145–147] Typically, the findings appeared gradually after an interval of 6 mo–3 y of parenteral nutrition and after an interval of 6 wk to several years of egg-white feeding. Thinning of hair often with loss of hair color was reported in most patients. A skin rash described as scaly (seborrheic) and red (eczematous) was present in the majority; in several, the rash was distributed around the eyes, nose, and mouth. Depression, lethargy, hallucinations, and paresthesias of the extremities were prominent neurologic symptoms in the majority of adults.

In infants who developed biotin deficiency, the signs and symptoms of biotin deficiency began to appear within 3–6 mo after initiation of total parenteral nutrition;[174] this earlier onset may reflect an increased biotin requirement as a consequence of rapid growth. The rash typically appeared first around the eyes, nose, and mouth; ultimately, the ears and perineal orifices were involved. The appearance of the rash was similar to that of cutaneous candidiasis (i.e., an erythematous base and crusting exudates) and *Candida* could be cultured from the lesions. The character and distribution of the rash are similar to the rash of zinc deficiency.[148,175] In infants, hair loss was noted after 6–9 mo of parenteral nutrition; within 3–6 mo of the onset of hair loss, two infants had lost all hair, including eyebrows and lashes. These cutaneous manifestations, in conjunction with an unusual distribution of facial fat, was called biotin deficiency facies.[148] The most striking neurologic findings in biotin-deficient infants were hypotonia, lethargy, and developmental delay. A peculiar withdrawn behavior was noted and may reflect the same CNS dysfunction diagnosed as depression in adult patients.

Pathogenesis of the Central Nervous System. Sander et al.[176] initially suggested that the CNS effects of biotinidase deficiency (and by implication biotin deficiency) might be mediated via deficiency of PC and the attendant CNS lactic acidosis. Because brain PC activity declined more slowly than did hepatic PC activity during progressive biotin deficiency in the rat, these investigators discounted this mecha-

nism; subsequent events suggest that their original hypothesis is correct. Diamantopoulos et al.[177] expanded the hypothesis by proposing that deficiency of brain biotinidase, which is quite low in normal brain,[91] combined with secondary biotin deficiency leads to a deficiency of brain pyruvate carboxylase and, in turn, to CNS accumulation of lactic acid. This CNS lactic acidosis is postulated to be the primary mediator of the hypotonia, seizures, ataxia, and delayed development seen in biotinidase deficiency. In two children with symptomatic biotinidase deficiency, Diamantopoulos et al.[177] demonstrated that concentrations of lactic acid in the CSF are greatly increased above normal and that CSF concentration of lactic acid was fourfold greater than the blood concentration of lactic acid. Similar observations were reported previously by De Rocco et al.[178] The fact that isolated, genetic deficiency of PC leads to lactic acidosis, seizures, ataxia, hypotonia, and developmental retardation[179] is consistent with their hypothesis; similar observations were made in other genetic causes of impaired pyruvate metabolism and CNS lactic acidosis.[180] Although the pathogenesis of biotinidase deficiency may not be identical to that of biotin deficiency, the observations of Mock et al.[146] in patients who developed biotin deficiency during parenteral nutrition are consistent with CNS lactic acidosis as a major pathogenetic factor. Mock et al. noted that with biotin therapy resolution of lactic acidemia coincided with a striking improvement of the CNS abnormalities.

Suchy et al.[181,182] addressed the question of whether the CNS dysfunction in biotin deficiency and biotinidase deficiency were caused by alterations in brain content of saturated fatty acids or cholesterol. They measured the effects of biotin deficiency and supplementation on composition of saturated fatty acids[181] and cholesterol content[182] in brain tissue of rats with biotin deficiency severe enough to produce striking CNS dysfunction and significant abnormalities in the composition of serum and hepatic saturated fatty acids. They found no effect on either fatty acid or cholesterol composition and concluded that abnormalities of cholesterol and saturated fatty acid metabolism do not play a major role in the neurologic abnormalities observed in biotin or biotinidase deficiency.

Pathogenesis of the Lipid Abnormalities and the Cutaneous Manifestations of Biotin Deficiency. Several studies demonstrated abnormalities in metabolism of fatty acids in biotin deficiency and pointed to the importance of these abnormalities in the pathogenesis of the skin rash and hair loss of biotin deficiency. The rate-limiting step in the elongation of fatty acids is catalyzed by acetyl-CoA carboxylase (ACC). Although there has been interest from the early 1940s in the relationship between biotin and lipid metabolism, the recognition by Wakil and Gibson[183] in 1960 that biotin is the essential cofactor in acetyl-CoA carboxylase led to investigation of the effect of biotin deficiency on hepatic fatty acid biosynthesis. Studies reported either decreased synthesis[184–186] or no effect.[187–189]

Recently, Kramer et al.,[190] Suchy et al.,[181] and Mock et al.[191] independently demonstrated an increase in the percent composition of odd-chain fatty acids in hepatic, cardiac, and/or serum phospholipid in biotin-deficient rats; similar accumulation was reported in livers of biotin-deficient chicks.[192,193] Further, Mock et al.[194] reported the accumulation of these odd-chain fatty acids in plasma of patients who developed biotin deficiency during parenteral nutrition. The accumulation of odd-chain fatty acids is thought to result from PCC deficiency because an isolated genetic deficiency of PCC also results in the accumulation of odd-chain fatty acids in plasma, red blood cells, and liver.[195–197] It was proposed that the accumulation of propionyl-CoA leads to the substitution of the propionyl-CoA moiety for acetyl-CoA in the ACC reaction and, hence, to the ultimate incorporation of a three-carbon rather than a two-carbon moiety during fatty acid elongation. This accumulation of odd-chain fatty acids currently is being investigated as a marker of biotin depletion in tissues.[191]

The cutaneous manifestations of biotin deficiency and essential fatty acid deficiency are similar.[198–200] This similarity in addition to the established role of biotin in lipid synthesis led to studies suggesting an abnormality of lipid metabolism in the pathogenesis of the cutaneous manifestations of biotin deficiency.[201–203] Three studies in rats support the possibility of abnormal polyunsaturated fatty acids (PUFA) metabolism as a result of biotin deficiency and as a cause of the cutaneous manifestations. Kramer et al.[190] and Mock et al.[191] reported significant abnormalities in the n − 6 phospholipids of blood, liver, and heart. Watkins and Kratzer[192] also found abnormalities of n − 6 phospholipids in liver and heart of biotin-deficient chicks.[192] It was speculated that these abnormalities might result in abnormal composition or metabolism of prostaglandins and related substances derived from these PUFAs.[6,191,204] However, these studies did not directly address the question of an etiologic role. To address that question, Mock et al.[205] examined the effect of supplementation of n − 6 PUFA (as Intralipid) on the cutaneous manifestations of biotin deficiency. Supplementation of n − 6 PUFA prevented the development of the cutaneous manifestation of biotin deficiency in a group of rats that were as biotin deficient as the control group that did not receive the supplemental n − 6 fatty acids and developed florid rashes and hair loss.

These investigators interpreted their results as providing evidence that an abnormality in n − 6 PUFA metabolism plays a pathogenetic role in the cutaneous manifestations of biotin deficiency and that the effect of the n − 6 PUFA cannot be attributed to biotin sparing.

Other Effects of Biotin Deficiency. Subclinical biotin deficiency was shown to be teratogenic in several species. Fetuses of mouse dams with subclinical degrees of biotin deficiency developed micrognathia, cleft palate, and micromelia.[206,207] The incidence of malformations increased with the degree of biotin deficiency to a maximum incidence of 91%. Pups of rat dams with subclinical biotin deficiency developed abnormally formed reproductive organs and a spectrum of congenital heart defects.[208,209] Differences in tetratogenic susceptibility among rodent species were reported; a corresponding difference in biotin transport from mother to fetus was proposed as the cause.[210] Hens with a subclinical degree of biotin deficiency produced eggs with higher embryonic mortality, reduced hatchability, chronodystrophy ("parrot beak" deformity), perosis (an abnormality of bone and tendon formation that results in a deformity similar to club foot), micromelia, and syndactyly.[211,212] Similar effects on hatchability and viability were observed in biotin-deficient turkey poults.[213] Recently, Bain et al.[214] hypothesized that biotin deficiency affects bone growth via effects on the synthesis of prostaglandins derived from n-6 fatty acid. This effect on bone growth may be the mechanism for the teratogenic effects of biotin deficiency.

On the basis of studies of both cultured lymphocytes and immune response in rats and mice in vivo, biotin is required for normal function of a variety of immunological cells. These functions include production of antibodies,[215,216] immunological reactivity,[217] macrophage function,[218–220] differentiation of T and B lymphocytes,[221] afferent immune response,[222] and cytotoxic T-cell response.[223] Okabe et al.[172] reported that patients with Crohn's disease have depressed killer-cell activity that is caused by biotin deficiency and is responsive to biotin supplementation. In patients with biotinidase deficiency, Cowan et al.[224] demonstrated defects in both T-cell and B-cell immunity.

Diagnosis of Biotin Deficiency. The diagnosis of biotin deficiency has been established by demonstrating reduced urinary excretion of biotin, increased urinary excretion of the characteristic organic acids, and resolution of the signs and symptoms of deficiency in response to biotin supplementation.[105] Plasma and serum concentrations of biotin, whether measured by bioassay[142,176] or avidin-binding assay,[144] did not uniformly reflect biotin deficiency. The response to administration of biotin has been dramatic in all documented cases. Healing of the rash was striking within a few weeks, and growth of healthy hair was generally present in 1–2 mo.

Treatment of Biotin Deficiency. Pharmacologic doses of biotin (e.g., 1–10 mg) were used to treat most patients, but observations reported on two patients suggest that parenteral administration of 100 μg biotin/d is adequate to cause resolution of the signs and symptoms of deficiency and to prevent recurrence.[174] However, abnormal organic aciduria persisted for at least 10 wk in one patient receiving 100 μg/d. In another patient who received 1 mg for 1 wk and 10 mg for 1 wk, organic acid excretion returned to normal.[174] A similar rapid decline was seen in a child who developed biotin deficiency during parenteral nutrition,[141] after 10 d of parenteral supplementation at 10 mg/d.

Could organic aciduria be an indication that biotin concentration in tissues has not been restored to normal? Could this degree of deficiency be less severe but sufficient to cause significant, subtle morbidity? Currently, there are no data on which to base answers to these questions. Studies to provide the needed data should examine organic aciduria as well as plasma and urinary biotin. Recent advances in organic acid analysis determination (e.g., authentic deuterated standards for determination of 3-hydroxyisovaleric acid excretion by gas chromatography/mass spectrometry[225–227] have stimulated interest in organic aciduria as an index of biotin status in tissues.

Requirements and Allowances

Few data providing an accurate estimate of the biotin requirement for infants, children, and adults are available.[228,229] The Food and Nutrition Board of the National Academy of Sciences recommended 10–100 μg/d with increasing age (Table 1). The German Nutrition Society recommended against dietary supplementation on the grounds that supplementation might diminish enteric synthesis.[2]

An important factor in the current uncertainty concerning the biotin requirement is lack of information on the nutritional significance of biotin synthesized by enteric bacteria.[2,5,22] Available data are conflicting;[31,121–126] interpretation is difficult because the analytical methods used did not distinguish between bound and free biotin in feces and could not identify and quantitate biotin and the various biotin metabolites in urine and feces.

Data providing an accurate estimate of the requirement for biotin administered parenterally also are lacking.[230,231] Uncertainty about the true metabolic requirement for biotin is compounded by lack of information concerning the effects of infusing biotin systemically and continuously. Despite these lim-

itations, recommendations for biotin supplementation were formulated in 1975.[231] However, for the preterm infant, the manufacturer's recommendation for use of the most common water-soluble vitamin supplement[105,232] did not take into account body weight, resulting in high doses of biotin and other water-soluble vitamins per kilogram body weight. These concerns led to a recent revision of recommendations for preterm infants;[230] recommendations for term infants were not changed (see Table 1). The only published study of parenterally supplemented infants reported normal plasma biotin concentrations in term infants supplemented with 20 μg/d and increased plasma concentrations of biotin in preterm infants supplemented at 12 $\mu g \cdot kg^{-1} \cdot d^{-1}$.[233]

There are substantial discrepancies between recommended and actual intakes that lead to questions about either the adequacy of biotin intakes or the accuracy of the recommendations. Breast-fed infants provide an example. Using the *L. plantarum* bioassay, Hamil et al.[234] measured urinary excretion of biotin from birth to age 7 d; urinary biotin decreased to undetectable amounts by age 7 d despite increasing biotin intake as a result of increased intake of human milk with increased biotin concentration. One interpretation of this observation is that the biotin available from colostrum and transitional milk plus that biotin available from intestinal flora (if any) was not adequate to maintain biotin nutritional status. Other studies suggested that the biotin intake of infants beyond the neonatal period also might be inadequate. In a study of infants 1–2 mo old, Salmenpera et al.[235] found that the average biotin intake of exclusively breast-fed infants (measured by *L. plantarum* bioassay) was only 4.4 μg/d, which is about one-tenth of the recommended safe and adequate intake (Table 1). These investigators also found that large variation in biotin concentrations in human milk would result in many infants receiving amounts that were unde-

Table 1. Recommended intake of biotin

Age	Safe and adequate biotin intakes*	Daily parenteral supplement†
	μg	μg/kg
Preterm infants	NA	8
Infants <6 mo	10	20
Infants up to 1 y	15	20
Children 1–3 y	20	20
Children 4–6 y	25	20
Older children 7–10 y	30	20
Older children >11 y and adults	30–100	60

* Reference 231.
† Reference 232.

tectable, which probably means <0.4 μg/d, which is <1% of the recommended intake.

However, overt findings of biotin deficiency have not been clearly documented in any breast-fed infant. If the intake of breast-fed infants is adequate, the recommended intake is too large by a factor greater than is usually allowed in calculating safe and adequate intakes.

Sources of Biotin

The great majority of measurements of biotin content of foods were made with bioassays. Despite the limitations because of interfering substances, protein binding, and lack of chemical specificity, there is reasonably good agreement among the published reports,[234-239] and some worthwhile generalizations can be made. (Note that in reference 237 biotin content should be μg/100 g rather than mg/100 g.)

Biotin is widely distributed in foodstuffs, but the content of even the richest sources is low when compared with the content of most other water-soluble vitamins. Foods relatively rich in biotin include egg yolk, liver, and some vegetables. On the basis of data of Hardinge and Crooks,[236] the average dietary biotin intake was estimated to be ~70 μg/d for the Swiss population.[2] These data are in reasonable agreement with the estimated dietary intake of biotin in a composite Canadian diet (62 μg/d) and the actual analysis of the diet (60 μg/d).[240] Calculated intake of biotin for the British population was 35 μg/d.[241,242]

Toxicity

Daily doses of ≤200 mg orally and ≤10 mg intravenously were given to treat biotin-responsive inborn errors of metabolism[49] and acquired biotin deficiency;[105] toxicity was not reported.

Many thanks to Don McCormick for his constructive criticism and also to Nell Mock for the artwork in Figure 1.

References

1. P.N. Achuta Murthy and S.P. Mistry (1977) Biotin. *Prog. Food Nutr. Sci.* 2:405–455.
2. J.P. Bonjour (1977) Biotin in man's nutrition and therapy—a review. *Int. J. Nutr. Res.* 47:107–118.
3. K.S. Roth (1981) Biotin in clinical medicine—a review. *Am. J. Clin. Nutr.* 34:1967–1974.
4. K. Dakshinamurti and H.N. Bhagavan, eds. (1985) Biotin. NY Academy of Sciences, New York.
5. L. Sweetman and W.L. Nyhan (1986) Inheritable biotin—treatable disorders and associated phenomena. *Annu. Rev. Nutr.* 6:317–343.
6. M.W. Marshall (1987) The nutritional importance of biotin—an update. *Nutr. Today* 22:26–30.
7. K. Dakshinamurti and Chuahan (1988) Regulation of biotin enzymes. *Annu. Rev. Nutr.* 8:211–233.
8. M.A. Boas (1927) The effect of desiccation upon the nutritive properties of egg-white. *Biochem. J.* 21:712–724.
9. N.M. Green (1975) Avidin. *Adv. Protein Chem.* 29:85–133.
10. P.C. Weber, D.H. Ohlendorf, J.J. Wendoloski, and F.R. Salemme (1989) Structural origins of high-affinity biotin binding to streptavidin. *Science* 243:85–88.
11. R.K. Garlick and R.W. Giese (1988) Avidin binding of radiolabeled biotin derivatives. *J. Biol. Chem.* 263:210–215.
12. N.M. Green (1970) Spectrophotometric determination of avidin and biotin. In: *Methods in Enzymology*, vol. 18, part A (D.B. McCormick and L.D. Wright, eds.), pp. 418–424, Academic Press, New York.
13. N.M. Green (1965) A spectrophotometric assay for avidin and biotin based on binding of dyes by avidin. *Biochem. J.* 94:23c–24c.
14. D.M. Mock and P. Horowitz (1989) A fluorometric assay for the interaction of biotin and avidin In: *Methods in Enzymology* (M. Wilchek and E.A. Bayer, eds.), Academic Press, Inc., San Diego.
15. D.M. Mock, G.L. Lankford, and P. Horowitz (1988) A study of the interaction of avidin with 2-anilinonaphthalene-6-sulfonic acid as a probe of the biotin binding site. *Biochim. Biophys. Acta* 956:23–29.
16. D.M. Mock, G. Lankford, D. DuBois, and P. Horowitz (1985) A fluorimetric assay for the biotin-avidin interaction based on displacement of the fluorescent probe 2-anilinonaphthalene-6-sulfonic acid. *Anal. Biochem.* 151:178–181.
17. L.D. Wright and H.R. Skeggs (1944) Determination of biotin with *Lactobacillus arabinosus. Proc. Soc. Exp. Biol. Med.* 56:95–98.
18. P. Gyorgy (1967) Biotin. In: *The Vitamins: Chemistry, Physiology, Pathology, Methods*, 7th ed. (P. Gyorgy and W.N. Pearson, eds.), pp. 263–359 Academic Press, New York.
19. M. Tanaka, Y. Izumi, and H. Yamada (1987) Biotin assay using lyophilized and glycerol-suspended cultures *J. Microbiol. Meth.* 6:237–246.
20. H. Baker and O. Frank (1968) *Clinical Vitaminology*, John Wiley and Sons, New York.
21. T.R. Guilarte (1985) Measurement of biotin levels in human plasma using a radiometric-microbiological assay. *Nutr. Rep. Int.* 31:1155–1163.
22. J.F. Borzelleca, H.G. Day, S.J. Fomon, et al. (1978) *Evaluation of the Health Aspects of Biotin as a Food Ingredient.* Life Sciences Research Office, FASEB, Bethesda, MD.
23. H.P. Broquist and E.E. Snell (1950) Biotin and bacterial growth. I. Relation to aspartate, oleate, and carbon dioxide. *J. Biol. Chem.* 188:431–444.
24. L. Drekter, J. Scheiner, E. DeRiter, and S.H. Rubin (1951) Utilization of d-biotinol by microorganisms, the rat and human. *Proc. Soc. Exp. Biol. Med.* 78:381–383.
25. L.D. Wright, H.R. Skeggs, and E.L. Cresson (1951) Amides and amino acid derivatives of biotin: microbiological studies. *J. Am. Chem. Soc.* 73:4144–4145.
26. M. Oshugi and Y. Imanishi (1985) Microbiological activity of biotin-vitamers. *J. Nutr. Sci. Vitaminol. (Tokyo)* 31:563–572.
27. E. DeMoll and W. Shive (1986) Assay for biotin in the presence of desthiobiotin with *Lactobacillus plantarum. Anal. Biochem.* 158:55–58.
28. L.D. Wright, E.L. Cresson, and C.A. Driscoll (1956) Biotin derivatives in human urine. *Proc. Soc. Exp. Biol. Med.* 91:248–252.
29. J.P. Bonjour, J. Bausch, T. Suormala, and E.R. Baumgartner (1984) Detection of biocytin in urine of children with congenital biotinidase deficiency. *Int. J. Vitam. Nutr. Res.* 54:223–231.
30. S.F. Suchy and B. Wolf (1982) Protein-bound biotin—a consideration in multiple carboxylase deficiency. *Lancet* 8263:108.
31. M. Frigg and G. Brubacher (1976) Biotin deficiency in chicks fed a wheat-based diet. *Int. J. Vitam. Nutr. Res.* 46:314–321.
32. R.P. Bhullar, S.H. Lie, and K. Dakshinamurti (1985) Isotope dilution assay for biotin. *Ann. NY Acad. Sci.* 447:279–287.

33. R. Hood (1979) Isotopic dilution assay for biotin: use of [^{14}C] biotin. In: *Methods in Enzymology: Vitamins and Coenzymes*, vol. 62 (D.B. McCormick and L.D. Wright, eds.), pp. 279–287, Academic Press, New York.

34. E. Livaniou, G.P. Evangelatos, and D.S. Ithakissios (1987) Biotin radioligand assay with an ^{125}I-labeled biotin derivative, avidin, and avidin antibody reagents. *Clin. Chem.* 33:1983–1988.

35. A.D. Landman (1976) A sensitive assay for biotin analogs and biotin-proteins. *Int. J. Vitam. Nutr. Res.* 46:310–313.

36. T. Horsburgh and D. Gompertz (1978) A protein-binding assay for measurement of biotin in physiological fluids. *Clin. Chim. Acta* 82:215–223.

37. R.S. Sanghvi, R.M. Lemons, H. Baker, and J.G. Thoene (1982) A simple method for determination of plasma and urinary biotin. *Clin. Chim. Acta* 124:86–90.

38. S.A. Yankofsky, R. Gurevitch, A. Niv, G. Cohen, and L. Goldstein (1981) Solid-phase assay for d-biotin on avidin cellulose disks. *Anal. Biochem.* 118:307–314.

39. P.W. Chan and K. Bartlett (1986) A new solid-phase assay for biotin and biocytin and its application to the study of patients with biotinidase deficiency. *Clin. Chim. Acta.* 159:185–196.

40. D.M. Mock (1989) A sequential, solid phase assay for biotin based on ^{125}I-avidin. In: *Methods in Enzymology* (M. Wilchek and E.A. Bayer, eds.), Academic Press, Inc., San Diego.

41. D.M. Mock and D.B. DuBois (1986) A sequential, solid-phase assay for biotin in physiologic fluids that correlates with expected biotin status. *Anal. Biochem.* 153:272–278.

42. R.S. Niedbala, F. Gergits, and K. Schray (1986) A spectrophotometric assay for nanogram quantities of biotin and avidin. *J. Biochim. Biophys. Methods* 13:205–210.

43. C.R. Gebauer and G.A. Rechnitz (1980) Ion selective electrode estimation of avidin and biotin using a lysozyme label. *Anal. Biochem.* 103:280–284.

44. H.J. Lin and J.F. Kirsch (1979) A rapid, sensitive fluorometric assay for avidin and biotin. *Methods Enzymol.* 62:287–289.

45. M. Al-Nakime, J. Landon, D.S. Simith, and R.D. Nargessi (1981) Fluorometric assays for avidin and biotin based on biotin-induced fluorescent enhancement of fluorescein-labeled avidin. *Anal. Biochem.* 116:264–267.

46. E.J. Williams and A.K. Campbell (1986) A homogeneous assay for biotin based on chemiluminescence energy transfer. *Anal. Biochem.* 155:249–255.

47. K.J. Schray and P.G. Artz (1988) Determination of avidin and biotin by fluorescence polarization. *Anal. Chem.* 60:853–855.

48. D.M. Mock (1987) A substantial percentage of the avidin-binding substances in human plasma is not biotin. *Fed. Proc.* 46:1159.

49. T. Suormala, E.R. Baumgartner, J. Bausch, W. Holick, and H. Wick (1988) Quantitative determination of biocytin in urine of patients with biotinidase deficiency using high-performance liquid chromatography (HPLC). *Clin. Chim. Acta* 177:253–270.

50. K. Hayakawa and J. Oizumi (1987) Determination of free biotin in plasma by liquid chromatography with fluorimetric detection. *J. Chromatogr.* 413:247–250.

51. M. Tanaka, Y. Izumi, and H. Yamada (1987) Enzymatic assay for biotin using biotinyl-CoA synthetase. *Agric. Biol. Chem.* 51:2585–2586.

52. S. Haarasilta (1978) Enzymatic determination of biotin. *Anal. Biochem.* 87:306–315.

53. P. Gyorgy, R. Kuhn, and E. Lederer (1939) The curative factor (vitamin H) for egg white injury, with particular reference to its presence in different foodstuffs and yeast. *J. Biol. Chem.* 131:733–744.

54. R.C. Thompson, R.E. Eakin, and R.J. Williams (1941) The extraction of biotin from tissues. *Science* 94:589–590.

55. J.O. Lampen, G.P. Bahler, and W.H. Peterson (1942) The occurrence of free and bound biotin. *J. Nutr.* 23:11–21.

56. B. Wolf, G.S. Heard, J.R. Secor McVoy, and H.M. Raetz (1984) Biotinidase deficiency: the possible role of biotinidase in the processing of dietary protein-bound biotin. *J. Inherited Metab. Dis.* 7(suppl. 2):121–122.

57. M.L.G. Gardner (1988) Intestinal absorption of peptides. In: *Nutritional Modulation of Neural Function* (J.E. Morley, M.B. Sterman, and J.H. Walsh, eds.), pp. 27–38, Academic Press, San Diego.

58. B. Wolf, R.E. Grier, J.R. Secor McVoy, and G.S. Heard (1985) Biotinidase deficiency: a novel vitamin recycling defect. *J. Inherited Metab. Dis.* 8(suppl. 1):53–58.

59. J.B. Turner and D.E. Hughes (1962) The absorption of some B-group vitamins by surviving rat intestine preparations. *Q. J. Exp. Physiol.* 47:106–123.

60. R.P. Spencer and K.R. Brody (1964). Biotin transport by small intestine of rat, hamster, and other species. *Am. J. Physiol.* 206:653–657.

61. E. Berger, E. Long, and G. Semenze (1972) The sodium activation of biotin absorption in hamster small intestine in vitro. *Biochim. Biophys. Acta.* 255:873–887.

62. B.B. Bowman, J. Selhub, and I.H. Rosenberg (1986) Intestinal absorption of biotin in the rat. *J. Nutr.* 116:1266–1271.

63. H.M. Said and R. Redha (1987) A carrier-mediated system for transport of biotin in rat intestine in vitro. *Am. J. Physiol.* 252:G52–G55.

64. H.M. Said and R. Redha (1988) Biotin transport in rat intestinal brush-border membrane vesicles. *Biochim. Biophys. Acta* 945:195–201.

65. H.M. Said and D.M. Mock (1989) Regulation of biotin intestinal transport in the rat: effect of biotin deficiency and supplementation. *Am. J. Physiol.* G306–G311.

66. K. Dakshinamurti, J. Chauhan, and H. Ebrahim (1987) Intestinal absorption of biotin and biocytin in the rat. *Biosci. Rep.* 7:667–673.

67. J. Gore, C. Hoinard, and P. Maingault (1986) Biotin uptake by isolated rat intestinal cells. *Biochim. Biophys. Acta* 856:357–361.

68. J. Gore and C. Hoinard (1987) Evidence for facilitated transport of biotin by hamster enterocytes. *J. Nutr.* 117:527–532.

69. B.B. Bowman and I.H. Rosenberg (1987) Biotin absorption by distal rat intestine. *J. Nutr.* 117:2121–2126.

70. H.M. Said and R. Redha (1988) Ontogenesis of the intestinal transport of biotin in the rat. *Gastroenterology* 94:68–72.

71. H.M. Said, D.W. Horne, and D. Mock (in press) Effect of aging on intestinal biotin transport in the rat. *Exp. Gerontol.*

72. T. Suormala, H. Wick, J.-P. Bonjour, and E.R. Baumgartner (1985) Intestinal absorption and renal excretion of biotin in patients with biotinidase deficiency. *Eur. J. Pediatr.* 144:21–26.

73. H.M. Said, R. Redha, and W. Nylander (1987) A carrier-mediated, Na$^+$ gradient-dependent transport for biotin in human intestinal brush border membrane vesicles. *Am. J. Physiol.* 253:G631–G636.

74. H.M. Said, R. Redha, and W. Nylander (1988) Biotin transport in the human intestine: site of maximum transport and effect of pH. *Gastroenterology* 95:1312–1317.

75. H.M. Said, R. Redha, and W. Nylander (1988) Biotin transport in basolateral membrane vesicles of human intestine. *Gastroenterology* 94:1157–1163.

76. M.F. Sorrell, O. Frank, A.D. Thompson, H. Aquino, and H. Baker (1971) Absorption of vitamins from the large intestine in vivo. *Nutr. Rep. Int.* 3:143–148.

77. T.W. Oppel (1948) Studies of biotin metabolism in man: IV. Studies of the mechanism of absorption of biotin and the effect of biotin administration on a few cases of seborrhea and other conditions. *Am. J. Med. Sci.* 76–83.

78. J. Chuahan and K. Dakshinamurti (1988) Role of human serum biotinidase as biotin-binding protein. *Biochem. J.* 256:265–270.

79. R. Spector and D. Mock (1988) Biotin transport and metabolism in the central nervous system. *Neurochem. Res.* 13(3):213–219.

80. O. Frank, A.V. Luisada-Opper, S. Feingold, and H. Baker (1970) Vitamin binding by human and some animal plasma proteins. *Nutr. Rep. Int.* 1:161–168.

81. R. Spector and D. Mock (1987) Biotin transport through the blood-brain barrier. *J. Neurochem.* 48:400–404.

82. G. Lankford and D.M. Mock (1988) The percent of biotin reversibly bound to plasma protein is small. *FASEB J.* 2:A440.

83. K. Dakshinamurti and L.E. Chalifour (1981) The biotin requirement of HeLa Cells. *J. Cell. Physiol.* 107:427–438.

84. L.E. Chalifour and K. Dakshinamurti (1982) The characterization of the uptake of avidin-biotin complex by HeLa cells. *Biochim. Biophys. Acta.* 721:64–69.

85. L.E. Chalifour and K. Dakshinamurti (1982) The biotin requirement of human fibroblasts in culture. *Biochem. Biophys. Res. Commun.* 104:1047–1053.

86. L.E. Chalifour and K. Dakshinamurti (1983) The partial characterization of the binding of avidin-biotin complex to rat liver plasma membrane. *Biochem. J.* 210:121–128.

87. N.D. Cohen and M. Thomas (1982) Biotin transport into fully differentiated 3T3-L1 cells. *Biochem. Biophys. Res. Commun.* 108:1508–1516.

88. D.M. Bowers-Komro and D.B. McCormick. (1985) Biotin uptake by isolated rat liver hepatocytes. In: *Ann. N.Y. Acad. Sci.* 447:350–358.

89. R.C. Rose, D.B. McCormick, T.-K. Li, L. Lumeng, J.G. Haddad, Jr., and R. Spector. (1986) Transport and metabolism of vitamins. *Fed. Proc.* 45:30–39.

90. R. Spector (1977) Vitamin homeostasis in the central nervous system. *N. Engl. J. Med.* 296:1393–1398.

91. S.F. Suchy, J. Secor McVoy, and B. Wolf (1985) Neurologic symptoms of biotinidase deficiency: possible explanation. *Neurology* 35:1510–1511.

92. H. Baker, O. Frank, B. DeAngelis, and S. Feingold (1983) Vitamins in human blood and cerebrospinal fluid after intramuscular administration of several B-vitamins. *Nutr. Rep. Int.* 27:661–670.

93. R.A. Podevin and B. Barbarat (1986) Biotin uptake mechanisms in brush-border and basolateral membrane vesicles isolated from rabbit kidney cortex. *Biochim. Biophys. Acta* 856:471–481.

94. G. Toggenburger, M. Hausermann, B. Mutsh, et al. (1981) Na⁺-dependent, potential-sensitive L-ascorbate transport across brush border membrane vesicles from kidney cortex. *Biochim. Biophys. Acta* 646:433–443.

95. E.F. Boumendil-Podevin and R.-A. Podevin (1981) Nicotinic acid transport by brush border membrane vesicles from rabbit kidney. *Am. J. Physiol.* 240:F185–F191.

96. P.D. Spencer and K.S. Roth (1988) On the uptake of biotin by the rat renal tubule. *Biochem. Med. Metab. Biol.* 40:95–100.

97. E.R. Baumgartner, T. Suormala, and H. Wick (1984) Biotin-responsive multiple carboxylase deficiency (MCD): deficient biotinidase activity associated with renal loss of biotin. *J. Inherited Metab. Dis.* 7(suppl 2):123–125.

98. E.R. Baumgartner, T. Suormala, and H. Wick (1985) Biotinidase deficiency: factors responsible for the increased biotin requirement. *J. Inherited Metab. Dis.* 8(suppl 1):59–64.

99. E.R. Baumgartner, T. Suormala, and H. Wick (1985) Biotinidase deficiency associated with renal loss of biocytin and biotin. *Ann. N.Y. Acad. Sci.* 447:272–287.

100. H. Baker, I.S. Thind, F. Oscar, B. DeAngelis, H. Caterini, and D.B. Louria (1977) Vitamin levels in low-birth-weight newborn infants and their mothers. *Am. J. Obstet. Gynecol.* 129:521–524.

101. R.L. Hood and A.R. Johnson (1980) Supplementation of infant formulations with biotin. *Nutr. Rep. Int.* 21:727–731.

102. D. Samois, C.G. Thornton, V.L. Murtif, G.K. Kumar, F.C. Haase, and H.G. Wood (1988) Evolutionary conservation among biotin enzymes. *J. Biol. Chem.* 263:6461–6464.

103. B. Wolf and G.L. Feldman (1982) The biotin-dependent carboxylase deficiencies. *Am. J. Hum. Genet.* 34:699–716.

104. B. Wolf, R.E. Grier, R.J. Allen, S.I. Goodman, and C.L. Kien (1983) Biotinidase deficiency: the enzymatic defect in late-onset multiple carboxylase deficiency. *Clin. Chim. Acta* 131:273–281.

105. D.M. Mock (1986) Water-soluble vitamin supplementation and the importance of biotin. In: *Textbook on Total Parenteral Nutrition in Children: Indications, Complications, and Pathophysiological Considerations* (E. Lebenthal, ed.), pp. 89–108, Raven Press, New York.

106. L. Sweetman, L. Surh, H. Baker, R.M. Peterson, and W.L. Nyhan (1981) Clinical and metabolic abnormalities in boy with dietary deficiency of biotin. *Pediatrics* 68:553–558.

107. C.S. Chandler and F.J. Ballard (1986) Multiple biotin-containing proteins in 3T3-L1 cells. *Biochem. J.* 237:123–130.

108. S.P. Mistry and K. Dakshinamurti (1964) Biochemistry of biotin. *Vitam. Horm.* 22:20–47.

109. R.P. Bhullar and K. Dakshinamurti (1985) The effects of biotin on cellular functions in HeLa cells. *J. Cell. Physiol.* 123:425–430.

110. F. Petrelli, P. Moretti, P. Sciarresi, and A.M. Dahir (1985) Relationships between biotin and DNA contents and DNA turnover in lymphoid organs: thymus, lymph nodes and spleen. *Acta Vitaminol. Enzymol.* 7:199–206.

111. D.L. Vesely (1982) Biotin enhances guanylate cyclase activity. *Science* 216:1329–1330.

112. J.T. Spence and A.P. Koudelka (1984) Effects of biotin upon the intracellular level of cGMP and the activity of glucokinase in cultured rat hepatocytes. *J. Biol. Chem.* 259:6393–6396.

113. D.L. Vesely, S.F. Kemp, and M.J. Elders (1987) Isolation of a biotin receptor from hepatic plasma membranes. *Biochem. Biophys. Res. Commun.* 143:913–916.

114. N. Singh and K. Dakshinamurti (1988) Stimulation of guanylate cyclase and RNA polymerase II activities in HeLa cells and fibroblasts by biotin. *Mol. Cell. Biochem.* 79:47–56.

115. S.P. Mistry, K. Dakshinamurti, and V.V. Modi (1962) Impairment of glucose utilization in biotin deficiency. *Arch. Biochim. Biophys.* 96:674–675.

116. K. Dakshinamurti, V.V. Modi, and S.P. Mistry (1968) Some aspects of carbohydrate metabolism in biotin-deficient rats. *Proc. Soc. Exp. Biol. Med.* 127:396–400.

117. A.D. Keodhar and S.P. Mistry (1970) Regulation of glycolysis in biotin-deficient rat liver. *Life Sci.* 9:581–588.

118. J.C. Coggeshall, J.P. Heggers, M.C. Robson, and H. Baker (1985) Biotin status and plasma glucose in diabetics. *Ann. NY Acad. Sci.* 447:389–392.

119. A. Reddi, B. DeAngelis, O. Frank, N. Lasker, and H. Baker (1988) Biotin supplementation improves glucose and insulin tolerances in genetically diabetic KK mice. *Life Sci.* 42:1323–1330.

120. J. Gardner, A.L. Neal, W.H. Peterson, and H.T. Parsons (1943) Biotin, pantothenic acid, and riboflavin balances of young women on a milk diet. *J. Am. Diet. Assoc.* 19:683–684.

121. J. Gardner, H.T. Parsons, and W.H. Peterson (1945) Human biotin metabolism on various levels of biotin intake. *Arch. Biochem.* 8:339–348.

122. J. Gardner, H.T. Parsons, and W.H. Peterson. Human utilization of biotin from various diets. *Am. J. Med. Sci.* 211:198–203.

123. C.W. Denko, W.E. Grundy, N.C. Wheeler, et al. (1946) The excretion of B-complex vitamins by normal adults on a restricted intake. *Arch. Biochem.* 11:109–117.

124. C.W. Denko, W.E. Grundy, J.W. Porter, G.H. Berryman, T.E. Friedemann, and J.B. Youmans (1946) The excretion of B-complex vitamins in the urine and feces of seven normal adults. *Arch. Biochem.* 10:33–40.

125. W.E. Grundy, M. Freed, H.C. Johnson, C.R. Henderson, and G.H. Berryman (1947) The effect of phthalylsulfathiazole (sul-

fathalidine) on the excretion of B-vitamins by normal adults. *Arch. Biochem.* 15:187–194.

126. H.P. Sarett (1952) Effect of oral administration of streptomycin on urinary excretion of B-vitamins in man. *J. Nutr.* 47:275–287.

127. H.M. Lee, L.D. Wright, and D.B. McCormick (1972) Metabolism of carbonyl-labeled ^{14}C-biotin in the rat. *J. Nutr.* 102:1453–1464.

128. H.M. Lee, L.D. Wright, and D.B. McCormick (1973) Metabolism, in the rat, of biotin injected intraperitoneally as the avidin-biotin complex. *Proc. Soc. Exp. Biol. Med.* 142:439–442.

129. J.L. Chastain, D.M. Bowers-Komro, and D.B. McCormick (1985) High-performance liquid chromatography of biotin and analogues. *J. Chromatogr.* 330:153–158.

130. T.S. Hudson, S. Subramanian, and R.J. Allen (1984) Determination of pantothenic acid, biotin, and vitamin B_{12} in nutritional products. *J. Assoc. Off. Anal. Chem.* 67:994–998.

131. S.L. Crivelli, P.F. Quirk, D.J. Steible, and S.P. Assenza (1987) A reversed-phase high-performance liquid chromatographic (HPLC) assay for the determination of biotin in multivitamin-multimineral preparations. *Pharm. Res.* 4:261–262.

132. E. Roder, U. Engelbert, and J. Troschutz (1984) High-pressure-liquid-chromatographic determination of biotin in pharmaceutics. *Z. Anal. Chem.* 319:426–427.

133. D.M. Mock and G.L. Lankford (1989) The concentration of biotin sulfoxide in human plasma is not negligible compared to biotin. *FASEB J.* 3:A1058.

134. V.P. Sydenstricker, S.A. Singal, A.P. Briggs, N.M. DeVaughn, and H. Isbell (1942) Observations on the 'egg white injury' in man and its cure with biotin concentrate. *JAMA* 118:1199–1200.

135. D. Scott (1958) Clinical biotin deficiency ('egg white injury'): report of a case with some remarks on serum cholesterol. *Acta Med. Scand.* 162:69–70.

136. C.M. Baugh, J.H. Malone, and C.E. Butterworth, Jr. (1968) Human biotin deficiency: a case history of biotin deficiency induced by raw egg consumption in a cirrhotic patient. *Am. J. Clin. Nutr.* 21:173–182.

137. S.F. Suchy, S.B. Brown, S.I. Goodman, and B. Wolf (1982) Diagnosis of biotin deficiency prior to the appearance of cutaneous symptoms. *Pediatr. Res.* 16:179A.

138. D.M. Mock, A.A. Delorimer, W.M. Liebman, L. Sweetman, and H. Baker (1981) Biotin deficiency: an unusual complication of parenteral alimentation. *N. Engl. J. Med.* 304:820–823.

139. Y. Mashima (1979) Translation: a skin lesion associated with biotin deficiency state during long-term total parenteral nutrition. *J. Jpn. Surg. Soc.* 80:141–146.

140. C.J. McClain, H. Baker, and G.R. Onstad (1982) Biotin deficiency in an adult during home parenteral nutrition. *JAMA* 247:3116–3117.

141. J. Gillis, F.R. Murphy, L.B.H. Boxall, and P.B. Pencharz (1982) Biotin deficiency in a child on long-term TPN. *JPEN* 6:308–310.

142. C.L. Kien, E. Kohler, D.I. Goodman, et al. (1981) Biotin-responsive in vivo carboxylase deficiency in two siblings with secretory diarrhea receiving total parenteral nutrition. *J. Pediatr.* 99:546–550.

143. S.M. Innis and D.B. Allardyce (1983) Possible biotin deficiency in adults receiving long-term total parenteral nutrition. *Am. J. Clin. Nutr.* 37:185–187.

144. N. Khalidi, J.R. Wesley, J.G. Thoene, W.M. Whitehouse, Jr., and W.L. Baker (1984) Biotin deficiency in a patient with short bowel syndrome during home parenteral nutrition. *JPEN* 8:311–314.

145. J.L. Levenson (1985) Biotin-responsive depression during hyperalimentation: a case report. *Ann. NY Acad. Sci.* 447:406.

146. D.M. Mock, D.L. Baswell, H. Baker, R.T. Holman, and L. Sweetman (1985) Biotin deficiency complicating parenteral alimentation: diagnosis, metabolic repercussions, and treatment. *J. Pediatr.* 106:762–769.

147. S. Matsusue, S. Kashihara, H. Takeda, and S. Koizumi (1985) Biotin deficiency during total parenteral nutrition: its clinical manifestation and plasma nonesterified fatty acid level. *JPEN* 9:760–763.

148. P. Lagier, P. Bimar, S. Seriat-Gautier, J.M. Dejode, T. Brun, and J. Bimar (1987) Zinc and biotin deficiency during prolonged parenteral nutrition in infants. *Presse Med.* 16:1795–1797.

149. B. Wolf, R.E. Grier, R.J. Allen, et al. (1983) Phenotypic variation in biotinidase deficiency. *J. Pediatr.* 103:233–237.

150. B. Wolf, G.S. Heard, K.A. Weissbecker, J.R. Secor McVoy, R.E. Grier, and R.T. Leshner (1985) Biotinidase deficiency: initial clinical features and rapid diagnosis. *Ann. Neurol.* 18:614–617.

151. G. Campana, G. Valentini, M.I. Legnaioli, M.L. Giovannucci-Uzielli, and E. Pavari (1987) Ocular aspects in biotinidase deficiency: clinical and genetic original studies. *Ophthalmic Paediatr. Genet.* 8:125–129.

152. G.S. Heard, M.L. Lenhardt, R.M. Bowie, A.M. Clarke, S.W. Harkins, and B. Wolf. (1989) Increased central conduction time (CCT) but no hearing loss (HL) in young biotin deficient rats. *FASEB J.* 3: A1242.

153. K.H. Krause, P. Berlit, and J.P. Bonjour (1982) Impaired biotin status in anticonvulsant therapy. *Ann. Neurol.* 12:485–486.

154. K.H. Krause, P. Berlit, J.P. Bonjour, H. Schmidt-Gayk, B. Schellenberg, and J. Gillen (1982) Vitamin status in patients on chronic anticonvulsant therapy. *Int. J. Vitam. Nutr. Res.* 52:375–385.

155. K.H. Krause, W. Kochen, P. Berlit, and J.P. Bonjour (1984) Excretion of organic acids associated with biotin deficiency in chronic anticonvulsant therapy. *Int. J. Vitam. Nutr. Res.* 54:217–222.

156. H.M. Said, R. Reyadh, and W. Nylander (1989) Biotin transport and anticonvulsant drugs. *Am. J. Clin. Nutr.* 49:127–131.

157. J. Messaritakis, C. Kattamis, C. Karabula, and N. Matsaniotis (1975) Generalized seborrheic dermatitis: clinical and therapeutic data of 25 patients. *Arch. Dis. Child.* 50:871–874.

158. A. Nisenson (1957) Seborrheic dermatitis of infants and Leiner's disease: a biotin deficiency. *J. Pediatr.* 51:537–548.

159. J. Svejcar and J. Homolka (1950) Experimental experiences with biotin in babies. *Ann. Paediatr.* 174:175–193.

160. M. Erlishman, R. Goldstein, E. Levi, A. Greenberg, and S. Freier (1981) Infantile flexural seborrhoeic dermatitis. Neither biotin nor essential fatty acid deficiency. *Arch. Dis. Child.* 56:560–562.

161. L.A. Barness (1972) Reply to treatment of seborrheic dermatitis with biotin and vitamin B complex. *J. Pediatr.* 81:630–631.

162. C.C. Whitehead, D.W. Bannister, A.F. Evans, W.G. Siller, and A.L. Wight (1976) Biotin deficiency and fatty liver and kidney syndrome in chicks given purified diets containing different fat and protein levels. *Br. J. Nutr.* 35:115–125.

163. C.C. Whitehead, D.W. Bannister, and M.E. Cleland (1978) Metabolic changes associated with the occurrence of fatty liver and kidney syndrome in chicks. *Br. J. Nutr.* 40:221–234.

164. C.C. Whitehead and D.W. Bannister (1980) Biotin status, blood pyruvate carboxylase (EC 6.4.1.1) activity and performance in broilers under different conditions of bird husbandry and diet processing. *Br. J. Nutr.* 43:541–549.

165. C.C. Whitehead, J.A. Armstrong, and D. Waddington (1982) The determination of the availability to chicks of biotin in feed ingredients by a bioassay based on the response of blood pyruvate carboxylase (EC 6.4.1.1) activity. *Br. J. Nutr.* 48:81–88.

166. A.R. Johnson, R.L. Hood, and J.L. Emery (1980) Biotin and the sudden infant death syndrome. *Nature* 285:159–160.

167. G.S. Heard, R.L. Hood, and A.R. Johnson (1983) Hepatic biotin and the sudden infant death syndrome. *Med. J. Aust.* 2:305–306.

168. H.N. Bhagavan (1969) Biotin content of blood during gestation. *Int. J. Vitam. Nutr. Res.* 39:235–237.

169. L. Dostalova (1984) Vitamin status during puerperium and lactation. *Ann. Nutr. Metab.* 28:385–408.

170. H. Baker, O. Frank, A.D. Thomson, et al. (1975) Vitamin profile

of 174 mothers and newborns at parturition. *Am. J. Clin. Nutr.* 28:59–65.

171. E. Livaniou, G.P. Evangelatos, D.S. Ithakissios, H. Yatzidis, and D.C. Koutsicos (1987) Serum biotin levels in patients undergoing chronic hemodialysis. *Nephron* 46:331–332.

172. N. Okabe, K. Urabe, K. Fujita, T. Yamamoto, and T. Yao (1988) Biotin effects in Crohn's disease. *Dig. Dis. Sci.* 33:1495–1496.

173. H. Yatzidis, D. Koutsicos, B. Agroyannis, C. Papastephanidis, M. Frangos-Plemenos, and Z. Delatola (1984) Biotin in the management of uremic neurologic disorders. *Nephron* 36:183–186.

174. D.M. Mock, D.L. Baswell, H. Baker, R.T. Holman, and L. Sweetman (1985) Biotin deficiency complicating parenteral alimentation: diagnosis, metabolic repercussions, and treatment. *Ann. NY Acad. Sci.* 447:314–334.

175. A.S. Prasad (1985) Clinical manifestations of zinc deficiency *Annu. Rev. Nutr.* 5:341–363.

176. J.E. Sander, S. Packman, and J.J. Townsend (1982) Brain pyruvate carboxylase and the pathophysiology of biotin-dependent diseases. *Neurology* 32:878–880.

177. N. Diamantopoulos, M.J. Painter, B. Wolf, G.S. Heard, and C. Roe (1986) Biotinidase deficiency: accumulation of lactate in the brain and response to physiologic doses of biotin. *Neurology* 36:1107–1109.

178. M. De Rocco, A. Superti-Furga, P. Durand, et al. (1984) Different organic acid patterns in urine and in cerebrospinal fluid in a patient with biotinidase deficiency. *J. Inherited Metab. Dis.* 7(suppl. 2): 119–120.

179. J.P. Blass (1983) Inborn errors of pyruvate metabolism. In: *The Metabolic Basis of Inherited Disease* (J.B. Stanbury, J.B. Wyngaarden, D.S. Fredrickson, J.L. Goldstein, and M.S. Brown, eds.), pp. 193–203, McGraw-Hill, New York.

180. G.K. Brown, E.A. Haan, D.M. Kirby, et al. (1988) 'Cerebral' lactic acidosis: defects in pyruvate metabolism with profound brain damage and minimal systemic acidosis. *Eur. J. Pediatr.* 147:10–14.

181. S.F. Suchy, W.B. Rizzo, and B. Wolf (1986) Effect of biotin deficiency and supplementation on lipid metabolism in rats: saturated fatty acids. *Am. J. Clin. Nutr.* 44:475–480.

182. S.F. Suchy and B. Wolf (1986) Effect of biotin deficiency and supplementation on lipid metabolism in rats: cholesterol and lipoproteins. *Am. J. Clin. Nutr.* 43:831–838.

183. S. Wakil and D.M. Gibson (1960) Studies on the mechanism of fatty acid synthesis. VIII. The participation of protein-bound biotin in the biosynthesis of fatty acids. *Biochim. Biophys. Acta* 41: 122–129.

184. K. Dakshinamurti and P.R. Desjardins (1978) Lipogenesis in biotin deficiency. *Can. J. Biochem.* 46:1261–1267.

185. P. Puddu, P. Zanetti, E. Turchetto, and M. Marchette (1976) Aspects of liver lipid metabolism in the biotin-deficient rat. *J. Nutr.* 91:509–513.

186. E.J. Masaro, H.M. Korchak, and E. Porter (1962) A study of the lipogenic inhibitory mechanisms induced by fasting. *Biochim. Biophys. Acta* 58:407–417.

187. K. Guggenhiem and R.E. Olson (1952) Studies of lipogenesis in certain B-vitamin deficiencies. *J. Nutr.* 48:345–358.

188. M.R. Gram and R. Okey (1958) Incorporation of acetate-2-[^{14}C] into liver and carcass lipids and cholesterol in biotin-deficient rats. *J. Nutr.* 64:217–228.

189. G.L. Curran (1950) Cholesterol and fatty acid synthesis in biotin-deficient rats. *Proc. Soc. Exp. Biol. Med.* 75:496–498.

190. T.R. Kramer, M. Briske-Anderson, S.B. Johnson, and R.T. Holman (1984) Effects of biotin deficiency on polyunsaturated fatty acid metabolism in rats. *J. Nutr.* 114:2047–2052.

191. D.M. Mock, N.I. Mock, S.B. Johnson, and R.T. Holman (1988) Effects of biotin deficiency on plasma and tissue fatty acid composition: evidence for abnormalities in rats. *Pediatr. Res.* 24: 396–403.

192. B.A. Watkins and F.H. Kratzer (1987) Effects of dietary biotin and linoleate on polyunsaturated fatty acids in tissue phospholipids. *Poult. Sci.* 66:2024–2031.

193. B.A. Watkins and F.H. Kratzer (1987) Tissue lipid fatty acid composition of biotin-adequate and biotin-deficient chicks. *Poult. Sci.* 66:306–313.

194. D.M. Mock, S.B. Johnson, and R.T. Holman (1987) Effects of biotin deficiency on serum fatty acid composition: evidence for abnormalities in humans. *J. Nutr.* 118:342–348.

195. F.A. Hommes, J.R.G. Kuipers, J.D. Elema, J.F. Janse, and J.J.P. Janxis (1968) Propionic-acidemia, a new inborn error of metabolism. *Pediatr. Res.* 2:519–524.

196. U. Wendel (1989) Abnormality of odd-numbered long-chain fatty acids in erythrocyte membrane lipids from patients with disorders of propionate metabolism. *Pediatr. Res.* 25:147–150.

197. D. Gomertz (1972) The distribution of 17 carbon fatty acids in the liver of a child with propionicacidaemia. *Lipids* 6:576–580.

198. R.T. Holman (1978) Essential fatty acid deficiency in humans. In: *Nutrition and Food* vol. 3, sect. E (M. Rechcigl, ed.), pp. 341–353, 355–357, CRC Press, Cleveland.

199. R. Postuma, P.W.B. Pease, R. Watts, S. Taylor, and F.A. McEvoy (1978) Essential fatty acid deficiency in infants receiving parenteral nutrition. *J. Pediatr. Surg.* 13:393–398.

200. R.T. Holman and S.B. Johnson (1983) Essential fatty acid deficiencies in man. In: *Dietary Fats and Health* (E.G. Perkins and W. Visek, eds.), pp. 247–266, American Oil Chemists Society, Champaign, IL.

201. M.L. Williams, S. Packman, and M.J. Cowan (1983) Alopecia and periorificial dermatitis in biotin-responsive multiple carboxylase deficiency. *J. Am. Acad. Dermatol.* 9:97–103.

202. M. Del, C. Gonzalez-Rios, S.C. Whitney, M.L. Williams, P.M. Elias, and S. Packman (1985) Lipid metabolism in biotin-responsive multiple carboxylase deficiency. *J. Inherited Metab. Dis.* 8:184–186.

203. A. Munnich, J.M. Saudubray, F.K. Coude, C. Charpentier, J.H. Saurat, and J. Frezal (1980) Fatty-acid-responsive alopecia in multiple carboxylase deficiency. *Lancet* 1:1080–1081 (letter).

204. B.A. Watkins and F.H. Kratzer (1987) Dietary biotin effects on polyunsaturated fatty acids in chick tissue lipids and prostaglandin E$_2$ levels in freeze-clamped hearts. *Poult. Sci.* 66:1818–1828.

205. D.M. Mock (1988) Evidence for a pathogenetic role of fatty acid (FA) abnormalities in the cutaneous manifestations of biotin deficiency. *FASEB J.* 2:A1204.

206. T. Watanabe (1983) Teratogenic effects of biotin deficiency in mice. *J. Nutr.* 113:574–581.

207. T. Watanabe and A. Endo (1984) Teratogenic effects of avidin-induced biotin deficiency in mice. *Teratology* 30:91–94.

208. W.A. Cooper and S.O. Brown (1958) Tissue abnormalities in newborn rats from biotin-deficient mothers. *Tex. J. Sci.* 10:60–68.

209. W.A. Cooper (1962) Congenital heart abnormalities in biotin-deficient and in pantothenic acid-deficient white rats. *Tex. J. Sci.* 14:278–288.

210. T. Watanabe and A. Endo (1989) Species and strain differences in teratogenic effects of biotin deficiency in rodents. *J. Nutr.* 119: 255–261.

211. J.R. Couch, W.W. Craven, C.A. Elvehjem, and J.G. Halpin (1948) Relation of biotin to congenital deformities in the chick. *Anat. Rec.* 100:29–48.

212. W.W. Cravens, W.H. McGibbon, and E.E. Sebesta (1944) Effect of biotin deficiency on embryonic development in the domestic fowl. *Anat. Rec.* 90:55–64.

213. T.M. Ferguson, T.H. Whiteside, C.R. Creger, M.L. Jones, A.L. Atkinson, and J.R. Couch (1961) B-vitamin deficiency in the mature turkey hen. *Poult. Sci.* 40:1151–1159.

214. S.D. Bain, J.W. Newbrey, and B.A. Watkins (1988) Biotin defi-

ciency may alter tibiotarsal bone growth and modeling in broiler chicks. *Poult. Sci.* 67:590–595.

215. A.E. Axelrod and J. Pruzansky (1955) The role of vitamins in antibody production. *Ann. NY Acad. Sci.* 63:202–209.

216. B.B. Carter and A.E. Axelrod (1948) Circulating antibodies in vitamin deficiency states: II. Thiamin and biotin deficiencies. *Proc. Soc. Exp. Biol. Med.* 67:416–417.

217. F. Petrelli and G. Marsili (1969) Research on the role of biotin in antibody production. *Acta Vitaminol. Enzymol.* 23:86–87 (in Italian).

218. F. Petrelli and G. Marsili (1971) Studies on the relationships between the function of biotin and activity of the RES in the rat. *J. Reticuloendothel. Soc.* 9:86–95.

219. F. Petrelli and G. Marsili (1973) Biotin and phagocitic activity of leucocytes. *Boll. Soc. Ital. Biol. Sper.* 49:1104–1108 (in Italian).

220. F. Petrelli, G. Marsili, and G. Centioni (1973) Biotin and phagocitic activity of leucocytes 'in vitro.' *Boll. Soc. Ital. Biol. Sper.* 49:1109–1113 (in Italian).

221. F. Petrelli, P. Moretti, and G. Campanati (1981) Studies on the relationships between biotin and the behavior of B and T lymphocytes in the guinea-pig. *Experientia* 37:1204–1205.

222. B.S. Rabin (1983) Inhibition of experimentally induced autoimmunity in rats by biotin deficiency. *J. Nutr.* 113:2316–2322.

223. J.T. Kung, C.G. MacKenzie, and D.W. Talmage (1979) The requirement for biotin and fatty acids in the cytotoxic T-cell response. *Cell Immunol.* 48:100–110.

224. M.J. Cowan, D.W. Wara, S. Packman, et al. (1979) Multiple biotin-dependent carboxylase deficiencies associated with defects in T-cell and B-cell immunity. *Lancet* 2:115–118.

225. C. Jakobs, L. Sweetman, N.Y. Nyhan, and S. Packman (1984) Stable isotope dilution of 3-hydroxyisovaleric acid in amniotic fluid: contribution to the prenatal diagnosis of inherited disorders of leucine catabolism. *J. Inherited Metab. Dis.* 7:15–20.

226. D.M. Mock, N.I. Mock, and S. Weintraub (1988) Abnormal organic aciduria in biotin deficiency: rat is similar to man. *J. Clin. Lab. Med.* 12:240–247.

227. D.M. Mock, H. Jackson, J.L. Lankford, N.I. Mock, and S.T. Weintraub (1989) Quantitation of urinary 3-hydroxyisovaleric acid as internal standard. *Biochem. Environ. Mass Spectrom.* (in press).

228. National Academy of Sciences (1989) *Recommended Dietary Allowances,* 10th ed., National Academy Press, Washington, DC.

229. Committee on Nutrition, American Academy of Pediatrics (1985) *Pediatric Nutrition Handbook,* 2nd ed. (G.B. Forbes, and C.W. Woodruff, eds.), pp. 352–353, American Academy of Pediatrics, Elk Grove Village, IL.

230. H.L. Greene, K.M. Hambidge, R. Schanler, and R.C. Tsang (1988) Guidelines for the use of vitamins, trace elements, calcium, magnesium, and phosphorus in infants and children receiving total parenteral nutrition: report of the Subcommittee on Pediatric Parenteral Nutrient Requirements from the Committee on Clinical Practice Issues of The American Society for Clinical Nutrition. *Am. J. Clin. Nutr.* 48:1324–1342.

231. American Medical Association, Department of Foods and Nutrition (1979) Multivitamin preparations for parenteral use—a statement by the Nutrition Advisory Group. *JPEN* 3:258–262.

232. M.G. MacDonald, A.B. Fletcher, E.L. Johnson, R.L. Boeck, P.R. Getson, and M.K. Miller (1987) The potential toxicity to neonates of multivitamin preparations used in parenteral nutrition. *JPEN* 11:169–171.

233. M.C. Moore, H.L. Greene, B. Phillips, et al. (1986) Evaluation of a pediatrics multiple vitamin preparation for total parenteral nutrition in infants and children: I. Blood levels of water-soluble vitamins. *Pediatrics* 77:530–538.

234. B.M. Hamil, M. Coryell, C. Roderuck, et al. (1947) Thiamine, riboflavin, nicotinic acid, panthothenic acid and biotin in the urine of newborn infants. *Am. J. Dis. Child.* 74:434–446.

235. L. Salmenpera, J. Perheentupa, J. Pispa, and M.A. Simes (1985) Biotin concentrations in maternal plasma and milk during prolonged lactation. *Int. J. Vitam. Nutr. Res.* 55:281–285.

236. M.G. Hardinge and H. Crooks (1961) Lesser known vitamins in foods. *J. Am. Diet. Assoc.* 8:240–245.

237. J. Wilson and K. Lorenz (1979) Biotin and choline in foods—nutritional importance and methods of analysis: a review. *Food Chem.* 4:115–129.

238. K. Hoppner and B. Lampi (1983) The biotin content of breakfast cereals. *Nutr. Rep. Int.* 28:793–798.

239. T.R. Guilarte (1985) Analysis of biotin levels in selected foods using a radiometric-microbiological method. *Nutr. Rep. Int.* 32:837–845.

240. K. Hoppner, B. Lampi, and D.C. Smith (1978) An appraisal of the daily intakes of vitamin B_{12}, pantothenic acid and biotin from a composite Canadian diet. *Can. Inst. Food Sci. Technol. J.* 11(2):71–74.

241. N.L. Bull and D.H. Buss (1982) Biotin, panthothenic acid and vitamin E in the British household food supply. *Hum. Nutr. Appl. Nutr.* 36A:190–196.

242. J. Lewis and D.H. Buss (1988) Trace nutrients: minerals and vitamins in the British household food supply. *Br. J. Nutr.* 60:413–424.

Pantothenic Acid

Pantothenic acid was recognized as a growth factor for yeast in 1933.[1] After its isolation in 1939[2,3] and synthesis in 1940 by R.J. Williams and coworkers,[4] D(+)-pantothenate was found to be an essential nutrient for a wide range of animals and birds. The deficiency syndromes in these animals are characterized by growth failure, dermatitis, achromotrichia (graying), adrenal necrosis and hemorrhage, spectacled eyes, spastic gait, anemia, leukopenia, impaired antibody production, infertility, and duodenal ulcer.

Chemistry

Pantothenic acid is an amide consisting of pantoic acid (α,γ-dihydroxy-β,β'-dimethylbutyric acid) joined to β-alanine. The biologically active coenzyme A (CoA), which was discovered by Lipmann and coworkers[5] in 1947 as a cofactor for acetylation, contains pantothenic acid as an essential component. Its structure is shown in Figure 1. In CoA the vitamin is derivatized at its carboxyl end by β-mercaptoethylamine and at its alcoholic end by phosphate to form a pseudodinucleotide-containing adenosine 3',5'-diphosphate. Pantotheine (N-pantothenyl-β-aminoethanethiol) is the functional group of CoA and acyl carrier protein. The vitamin is essential for all living forms and, hence, is widely distributed in nature. Liver, meat, cereal, milk, eggs, fresh vegetables, and many other foods are good sources. The vitamin is measured either by microbiologic assay or radioimmunoassay.

Absorption and Transport

Dietary pantothenate occurs primarily in the form of CoA and pantetheine derivatives. In tomatoes a glycoside of pantothenate exists that was characterized as 4'O-(β-D-glucopyranosyl)-D-pantothenic acid. CoA is hydrolyzed to pantetheine and then to pantothenate by enzymes in the intestinal lumen. Pantothenate is then absorbed in the jejunum by a specific transport system that is saturable and sodium ion dependent.[6] After absorption, the free vitamin is transported to various tissues in the plasma from which it is taken up by most cells via another active-transport process involving cotransport of pantothenate and sodium in a 1:1 ratio.[7] Pantothenic acid is taken up by brain, adipose, and kidney cells by facilitated diffusion and is rapidly phosphorylated. Plasma concentrations of pantothenic acid range from 0.15 to 0.73 μmol/L in various species. Because of the CoA present in blood cells, total pantothenate concentrations in blood range from 0.91 to 2.74 μmol/L.

Biochemical Functions of Coenzyme A

CoA, an acyl carrier protein, and other pantetheine-containing enzymes all employ the free sulfhydryl group of pantetheine as the site for acyl transfer reactions. All known acyl derivatives of CoA and related pantetheine derivatives are thiol esters. These acyl derivatives participate in a number of metabolic reactions involving condensation and addition reactions, acyl group exchange, acyl group transfers, and nucleophilic reactions. In this manner CoA is enzymatically involved in acylation of alcohols, amines, and amino acids (including choline, sulfonamides, p-aminobenzoate, and proteins); oxidation of pyruvate and α-ketoglutarate; and fatty acid β-oxidation. Pantetheine derivatives also are involved in the synthesis of fatty acids, cholesterol, sphingosine, citrate, acetoacetate, 3-hydroxy-3-methylglutarate (HMG), and porphyrins.

4'-Phosphopantetheine is incorporated into acyl carrier protein (molecular weight 10,000), which acts as an acyl carrier in fatty acid synthesis. 4'-Phosphopantetheine also is the prosthetic group of an enzyme system that synthesizes peptide antibiotics, such as gramicidin in bacteria. In the transport of fatty acyl

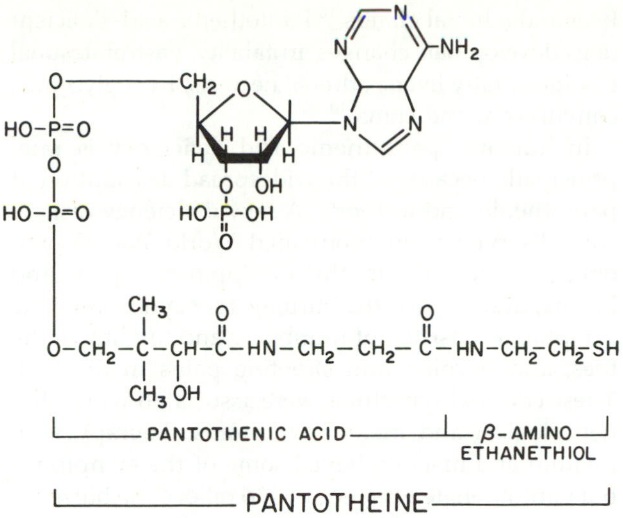

Figure 1. Structure of coenzyme A.

groups across the mitochondrial membrane, fatty acyl coenzyme esters in the cytoplasm react with carnitine to form fatty acyl carnitine esters that reacylate CoA in the mitochondrial matrix where β-oxidation occurs. Some of these reactions are detailed in Table 1.

Biosynthesis and Degradation of Coenzyme A

The currently accepted pathway for the biosynthesis of CoA begins with the phosphorylation of pantothenic acid by a kinase.[8] This reaction appears to be the rate-limiting reaction in CoA synthesis. The 4'-phosphopantothenate then is converted to 4'-phosphopantothenyl cysteine by an ATP-requiring synthetase. The product is decarboxylated to 4'-phosphopantetheine, which is coupled with ATP to generate dephospho-CoA. The dephospho-CoA then is phosphorylated in the 3' position of ribose by ATP to yield CoA. CoA is also the source of pantetheine for acyl carrier protein.

In plants pantothenic acid is derived from α-ketoisovaleric acid, which is converted to ketopantoic acid and to pantoic acid. Pantoic acid is then phosphorylated to yield pantoyl-AMP, which, in the presence of an appropriate enzyme and β-alanine, is converted to pantothenate.

In animal tissues CoA undergoes constant turnover. The degradation of CoA is accomplished by phosphatases, an amidase, and an oxygenase to yield pantothenic acid and hypotaurine. The steps in the catabolism represent a reversal of the steps in the synthesis of CoA.

Antimetabolites of Pantothenic Acid

Omega-methyl PA was used to induce pantothenic acid deficiency in both animals and humans. In this compound the terminal hydroxymethyl group is replaced by a methyl group, which prevents phosphorylation of the analogue and inhibits the action of pantothenic acid kinase. Desthio-CoA, in which the terminal sulfhydryl group is replaced by a hydroxyl, is also inactive as a coenzyme.

Another homologue of pantothenic acid is hopantenate, in which the β-alanine moiety containing three carbons is replaced by the four-carbon γ-aminobutyric acid (GABA) to produce pantoyl-GABA. This compound was synthesized first in 1964 by Fuerst and Li[9] and shortly thereafter was discovered to be a pantothenic acid antagonist, which produced pantothenic acid deficiency in animals.[10] GABA is a central inhibitory neurotransmitter. Mitsuma and Nogimori[11] found that hopantenate inhibited the se-

Table 1. Selected biochemical reactions catalyzed by coenzyme A

Enzyme	Pantothenate derivative	Reactant	Product	Site
Pyruvic dehydrogenase	CoA	Pyruvate	Acetyl CoA	Mitochondria
α-Ketoglutarate dehydrogenase	CoA	α-Ketoglutarate	Succinyl CoA	Mitochondria
Fatty acid oxidase	CoA	Palmitate	Acetyl CoA	Mitochondria
HMG CoA synthetase	CoA	Acetyl CoA Acetoacetyl CoA	HMG CoA	Microsomes
Acyl CoA transferase	CoA	Protein + acyl CoA	Acylproteins + CoA	Cytoplasm
Propionyl CoA carboxylase	CoA	Propionyl CoA Carbon dioxide	Methylmalonyl CoA	Microsomes
(ATP) Acyl CoA synthetase	CoA	ATP + acetate + CoA	Acetyl CoA + ADP + P_i	Cytoplasm
(GTP) Acyl CoA synthetase	CoA	Succinate GTP + CoA	Succinyl CoA GDP + P_i*	Mitochondria
Fatty acid synthetase	Acyl carrier protein	Acetyl CoA Malonyl CoA	Palmitate	Microsomes

* Reaction moves in the opposite direction in tricarboxylic acid cycle.

cretion of the thyrotropin-releasing hormone from rat hypothalmus in vivo.

Nakahiro et al.[12] reported that hopantenate administered intraperitoneally inhibited scopolamine- and atropine-induced locomotor activities in mice but did not inhibit methamphetamine- and apomorphine-induced locomotor activities. In radiolabeled ligand-binding experiments, hopantenate inhibited only that of the GABA agonist [^{3}H]muscimol. These results suggest that hopantenate binds to GABA receptors as a GABA agonist and stimulates cholinergic transmission in the central nervous system.

Schaefer et al.[13] reported that pantothenic acid deficiency in dogs is characterized by sudden prostration, vomiting, convulsions, hypoglycemia, and fatty liver. These symptoms are typical of Reye's syndrome. Reye's syndrome also was noted in three elderly patients who were treated with hopantenate for 4 mo as an aid to memory.[14] Whether Reye's syndrome is a manifestation of pantothenic acid deficiency in humans is open to further study.

Acylation of Tissue Proteins

Plesofsky-Vig and Brambl[15] explored the extent to which CoA-dependent reactions modify protein structure and function. It was estimated that 80% of soluble proteins of Ehrlich ascites cells are acetylated at their amino termini, which occurs cotranslationally. The acetylated proteins are specifically resistant to ubiquitin-dependent proteolysis. The processing of mammalian peptide hormones from polyprotein precursors is accompanied by amino-terminal acetylation of the products. One such compound is pro-opiomelanocortin, which gives rise to adrenocorticotrophic hormone (ACTH), which in turn leads to synthesis of β-lipotropin, α-melanocyte-stimulating hormone, and β-endorphin. All are N-acetylated. Internal amino acids also are acetylated, particularly lysine. These acetylated amino acids influence the organization and stability of such proteins as histones and α-tubulin. Myristate was identified as an aminoterminal amide-linked fatty acid, and palmitate was found in ester linkage with serine.

Pantothenic Acid Deficiency

In rodents, restriction of pantothenic acid in the diet results in growth failure, dermatitis, achromotrichia, bloody whiskers from release of protoporphyrins by the Harderian gland, hemorrhage, necrosis of the adrenals, and impaired antibody production. These pathophysiological effects are accompanied by a reduction in plasma and urinary concentrations of pantothenic acid and are accompanied by a decrease in CoA concentrations in most tissues, particularly the liver and adrenal glands.[16] Pantothenic acid–deficient dogs develop hair changes, irritability, gastrointestinal disorders, fatty livers, adrenal necrosis, hypoglycemia, convulsions, and coma.[13]

In humans, pantothenic acid deficiency is rare, principally because of the widespread distribution of pantothenic acid in foods. A new deficiency disease was observed in malnourished World War II prisoners, particularly in the Philippines, Japan, and Burma, described as the burning-foot syndrome. The symptoms consisted of numbness and tingling in the toes, and burning and shooting pains in the feet. These cardinal symptoms were associated with other neurological and mental symptoms. Therapy with thiamin and niacin relieved some of the symptoms, but pantothenate was required to relieve the burning-foot syndrome, which was later called nutritional erythromelalgia.[17] Furthermore, subjects with this disorder had reduced ability to acetylate p-aminobenzoic acid and a low urinary concentration of pantothenic acid, both of which are suggestive of pantothenic acid deficiency.

Human volunteers fed 1–4 g/d of the antimetabolite ω-methyl pantothenic acid for 12 wk developed vomiting, malaise, abdominal distress, burning cramps, fatigue, insomnia, and paresthesia of hands and feet. The eosinopenic response to ACTH was reduced in these subjects, but adrenocortical function remained within normal limits.[18,19] Three elderly patients receiving 37 mg$\cdot$kg$^{-1}\cdot$d^{-1} of hopantenate developed Reye's syndrome, which includes hepatomegaly, fatty liver, and encephalopathy with coma.[13]

The administration of a purified diet containing no pantothenate to 10 adult human volunteers for 9 wk caused no symptoms or signs related to pantothenate deficiency, although urinary excretion of pantothenic acid decreased from 14.1 to 3.6 μmol/d.[20]

Humans are resistant to pantothenic acid deficiency of dietary origin and require periods of deprivation >12 wk to show signs and symptoms despite low urinary excretion of the vitamin. With antimetabolites to pantothenic acid, however, various syndromes related to nutritional erythromelalgia were produced.

Requirements and Allowances for Pantothenic Acid

Although no Recommended Dietary Allowances (RDA) have been set for pantothenic acid, the 1989 report of the Food and Nutrition Board of the National Research Council[21] on RDA set 4–7 mg/d for adults and 2–5 mg/d for infants and children as safe and adequate daily intakes. These recommendations are based on studies of healthy persons whose intakes, blood levels, and urinary excretion of the vitamin were measured.

Eissenstat et al.[22] studied the nutritional status of 63 healthy adolescents. Dietary intakes of pantothenic acid, which ranged from 1.7 to 12.7 mg/d, were calculated from 4-d diet records. Pantothenic acid concentrations in urine, whole blood, and erythrocytes were determined by radioimmunoassay. Although 49% of females and 15% of males consumed <4 mg/d of pantothenate, average blood concentrations for both groups were in the normal range of 0.91–2.74 μmol/L. Urinary excretion varied from 9.13 to 36.5 μmol/d and was highly correlated with dietary intake.

Song et al[23] studied 17 lactating women who delivered preterm infants between 28 and 34 wk of gestation and 26 nursing mothers of term infants. The average pantothenate concentrations in fore and hind samples of preterm milk (15.0 and 16.9 mmol/L) were higher than those of term milk (11.9 and 11.4 mmol/L).

On intakes of 1.2–9.9 mg/d the concentration of pantothenic acid in human mature milk varied from 6.4 to 30.6 mmol/L. Blood values of pantothenic acid ranged from 1.32 to 3.15 μmol/L. The concentrations of pantothenic acid in milk correlated best with intake and less well with blood values. In a second paper, Song et al.[24] studied 26 pregnant and ultimately lactating women whose dietary pantothenate intake averaged 2.75 mg/1000 kcal. Blood values were in the same range as previously reported.

Summary

Pantothenic acid is a widely distributed vitamin whose biochemical function is expressed in CoA or other pantetheine derivatives. CoA functions as an acyl transfer cofactor in many enzymatic reactions, including those in which the acyl group is enolized to produce unique condensations, such as in citrate synthesis.

Pantothenic acid deficiency can be produced easily in experimental animals but only with difficulty in humans, who require long-term deprivation to manifest nutritional erythromelalgia. Recommended safe and adequate intakes of pantothenic acid set by the Food and Nutrition Board are 4–7 mg/d, which will maintain blood pantothenic acid concentrations of 1.37–2.74 μmol/L. The recommended lower amount of 4 mg/d may be too high because many persons, including pregnant females, appear to remain healthy on intakes <4 mg/d. No RDA for pantothenic acid has yet been set.

References

1. R.J. Williams, C.M. Lyman, G.H. Goodyear, J.H. Truesdail, and D. Holaday (1933) "Pantothenic acid," a growth determinant of universal biological occurrence. J. Am. Chem. Soc. 55:2912–2927.

2. R.J. Williams (1939) Pantothenic acid—a vitamin. Science 89:486.

3. R.J. Williams, H.H. Weinstock, Jr., E. Rohrmann, J.H. Truesdail, H.K. Mitchell, and C.E. Meyer (1939) Pantothenic acid. III. Analysis and determination of constituent groups. J. Am. Chem. Soc. 61:454–457.

4. R.J. Williams and R.T. Major (1940) The structure of pantothenic acid. Science 91:246.

5. F. Lipmann, N.O. Kaplan, G.D. Novelli, L.C. Tuttle, and B.M. Guirard (1947) Coenzyme for acetylation, a pantothenic acid derivative. J. Biol. Chem. 167:869–870.

6. D.K. Fenstermacher and R.C. Rose (1986) Absorption of pantothenic acid in rat and chick intestine. Am. J. Physiol. 250:G155–G160.

7. C.M. Smith and R.E. Milner (1985) The mechanism of pantothenate transport by rat liver parenchymal cells in primary culture. J. Biol. Chem. 260:4823–4831.

8. J.D. Robishaw and J.R. Neely (1985) Coenzyme A metabolism. Am. J. Physiol. 248:E1–E9.

9. R. Fuerst and L. Li (1964) A study of the synthesis of γ-pantothenate by Neurospora. Biochim. Biophys. Acta 86:26–32.

10. F. Matsuzaki (1965) Antagonistic action of homopantothenate against pantothenic acid. Vitamin (Japan) 32:245–259.

11. T. Mitsuma and T. Nogimori (1983) Effects of calcium hopantenate on the hypothalamic-pituitary-thyroid axis in rats. Horm. Res. 18:210–214.

12. M. Nakahiro, N. Fujita, I. Fukuchi, K. Saito, T. Nishimura, and H. Yoshida (1985) Pantoyl-γ-aminobutyric acid facilitates cholinergic function in the central nervous system. J. Pharmacol. Exp. Ther. 232:501–506.

13. A.E. Schaefer, J.M. McKibbin, and C.A. Elvehjem (1942) Pantothenic acid deficiency studies in dogs. J. Biol. Chem. 143:321–330.

14. S. Noda, H. Umezaki, K. Yamamoto, T. Araki, T. Murakami, and N. Ishii (1988) Reye-like syndrome following treatment with the pantothenic acid antagonist, calcium hopantenate. J. Neurol. Neurosurg. Psychiatry 51:582–585.

15. N. Plesofsky-Vig and R. Brambl (1988) Pantothenic acid and coenzyme A in cellular modification of proteins. Annu. Rev. Nutr. 8:461–482.

16. R.E. Olson and N.O. Kaplan (1948) The effect of pantothenic acid deficiency upon coenzyme A content and pyruvate utilization of rat and duck tissues. J. Biol. Chem. 175:515–529.

17. M. Glusman (1947) The syndrome of "burning feet" (nutritional melalgia) as manifestation of nutritional deficiency. Am. J. Med. 3:211–223.

18. R.E. Hodges, M.A. Ohlson, and W.B. Bean (1958) Pantothenic acid deficiency in man. J. Clin. Invest. 37:1642–1657.

19. R.E. Hodges, W.B. Bean, M.A. Ohlson, and R. Bleiler (1959) Human pantothenic acid deficiency produced by omega-methyl pantothenic acid. J. Clin. Invest. 38:1421–1425.

20. P.C. Fry, H.M. Fox, and H.G. Tao (1976) Metabolic response to a pantothenic-acid-deficient diet in humans. J. Nutr. Sci. Vitaminol. (Tokyo) 22:339–346.

21. National Research Council (1989) Recommended Dietary Allowances, 10th ed., National Academy Press, Washington, DC.

22. B.R. Eissenstat, B.W. Wyse, and R.G. Hansen (1986) Pantothenic acid status of adolescents. Am. J. Clin. Nutr. 44:931–937.

23. W.O. Song, G.M. Chan, B.W. Wyse, and R.G. Hansen (1984) Effect of pantothenic acid status on the content of the vitamin in human milk. Am. J. Clin. Nutr. 40:317–324.

24. W.O. Song, B.W. Wyse, and R.G. Hansen (1985) Pantothenic acid status of pregnant and lactating women. J. Am. Diet. Assoc. 85:192–198.

Chapter **24**   Claude D. Arnaud and Sarah D. Sanchez

Calcium and Phosphorus

Calcium and phosphorus occupy central places in biology. They are responsible for structural functions involving the skeleton and soft tissues and for such regulatory functions as neuromuscular transmission of chemical and electrical stimuli, cellular secretion, blood clotting, oxygen transport, and enzymatic activity. Calcium is the most abundant divalent cation in the human body, making up 1.5–2% of its total weight. More than 99% of body calcium and 85% of body phosphorus is present in the skeleton.

All living things possess powerful mechanisms both to conserve calcium and to maintain constant cellular and extracellular fluid (ECF) concentrations.[1-3] In fact, the physiologic functions subserved by calcium are so vital to survival that in the face of severe dietary deficiency or abnormal losses from the body these same mechanisms are capable of demineralizing bone to prevent even minor degrees of hypocalcemia. Bone provides a vital and readily available source of calcium for the maintenance of normal ECF calcium concentrations, ~50% of which is ionized (Ca^{2+}) and physiologically active.

The endocrine system that helps maintain calcium and phosphorus homeostasis in vertebrates is highly integrated and complex.[4,5] It involves an interplay between the actions of two polypeptide hormones, parathyroid hormone (PTH)[6] and calcitonin (CT),[7] and a sterol hormone, 1,25-dihydroxycholecalciferol [1,25$(OH)_2D_3$].[8] Biosynthesis and secretion of the polypeptide hormones are regulated by a negative feedback mechanism that involves the activity of ionic calcium in the extracellular fluid. The biosynthesis of 1,25$(OH)_2D_3$ from the major circulating metabolite of vitamin D, 25-hydroxycholecalciferol (25OHD$_3$), takes place in the kidney and is regulated by PTH and CT as well as by the extracellular fluid concentrations of calcium and phosphate. Other hormones, such as insulin, cortisol, growth hormone, thyroxine, epinephrine, estrogen, testosterone, and somatomedin, together with some compounds not yet identified and certain physical phenomena, undoubtedly have roles in modifying and regulating organ responses to PTH, CT, and 1,25$(OH)_2D_3$.[9]

The relationships among the several components involved in maintaining mineral homeostasis are illustrated in Figure 1.[2] Each of the three overlapping feedback loops involves one of the target organs of the calciotropic hormones and the four controlling elements, i.e., plasma calcium, PTH, CT, and 1,25$(OH)_2D_3$. The left limbs of the loops depict physiologic events that increase plasma calcium, and the right limbs, events that decrease plasma calcium. Under physiologic conditions there are small fluctuations in plasma calcium. Decreases in plasma calcium increase PTH secretion and decrease CT secretion. These changes in hormone secretion lead to increased bone resorption, decreased renal excretion of calcium, and increased intestinal calcium absorption via PTH stimulation of 1,25$(OH)_2D_3$ production (left side of figure). As a consequence of these events, plasma calcium increases slightly above its physiologic concentrations, inhibiting PTH secretion and stimulating CT secretion. These changes in plasma hormone concentrations decrease bone resorption, increase renal excretion of calcium, and decrease intestinal absorption of calcium (right side of figure), causing plasma calcium to decrease slightly below the physiologic concentration. This sequence of events occurs within milliseconds and is constantly repeated so that plasma calcium is maintained at physiologic concentrations with minimal oscillation. The "butterfly" scheme in the figure not only demonstrates the relationships among elements that control mineral homeostasis under physiologic conditions but also illustrates adaptive responses to various specific perturbations.

Plasma Calcium and Phosphate

Plasma calcium is distributed in three major fractions: ionized, protein bound, and complexed.[10] The

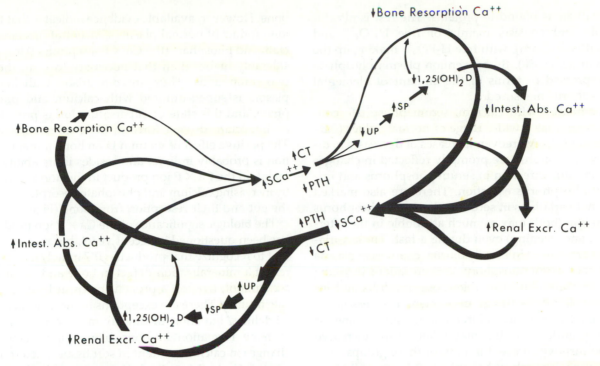

Figure 1. Regulation of calcium homeostasis. Three overlapping control loops interlock and relate to one another through the level of blood concentrations of ionic calcium, PTH and CT. Each loop involves a calciotropic hormone target organ (bone, intestine, kidney). The limbs on the left depict physiologic events that increase the blood concentration of calcium (SCa^{2+}), and the limbs on the right, events that decrease this concentration. UP, urine phosphorus; SP, serum phosphorus. From reference 2. (Used with permission.)

ionized form (Ca^{2+}), the only biologically active species, constitutes 46–50% of the total calcium. The protein-bound fraction, roughly equivalent to the ionized fraction in amount, is biologically inert. However, the calcium bound to albumin (80%) and globulin (20%) is important because it provides a readily available reservoir for this important cation. Because the binding of calcium to these proteins obeys the mass-law equation, calcium can dissociate from its binding sites as a first-line defense against hypocalcemia. Moreover, hyperproteinemia (e.g., hyperglobulinemia in myelomatosis) can increase and hypoproteinemia (e.g., hypoalbuminemia in cirrhosis of the liver and nephrosis) can decrease total plasma calcium without changing the concentration of ionized calcium. The only means of accurately determining the plasma concentration of ionized calcium in hypoproteinemic or hyperproteinemic states is to measure it directly by an ion-sensitive electrode procedure. The fraction of calcium that is complexed to organic (e.g., citrate) and inorganic (e.g., phosphate or sulfate) acids is small (~8%) and like the ionized fraction it is ultrafiltrable (diffusible). Complexed calcium probably has little quantitative importance as a reservoir for ionized calcium, but in states of hyperphosphatemia such as may exist in chronic renal failure, excessive complexing of calcium with

phosphate may contribute to the decrease in plasma ionized calcium observed in this condition.

The normal range for total serum calcium is narrow (2.2–2.5 mmol/L), and the same is true for the ionized fraction. Thus values for total calcium below 2.2 mmol/L, assuming that plasma protein concentrations are normal, reflect clinically significant hypocalcemia, and values >2.5 mmol/L reflect hypercalcemia. Hypocalcemia produces a myriad of symptoms and when severe can result in tetany and possibly convulsions.[11] Hypercalcemia can produce functional changes in most organ systems, and these changes may lead to a confusing variety of symptoms and objective findings.[12]

The serum calcium concentration varies little in spite of large changes in dietary calcium because of the adaptive alteration in the endocrine system regulating this mineral (Figure 1). Minor diurnal changes (decreases in the afternoon) have been recorded. In addition, serum calcium concentration decreases with age in men but not in women, probably because of a decrease in serum albumin concentration in men. Total (but not ionized) serum calcium concentration also decreases in pregnancy, and this change may be due to the decrease in serum albumin concentration caused by plasma volume expansion.

In contrast to plasma calcium, only 15% of plasma

phosphate is bound to proteins. The rest is ultrafiltrable and consists mainly of free HPO_4^{2-} and $NaHPO_4^{1-}$ (85%), with free $H_2PO_4^{1-}$ making up the remainder (15%). By convention plasma phosphate is expressed in terms of the amount of elemental phosphorus measured.

Compared with calcium, serum phosphate concentration has a wider range of normal values (0.8–1.0 mmol/L). Moreover, increases or decreases in dietary phosphorus are promptly reflected in changes in the same direction in serum phosphorus and urinary phosphorus excretion. There are also marked diurnal variations in serum and urinary phosphorus excretion (both may as much as double in the afternoon and evening) even during a fast. These variations are caused in part by diurnal changes in plasma cortisol. Serum phosphorus concentrations in young children are almost double those in adults and increase slightly with age in women. The reason for these differences in children and in aging women is poorly understood but may relate to the increased bone turnover present in both of these groups.

Severe hypophosphatemia (<0.5 mmol/L) can cause both skeletal myopathy and cardiomyopathy.[10] These conditions may lead to rhabdomyolysis. The levels of 2,3-diphosphoglyceric acid and adenosine triphosphate (ATP) in erythrocytes may also decrease; the decrease in 2,3-diphosphoglyceric acid in turn may decrease oxygen delivery to tissues, and the decrease in ATP may cause hemolytic anemia. Chronic moderate hypophosphatemia frequently results in osteomalacia or rickets. Generally, restoration of serum phosphate concentration to normal corrects abnormal organ function in hypophosphatemic conditions.

Acute, severe hyperphosphatemia as might be induced by intravenous phosphate infusion can cause hypocalcemia sufficiently severe as to result in tetany and even death.[10] The less severe hyperphosphatemia induced by phosphate ingestion rarely causes symptoms; however, if patients have associated disorders in which there is a tendency toward hypocalcemia (e.g., mild hypoparathyroidism or chronic renal failure), frank hypocalcemia can be precipitated.

Interrelation of Plasma Calcium and Phosphorus

The physiologic importance of the relationship between the circulating concentrations of ionized calcium and diffusible (free) phosphate is poorly understood especially with regard to the formation and dissolution of amorphous calcium phosphate [$Ca_3(PO_4)_2$] and hydroxyapatite [$Ca_{10}(PO_4)_6(OH)_6$] in bone. However, available evidence indicates that the ion product of normal plasma concentrations of calcium and phosphate (the Ca × P ion product) is considerably higher than that necessary to form these two compounds. Thus, in comparison with bone, plasma is supersaturated with calcium and phosphate, and this state of supersaturation is probably an important driving force in bone mineralization. The positive effect of vitamin D on bone mineralization is probably indirect and resides in its ability to maintain the Ca × P ion product in the normal range by increasing calcium and phosphate absorption from the gut and their resorption from bone (Figure 1).

The biologic significance of the Ca × P ion product has been questioned in recent years, but it is important to recognize that products <0.7 mmol/L usually reflect a mineralization defect in bone and products >2.2 mmol/L reflect a propensity toward soft tissue calcification. There are exceptions to these numerical guidelines, but short of directly measuring changes in bone formation in bone biopsy specimens or changes in calcium content in soft tissues, determining the Ca × P ion product may provide the best indirect indication of the presence of these pathologic changes.

Calcium and Phosphate Economy

The amounts of dietary calcium and phosphate required to maintain metabolic balance (dietary intake equal to urinary and fecal excretion) vary with the physiologic need for these minerals, the ability of the intestine to absorb them, and the ability of the kidneys to conserve them.[10]

Dietary deprivation of calcium or phosphorus induces adaptive changes in the production and secretion of the calciotropic hormones that minimize the development of negative balance of these two ions (Figure 1). In the case of calcium, only 30–50% of ingested calcium is normally absorbed (fractional absorption). With decreased intake serum calcium decreases slightly, and the sequence of events depicted in the left limbs of the feedback loops in the figure is activated. In severe chronic dietary deficiency of calcium in normal subjects, PTH stimulates an increase in plasma $1,25(OH)_2D_3$ concentration, which can increase fractional intestinal calcium absorption up to 75%. It also reduces renal calcium excretion to low concentrations, but this response is quantitatively less important because of the relatively small percentage of filtered calcium that is excreted. Such changes reduce the overall consequences of this perturbation on overall body calcium economy. However, the tradeoff for this adaptive response is chronic hyperparathyroidism, a condition that can induce progressive demineralization of bones. Thus, as is the case for most adaptive mechanisms in biology, they are beneficial when applied over a relatively short period of time, but when applied chronically, they can have destructive effects of considerable consequence.

Whereas the intestine plays the major role in the body's adaptation to a dietary deficiency of calcium, the kidney plays the major role in maintaining phosphate balance during dietary deficiency of this mineral. This is because 70–80% of dietary phosphorus is normally absorbed and practically all (≥80%) of absorbed phosphorus is excreted by the kidney. Thus, any increase in intestinal absorption of phosphorus in response to dietary deprivation would have little influence in preventing negative balance, but reducing its renal excretion by only 50%, for example, would have an effect comparable to that of almost tripling dietary intake. Reductions of this magnitude and greater occur rapidly and are sustained for long periods of time in response to dietary deprivation of phosphorus. The mechanism involved in this response is not entirely understood. The hypophosphatemia that occurs in phosphate deficiency is associated with increased production of $1,25(OH)_2D_3$, increased intestinal absorption of calcium, mild hypercalcemia, and a decrease in PTH secretion (Figure 1, left, middle limb), increased renal tubular reabsorption of phosphate, and hypophosphaturia. However, it is well established that efficient renal phosphate conservation in response to dietary phosphate deprivation occurs in parathyroidectomized animals, a finding that casts doubt upon whether the calciotropic hormone response to phosphorus deprivation is singularly responsible for the observed hypophosphaturia in this condition.

Bone

As a living tissue bone is unique in that it is not only rigid and resists forces that would ordinarily break brittle materials but is also light enough to be moved by coordinated muscle contractions.[13] These characteristics are functions of the strategic locations of two major types of bone. Cortical bone, composed of densely packed mineralized collagen laid down in layers, provides rigidity and is the major component of tubular bones. Trabecular (cancellous) bone is spongy in appearance, provides strength and elasticity, and constitutes the major portion of the axial skeleton. Disorders in which cortical bone is defective or scanty lead to fractures of the long bones, whereas disorders in which trabecular bone is defective or scanty lead to vertebral fractures. Fractures of long bones also may occur because normal trabecular bone reinforcement is lacking.

Two-thirds of the weight of bone is due to mineral and the remainder to water and collagen. Minor organic components, such as proteoglycans, lipids, noncollagenous proteins, and acidic proteins containing γ-carboxyglutamic acid, are probably very important, but their functions are poorly understood.

The mineral of bone is present in two forms. The major form consists of hydroxyapatite in crystals of various maturity. The remainder is amorphous calcium phosphate, which lacks a coherent x-ray diffraction pattern, has a lower calcium-to-phosphate ratio than pure hydroxyapatite, occurs in regions of active bone formation, and is present in larger quantities in young bone.

Bone is resorbed and formed continuously throughout life, and these important processes are dependent upon three major types of bone cells, each with different functions. Osteoblasts form new bone on surfaces of bone previously resorbed by osteoclasts. The osteoblasts are thought to be derived from a population of dividing cells on bone surfaces that arise from mesenchymal cells in bone connective tissue. Osteoblasts are actively involved in the synthesis of matrix components of bone (primary collagen) and probably facilitate the movement of mineral ions between extracellular fluid and bone surfaces. The physiologic importance of such ion transport by osteoblasts, if it occurs at all, is controversial, but there is widespread agreement that osteoblast-mediated transport of calcium and phosphate is involved in the mineralization of collagen, which in turn is crucial to the formation of bone. In the process of bone formation, osteoblasts gradually become encased in the bone matrix that they have produced.

Once osteoblasts are trapped in the mineralized matrix, their functional and morphologic characteristics change, and they are then called osteocytes. Protein synthetic activity decreases markedly, and the cells develop multiple processes that reach out through lacunae in bone tissue to "communicate" with processes of other osteocytes within a unit of bone (osteon) and also with the cell processes of surface osteoblasts. The physiologic importance of osteocytes is controversial, but they are believed to act as a cellular syncytium that permits translocation of mineral in and out of regions of bone removed from surfaces.

The osteoclast is a multinucleated giant cell that is responsible for bone resorption. It is probably derived from circulating mononucleated macrophages, which differentiate into the mature osteoclasts by fusion in the bone environment. These cells contain all of the enzymatic components that, when secreted into their environs, are capable of solubilizing matrix and releasing calcium and phosphate. Once released, mineral is transported through the osteoclast into the extracellular fluid and ultimately into blood. Opinion has varied over the years concerning the relative importance to extracellular mineral homeostasis of resorption of bone by osteoclasts and of the translocation of mineral from the surface of bone into the extracellular space by surface osteoblasts.

Microscopically, there are two types of bone structure: woven and lamellar. Both may be found in either cortical or trabecular bone. However, whereas woven bone is a normal constituent of embryonic bone, it usually reflects the presence of disease in adult bone. Lamellar bone is stronger than woven bone and is formed more slowly. It progressively replaces woven bone as the skeleton develops after birth. Whereas woven bone is characterized by nonparallelism of collagen fibers, many osteocytes per unit area of matrix, and mineral that is poorly incorporated into collagen fibrils, lamellar bone has a parallel arrangement of collagen fibers, few osteocytes per unit area of matrix, and a mineral phase that is within the collagen fibrils. Cortical lamellar bone is present in concentric layers surrounding vascular channels that comprise the haversian systems of cortical bone (osteons). By contrast, the lamellar bone of trabeculae is present in layers and is laid down in long sheaves and sheets.

The term *modeling* as applied to bone denotes processes involved in formation of the macroscopic skeleton. Thus, modeling ceases at maturity (age 18–20 y). The term *remodeling* denotes processes occurring at bone surfaces before and after adult development that are required to maintain the structural integrity of bone. Abnormalities of remodeling are responsible for metabolic bone diseases. These abnormalities involve alterations in the balance between bone formation and bone resorption that lead to diminished structural integrity of bone and ultimately compromise its functions.

Normally, in spite of continuous bone remodeling, there is no net gain or loss of skeletal mass after longitudinal growth has ceased. This finding led to the view that bone resorption and formation are closely coupled and that coupling is the result of the coordinated activity of packets of interacting osteoblasts and osteoclasts. These packets have been called basic multicellular units. The temporal activity of such a unit is characterized by osteoclastic resorption of a defined quantity of bone (on the surface in trabecular bone and by actual excavation in cortical bone) followed by repair of the defect by osteoblasts. Such repair occurs as a result of laying down of collagen (osteoid) and its subsequent mineralization.

Thus, the driving force for changing net bone mass is intrinsic to the cellular processes that govern bone resorption and formation, and functional uncoupling of these cellular processes is required to either increase or decrease bone mass. By contrast, the major mineral ions of bone (calcium, phosphorus, and magnesium) play a more passive role in any mass changes that occur in bone. They must be present at physiologic concentrations in extracellular fluids for bone mineralization (formation) to occur normally. Dietary minerals contribute to this physiologic state by helping to replace minerals that have been lost either by obligatory processes (in urine, stool, and sweat) or by normal distribution to bone and soft tissues. Hence, calcium balance generally reflects the degree of coupling of bone formation and resorption. Negative balances are recorded when bone resorption exceeds formation, and positive balances are recorded when bone formation exceeds bone resorption.

Osteoporosis

Osteoporosis is a disease characterized by an absolute decrease in bone mass that results in an increased susceptibility to fracture especially at the wrist, spine, and hip. It is common in postmenopausal women and in elderly persons of both sexes and constitutes an important public health problem.[14–21]

The level of bone mass achieved at skeletal maturity (peak or maximal bone mass) is one major factor modifying the risk of development of osteoporosis. The more bone mass that is available before the period of age-related bone loss, the less likely it will decrease to a level at which fracture will occur.[22–24] Normally, longitudinal bone growth is complete sometime during the second decade of life. It is axiomatic that positive calcium balance is needed for growth to occur normally, and it is easy to calculate that the required average daily body retention of calcium during this 20-y period is in the range of 110 mg/d for females and 140 mg/d for males. During the adolescent growth spurt, the required calcium retention is two to three times higher than the average value.[25,26] To achieve such retention, the Food and Nutrition Board[27] recommends intakes of 1200 mg/d for persons 11–18 y of age. If obligate losses of calcium (in the urine, stool, and sweat) are not greater than average, such calcium intakes are adequate assuming that fractional absorption of calcium in these individuals is in the range of 50%. Fractional absorption below this percentage or calcium intakes <1200 mg/d without appropriate increases in fractional absorption would not provide adequate quantities of calcium to achieve peak longitudinal bone growth. It is not known whether teenagers have such levels of calcium absorption or whether they can routinely attain the increased absorption levels that would be required if calcium intakes were low.

Opinion is mixed as to the age at which peak bone mass is achieved. Data concerning this issue are available only from studies using cross-sectional designs. These studies show that values for measurements of metacarpal cortical area,[25] phalangeal density,[28] combined cortical thickness,[29] and bone mineral content of the spine[30] do not appear to reach maximum levels until sometime during the middle of the third or early in the fourth decade of life. Such data suggest that peak bone mass may not be achieved until 5–10 y after longitudinal bone growth has ceased. It is thought that cortical porosity, which is increased during the adolescent growth spurt, is filled in and that the bone cortices become thicker during this period. The quantity of bone mass that can be added is not known, but it is variously estimated to be in the range of 5–10%.[23] The optimum calcium retention needed to achieve this apparent increment in bone mass is not yet known but is probably in the range of 0.99–1.50 mmol/d. That this increment in bone mass may be related to calcium intake is suggested by the results of a Yugoslavian study in which there was a 5–10% higher metacarpal bone mass in the inhabitants of the high-calcium district starting at age 30 y and extending throughout the age range of the investigation, that is, 30–75 y of age.[29]

As is the case with the need to maintain positive calcium balance to complete longitudinal bone growth, it is logical that the quantity of calcium derived from the diet that might be required to achieve peak bone mass would be greater than that required to replace obligatory losses of this ion in urine, stool, and sweat (~50–75 mmol/d). Thus, the period during which positive calcium balance needs to be maintained to achieve peak bone mass has been extended in the 1989 RDA to include the 19–24-y age group.

The other major factor modifying osteoporosis risk is the rate at which bone is lost as life progresses. After peak bone mass is achieved, bone mass appears to be maintained without much change until age 40–45 y. Subsequently, bone is lost at a rate of 0.2–0.5%/y in both men and women until the eighth or ninth decade of life. However, bone loss accelerates to 2.0–5.0%/y immediately before and for ~10 y after menopause, after which time the rate of bone loss returns to the 0.2–0.5%/y rate.[24]

Intestinal calcium absorption and the ability to adapt to low-calcium diets are impaired in many postmenopausal women[24,31,32] and elderly persons.[33–38] The pathogenesis of these abnormalities is controversial, but available evidence suggests that they may be due to a functional decrease in the ability of the kidney to produce $1,25(OH)_2D_3$ in postmenopause[38,39] and an absolute decrease in old age.[40] The findings that serum immunoreactive parathyroid hormone[41–45] and bioactive parathyroid hormone[46] increase with age imply that these defects in calcium absorption are functionally important in that they result in sufficient degrees of hypocalcemia to produce chronic hyperparathyroidism (secondary hyperparathyroidism). It is well established that hyperparathyroidism increases the bone remodeling rate and that a high remodeling rate leads to accelerated bone loss whenever intrinsic imbalance in the remodeling apparatus favors the process of resorption over formation.[47,48]

Thus, it appears that the ability of the intestine to support calcium homeostasis progressively declines with age and that elderly persons are forced, more and more, to rely on their own bones rather than the external environment as a source of calcium for maintaining normal ECF Ca^{2+}.[49] The degree to which this tradeoff (bone demineralization for calcium homeostasis) is needed depends upon the severity of the described defects in calcium absorption, the amount and bioavailability of dietary calcium, and whether specific therapeutic means are taken to correct defects in calcium absorption. The quantitative contribution, if any, of the tradeoff to decreased bone mass and increased incidence of fractures seen in elderly persons is not known and is the subject of intensive investigation.

Calcium Intake and Bone Mass

A number of published reports showed either no relationship or only a modestly positive relationship between dietary calcium and cortical bone mass. Garn et al.[50] found the same rate of loss of metacarpal cortical mass in >5,800 subjects from seven countries despite wide variations in calcium intake among groups. In fact, low calcium intakes in some ethnic groups were associated with bone mass values higher than in others ingesting high lifelong calcium intakes. On the other hand, in the Ten-State Nutrition Survey, Garn et al.[51] found a statistically significant increase in metacarpal cortical area in persons determined to be in the highest as compared with the lowest percentile of calcium intake. In a similar analysis using data available from the HANES I study,[52,53] Stanton (M.F. Stanton, unpublished observation, 1980) found a significant positive correlation between calcium intake and metacarpal cortical width for all subjects (n = 2250). When white women (n = 960) were excluded, the significance of the correlation disappeared.

Matkovic et al.[29] investigated metacarpal bone mass and the incidence of hip fracture in two regions of Yugoslavia whose inhabitants ingested greatly different quantities of calcium (500 vs. 1100 mg/d, contained largely in dairy products). The inhabitants of the high-calcium district ingested more calories, fat, and protein and less carbohydrate than did inhabitants of the low-calcium district. However, the regions were similar in their agrarian economy and, except for a significantly longer lower limb length in the high-calcium district, the inhabitants' age, weight, and other anthropomorphic indices were identical. The inhabitants of the high-calcium district had a 50% lower incidence of hip fractures and a significant increase in metacarpal cortical bone volume than did the inhabitants of the low-calcium district. Because the differences in bone mass as a function of age were constant, it is likely that high lifelong intakes of calcium in this population increased peak cortical bone mass rather than preventing bone loss. In contrast to the decreased incidence in hip fractures observed in the high-calcium district, the incidence of fractures of the distal forearm (distal 3 cm of the radius or ulna) was the same in the two regions. This finding is of interest because the sites of fracture at the hip generally are considered to be composed mainly of cortical bone whereas those at the wrist are mainly of trabecular bone. The results of a study reported by Anderson and Tylavsky[54] are highly relevant in this regard. These investigators related current and lifelong calcium intake to bone mineral content (BMC) measured by single-photon absorptiometry (SPA) at the distal radius (mixture of cortical and trabecular bone) and at the midshaft of the radius (largely cortical bone) in residents of four North Carolina communities. They found a positive correlation of BMC with calcium intake at the midshaft site but no correlation at the distal site.

Several clinical studies examined the relationship of calcium intake to bone mass. Using radiogrammetry, Smith and Frame,[55] Smith and Rizak,[56] and Garn[25] found no relation between current calcium intake and current bone mass. Similarly, Laval-Jeanet et al.[57] and Pacifici et al.[58] showed no correlation of calcium intake to vertebral density as measured by quantitative computed tomography (QCT). Most recently, Riggs et al.[59] found no relationship between calcium intakes (range 260–2003 mg/d, mean 922 mg/d) of 106 normal women, aged 23–84 y, and the rates of change in bone mineral density at the midradius (determined by SPA) and the lumbar spine [determined by dual-photon absorptiometry (DPA)] over a mean period of 4.1 y.

In contrast to the negative observations made by Laval-Jeanet et al.[57] and by Pacifici et al.[58] using QCT of the spine, Kanders et al.[60] found an increase in the BMC of L2–L4 vertebrae by using DPA in young women with a high calcium intake as compared with those with a low intake. In addition, in a longitudinal study of 76 healthy postmenopausal women, Dawson-Hughes et al.[61] found that women with dietary intakes of <405 mg/d lost spinal bone density (DPA) at a significantly greater rate than those with an intake of >777 mg/d ($p < 0.026$).

Calcium Intake and Osteoporosis

Nordin[62] reported the results of an international investigation of calcium intake and osteoporotic fractures. In spite of inconsistent methods in the reporting of calcium intakes by the countries involved in the study, it was possible to demonstrate an inverse rank-order relation between calcium intakes and osteoporotic vertebral fracture frequency (spine x ray). Japanese women, whose calcium intake averaged 400 mg/d, had the highest frequency of fracture, whereas Finnish women, with the highest intake (1300 mg/ d), had the lowest fracture frequency. This relationship did not hold for some countries. Although calcium intakes in Gambia and Jamaica were low, osteoporotic fractures were rare. As noted in the study reported by Matkovic et al.,[29] the hip fracture incidence in the Yugoslav district with a high-calcium intake was 50% lower than in the low-calcium district. However, no difference was detected in the incidence of fractures about the wrist.

Most clinical studies of dietary calcium in osteoporotic patients show lower intakes than in age-matched control subjects.[63–67] Although dietary calcium was <800 mg/d in both patients and controls in all of these investigations, intakes were >800 mg/ d in a study in which no differences in calcium intake between osteoporotic patients and controls were demonstrated.[26] The results of this latter study support Heaney's view[24] that low dietary calcium may play a permissive rather than a causative role in the development of osteoporosis and that this role can be demonstrated best when dietary calcium is below a saturation level.

Effect of Calcium Supplementation on Bone Mass

The long-term effects of calcium supplementation on bone mass have not been established. The results of short-term investigations (≤2 y) are mixed. In general, they show a slowing of bone loss measured at sites comprised mostly of cortical bone but not at sites comprised of trabecular bone. All studies using estrogen treatment as a companion protocol showed that calcium supplementation is inferior to estrogen in slowing cortical bone loss and that estrogen prevents trabecular bone loss completely. Some of these studies were randomized[68–72] but only two were double blind.[70,72] The Smith study[70] lost 40% of the subjects to follow-up. The results of a study performed by Recker et al.[68] reflects those of the others. It showed that after 2 y, a supplement of 1.04 g elemental calcium, given as the carbonate salt, to 22 women between 55 and 65 y of age resulted in a 0.22% decrease in metacarpal cortical bone area as compared with a 1.18% decrease in 20 placebo-treated, age-matched women ($p < 0.05$). By contrast, there was no difference in bone mineral content of the distal radius (mixture of trabecular and cortical bone). The effect of calcium supplementation to prevent metacarpal cortical bone loss was less than the effect of estrogen treatment in 18 age-matched women, and estrogen completely prevented bone loss at the distal radius. In a similar but nonrandomized study, Horsman et al.[73] administered 800 mg elemental calcium as the gluconate salt to 24 postmenopausal women over a 2-y period and found a significant decrease in bone loss from the ulna (cortical bone) as compared with 18 placebo-treated control subjects. However, calcium treatment caused little if any diminution of the bone loss observed at the distal radius or in metacarpal cortices. Similarly, Nilas et al.[74] found no change in bone mineral content at the distal radius when three groups of women with calcium intakes varying from <550 to >1150 mg/d were administered a 500 mg elemental calcium supplement daily. However, an investigation performed by the same group,[72] which was both randomized and double blind, found that the administration of 2000 mg/d elemental calcium as the carbonate salt for 2 y to postmenopausal women slowed bone loss at the proximal forearm and slowed calcium loss from the total skeleton, whereas the loss of bone from sites composed predominantly of trabecular bone was no different from that of placebo-treated control subjects. As in previous studies bone mineral content remained constant at all measurement sites in subjects receiving estrogen. In a nonrandomized study Ettinger et al.[75] found no effect of calcium supplementation up to 1500 mg/d as the carbonate salt on bone mineral content in the spine as assessed by QCT, distal radius, or metacarpal cortical bone mass in 44 postmenopausal women as compared with 25 age-matched women who elected not to receive treatment. By contrast, 15 women who elected to take low-dose conjugated estrogen (0.3 mg/d) combined with 1500 mg calcium/d demonstrated complete protection against bone loss. This latter observation is of considerable theoretical and practical interest because these investigators[76] previously demonstrated that conjugated estrogen at the same low dose, given without calcium, failed to prevent vertebral bone loss. Thus, it is possible that dietary calcium may play a permissive role in the maintenance of bone mass that is sex-hormone dependent.

Riggs et al.[77] showed that the increased bone resorption surface observed in iliac crest bone biopsies from osteoporotic patients are restored toward normal by combined calcium and vitamin D supplementation. This effect was associated with a decrease in serum immunoreactive parathyroid hormone (iPTH) within the normal range, an event the authors justifiably speculated was responsible for the decrease in resorption surfaces. The results of several other investigations, not involving bone histomorphometry, are consistent with this apparent antiresorption effect of calcium supplementation. Recker et al.[68] showed that bone resorption, as assessed by kinetic analysis of plasma ^{45}Ca-decay curves, was decreased by supplementation of postmenopausal women with calcium carbonate. Horowitz et al.[78] reported that oral calcium suppresses hydroxyproline excretion, a well-established index of bone resorption, in osteoporotic postmenopausal women.

The evidence relating calcium supplementation to fracture prevalence is scanty. The only study of substance comes from the Mayo Clinic,[79] which reported a nonrandomized but prospective assessment of the effect of various treatments of patients with generalized osteopenia on the occurrence of future vertebral fractures. In the study 8 individuals received calcium carbonate (1500–2500 mg/d) and 19 received calcium plus vitamin D (50,000 U once or twice a week). Both groups had 50% fewer vertebral fractures than did 27 placebo-treated and 18 untreated patients.

Calcium treatment is safe in the absence of conditions that cause hypercalcemia or nephrolithiasis.[80] Thus, in normal individuals calcium intakes ranging from 1000 to 2500 mg/d do not result in hypercalcemia[81] and extremely high intakes (>2500 mg/d) are required to produce hypercalciuria (>75 mmol/d).[82] Elemental calcium intakes in excess of 3.0–4.0 g/d should be avoided because they will cause hypercalcemia in most subjects.[83] Constipation can be a limiting side effect of calcium supplementation in many persons and is particularly bothersome in elderly persons. Calcium carbonate is currently the favored and cheapest form of supplemental calcium. There are other anionic forms that are equally effective but these supplements generally are more expensive.

Interactions of Calcium with Other Nutrients and Drugs

Lack of or diminished concentrations of estrogen are a risk factor for osteoporosis. Estrogen-replacement therapy reduces the loss of bone mass associated with oophorectomy[68,72,73,84–87] and markedly reduces risk of hip and vertebral fracture.[88,89] It is not clear if addition of calcium supplements to hormone replacement therapy results in added benefit. Increased amounts of dietary phosphorus were shown to promote fecal calcium loss but to have an equal but opposite effect on the urinary excretion of calcium. This finding explains why calcium balance is maintained in most normal subjects on a high-phosphorus diet.[90,91] The mechanism whereby increased dietary phosphorus decreases intestinal absorption of calcium was investigated by Portale et al.[92] These investigators showed that increasing dietary phosphorus from a low intake of <500 mg/d to an intake of 3000 mg/d decreased the production rate of $1,25(OH)_2D_3$ so that its serum concentrations fell from 80% greater than normal into the low-normal range. This observation strongly suggests that the ability to adapt to decreases or increases in dietary phosphorus depends upon the ability of the kidney to respond by increasing or decreasing its production of $1,25(OH)_2D_3$, respectively.

The question arises, therefore, whether increases in dietary phosphorus might have an adverse influence on calcium economy in individuals whose kidneys have a limited capacity to produce $1,25(OH)_2D_3$ or in individuals who need to be in positive calcium balance. In this regard, Portale et al.[93] reported that normal dietary phosphorus amounts were sufficient to suppress plasma concentrations of $1,25(OH)_2D_3$ in children with moderate renal insufficiency. No studies of the influence of dietary phosphorus on calcium and bone metabolism have been reported in other populations that may be unduly sensitive to increments in dietary phosphorous above the RDA (e.g., the young who are building bone or those with a decreased ability to absorb or conserve calcium, as might be the case in elderly persons) even though concern was expressed previously that high phosphorus intakes may contribute to age-related bone loss in humans.[94,95]

Although studies over the last half century established that high amounts of dietary protein taken as an isolated nutrient increase the renal excretion of calcium,[96,97] epidemiologic studies showed no adverse effect of high amounts of dietary protein on either rate of hip fracture[29] or metacarpal cortical bone mass.[51]

Dietary fiber was reported to chelate calcium and other minerals in the gastrointestinal tract,[98–100] and this observation led to concern that high-fiber diets may increase risk of bone loss and osteoporotic fracture. Although there is evidence in some[101–103] but not all[104] studies that consumption of high dietary fiber (in particular wheat bran) may interfere with the absorption of calcium, there is little evidence that high-fiber diets alone induce calcium deficiency in individuals who otherwise consume a balanced diet.

Although some drugs (e.g., thiazide diuretics) increase renal tubular reabsorption of calcium, they do not appear to influence calcium balance or changes in bone mass.[105] It was reported that phosphate-binding antacids, such as the nonprescription aluminum hydroxide gels, if taken chronically even at low doses, can cause phosphate depletion and an accompanying increase in bone resorption and urinary calcium excretion.[92,106–108] However, the relevance of use of antacids of the phosphate-binding type to age-related bone loss, particularly in individuals who are calcium deficient, is unknown.

Summary

The quantity of calcium derived from the diet that is required to achieve peak bone mass is greater than that required to replace obligatory losses of this ion in urine, stool, and sweat. Thus, persons under 25–30 y of age probably need to ingest sufficient calcium so that they absorb more calcium than they excrete. This quantity will vary depending upon individual efficiencies of intestinal calcium absorption, but 1200 mg/d is probably more than adequate and <600 mg/d is probably inadequate.

Once maximum bone mass is achieved (age 25–30 y), it is maintained without much change for 10–20 y. Calcium intake need not be >800 mg/d during this relatively short period of time because bone building is completed and intestinal absorption of calcium is normal. However, both men and women lose bone at a constant rate of 0.3–0.5%/y starting at age 40–45 y, and during a period of time (~10 y) immediately before and after menopause, women lose bone more rapidly than men (2–5%/y). This rapid rate of bone loss in menopausal women returns to the slower rate shared by the sexes after this 10-y period.

Women taking estrogen replacement to prevent bone loss should be provided the RDA for calcium (800 mg/d).[27] Those menopausal women who for some reason are unable or refuse to take estrogen should be asked to ingest at least 1000–1500 mg calcium/d with the idea that loss of cortical bone might be delayed and chronic secondary hyperparathyroidism prevented. For similar reasons it would seem prudent that these amounts of dietary calcium be provided to both women and men throughout the period of life after age 45–50 y. Ingestion of ≤2000 mg/d of calcium is safe in teenage children and adults.

Supported in part by a grant from the USPHS, 5P01DK39964, entitled Center of Excellence of Research on Osteoporosis.

References

1. J.H. Exton (1986) Mechanisms involved in calcium-mobilizing agonist responses. In: *Advances in Cyclic Nucleotide and Protein Phosphorylation Research* (P. Greengard and G.A. Robison, eds.), pp. 211–262, Raven Press, New York.

2. C.D. Arnaud (1978) Calcium homeostasis: regulatory elements and their integration. *Fed. Proc.* 37:2557–2560.

3. C.D. Arnaud (1988) Mineral and bone homeostasis. In: *Cecil Textbook of Medicine,* 18th ed. (J.B. Wyngaarden, L.H. Smith, and F. Plum, ed.), pp. 1469–1479, W.B. Saunders Company, Philadelphia.

4. G.D. Aurbach, S.J. Marx, and A.M. Spiegel (1985) Parathyroid hormone, calcitonin and the calciferols. In: *Williams Textbook of Endocrinology,* 7th ed. (J.D. Wilson and D.W. Foster, eds.), pp. 1137–1217, W.B. Saunders Company, Philadelphia.

5. R.M. Neer (1989) Calcium and inorganic phosphate homeostasis. In: *Endocrinology,* vol. 2, 2nd ed. (L.J. DeGroot, G.M. Besser, G.F. Cahill, et al., eds.), pp. 927–953, W.B. Saunders, Philadelphia.

6. M. Rosenblatt, H.M. Kronenberg, and J.T. Potts, Jr. (1989) Parathyroid hormone: physiology, chemistry, biosynthesis, secretion, metabolism, and mode of action. In: *Endocrinology,* vol. 2, 2nd ed. (L.J. DeGroot, G.M. Besser, G.F. Cahill, et al., eds.), pp. 848–891, W.B. Saunders, Philadelphia.

7. I. MacIntyre (1989) Calcitonin: physiology, biosynthesis, secretion, metabolism, and mode of action. In: *Endocrinology,* vol. 2, 2nd ed. (L.J. DeGroot, G.M. Besser, G.F. Cahill, et al., eds.), pp. 892–901, W.B. Saunders, Philadelphia.

8. M.F. Holick (1989) Vitamin D: biosynthesis, metabolism, and mode of action. In: *Endocrinology,* vol. 2, 2nd ed. (L.J. DeGroot, G.M. Besser, G.F. Cahill, et al., eds.), pp. 902–926, W.B. Saunders, Philadelphia.

9. M. Centrala and E. Canalis (1985) Local regulators of skeletal growth: a perspective. *Endocrinol. Rev.* 6:544–551.

10. F.R. Bringhurst (1989) Calcium and phosphate distribution, turnover and metabolic actions. In: *Endocrinology,* vol. 2, 2nd ed. (L.J. DeGroot, G.M. Besser, G.F. Cahill, et al., eds.), pp. 805–843, W.B. Saunders, Philadelphia.

11. A.M. Parfitt (1989) Surgical, idiopathic and other varieties of parathyroid hormone-deficient hypoparathyroidism. In: *Endocrinology,* vol. 2, 2nd ed. (L.J. DeGroot, G.M. Besser, G.F. Cahill, et al., eds.), pp. 1049–1064, W.B. Saunders, Philadelphia.

12. J.F. Habener and J.T. Potts, Jr. (1989) Primary hyperparathyroidism clinical features. In: *Endocrinology,* vol. 2, 2nd ed. (L.J. DeGroot, G.M. Besser, G.F. Cahill, et al., eds.), pp. 954–966, W.B. Saunders, Philadelphia.

13. S.M. Krane and A.L. Schiller (1989) Metabolic bone disease: introduction and classification. In: *Endocrinology,* vol. 2, 2nd ed. (L.J. DeGroot, G.M. Besser, G.F. Cahill, et al., eds.), pp. 1151–1164, W.B. Saunders, Philadelphia.

14. J.C. Gallagher, J.L. Melton, B.L. Riggs, and F. Bergstrahl (1980) Epidemiology of fractures of the proximal femur in Rochester, Minnesota. *Clin. Orthop.* 150:163–171.

15. J.L. Melton and B.L. Riggs (1983) Epidemiology of age-related fractures. In: *The Osteoporotic Fracture Syndrome* (L.V. Avioli, ed.), pp. 45–72, Grune & Stratton, New York.

16. J.F. Kelsey (1984) Osteoporosis: prevalence and incidence. *Osteoporosis* 5:25–28.

17. T.L. Holbrook, K. Grazier, J.L. Kelsey, and R.N. Stauffer (1984) *The Frequency of Occurrence, Impact and Cost of Selected Musculoskeletal Conditions in the United States,* American Academy of Orthopedic Surgeons, Chicago.

18. S.R. Cummings, J.L. Kelsey, M.C. Nevitt, and K.J. O'Dowd (1985) Epidemiology of osteoporosis and osteoporotic fractures. *Epidemiol. Rev.* 7:178–208.

19. J. Mangaroo, J.H. Glasser, L.H. Roht, and A.S. Kapadia (1985) Prevalence of bone demineralization in the United States. *Bone* 6:135–139.

20. B.L. Riggs and L.J. Melton III (1986) Involutional osteoporosis. *N. Engl. J. Med.* 314:1676–1686.

21. J.F. Kelsey (1987) Epidemiology of osteoporosis and associated fractures. In: *Bone and Mineral Research,* vol. 5 (W.A. Peck, ed.), pp. 409–444, Elsevier, New York.

22. R. Marcus (1982) The relationship of dietary calcium to the maintenance of skeletal integrity in man: an interface of endocrinology and nutrition. *Metabolism* 31:93–102.

23. A.M. Parfitt (1983) Dietary risk factors for age-related bone loss and fractures. *Lancet* 2:1181–1185.

24. R.P. Heaney (1986) Calcium, bone health and osteoporosis. In: *Bone and Mineral Research,* vol. 4 (W.A. Peck, ed.), pp. 255–301, Elsevier, New York.

25. S.M. Garn (1970) *The Earlier Gain and Later Loss of Cortical Bone,* Charles C. Thomas, Springfield, IL.

26. B.E.C. Nordin, A. Horsman, D.H. Marshall, M. Simpson, and G.M. Waterhouse (1979) Calcium requirement and calcium therapy. *Clin. Orthop.* 140:216–239.

27. National Research Council (1989) *Recommended Dietary Allowances,* 10th ed., National Academy Press, Washington, DC.

28. A.A. Albanese, A.H. Edelson, E.J. Lorenze, Jr., M.L. Woodhull, and E.H. Wein (1975) Problems of bone health in the elderly. *N.Y. State J. Med.* 75:326–336.

29. V. Matkovic, K. Kostial, I. Simonovic, R. Buzin, A. Brodarec, and B.E.C. Nordin (1979) Bone status and fracture rates in two regions of Yugoslavia. *Am. J. Clin. Nutr.* 32:540–549.

30. B. Krolner and S. Pors Nielsen (1982) Bone mineral content of the lumbar spine in normal and osteoporotic women: cross-sectional and longitudinal studies. *Clin. Sci.* 62:329–336.

31. R.P. Heaney, R.R. Recker, and P.D. Saville (1977) Calcium balance and calcium requirements in middle-aged women. *Am. J. Clin. Nutr.* 30:1603–1611.

32. R.P. Heaney (1985) The role of calcium in osteoporosis. *J. Nutr. Sci. Vitaminol. Tokyo* 31(suppl.):S21–26.

33. L.V. Avioli, J.E. McDonald, and S.W. Lee (1965) The influence of age on the intestinal absorption of ^{47}Ca in women and its relation to ^{47}Ca absorption in postmenopausal osteoporosis. *J. Clin. Invest.* 44:1960–1967.

34. J.R. Bullamore, R. Wilkinson, J.C. Gallaher, B.E.C. Nordin, and D.H. Marshall (1970) Effect of age on calcium absorption. *Lancet* 2:535–537.

35. C.C. Alevizaki, D.C. Ikkos, and P.J. Singhelakis (1973) Progressive decrease of true intestinal calcium absorption with age in normal man. *Nucl. Med.* 14:760–762.

36. P. Ireland and J.S. Fordtran (1973) Effect of dietary calcium and age on jejunal calcium absorption in humans studied by intestinal perfusion. *J. Clin. Invest.* 52:2672–2681.

37. B.E.C. Nordin, R. Williams, D.H. Marshall, J.C. Gallagher, A. Wil-

liams, and M. Peacock (1975) Calcium absorption in the elderly. *Calcif. Tissue Res.* 21(suppl.):422–451.

38. J.C. Gallagher, B.L. Riggs, J. Eisman, A. Hamstra, S.B. Arnaud, and H.F. Deluca (1979) Intestinal absorption and vitamin D metabolites in normal subjects and osteoporotic patients: effect of age and dietary calcium. *J. Clin. Invest.* 64:729–736.

39. B.L. Riggs, A. Hamstra, and H.F. DeLuca (1981) Assessment of 25 hydroxyvitamin D alpha-hydroxylase reserve in postmenopausal osteoporosis by administration of parathyroid extract. *J. Clin. Endocrinol. Metab.* 53:833–835.

40. K.S. Tsai, H. Heath III, R. Kumar, and B.L. Riggs (1984) Impaired vitamin D metabolism with aging in women: possible role in pathogenesis of senile osteoporosis. *J. Clin. Invest.* 73:1668–1672.

41. P.S. Wiske, S. Epstein, N.H. Bell, S.F. Queener, J. Edmonson, and C.C. Johnston, Jr. (1979) Increases in immunoreactive parathyroid hormone with age. *N. Engl. J. Med.* 300:1419–1421.

42. J.C. Gallagher, B.L. Riggs, C.M. Jerpbak, and C.D. Arnaud (1980) The effect of age on serum immunoreactive parathyroid hormone in normal and osteoporotic women. *J. Lab. Clin. Med.* 95:373–385.

43. K.L. Insogna, A.M. Lewis, B.A. Lipinski, C. Bryant, and D.T. Baran (1981) Effect of age on serum immunoreactive parathyroid hormone and its biological effects. *J. Clin. Endocrinol. Metab.* 53:1072–1075.

44. R. Marcus, P. Madvig, and G. Young (1984) Age-related changes in parathyroid hormone and parathyroid hormone action in normal humans. *J. Clin. Endocrinol. Metab.* 58:223–230.

45. E.S. Orwoll and D.E. Meier (1986) Alterations in calcium, vitamin D, and parathyroid hormone physiology in normal men with aging: relationship to the development of senile osteoporosis. *J. Clin. Endocrinol. Metabol.* 63:1262–1269.

46. M.S. Forero, R.F. Klein, R.A. Nissenson, et al. (1987) Effect of age on circulating immunoreactive and bioactive parathyroid hormone levels in women. *J. Bone Miner. Res.* 2:363–366.

47. A.M. Parfitt (1980) Morphologic basis of bone mineral measurements: transient and steady state effects of treatment of osteoporosis. *Miner. Electrolyte Metab.* 4:273–287.

48. K. Sakhaee, M.J. Nicar, K. Glass, J.E. Zerwekh, and C.Y.C. Pak (1985) Postmenopausal osteoporosis as a manifestation of renal hypercalciuria with secondary hyperparathyroidism. *J. Clin. Endocrinol. Metab.* 61:368–373.

49. C.D. Arnaud, J.C. Gallagher, C.M. Jerpbak, and B.L. Riggs (1980) On the role of parathyroid hormone in the osteoporosis of aging. In: *Osteoporosis: Recent Advances in Pathogenesis and Treatment* (H.F. DeLuca, ed.), pp. 215–225, University Park Press, Baltimore.

50. S.M. Garn, C.G. Rohmann, B. Wagner, G.H. Davila, and W. Ascoli (1969) Population similarities in the onset and rate of adult endosteal bone loss. *Clin. Orthop.* 65:51–60.

51. S.M. Garn, M.A. Solomon, and J. Friedl (1981) Calcium intake and bone quality in the elderly. *Ecol. Food Nutr.* 10:131–133.

52. S. Abraham, M.D. Carroll, C.N. Dresser, and C.L. Johnson (1977) Dietary intake findings, United States 1971–1974, HEW Publication no. (HRA) 77-1647, National Center for Health Statistics, Hyattsville, MD.

53. National Center for Health Statistics (1978) *Dietary intake source data, United States, 1971–1974,* HEW Publication no. (PHS) 79-1221, National Center for Health Statistics, Hyattsville, MD.

54. J.J.B. Anderson and F.A. Tylavsky (1984) Diet and osteopenia in elderly Caucasian women. In: *Proceedings of the Copenhagen International Symposium on Osteoporosis* (C. Christiansen, C.D. Arnaud, B.E.C. Nordin, A.M. Parfitt, W.A. Peck, and B.L. Riggs, eds.), pp. 299–304, Department of Clinical Chemistry, Glostrup Hospital, Copenhagen, Denmark.

55. R.W. Smith, Jr., and B. Frame (1965) Concurrent axial and ap- pendicular osteoporosis. Its relation to calcium consumption. *N. Engl. J. Med.* 273:72–78.

56. R.W. Smith, Jr., and J. Rizak (1966) Epidemiologic studies of osteoporosis in women of Puerto Rico and Southwest Michigan with special reference to age, race, nationality and to other associated findings. *Clin. Orthop.* 45:31–48.

57. A.M. Laval-Jeanet, G. Paul, C. Bergot, J.L. Lamarque, and M.D. Ghiania (1984) Correlation between vertebral bone density measurement and nutritional status. In: *Proceedings of the Copenhagen International Symposium on Osteoporosis* (C. Christiansen, C.D. Arnaud, B.E.C. Nordin, A.M. Parfitt, W.E. Peck, and B.L. Riggs, eds.), pp. 305–309, Department of Clinical Chemistry, Glostrop Hospital, Copenhagen, Denmark.

58. R. Pacifici, D. Droke, S. Smith, N. Susman, and L.V. Avioli (1985) Quantitative computer tomographic (QCT) analysis of vertebral bone mineral (VBM) in a female population. *Clin. Res.* 33:615A (abstr).

59. B.L. Riggs, H.W. Wahner, L.J. Melton III, L.S. Richelson, H.L. Judd, and W.M. O'Fallon (1987) Dietary calcium intake and rates of bone loss in women. *J. Clin. Invest.* 80:979–982.

60. B. Kanders, R. Lindsay, D. Dempster, L. Markhard, and G. Valiquette (1984) Determinants of bone mass in young healthy women. In: *Proceedings of the Copenhagen International Symposium on Osteoporosis* (C. Christiansen, C.D. Arnaud, B.E.C. Nordin, A.M. Parfitt, W.E. Peck, and B.L. Riggs, eds.), pp. 337–340, Department of Clinical Chemistry, Glostrop Hospital, Copenhagen, Denmark.

61. B. Dawson-Hughes, P. Jacques, and C. Shipp (1987) Dietary calcium intake and bone loss from the spine in healthy postmenopausal women. *Am. J. Clin. Nutr.* 46:685–687.

62. B.E.C. Nordin (1966) International patterns of osteoporosis. *Clin. Orthop.* 45:17–30.

63. N. Vintner-Paulsen (1953) Calcium and phosphorus intake in senile osteoporosis. *Geriatrics* 8:76–79.

64. B.E.C. Nordin (1961) The pathogenesis of osteoporosis. *Lancet* 1:1011–1014.

65. L. Lutwak and G.D. Whedon (1963) *Osteoporosis: Disease-a-Month (April),* Yearbook of Medical Publications Inc., Chicago.

66. B.L. Riggs, P.J. Kelley, V.R. Kinney, D.A. Scholz, and A.J. Bianco, Jr. (1967) Calcium deficiency and osteoporosis. *J. Bone Joint Surg.* 49A:915–924.

67. L.M. Hurxthal and G.P. Vose (1969) The relationship of dietary calcium intake to radiographic bone density in normal and osteoporotic persons. *Calcif. Tissue Res.* 4:245–256.

68. R.R. Recker, P.D. Saville, and R.P. Heaney (1977) Effect of estrogens and calcium carbonate on bone loss in postmenopausal women. *Ann. Intern. Med.* 87:649–655.

69. B. Lamke, H.E. Sjoberg, and M. Sylven (1978) Bone mineral content in women with Colle's fracture: effect of calcium supplementation. *Orthop. Scand.* 49:143–149.

70. E.L. Smith, Jr., W. Reddan, and P.E. Smith (1981) Physical activity and calcium modalities for bone mineral in aged women. *Med. Sci. Sports Exerc.* 13:60–64.

71. R.R. Recker and R.P. Heaney (1985) The effect of milk supplements on calcium metabolism, bone metabolism, and calcium balance. *Am. J. Clin. Nutr.* 42:254–263.

72. B. Riis, K. Thomsen, and C. Christiansen (1987) Does calcium supplementation prevent postmenopausal osteoporosis? *N. Engl. J. Med.* 316:173–177.

73. A. Horsman, J.C. Gallagher, M. Simpson, and B.E.C. Nordin (1977) Prospective trial of oestrogen and calcium in postmenopausal women. *Br. Med. J.* 2:789–792.

74. L. Nilas, C. Christiansen, and P. Rodbro (1984) Calcium supplementation and postmenopausal bone loss. *Br. Med. J.* 289:1103–1106.

75. B. Ettinger, H.K. Genant, and C.E. Cann (1987) Postmenopausal

bone loss is prevented by treatment with low-dosage estrogen with calcium. *Ann. Intern. Med.* 106:40–45.

76. C.E. Cann, H.K. Genant, B. Ettinger, and G.S. Gordan (1980) Spinal mineral loss in oopherectomized women. *JAMA* 244:2056–2059.

77. B.L. Riggs, J. Jowsey, P.J. Kelly, D.L. Hoffman, and C.D. Arnaud (1976) Effects of oral therapy with calcium and vitamin D in primary osteoporosis. *J. Clin. Endocrinol. Metab.* 42:1139–1144.

78. M. Horowitz, A.J. Need, J.C. Philcox, and B.E.C. Nordin (1984) Effect of calcium supplementation on urinary hydroxyproline in osteoporotic postmenopausal women. *Am. J. Clin. Nutr.* 39:857–859.

79. B.L. Riggs, E. Seaman, S.F. Hodgson, D.R. Taves, and W.M. O'Fallon (1982) Effect of the fluoride/calcium regimen on vertebral fracture occurrence in postmenopausal osteoporosis. *N. Engl. J. Med.* 306:446–450.

80. H. Heath III and C.W. Callaway (1985) Calcium tablets for hypertension? *Ann. Intern. Med.* 103:946–947.

81. Food and Drug Administration (1979) Report on over the counter preparations. *Fed. Regist.* 44:16175–16178.

82. E.L. Knapp (1947) Factors influencing the urinary excretion of calcium. *J. Clin. Invest.* 26:182–202.

83. P. Ivanovich, H. Fellows, and C. Rich (1967) The absorption of calcium carbonate. *Ann. Intern. Med.* 66:917–923.

84. C. Christiansen, M.J. Christiansen, P. McNair, C. Hagen, E.E. Stocklund, and I. Transbol (1980) I. Prevention of early postmenopausal bone loss: controlled 2-year study in 315 normal females. *Eur. J. Clin. Invest.* 10:273–279.

85. H.K. Genant, C.E. Cann, B. Ettinger, and G.S. Gordon (1982) Quantitative computed tomography of vertebral spongiosa: a sensitive method for detecting early bone loss after oopherectomy. *Ann. Intern. Med.* 97:699–705.

86. R. Lindsay, J.M. Aitken, J.B. Anderson, D.M. Hart, E.B. MacDonald, and A.C. Clarke (1976) Long term prevention of postmenopausal osteoporosis by oestrogen. Evidence for an increased bone mass after delayed onset of oestrogen treatment. *Lancet* 1:1038–1041.

87. L.E. Nachtigall, R.H. Nachtigall, R.D. Nachtigall, and E.M. Beckman (1979) Estrogen replacement therapy. I. A 10-year prospective study of the relationship to osteoporosis. *Obstet. Gynecol.* 53:277–281.

88. A. Paganini-Hill, R.K. Ross, V.R. Gerkins, B.E. Henderson, M. Arthur, and T.M. Mack (1981) Menopausal estrogen therapy and hip fractures. *Ann. Intern. Med.* 95:28–31.

89. N.S. Weiss, C.L. Ure, J.H. Ballard, A.R. Williams, and J.R. Daling (1980) Decreased risk of fractures of the hip and lower forearm with postmenopausal use of estrogen. *N. Engl. J. Med.* 303:1195–1198.

90. R.P. Heaney and R.R. Recker (1982) Effects of nitrogen, phosphorus and caffeine on calcium balance in women. *J. Lab. Clin. Med.* 99:46–55.

91. H. Spencer, L. Kramer, D. Osis, and C. Norris (1978) Effect of phosphorus on the absorption of calcium and on the calcium balance in man. *J. Nutr.* 108:447–457.

92. A.A. Portale, B.P. Halloran, M.M. Murphy, and R.C. Morris (1986) Oral intake of phosphorus can determine the serum concentration of 1,25-dihydroxyvitamin D by determining its production rate in humans. *J. Clin. Invest.* 77:7–12.

93. A.A. Portale, B.E. Booth, B.P. Halloran, and R.C. Morris, Jr. (1984) Effect of dietary phosphorus on circulating concentrations of 1,25-dihydroxyvitamin D and immunoreactive parathyroid hormone in children with moderate renal insufficiency. *J. Clin. Invest.* 73:1580–1589.

94. L. Lutwak (1975) Metabolic and diagnostic considerations of bone. *Ann. Lab. Clin. Sci.* 5:185–194.

95. R.R. Bell, H.H. Draper, D.Y.M. Tszeng, H.K. Shin, and G.R. Schmidt (1977) Physiological responses of human adults to foods containing phosphate additives. *J. Nutr.* 107:42–50.

96. L.H. Allen, E.A. Oddoye, and S. Margen (1979) Protein-induced hypercalciuria: A longer term study. *Am. J. Clin. Nutr.* 32:741–749.

97. J.J.B. Anand and H.M. Linkswiler (1974) Effect of protein intake on calcium balance of young men given 500 mg calcium daily. *J. Nutr.* 104:695–700.

98. R.J. Dobbs and I.M. Baird (1977) The effect of whole meal and white bread on iron absorption in normal people. *Br. Med. J.* 1:1641–1642.

99. F. Ismail-Beigi, J.G. Reinhold, B. Faraji, and P. Abadi (1977) Effects of cellulose added to diets of low and high fiber content upon the metabolism of calcium, magnesium, zinc and phosphorus in man. *J. Nutr.* 107:510–518.

100. R.A. McCance and E.M. Widdowson (1942) Mineral metabolism of healthy adults on white and brown bread dietaries. *J. Physiol.* 101:44–85.

101. J.H. Cummings, M.J. Hill, T. Jivraj, H. Houston, W.J. Branch, and D.J.A. Jenkins (1979) The effect of meat protein and dietary fiber on colonic function and metabolism. I. Changes in bowel habit, bile acid excretion and calcium absorption. *Am. J. Clin. Nutr.* 32:2086–2093.

102. J.G. Reinhold, B. Faradji, P. Abadi, and F. Ismail-Beigi (1976) Decreased absorption of calcium, magnesium, zinc and phosphorus by humans due to fiber and phosphorus consumption as wheat bread. *J. Nutr.* 106:493–503.

103. H.H. Sandstead, L.M. Klevay, R.A. Jacob, J.M. Munoz, G.M. Logan, and S.L. Reck (1979) Effects of dietary fiber and protein level on mineral element metabolism. In: *Dietary Fibers, Chemistry and Nutrition* (G.E. Inglett, S.I. Falkehaged, eds.), pp. 147–156, Academic Press, New York.

104. M. Stasse-Wolthius, H.F. Albers, J.G. van Jeveren, et al. (1980) Influence of dietary fiber from vegetables and fruits, bran or citrus pectin on serum lipids, fecal lipids, and colonic function. *Am. J. Clin. Nutr.* 33:1745–1756.

105. K. Sakhaee, M.J. Nicar, K. Glass, E. Zerwekh, and C.Y.C. Pak (1985) Reduction in calcium absorption by hydrochlorthiazide in postmenopausal osteoporosis. *J. Clin. Endocrinol. Metab.* 59:1037–1043.

106. W.J. Maierhofer, R.W. Gray, and J. Lemann Jr. (1984) Phosphate deprivation increases serum 1,25-(OH)$_2$-vitamin D concentrations in healthy men. *Kidney Int.* 25:571–575.

107. H. Spencer and M. Lender (1979) Adverse effects of aluminum-containing antacid on mineral metabolism. *Gastroenterology* 76:603–606.

108. H. Spencer, L. Kramer, C. Norris, and D. Osis (1982) Effect of small doses of aluminum-containing antacids on calcium and phosphorus metabolism. *Am. J. Clin. Nutr.* 36:32–40.

Chapter 25

Maurice E. Shils

Magnesium

Magnesium plays an essential role in a very wide range of fundamental cellular reactions. Hence, it is not surprising that deficiency in the organism may lead to serious biochemical and symptomatic changes. McCollum and associates[1] made the first systematic observations of magnesium deficiency in rats and dogs in the early 1930s. The first description of clinical depletion in man was published in 1934 in a small number of patients with various underlying diseases. Flink and associates[1] in the early 1950s documented depletion of this ion in alcoholics and in patients on magnesium-free I.V. solutions. Although magnesium deficiency does not appear to be a problem in healthy persons, increasing numbers of clinical disorders associated with magnesium depletion have been recognized. Experimental and clinical observations revealed fascinating interrelations of this ion with other electrolytes, second messengers, hormone receptors, parathyroid hormone secretion and action, vitamin D metabolism, and bone functions.

Body Compartments[1]

The adult human weighing 70 kg contains ~834–1200 mmol (~20–28 g) magnesium. About 60–65% of the total is present in bone, ~27% is in muscle, another 6–7% is in other cells, and only ~1% is in extracellular fluid. Muscle, liver, heart, and other soft tissues contain about the same amount (~7–10 mmol). Erythrocyte content varies from 2.2 to 3.1 mmol/L, depending on the age of the cells and the analytic measurement used. As the red cells age, the magnesium content slowly drops. Normal serum concentrations vary somewhat depending on analytic methods. With atomic absorption spectrophotometry, the usual range for neonates, older children, and adults is 0.7–0.75 mmol/L. Magnesium ion in erythrocytes and plasma exists as free, complexed (with citrate, phosphate, and other ions), and protein-bound forms; in plasma the approximate percentages are 55% free, 13% complexed, and 32% protein bound. Thirty percent of bone magnesium is in a surface-limited pool present either within the hydration shell or on the crystal surface. In adult men the large fraction of bone magnesium does not appear to be associated with bone matrix but, rather, is an integral part of the bone crystal.

Magnesium as well as calcium forms complexes with phospholipids of various cell membranes (e.g., plasma, endoplasmic, and mitochondrial) and with nucleic acids. Total intracellular magnesium concentration varies from ~6 to 10 mmol/kg wet weight, depending on the tissue, with the exception of the erythrocyte, which has less. The range often given for free Mg^{2+} in many cells is 0.3–0.6 mmol.

Analytic Procedures

A review of the development of methods for determining total magnesium in biologic fluids, cells and isolates of cells, foods, and other materials was reported by Alcock.[2] Atomic absorption spectrophotometry currently is the procedure usually employed in clinical chemistry laboratories.

Isotopes of magnesium have been used as biologic tracers in analyzing absorption and distribution of this ion. The radioisotope ^{28}Mg with a short half-life (21.3 h) has been used in human subjects. It disappears from the circulation rapidly after injection and initially is concentrated in soft tissues; however, >80% of the ^{28}Mg in the body appears to be in slowly exchanging components.[3] Naturally occurring magnesium contains 78.99 atom % ^{24}Mg, 10.0% ^{25}Mg, and 11.01% ^{26}Mg. ^{26}Mg has been used as a tracer in biomedical research, including absorption studies in man.[4]

Dietary Sources

Magnesium is widely distributed in foods. It is the mineral ion of chlorophyll; hence, vegetables are an important source. Similarly, ingestion of animal products, legumes, and cereals helps to assure a good intake. Intakes of adult females and males in a national survey in 1977–1978 averaged 230 and 310 mg, respectively.[5] These values are similar to average intakes of free-living healthy adult men and women whose customary diets were analyzed periodically over 1 y; however, individual daily intakes varied greatly.[6]

Absorption

Magnesium is absorbed primarily in the small intestine. The usual enteric conditions with contraction or expansion of luminal volume tend to increase or decrease luminal magnesium concentration, and absorption is influenced significantly by water movement (i.e., solvent drag). Two separate transport systems appear to participate in absorption from the proximal small intestine. One is a carrier-mediated system that becomes saturated at low intraluminal concentrations (1–2 mmol/L); this system appears to be defective in primary (or idiopathic) hypomagnesemia, which is a rare genetically determined disorder.[7] The other system is that of simple diffusion and occurs at higher concentrations of magnesium (e.g., 10 mmol/L). Free-living adults, who had periodic evaluations over the course of a year during which they consumed self-selected diets, had average absorptions of 21% for males and 27% for females.[6] In various metabolic studies done with usual diets, average absorptions were in the range of ≥50–70%.[1]

The influence of vitamin D on magnesium absorption is not known because of contradictory reports of either no effect[8,9] or of a positive effect of calcitriol in the jejunum but not in the ileum.[10] In the latter study[10] segmental perfusion techniques were used and the data have been questioned.[1] Intestinal absorption of magnesium is reduced in a variety of malabsorption syndromes, particularly those associated with steatorrhea (Table 1).

Renal Regulation[1]

Absorbed magnesium is either retained for tissue growth (including bone) or as turnover replacement; the remainder is excreted in the urine. Eighty percent of serum magnesium is ultrafiltrable, and 20–30% is absorbed in the proximal convoluted tubule. The thick ascending limb of the loop of Henle appears to be the major site of magnesium reabsorption in the kidney, and the major site of control of excretion (50–60% of filtered magnesium being reabsorbed) is between the thin descending limb and the early distal tubule. Changes in concentration of magnesium in the tubular lumen and in the plasma affect renal ab-

Table 1. Clinical conditions associated with magnesium depletion*

Gastrointestinal disorders—malabsorption
  Inflammatory bowel disease
  Gluten enteropathy, sprue
  Intestinal fistulas or bypass
  Ileal dysfunction with steatorrhea
  Immune diseases with villous atrophy
  Short-bowel syndrome
  Radiation enteritis
  Miscellaneous other disorders
Renal tubular dysfunction†
  Metabolic
  Hormonal
  Drugs
Endocrine disorders†
  Hyperaldosteronism
  Hyperparathyroidism with hypercalcemia
  Postparathyroidectomy
  Hyperthyroidism
Pediatric genetic and familial disorders
  Primary idiopathic hypomagnesemia
  Renal wasting syndrome†
  Bartter's syndrome†
  Infants born of diabetic or hyperparathyroid mothers
  Transient neonatal hypomagnesemic hypocalcemia
Inadequate intake or provision of magnesium
  Alcoholism
  Protein-calorie malnutrition (usually with infection)
  Prolonged infusion or ingestion of magnesium-low nutrient solutions or diets
  Hypercatabolic states (burns, trauma) usually associated with above item
  Excessive lactation

---

* Reproduced with modification from reference 1 with permission.
† See Table 2.

sorption in this segment. The distal convoluted tubule has limited reabsorption ability (<5% of the filtered load), and the collecting tubules and ducts normally absorb very little. Tubular secretion, if it occurs, must be a minor factor.

Drug and Hormonal Influences on Renal Regulation

Magnesium reabsorption in the nephron is influenced by a number of physiologic and metabolic factors as well as by drugs and disease states (Table 2). Of particular clinical significance with respect to renal losses are the loop diuretics, such as furosemide and ethacrinic acid, and certain nephrotoxic drugs. The diuretics triamterene and amiloride exert a magnesium-sparing effect as they do for potassium. The cancer chemotherapeutic agent, cisplatin, may cause serious losses of magnesium that may persist for many months after the drug is discontinued. Although it is known that a number of hormones may

Table 2. Metabolic, hormonal, and drug influences
on renal magnesium excretion*

Increased excretion
　Hypermagnesemia†
　Hypercalciuria
　Hyperaldosteronism
　Hyperparathyroidism‡
　Renal tubular dysfunction
　　Familial renal wasting syndromes
　　　Primary magnesuric hypomagnesemia, Bartter's and
　　　　related syndromes
　　　Postrenal obstruction
　　　Postrenal transplantation
　　　Acute tubulointerstitial nephritis
　　Nephrotoxic drugs
　　　Amphotericin, cisplatin
　　　Aminoglycosides, cyclosporin
　Potassium depletion
　Alcoholism
　Increased extracellular fluid volume
　Phosphate depletion
　Diuresis
　　Diuretics
　　Osmotic (diabetes, glucose, mannitol)
　Acidosis
　　Fasting, diabetic ketoacidosis, NH_4Cl administration
　Mineralocorticoids§
　Hyperthyroidism
Decreased excretion
　Hypomagnesemia
　Parathyroid hormone
　Hypocalcemia
　Alkalosis
　Hypothyroidism
　Contracted extracellular fluid volume
　Andidiuretic hormone
　Calcitonin
　Glucagon
　K^+-, Mg^{2+}-sparing diuretics

* Reproduced with modification from reference 1 with permission.
† When associated with magnesium infusion or injection.
‡ Secondary to hypercalcemia; transient negative balance.
§ Secondary to increased extracellular fluid volume.

influence magnesium reabsorption in the rat kidney tubule (Table 2), their roles and quantitative effects in the human kidney are still speculative.[11]

Summary of Homeostatic Factors

When magnesium intake is severely restricted in human subjects with normal kidney function, magnesium output becomes very low (i.e., <0.25 mmol/d) within 5–7 d.[12] Supplementing a normal intake increases urinary excretion without altering serum concentrations provided that renal function is normal and that the amounts given are not excessive. The intestinal and renal conservation and excretory mechanisms in normal individuals permit homeostasis over a wide intake of dietary magnesium.

Requirement for Healthy Individuals

A large number of balance studies have been performed over the years in an effort to obtain quantitative data on magnesium requirements. For a number of methodologic reasons, including metabolic and analytic problems, caution is indicated in accepting the older data.[1,13] The possible influence of types of protein and of the amounts of protein, fiber, calcium, and phosphate on magnesium balance has been studied; however, the results are often contradictory.[1]

Serum magnesium concentrations were determined by atomic absorption spectrophotometry on a U.S. population sample of 15,820 persons 1–74 y of age who were examined between 1971 and 1974 in the first National Health and Nutrition Examination Survey (NHANES I).[14] Ninety-five percent of adults aged 18–74 y had serum concentrations in the range 0.75–0.96 mmol/L. The values of the fifth percentile were at or above the lower values of normal generally used in clinical laboratories (i.e., 0.70–0.75 mmol/L). In this author's opinion, serum magnesium concentrations in healthy individuals are a good index of magnesium nutriture; hence, these data indicate that magnesium deficiency in the U.S. population in 1970–1974 and presumably now is very uncommon from childhood to older age.

There is some question as to the reliability of the 1989 RDA for magnesium,[15] which are based on human milk content consumption for infants and older balance studies for other age groups.

Magnesium Deficiency

Laboratory Species. Although most studied, the rat is not representative of other species with respect to certain deficiency signs, e.g., hyperemia and repetitive (and usually acutely fatal) tonic-clonic convulsions, and to associated normal to high concentrations of serum calcium and decreased concentrations of parathyroid hormone (PTH). Mice on the same diet developed no hyperemia, became hypocalcemic in association with hypomagnesemia, and often died with a single abrupt and massive convulsion.[16] Deficient dogs and monkeys—also on diets of the same composition—developed spasticity, tremors, and occasionally nonfatal convulsions with hypocalcemia; increasing calcium intake did not increase serum calcium nor prevent the neuromuscular changes.[17]

Human Magnesium Deficiency. Symptomatic human deficiency usually develops in a setting of predisposing and complicating disease states (Table 1) that often reduce intestinal absorption or are associated with impaired renal tubular reabsorption (Table 2). Decreased magnesium intake or inadequate amounts of magnesium in parenteral or enteral preparations may be a complicating factor.

Experimental Human Studies. Four groups of investigators recorded efforts to induce magnesium deficiency experimentally in human volunteers.[1] In the one study in which symptomatic depletion occurred,[12] the experimental diet provided ~0.4 mmol magnesium/d and the following changes occurred. Plasma magnesium decreased progressively to concentrations that were 10–30% those of control periods. Erythrocyte magnesium decreased more slowly and to a lesser degree. Urine and fecal magnesium decreased to extremely low concentrations within 7 d. Hypomagnesemia, hypocalcemia, and hypokalemia were present in all of the consistently symptomatic patients. Good intestinal absorption of calcium and low urinary calcium output resulted in positive calcium balance. Serum phosphate values varied among the subjects. Most subjects developed hypokalemia and negative potassium balance that resulted from increased urinary losses. Serum sodium remained normal, and the subjects were in positive sodium balance. Abnormal neuromuscular function occurred in five of the seven subjects after deficiency periods ranging from 25 to 110 d.

All symptoms and signs (including personality changes and gastrointestinal symptoms) reverted to normal with reinstitution of magnesium. A characteristic finding (which has been confirmed repeatedly in cases of clinical magnesium depletion) was the delayed increase in serum calcium despite the rapid return of serum magnesium to normal; a week or longer intervened before calcium returned to baseline concentrations. Potassium balances became strongly positive as sodium balances became negative. The return of serum potassium to normal also required ≥5 d.

The signs and symptoms noted above in experimental deficiency were described individually or in various combinations in clinical cases of hypomagnesemia. They included Trousseau and Chvostek signs, muscle fasciculations, tremor, muscle spasm, personality changes, anorexia, nausea, and vomiting. Frank tetany, myoclonic jerks, convulsions, and coma also were reported. Convulsions with or without coma occur more frequently in acutely deficient infants than in adults.

Clinical Deficiency. In humans the closest related condition to experimental magnesium deficiency is an uncommon congenital primary hypomagnesemia related to a specific defect in intestinal absorption of this ion.[18] Hypomagnesemia, hypomagnesuria, hypocalcemia, and hypokalemia with tetany and often with convulsions were corrected with magnesium supplements. Calcium and vitamin D supplements were ineffective in maintaining normocalcemia.

Comparison of Human Experimental and Clinical Depletion States

Variability in Distribution of Magnesium in Body Compartments. An early and progressive decrease in serum or plasma magnesium is found uniformly in all of the many species in which experimental depletion has been induced. In contrast, there are reports that serum or plasma magnesium concentrations may be normal or only slightly low in patients (particularly those with myocardial abnormalities) who have depressed muscle magnesium (many of whom have been on diuretics and other drugs).[1,19] On the other hand, symptomatic patients with difficulties absorbing magnesium from either the intestinal tract or kidney tubules usually have hypomagnesemia of serious degree. The clinical literature contains contradictory reports of the levels of magnesium in serum, muscle, and bone in patients claimed to be magnesium deficient.[1] It has been claimed that serum magnesium is not a good indicator of systemic magnesium depletion in clinical states. This issue has been discussed.[1] Claims were made that magnesium in mononuclear cells is a better guide to magnesium nutriture in clinical situations than is the serum concentration;[19] this suggestion contrasts with the report that during magnesium deficiency in the rat, the losses of this ion from lymphocytes (9%) were about the same as those from cardiac muscle (10%) and skeletal muscle (6%) but far less than those in serum (71%) and erythrocytes (33%).[20]

The rather bewildering combinations of contradictory variations reported in the clinical literature with respect to concentrations of blood and tissue magnesium and other electrolytes emphasize the difficulty in ascribing cause and effect to a specific nutrient deficiency in uncontrolled clinical situations. It is important to recognize that deficiency of one or more critical nutrients may have an impact on utilization or retention of other nutrients. For example, magnesium deficiency can deplete serum and cellular potassium, and potassium depletion can reduce cellular magnesium content. Starvation in obese subjects caused protein catabolism, acidosis, loss of cellular constituents, and decrease in bone and muscle magnesium.[21] Serum magnesium was well maintained presumably by a fairly constant input of magnesium into the blood from chronic acidosis and from catabolizing tissues.

Reports of medical cases believed to involve magnesium deficiency should include sufficient clinical and biochemical data to permit evaluation of whether the observed alterations (or lack of changes) in magnesium concentrations in tissues and serum reflect primary or secondary causes of magnesium depletion.

Sequence of Changes in Magnesium Deficiency and Repletion in Humans

Initiation of Hypocalcemia. The factor that initiates hypocalcemia appears to be failure of the normal heterionic exchange of bone calcium for magnesium at the labile bone mineral surface.[22] Impairment of receptor responsiveness to PTH of the osteoclasts then occurs with reduction of active bone resorption,[23] and hypocalcemia progresses despite increased concentrations of circulating PTH.[24]

Perpetuation of Electrolyte, PTH, and Clinical Abnormalities. As depletion progresses, secretion of PTH diminishes to very low amounts despite adequate intraparathyroid gland hormonal reserves.[24,25] The signs of severe magnesium depletion are present at this stage, i.e., very low circulating PTH, unresponsive bone, hypocalcemia, hypercalciuria, hypokalemia, sodium retention, and neuromuscular and other clinical signs and symptoms.

Regression of Magnesium Depletion and Associated Changes. After administration of adequate magnesium, serum magnesium rapidly increases, permitting heterionic calcium exchange to begin, with little or no detectable change in circulating calcium. There is an increase in circulating PTH.[24,25] Receptors for PTH on osteoclasts eventually regain responsiveness, serum calcium increases, and plasma PTH concentrations decrease appropriately. Electrolyte abnormalities recede and clinical signs and symptoms disappear with various degrees of rapidity.

Vitamin D Concentrations and Resistance in Magnesium Deficiency. The calcemic effect of vitamin D—even in high doses—is blunted in the presence of magnesium depletion in rickets,[26] malabsorption,[27] and idiopathic[28] or surgically induced hypoparathyroidism.[29] PTH is necessary for the formation of calcitriol [1,25(OH)$_2$D], and calcitriol is necessary for PTH to exert its effect on calcium mobilization from bone.[30] However, despite low concentrations of calcitriol in the majority of reported cases with magnesium depletion, serum calcium increased after magnesium repletion.[29–32] Thus, normal calcitriol concentrations do not appear to be necessary for the PTH-mediated response to magnesium.

Citrate Concentrations. Magnesium-deficient patients (depleted chronically as the result of intestinal malabsorption or acutely by low magnesium concentrations in total-parenteral-nutrition solutions) had a markedly decreased content of citrate in their urine; this decrease was secondary to increased renal tubular citrate reabsorption.[33]

Magnesium Depletion in Various Disease States

Prevalence. The list of causes of magnesium depletion (Table 1) emphasizes that this condition is unlikely to be a rare occurrence in acutely or chronically ill patients.

Alcoholism. Magnesium depletion in acute and chronic alcoholism has been documented over many years. Causes include poor magnesium intake, increased urinary losses, vomiting, diarrhea, and ketosis.[34]

Diabetes. Loss of magnesium in diabetic ketoacidosis has been appreciated for many years.[35] A significant negative correlation was noted between serum or plasma magnesium and blood glycohemoglobin in insulin-dependent pregnant women and was significantly related to rates of spontaneous abortion and fetal malformation.[36] About one-third of infants born to diabetic mothers were hypomagnesemic during the first 3 d of life. Similar negative correlations were noted between serum[37] or plasma and muscle[38] magnesium and glycohemoglobin in insulin-dependent (type I) diabetics. Children with insulin-dependent diabetes tended to have lower serum magnesium values than did nondiabetic control subjects;[37] serum magnesium values increased significantly with improved diabetes control. Non-insulin-dependent (type II) diabetics, most of whom were on insulin or oral hypoglycemics, had decreased amounts of magnesium in plasma, mononuclear cells, and skeletal muscle and increased amounts in urine compared with healthy control subjects.[39] Such depletion has been attributed to increased urinary losses with poor diabetes control.

Malabsorption. Serum magnesium is often subnormal in patients with malabsorption syndromes of various etiologies (Table 1). Increased amounts of fatty acids in the intestinal lumen form insoluble soaps with Mg^{2+}, leading to loss from both dietary and endogenous sources. This well-established finding was reconfirmed in malnourished adolescents with Crohn's disease given nutritional supplementation that further increased fecal magnesium but not fecal nitrogen or calcium.[40] Restriction of dietary fat plays a role in managing magnesium-losing steatorrhea.[41]

Protein-energy Malnutrition. Magnesium depletion occurs in children with inadequate food intakes in association with malabsorption, persistent vomiting and/or diarrhea, and infection. Serum or plasma magnesium was low in a significant proportion of such children in various studies in Africa.[42] In a study in Central America, 50% of serum magnesium values were below 0.65 mmol/L.[43]

Kidney Disease and Nephrotoxic Drugs. A number of factors may modify adversely the critical role of the kidney in magnesium homeostasis (Table 2). When glomerular filtration is impaired or there is tubular obstruction, hypermagnesemia is usual. However, hypomagnesemia may occur in patients with renal failure because of poor food intake and concomitant losses associated with vomiting, diarrhea, malabsorption, use of diuretics or nephrotoxic drugs, acidosis, and/or use of a magnesium-free dialysate. Increased excretion is also associated with postobstructive nephropathy, chronic glomerulonephritis, acute tubulointerstitial nephritis, postrenal transplantation, and familial urinary magnesium-wasting syndromes.[1]

The risk of stone formation and nephrocalcinosis in magnesium-depleted rats is well documented. There is an added risk of kidney stone formation in humans associated with the hypocitraturia that can occur within a matter of days in magnesium-depleted patients.[33] Because both citrate and magnesium tend to keep calcium from precipitating in urine, there is value in maintaining adequate urine concentrations of both.

Hypomagnesemia after Parathyroidectomy. Symptomatic hypomagnesemia may follow parathyroidectomy for primary hyperparathyroidism in association with the expected hypocalcemia, presumably as part of the "hungry bone" syndrome after removal of the parathyroid adenoma. Symptoms of muscle weakness, tremor, and mental changes were reversed by magnesium supplementation despite continuing low calcium blood concentrations.[44]

Magnesium Repletion

When a patient presents for the first time with hypomagnesemia, the etiology should be determined. If it is uncertain, same-day measurement of serum and urine magnesium concentrations is indicated. If the serum magnesium is consistently subnormal (i.e., <0.6 mmol/L), the normal kidney will usually excrete only small amounts of magnesium (i.e., <1 mmol/d). If renal tubular insufficiency is present, urinary magnesium will be appreciably higher so that it may equal or exceed the magnesium absorbed from the intestine or that given parenterally.

The amount and the route of magnesium administration will depend upon the severity of depletion, its etiology, and intestinal and kidney functions. Specific management of acute and chronic magnesium depletion in adults and children was reviewed.[1]

Hypermagnesemia and Magnesium Toxicity

Hypermagnesemia with Normal Renal Function. The normal kidney is capable of excreting large amounts of absorbed or injected magnesium ion so rapidly that serum concentrations usually do not increase to dangerous values. For example, in the treatment of preeclampsia, eclampsia, and premature labor with magnesium salts, relatively massive doses have been given as a loading dose followed by maintenance doses with the objective of maintaining the serum concentration at 2.5–4 mmol/L.[45] Patients with normal kidneys are able to excrete 40–60 g magnesium sulfate/d when it is given by persistent infusion.[46] With acute excess infusion, serum magnesium increases and is followed by a decrease in PTH[45,47] and an associated decrease in total and ionized calcium[45] accompanied by hypercalcuria and an increase in plasma renin activity and renin.[47]

Hypermagnesemia with Renal Insufficiency. Hypermagnesemia may develop in other clinical situations when magnesium-containing drugs, usually antacids or cathartics, are given to individuals with renal insufficiency, because ≥20% of Mg^{2+} in the form of sulfate, hydroxide, or citrate may be absorbed. In acute renal failure with oliguria—especially in the presence of acidosis—tissue release in association with the usual intake of magnesium will result in some degree of hypermagnesemia. The effects of magnesium excess are multiple and potentially lethal especially when serum concentrations are >4 mmol/L.[48] Uremic syndromes may mask those of hypermagnesemia.

Magnesium Alterations and Possible Disease Development

Coronary Artery Disease. It has been suggested that there is an inverse relation between magnesium intake and nutriture and the development of coronary artery disease and its sequelae.[49–51] The prevalence, morbidity, and mortality of this disease are such that these claims merit review here.

Some reports noted decreased prevalence of deaths from coronary artery disease in areas where the water is hard (i.e., high in calcium, magnesium, and fluoride). However, because of sufficient conflicting data, there is no consensus regarding the role of hard water as a factor in the prevalence of coronary artery disease.[1]

Serum Magnesium Concentrations in Acute Myocardial Infarction. The majority of older reports noted decreased serum or plasma values soon after or upon admission to hospital of patients with acute myocardial infarction. More recent data contradict these claims.[52–54] They also emphasize (1) that the time of drawing blood is critical in detecting changes[55] and (2) that complications such as congestive heart failure[56] and arrythmias[53,56] and the use of diuretics or digitalis drugs influence serum magnesium concentrations,[53,54] as do the degree of host infarction lipolysis,[57] and the degree of pain.[58]

A moderate number of reports from 1950 to 1980 suggested decreased magnesium in the myocardium of patients dying from ischemic heart disease.[49,50] More recent data indicate the variability of magnesium distribution in the heart.[59] The left ventricle in individuals dying from acute trauma had 11% more magnesium than did the right ventricle. Noninfarcted areas in patients dying from acute myocardial infarction had 20–28% less magnesium in both ventricles than did control subjects. Infarcted areas had decreased concentrations of calcium, potassium, and sodium as well as magnesium in addition to changes in various electrolyte ratios.

Positive correlations between plasma and erythrocyte magnesium and creatine kinase isoenzyme MB (an indicator of infarct size) suggested that magnesium left the heart at the time of the infarction and entered the extracellular compartment in proportion to cardiac enzyme activities.[54] A larger decrease in myocardial magnesium was noted in men with a prior history of angina who died suddenly of heart disease as compared with those without prior angina.[60]

In summary, the causes and significance of the decreased magnesium content in ischemic hearts are not clear because there are many complicating factors that are not included in most of the published reports. These factors include duration of heart disease; prior medications; dietary intakes and therapies; elapsed time between the infarction, death, and tissue sampling; areas of sampling; and variability in sampling. Whether the reported changes in magnesium content of heart are related to prior state of magnesium nutrition is uncertain.

Cardiac Arrhythmias and Spasms. Magnesium salts have been used empirically for some 50 y in the treatment of various tachyarrhythmias occurring with ischemia, digitalis toxicity, and diuretic therapy.[61] Increased understanding of the close physiologic, biochemical, and clinical interrelations of magnesium and potassium as well as of calcium and sodium makes it apparent that either magnesium or potassium depletion can influence serum and cellular concentrations of the other and that certain drugs adversely affect serum and tissue concentration of both. Hypokalemia and hypomagnesemia in seriously ill hospitalized patients are frequently associated.[1] Mean plasma concentrations of both potassium and magnesium were lower in diuretic-treated patients than in a nontreated control group.[62]

Hypokalemia in patients with acute myocardial infarction is associated with increased risk of ventricular arrhythmias.[63] An increase in sudden death was noted in the Multiple Risk Factor Intervention Trial (MRFIT) in a subgroup of hypertensive patients with baseline electrocardiographic abnormalities who received higher doses of diuretics and developed a greater degree of hypokalemia.[64] Ventricular arrhythmias occurred in 10 of 13 patients with infarction who were hypomagnesemic; 8 of these patients also were hypokalemic. The occurrence of serious arrhythmias was more common in those with hypokalemia. The incidence of serious ventricular ectopic beats, ventricular tachycardia, and ventricular fibrillation was higher in hypomagnesemic patients with acute myocardial infarction. The incidence of atrial fibrillation and supraventricular tachycardia also was higher in such patients.[53]

The effectiveness of supplementary magnesium administration in ameliorating or preventing arrhythmias was tested in patients who were eumagnesemic or mildly hypomagnesemic; several short-term studies of 12–18 h duration suggested a decrease in arrhythmias.[65,66] Randomized double-blind placebo studies were performed with patients suffering acute infarctions. Either isotonic glucose (74 patients) or magnesium chloride in glucose (56 patients) was started intravenously within 3 h of admission. Mean serum magnesium and potassium concentrations were within normal limits initially but ranged from moderately low to high normal.[67] Patients were monitored for 7 d and mortality recorded for 4 wk. The incidence of arrhythmias was 47% in the placebo group and 21% in the magnesium-treated group. However, supraventricular but not ventricular tachyarrhythmias were significantly reduced.[67] Mortality was reduced from 26% to 12.5% by administration of magnesium.[68] Of interest was the fact that the percentages of male deaths were similar with the two treatments, but none of the 17 women given magnesium died whereas 9 of 31 on placebo died—a statistic which, if verified, indicates a gender specificity.

Hypertension. Older studies reported conflicting data on serum magnesium concentrations in hypertensive as compared with normal subjects: lower values in both sexes,[69] in men but not women,[70] or similar to control subjects.[71] In an intervention study hypertensive patients on diuretic therapy were given magnesium aspartate-HCl, which resulted in a subsequent decrease in blood pressure over 6 mo without changes in plasma magnesium or other electrolytes.[72] There are a limited number of reports on magnesium intake in relation to hypertension, and results are conflicting.[73,74]

In patients with essential hypertension (without medications for ≥2 wk) and with essentially normal serum blood urea nitrogen and creatinine values, those with low-renin hypertension had an average serum magnesium of 1.04 ± 0.015 mmol/L. Those with normal renin had an average value of 0.97 ± 0.01 mmol/L, and those with high renin had 0.92 ± 0.01 mmol/L.[75] Each group was significantly different from the other and the high- and low-renin groups differed significantly from the normotensive control group, which had a magnesium value of 0.96 ± 0.01 mmol/L. Reciprocal relations were noted for serum ionized calcium in these patients. The range of variability within all groups covered essentially the normal clinical range. Concentrations of calcitonin, PTH, and calcitriol varied appropriately with calcium concentrations.[76] The physiologic and biochemical relevance of these relatively small but statistically significant changes is unclear but may be related to changes in intracellular Ca^{2+}.

With the increasing armamentarium of antihypertensive drugs, the state of magnesium nutriture on the effectiveness of the newer drugs and on their influence on magnesium excretion needs to be better documented. As an example, it was reported that normal or increased amounts of magnesium in the diet of spontaneously hypertensive rats did not appear to play an important role in the long-term regulation of blood pressure.[77] However, a response to the calcium channel blocker nifedipine was most pronounced in the rats on the normal (0.1%) diet and was significantly decreased in those on the magnesium-deficient diet.

References

1. M.E. Shils (1988) Magnesium. In: *Modern Nutrition in Health and Disease,* 7th ed. (M.E. Shils and V.R. Young, eds.), pp. 159–192, Lea and Febiger, Philadelphia.

2. N.W. Alcock (1969) Development of methods for the determination of magnesium. *Ann. N.Y. Acad. Sci.* 162:707–716.

3. J.K. Aikawa, G.S. Gordon, and E.L. Rhoades (1960) Magnesium metabolism in human beings: studies with Mg 28. *J. Appl. Physiol.* 15:503–507.

4. R. Schwartz (1982) ^{26}Mg as a probe in research in the role of magnesium in nutrition and metabolism. *Fed. Proc.* 41:2709–2713.

5. U.S. Department of Health and Human Services, Department of Agriculture (1986) *Nutrition Monitoring in the U.S.* DHHS Publication No. 86-1255. U.S. Government Printing Office, Washington, DC.

6. F.L. Lakshmanan, R.B. Rao, W.W. Kim, and J.L. Kelsay (1984) Magnesium intakes, balances, and blood levels of adults consuming self-selected diets. *Am. J. Clin. Nutr.* 40:1380–1389.

7. P.J. Milla, P.J. Aggett, O.H. Wolff, and J.T. Harries (1979) Studies in primary hypomagnesaemia: evidence for defective carrier-mediated small intestinal transport of magnesium. *Gut* 20:1028–1033.

8. A. Hodgkinson, D.H. Marshall, and B.E. Nordin (1979) Vitamin D and magnesium absorption in man. *Clin. Sci.* 57:121–123.

9. D.R. Wilz, R.W. Gray, J.H. Dominguez, and J. Lemann, Jr. (1979) Plasma 1,25-$(OH)_2$ vitamin D concentrations and net intestinal calcium, phosphate, and magnesium absorption in humans. *Am. J. Clin. Nutr.* 32:2052–2060.

10. G.J. Krejs, M.J. Nicar, J.E. Zewekh, et al. (1983) Effect of 1,25-dihydroxyvitamin D_3 on calcium and magnesium absorption in the healthy human jejunum and ileum. *Am. J. Med.* 75:973–976.

11. C. DeRouffignac, J.M. Elalouf, and N. Roinel (1987) Physiological control of the urinary concentrating mechanism by peptide hormones. *Kidney Int.* 31:611–620.

12. M.E. Shils (1969) Experimental human magnesium depletion. *Medicine (Baltimore)* 48:61–85.

13. H. Spencer, M. Lesniak, C.A. Gatza, D. Osis, and M. Lender (1980) Magnesium absorption and metabolism in patients with chronic renal failure and in patients with normal renal function. *Gastroenterology* 79:26–34.

14. F.W. Lowenstein and M.F. Stanton (1986) Serum magnesium levels in the United States, 1971–74. *J. Am. Coll. Nutr.* 5:399–414.

15. National Research Council (1989) *Recommended Dietary Allowances,* 10th ed., National Academy Press, Washington, DC.

16. N.W. Alcock and M.E. Shils (1974) Comparison of magnesium deficiency in the rat and mouse. *Proc. Soc. Exp. Biol. Med.* 146:137–141.

17. M.E. Shils (1976) Magnesium deficiency and calcium and parathyroid hormone interrelation. In: *Trace Elements in Human Health and Disease,* vol. 2 (A. Prasad, ed.), pp. 23–46, Academic Press, New York.

18. T. Yamamoto, H. Kabata, R. Yagi, M. Takashima, and Y. Itokawa (1985) Primary hypomagnesemia with secondary hypocalcemia. Report of a case and review of the world literature. *Magnesium* 4:153–164.

19. R.A. Reinhart (1988) Magnesium metabolism. A review with special reference to the relationship between intracellular content and serum levels. *Arch. Intern. Med.* 148:2415–2420.

20. M.F. Ryan and M.P. Ryan (1979) Lymphocyte electrolyte alterations during magnesium deficiency in the rat. *Isr. J. Med. Sci.* 148:108–109.

21. E.J. Drenick, I.F. Hunt, and M.E. Swendseid (1969) Magnesium depletion during prolonged fasting of obese males. *J. Clin. Endocrinol. Metab.* 29:1341–1348.

22. A.J. Johannesson and L.G. Raisz (1983) Effects of low medium magnesium concentration on bone resorption in response to parathyroid hormone and 1,25-dihydroxyvitamin D in organ culture. *Endocrinology* 113:2294–2298.

23. J.J. Freitag, K.J. Martin, M.E. Conrades, et al. (1979) Evidence for skeletal resistance to parathyroid hormone in magnesium deficiency. Studies in isolated perfused bone. *J. Clin. Invest.* 64:1238–1244.

24. R.K. Rude, S.B. Oldham, C.F. Sharp, Jr., and F.R. Singer (1978) Parathyroid hormone secretion in magnesium deficiency. *J. Clin. Endocrinol. Metab.* 47:800–806.

25. C.S. Anast, J.L. Winnacker, L.R. Forte, and T.W. Burns (1976) Impaired release of parathyroid hormone in magnesium deficiency. *J. Clin. Endocrinol. Metab.* 42:707–717.

26. F. Reddy and B. Sivakumar (1974) Magnesium dependent vitamin D resistant rickets. *Lancet* 1:963–965.

27. R. Medalle, C. Waterhouse, and T.J. Hahn (1976) Vitamin D resistance in magnesium deficiency. *Am. J. Clin. Nutr.* 29:854–858.

28. A. Rosler and D. Rabinowitz (1973) Magnesium-induced reversal of vitamin-D resistance in hypoparathyroidism. *Lancet* 1:803–804.

29. M.L. Graber and G. Schulman (1986) Hypomagnesemic hypocalcemia independent of parathyroid hormone. *Ann. Intern. Med.* 104:804–805.

30. M. Garabedian, Y. Tanaka, M.F. Holick, and H.F. DeLuca (1974) Response of intestinal calcium transport and bone calcium mobilization to 1,25-dihydroxyvitamin D_3 in thyroparathyroidectomized rats. *Endocrinology* 94:1022–1027.

31. R.K. Rude, J.S. Adams, E. Ryzen, et al. (1985) Low serum concentrations of 1,25-dihydroxy vitamin D in human magnesium deficiency. *J. Clin. Endocrinol. Metab.* 61:933–940.

32. M. Fuss, E. Cogan, C. Gillet, et al. (1985) Magnesium administration reverses the hypocalcemia secondary to hypomagnesemia despite low circulating levels of 25-hydroxyvitamin D and 1,25-dihydroxyvitamin D. *Clin. Endocrinol. Metab.* 22:807–815.

33. D. Rudman, J.L. Dedonis, M.T. Fountain, et al. (1980) Hypocitraturia in patients with gastrointestinal malabsorption. *N. Engl. J. Med.* 303:657–661.

34. E.B. Flink (1986) Magnesium deficiency in alcoholism. *Alcoholism* 10:590–594.

35. A.M. Butler (1950) Diabetic coma. *N. Engl. J. Med.* 234:648–656.

36. F. Mimouni, M. Miodovnik, R.C. Tsang, et al. (1987) Polycythemia, hypomagnesemia, and hypocalcemia in infants of diabetic mothers. *Obstet. Gynecol.* 70:85–88.

37. P. Fort and F. Lifshitz (1986) Magnesium status in children with insulin dependent diabetes mellitus. *J. Am. College. Nutr.* 5:69–78.

38. A. Sjögren, C.H. Floren, and A. Nilsson (1986) Magnesium deficiency in IDDM related to levels of glycosolated hemoglobin. *Diabetes* 35:459–463.

39. A. Sjögren, C.H. Floren, and A. Nilsson (1988) Magnesium, potassium and zinc deficiency in subjects with Type II diabetes mellitus. *Acta. Med. Scand.* 224:461–465.

40. K.J. Motil, S.I. Altschuler, and R.J. Grand (1985) Mineral balance during nutritional supplementation in adolescents with Crohn's disease and growth failure. *J. Pediatr.* 107:473–479.

41. C.C. Booth, N. Barbouris, S. Hanna, and I. MacIntyre (1963) Incidence of hypermagnesemia in intestinal malabsorption. *Br. Med. J.* 2:141–144.

42. E.U. Rosen, P.G. Campbell, and G.M. Moosa (1970) Hypomagnesemia and magnesium therapy in protein-calorie malnutrition. *J. Pediatr.* 77:709–714.

43. B.L. Nichols, J. Alvarado, C.F. Hazlewood, and F. Viteri (1978) Magnesium supplementation in protein-calorie malnutrition. *Am. J. Clin. Nutr.* 31:176–188.

44. C.T. Jones, R.A. Sellwood, and J.M. Evanson (1973) Symptomatic hypomagnesaemia after parathyroidectomy. *Br. Med. J.* 3:391–392.

45. I.N. Cholst, S.F. Steinberg, P.J. Tropper, et al. (1984) The influence of hypermagnesemia on serum calcium and parathyroid hormone levels in human subjects. *N. Engl. J. Med.* 310:1221–1225.

46. E.B. Flink (1969) Therapy of magnesium deficiency. *Ann. N.Y. Acad. Sci.* 162:901–905.

47. M. Dechaux, C. Kindermans, K. Laborde, I. Blazy, and C. Sachs (1988). Magnesium and plasma renin concentration. *Kidney Int.* 34(suppl. 25):512–513.

48. J.P. Mordes and W.E. Wacker (1977) Excess magnesium. *Pharmacol. Rev.* 29:273–300.

49. M.S. Seelig and H.A. Heggtveit (1974) Magnesium interrelations in ischemic heart disease: a review. *Am. J. Clin. Nutr.* 27:59–79.

50. J.R. Marier (1982) Quantitative factors regarding magnesium status in the modern-day world. *Magnesium* 1:3–15.

51. B.M. Altura and B.T. Altura (1985) New perspectives on the role of magnesium in the pathophysiology of the cardiovascular system, I. Clinical aspects. *Magnesium.* 4:226–244.

52. A.S. Abraham, U. Eylath, M. Weinstein, and E. Czaczkes (1977) Serum magnesium levels in patients with acute myocardial infarction. *N. Engl. J. Med.* 296:862–863.

53. T. Dyckner (1980) Serum magnesium in acute myocardial infarction. Relations to arrhythmias. *Acta. Med. Scand.* 207:59–66.

54. J. Manthey, M. Stoeppler, W. Morgenstern, et al. (1981) Magnesium and trace metals: risk factors for coronary heart disease? Association between blood levels and angiographic findings. *Circulation* 64:722–729.

55. M. Speich (1987) Magnesium and creatinine kinase in myocardial failure: new data. *Clin. Chem.* 33:739–740.

56. W.G. Rector, Jr., M.A. DeWood, R.V. Williams, and J.F. Sullivan (1981) Serum magnesium and copper levels in myocardial infarction. *Am. J. Med. Sci.* 281:25–29.

57. E.B. Flink, J.E. Brick, and S.R. Shane (1981) Alterations of long-chain free fatty acid and magnesium concentrations in acute myocardial infarction. *Arch. Intern. Med.* 141:441–443.

58. A.S. Abraham, R. Shaoul, E. Shimonovitz, U. Eylath, and M. Weinstein (1980) Serum magnesium levels in acute medical and surgical conditions. *Biochem. Med.* 24:21–26.

59. M. Speich, B. Bousquet, and G. Nicholas (1980) Concentrations of magnesium, calcium, potassium, and sodium in human heart muscle after acute myocardial infarction. *Clin. Chem.* 26:1662–1665.

60. C.J. Johnson, D.R. Peterson, and E.K. Surith (1979) Myocardial tissue concentrations of magnesium and potassium in men dying suddenly from ischemic heart disease. *Am. J. Clin. Nutr.* 32:967–970.

61. M.J. Eisenberg (1986) Magnesium deficiency and cardiac arrhythmias. *N.Y. State J. Med.* 86:133–136.

62. J.C. Boyd, E.E. Bruns, and M.R. Wills (1983) Frequency of hypomagnesemia in hypokalemic states. *Clin. Chem.* 29:178–179.

63. H. Kafka, L. Langevin, and P.W. Armstrong (1987) Serum magnesium and potassium in acute myocardial infarction. Influence on ventricular arrhythmias. *Arch. Intern. Med.* 147:465–469.

64. R. Sherwin (1984) Sudden death in men with increased risk of myocardial infarction. The MRFIT programme. *Drugs* 28(suppl. 1):46–53.

65. T. Dyckner and P.O. Wester (1979) Ventricular extrasystoles and intracellular electrolytes before and after magnesium infusion in patients on diuretic treatment. *Am. Heart J.* 97:12–18.

66. L.T. Iseri, R.D. Fairshter, J.L. Hardemann, and M.A. Brodsky (1985) Magnesium potassium therapy in multifocal atrial tachycardia. *Am. Heart J.* 110:789–794.

67. H.S. Rasmussen, M. Suenson, P. McNair, P. Norregard, and S. Balslev (1987) Magnesium infusion reduces the incidence of arrhythmias in acute myocardial infarction. A double-blind placebo-controlled study. *Clin. Cardiol.* 10:351–356.

68. H.S. Rasmussen, P. McNair, P. Norregard, V. Backer, O. Lindeneg, and S. Balslev (1986) Intravenous magnesium in acute myocardial infarction. *Lancet* 1:234–236.

69. D.G. Albert, Y. Morita, and L.T. Iseri (1958) Serum magnesium and plasma sodium levels in essential vascular hypertension. *Circulation* 17:761–763.

70. F.K. Bauer, H.E. Martin, M.R. Mickey (1965) Exchangeable magnesium in hypertension. *Proc. Soc. Exp. Biol. Med.* 120:466–468.

71. D.W. Tillman, P.F. Semple (1988) Calcium and magnesium in essential hypertension. *Clin. Sci.* 75:395–402.

72. T. Dyckner, P.O. Wester (1983) Effect of magnesium on blood pressure. *Br. Med. J.* 286:1847–1849.

73. T. Thulin, M. Abdulla, I. Dencker, et al. (1980) Comparison of energy and nutrient intakes in women with high and low blood pressure levels. *Acta Med. Scand.* 208:367–373.

74. D.A. McCarron, C.D. Morris, and C. Cole (1982) Dietary calcium in human hypertension. *Science* 217:267–269.

75. L.M. Resnick, J.H. Laragh, J.E. Sealey, and M.H. Alderman (1983) Divalent cations in essential hypertension. Relations between serum ionized calcium, magnesium, and plasma renin activity. *N. Engl. J. Med.* 309:888–889.

76. L.M. Resnick, F.B. Miller, and J.H. Laragh (1986) Calcium regulating hormones in essential hypertension. *Ann. Intern. Med.* 105:649–654.

77. A. Overlack, J.G. Zenzen, C. Ressel, H.M. Muller, and K.O. Stumpe (1987) Influence of magnesium on blood pressure and effect of nifedipine in rats. *Hypertension* 9:139–143.

Chapter 26

Friedrich C. Luft

Sodium, Chloride, and Potassium

Claude Bernard was the first to appreciate and draw attention to the body's compartments in terms of an internal environment (*milieu intérieur*). He suggested that the extracellular fluid provided an internal environment, a medium in which all cells are bathed.[1] The internal environment constitutes the extracellular compartment. Its solute constituents and their concentrations are tightly regulated to permit cell growth, function, and survival. Indeed, the volume of the cells themselves (intracellular compartment), their cytosolic solute concentrations, and their water content are dictated by the constituents of the extracellular compartment and their respective concentrations. Bernard was aware that the extracellular compartment consisted of a solution of approximately 0.9% sodium chloride and that the predominant cation in intracellular fluid was potassium.

Homer Smith pointed out the crucial role of the kidneys in the regulation of the constituents and the volume of both the extracellular and intracellular compartments.[2] He presented a convincing teleological argument that the extracellular compartment contains constituents and concentrations similar to the Precambrian seas, which presumably bathed the earliest primordial unicellular organisms. Further, he suggested that eons earlier the prototype molecules and organelles of cells may have developed in solutions more akin to today's intracellular compartment, that is, a solution that was relatively high in potassium and phosphate and low in sodium and chloride. Smith argued that the maintenance of the extracellular compartment dictated the evolutionary changes observed in both kidney structure and function. Kidneys of diverse organisms, existing in either aquatic environments, fresh water, or sea water, as well as kidneys of animals living in various terrestrial environments have in common the task of guarding and regulating the external and the internal compartment. They perform this function by regulating the sodium, chloride, and potassium content and concentration in the body. Further, they regulate the concentration of solutes in both compartments within extremely narrow limits. This function permits the body's cells to thrive and perform their various functions, a process and a concept termed *homeostasis* by Claude Bernard.[1]

Body Compartments

The total body water (TBW) in the ideal, prototypic, 70-kg human is ~0.6 of the body's weight or 40 L.[3] Two-thirds of this water resides inside cells (intracellular fluid compartment) and one-third exists outside cells (extracellular fluid compartment). A minor portion of the TBW exists in the intestines, the anterior chamber of the eye, and the subarachnoid space and is termed the transcellular compartment. This compartment makes up <1 L of the TBW. By far the most important solutes of the extracellular fluid compartment (ECF) are the electrolytes sodium (135–145 mmol/L) and chloride (98–108 mmol/L). The concentration of potassium in the ECF is much less (3.5–4.5 mmol/L). In the intracellular fluid compartment (ICF), potassium is the predominant cation (150 mmol/L) whereas the concentrations of sodium and chloride are negligible. The water content of cells varies as to their type. Muscle cells have a much higher water content than fat cells have. Therefore, the ICF and the TBW are closely related to lean body mass.[3]

Sodium, chloride, and potassium are important constituents of the diet. They are virtually completely absorbed in the upper small intestine, and they are eliminated in the urine. If sweating is not excessive and if diarrhea is not present, >98% of the ingested sodium and chloride appear in the urine.[3] More than 85% of ingested potassium appears in the urine as well.[3] A diagrammatic representation is shown in Figure 1. The TBW, ICF, and ECF are represented as a box. The mouth provides an entrance and the kid-

BODY WATER DISTRIBUTION

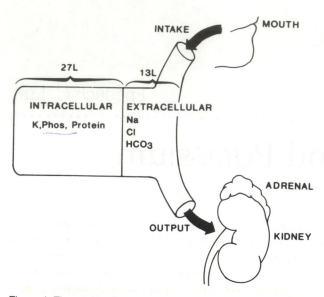

Figure 1. The total body water (40 L) is distributed as intracellular (27 L) and extracellular (13 L) fluid. Fluids and electrolytes enter via the mouth and are excreted via the kidneys.

neys provide an exit. Immediately apparent is the concept of homeostasis in terms of "what goes in must come out." Violation of this principal results in either expansion (more in than out) or contraction (more out than in) of the boxes (Figures 2 and 3). As illustrated in Figure 2, renal disease may decrease the capacity of the body to eliminate sodium, chloride, and water. As a result, the ECF will expand; hypertension, edema, eventually pulmonary edema, and death will result. Figure 3 illustrates the result of sodium, chloride, and water losses as may occur in Addison's disease, a condition in which mineralocorticoid hormones are not produced because of failure of the adrenal cortex. Although mineralocorticoids influence <2% of sodium and chloride reabsorption, gradual decreases in the ECF result. The consequences of volume contraction are hypotension, shock, and death.

The methods of analyses for sodium, potassium, and chloride are well established and include flame photometry or ion-specific electrodes in the case of sodium and potassium.[4] Chloride is measured by silver nitrate titration or more commonly by automated methods.[4]

The absorption of these electrolytes, their transport across cell membranes, and their transport across the renal epithelium occur via active and passive transport involving energy-dependent enzymatic mechanisms and physical forces that are beyond the scope of this chapter but are reviewed in detail elsewhere.[4] Rather than concentrating on details of transcellular

transport and biochemical function, this discussion will be concerned with the volume-regulating functions of sodium and chloride, internal potassium balance, and the control of plasma potassium concentration.

Sodium, Chloride, and Volume-regulating Systems

The predominant cation and anion in the ECF are sodium and chloride. Normally they cannot be replaced to a great extent by other cations or anions. Therefore, regulation of both sodium and chloride, in terms of both total amount and concentration, is responsible for the regulation of the ECF. Restriction of dietary chloride without restriction of sodium prevents expansion of the ECF. Similarly, administration of sodium with a concomitant anion other than chloride fails to expand the ECF. The interdependence of sodium and chloride in the process of regulating the ECF is outlined in detail elsewhere.[5] (Because this discussion will concern itself primarily with compartment regulation, the ions sodium and chloride will be discussed together.)

The intake of sodium and chloride is mainly derived from salt and varies greatly among countries. For example, the mean daily intake per person is >240 mmol/d in certain parts of northern China, 200 mmol/d in Finland, 150 mmol/d in the United States and western Europe, and <30 mmol/d in the Amazon Jungle, the New Guinea Highlands, and the

VOLUME EXPANSION

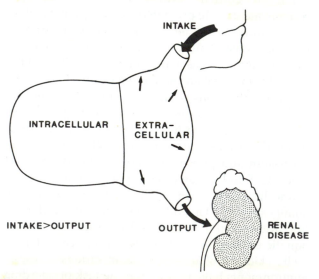

Figure 2. If intake cannot be eliminated, as is the case in certain forms of renal disease, the volume of the compartments must necessarily increase. If sodium, chloride, and water are retained, edema, hypertension, and eventual pulmonary edema develop.

VOLUME CONTRACTION

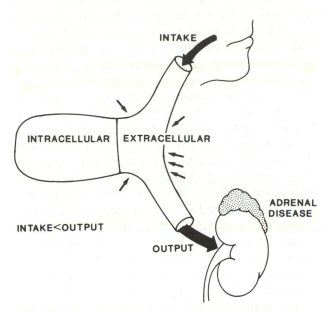

Figure 3. If the excretion of water and electrolytes exceeds intake, as may occur if sweating is excessive, diarrhea is present, or the kidneys are unable to retain sodium and chloride (e.g., Addison's disease), volume contraction will occur. Blood pressure will fall until shock results.

Kalahari Desert.[6] The range in sodium and chloride intake is vast; the Yanamamo Indians of Brazil ingest <1 mmol/d of sodium and chloride. In experimental settings, intakes in excess of 1500 mmol/d have been tolerated by normal human subjects for short periods without apparent ill effects.[7] Thus, the kidneys are able to cope with widely differing intakes of sodium and chloride as well as with sudden changes in intake.

The overall control system of sodium and chloride is by no means clear. Adaptation to different levels of sodium chloride intake is physiologically quite complicated with well-documented changes in plasma renin activity (PRA), plasma angiotensin II, aldosterone production, atrial natriuretic peptide, sympathetic nervous system tone, substances of gut origin, and perhaps the elusive natriuretic hormone (sodium-potassium-dependent ATPase [Na$^+$, K$^+$-ATPase] inhibitor), which is thought to be produced in the hypothalamus. These and probably other adaptations help to minimize the effect of changes in sodium intake on ECF and total body sodium. The effects are minimized but not eliminated completely. Thus, the greater the sodium chloride intake, the greater the ECF, plasma volume, blood volume, and cardiac output. However, the principles of Figures 2 and 3 apply. Whatever goes in must come out.

Strauss and colleagues[8] observed that when sodium chloride intake is suddenly reduced to very low

levels, urinary sodium and chloride excretion decrease in an exponential fashion over 4 or 5 d to virtually zero (to match the intake). They showed that if even a small amount of salt is ingested, sodium and chloride are immediately excreted. However, if extra sodium and chloride are forced from the body, either through sweating or diuretic administration, any ingested sodium and chloride is retained in the body until the added deficit is restored. Hollenberg[9] refined this observation and coined the term homeostatic set point, a state between surfeit and deficit or a level of sodium and chloride in the body that is defended. Simpson[10] has termed this point the basal level of body sodium and chloride. He proposed the following model for body sodium and chloride based on the principles first described by Strauss:

1. The basal level of sodium and chloride is maintained when intake is very low, just sufficient to cover obligatory losses from the skin and bowel. Urinary excretion rates at this state are also very low but must approximate intake.

2. If the body sodium and chloride decrease below the basal level for any reason, the body will exist in a state of true sodium chloride deficit. Any ingested salt will be retained in the body until the deficit of sodium chloride is made up.

3. When body sodium lies above the basal level (which it does in the majority of the world's peoples), the body is in a state of surfeit, and the extra sodium and chloride (amount in the body above basal levels) is excreted. The rate of excretion of sodium and chloride is exponentially related to the amount of extra sodium and chloride in the body. As emphasized by Hollenberg,[9] the body sodium and chloride is running downhill all the time toward the basal level and is constantly being increased by further intake of sodium and chloride.

The Yanamamo Indians of Brazil are able to maintain homeostasis with a salt intake barely sufficient to maintain the basal level of body sodium and chloride (<1 mmol/d).[6] However, this ability is a function of the development of a number of homeostatic mechanisms and of normal kidney function. Healthy Americans can maintain homeostasis at intakes of sodium and chloride of <10 mmol/d. Whether or not such a low intake is either healthy or desirable for acculturated man is a matter of debate.[11]

Mechanisms of Volume Control (Basal Body Sodium and Chloride)

Control of the ECF is essential to maintenance of the internal environment in terms of both ECF constituents and blood pressure. The basic paradigm of redundancy in biological control systems has resulted in several control systems that may be distinguished in a hierarchical fashion as follows:

1. Behavioral central mechanisms exist that control solute and water intake. Particularly relevant to this discussion are salt appetite and thirst.[12,13]

Salt appetite is an overriding driving force for sodium and chloride intake in omnivores and particularly in herbivores. A body of evidence indicates that the brain renin-angiotensin system is important in this regard.[14] Intracerebroventricular injection of angiotensin II stimulates salt appetite whereas the central administration of captopril, a drug that inhibits the formation of angiotensin II, diminishes salt appetite.

The thirst center influences not only the TBW but also the concentration of the solutes in the body. This concentration is maintained within incredibly narrow limits. An increase in plasma osmolality >288 mmol/L (increase in sodium >140 mmol/L) stimulates the thirst center. Drinking behavior or the search for water ensues. A decrease in plasma osmolality below this level causes a cessation of drinking behavior. In response to these changes in osmolality, arginine vasopressin, the antidiuretic hormone, is either released (>288 mmol/L) or inhibited (<288 mmol/L). This hormone acts on the renal collecting duct and increases its permeability to water thereby affecting the excretion of a concentrated urine and maintaining water inside the body. However, the body's volume status also influences the threshold of the osmoregulatory system.[15] Hemodynamic influences either raise or lower the set point of the osmoreceptor mechanism, which is normally situated at 288 mmol/L. Robertson showed that resetting the osmoreceptor requires the participation of opioid-secreting neurons.[16]

2. Hormonal systems, such as the renin-angiotensin-aldosterone axis, vasopressin, atrial natriuretic peptide, intestinal vasoactive peptides, and the putative inhibitor of Na^+, K^+-ATPase, all control or influence renal sodium and chloride excretion and have in addition other homeostatically relevant extrarenal sites of action.[17]

The circulating renin-angiotensin-aldosterone axis plays a critical role in regulating the basal body sodium and chloride levels. Its suppression enables sodium and chloride to be eliminated from the body. Circulating renin is an enzyme released into the circulation by the juxtaglomerular apparatus of the nephron. The enzyme cleaves angiotensinogen, a peptide of hepatic origin, into angiotensin I, which is in turn cleaved into angiotensin II by kininase II, the converting enzyme. Angiotensin II, a potent vasoconstrictor, operates on the nephron directly to promote sodium and chloride retention but also stimulates the adrenal cortex to release aldosterone

into the circulation. Aldosterone has its main action on the collecting duct and the most distal part of the distal tubule. The maintenance of basal body sodium and chloride is dependent on sodium and chloride reabsorption from these structures. Adrenalectomized persons or those with Addison's disease are unable to tolerate a very low sodium chloride intake. Their basal body sodium chloride content may fall too low to sustain life. On the other end of the scale is primary aldosteronism, the inappropriate release of aldosterone by an adrenal adenoma. Patients with this disorder have arterial hypertension and a total body sodium and chloride content ~16% above normal values.[10] Any increased intake of sodium or chloride by such individuals is characterized by very rapid excretion, termed *exaggerated natriuresis*. Aldosterone (the renin-angiotensin-aldosterone axis) plays a dominant role in the maintenance of the basal body sodium and chloride content. A potential role for atrial natriuretic peptide and other natriuretic factors, either identified or putative, is not as well defined.

3. The sympathetic nervous system is a major regulatory mechanism controlling the excretion of sodium and chloride by the kidneys.[18]

The sympathetic nervous system may cause sodium and chloride retention by at least three mechanisms: alterations in renal blood flow; initiation of release of renin by the juxtaglomerular apparatus, an innervated structure; and direct effects on the renal tubule via either α or β receptors or both. The role of the sympathetic nervous system in sodium and chloride homeostasis was reviewed by DiBona.[18] The sympathetic nervous system is activated in states of sodium depletion and suppressed in states of sodium excess.[19] It is possible that disturbances in sympathetic nervous system tone may lead to hypertension by influencing the basal sodium and chloride content of the body.

4. Intrarenal mechanisms exist that influence sodium and chloride excretion independent of neural and humoral signals from elsewhere.

Intrarenal mechanisms of sodium and chloride handling are also important in the control of basal body sodium and chloride. These mechanisms include locally released autocoid tissue hormones, including intrarenal tissue angiotensin, prostaglandins, kinins, endothelial relaxing factor, endothelin, and lesser well-defined factors.[17] Physical factors, including the oncotic pressure of plasma proteins in the blood bathing the renal tubules, are important as well. A high filtration fraction results in a higher oncotic pressure of the plasma exiting the glomerulus and therefore an increase in sodium and chloride reabsorption (glomerular-tubular balance).

ECF and Arterial Blood Pressure

Selkurt et al.[20] showed that sodium and chloride excretion is a function of renal perfusion pressure. Guyton[21] examined this phenomenon in detail and formulated a computerized model framework relating renal sodium and chloride handling to arterial blood pressure. According to their concept, renal sodium and chloride excretion is of overriding importance for long-term control of volume status and blood pressure. They termed the relationship between sodium and chloride intake (and excretion) and blood pressure the renal function curve. The vast ranges in which sodium and chloride are ingested result in very minor alterations in arterial blood pressure. Guyton reasoned that patients with hypertension have renal function curves different from normal. Some individuals might exhibit greater changes in blood pressure with changes in dietary sodium and chloride intake than others. Recent work by Kimura[22] in patients with surgically correctable forms of hypertension corroborates his viewpoint.

Requirements and Allowances for Sodium and Chloride

It is impossible to determine a minimum daily requirement for sodium or chloride. Although the Yanamamo Indians are able to regulate their internal environments with an extremely low sodium chloride intake, it is by no means established that such an intake is advisable for acculturated peoples. As the above discussion indicates, the regulation of basal body sodium and chloride requires normal kidneys as well as intact central, humoral, and intrarenal mechanisms. The regulatory systems also are influenced by age. The Intersalt study indicates that salt intake of the world's populations (with the exception of four unacculturated centers) ranges from 100 to 240 mmol sodium and chloride per day.[6] Some authorities have recommended that dietary sodium and chloride intake should be curtailed to <100 mmol/d in the hope that the development of hypertension, increase in blood pressure with age, and cardiovascular disease morbidity and mortality may be alleviated. The wisdom of such an approach in terms of a public health strategy for nonhypertensive normal individuals is currently under debate and is not yet thoroughly established.[11]

Internal Potassium Balance and Potassium Concentration

The potassium concentration in the ECF represents only ~2% of the total body potassium. Therefore 98% of the potassium in the body (3–4 mol depend-ing on muscle mass) must reside inside cells.[4] However, because the concentration of potassium in the ECF is a critical determinant of neuromuscular excitability,[23] the control of the potassium concentration in the ECF is of major biological importance. According to the Nernst equation, the potential difference across cell membranes is proportional to the intracellular potassium concentration divided by the extracellular potassium concentration. For the purposes of this discussion, the relationship may be simplified accordingly: $E \alpha K_i/K_e$. E is the potential difference across the cell membrane, normally about −90 mV, K_i is the concentration of potassium inside cells (intracellular), and K_e is the potassium concentration outside cells (extracellular). An increase in the extracellular potassium concentration (hyperkalemia) decreases the potential difference, which defines the resting potential of the cell. When the resting potential approaches threshold, the cell depolarizes and may not be able to repolarize (repolarization block). Such a cell is rendered nonfunctional. Similarly, when the extracellular potassium concentration decreases (hypokalemia), the potential difference across the membrane becomes greater thereby increasing the stimulus required to bring about depolarization (depolarization block). In either event (hyperkalemia or hypokalemia) the cell becomes nonfunctional. It will come as no surprise that the symptoms of hyperkalemia and hypokalemia are similar, i.e., weakness, lethargy, gastric hypomotility, cardiac arrhythmias, and conduction disturbances. Both disorders may be life threatening.

The extracellular potassium concentration is a function of two variables: the total body potassium content and the relative distribution of potassium between the ECF and the ICF. The total body potassium content is determined by the difference between potassium intake and excretion. The second variable is a function of internal potassium balance. Figures 4 and 5 display potassium homeostasis. They outline how either hyperkalemia or hypokalemia may come about.

As mentioned earlier, potassium enters the body through the diet and is eliminated almost exclusively by the kidneys under normal circumstances. A review of the figures permits a rapid assessment of either hyperkalemia or hypokalemia. An increase in the ECF potassium concentration may occur either because of increased potassium intake, decreased renal excretion of potassium, or a shift in potassium balance across cell membranes from inside to outside cells. Similarly, a decrease in the ECF potassium concentration can result only from a decrease in potassium intake, an increase in potassium excretion, or a shift of potassium from outside to inside cells. Clearly,

HYPERKALEMIA

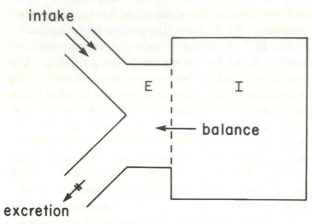

Figure 4. Potassium is almost all (98%) intracellular. The relationship between intracellular and extracellular potassium determines the potential difference across cell membranes. Hyperkalemia can develop if intake exceeds excretion, excretion is impaired, or if potassium moves from inside to outside cells.

combinations of these disorders may exist simultaneously.

Because only 2% of the total body potassium is outside cells, measurement of the ECF potassium concentration is a relatively crude estimate of the total body potassium, and serious errors in interpretation may result. Unfortunately, measurement of the total body potassium content is difficult and cumbersome. Sterns et al.[24] plotted the results of several studies and found that despite considerable variability, a crude estimate of total body potassium deficits can be made if hypokalemia is present. According to their estimate, a decrease in the serum concentration of 0.27 mmol/L represents a decrease in total body potassium of ~100 mmol.

The American diet contains ~50–80 mmol potassium/d.[6] Societies across the world differ in their potassium intake depending upon their diets.[6] Urinary excretion approaches intake albeit in a somewhat less accurate fashion than for sodium and chloride. Potassium is freely filtered at the glomerulus, reabsorbed in the proximal tubule, and secreted in the distal tubule, a process facilitated by the hormone aldosterone. Details on this process are outlined elsewhere.[4] (In the remainder of this discussion, we will concentrate on factors that alter internal balance.)

Factors Altering Internal Potassium Balance

Changes in Cell Mass. Changes in the size of the ICF may alter the internal potassium balance. For example, during chronic starvation cell mass decreases as a result of cellular protein and potassium losses from the body. Similarly, if cell mass were to increase as a result of growth or refeeding, potassium would be retained by the body in proportion to the retention of nitrogen. Many chronically starved individuals are hypokalemic, suggesting that potassium losses in these patients are out of proportion to nitrogen losses so that true potassium depletion as well as decreased cell mass may result. Refeeding of protein with resultant anabolism and cell growth and recovery may increase potassium requirements and aggravate hypokalemia if the requirements are not met. The same may occur if a chronic vitamin deficiency is treated in patients who are depleted in total body potassium. Examples include the treatment of vitamin B-12 or folic acid deficiency. Acute changes in cell mass from cell destruction, such as may occur from rhabdomyolysis or from hemolysis, may result in large endogenous potassium infusions, which may overwhelm the renal excretory capacity. Hyperkalemia, which may be life-threatening, may result.

Changes in Tonicity. When hypertonic solutions are infused intravenously, the resulting increase in osmolality of the ECF results in a shift of fluid from the ICF to the ECF. The resulting cellular dehydration results in a shift of potassium from inside cells to outside cells, thereby increasing the concentration of potassium in the ECF.[25] This effect may be clinically important. Hypertonic solutions both of glucose and of sodium bicarbonate are frequently given to treat hyperkalemia. If these solutions are infused quickly, the resulting cellular dehydration may obviate the desired clinical response.

Acid-base Disturbances. Under most circumstances, when extracellular pH decreases, potassium

HYPOKALEMIA

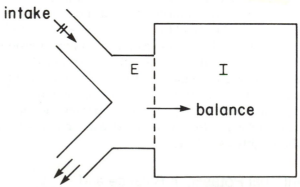

Figure 5. Hypokalemia can develop only if the intake of potassium is less than the losses, if potassium losses (e.g., renal losses, diarrhea, etc.) exceed intake, or if potassium moves from outside to inside cells.

exits from cells and the plasma potassium concentration increases. The converse occurs when extracellular pH increases. However, metabolic and respiratory acidoses differ in regard to their effect on ECF potassium.[24] Chronic respiratory acidosis does not influence internal potassium balance whereas effects of acute respiratory acidoses depend upon the duration of the disturbance.[26] Further, the effect of metabolic acidosis on internal potassium balance depends on the type of metabolic acidosis. The effects of mineral acids, such as hydrochloric acid, are greater than the effects of organic acids, such as lactic acid.[24] Metabolic alkalosis is almost invariably associated with a negative internal potassium balance. Hyperkalemia may be treated by precipitating metabolic alkalosis via the administration of sodium bicarbonate.

The effects of acid-base disturbance on internal potassium balance are complex and variable. The following generalizations are of clinical significance: (1) Patients with metabolic alkalosis are usually hypokalemic; however, the primary cause is total body potassium depletion rather than a redistribution of potassium within the body. (2) If renal function is adequate, metabolic acidosis also results in total body potassium depletion. Internal shifts of potassium from inside to outside cells are accompanied by increases in urinary potassium excretion. (3) Respiratory acid-base disturbances generally do not cause much of a change in internal potassium balance. (4) In hyperkalemic patients, the administration of alkali should cause a prompt movement of potassium from outside to inside cells regardless of the plasma pH. Such therapy should be accompanied by the administration of glucose and insulin, which also moves potassium to inside cells, as well as calcium gluconate infusion, which directly counteracts the cardiac toxicity of hyperkalemia. Potassium should also be removed from the body with the administration of cationic exchange resins or dialysis.

Hormones. Insulin directly stimulates net potassium uptake by skeletal muscle and hepatic cells.[27] Aldosterone promotes renal potassium excretion.[4] Catecholamines have direct effects on internal potassium balance. Beta-adrenergic agonists and epinephrine promote hypokalemia by enhancing the uptake of potassium by muscle, whereas α-agonists promote hyperkalemia by promoting the release of potassium from liver.[28,29] Thus, the effect of epinephrine may be biphasic, i.e., hyperkalemia followed by hypokalemia.

Drugs. Cardiac glycosides inhibit Na^+, K^+-ATPase. These drugs inhibit the net uptake of potassium. Succinylcholine induces a prolonged dose-related increase in the ionic permeability of muscle cells and consequently a prolonged efflux of potassium.[30] Beta-

blockers interfere with the deposition of potassium into muscle cells by epinephrine or other β-agonists.

Exercise. Exercise causes release of potassium from skeletal muscle. As a result, the systemic plasma potassium concentration increases to a degree determined by the extent of the exercise.

Requirements and Allowances for Potassium

The kidneys are responsible for potassium elimination and retention. However, the range in which the kidneys operate to maintain homeostasis of this cation is not as great as for sodium. Potassium ingestion throughout the world ranges from 50 to 200 mmol/d. An intake <50 mmol/d markedly impairs the palatability of food. An intake >200 mmol/d may cause hyperkalemia, although with adaptation potassium elimination by the kidneys is enhanced.[4]

Authorities have argued that a diet high in potassium and low in sodium (low urinary sodium-potassium ratio) favors lower blood pressure. Increase in dietary potassium (as the chloride salt) has been shown to decrease blood pressure in some hypertensive individuals. Finally, an increase in dietary potassium may result in a decrease in the susceptibility to stroke independent of blood pressure. Tobian reasons that primordial hunter-gatherer man ingested a diet low in sodium and chloride and high in potassium. It is possible that such a diet would decrease the development of cardiovascular disease.[31]

References

1. C. Bernard (1865) *An Introduction to the Study of Experimental Medicine* (translated by H.C. Green, 1957), Dover Publications, Inc., New York.
2. H.W. Smith (1959) *From Fish to Philosopher: the Story of Our Internal Environment,* CIBA Pharmaceutical Products Inc., Summit, NY.
3. R.F. Pitts (1974) *Physiology of the kidney and body fluids,* Year Book Medical Publishers Inc., Chicago, IL.
4. M.H. Maxwell, C.R. Kleeman, and R.G. Narins (1987) *Clinical Disorders of Fluid and Electrolyte Metabolism,* McGraw-Hill Book Company, New York.
5. M.P. Blaustein (1985) Sodium chloride, extracellular fluid volume, and hypertension. *Hypertension* 7:834–835.
6. The Intersalt Cooperative Research Group (1988) Intersalt: an international study of electrolyte excretion and blood pressure. Results for 24 hour urinary sodium and potassium excretion. *Br. Med. J.* 297:319–328.
7. F.C. Luft, L.I. Rankin, R. Bloch, et al. (1979) Cardiovascular and humoral responses to extremes of sodium intake in normal white and black men. *Circulation* 60:697–706.
8. M.B. Strauss, E. Lamdin, W.P. Smith, and D.J. Bleifer (1958) Surfeit and deficit of sodium. A kinetic concept of sodium excretion. *Arch. Intern. Med.* 102:527–536.
9. N.K. Hollenberg (1980) Set point for sodium homeostasis: surfeit, deficit, and their implications. *Kidney Int.* 17:423–429.

10. F.O. Simpson (1988) Sodium intake, body sodium, and sodium excretion. *Lancet* 2:25–28.
11. J.D. Swales (1988) Salt has only small importance in hypertension. *Br. Med. J.* 297:307–308.
12. A.N. Epstein (1986) Hormonal synergy as the cause of salt appetite. In: *The Physiology of Thirst and Sodium Appetite,* Series A: Life sciences, vol. 105 (G. De Caro, A.N. Epstein, and M. Massi, eds.), Plenum, New York.
13. J.T. Fitzsimons (1986) Endogenous angiotensin and sodium appetite. In: *The Physiology of Thirst and Sodium Appetite,* Series A: Life sciences, vol. 105 (G. De Caro, A.N. Epstein, and M. Massi, eds.), Plenum, New York.
14. J.L.S. Robertson (1984) The Franz Gross memorial lecture. The renin-aldosterone connection: past, present and future. *J. Hypertens.* 2(suppl. 3):1–14.
15. J.L.S. Robertson and R. Fraser (1987) Salt, volume, and hypertension: causation or correlation? *Kidney Int.* 32:590–602.
16. G.L. Robertson (1987) Physiology of ADH secretion. *Kidney Int.* 32(suppl. 21):S-20–S-26.
17. E. Ritz, J. Mann, and M. Schmid (1988) Salt and volume-regulating systems. In: *Salt and Hypertension* (R. Rettig, D. Ganten, and F.C. Luft, eds.), pp. 12–17, Springer Verlag, Berlin.
18. G.F. DiBona (1982) The renal nerves in renal adaptation to dietary Na restriction. *Am. J. Physiol.* 245:F322–F328.
19. F.C. Luft, L.I. Rankin, D.P. Henry, et al. (1979) Plasma and urinary norepinephrine values at extremes of sodium intake in normal man. *Hypertension* 1:261–266.
20. E.E. Selkurt, P.W. Hall, and M.P. Spencer (1949) Influence of graded arterial pressure decrement on renal clearance of creatinine, p-aminohippurate, and sodium. *Am. J. Physiol.* 159:369–376.
21. A.C. Guyton (1987) Renal function curve: a key to understanding the pathogenesis of hypertension. *Hypertension* 10:1.
22. G. Kimura (1987) Renal function curve in patients with secondary forms of hypertension. *Hypertension* 10:11–15.
23. M. Weiner and F.H. Epstein (1970) Signs and symptoms of electrolyte disorders. *Yale J. Biol. Med.* 43:76–109.
24. R.H. Sterns, C. Malcolm, P.U. Feig, and I. Singer (1981) Internal potassium balance and the control of the plasma potassium concentration. *Medicine* 60:339–354.
25. M. Moreno, C. Murphy, and C. Goldsmith (1969) Increase in serum potassium resulting from the administration of hypertonic mannitol and other solutions. *J. Lab. Clin. Med.* 73:291–298.
26. W.B. Schwartz, N.C. Brackett, and J.J. Cohen (1965) The response of extracellular hydrogen ion concentration to graded degrees of chronic hypercapnia: the physiologic limits of the defence of pH. *J. Clin. Invest.* 36:373–382.
27. R. DeFronzo, P. Felig, E. Ferrannini, and J. Wahren (1980) Effects of graded doses of insulin on splanchnic and peripheral potassium metabolism in man. *Am. J. Physiol.* 238:E421–E427.
28. E.P. Todd and R.L. Vick (1971) Kalemotropic effect of epinephrine: analysis with adrenergic agonists and antagonists. *Am. J. Physiol.* 220:1963–1969.
29. J. Castro-Tavares (1976) A comparison between the influence of pindolol and propranolol on the response of plasma potassium to catecholamines. *Arzneim. Forsch. Drug Research* 26:238–241.
30. G.A. Gronert and R.A. Theye (1975) Pathophysiology of hyperkalemia induced by succinylcholine. *Anesthesiology* 43:89–99.
31. R. Rettig, D. Ganten, and F.C. Luft (1988) *Salt and Hypertension,* Springer Verlag, Berlin.

Chapter 27

Peter R. Dallman

Iron

Iron is one of the most investigated and best understood of nutrients. Interest in iron deficiency has been stimulated by evidence that it is the most common nutritional deficiency in the United States[1,2] and worldwide[3] and by the demonstration that it can be successfully prevented on a large scale.[4,5] Research on iron nutrition has been facilitated by the relative ease with which the major iron pools of the body can be studied with blood samples and bone marrow aspirates. Furthermore, body iron homeostasis is regulated primarily by absorption, and the factors that alter and regulate iron absorption have been elucidated with the use of radioactive isotopes.[5]

Historical Background

The application of the scientific method to the study of iron nutrition probably began with the demonstration early in the 18th century that iron was a major constituent of blood.[6,7] Menghini, for example, drew attention to the iron content of blood by the simple experiment of showing that particles from dried, powdered blood could be lifted with a magnet. The widespread therapeutic use of iron tablets began in 1832 with a report by Blaud on the efficacy of treating young women in whom "coloring matter is lacking in the blood." About 50 years later, Bunge, professor of medicine at Basle and one of the first to quantify the iron content of the body and of foods, ridiculed Blaud's pills, which by then were in worldwide use. He interpreted the appearance of iron in the stools as showing that it could not be absorbed, and he believed with many other scientists of his time that no form of inorganic iron could serve as a precursor of hemoglobin. Although such vitalist views came under attack before the turn of the century, they persisted and were given a boost in the 1920s when Whipple and coworkers reported that cooked liver was more effective than ferrous carbonate in promoting the regeneration of blood. Convincing proof that inorganic iron could be used for hemoglobin synthesis came in 1932 from Castle and coworkers.[8] They found that the amount of iron given parenterally to patients with hypochromic anemia corresponded closely to the amount of iron gained in the circulating hemoglobin. The realization that dietary inorganic iron had to be in a soluble form in the intestine to be well absorbed became fully established only in the past few decades through absorption studies using radioactive isotopes of iron.

The special vulnerability of infants to iron deficiency was described by Bunge in 1892. He found that milk was an unusually poor source of iron and predicted that excessive feeding of milk could lead to iron deficiency after the depletion of neonatal iron reserves at the end of the suckling period. In 1928, Mackay[9] was among the first to demonstrate a high prevalence of iron-deficiency anemia in a large group of infants in East London and showed that the anemia could be alleviated by providing iron-fortified powdered milk. The widespread iron fortification of cereal products did not begin until World War II.

Iron Compounds in the Body: Distribution and Metabolic Functions[5,10]

Total body iron averages ~3.8 g in men and ~2.3 g in women. The iron-containing compounds in the body are grouped into two categories: those known to serve a metabolic or enzymatic function and those associated with iron storage and transport. The first category of so-called essential iron compounds consists primarily of heme proteins, i.e., proteins with an iron-porphyrin prosthetic group. The function of heme proteins is related to oxidative energy metabolism.

Essential Iron Compounds. Hemoglobin is the most abundant and easily sampled of the heme proteins and accounts for >65% of body iron. The function of hemoglobin is to transport oxygen via the bloodstream from the lungs to the tissues. Hemoglobin is a tetramer made up of four globin chains, each of which is associated with a heme group that contains one iron atom. Hemoglobin makes up >95% of the protein of the red cell and accounts for >10% of the weight of whole blood (mean values of 100–150 g/L, depending on age and sex).

Myoglobin, the red pigment of muscle, transports and stores oxygen for use during muscle contraction. This protein accounts for ~10% of total body iron. Its structure is similar to the monomeric units of hemoglobin; i.e., it is made up of one globin chain attached to one heme group containing a single iron atom. The myoglobin concentration in human muscle is ~5 mg/g of tissue.

Cytochromes are enzymes involved in electron transport and are located in the mitochondria and in other organelles. Cytochromes a, b, and c are present within the cristae of mitochondria in all aerobic cells and are essential for the oxidative production of cellular energy in the form of adenosine triphosphate (ATP). Cytochrome c, the most easily isolated and best characterized of the cytochromes, is a pink protein, and like myoglobin, it is made up of one globin chain and one heme group containing one atom of iron. Its concentration in man ranges from 5 to 100 μg/g of tissue. The highest concentrations are in tissues such as heart muscle that have a high rate of oxygen utilization. Cytochrome P-450 is located primarily within the microsomal membranes of liver cells and is involved in oxidative degradation of drugs and endogenous substrates. Cytochrome b_5 is a component of many membranes and is also present in the matrix of the red blood cell. In the latter it is believed to function in the reduction of methemoglobin. Other heme enzymes are catalase and peroxidase, including the myeloperoxidase of the granulocyte.

Another important group of iron enzymes is involved in oxidative metabolism in which iron is not in the form of heme. These compounds include the iron-sulfur proteins and metalloflavoproteins that account for more iron in the mitochondria than do the cytochromes. Examples are reduced nicotinamide adenine dinucleotide (NADH) dehydrogenase and succinic dehydrogenase. Heme and nonheme iron enzymes together account for ~3% of total body iron.

There is also a group of enzymes in which a supply of exogenous iron is required for enzymatic function. This group includes aconitase, an enzyme of the tricarboxylic acid cycle; phosphoenolpyruvate carboxykinase, a rate-limiting enzyme in the gluconeogenic pathway; and ribonucleotide reductase, an enzyme required for DNA synthesis.

Iron Storage Compounds. The major iron storage compounds are ferritin and hemosiderin, which are present primarily in the liver, reticuloendothelial cells, and bone marrow.[11,12] The total amount of storage iron varies over a wide range without apparent impairment of body function. Storage iron may be almost entirely depleted before iron-deficiency anemia develops. Conversely, a more than 20-fold increase over normal average iron stores may occur before there is evidence of tissue damage. Apoferritin, the protein portion of ferritin, consists of 24 polypeptide chains that form a raspberry-like spherical cluster around hydrated ferric phosphate that is contained within the hollow center. Ferritin contains varying amounts of iron ≤25% iron by weight. Hemosiderin, which makes up the other half of storage iron in the liver, is a heterogeneous group of large iron-salt-protein aggregates. Hemosiderin is believed to represent ferritin in various stages of degradation, because hemosiderin will react with antibodies to ferritin. As liver iron stores become abnormally large, hemosiderin makes up an increasingly greater proportion of total iron.

The contribution of storage iron to total body iron varies widely and averages ~12% in women and ~25% in men. The amount of storage iron influences iron absorption; as stores decrease, absorption increases. This autoregulatory response helps to maintain iron homeostasis and in large measure protects against both iron deficiency and iron overload.

Synthesis and Turnover of Iron Compounds.[5,10] Hemoglobin has a life span that corresponds to the roughly 120-d survival of the circulating red cell. Thus, <1% of total red cell iron is released each day from senescent red cells. Because of the large size of the hemoglobin iron pool, this small percentage of iron nevertheless accounts for the major flux of iron within the body. The iron released from hemoglobin breakdown is almost completely reutilized as are the amino acids. Heme, on the other hand, is degraded to bilirubin and is largely lost via the bile.

In contrast to hemoglobin in the red cell, tissue iron compounds are very heterogeneous with respect to lifespan. Furthermore, these compounds are subject to random degradation at an exponential rate similar to the rate of turnover of the subcellular structure with which they are associated. In rats, skeletal muscle cytochrome c, for example, has a half-life of ~6 d.[13] The implication of the dynamic state of most body iron constituents is that tissue deficits should be largely reversible by treatment with iron. However, the rates at which deficiencies of individual iron compounds are corrected often will differ markedly from the rate at which anemia is reversed.[14] Correction is most rapid in cell populations with a high turnover, such as intestinal mucosa. Deficiencies of muscle myoglobin and iron-containing electron-transport compounds are corrected more slowly than deficiencies of hemoglobin; depleted brain nonheme iron in the rat is replenished at such an extremely slow rate that the abnormality may not be completely reversible. In the case of some iron enzymes such as ribonucleotide reductase, a decrease in activity because of a lack of iron can probably be corrected within 1 h when increased iron becomes available without requiring the synthesis of the entire molecule.[15]

In an individual with iron deficiency anemia who is treated with iron, the rate of hemoglobin synthesis can increase severalfold, as indicated by the reticulocyte response and by a hemoglobin concentration that has increased about two-thirds toward the normal value within 1 mo of starting iron treatment.[5]

Iron Metabolism and Iron Absorption.

Iron metabolism is unusual in the degree to which dietary iron absorption differs and in the efficiency with which iron is retained once it has been absorbed. The bioavailability of iron—that is, the amount absorbed from food—can vary from <1% to >50%.[16,17] The percentage that is absorbed depends both on the nature of the diet and on regulatory mechanisms in the intestinal mucosa that reflect the body's physiologic need for iron.

Nonheme Iron.

Two types of iron are present in food: heme iron, which is found principally in animal products, and nonheme iron, which is found mainly in plant products. Most of the iron in the diet, usually >85%, is present as nonheme iron and consists primarily of iron salts. The absorption of nonheme iron is strongly influenced by its solubility in the upper part of the small intestine, which, in turn, depends on how the composition of the meal as a whole affects iron solubility. For example, nonheme iron absorption from a representative meal containing enhancers of absorption, such as meat, fish, or chicken, is about four times greater than it would be if the major protein source were equivalent portions of milk, cheese, or eggs.[18] Iron absorption tends to be poor from meals in which whole grain cereals and legumes predominate, but the addition of even relatively small amounts of meat or a source of vitamin C (ascorbic acid) substantially increases iron absorption from the entire meal. In comparison with water, orange juice or other beverages containing vitamin C will increase absorption of nonheme iron from a meal. Tea and coffee, on the other hand, decrease absorption of nonheme iron as compared with water.[16,19]

Human milk is low in iron, but its iron is relatively well absorbed in comparison with that in unfortified cow-milk formula.[20] This increased absorption may explain why breast-fed infants are less vulnerable to iron deficiency than infants fed unfortified cow-milk formula.

Heme Iron.

Heme iron is derived primarily from the hemoglobin and myoglobin in meat, poultry, and fish. Although heme iron accounts for a smaller proportion of iron in the diet than nonheme iron, it plays a quantitatively important role; a much greater percentage of heme iron is absorbed, and its absorption is less affected by other dietary constituents than is the absorption of nonheme iron.[16]

When both forms of iron in the diet are considered, an average of ~6% of total dietary iron is absorbed by men and ~13% by women in their childbearing years.[17] The higher absorption of iron by women is related to their lower body iron stores and helps to compensate for losses of iron associated with menstruation.

Intestinal Regulation.

The regulation of iron entry into the body takes place at the mucosal cell of the small intestine,[17] but the mechanism by which iron absorption is regulated remains in dispute.[21-23] If iron stores are low, as is true for most women and children, the intestinal mucosa readily takes up iron and increases the proportion absorbed from the diet. Conversely, the high-iron stores typical of men and postmenopausal women reduce the percentage of iron absorbed thereby offering some protection against iron overload (which is discussed later in this chapter). In infancy the abundance of lactoferrin, an iron-binding protein in human milk, and the presence of lactoferrin receptors on the surface of the intestinal mucosa may explain why iron is so well absorbed from human milk.[23]

Iron Transport.

The delivery of iron to the tissues of the body involves transferrin in the plasma and a system of cell-membrane receptors that are specific for transferrin.[21] The receptors bind the transferrin-iron complex at the cell surface and carry it into the cell where iron is released. The genes for both transferrin and the transferrin receptor are located on chromosome 3. The affinity of transferrin receptors for transferrin appears to be constant in various tissues. However, tissues such as erythroid precursors, placenta, and liver that have a high uptake of iron contain large numbers of transferrin receptors. The number of receptors is highly regulated.[24,25] When cells are in an iron-rich environment, the number of receptors decreases. Conversely, in iron-poor surroundings the number of transferrin receptors increases. These changes in receptor number can be accounted for by corresponding alterations in the level of messenger RNA, which, in turn, are mediated by two regions of the gene. These two gene regions can produce more than 20-fold differences in transcription levels according to iron availability.

Iron Requirements

Estimates of average requirements for absorbed iron in adults are based on careful experimental measurements of iron losses. The quantity of additional iron needed by growing infants and children is derived from the average weight gain and from estimates of iron needed to supply that gain with iron as hemoglobin, myoglobin, and iron enzymes. Such calculations are fairly straightforward. However, the derivation of recommendations for dietary iron intake requires some assumptions for which there is less quantitative support, i.e., (1) the amount of storage iron considered normal, (2) the figures used for the percentage of iron absorbed, and (3) the margin of safety allowed to accommodate for variations in iron requirements among individuals of the same age-sex group.

Iron losses occur primarily in the feces (0.6 mg/d): from bile, desquamated mucosal cells, and the loss of minute amounts of blood.[26] Smaller amounts of iron are lost in desquamated skin cells and in sweat (0.2–0.3 mg/d). Urinary losses are minor (<0.1 mg/d). For males, the total losses average 0.9 mg/d (with a range of ~0.5–2.0 mg/d). In addition to the above-mentioned losses, females during the childbearing years must replace the iron lost in menstrual blood, which over the month averages about 0.4 mg/d, making a total average loss of 1.3 mg/d.

During infancy and childhood, ~40 mg iron is required for the production of essential iron compounds (hemoglobin, myoglobin, and enzyme iron) for each kilogram of weight gain. If an allowance is made for the accumulation of iron stores, equivalent to the average iron stores of 300 mg/kg in women, an extra 5 mg/kg weight gain is required, making a total of 45 mg/kg of body weight gain. Iron needs for growth are greatest in infants and in adolescents.

Accurate measurements of iron losses are not available for children. However, because the major losses are from body surfaces (i.e., intestinal mucosa and skin), it seems reasonable to extrapolate on the basis of body surface area from the value of 1.0 mg/d in men. By this approach losses average ~0.2 mg/d for infants and 0.5 mg/d for children aged 6–11 y.

Once the needs for absorbed iron for growth and replacement of losses have been estimated, it is necessary to make an assumption about the percentage of iron absorbed from the diet. This will depend very much on the nature of the diet. A figure of 5% has been used for diets in which cereals and legumes predominate and that are low in tissue protein and ascorbic acid;[27] such diets are typical of many developing countries. A value of 15% is proposed for more varied diets that are rich in meat and ascorbic acid; 10% is used as an intermediate figure.[27] For the United States a working figure of 12.5% seems reasonable. Thus, multiplying the iron needs for growth

plus replacement of losses by eight provides an estimate for mean dietary iron requirements.

Lastly, recommendations for dietary iron, such as the RDA, make an allowance for individuals whose needs are greater than average. A factor of 1.25 (based on a coefficient of variation of 15%) has been used for this purpose.[28] The latter theoretically would provide sufficient iron to meet the needs of most of the population. However, the roughly 10% of women with menstrual blood loss >80 mL/mo might develop iron deficiency despite the consumption of a good diet and might require supplemental iron.[29]

Iron Deficiency and Iron-deficiency Anemia

Because iron is one of the earth's most abundant elements, it may seem surprising that iron deficiency should be a nutritional problem. One explanation is that the most common forms of iron in food are relatively insoluble and poorly absorbed from the intestine. Other factors predisposing to iron deficiency are related to evolving changes in the diet, not only during past millennia, but also within the last century.[30] To avoid obesity, energy intake should decline to accommodate a more sedentary lifestyle. However, a decreased energy intake is also likely to curtail iron intakes to a degree that may result in anemia in some children and young women.

Iron is poorly absorbed from diets consisting primarily of whole-grain cereals and legumes,[16,17] even though these relatively inexpensive foods contain substantial amounts of iron. This problem may be one reason that iron-deficiency anemia remains more common in developing countries in which cereals and legumes dominate the diet than in the United States.[1–3]

Stages of Iron Depletion. In theory iron depletion occurs in three stages.[31] The first involves only *decreased iron stores* (as measured by a decrease in serum ferritin) without loss of essential iron compounds. This stage is not associated with adverse physiologic consequences, but it does represent a condition of vulnerability. In the United States, women of childbearing age, for example, may characteristically have low iron stores, but in only a small percentage is there progression to anemia.[1] The risk of developing anemia is lessened by the body's ability to increase iron absorption as iron stores diminish.

The second stage is characterized by biochemical changes that reflect the lack of iron sufficient for normal production of hemoglobin and other essential iron compounds and is indicated by a decrease in transferrin saturation levels and an increase in erythrocyte protoporphyrin. Because the hemoglobin concentration does not yet fall below levels considered indicative of anemia, this stage is regarded as *iron deficiency without anemia.*

The third stage is frank *iron-deficiency anemia,* which occurs when hemoglobin production has been sufficiently depressed to result in a hemoglobin concentration (and often mean corpuscular volume) below the normal reference range for individuals of the same age and sex. It is important to make the distinction between anemia and iron-deficiency anemia. Anemia refers to a concentration of hemoglobin or a hematocrit below the central 95% range for healthy individuals of the same age and sex. A corollary of this definition is that 2.5% of healthy individuals will be termed anemic. Furthermore, it should be realized that there are many causes of anemia other than iron deficiency; infection and inflammatory disease, even if mild, are particularly common causes. A diagnosis of iron-deficiency anemia is customarily made if anemia is accompanied by another laboratory abnormality, such as low serum ferritin or anemia corrected by treatment with iron.

Causes of Iron Deficiency. The major causes of iron deficiency are insufficient assimilation of iron from the diet, dilution of body iron by rapid growth, and loss of blood.[5,28] Because the manifestations of iron deficiency are rarely obvious, most cases are detected by laboratory tests. The groups at highest risk for iron deficiency are infants, adolescents, and women, especially pregnant women, between the ages of menarche and menopause.[1]

Age-related Factors in Susceptibility to Iron Deficiency

Infants. The prevalence of iron deficiency in infants is highest between ~4 mo, when neonatal iron stores are first likely to become depleted, and 3 y of age.[32] During this period total iron in the body should more than double to accommodate a rapid rate of growth and an increase in red cell mass. Excessive consumption of milk is commonly associated with iron deficiency in young infants. Milk is a poor source of iron and is frequently associated with occult intestinal blood loss in early infancy.[33] In premature infants and in twins, iron-deficiency anemia may develop as early as 3 mo after birth, because neonatal iron stores are smaller and infant weight gain is proportionately greater than that of full-term or single infants. In children of all age groups, iron deficiency results from diets that are poor sources of absorbable iron and is associated with poverty.[1]

Adolescents. Iron deficiency is common during and after the period of rapid growth during adolescence.[1,2] Boys gain an average of 10 kg during the peak year of their growth spurt, i.e., sometime between ~12 and 15 y of age. At about the same age as the growth spurt and in response to sexual maturation, the concentration of hemoglobin increases between 5 and 10 $g \cdot L^{-1} \cdot y^{-1}$ toward values that are characteristic of adult men.[32] The double burden of providing iron for an increased red cell mass and increased hemoglobin concentration requires an increase of ~25% in total body iron during the year of peak growth. The iron need of adolescent girls is also large. Their average weight gain of 9 kg during the peak year of the growth spurt, i.e., sometime between ~10 and 12 y of age, is almost as great as in boys. Although the concentration of hemoglobin changes very little during this period, the onset of menstruation imposes additional iron needs.

Women During the Childbearing Years. The major factors that predispose to iron-deficiency anemia in this group are menorrhagia (excessive loss of blood during menstruation) and pregnancy.[5] Heavy blood loss (>80 mL/mo) has been reported to occur in ~10% of women and frequently lends to anemia.[29] The use of intrauterine contraceptive devices increases the prevalence of menorrhagia to ~30–50% of women, depending on the type used.[34] Oral contraceptives, on the other hand, decrease menstrual blood loss by about half and are rarely associated with menorrhagia.[35] Women with menorrhagia are characteristically unaware of their greater than normal menstrual blood loss.[29] For this reason blood tests at the time of routine health examinations sometimes detect an anemia that is most frequently related to menorrhagia, even when the woman does not consider menstrual blood loss to be unusual.

Iron-deficiency anemia may develop during pregnancy[32] because of the increased requirements for iron to supply the expanding blood volume of the mother as well as the rapidly growing fetus and placenta.[5,36–39] True anemia, however, must be distinguished from the decline in hemoglobin concentration that normally occurs as a result of the disproportionate expansion of plasma to red cell volume. Anemia during pregnancy, therefore, must be diagnosed with the use of appropriate standards, e.g., a lower limit of normal of 110 g/L between 20 and 30 wk of gestation rather than the 120 g/L for nonpregnant women. Hemoglobin concentration normally increases during the last 6–8 wk of a full-term gestation.

Healthy women who are not pregnant average ~2.3 g of total body iron; only ~0.3 g of this amount is storage iron. The total iron requirement during the entire course of pregnancy averages 1 g and, therefore, exceeds the amount of storage iron in most women.[36] However, an increase in efficiency of dietary iron absorption compensates in part for the limited iron stores. Most of the additional iron is needed during the last half of pregnancy.

Even with the normal adaptive increase in iron absorption that takes place during pregnancy, iron stores are likely to become depleted, and some women will develop anemia.[37,39] Therefore, it is reasonable to recommend an iron supplement that provides the equivalent of ~30 mg/d of elemental iron during the second and third trimesters of pregnancy. After delivery the iron requirement of the mother is reduced as the expanded mass of red cells decreases to prepregnancy levels. Mild iron deficiency in the pregnant woman has no detectable effect on hemoglobin concentration in the newborn but may result in a moderate decrease in serum ferritin.[32]

Men and Postmenopausal Women. Normally, iron stores increase throughout adult life in men and after menopause in women,[1] and nutritional iron deficiency rarely develops in these groups. In elderly people anemia is more commonly associated with chronic inflammatory conditions (e.g., arthritis) than with iron deficiency.[40] However, factors that could predispose to iron-deficiency anemia in these groups are frequent blood donations (three or more times a year), blood loss from chronic aspirin ingestion, and such conditions as bleeding ulcers and colorectal cancers. Aspirin consumption results in intestinal blood loss by impairing platelet aggregation. In one study, it was found that an aspirin (300 mg) taken three times a day for a week increased intestinal blood loss to 5 mL/d from a normal average of 0.5 mL/d.[41] When there is no known basis for iron-deficiency anemia, chronic and inapparent loss of blood from the intestine because of lesions such as a peptic ulcer or carcinoma may prove to be responsible. Parasitic infestation, particularly hookworm, is also a common cause of inapparent intestinal blood loss in some developing countries but is rare in the United States.

Consequences of Iron Deficiency

The manifestations of iron-deficiency anemia are usually subtle. The degree of functional impairment generally increases as the essential iron compounds become more depleted.[42] Some manifestations are related to anemia itself, some to the effects of iron deficiency on tissues, and some to a combination of the two.[10]

Work Performance. Studies in humans as well as in rats show that anemia causes a substantial reduction in work capacity. This is particularly evident when the concentration of hemoglobin falls below 100 g/L, which is 20–40 g/L below the lower limit of normal for adults. Some studies in humans indicate that even milder anemia can decrease performance in brief, hard exercise.[43] The practical significance of

these findings in regard to productivity has been investigated in studies in developing countries of manual laborers suffering from iron-deficiency anemia. For example, for men on a rubber plantation in Indonesia[44] and women on a tea plantation in Sri Lanka,[45] the productivity of iron-deficient individuals was significantly less than that of workers with normal hemoglobin concentrations. After supplementation with iron, the performance of the iron-deficient subjects improved; the greatest improvement occurred in those who had the lowest initial hemoglobin concentrations.

In humans, impaired work performance certainly can be related to anemia per se, but it is uncertain to what extent tissue abnormalities are also responsible. Experiments with rats show that dietary iron deficiency in addition to anemia results in a marked impairment in the oxidative production of cellular energy in skeletal muscle.[46–48] A major consequence of this muscle impairment is a lessened capacity for prolonged exercise, increased glucose oxidation, and greater use of the gluconeogenic pathway by which lactate from the muscle is converted to glucose in the liver.[10]

Body Temperature Regulation. An impaired capacity to maintain body temperature in a cold environment is characteristic of iron-deficiency anemia. This abnormality appears to be related to decreased secretion of thyroid-stimulating hormone and thyroid hormone.[49] Impaired heat production appears to result from the anemia itself; a transfusion of red blood cells in the iron-deficient rat corrects the abnormality. Furthermore, rats fed adequate diets develop impaired heat production when they are made anemic by bleeding.

Behavior and Intellectual Performance. Increasing evidence indicates that impaired psychomotor development and intellectual performance and changes in behavior result from iron deficiency.[50] Most studies have evaluated infants between 6 mo and 2 y of age using the Bayley Scale of Infant Development, a test for sensory development, fine and gross motor skills, and language development. Using this test, infants who are even mildly iron deficient (the second and third stages of iron depletion) are found to exhibit a statistically significant decrease in responsiveness and activity and increased body tension, fearfulness, and tendency to fatigue.[51] The long-term significance of these changes has not been determined. Of particular interest is the observation that abnormalities are most profound in older infants (19–24 mo) in whom iron deficiency can be presumed to have been present for the longest period.[52] Another important finding is that even infants with very mild iron-deficiency anemia do not score as well as infants with no laboratory evidence of iron deficiency or evidence merely of depleted iron stores.[51,53,54] The possibility of behavioral abnormalities assumes importance because the rapid rate of growth and differentiation of brain cells during infancy might be expected to make the brain particularly vulnerable to deficiencies in the supply of nutrients. Furthermore, there is evidence that the abnormalities are not corrected after 1–3 mo of iron treatment.[50]

Resistance to Infections. Laboratory evidence of decreased resistance to infection is a characteristic of iron deficiency in both humans and experimental animals.[55] Iron-deficient children have abnormalities in the function of lymphocytes and neutrophils, two types of white blood cells that play important roles in the defense against infection. Despite numerous studies that show an impaired resistance to infection under laboratory conditions, there is no conclusive evidence for an increased rate of infections caused by iron deficiency per se. Iron-deficiency anemia and infections are both common among poor populations, but a cause-and-effect relationship, although plausible, has not been established.[55]

Lead Poisoning. Iron deficiency substantially increases the risk of lead poisoning, particularly in young children. Iron-deficient individuals absorb increased amounts of lead,[56] and elevated blood lead concentrations are most common in young children with laboratory evidence of iron deficiency.[57]

Prevention of Iron Deficiency

Iron deficiency can be prevented by increasing the content and bioavailability of iron in the diet. Iron absorption can be improved by including meat, fish, or poultry and/or ascorbic acid–rich foods in meals and by decreasing consumption of tea and milk with meals. Iron-fortified cereal products augment iron intake. Parental awareness of appropriate diet is especially important for infants, whose diet is relatively simple. Iron nutrition can be improved by breast-feeding and by using iron-fortified formula during the first year for infants who are not breast-fed. Iron-fortified infant cereals are used when solid foods become part of the diet after ~4–6 mo of age. These infant-feeding practices have been widely adopted over the past 10–15 y, a change that helps to explain the striking decline in prevalence of anemia over this period.[58,59]

Fortification of infant formula and of cereal and grain products is a relatively inexpensive and effective means of increasing iron intake.[60,61] These foods can reach a large segment of the population in amounts adequate to decrease the prevalence of iron deficiency. The use of supplements, on the other hand, involves less certainty of compliance. However, iron supplements are appropriate for certain groups with unusually large iron requirements, such as women with menorrhagia, women during the last half of pregnancy, and breast-fed low-birth-weight infants.

Decline in Prevalence and Severity of Iron Deficiency in the United States

The striking decline in prevalence of anemia in infants and children over the past 10–15 y[59,60] can be attributed partly to the increased use of bioavailable iron compounds to fortify cereal products in addition to the dietary trends already described. There has probably been a substantial decline in prevalence of anemia among women of childbearing years as well.[1,2] The best evidence regarding trends has come from Gothenburg, Sweden, where 30% of women of fertile age were anemic in 1965 compared with 7% in 1975.[4] The difference was attributed to several causes including the increased use of iron supplements, increased iron fortification of foods, increased use of birth-control pills, and increased intake of ascorbic acid. Some of these factors should also apply to the United States.

Diagnosis of Iron Deficiency[5,62]

The manifestations of iron deficiency are usually too subtle to initiate a visit to the doctor.[42] Typically, iron deficiency is suspected on the basis of the dietary history and a low hemoglobin concentration or hematocrit (Table 1) obtained on a routine health-maintenance visit. If the hemoglobin concentration is determined by electronic counter, the red blood cell indices are also provided and are helpful; a low mean corpuscular volume (MCV) and/or mean cor-

Table 1. Screening tests for iron deficiency: lower limits of the 95% reference range*

Age	Hemo-globin	Hemato-crit	Mean corpuscular volume	Mean corpuscular hemoglobin
	g/L		fL	pg
0.5–4 y	110	0.32	72	24
5–10 y	110	0.33	75	25
11–14 y				
Female	115	0.34	78	26
Male	120	0.35	78	26
15–19 y				
Female	120	0.35	79	27
Male	130	0.39	79	27
20–44 y				
Female	120	0.35	80	27
Male	135	0.40	80	27

* From reference 62.

puscular hemoglobin (MCH) provides strong supportive evidence for iron deficiency. If the history and the blood count seem in accord with iron deficiency, a therapeutic trial with iron may be indicated without further confirmatory tests, especially if the anemia is mild (hemoglobin within 10 g/L of the lower limit of normal). However, hemoglobin and hematocrit determinations on skin puncture blood have a substantial sampling error. If the results are borderline or only slightly below the normal range, a repeat hemoglobin analysis on venous blood will often be normal. Therefore, a finding of anemia on venous blood is a sounder basis for either a therapeutic trial or a decision on the necessity for additional laboratory tests.

An alternative to a therapeutic trial with iron is to select an additional laboratory test to strengthen the presumptive diagnosis of iron deficiency. The tests that are used most commonly are erythrocyte protoporphyrin, serum ferritin, and transferrin saturation (Table 2). The choice of tests depends on local circumstances, convenience, and availability. The most common source of diagnostic error is a recent or concurrent infection or an inflammatory condition (such as arthritis) that typically causes anemia and results in confusing abnormalities in other laboratory tests used in the diagnosis of iron deficiency, i.e., a decrease in transferrin saturation and an increase in serum ferritin.

Treatment[5,62]

The most common problem encountered in the treatment of iron deficiency is gastrointestinal side effects, usually resulting from larger-than-necessary doses of iron compounds in excess of 120 mg/d of elemental iron. Ferrous sulfate is the least expensive and most widely used oral form of iron. A dose equivalent to 60 mg of elemental iron (300 mg ferrous sulfate) once or twice a day is ample for an adult if given between meals, first thing in the morning, or at bedtime. In infants at ~1 y of age, 30 mg/d as elemental iron first thing in the morning rarely causes side effects; this dose is also appropriate and adequate for older children and adolescents. Fortunately, the smaller the dose and the more severe the anemia, the greater will be the percentage of iron absorbed. A response to treatment of anemia should be evident after 1 mo when, on average, the deficit in hemoglobin is two-thirds corrected. Iron treatment then should be continued for another 2–3 mo. If there is no correction of anemia after 1 mo despite good compliance in taking iron medication, other diagnoses, including iron deficiency from chronic blood loss, should be considered. The continued administration of iron for an unresponsive anemia obscures

Table 2. Confirmatory tests for iron deficiency: recommended cutoff values*

Age	Serum ferritin	Transferrin saturation	Erythrocyte protoporphyrin*
	µg/L	%	µmol/L RBC
0.5–4 y	<10	<12	>1.42
5–10 y	<10	<14	>1.24
11–14 y	<10	<16	>1.24
≥15 y	<12	<16	>1.24

* From reference 62.

the real cause of the abnormality and risks the accumulation of excess iron.

Iron Toxicity and Excess

Acute iron toxicity is one of the most common forms of poisoning, particularly among preschool-age children.[63] The most effective form of prevention is to keep iron supplements out of reach of children. Severe iron poisoning is characterized by damage to the intestinal lining, which can cause bloody diarrhea and vomiting. Acidosis, liver failure, and shock may follow. Effective treatment by induced emesis, fluid and electrolyte treatment to prevent shock, and use of iron-chelating agents has substantially decreased the mortality from ~50% in the 1950s to less than a few percent in recent years.

Chronic iron overload results primarily from a genetic disorder, hemochromatosis, which is characterized by increased iron absorption, and from relatively rare diseases that require frequent transfusions, such as thalassemia and aplastic anemia.[5] Hemochromatosis is a homozygous disorder that results in clinical abnormalities primarily among men after their 50s. These manifestations include diabetes, liver failure, and heart failure caused by excess iron deposition and cell damage in the pancreas, liver, and heart. The frequency of the homozygous state is estimated to be between 1 per 125 and 1 per 300 but only a fraction of this number develops clinically apparent disease, which is present in a frequency between 1 per 500 and 1 per 1000.[64] Because increased dietary iron could aggravate hemochromatosis, the existence of this problem argues against a substantial increase in the level of iron fortification of foods above current levels. However, the degree of risk should not be exaggerated. In Sweden where iron fortification of cereal products is about three times that in the United States, clinically apparent disease is present in fewer than 1 in 1000 men.[65]

Homozygous thalassemia is a relatively rare hereditary hemolytic anemia seen primarily in individuals of Mediterranean or Southeast Asian origin and requires treatment with repeated blood transfusions for survival. Iron fortification of foods adds an undesirable additional iron load but one that is relatively small compared with the >200 mg iron that is supplied in each unit of packed red blood cells.

Excessive iron intake may affect the absorption of other trace elements. Although a high dose of iron medication will impair the absorption of zinc or copper administered at the same time,[66] it is doubtful that this interaction is important with ordinary diets. Of greater concern is the possibility of compromised zinc or copper absorption when iron supplements are administered in very large doses.[67,68]

Excessive iron administration, particularly when given parenterally, may increase the risk of infection.[69,70] The basis for this concern is that a high degree of saturation of the iron-binding protein transferrin enhances the growth of many bacteria. Conditions of iron overload are associated with very high levels of transferrin saturation. Although this issue may be important for patients with iron overload, recent U.S. survey data indicate that an abnormally high transferrin saturation is rare in the general population.[1]

References

1. S.M. Pilch and F.R. Senti (1984) *Assessment of the Iron Nutritional Status of the U.S. Population Based on the Data Collected in the Second National Health and Nutrition Examination Survey, 1976–1980*, p. 65, Federation of American Societies for Experimental Biology, Bethesda, MD.
2. P.R. Dallman, R. Yip, and C. Johnson (1984) Prevalence and causes of anemia in the United States, 1976–1980. *Am. J. Clin. Nutr.* 39:437–445.
3. E. DeMaeyer, M. Adiels-Tegman, and E. Rayston (1985) The prevalence of anemia in the world. *World Health Stat. Q.* 38:302–316.
4. L. Hallberg, C. Bengtsson, L. Garby, J. Lennartsson, L. Rossander, and E. Tibblin (1979) An analysis of factors leading to a reduction in iron deficiency in Swedish women. *Bull WHO* 57:947–954.
5. T.H. Bothwell, R.W. Charlton, J.D. Cook, and C.A. Finch (1979) *Iron Metabolism in Man,* Blackwell, Oxford.
6. C.M. McCay (1973) *Notes on the History of Nutrition Research,* pp. 138–144 and 156–171, Huber, Bern.
7. E.V. McCollum (1957) *A History of Nutrition,* pp. 334–358, Houghton Mifflin, Boston.
8. C.W. Heath, M.B. Strauss, and W.B. Castle (1932) Quantitative aspects of iron deficiency in hypochromic anemia. *J. Clin. Invest.* 11:91–110.
9. H.M. Mackay (1928) Anaemia in infancy; prevalence and prevention. *Arch. Dis. Child.* 3:117–146.
10. P.R. Dallman (1986) Biochemical basis for the manifestations of iron deficiency. *Annu. Rev. Nutr.* 6:13–40.
11. C. Hershko (1977) Storage iron regulation. *Prog. Hematol.* 10:105–148.
12. A. Deiss (1983) Iron metabolism in reticuloendothelial cells. *Semin. Hematol.* 20:81–90.
13. F.W. Booth and J.O. Holloszy (1977) Cytochrome c turnover in rat skeletal muscles. *J. Biol. Chem.* 252:416–419.
14. P.R. Dallman (1974) Tissue effects of iron deficiency. In: *Iron in Biochemistry and Medicine* (A. Jacobs and M. Worwood, eds.), pp. 437–476, Academic Press, London.
15. L. Thelander, A. Gräslund, and M. Thelander (1983) Continual presence of oxygen and iron required for mammalian ribonucleotide reduction: possible regulation mechanism. *Biochem. Biophys. Res. Commun.* 110:859–865.
16. L. Hallberg (1981) Bioavailability of iron in man. *Annu. Rev. Nutr.* 1:123–147.
17. R.W. Charlton and T.H. Bothwell (1983) Iron absorption. *Annu. Rev. Med.* 34:55–68.
18. J.D. Cook and E.R. Monsen (1976) Food iron absorption in human subjects. III. Comparison of the effect of animal proteins on nonheme iron absorption. *Am. J. Clin. Nutr.* 29:859–867.
19. L. Rossander, L. Hallberg, and E. Björn-Rasmussen (1979) Absorption of iron from breakfast meals. *Am. J. Clin. Nutr.* 32:2484–2489.
20. U.M. Saarinen, M.A. Siimes, and P.R. Dallman (1977) Iron absorption in infants: high bioavailability of breast milk iron as indicated by the extrinsic tag method of iron absorption and by the concentration of serum ferritin. *J. Pediatr.* 91:36–39.
21. H.A. Huebers and C.A. Finch (1987) The physiology of transferrin and transferrin receptors. *Physiol. Rev.* 67:520–581.
22. T.J. Peters, K.B. Raja, R.J. Simpson, and S. Snape (1988) Mechanisms and regulation of iron absorption. *Ann. N.Y. Acad. Sci.* 526:141–147.
23. L.A. Davidson, and B. Lönnerdal (1988) Specific binding of lactoferrin to brush-border membrane: ontogeny and effect of glycon chain. *Am. J. Physiol.* 254:G580–G585.
24. J.L. Casey, M.W. Hentze, D.M. Koeller, et al. (1988) Iron-responsive elements: regulatory RNA sequences that control in RNA levels and translation. *Science* 240:924–928.
25. J.L. Casey, B. DiJeso, K. Rao, T.A. Rouault, R.D. Klausner, and J.B. Harford (1988) The promoter region of the human transferrin receptor gene. *Ann. N.Y. Acad. Sci.* 526:54–64.
26. R. Green, R.W. Charlton, H. Seftel, et al. (1968) Body iron excretion in man. A collaborative study. *Am. J. Med.* 45:336–353.
27. E.R. Monsen, L. Hallberg, M. Layrisse, et al. (1978) Estimation of available dietary iron. *Am. J. Clin. Nutr.* 31:134–141.
28. FAO/WHO (Food and Agriculture Organization/ World Health Organization). (1989 in press) Requirements of Vitamin A, Iron, Folate and Vitamin B$_{12}$. Report of a Joint FAO/WHO Expert Group, WHO, Geneva.
29. L. Hallberg, A. Högdahl, L. Nilsson, and G. Rybo (1966) Menstrual blood loss—a population study. *Acta Obstet. Gynecol. Scand.* 45:320–351.
30. S.B. Eaton and M. Konner (1985) Paleolithic nutrition. A consideration of its nature and current implications. *N. Engl. J. Med.* 312:283–289.
31. J.D. Cook and C.A. Cook (1979) Assessing iron status of a population. *Am. J. Clin. Nutr.* 32:2115–2119.
32. P.R. Dallman, M.A. Siimes, and A. Stekel (1980) Iron deficiency in infancy and childhood. *Am. J. Clin. Nutr.* 33:86–118.
33. S.J. Fomon, E.E. Ziegler, S.E. Nelson, and B.B. Edwards (1981) Cow milk feeding in infancy: gastrointestinal blood loss and iron nutritional status. *J. Pediatr.* 98:540–545.
34. R. Israel, S.T. Shaw, and M.A. Martin (1974) Comparative quantitation of menstrual blood loss with the Lippes loop, Dalkon shield, and Copper T intrauterine devices. *Contraception* 10:63–71.
35. F. Hefnawi, H. Askalani, and K. Zaki (1974) Menstrual blood loss with copper intrauterine devices. *Contraception* 9:133–139.
36. L. Hallberg (1988) Iron balance in pregnancy. In: *Vitamins and Minerals in Pregnancy and Lactation,* vol. 16, (H. Beyer, ed.), pp. 115–126, Nestle Nutrition Workshop Series, Rouen Press, New York.
37. B. Svanberg, B. Arvidsson, A. Norrby, G. Rybo, and L. Solvell (1975) Absorption of supplemental iron during pregnancy. *Acta Obstet. Gynecol. Scand. [Suppl.]* 48:87–108.

38. J. Puolakka (1980) Serum ferritin as a measure of iron stores during pregnancy. *Acta Obstet. Gynecol. Scand.* [*Suppl.*] 95:1–63.

39. D.J. Taylor, C. Mallen, N. McDougall, and T. Lind (1982) Effect of iron supplementation on serum ferritin levels during and after pregnancy. *Br. J. Obstet. Gynaecol.* 89:1011–1017.

40. R. Yip and P.R. Dallman (1988) The roles of inflammation and iron deficiency as causes of anemia. *Am. J. Clin. Nutr.* 48:1295–1300.

41. R.N. Pierson, Jr., P.R. Holt, R.M. Watson, and R.P. Keating (1961) Aspirin and gastrointestinal bleeding. Chromate 51 blood loss studies. *Am. J. Med.* 31:259–265.

42. P.R. Dallman (1982) Manifestations of iron deficiency. *Semin. Hematol.* 19:19–30.

43. F.E. Viteri and B. Torun (1974) Anemia and physical work capacity. *Clin. Hematol.* 3:609–626.

44. S.S. Basta, M.S. Soekirman, D. Karyadi, and N.S. Scrimshaw (1979) Iron deficiency anemia and the productivity of adult males in Indonesia. *Am. J. Clin. Nutr.* 32:916–925.

45. V.R. Edgerton, G.W. Gardner, Y. Ohira, K.A. Gunawardena, and B. Senewiratne (1979) Iron-deficiency anemia and its effect on worker productivity and activity patterns. *Br. Med. J.* 2:1546–1549.

46. C.A. Finch, L.R. Miller, A.R. Inamdar, R. Person, K. Seiler, and B. Mackler (1976) Iron deficiency in the rat: physiological and biochemical studies of muscle dysfunction. *J. Clin. Invest.* 58:447–453.

47. J.A. McLane, R.D. Fell, R.H. McKay, W.W. Winder, E.B. Brown, and J.O. Holloszy (1981) Physiological and biochemical effects of iron deficiency on rat skeletal muscle function. *Am. J. Physiol.* 241:C47–C54.

48. K.J.A. Davies, C.M. Donovan, C.A. Refino, G.A. Brooks, L. Packer, and P.R. Dallman (1984) Distinguishing effects of anemia and muscle iron deficiency on exercise bioenergetics in the rat. *Am. J. Physiol.* 246:E535–E543.

49. J. Beard, W. Green, L. Miller, and C.A. Finch (1984) Effect of iron-deficiency anemia on hormone levels and thermoregulation during cold exposure. *Am. J. Physiol.* 247:R114–R119.

50. B. Lozoff (1988) Behavioral alterations in iron deficiency. *Adv. Pediatr.* 35:331–359.

51. B. Lozoff, G.M. Brittenham, F.E. Viteri, A.W. Wolf, and J.J. Urrutia (1982) The effects of short-term oral iron therapy on developmental deficits in iron-deficient anemic infants. *J. Pediatr.* 100:351–357.

52. B. Lozoff, G.M. Brittenham, F.E. Viteri, A.W. Wolf, and J.J. Urrutia (1982) Developmental deficits in iron-deficient infants: effects of age and severity of iron lack. *J. Pediatr.* 101:948–952.

53. F.A. Oski, A.S. Honig, B. Helu, and P. Howanitz (1983) Effect of iron therapy on behavior performance in nonanemic, iron-deficient infants. *Pediatrics* 71:877–880.

54. T. Walter, J. Kovalskys, and A. Stekel (1983) Effect of mild iron deficiency on infant mental development scores. *J. Pediatr.* 104:710–713.

55. P.R. Dallman (1987) Iron deficiency and the immune response. *Am. J. Clin. Nutr.* 46:329–334.

56. W.S. Watson, J. Morrison, M.I.F. Bethel, et al. (1986) Food iron and lead absorption in humans. *Am. J. Clin. Nutr.* 44:248–256.

57. R. Yip and P.R. Dallman (1984) Developmental changes in erythrocyte protoporphyrin: roles of iron deficiency and lead toxicity. *J. Pediatr.* 104:710–713.

58. R. Yip, N.J. Blinkin, L. Fleshood, and F.L. Trowbridge (1987) Declining prevalence of anemia among low-income children in the United States. *JAMA* 258:1619–1623.

59. R. Yip, K.M. Walsh, M.G. Goldfarb, and N.V. Binkin (1987) Declining prevalence of anemia in childhood in a middle class setting: a pediatric success story? *Pediatrics* 80:330–334.

60. International Nutritional Anemia Consultative Group (1982) *The Effects of Cereals and Legumes on Iron Absorption,* Nutrition Foundation, New York.

61. F.M. Clydesdale and K.L. Wiemer, eds. (1985) *Iron Fortification of Foods,* Academic Press, Orlando, FL.

62. P.R. Dallman (1987) Iron deficiency and related nutritional anemias. In: *Hematology of Infancy and Childhood,* 3rd ed. (D.G. Nathan and F.A. Oski, eds.), pp. 274–296, Saunders, Philadelphia.

63. W. Banner, Jr., and T.G. Tong (1986) Iron poisoning. *Pediatr. Clin. North Am.* 33:393–409.

64. C.Q. Edwards, L.M. Griffen, D. Goldgar, C. Drummond, M.H. Skolnick, and J.P. Kushner (1988) The prevalence of hemachromatosis among 11,065 presumably healthy blood donors. *N. Engl. J. Med.* 318:1355–1362.

65. B. Lindmark and S. Eriksson (1985) Regional differences in the idiopathic hemochromatosis gene frequency in Sweden. *Acta Med. Scand.* 218:299–304.

66. N.W. Solomons and R.A. Jacobs (1981) Studies of the bioavailability of zinc in man. IV. Effects of heme and non-heme iron on absorption of zinc. *Am. J. Clin. Nutr.* 34:475–482.

67. M.W. Breskin, B.S. Worthington-Roberts, R.H. Knopp, et al. (1983) First trimester serum zinc concentrations in human pregnancy. *Am. J. Clin. Nutr.* 38:943–953.

68. K.M. Hambidge, N.F. Krebs, L. Sibley, and J. English (1987) Acute effects of iron therapy on zinc status during pregnancy. *Obstet. Gynecol.* 70:593–596.

69. R.G. Strauss (1978) Iron deficiency, infections, and immune function: a reassessment. *Am. J. Clin. Nutr.* 31:660–666.

70. E.D. Weinberg (1984) Iron withholding: a defense against infection and neoplasia. *Physiol. Rev.* 64:65–102.

Chapter **28**   Robert J. Cousins and James M. Hempe

Zinc

The current focus of zinc nutrition research includes assessment of requirements, evaluation of factors affecting absorption and metabolism, determination of metabolic pathways, identification and characterization of zinc metalloenzymes and metal-protein complexes, and elucidation of the molecular biology of zinc, particularly zinc-dependent DNA-binding proteins. This chapter is intended to be a condensation of the vast recent literature related to these subjects. In-depth reviews are available for more detailed information.[1-10]

Discovery of Essentiality

Because of its unique chemistry, zinc serves essential structural, catalytic, and regulatory functions in many biological systems.[11] Essentiality was demonstrated first in plants in 1869.[12] Evidence of essentiality in animals, reported in 1934, required the use of low-zinc semipurified diets.[13] Because of the ubiquitous presence of zinc in foods, naturally occurring zinc deficiency was thought unlikely until 1957 when zinc was shown to alleviate parakeratosis in swine fed practical-type, vegetable-protein diets high in calcium.[14]

The essentiality of zinc in human nutrition was first documented in the early 1960s.[3] Growth depression and delayed sexual development in young Iranian and Egyptian men consuming vegetable-protein-based diets was alleviated by supplemental zinc. Classical symptoms of severe zinc deficiency are observed rarely. However, nutrition surveys and recent clinical findings with human patients suggest that marginal or mild zinc deficiency may be widespread in developed nations.[1,15,16] Consequently, human zinc deficiency may represent a significant health concern throughout the world particularly during adolescence, pregnancy, old age, stress, or disease.

Body Compartments

Zinc is present in virtually all cells, but certain tissues in animals have a higher abundance.[1] Moreover, zinc distribution among tissues is similar in different animal species. Concentrations typically are between 10 and 100 $\mu g/g$ wet weight. The zinc concentrations of most soft tissues, e.g., muscle, brain, lung, and heart, are relatively stable and unresponsive to amounts of dietary zinc over most ranges of intake. Zinc concentration in other tissues, especially bone, testes, hair, and blood, tend to reflect dietary zinc intake. The highest concentrations of zinc in the body are typically found in bone, prostate, and the choroid of the eye. Despite its moderate zinc concentration, skeletal muscle usually represents the greatest proportion (60%) of total body zinc because it comprises the largest part of total body mass. Skeletal muscle and bone (calcified bone and marrow) together account for ~90% of total body zinc. Some redistribution of body zinc occurs as animals age. For example, liver zinc may represent as much as 25% of total body zinc in neonates but only 6% in adults.[17] Although extracellular fluids represent a metabolically important body zinc compartment, <0.5% of total body zinc is found in blood.[18] Therefore, zinc is primarily an intracellular ion.

Membrane-bound zinc represents a large proportion of cellular zinc and may serve a role in membrane function and stability.[19] Most of the subcellular zinc in liver cells (60%) is associated with the supernatant fraction,[20] although nuclear, mitochondrial, and microsomal fractions also contain significant amounts of zinc (23%, 5%, and 12%, respectively). On a protein basis, however, microsomes and the cytosol have the highest concentrations. Redistribution of zinc between compartments may occur during illness and stress or in response to changes in dietary zinc intake.

Functional and metabolic significance may not be directly related to tissue zinc concentration. Rather, the kinetic distribution of zinc atoms among cellular ligands is more likely to reflect the biological roles of this nutrient. For example, the zinc content of liver and bone marrow is comparable to that of numerous other tissues, but kinetic experiments with [65]Zn indicate these organs comprise more metabolically active pools of body zinc.[21–23]

Methods of Analysis

The standard method of measuring zinc for nutritional, clinical, or biochemical studies is air-acetylene flame atomic absorption spectrophotometry. A characteristic absorption at 213.8 nm provides sensitivity to <1.5 μmol/L (0.1 mg/L) with excellent accuracy and precision. Preparation of samples for analysis involves combustion of organic material (wet or dry ashing) followed by solubilization of the ash in acid.[24,25] Cells and organelles can be hydrolyzed with base, e.g., 0.2 mol NaOH/L in 0.2% sodium dodecyl sulfate before atomic absorption analysis.[26] Fluids usually are diluted with H_2O or dilute acid to appropriate concentrations, without ashing, before analysis. Standardization is usually against National Institute of Standards and Technology biological reference materials, viz. bovine liver and human serum. Standards of similar viscosity and with a matrix composition (presence of other minerals) comparable with the assay samples are used for instrument calibration.

Compared with flame atomic absorption spectrophotometry, the extreme sensitivity of flameless atomic absorption and the ubiquitous presence of zinc as background contamination precludes wide application of graphite furnace techniques for zinc assays. Inductively coupled plasma emission spectrophotometry can be used as an alternative to atomic absorption. Although the instrumentation is more expensive and the sensitivity is somewhat less, plasma emission is excellent for simultaneous determination of zinc and other metals. X-ray emission spectrometry is gaining increased attention as a semiquantitative approach to subcellular zinc localization and measurement.

Metabolic studies with zinc use principally either the radioisotope [65]Zn, assayed by liquid or solid scintillation techniques, or the stable isotopes [68]Zn and [70]Zn. For human subjects the stable isotope approach with thermal ionization detection is gaining increased research use.

Absorption

Knowledge of the biochemical basis of zinc absorption has relevance toward understanding zinc requirements, factors affecting zinc bioavailability, and zinc malabsorption associated with disease.

Similarly, congenital zinc malabsorption syndromes, such as acrodermatitis enteropathica in humans,[27] Adema disease (lethal trait A 46) in cattle,[28] and lethal milk mutation in mice,[29] can be understood more easily. Despite considerable research (see reviews 4, 5, 30), neither the site nor the mechanism of zinc absorption has been fully delineated.

Zinc is absorbed primarily in the mammalian small intestine although the relative contribution of the duodenum, jejunum, and ileum toward overall zinc absorption is not clear.[4] Regardless of which segment has the highest capacity to absorb zinc, the duodenum has first access to ingested zinc and to endogenously secreted zinc. Zinc may become more accessible in the latter segments of the intestine through the action of digestive processes. Thus all parts of the small intestine may have functional importance in zinc absorption. Zinc absorption is rapid[31,32] and the transport process may be energy dependent.[5]

There is general consensus that absorption involves two kinetic processes, a carrier-mediated component (saturable at higher luminal zinc concentrations) and a nonsaturable diffusion component.[32–34] The sites of the two kinetic processes and their interrelationships remain unclear. The carrier-mediated and diffusion processes may represent components of a single transport step, e.g., uptake at the brush border membrane.[35] Alternatively, luminal-to-vascular zinc transport may occur by two independent routes, e.g., transcellular and paracellular. Transcellular zinc absorption could involve a recently identified low-molecular-weight component of intestinal mucosal cytosol[36] that may serve as an intracellular zinc carrier analogous to calcium-binding protein (calbindin) in calcium absorption.

Carrier-mediated zinc absorption may account for a greater proportion of total absorption at low luminal zinc concentrations.[33,34] In studies using intact rats, estimates of the half-saturation luminal zinc concentration (K_m) for the carrier-mediated process ranged from 32 μmol/L[34] to 2.1 μmol/L[32] and were unaffected by zinc deficiency.[34] However, the maximal transport rate (V_{max}) was reported to increase more than threefold (to 183 nmol Zn $\cdot$ g tissue$^{-1} \cdot$ 30 min^{-1}) in rats fed a zinc-deficient diet. This finding suggests that zinc absorption by the carrier-mediated process is enhanced during periods of low zinc intake. In contrast, the diffusion component of zinc absorption is unaffected by zinc deficiency, and absorption via this process is proportional to luminal zinc concentration.

There has been much speculation regarding the roles of intraluminal zinc-binding ligands in the zinc absorption process.[4,5] Agents advanced as having functional significance include fatty acids, prostaglandins, picolinic acid, and citric acid. There is little doubt that zinc-binding ligands of exogenous (dietary) or endogenous (e.g., pancreatic, biliary, or mucosal) origin affect zinc absorption from a meal. It is unlikely, however, that the presence of intraluminal ligands is required for zinc to be absorbed.

Homeostatic regulation of zinc absorption appears to be related to the synthesis of intestinal metallothionein, a small cysteine-rich metalloprotein that binds zinc, copper, and other divalent cations. Expression of the metallothionein gene is induced by certain hormones[37] and by high dietary zinc, particularly when copper intake is low.[38] Metals bound to metallothionein exchange rapidly, on the order of seconds to minutes,[39] suggesting that metallothionein acts as an inducible ligand that buffers zinc absorption. For example, release of zinc from the intestine to portal circulation increases when cellular metallothionein concentrations are low as occurs in zinc deficiency.[40] Conversely, zinc absorption decreases and intestinal metallothionein increases during periods of high zinc intake or fasting. This finding suggests that dietary and hormonally responsive processes that induce metallothionein synthesis may buffer zinc uptake or release by enterocytes thus allowing for efficient regulation of zinc transfer to the circulatory system.

Intestinal metallothionein is also a site of interaction between copper and zinc.[4,41] Copper is much more tenaciously bound to metallothionein than is zinc. This relationship is used to alleviate excess copper accumulation in patients suffering from Wilson's disease.[42] Wilson's disease patients given daily zinc supplements exhibited negative copper balance because of reduced copper absorption. Intestinal biopsies collected after zinc therapy showed elevated metallothionein concentrations as determined by enzyme-linked immunosorbent assay (ELISA) (A. Grider, G.J. Brewer, and R.J. Cousins, unpublished observations, 1989). Intestinal metallothionein, induced in response to high zinc intake, may preferentially bind dietary and/or endogenous copper and account for the beneficial reduction in copper accumulation.

A link between the pancreas and zinc absorption may exist during bowel or pancreatic disease. Malabsorption arising from a variety of factors can alter water and electrolyte balance and influence the absorption of zinc and other cations. Pancreatic insufficiency will reduce the enzymatic hydrolysis of food components, which then limits zinc release and availability for cellular uptake. Pancreatic secretions may contain constituents that increase zinc uptake by the intestine.[4,5] Furthermore, zinc secretion from enterocytes to the lumen has been shown experimentally.[34] Osmotic changes in the gastrointestinal environment may alter the absorption-secretion balance for zinc.

Transport

Zinc is rapidly transported to and concentrates in the liver after transfer from the intestine into portal circulation.[18] Albumin was identified as the plasma protein that transports zinc in portal blood.[43] Furthermore, there is some indication that plasma albumin concentration may in part determine zinc absorption possibly by affecting the rate of zinc transfer from enterocytes. Distribution to extrahepatic tissues occurs primarily via the plasma, which comprises ~10–20% of the zinc in whole blood.[18] The major portion of zinc in blood is contained in erythrocytes and is associated primarily with the isoenzymes of carbonic anhydrase and to a much lesser extent with superoxide dismutase and metallothionein. Albumin appears to be the principal metabolically active, exchangeable zinc pool in blood and comprises ~80% of the zinc in plasma depending upon the species. Other zinc-containing components of plasma include α2-macroglobulin, transferrin, and amino acids, especially cysteine and histidine.

Serum or plasma zinc concentrations tend to reflect intake when dietary zinc amounts are low but are maintained between 10–23 μmol/L in animals fed adequate amounts of zinc over a fairly wide range of intakes.[1] Nevertheless, the plasma zinc concentration exhibits circadian variations, decreases during stress, and is subject to transitory postprandial depression. Mechanisms regulating plasma zinc concentrations appear to be related to protein synthesis in certain organs.[23] Excessive zinc intake can increase blood zinc concentrations severalfold.[18] The response of plasma zinc to oral zinc supplementation of human subjects, termed the zinc tolerance test, has been used as an indicator of zinc status.[44] Presumably, homeostatic mechanisms that may include intestinal metallothionein expression are depressed when dietary zinc is low. This depression may result in higher transitory increases in plasma zinc after an oral zinc dose (usually 50 mg) in zinc-depleted subjects. Although this technique is used widely in research, it has not received universal acceptance as a means of assessing zinc nutritional status.[1]

Plasma and blood cell concentrations of metallothionein were shown to correlate with dietary zinc intake in rats[45] and may reflect the direct involvement of zinc in metallothionein gene expression. Plasma metallothionein concentrations may be useful indicators of dietary status assessment. In humans, erythrocyte metallothionein is increased during zinc supplementation and is decreased during dietary zinc restriction.[46] These changes may reflect metallothionein synthesis during hematopoietic development in the bone marrow. Serum metallothionein concentrations are less responsive to dietary zinc intake in humans than are those found in erythrocytes.

Metabolism

Radioisotope studies in animals and human subjects as well as in vitro cell uptake studies provide a fairly defined characterization of zinc metabolism after absorption. A large portion of zinc initially is taken up by the liver where it interacts with a variety of intracellular ligands including metallothionein. Both zinc and copper bind to metallothionein in ratios that somewhat reflect dietary intake amounts.[37] Expression of the metallothionein gene may be regulated by these metals through a specific nuclear metal-binding protein that also binds to unique DNA sequences in the promoter region.[47,48]

Kinetic studies in rats showed that the initial rate of tissue uptake of ^{65}Zn from an ingested dose is most rapid in liver followed by bone marrow, bone, skin, kidney, and thymus, respectively.[22,23] Tissues with the greatest rates of uptake presumably have correspondingly higher rates of zinc turnover and perhaps greater functional importance. Intact animal and cellular models showed that hepatic zinc turnover occurs approximately every 15 h.[23,49] Kidney has a fairly high, intake-dependent rate of zinc exchange with newly absorbed ^{65}Zn. Renal nuclear zinc concentrations were shown to have a half-life of 2 h.[48] Rapid turnover indicates that zinc exchange between cells and systemic circulation is also rapid.

A kinetic model of zinc metabolism in humans showed how rate constants for zinc uptake by various tissues respond to an oral zinc load and glucocorticoid hormones.[50,51] In the model, glucocorticoids enhance plasma clearance and apparent hepatic ^{65}Zn uptake. Analysis of comparable rate constants in detailed kinetic experiments with rats showed that the reduction in plasma ^{65}Zn concentration (increased plasma clearance) was associated with enhanced synthesis of metallothionein.[23] Glucocorticoid hormones, interleukin 1 (via interleukin 6), glucagon, and epinephrine all were shown to increase hepatic metallothionein gene expression concomitantly with plasma zinc depression. Tissue-specific hormonal induction of metallothionein during periods of acute disease (e.g., infection), stress, and inflammation can cause a redistribution of body zinc. For example, the distribution of injected ^{65}Zn in rats given interleukin 1 or dibutyryl cAMP is characterized by enhanced ^{65}Zn accumulation in liver and bone marrow and reduced accumulation in bone, skin, and intestine.[21-23]

Zinc excretion occurs primarily via the feces, orig-inating from pancreatic, biliary, and mucosal secretions or from desquamated mucosal cells.[1,4] Transepithelial zinc transfer from the vascular system into the intestinal lumen may occur through mucosal cells or intracellular junctions.[34] Meal-stimulated endogenous zinc secretion can account for over half the zinc contained in the intestinal lumen.[52] A portion of secreted zinc represents digestive metalloenzymes such as carboxypeptidase A. Reabsorption of endogenously secreted zinc is normally very efficient; however, luminal factors such as phytic acid can limit endogenous zinc reabsorption. Zinc also is excreted from the body surface in sloughed epithelial tissues.[1] Surface zinc loss can represent a significant proportion of total zinc excretion determined by balance studies.[53] Little zinc normally is excreted in urine although the amount may increase markedly in response to diseases that result in excessive muscle catabolism or proteinuria from kidney dysfunction.

Zinc homeostasis is regulated in part by changes in absorption and excretion in response to changes in dietary zinc intake. Cotzias et al.[54] suggested that zinc homeostasis was maintained by increased absorption in zinc-deficient animals and by increased excretion in animals fed excess zinc. A recent study showed that ^{65}Zn absorption was inversely related to dietary zinc amount in rats fed between 5 and 40 mg zinc/kg diet but was unaffected by further increases up to 160 mg/kg.[55] In contrast, zinc excretion measured as the rate of ^{65}Zn turnover increased steadily over the entire range of zinc intakes. These data suggest that zinc homeostasis is optimal during periods of low zinc intake as a result of more efficient absorption and retention of dietary zinc. At higher intakes of zinc, regulation of absorption plays a progressively less important role in the maintenance of zinc homeostasis, whereas the role of zinc excretion becomes more pronounced.

Biochemical Functions

Zinc is a ubiquitous component in all cells and is the most abundant transition metal. It is well suited for regulatory functions, because its intracellular concentration can be homeostatically controlled in a tissue-specific fashion.[21,38] Structural and functional roles for many metalloenzymes, encompassing each enzyme class, as well as a role in stabilization of macromolecules (including receptor molecules) have been described.[1] Furthermore, the interaction of zinc with nuclear proteins that bind to promoter sequences of specific genes and thus regulate transcription suggests another broad spectrum of biological effects for the nutrient.

Zinc is a component of many enzymes that catalyze nucleotide phosphate ester formation. This metal is well suited for a role in nucleic acid metabolism because it does not exhibit any direct redox chemistry thus precluding generation of DNA-damaging free radicals and reactive oxygen species.[11] The growth-promoting effects of zinc would suggest a role in DNA polymerase. However, recent evidence suggests that in *E. coli*, DNA polymerase is not a zinc metalloenzyme.[56] Thymidine kinase activity is affected by dietary zinc intake; therefore, it could be a zinc-dependent enzyme.[57] Changes in histones could affect chromatin structure and relate to the growth limitation associated with zinc deficiency. These topics were reviewed.[6,7]

There is convincing evidence that RNA polymerases I, II, and III are zinc metalloenzymes.[6] Zinc-related effects on protein synthesis could occur through changes in ribosomal, messenger, or transfer RNA pools. Most evidence comes from *Euglena* (a eucaryote),[6] but data from zinc-deficient animals support the notion that RNA synthesis may be sensitive to very low zinc intakes in multicellular systems.[7]

Zinc dependency in the control of gene transcription also can be explained through *zinc fingers* of transcription factors.[58] Zinc fingers are repeated cysteine- and histidine-containing domains of DNA-binding proteins that tenaciously bind zinc in a tetrahedral configuration. Zinc provides a structural role required for binding to DNA. These unique zinc-binding motifs have been identified in nuclear transcription factors from many mammalian cells.[59] The effect of dietary zinc on zinc fingers needs to be investigated. In this regard it is of interest that nuclear zinc concentrations reflect dietary zinc intake.[48] This intranuclear-dietary communication could affect expression of genes and account for some of the specific metabolic dysfunctions observed in zinc deficiency.

The estimated number of zinc-requiring enzymes varies depending on species and tissues examined, but 60 is probably a conservative estimate. This number is small considering that mammalian cells can contain thousands of different mRNA molecules. Data from nutrition experiments have not provided unequivocal evidence for a direct zinc-enzyme effect for individual enzymes.[60] Hence, alternative physiologic roles were proposed. For example, zinc may affect the binding of proteins to membranes. Zinc was shown to increase the binding of protein kinase C to plasma membranes in Ca^{2+} or antigen-induced T lymphocytes.[61] Increased protein binding is accompanied by cellular redistribution of zinc to the microsomes and cytosol with increased activity of the protein kinase C signal transduction pathway. Many physiological functions of zinc could be related to this type of biochemical role.

Zinc also may have a role in membrane function. An underlying mechanism has not been elucidated, however. Many of the signs of zinc deficiency could be explained on the basis of membrane dysfunction.[19] Stabilization of cellular membranes via thiol groups or phospholipids and inhibition of ATPases or receptors or NADPH oxidation were proposed.[62] Numerous studies showed that certain tissues undergo lipid peroxidation during zinc deficiency.[63,64] This finding is of interest because many pathological conditions may relate to oxidative damage caused by free radicals. Zinc was shown to suppress free radicals in isolated cells after initiation of lipid peroxidation by a variety of mechanisms.[26] Metallothionein induction by zinc has been correlated with free-radical suppression. Hydroxyl radicals are reported to be scavenged by this metalloprotein in vitro.[65] The protein protects red cell membranes from in vitro oxidative conditions that produce lipid peroxidation.[66]

Deficiency Symptoms

Clinical manifestations of dietary zinc deficiency are ultimately the result of altered zinc metabolism and/or biochemical functions. Overt signs of severe zinc deficiency are similar in humans and animals. These signs include retarded growth, depressed immune function, anorexia, dermatitis, altered reproductive performance, skeletal abnormalities, diarrhea, and alopecia.[1,2] Skeletal abnormalities in zinc-deficient animals may be related to impaired development of epiphyseal cartilage[67] or defective collagen synthesis.[68] Defective collagen synthesis or cross-linking also may contribute to the dermatitis and impaired wound healing observed in severe deficiency.[1,3,14]

Impaired reproductive performance in zinc deficiency is manifested by congenital abnormalities, poor pregnancy outcome, and gonadal dysfunction.[69] Altered immune function in zinc-deficient animals results in thymus gland atrophy and abnormal leukocyte differentiation.[70] In both mice and humans zinc deficiency reduces concentrations of thymic hormones that transform thymocytes into active T lymphocytes.[71] Altered taste acuity and behavioral disturbances, perhaps related to depressed zinc status, were reported in human subjects.[1,2]

Lesions resulting from severe zinc deficiency are manifestations of altered physiological processes. It is likely that less-essential systems are affected first. Many of these lesions occur in tissues that contain some of the highest levels of zinc in the body, such as skin, bone, and reproductive organs. Redistribution of zinc away from these tissues may reflect conservation of zinc for more essential biochemical functions. Numerous diseases have been shown to include events mediated by the cytokines.[72] Therefore, it is of note that interleukin 1, which influences metallothionein synthesis, causes redistribution of circulating zinc away from skin, bone, and intestine with redirection to liver, bone marrow, and thymus.[21,22]

Behavioral modifications also may enhance survival during zinc deficiency. For example, rats fed zinc-deficient diets develop a cyclic pattern of food intake[73] that may be related to the catecholaminergic mechanism in the hypothalamus, which controls feeding behavior.[74] Zinc-deficient diets are toxic when force-fed to rats and result in decreased weight gain and high mortality if not alleviated by parenteral zinc.[75] Thus, voluntary food restriction may represent a physiologically mediated behavioral adaptation that enhances survival during short-term zinc deprivation.

Diagnosis of zinc deficiency in humans is difficult because the condition produces a range of nonspecific clinical symptoms. As was shown in animals, human zinc deficiency is not an all-or-none condition, and progressive degrees of zinc deficiency probably produce a graded response in the severity of the effects.[16] The occurrence of severe zinc deficiency is rare and primarily associated with abnormal dietary practices or disease states, particularly hepatic and gastrointestinal disorders with associated zinc malabsorption. Evidence of low plasma zinc in conjunction with some of the symptoms mentioned above may be indicative of severe clinical zinc deficiency. The condition can be confirmed by amelioration of symptoms in response to increased zinc intake. Because there is no major body store of zinc, response to repletion can be rapid.[76]

Mild chronic zinc deficiency may be indicated by impaired immune function and reduced rate and/or quality of growth in children.[16] Lacking a reliable index of human zinc deficiency and obvious clinical features, the occurrence of mild zinc deficiency or its significance to human health is uncertain. Those most at risk primarily include pregnant women, children, and elderly people, especially those from lower socioeconomic groups.

Zinc Requirement and Allowances

The dietary zinc requirement is defined as the minimum zinc intake that will support optimal growth and metabolism.[77] The required intake is affected by physiological and dietary factors that influence zinc absorption and utilization. Physiological factors include age, growth, pregnancy, and lactation. Diseases resulting in intestinal malabsorption and/or enhanced excretion may increase the zinc requirement. Dietary factors include the chemical form of zinc in foods, interactions between zinc and other nutrients, and the presence or absence of dietary inhibitors or enhancers of zinc absorption.

In theory, each individual's dietary zinc requirement can be calculated by dividing the individual's true requirement by the bioavailability of zinc in the diet.[78] Zinc bioavailability will be discussed in detail in the next section. Briefly, it represents the proportion of dietary zinc that can be absorbed and utilized, thus having direct effect on the total amount that must be ingested to meet the body's need for zinc. Zinc bioavailability varies in foods and is difficult to measure accurately. The true zinc requirement, i.e., that amount of absorbed zinc needed for optimal growth and metabolism, also is difficult to determine partly because adequate indices of zinc status are unavailable. In practice, the true requirement can be estimated based on the amount of zinc needed to replace all endogenous losses plus supply zinc for production of a viable fetus during pregnancy, milk during lactation, or body mass during growth.[78] Obviously, the range of zinc requirements among individuals within a population can vary widely depending on dietary habit and physiological state.

In laboratory animals or livestock, the true zinc requirement can be determined empirically by assessing indices of physiological normality in animals fed graded amounts of zinc ranging from insufficient to excess.[79] Zinc intake must be limited to a highly available source to minimize bioavailability effects. Indices can include growth rate, tissue zinc concentration, or biochemical measures, such as zinc-dependent enzyme activity or tissue concentrations of a zinc metalloprotein. Data from animal models can be extrapolated to human requirements, especially for evaluation of dietary or physiological factors that influence dietary zinc requirements. Direct measurements of human zinc requirements are preferred but are severely limited by the lack of adequate indices of status.

Present methods of determining zinc status in humans are unreliable. For example, plasma zinc concentration is a commonly used index but is subject to fluctuations caused by circadian variations, food intake or fasting, stress, or complicating disease.[5,18] The zinc tolerance test described above is not a generally accepted index of zinc status. In contrast, expression of the metallothionein gene is proportional to zinc intake.[38] Furthermore, a recent report suggests that circulating concentrations of metallothionein may reflect zinc intake in rats.[45] If so, human serum or red blood cell metallothionein determined by sensitive radioimmunoassay[45] or ELISA[46,80] may serve as the indicator of zinc status needed to confidently assess the human zinc requirement.

The 1989 Recommended Dietary Allowance (RDA) of zinc for healthy Americans established by the National Research Council is (in mg/d): 5 for infants, 10 for children 1–10 y, 15 for males >10 y, 12 for females >10 y, 15 for pregnant women, and 19 and 16 for women during the first and second months of lactation, respectively.[81] Adult zinc intakes recommended by the World Health Organization and countries other than the United States range from 8 to 16 mg/d.[78] Adult RDA are based on an assumed average requirement for absorbed zinc of 2.5 mg/d. Absorption efficiency is assumed to be 20% since zinc bioavailability from different foods can vary significantly. The recommended amount for adult men contains an additional 2.5 mg/d to meet the needs of most healthy individuals, including those whose diets typically contain foods with low zinc bioavailability. The lower requirement for adult women is based on their lower body weight. A compilation of data on fractional absorption of zinc in human subjects showed a range of 12–59% when zinc was consumed with meals.[4] Thus in some cases the RDA might underestimate the dietary requirement.

Survey data on customary zinc intakes by different population subclasses suggest that average intakes range from only 47% to 67% of the RDA.[9] Elderly persons also may have a higher zinc requirement than previously thought because of a reduced ability to absorb and utilize zinc.[82,83] This would suggest a high incidence of marginal (mild) zinc deficiency in the United States and validate concerns regarding current human zinc status.[15,16] However, data compiled from absorption studies suggest that the amount of zinc required by healthy human adults may be closer to 2.5–4 mg/d if the zinc is obtained from a highly available source.[9,78] Further refinement of the RDA and better assessment of the adequacy of normal dietary zinc intakes will require technological advances in the determination of human zinc status and zinc bioavailability.

Sources

Foods vary widely in zinc content. Zinc is particularly abundant in red meats, some seafoods, and the embryo portion of grains. Zinc in plant products is generally less available than that supplied by most animal proteins or zinc salts.[10] A major contributing factor is the presence of phytic acid, which forms an insoluble zinc-chelate complex that is not absorbed from the gastrointestinal tract.[4] High dietary calcium has been shown to enhance the adverse effect of phytic acid. Processing also can markedly alter zinc availability from that present in the unaltered food.[84]

Zinc in foods is primarily associated with proteins and nucleic acids.[4] The nature of these associations, i.e., relative zinc-binding affinity and complex solubility in the intestinal milieu, can influence zinc ab-

sorption markedly. Inhibitory ligands appear to reduce the size of the absorbable zinc pool in the intestinal tract by forming zinc-ligand complexes that make zinc unavailable to the absorption mechanisms. These complexes presumably are unabsorbable and have a greater affinity for zinc than for mucosal factors that are involved in the zinc absorption process. In contrast, compounds that enhance zinc absorption may do so by facilitating zinc binding to mucosal receptors or by forming absorbable zinc complexes especially in competition with inhibitors of zinc absorption.

Data on the zinc content of foods can be used to provide a gross estimate of intake for humans and domestic animals.[1,85] However, total zinc intake is a poor indicator of zinc supply, because much of the zinc in a food may be in an unavailable form. A more accurate indicator is the amount of bioavailable zinc in the diet, defined as the proportion of zinc in a food that is absorbed and utilized.[10] Zinc bioavailability is difficult to measure because zinc status and nutrient interactions can markedly influence these estimates, especially from composite meals. Thus estimates of zinc bioavailability from foods vary widely depending on experimental methods. Lack of reliable information about zinc bioavailability from human foods is a major impediment toward better understanding of human zinc requirements and adequacy of normal dietary zinc intakes.

Zinc absorption sometimes is used as an approximation of zinc bioavailability, although the two measurements differ depending on the efficiency with which absorbed zinc is utilized.[10] Methods used to measure bioavailability include absorption or retention of stable or radioactive zinc isotopes from extrinsically or intrinsically labeled foods, balance estimates, and slope ratio assays of growth rate or tissue zinc concentration in animal models. Many dietary factors were shown to affect zinc bioavailability.[4] These include amino acids (histidine, cysteine, lysine, and glycine) and natural or synthetic chelators (citrate, picolinate, and EDTA) that appear to enhance zinc bioavailability. Other chelators (phytic acid, oxalic acid, and high levels of EDTA), fiber, and some minerals (copper, iron, and calcium) tend to reduce zinc bioavailability.

Milk is an important source of zinc in the human diet.[84,85] Zinc in human milk was shown to be more available than that in cow milk or infant formula. A greater percentage of the zinc in human milk compared with cow milk was found associated with low-molecular-weight zinc-binding components.[86] This finding led to the hypothesis that these zinc-binding components enhance zinc absorption and thus bioavailability from human milk. However, data from a variety of sources demonstrated that protein composition is a major determinant of zinc bioavailability from milk.[87–89] Casein, the major protein component of cow milk, is not readily digested by humans. Thus, much of the zinc in cow milk cannot be released during digestion and is unavailable. In contrast, human milk proteins (primarily lactalbumin) are readily digestible so that bound zinc is more available for absorption.

Toxicity

The range between deficient and toxic zinc intakes appears fairly wide, suggesting that dietary fortification with zinc would be a simple solution to low zinc bioavailability. Unfortunately, information regarding the deleterious effects of excess zinc is insufficient especially when copper intake is marginal.[1,2]

The principal toxic effect of zinc apparently results from its interference with normal copper metabolism, leading to copper-deficiency anemia during total parenteral nutrition in persons with prolonged intakes of >150 mg zinc/d.[90] Mild gastric erosion,[4] depressed immune function,[91] and reduced plasma high-density-lipoprotein cholesterol[92] also may result from zinc excess. Nevertheless, there would appear to be a reasonable margin of safety allowing the addition of moderate amounts of zinc to the normal human diet. Future research must evaluate whether or not zinc supplementation at amounts above those found in a well-balanced diet has consequences as serious as those associated with low zinc intake or whether in some specific situations supplemental zinc is of therapeutic value.[2,4]

References

1. K.M. Hambidge, C.E. Casey, and N.F. Krebs (1986) Zinc. In: *Trace Elements in Human and Animal Nutrition,* vol. 2, 5th ed. (W. Mertz, ed.), pp. 1–137, Academic Press, Orlando, FL.
2. C.F. Mills, ed. (1989) *Zinc in Human Biology,* Springer-Verlag, New York.
3. A.S. Prasad, A.O. Cavdar, G.J. Brewer, and P.J. Aggett (1983) *Zinc Deficiency in Human Subjects,* Alan R. Liss, Inc., New York.
4. N.W. Solomons and R.J. Cousins (1984) Zinc. In: *Absorption and Malabsorption of Mineral Nutrients* (N.W. Solomons and I.H. Rosenberg, eds.), pp. 125–197, Alan R. Liss, Inc., New York.
5. R.J. Cousins (1985) Absorption, transport, and hepatic metabolism of copper and zinc: special reference to metallothionein and ceruloplasmin. *Physiol. Rev.* 65:238–309.
6. F.Y.-H. Wu and C.-W. Wu (1987) Zinc in DNA replication and transcription. *Annu. Rev. Nutr.* 7:251–272.
7. R.J. Cousins (1986) Molecular biology of zinc. In: *Biotechnology for Solving Agricultural Problems,* Beltsville Symposium on Agricultural Research, vol. X (D.C. Augustine, H.D. Danforth, and M.R. Bakst, eds.), pp. 207–219, Martinus Nijhoff Publishers, Boston.
8. B.L. Vallee and A. Galdes (1984) The metallobiochemistry of zinc enzymes. In: *Advances in Enzymology* (A. Meister, ed.), pp. 283–429, John Wiley and Sons, New York.
9. N.W. Solomons (1982) Biological availability of zinc in humans. *Am. J. Clin. Nutr.* 35:1048–1075.
10. B.L. O'Dell (1985) Bioavailability of and interactions among trace elements. In: *Trace Elements in Nutrition of Children* (G.E. Chandra, ed.), pp. 41–62, Vevey/Raven Press, New York.
11. R.J.P. Williams (1984) Zinc: what is its role in biology? *Endeavor* 8:65–70.
12. M.J. Raulin (1869) Chemical studies on vegetation. *Ann. Sci. Nat. Bot. Biol. Veg.* (Ser. 5) 11:93–299 (in French).
13. W.R. Todd, C.A. Elvehjem, and E.B. Hart (1934) Zinc in the nutrition of the rat. *Am. J. Physiol.* 107:146–156.
14. H.F. Tucker and W.D. Salmon (1955) Parakeratosis or zinc deficiency disease in the pig. *Proc. Soc. Exp. Biol. Med.* 88:613–616.
15. A.S. Prasad (1984) Discovery and importance of zinc in human nutrition. *Fed. Proc.* 43:2829–2834.
16. K.M. Hambidge (1989) Mild zinc deficiency in human subjects. In: *Zinc in Human Biology* (C.F. Mills, ed.), pp. 281–296, Springer-Verlag, New York.
17. M.J. Jackson (1989) Physiology of zinc: general aspects. In: *Zinc in Human Biology* (C.F. Mills, ed.), pp. 1–13, Springer-Verlag, New York.
18. R.J. Cousins (1988) Systemic transport of zinc. In: *Zinc in Human Biology* (C.F. Mills, ed.), pp. 79–93, Springer-Verlag, New York.
19. W.J. Bettger and B.L. O'Dell (1981) A critical physiological role of zinc in the structure and function of biomembranes. *Life Sci.* 28:1425–1438.
20. J. Smeyers-Verbeke, C. May, P. Drochmans, and D.L. Massart (1977) The determination of Cu, Zn, and Mn in subcellular rat liver fractions. *Ann. Biochem.* 83:746–753.
21. R.J. Cousins and Annette S. Leinart (1988) Tissue-specific regulation of zinc metabolism and metallothionein genes by interleukin-1. *FASEB J.* 2:2884–2890.
22. K.L. Huber and R.J. Cousins (1988) Maternal zinc deprivation and interleukin-1 influence fetal metallothionein gene expression and zinc metabolism. *J. Nutr.* 118:1570–1576.
23. M.A. Dunn and R.J. Cousins (1989) Kinetics of zinc metabolism in the rat: effect of dibutyryl cyclic AMP. *Am. J. Physiol.* 256:E420–E430.
24. M.S. Clegg, C.L. Keen, B. Lonnerdal, and L.S. Hurley (1981) Influence of ashing techniques on the analysis of trace elements in animal tissue. I. Wet ashing. *Biol. Trace Element Res.* 3:107–115.
25. E.E. Menden, D. Brockman, H. Choudhury, and H.G. Petering (1977) Dry ashing of animal tissues for atomic absorption spectrometric determination of zinc, copper, cadmium, lead, iron, manganese, magnesium and calcium. *Anal. Chem.* 49:1644–1645.
26. D.E. Coppen, D.E. Richardson, and R.J. Cousins (1988) Zinc suppression of free radicals induced in cultures of rat hepatocytes by iron, t-butyl hydroperoxide, and 3-methylindole. *Proc. Soc. Exp. Biol. Med.* 189:100–109.
27. I. Lombeck, H.G. Schnippering, F. Ritzl, L.E. Feinendegen, and H.J. Bremer (1975) Absorption of zinc in acrodermatitis enteropathica. *Lancet* 1:855.
28. T. Flagstad (1976) Lethal trait A 46 in cattle. *Nord. Vet. Med.* 28:160–169.
29. A. Grider, Jr. and L.C. Erway (1986) Intestinal metallothionein in lethal-milk mice with systemic zinc deficiency. *Biochem. Genet.* 24:635–642.
30. B. Lonnerdal (1989) Intestinal absorption of zinc. In: *Zinc in Human Biology* (C.F. Mills, ed.), pp. 33–55, Springer-Verlag, New York.
31. K.T. Smith, R.J. Cousins, B.L. Silbon, and M.L. Failla (1978) Zinc absorption and metabolism by isolated vascularly perfused rat intestine. *J. Nutr.* 108:1849–1857.
32. N.T. Davies (1980) Studies on the absorption of zinc by rat intestine. *Br. J. Nutr.* 43:189–203.
33. L. Steel and R.J. Cousins (1985) Kinetics of zinc absorption by luminally and vascularly perfused rat intestine. *Am. J. Physiol.* 248:G46–G53.

34. J.E. Hoadley, A.S. Leinart, and R.J. Cousins (1987) Kinetic analysis of zinc uptake and serosal transfer by vascularly perfused rat intestine. *Am. J. Physiol.* 252:G825–G831.

35. M.P. Menard and R.J. Cousins (1983) Zinc transport by brush border membrane vesicles from rat intestine. *J. Nutr.* 113:1434–1442.

36. J.M. Hempe and R.J. Cousins (1989) Identification of a low molecular weight zinc-binding component from rat intestinal mucosa. *FASEB J.* 3:A457(abstr.).

37. M.A. Dunn, T.L. Blalock, and R.J. Cousins (1987) Metallothionein. *Proc. Soc. Exp. Biol. Med.* 185:107–119.

38. T.L. Blalock, M.A. Dunn, and R.J. Cousins (1988) Metallothionein gene expression in rats: tissue-specific regulation by dietary copper and zinc. *J. Nutr.* 118:222–228.

39. D.G. Nettesheim, H.R. Engeseth, and J.D. Otvos (1985) Products of metal exchange reactions of metallothionein. *Biochemistry* 24:6744–6751.

40. J.E. Hoadley, A.S. Leinart, and R.J. Cousins (1988) Relationship of ^{65}Zn absorption kinetics to intestinal metallothionein in rats: effects of zinc depletion and fasting. *J. Nutr.* 118:497–502.

41. P. Oestreicher and R.J. Cousins (1985) Copper and zinc absorption in the rat: mechanism of mutual antagonism. *J. Nutr.* 115:159–166.

42. G.J. Brewer, G.M. Hill, A.S. Prasad, Z.T. Cossack, and P. Rabbani (1983) Oral zinc therapy for Wilson's disease. *Ann. Intern. Med.* 99:314–320.

43. K.T. Smith, M.L. Failla, and R.J. Cousins (1979) Identification of albumin as the plasma carrier for zinc absorption by perfused rat intestine. *Biochem. J.* 184:627–633.

44. J.F. Sullivan, M.M. Jetton, and R.E. Burch (1979) A zinc tolerance test. *J. Lab. Clin. Med.* 93:485–492.

45. I. Bremner, J.N. Morrison, A.M. Wood, and J.R. Arthur (1987) Effects of changes in dietary zinc, copper and selenium supply and of endotoxin administration on metallothionein I concentrations in blood cells and urine in the rat. *J. Nutr.* 117:1595–1602.

46. A. Grider, L.B. Bailey, and R.J. Cousins (1990) Erythrocyte metallothionein as an index of zinc status in humans. *Proc. Natl. Acad. Sci. USA* 87:1259–1262.

47. R.J. Cousins, M.A. Dunn, T.L. Blalock, and A.S. Leinart (1988) Coordinate regulation of zinc metabolism and metallothionein gene expression by cAMP, interleukin-1 and dietary copper and zinc. In: *Trace Elements in Man and Animals 6* (L.S. Hurley, C.L. Keen, B. Lonnerdal, and R.B. Rucker, eds.), pp. 281–285, Plenum Publishing, New York.

48. R.J. Cousins and L.M. Lee-Ambrose (1989) Nuclear zinc binding factors interact with dietary zinc. *FASEB J.* 3:A458(abstr.).

49. S.E. Pattison and R.J. Cousins (1986) Kinetics of zinc uptake and exchange by primary cultures of rat hepatocytes. *Am. J. Physiol.* 250:E677–E685.

50. A.K. Babcock, R.I. Henkin, R.L. Aamodt, D.M. Foster, and M. Berman (1982) Effects of oral zinc loading on zinc metabolism in humans. II: In vivo kinetics. *Metabolism* 31:335–347.

51. R.I. Henkin, D.M. Foster, R.L. Aamodt, and M. Berman (1984) Zinc metabolism in adrenal cortical insufficiency: effects of carbohydrate active steroids. *Metabolism* 33:491–501.

52. J.W. Matseshe, S.F. Phillips, J.R. Malagelada, and G.T. McCall (1980) Recovery of dietary iron and zinc from the proximal intestine of healthy man: studies of different meals and supplements. *Am. J. Clin. Nutr.* 33:1946–1953.

53. D.B. Milne, W.K. Canfield, J.R. Mahalko, and H.H. Sandstead (1983) Effect of dietary zinc on whole body surface loss of zinc: impact on estimation of zinc retention by balance method. *Am. J. Clin. Nutr.* 38:181–186.

54. G.C. Cotzias, D.C. Borg, and B. Sellect (1962) Specificity of zinc pathway through the body: turnover of Zn^{65} in the mouse. *Am. J. Physiol.* 202:359–363.

55. D.E. Coppen and N.T. Davies (1987) Studies on the effects of dietary zinc on ^{65}Zn absorption in vivo and on the effects of Zn status on ^{65}Zn absorption and body loss in young rats. *Br. J. Nutr.* 57:35–44.

56. I. Sloby, B. Kind, and A. Holmgren (1984) T7 DNA polymerase is not a zinc-metalloenzyme and the polymerase and exonuclease activities are inhibited by zinc ions. *Biochem. Biophys. Res. Commun.* 122:1410–1417.

57. I.E. Dreosti and L.S. Hurley (1975) Depressed thymidine kinase activity in zinc-deficient rat embryos. *Proc. Soc. Exp. Biol. Med.* 150:161–165.

58. A. Klug and D. Rhodes (1987) Zinc fingers: a novel protein motif for nucleic acid recognition. *Trends Biochem. Sci.* 12:464–469.

59. P. Chavrier, P. Lemaire, O. Relevant, R. Bravo, and P. Charnay (1988) Characterization of a mouse multigene family that encodes zinc finger structures. *Mol. Cell. Biol.* 8:1319–1326.

60. M. Kirchgessner, H.P. Roth, and E. Weigand (1976) Biochemical changes in zinc deficiency. In: *Trace Elements in Human Health and Disease* (A.S. Prasad and D. Oberleas, eds.), pp. 189–225, Academic Press, New York.

61. P. Csermely, M. Szamel, K. Resch, and J. Somogy (1988) Zinc can increase the activity of protein kinase C and contributes to its binding to plasma membranes in T lymphocytes. *J. Biol. Chem.* 263:6487–6490.

62. M. Chvapil (1976) Effect of zinc on cells and biomembranes. *Med. Clin. North Am.* 60:799–812.

63. J.F. Sullivan, M.M. Jetton, H.J.K. Hahn, and R.E. Burch (1980) Enhanced lipid peroxidation in liver microsomes of zinc deficient rats. *Am. J. Clin. Nutr.* 110:51–56.

64. J.P. Burke and M.R. Fenton (1985) Effect of a zinc-deficiency diet on lipid peroxidation in liver and tumor subcellular membranes. *Proc. Soc. Exp. Biol. Med.* 179:187–191.

65. P.J. Thornalley and M. Vasak (1985) Possible role for metallothionein in protection against radiation-induced oxidative stress. Kinetics and mechanism of its reaction with superoxide and hydroxyl radicals. *Biochim. Biophys. Acta* 827:36–44.

66. A.W. Girotti, J.P. Thomas, and J.E. Jordan (1985) Inhibitory effect of zinc (II) on free radical lipid peroxidation in erythrocyte membranes. *J. Free Radic. Biol. Med.* 1:395–401.

67. F.H. Nielsen, R.P. Dowdy, and Z.Z. Ziporin (1970) Effect of zinc deficiency on sulfur-35 and hexosamine metabolism in the epiphyseal plate and primary spongiosa of the chick. *J. Nutr.* 100:903–908.

68. P.E. McClain, E.R. Wiley, G.T. Beecher, W.L. Anthony, and J.M. Hsu (1973) Influence of zinc deficiency on synthesis and cross-linking of rat skin collagen. *Biochim. Biophys. Acta* 304:457–465.

69. J. Apgar (1985) Zinc and reproduction. *Annu. Rev. Nutr.* 5:43–68.

70. P.J. Fraker, M.E. Gershwin, R.A. Good, and A. Prasad (1986) Interrelationships between zinc and immune function. *Fed. Proc.* 45:1474–1479.

71. M. Dardenne, W. Savino, S. Berrih, and J.F. Bach (1985) A zinc-dependent epitope on the molecule of thymulin, a thymic hormone. *Proc. Natl. Acad. Sci. USA* 82:7035–7038.

72. C.A. Dinarello (1987) Biology of interleukin 1. *FASEB J.* 2:108–115.

73. J.K. Chesters and J. Quarterman (1970) Effects of zinc deficiency on food intake and feeding patterns of rats. *Br. J. Nutr.* 24:1061–1069.

74. B.L. O'Dell and P.G. Reeves (1989) Zinc status and food intake. In: *Zinc in Human Biology* (C.F. Mills, ed.), pp. 173–181, Springer-Verlag, New York.

75. P.R. Flanagan (1984) A model to produce pure zinc deficiency in rats and its use to demonstrate that dietary phytate increases the excretion of endogenous zinc. *J. Nutr.* 114:493–502.

76. M.H.N. Golden (1989) The diagnosis of zinc deficiency. In: *Zinc in Human Biology* (C.F. Mills, ed.), pp. 322–333, Springer-Verlag, New York.

77. J.C. Smith, Jr., E.R. Morris, and R. Ellis (1983) Zinc: requirements, bioavailabilities and recommended dietary allowances. In: *Zinc Deficiency in Human Subjects* (A.S. Prasad, A.O. Cavdar, G.J. Brewer, and P.J. Aggett, eds.), pp. 147–169, Alan R. Liss, Inc., New York.

78. J.C. King and J.R. Turnlund (1989) Human zinc requirements. In: *Zinc in Human Biology* (C.F. Mills, ed.), pp. 335–350, Springer-Verlag, New York.

79. M.R.S. Fox, R.M. Jacobs, O.L. Jones, et al. (1981) Animal models for assessing bioavailability of essential and toxic elements. *Cereal Chem.* 58:6–11.

80. A. Grider, K.J. Kao, P.A. Klein, and R.J. Cousins (1989) Enzyme linked immunosorbent assay for human metallothionein: correlation of induction with infection. *J. Lab. Clin. Med.* 113:221–228.

81. National Research Council (1989) *Recommended Dietary Allowances,* 10th ed., National Academy Press, Washington, DC.

82. J.R. Turnlund, N. Durkin, F. Costa, and S. Margen (1986) Stable isotope studies of zinc absorption and retention in young and elderly men. *J. Nutr.* 116:1239–1247.

83. R.L. Aamodt, W.F. Rumble, and R.I. Henkin (1983) Zinc absorption in humans: effect of age, sex, and food. In: *Nutritional Bioavailability of Zinc,* ACS Symposium Series 210 (G.E. Inglett, ed.), pp. 61–82, American Chemical Society, Washington, DC.

84. B. Sandstrom (1989) Dietary pattern and zinc supply. In: *Zinc in Human Biology* (C.F. Mills, ed.), pp. 351–363, Springer-Verlag, New York.

85. S.O. Welsh and R.M. Marston (1982) Zinc levels of the U.S. food supply 1909–1980. *Food Technol.* 36:70–76.

86. C.D. Eckhert, M.V. Sloan, J.R. Duncan, and L.S. Hurley (1977) Zinc binding: a difference between human and bovine milk. *Science* 195:789–790.

87. R.J. Cousins and K.T. Smith (1980) Zinc-binding properties of bovine and human milk in vitro: influence of changes in zinc content. *Am. J. Clin. Nutr.* 33:1083–1087.

88. B. Sandstrom, A. Cederblad, and B. Lonnerdal (1983) Zinc absorption from human milk, cow's milk, and infant formulas. *Am. J. Dis. Child.* 137:726–729.

89. H.P. Roth and M. Kirchgessner (1985) Utilization of zinc from picolinic or citric acid complexes in relation to dietary protein source in rats. *J. Nutr.* 115:1641–1649.

90. A.S. Prasad, G.J. Brewer, E.B. Schoomaker, and P. Rabbani (1984) Hypocupremia induced by zinc therapy in adults. *JAMA* 240:2166–2168.

91. R.K. Chandra (1984) Excess intake of zinc impairs immune responses. *JAMA* 252:1443–1446.

92. P.L. Hooper, L. Visconti, P.J. Garry, and G.E. Johnson (1980) Zinc lowers high-density lipoprotein cholesterol levels. *JAMA* 224:1960–1961.

Chapter 29

Copper

History

The nutritional essentiality of copper was first clearly demonstrated when it was shown to be required, in addition to iron, for the prevention of anemia in rats.[1] Other pathological signs of deficiency followed: enzootic ataxia in sheep,[2] myocardial disease in cattle,[3] and vascular disease in chicks[4] and pigs.[5] An understanding of the catalytic functions of copper began to unfold with the discovery that nutritional deficiency leads to decreased cytochrome *c* oxidase activity in rat liver.[6] The copper metalloprotein, hemocuprein, was isolated in 1939,[7] but not until 30 y later was it found to possess an important enzymatic activity; it is a superoxide dismutase.[8] Lysyl oxidase, which catalyzes the crosslinking of collagen and elastin in connective tissue, is also a copper metalloenzyme.[9] The activities of these enzymes are decreased by copper deprivation whether because of dietary deficiency or a genetic defect in copper metabolism.

The first evidence of copper deficiency in humans was observed in malnourished infants repleted with modified cow milk.[10] Similar signs of deficiency were observed in an infant during extended total parenteral nutrition.[11] Unequivocal evidence that copper is essential for humans arose from study of Menkes' disease, a genetic disease that results from a primary defect in copper absorption and metabolism.[12] A similar pathology is associated with the mottled mouse mutant.[13]

This chapter is concerned primarily with the literature published since the last review in this publication.[14] For more in-depth coverage the reader is referred to other reviews.[15–17]

Metabolism

Body Compartment. The adult (70 kg) human body contains ~80 mg copper, but reported analytical values range from 50 to 120 mg.[17] The highest tissue concentration in most animals occurs in liver, followed closely by brain. Human liver contains ~15% and brain 10%. Other organs contain lower concentrations (16–32 mmol/g wet weight), but muscle content approaches 40% of the total.[16,17] Liver and spleen appear to serve as copper-storage organs, and the copper concentrations of these organs are much higher in the fetus and infant than in the adult.[18] The ileum of the neonatal rat contains a heterogeneous copper complex that increases during the suckling period, with copper exceeding 6300 mmol/g at age 14 d and decreasing to ~315 mmol/g at age 20 d.[19] The major portion of copper in liver cells is found in the cytosol associated with superoxide dismutase and metallothionein or related protein.[16]

Absorption and Utilization. Copper is absorbed from all segments of the gastrointestinal tract including the stomach and large intestine.[16,17] Although the sites of absorption are species dependent, the duodenum appears to be the major site for all species. The mechanism of copper absorption is not clear, but absorption is regulated at the level of the intestinal mucosa. At the molecular level most attention has been focused on metallothionein, which is an inducible protein of low molecular weight with a high affinity for several mineral ions. Metallothionein appears to serve primarily as a negative rather than a positive regulator of copper absorption. However, much of the copper in the mucosal-cell cytosol is associated with high-molecular-weight proteins.[20]

Recent research has added materially to our knowledge of copper bioavailability. Several dietary factors negatively affect copper bioavailability, notably zinc, thiomolybdate, ascorbic acid, and fructose.

Of all the known metal interactions, the antagonistic effect of zinc on copper bioavailability is perhaps of greatest practical significance.[21] Excess dietary zinc aggravates the signs of low copper status.[22] Zinc levels of 120 and 240 µg/g significantly lower the activities of important copper-dependent enzymes, including liver Cu,Zn-superoxide dismutase and heart cytochrome *c* oxidase, even when the diet contains a normally adequate level of copper (6 μg/g). Serum and tissue copper concentrations in rats increase during zinc deficiency, showing the extremely sensitive interaction of these ions.[21]

Even Recommended Dietary Allowances (RDA) levels of zinc increase the fecal excretion of copper in humans adapted to a low zinc intake and induce negative copper balance.[23] Although copper deficiency in the adult human is rare, it has been induced by ingestion of $\geq$150 mg Zn^{2+}/d.[24,25] The signs included hypocupremia, hypochromic-microcytic anemia, leucopenia, and neutropenia. A practical application of the zinc-copper antagonism was made in the treatment of Wilson's disease patients, who accumulate toxic levels of copper.[26] Oral zinc, as the sole therapy, prevents reaccumulation of copper in patients who have been treated with penicillamine.[27] (*See* references 26 and 27 for related literature.) Because excess zinc antagonizes copper and because phytate impairs zinc bioavailability, it is interesting that phytate actually increases the absorption and utilization of copper.[28]

The antagonistic effect of zinc on copper metabolism appears to be mediated primarily at the level of the intestinal mucosa via metallothionein (MT).[20] Hall et al.[29] suggested that zinc induces MT synthesis and, because MT binds copper much more strongly than it does zinc, copper is bound in a nonabsorbable form. The high susceptibility of sheep to copper toxicity may relate to their limited capacity to synthesize MT in the intestinal mucosa.[30]

That a three-way interaction of copper, molybdenum, and sulfur decreases the bioavailability of copper in ruminants has been recognized for more than 30 y. In the rumen, sulfur is reduced to sulfide, which reacts with ingested molybdenum to form tetrathiomolybdate $(MoS_4)^{2-}$ or oxythiomolybdates $(MoO_nS_{4-n})^{2-}$. These products react with copper to yield a physiologically unavailable form of copper. Low concentrations of $(MoS_4)^{2-}$ in the diet of rats induce clinical signs of copper deficiency by inhibiting absorption and modifying copper metabolism.[31,32] Absorbed $(MoS_4)^{2-}$ forms an insoluble complex with copper so that the concentration of total copper in the plasma is increased but is unavailable. A fraction of the complex is bound to plasma proteins even in the presence of trichloroacetic acid. In sheep the solid phase of the rumen digesta plays a major role in the copper-molybdenum-sulfur interaction.[33]

A high dietary intake of ascorbic acid decreases copper bioavailability and aggravates deficiency signs in avian species, impairs copper absorption from ligated intestinal segments of the rat, and lowers blood and liver copper concentrations in guinea pigs.[21] Ascorbate affects not only intestinal absorption of copper but also its utilization.[34] Intraperitoneal administration of ascorbate before copper injection impairs the restoration of aortic lysyl oxidase activity in deficient animals. Administration after copper treatment increases the restoration of both lysyl oxidase and ceruloplasmin oxidase activities. Consumption of 1500 mg ascorbic acid/d for 2 mo reduced serum ceruloplasmin in young adult men.[35] In the rat high intakes of dietary ascorbic acid and iron decreased the hematocrit levels when copper was limited.[36] Under these circumstances ascorbate and iron also interacted to decrease copper concentration and superoxide dismutase activity in heart. This interaction is interesting in view of the beneficial effect of ascorbate on iron absorption.

That the source of dietary carbohydrate affects the development of clinical signs of deficiency when dietary copper is limiting has been shown in rats but not in humans. Compared with starch, fructose and sucrose aggravate the signs of deficiency, suggesting that copper bioavailability is less in the presence of fructose-containing sugars than in the presence of glucose and its polymers.[37-39] In weanling male rats fed a low level of copper (1 μg/g), Fields et al.[37] observed lower liver copper concentration and higher mortality in rats whose diet contained sucrose than in those fed starch. If one considers starch-based diets as the norm, the detrimental effect of sucrose is largely related to the fructose moiety.[40] However, glucose as a simple sugar has an intermediary effect in aggravating copper deficiency. The effect of fructose on copper bioavailability appears to be primarily due to lower absorption of copper. After intubation of ^{67}Cu-labeled diets into copper-deficient rats, there was higher retention in the gastrointestinal tract of the fructose-fed rats than in starch-fed rats.[41] This effect did not occur in controls consuming adequate copper. However, in rats fed a minimal level of copper, Johnson et al.[42] found no effect of carbohydrate source on copper absorption from a single meal. These results suggest a possible interaction between copper nutritional status and fructose affecting copper absorption. Both fructose and ascorbic acid are strong reducing compounds and may convert copper to the cuprous state, thereby impairing utilization as well as absorption.

Transport and Cellular Uptake. Newly absorbed copper is bound primarily to serum albumin.[17,20] Much of this copper is taken up by the liver and converted to ceruloplasmin. The latter is released into the blood where it normally constitutes 90% of the plasma copper pool, 15.7 μmol/L. Copper is bound tightly to ceruloplasmin, whereas it is bound loosely to albumin and some free amino acids such as his-

Table 1. Cuproenzymes and associated pathology of copper deficiency*

Enzyme	Catalytic function	Known (or possible) pathology
Cytochrome c oxidase	Electron transport; terminal oxidase	(Cardiomyopathy)
Superoxide dismutase, cytosolic	Decomposition of superoxide free radical	(Membrane damage and cell death)
Dopamine-B-hydroxylase	Dopamine → norepinephrine	(Neuropathology; cardiac hypertrophy)
Lysyl oxidase	Deamination of lysyl residues; collagen and elastin crosslinking	Vascular rupture, osteoporosis, emphysema
Tyrosinase	Melanin formation	Lack of pigmentation
Ceruloplasmin	Ferroxidase, amine oxidase	(Anemia; impaired iron metabolism)
Factor IV	Blood coagulation	—
Thiol oxidase	Disulfide-bond formation	(Steely wool, pili torti)

* From reference 15 except for thiol oxidase, from reference 49.

tidine. By use of high–specific-activity [67]Cu, Weiss and Linder[43] found evidence for another copper-transport protein, which they termed transcuprein. This 270-kDa protein readily gave up [67]Cu to the liver and rapidly appeared in ceruloplasmin. Others were unable to detect this protein and support the older concept that albumin is primarily responsible for the initial transport of copper.[44] The basis of the differing observations is not clear, but it should be noted that one group administered the isotope intraperitoneally and studied blood from the vena cava,[43] whereas the other group administered it intraduodenally and studied portal blood.[44]

Ceruloplasmin donates copper to nonhepatic tissues for synthesis of cuproenzymes such as cytochrome c oxidase, superoxide dismutase, and lysyl oxidase.[20] However, the mechanism by which ceruloplasmin copper is made available to cells is unclear. Intravenously infused ceruloplasmin restores cytochrome c oxidase activity in rats more readily than does an albumin-copper complex.[45] Ceruloplasmin may enter the cell intact or ceruloplasmin copper may be reduced to Cu^+ and transferred to an intracellular protein. If ceruloplasmin serves as a direct donor of copper, there should be receptors on the cell plasma membrane. Stevens et al.[46] showed that chick aorta and heart-tissue membranes contain specific binding sites for ceruloplasmin. Furthermore, in copper-deficient animals both ceruloplasmin and lysyl oxidase activities respond rapidly and correlatively to copper repletion. Although these studies provide only circumstantial evidence that ceruloplasmin transports copper directly to cells, they support the concept. Interleukin 1 stimulates the synthesis of apoceruloplasmin leading to increased amine oxidase activity in copper-sufficient rats but not in deficient rats.[47] Whether or not increases in this acute phase protein affect copper utilization is not known.

Excretion. Copper is excreted primarily via the gastrointestinal tract with <3% of the intake appearing in the urine.[17] Bile contributes the major portion of endogenous fecal copper. Bile from normal humans contains a high-molecular-weight substance that is absent in Wilson's disease.[48] The role of this protein is unknown, but it may normally decrease copper reabsorption.

Biochemical Functions

Several cuproenzymes play critical metabolic roles. To a greater extent than for most catalytic nutrients, derangement of the biochemical functions of copper can be identified with specific pathology. A list of cuproenzymes, their catalytic functions, and the pathology associated with deficiency of the enzyme are presented in Table 1. Although specific pathology has not been identified for all cuproenzymes, their activities are generally depressed by copper deprivation.

The decreased lysyl oxidase activity associated with copper deficiency results in failure of collagen and elastin crosslinking and ultimately leads to vascular disease and spontaneous rupture of major vessels as well as defective bone matrices and osteoporosis. Decreased tyrosinase activity leads to achromotrichia of hair, wool, and feathers, because melanin formation is impaired. Although cytochrome c oxidase activity is markedly decreased by copper deficiency, it is not clear whether its activity becomes limiting in metabolism. Mitochondrial morphology and function are adversely affected by copper deficiency.[50] Oxygen consumption in the presence of exogenous ADP is impaired but is not due to decreased cytochrome c oxidase activity.[50,51] The primary defect appears to be reduced activity of adenine nucleotide translocase.[50]

Superoxide dismutase (SOD) along with glutathione peroxidase and catalase constitute the primary catalytic defense against metabolically generated free radicals.[52] Dietary copper deficiency leads to low SOD activity in liver, aorta, lung, and erythrocytes. Lung

SOD activity is only marginally decreased.[52] (See references 52 and 53 for earlier literature.) Although aortic SOD activity is dramatically lower in copper deficiency than under normal conditions, the immunoreactive apoenzyme is present and is readily reactivated by copper in vivo but not in vitro.[53] Copper deficiency deprives SOD of its essential copper component but does not prevent SOD apoprotein synthesis.

Physiological Functions and Deficiency Signs

Iron Metabolism and Anemia. Anemia was the first described sign of copper deficiency. In spite of multiple suggestions, the biochemical mechanism by which copper prevents anemia is still unclear. There is evidence that copper deficiency shortens the life span of the erythrocyte.[18] This finding may relate to changes in the plasma membrane because of free radical accumulation when SOD activity is low. Osmotic fragility is decreased by copper deficiency, and there is an increased concentration of phospholipid-derived malondialdehyde in the membranes.[54] Red blood cell viscosity is increased as well, suggesting crosslinking of membrane components. Another laboratory observed an increased concentration of a 170-kDa protein in erythrocyte membranes from copper-deficient rats.[55] This large cytoskeletal protein may arise from protein crosslinking because of oxygen free radicals. Such a process could account for the shorter survival time of red cells.

Copper also plays a key role in iron metabolism and thereby in hemoglobin biosynthesis. Serum iron tends to be low whereas liver and intestinal mucosa iron levels are elevated. These data suggest failure of iron mobilization. Frieden and Hsieh[56] proposed that circulating ferroxidase (ceruloplasmin), which is low in both dietary and genetic copper deficiency, is limiting in the oxidation of ferrous iron for transferrin transport. This theory is not entirely adequate because brindled mice, Menkes' patients, and Wilson's patients have low ceruloplasmin but do not develop anemia. The level of iron in the diet and the sex of the animal have a direct effect on the hematologic response to copper deficiency.[55,57] The maximal effect occurs in males fed a marginal level of iron. The precise role of copper in iron metabolism and anemia prevention requires additional research.

Connective Tissue Protein Crosslinking. Collagen and elastin constitute ∼30% of total body protein, and their maturation is dependent upon the copper-dependent enzyme lysyl oxidase.[58] Copper deficiency results in low lysyl oxidase activity and consequent failure of elastin and collagen crosslinking. Major blood vessels, such as the aorta, rupture spontaneously in many species and in individuals with Menkes' disease.

Osteoporosis and bone abnormalities were reported in dogs, rabbits, pigs, and children.[16] Bones of copper-deficient animals are more fragile than bones of normal animals, and they fracture with low deformation and torque.[59] The collagen in copper-deficient bone is more soluble than in control bone, indicating impaired crosslinking.

Lung tissue contains both collagen and elastin, and failure of crosslinking in copper-deficient rats[60] and pigs[61] leads to emphysema. A similar pathology was observed in the avian lung.[62]

Cardiac Disease. Hypertrophy of the heart results from severe copper deficiency, but the biochemical defect is unknown. Cardiac enlargement in rats was reported in the 1930s and has been studied since in several laboratories. Not only are the hearts of copper-deficient rats greatly enlarged, but ventricular aneurysms are common, occurring most commonly at the apex of the heart. The norepinephrine content of the copper-deficient heart is greatly decreased, and this defect may be related to cardiac malfunction.[63] Electrocardiography of copper-deficient rats has revealed abnormalities of the ST segment and occurrence of bundle-branch block.[64] There is also evidence of abnormal electrocardiographs in humans who consumed low-copper diets.[65,66]

Central Nervous System. Ataxia and related neurological disorders have long been associated with copper deficiency under field conditions as well as in experimental animals. Although the biochemical defects underlying the central nervous system pathology are unclear, current information was reviewed.[67,68] Impaired myelination or demyelination is associated with ataxia in lambs, but this condition does not occur in all species. It appears that the role of copper in myelination has been overemphasized. Clearly, copper deficiency affects the brain catecholamine pool size. Norepinephrine levels are decreased but readily restored by copper therapy. Whether norepinephrine levels relate to the neurological signs is unknown.

In severely copper-deficient rats, the striatal dopamine concentration is also depressed, but it is not readily reversed by copper therapy. This situation is analogous to the pathology of Parkinson's disease and is associated with neurological disorders in rats and sheep. Low dopamine is probably the result of brain-cell death, but the basis of copper's effect on these specific cells is unknown. It appears that a genetic component is involved, because not all severely copper-deficient rats develop neurological signs and low striatal dopamine.[69] There seem to be two populations of rats: one with a familial trait predisposed to develop low striatal dopamine when copper deficiency is imposed and another that is without this trait.

Lipid Metabolism. Whether copper status has a direct effect on the interconversion of fatty acids is controversial, but there is strong evidence that copper deficiency leads to increased lipid peroxidation of cell membranes.[16] Peroxidation correlates with decreased SOD and glutathione peroxidase activities. The latter enzyme contains selenium and its activity is affected markedly by selenium status. Evidence suggests that copper plays a role in selenium metabolism.[70] Copper deficiency decreased glutathione peroxidase activity in liver, but the effect of reduced food intake associated with copper deficiency on the activity of this enzyme has not been clarified.

In 1973 Klevay[71] produced hypercholesterolemia in rats by feeding a high ratio of zinc to copper. The hypercholesterolemia proved to be the result of copper deficiency and has been confirmed in numerous laboratories and species, including the mouse, monkey, and human.[16] Although the biochemical function of copper in cholesterol metabolism remains unclear, cholesterol synthesized from labeled mevalonate appears in the plasma more rapidly and to a greater extent in copper-deficient than in control rats.[72,73] The cholesterol in liver tissue is inversely related to that in plasma. High-density lipoprotein (HDL) is thought to play a key role in removing peripheral cholesterol. In copper-deficient rats both the HDL cholesterol and the apolipoprotein E associated with HDL are significantly higher than normal.[74] However, in human subjects who consumed a low-copper diet for 11 wk (but were not shown to be copper deficient), HDL cholesterol decreased.[75] The accumulation of HDL cholesterol in rat plasma could be the result of defective plasma-membrane receptors. Contrary to this hypothesis, a recent study shows greater total and specific binding of ^{125}I-ApoE-rich HDL to hepatic membranes from copper-deficient rats.[76] Further research is needed to explain the abnormal distribution of cholesterol in copper deficiency; exploration of events beyond the binding step deserves attention.

Immune Competence. The mouse is the most commonly used species for immunology investigation, and copper deficiency was shown to impair both humoral and cell-mediated immunity in mice and rats.[77,78] Importantly, the extent of impairment is related to the degree of copper deficiency. Thymus weights are decreased and natural killer-cell cytotoxicity is suppressed. There is a decrease in helper T cells. In copper-deficient rats antibody titers after immunization with sheep erythrocytes are lower than normal, and thymic hypogenesis occurs.[78] Copper repletion rapidly restores immunocompetence. Thus,

copper appears to exert a specific function in regard to the immune system. Cytochrome *c* oxidase and SOD activities are depressed in both spleen and thymus tissue of copper-deficient mice. Not only does copper status affect immune competence, but the latter may serve as a sensitive index of copper status.

Requirement

Apart from the bioavailability aspect discussed above, little new information relative to copper requirement has become available since the earlier chapter.[14] More complete discussion of the subject is presented elsewhere.[16,17]

Summary

The liver is the major storage organ for copper; its copper concentration is approached by that of the brain. Copper absorption occurs chiefly in the duodenum, and the process is regulated in part by the negative effect of metallothionein. Two dietary components of high reducing capacity, ascorbic acid and fructose, decrease the bioavailability of copper. High levels of dietary zinc have a similar effect via negative interaction. Ceruloplasmin, which is synthesized in the liver, is the major transport protein for copper, and there is evidence that peripheral cells possess specific binding sites for this protein.

Copper plays key metabolic roles in several organ and tissue systems as shown by the effects of copper deprivation. The signs of deficiency include anemia; failure of collagen and elastin crosslinking resulting in vascular rupture, emphysema, and osteoporosis; cardiac disease, achromotrichia; central nervous system and neurological disorders; hypercholesterolemia; and impaired immune competence.

The biochemical bases of the specific pathologies are only partially known. It is clear that lack of lysyl oxidase activity is responsible for failure of crosslink formation and that low tyrosinase activity leads to lack of melanin formation. Anemia results, at least in part, from faulty iron metabolism and may relate to impaired ferroxidase activity in some body compartment. Approximately 3 mg copper/kg dry diet (0.6–0.7 mg/1000 kcal) meets the requirement for most species and functions.

References

1. E.B. Hart, H. Steenbock, J. Waddell, and C.A. Elvehjem (1928) Iron in nutrition. VII. Copper as a supplement to iron for hemoglobin building in the rat. *J. Biol. Chem.* 77:797–812.
2. H.W. Bennetts and F.E. Chapman (1937) Copper deficiency in sheep in Western Australia: a preliminary account of the aetiology of enzootic ataxia of lambs and anemia of ewes. *Aust. Vet. J.* 13: 138–149.

3. H.W. Bennetts and H.T.B. Hall (1939) "Falling disease" of cattle in the southwest of Western Australia. *Aust. Vet. J.* 15:152–159.

4. B.L. O'Dell, B.C. Hardwick, G. Reynolds, and J.E. Savage (1961) Connective tissue defect in the chick resulting from copper deficiency. *Proc. Soc. Exp. Biol. Med.* 108:402–405.

5. G.S. Shields, W.F. Coulson, D.A. Kimball, W.H. Carnes, G.E. Cartwright, and M.M. Wintrobe (1962) Studies on copper metabolism. *Am. J. Pathol.* 41:603–621.

6. E. Cohen and C.A. Elvehjem (1934) The relation of iron and copper to the cytochrome and oxidase content of animal tissue. *J. Biol. Chem.* 107:97–105.

7. T. Mann and D. Keilin (1939) Haemocuprein and hepatocuprein, copper-protein compounds of blood and liver in mammals. *Proc. R. Soc. Lond.* [*Biol.*] 126:303–315.

8. J.M. McCord and I. Fridovich (1969) Superoxide dismutase. An enzymatic function for erythrocuprein (hemocuprein). *J. Biol. Chem.* 244:6049–6055.

9. E.D. Harris, W.A. Gonnerman, J.E. Savage, and B.L. O'Dell (1974) Connective tissue amine oxidase. II. Purification and partial characterization of lysyl oxidase from chick aorta. *Biochim. Biophys. Acta* 341:332–344.

10. A. Cordano, J.M. Baertl, and G.G. Graham (1964) Copper deficiency in infancy. *Pediatrics* 34:324–326.

11. J.T. Karpel and V.H. Peden (1972) Copper deficiency in long-term parenteral nutrition. *J. Pediatr.* 80:32–36.

12. D.M. Danks, P.E. Campbell, B.J. Stevens, V. Mayne, and E. Cartwright (1972) Menkes' kinky hair syndrome: an inherited defect in copper absorption with widespread effects. *Pediatrics* 50:188–201.

13. D.M. Hunt (1974) Primary defect in copper transport underlies mottled mutants in the mouse. *Nature* 249:852–854.

14. B.L. O'Dell (1984) Copper. In: *Present Knowledge in Nutrition* (R.E. Olson, H.P. Broquist, C.O. Chichester, W.J. Darby, A.C. Kolbye, Jr., and R.M. Stalvey, eds.) pp. 506–518, The Nutrition Foundation, Inc., Washington, DC.

15. D.M. Danks (1988) Copper deficiency in humans. *Annu. Rev. Nutr.* 8:235–237.

16. G.K. Davis and W. Mertz (1986) Copper. In: *Trace Elements in Human and Animal Nutrition,* 5th ed. (W. Mertz, ed.) pp. 301–364. Academic Press, New York.

17. K. Mason (1979) A conspectus of research on copper metabolism and requirements of man. *J. Nutr.* 109:1979–2066.

18. D.M. Williams (1983) Copper deficiency in humans. *Semin. Hematol.* 20:118–128.

19. D. Holt, D. Dinsdale, and M. Webb (1986) Intestinal uptake and retention of copper in the suckling rat, *Rattus rattus*. I. Distribution and binding. *Comp. Biochem. Physiol.* 83C:313–316.

20. R.J. Cousins (1985) Absorption, transport and hepatic metabolism of copper and zinc: special reference to metallothionein and ceruloplasmin. *Physiol. Rev.* 65:238–309.

21. B.L. O'Dell (1985) Bioavailability of and interactions among trace elements. In: *Trace Elements in Nutrition of Children* (R.K. Chandra, ed.), pp. 41–62, Nestle Nutrition, Vevey/Raven Press, New York.

22. M.R. L'Abbe and P.W.F. Fischer (1984) The effects of dietary zinc on the activity of copper-requiring metalloenzymes in the rat. *J. Nutr.* 114:823–828.

23. M.D. Festa, H.L. Anderson, R.P. Dowdy, and M.R. Ellersieck (1985) Effect of zinc intake on copper excretion and retention in men. *Am. J. Clin. Nutr.* 41:285–292.

24. A.S. Prasad, G.J. Brewer, E.B. Schoomaker, and P. Rabbini (1978) Hypocupremia induced by zinc therapy in adults. *JAMA* 240:2166–2168.

25. H.N. Hoffman, R.L. Phyliky, and C.R. Fleming (1988) Zinc-induced copper deficiency. *Gastroenterology* 94:508–512.

26. G.J. Brewer, G.H. Hill, A.S. Prasad, Z.T. Cossack, and P. Rabbani (1983) Oral zinc therapy in Wilson's disease. *Ann. Intern. Med.* 99:314–320.

27. G.J. Brewer, G.M. Hill, R.D. Dick, et al. (1987) Treatment of Wilson's disease with zinc. III. Prevention of reaccumulation of hepatic copper. *J. Lab. Clin. Med.* 109:526–531.

28. D.Y. Lee, J. Schroeder, and D.T. Gordon (1988) Enhancement of Cu bioavailability in the rat by phytic acid. *J. Nutr.* 118:712–717.

29. A.C. Hall, B.W. Young, and I. Bremner (1979) Intestinal metallothionein and the mutual antagonism between copper and zinc in the rat. *J. Inorg. Biochem.* 11:57–66.

30. W.W. Saylor, F.D. Morrow, and R.M. Leach (1980) Copper- and zinc-binding proteins in sheep liver and intestine: effects of dietary levels of the metals. *J. Nutr.* 110:460–468.

31. A.T. Dick, D.W. Dewey, and J.M. Gawthorne (1975) Thiomolybdates and the copper-molybdenum-sulphur interaction in ruminant nutrition. *J. Agric. Sci.* 85:567–568.

32. C.F. Mills, T.T. El-Gallad, and I. Bremner (1981) Effects of molybdate, sulfide and tetrathiomolybdate on copper metabolism in rats. *J. Inorg. Biochem.* 14:189–207.

33. J.D. Allen and J.M. Gawthorne (1987) Involvement of the solid phase of rumen digesta in the interaction between copper, molybdenum and sulfur in sheep. *Br. J. Nutr.* 58:265–276.

34. R.A. DiSilvestro and E.D. Harris (1981) A postabsorption effect of L-ascorbic acid on copper metabolism in chicks. *J. Nutr.* 111:1964–1968.

35. E.B. Finley and F.L. Cerklewski (1983) Influence of ascorbic acid supplementation on copper status in young adult men. *Am. J. Clin. Nutr.* 37:553–556.

36. M.A. Johnson and C.L. Murphy (1988) Adverse effects of high dietary iron and ascorbic acid on copper status in copper-deficient and copper-adequate rats. *Am. J. Clin. Nutr.* 47:96–101.

37. M. Fields, O.E. Michaelis, J. Hallfrisch, S. Reiser, and J.C. Smith (1983) Effect of copper deficiency on intestinal hexose uptake and hepatic enzyme activity in the rat. *Nutr. Rep. Int.* 28:123–131.

38. M.A. Johnson and E.W. Flagg (1986) Effect of sucrose and cornstarch on the development of copper deficiency in rats fed high levels of zinc. *Nutr. Res.* 6:1307–1319.

39. H.G. Petering, L. Murthy, K.L. Stemmer, V.N. Finellia, and E.E. Menden (1986) Effects of copper deficiency on the cardiovascular system of the rat. *Biol. Trace Element Res.* 9:251–270.

40. M. Fields, R.J. Ferretti, J.C. Smith, and S. Reiser (1984) The interaction of type of dietary carbohydrates with copper deficiency. *Am. J. Clin. Nutr.* 39:289–295.

41. M. Fields, J. Holbrook, D. Scholfield, J.C. Smith, S. Reiser, and Los Alamos Medical Research Group (1986) Effect of fructose or starch on copper-67 absorption and excretion by the rat. *J. Nutr.* 116:625–632.

42. P.E. Johnson, M.A. Stuart, and T.D. Bowman (1988) Bioavailability of copper to rats from various foodstuffs and in the presence of different carbohydrates. *Proc. Soc. Biol. Med.* 187:44–50.

43. K.C. Weiss and M.C. Linder (1985) Copper transport in rats involving a new plasma protein. *Am. J. Physiol.* 249:E77–E88.

44. D.T. Gordon, A.S. Leinart, and R.J. Cousins (1987) Portal copper transport in rats by albumin. *Am. J. Physiol.* 252:E327–E333.

45. H.S. Hsieh and E. Frieden (1975) Evidence for ceruloplasmin as a transport protein. *Biochim. Biophys. Res. Commun.* 67:1326–1330.

46. M.D. Stevens, R.A. Di Silvestro, and E.D. Harris (1984) Specific receptor for ceruloplasmin in membrane fragments from aortic and heart tissues. *Biochemistry* 23:261–266.

47. E.F. Barber and R.J. Cousins (1988) Interleukin-1-stimulated induction of ceruloplasmin synthesis in normal and copper deficient rats. *J. Nutr.* 118:375–381.

48. V. Iyengar, G.J. Brewer, R.D. Dick, and C. Owyang (1988) Studies of cholecystokinin-stimulated biliary secretions reveals a high molecular weight substance in normal subjects that is absent in patients with Wilson's disease. *J. Lab. Clin. Med.* 111:267–274.

49. L.L. Lash and D.P. Jones (1986) Purification and properties of the

membranal thiol oxidase from porcine kidney. *Arch. Biochem. Biophys.* 247:120–130.

50. N.T. Davies and C.B. Lawrence (1986) Studies on the effect of copper deficiency on rat liver mitochondria III. Effects on adenine nucleotide translocase. *Biochim. Biophys. Acta* 848:294–304.

51. N. Rusinko and J.R. Prohaska (1985) Adenine nucleotide and lactate levels in organs from copper-deficient mice and brindled mice. *J. Nutr.* 115:936–943.

52. C.G. Taylor, W.J. Bettger, and T.M. Bray (1988) Effect of dietary zinc or copper deficiency on the primary free radical defense system. *J. Nutr.* 118:613–621.

53. C.T. Dameron and E.D. Harris (1987) Regulation of aortic Cu,Zn-superoxide dismutase with copper. Effects in vivo. *Biochem. J.* 248:663–668.

54. S.K. Jain and D.M. Williams (1988) Copper deficiency anemia: altered red blood cell lipids and viscosity in rats. *Am. J. Clin. Nutr.* 48:637–640.

55. W.T. Johnson and T.R. Kramer (1987) Effect of copper deficiency on erythrocyte membrane proteins of rats. *J. Nutr.* 117:1085–1090.

56. E. Frieden and H.S. Hsieh (1976) Ceruloplasmin: the copper transport protein with essential oxidase activity. *Adv. Enzymol.* 44:187–236.

57. N.L. Cohen, C.L. Keen, L.S. Hurley, and B. Lönnerdal (1985) Determinants of copper-deficiency anemia in rats. *J. Nutr.* 115:710–725.

58. B.L. O'Dell (1981) Roles for iron and copper in connective tissue biosynthesis. *Philos. Trans. R. Soc. Lond.* [Biol.] 294:91–104.

59. R.B. Rucker, R.S. Riggins, R. Laughlin, M.M. Chan, M. Chen, and K. Tom (1975) Effects of nutritional copper deficiency on the biomechanical properties of bone and arterial metabolism in the chick. *J. Nutr.* 105:1062–1070.

60. B.L. O'Dell, K.H. Kilburn, W.N. McKenzie, and R.J. Thurston (1978) The lung of the copper-deficient rat. A model for developmental pulmonary emphysema. *Am. J. Pathol.* 91:413–432.

61. N.T. Soskel, S. Watanabe, E. Hammond, L.B. Sandberg, A.D. Renzetti, and J.D. Crapo (1982) A copper-deficient, zinc-supplemented diet produces emphysema in pigs. *Am. Rev. Respir. Dis.* 126:316–325.

62. K. Buckingham, C.S. Heng-Khoo, M. Dubick, et al. (1981) Copper deficiency and elastin metabolism in avian lung. *Proc. Soc. Exp. Biol. Med.* 166:310–319.

63. J.R. Prohaska and L.J. Heller (1982) Mechanical properties of the copper-deficient rat heart. *J. Nutr.* 112:2142–2150.

64. K.E. Viestenz and L.M. Klevay (1982) A randomized trial of copper therapy in rats with electrocardiographic abnormalities due to copper deficiency. *Am. J. Clin. Nutr.* 35:258–266.

65. L.M. Klevay, L. Inman, L.K. Johnson, et al. (1984) Increased cholesterol in plasma in a young man during experimental copper depletion. *Metabolism* 33:1112–1118.

66. S. Reiser, J.C. Smith, W. Mertz, et al. (1985) Indices of copper status in humans consuming a typical American diet containing either fructose or starch. *Am. J. Clin. Nutr.* 42:242–251.

67. B.L. O'Dell and J.R. Prohaska (1983) Biochemical aspects of copper deficiency in the nervous system. In: *Neurobiology of the Trace Element* (I.E. Dreosti and R.M. Smith, eds.), pp. 41–81, Humana Press, Clifton, NJ.

68. J.R. Prohaska (1987) Functions of trace elements in brain metabolism. *Physiol. Rev.* 67:858–901.

69. D.S. Miller and B.L. O'Dell (1987) Milk and casein-based diets for the study of brain catecholamines in copper-deficient rats. *J. Nutr.* 117:1890–1897.

70. S.G. Jenkinson, R.A. Lawrence, R.F. Burk, and D.M. Williams (1982) Effects of copper deficiency on the activity of the selenoenzyme glutathione peroxidase and on excretion and tissue retention of $^{75}SeO_3^{2-}$. *J. Nutr.* 112:197–204.

71. L.M. Klevay (1973) Hypercholesterolemia in rats produced by an increase in the ratio of zinc to copper ingested. *Am. J. Clin. Nutr.* 26:1060–1068.

72. K.G.D. Allen and L.M. Klevay (1978) Copper deficiency and cholesterol metabolism in the rat. *Atherosclerosis* 31:259–271.

73. M.J.S. Shao and K.Y. Lei (1980) Conversion of [2-^{14}C] mevalonate into cholesterol, lanosterol and squalene in copper-deficient rats. *J. Nutr.* 110:859–867.

74. K.Y. Lei (1983) Alterations in plasma, lipid, lipoprotein and apolipoprotein concentrations in copper deficient rats. *J. Nutr.* 113:2178–2183.

75. S. Reiser, A. Powell, C-Y. Yang, and J.J. Canary (1987) Effect of copper intake on blood cholesterol and its lipoprotein distribution in men. *Nutr. Rep. Int.* 36:641–649.

76. C.A. Hassel, T.P. Carr, J.A. Marchello, and K.Y. Lei (1988) Apolipoprotein E-rich HDL binding to liver plasma membranes in copper-deficient rats. *Proc. Soc. Exp. Biol. Med.* 187:296–308.

77. J.R. Prohaska and O.A. Lukasewycz (1981) Copper deficiency suppresses the immune response of mice. *Science* 213:559–561.

78. M.L. Failla, U. Babu, and K.E. Seidel (1988) Use of immunoresponsiveness to demonstrate that the dietary requirement for copper in young rats is greater with dietary fructose than dietary starch. *J. Nutr.* 118:487–496.

Chapter 30

Orville A. Levander and Raymond F. Burk

Selenium

In 1957 Schwarz and Foltz[1] showed that traces of dietary selenium prevented nutritional liver necrosis in rats deficient in vitamin E. Soon thereafter selenium was used widely in agriculture to prevent a variety of selenium- and vitamin E-responsive conditions in livestock and poultry, such as white muscle disease in sheep and cattle, hepatosis dietetica in swine, exudative diathesis in chickens, and gizzard myopathy in turkeys.[2] Supplementation of feeds with selenium resulted in great economic gains for animal producers.

Signs of selenium deficiency have not been observed in free-living animals adequate in vitamin E. A "pure" deficiency of selenium uncomplicated by simultaneous vitamin E deficiency has been seen only in laboratory animals under experimental conditions. Rats fed a low-selenium diet adequate in vitamin E through two generations exhibited poor growth, sparse hair coats, cataracts, and reproductive failure.[3] Nutritional pancreatic atrophy (NPA) was produced in chicks fed amino acid-based diets severely deficient in selenium.[4] NPA was originally considered the only well-documented specific organ lesion resulting from uncomplicated selenium deficiency in any species, but the atrophy now has been found to respond also to high levels of dietary vitamin E and other antioxidants.[5] NPA can be produced in chicks by feeding a practical-type diet composed of ingredients from a selenium-deficient region of China, but the severity of the atrophy is reduced, thereby suggesting that a factor associated with the practical diet may provide partial protection from NPA in the selenium-deficient chick.[6]

Despite the difficulties encountered in producing a pure selenium deficiency in animals, selenium is considered an essential element for humans. It is a constituent of the enzyme glutathione peroxidase isolated from human red blood cells,[7] and selenium deficiency has been associated with two diseases of childhood in China.[8]

Body Compartments

Most selenium in animal tissues is present in two compartments or forms (Figure 1). One is selenocysteine in selenoproteins, such as glutathione peroxidase and selenoprotein P, and the other is selenomethionine, which is incorporated in place of methionine in a variety of proteins. Other forms may be present because tissue selenium has not been fully characterized.

Selenomethionine in tissues is derived from the diet; it cannot be synthesized in the body. As discussed below, this form of selenium is not regulated by the selenium status of the animal and can be regarded as an unregulated storage compartment. When dietary selenium supply is interrupted, turnover of the selenomethionine pool provides selenium to the organism. This adjustment has been demonstrated in human beings who moved from areas of high selenium intake to areas of low intake. Blood selenium levels declined slowly for a year before reaching levels typical of the low-selenium area.[9] Glutathione peroxidase activity in red blood cells was similar in subjects residing in the two areas, suggesting that selenium was transferred from the selenomethionine compartment to the regulated selenocysteine compartment.

Selenocysteine is the form of selenium that accounts for its biological activity. Most evidence suggests that the selenocysteine compartment is tightly regulated. Such regulation is necessary because this reactive compound could interfere with biochemical function if it were free in the cell. Selenocysteine is incorporated into proteins by a specific mechanism, and there is no evidence that it substitutes for cysteine in animal systems. The regulation of selenocysteine synthesis and insertion into proteins is currently under investigation. It appears to be coordinated with production of excretory metabolites so that when more selenium is available than is needed for selenocysteine formation, the element is excreted.

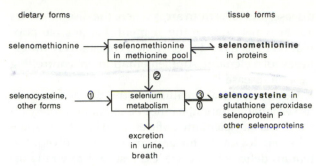

Figure 1. Outline of selenium metabolism. Dietary forms of the element are shown on the left and tissue forms are shown on the right. ① indicates selenocysteine β-lyase, which catabolizes selenocysteine, and ② indicates processes that catabolize selenomethionine. Both processes make selenium available to the organism. ③ indicates incorporation of selenium into serine during translation with formation of selenocysteine in selenoproteins.

Methods of Analysis and Assessment of Selenium Status

Selenium concentration can be determined with great accuracy by a variety of methods. Fluorometry, neutron activation analysis, atomic absorption, and mass spectrometry have been used to measure the element in fluids and tissues. Biologically active selenium can be estimated by measuring glutathione peroxidase activity[10] and selenoprotein P concentration.[11]

The use of these measurements in the assessment of selenium status requires an understanding of selenium metabolism. As indicated above and illustrated in Figure 1, intake of the element as selenomethionine results in a higher tissue selenium concentration than will intake of the same amount of the element in other forms, because some of the selenomethionine is present in proteins substituting for methionine. Selenium thus released by catabolism of selenomethionine then will be present as selenocysteine in selenoproteins.

Intake of the element in inorganic form or in the form of selenocysteine affects only the selenocysteine compartment. This compartment is regulated and is useful in detecting selenium deficiency. It is not useful in assessing selenium status, however, once the selenium requirement has been met.

Additional biochemical changes can be used to judge the severity of selenium deficiency in experimental animals. In the rat, plasma glutathione concentration and liver glutathione S-transferase activity increase in severe selenium deficiency.[10] These changes have not been described in human beings.

Metabolism

Seleno amino acids are the principal dietary forms of the element for free-living animals (Figure 1). Se-lenomethionine is derived from plants[12] and selenocysteine from animals.[13] Other forms occur, but their quantitative importance has not been established. Selenium is often supplied in inorganic form in experimental diets and in supplements.

Absorption of selenium does not appear to be regulated, and most studies have shown it to be high (>50%). Selenomethionine is absorbed by the same mechanism as methionine,[14] but little is known about selenocysteine absorption. Absorption of inorganic selenium is very efficient and is unaffected by selenium status.[15]

Available evidence suggests that selenomethionine follows some of the methionine metabolic pathways. It is incorporated into proteins in place of methionine and in this way contributes to tissue selenium. This form of selenium is not known to have a physiological function, nor does it appear to be recognized by the organism as selenium. Only when the selenomethionine is catabolized is its selenium released for specific utilization.

The rate of selenomethionine catabolism appears to be determined by methionine intake.[16] Consequently a low methionine intake can lead to low glutathione peroxidase activity (selenium deficiency), because dietary selenomethionine is sequestered in protein. Thus, lowered glutathione peroxidase activity can occur despite adequate selenium intake and tissue selenium levels. Higher methionine intakes lead to catabolism of methionine and selenomethionine with release of selenium and repair of the selenium deficiency.[16]

Bacterial systems incorporate selenium into serine in place of oxygen to form selenocysteine,[17] and there is evidence that this reaction occurs in animal cells as well.[18] Incorporation takes place while serine is attached to a unique tRNA that recognizes the stop codon TGA in animal systems.[19] Selenocysteine then is incorporated into a selenoprotein such as glutathione peroxidase. Free selenocysteine has not been found because selenocysteine β-lyase catabolizes it and prevents its accumulation.[20] This enzyme is presumably responsible for releasing selenium from dietary selenocysteine as well (Figure 1).

Homeostasis of selenium is achieved by regulation of its excretion. Excretion takes place via the urine, but very high selenium intake leads to exhalation of volatile forms.[21] There are several urinary metabolites, but only one, trimethylselenonium ion, has been identified.[22] It is a minor metabolite in human beings.

Biochemical Functions

Selenium defends the organism against oxidant stress. The selenoenzyme glutathione peroxidase, which is present in cells and in plasma, removes hydrogen peroxide and other free hydroperoxides.[23] A selenium-containing phospholipid hydroperoxide glutathione peroxidase metabolizes fatty acid hydroperoxides that are present in phospholipids.[24] There is evidence that the element may have additional antioxidant effects.[25]

Selenium has a number of biochemical effects that have not been characterized fully. Deficiency of the element causes changes in the activities of many drug-metabolizing enzymes.[26] As a result some toxicities are worsened and some are ameliorated.[27] In the rat, selenium deficiency leads to increased hepatic heme turnover, increased hepatic glutathione synthesis, and changes in glucose utilization.[28]

The biological activity of selenium is mediated by selenoenzymes. Several bacterial selenoenzymes have been characterized, and they all have redox functions as does glutathione peroxidase.[29] Thus, it can be predicted that redox selenoenzymes account for some of the unexplained effects of the element. In addition to the selenium-dependent glutathione peroxidases, a rat plasma protein containing selenocysteine has been purified and quantitated.[11] It was designated selenoprotein P, and its concentration falls to <10% of control in selenium deficiency. The function of selenoprotein P is unknown, but it has been suggested that it is an extracellular oxidant defense enzyme[11] and that it transports selenium from the liver to the testis.[30]

There is clear evidence that additional selenoproteins exist.[31] Characterization of these proteins undoubtedly will lead to understanding some of the nonglutathione peroxidase effects of selenium.

Molecular biology studies of selenium are beginning to unravel the role of the element in the control of biochemical processes. Recently, the effect of selenium deficiency on rat liver glutathione peroxidase mRNA levels was determined. Enzyme activity and its mRNA levels were low in selenium deficiency, implying that selenium has an effect on transcription of the glutathione peroxidase gene.[32,33] Administration of selenium led to a rapid increase in mRNA to control levels followed by a gradual increase in enzyme activity. This finding suggests that some control over selenium incorporation into proteins may be exerted at the level of translation. Further studies should delineate the control mechanisms in selenium utilization and function.

Deficiency

Selenium deficiency has been associated with Keshan disease, an endemic cardiomyopathy that primarily affects children and women of child-bearing age in some areas of China.[8] A variety of indices of selenium status are depressed in patients with Keshan disease, and diets from areas where the disease occurs are extremely low in the element. Large-scale population trials have demonstrated conclusively the efficacy of selenium supplementation in controlling Keshan disease.[34]

However, certain features of the disease, such as its seasonal variation, cannot be explained solely on the basis of selenium deficiency. Therefore, some other etiological factor appears to be involved. Selenium-deficient mice are less resistant to virally induced cardiac damage,[35] so the disease may have an infectious component. Nonetheless, the Chinese investigators believe that selenium deficiency is the underlying condition that predisposes an individual to the disease and concluded that the role of any other causal agents (infectious, environmental, nutritional, etc.) is secondary.

Kashin-Beck disease, an endemic osteoarthritis that occurs during the preadolescent or adolescent years,[36] is another disease that has been linked to low-selenium status in China.[8] However, the selenium deficiency hypothesis does not seem to be as widely accepted for Kashin-Beck disease as for Keshan disease, and other etiological theories (mycotoxins in grain, mineral imbalance, organic contaminants in drinking water) have been proposed.[37]

In past years selenium was not generally added to fluids used for total parenteral nutrition (TPN). As a result, several cases of biochemical selenium deficiency (low plasma or blood selenium levels, depressed glutathione peroxidase activity) were reported. Despite these reports of impaired selenium status, no clinical syndrome characteristic of selenium deficiency was seen in such patients.[38] Cardiomyopathy and skeletal muscle weakness have been observed in a few intravenously fed individuals who were not supplemented with selenium.[39-41] Currently, there are no official guidelines for the doses or forms of selenium supplements to be administered to TPN patients.[42]

A number of epidemiological studies have been published that suggest that poor selenium status may be associated with an increased risk of developing cancer or heart disease.[43] In the case of cancer, several experiments with rodent models also indicate a protective effect of selenium against tumorigenesis,[44] although high (i.e., nonnutritional, >0.25 $\mu g/g$ dry diet) doses of selenium are generally used and, at least in one instance, selenium increased rather than decreased tumor formation.[45] A recent evaluation of the selenium-cancer relationship concluded that the protective effect of selenium against cancer in humans still is not proved and recommended against the use of dietary selenium supplements except in Keshan disease areas of China.[46] Likewise, evaluation of five prospective epidemiological studies from

Scandinavia could establish no causal relationship between selenium status and the risk of ischemic heart disease.[47] Clarification of any role for selenium in the etiology of these two human degenerative diseases must await additional research.

Requirements and Allowances

During the past decade our quantitative knowledge of human selenium requirements has increased markedly.[43] In 1980 the Food and Nutrition Board of the U.S. National Academy of Sciences proposed an Estimated Safe and Adequate Daily Dietary Intake of selenium of 50–200 μg for adults.[48] This range was based on extrapolation from animal experiments because few data about selenium in human nutrition were available. Most mammals appear to require ~0.1 μg selenium/g dry diet. Thus, if humans consumed 500 g of diet daily (dry basis) then they would require 50 μg of selenium per day, the lower limit of the safe and adequate range. However, some workers have found that the young of certain species of animals need >0.1 μg/g diet.[49] Therefore, the validity of human requirements based on extrapolation from animal studies is uncertain.

Balance studies often have been used in the past to estimate human requirements for various minerals, but the pitfalls in the use of balance data for this purpose are well known.[50] A comparison of balance studies from China, New Zealand, and the United States revealed that metabolic balance could be achieved over a wide range of selenium intakes (9–80 μg/d).[51] Balance was maintained in persons with low selenium intakes by a decreased urinary and fecal excretion of selenium. Thus, this time-honored technique does not appear to be particularly helpful in delineating human requirements for selenium.

On the basis of dietary surveys, scientists in China determined the dietary selenium intake needed to prevent Keshan disease. The disease is absent in areas where the dietary intake averages 19 and 14 μg/d for adult men and women, respectively.[52] This intake is very low and could be considered a "minimum daily requirement" for selenium.

Chinese scientists also have estimated what they called a "physiological" selenium requirement based on saturation of plasma glutathione peroxidase activity. Men living in a Keshan disease area (average dietary selenium intake of 10 μg/d) were supplemented with graded doses of selenomethionine for several months. Individuals consuming a total of ≥40 μg selenium/d had similar enzyme values, and this intake was considered the physiological requirement under these conditions.[52]

The Food and Nutrition Board used the above experiment as the basis for its 1989 Recommended Dietary Allowance (RDA) for selenium.[53] The Chinese value was adjusted to account for differences in body weight and to incorporate an appropriate safety factor. RDAs for selenium of 70 and 55 μg/d were calculated for adult men and women, respectively.[43] The selenium RDA for younger age groups was extrapolated downward on the basis of metabolic body size.

Sources

The selenium content of foods varies widely (μg/g fresh weight): organ meats and seafoods, 0.4–1.5; muscle meats, 0.1–0.4; cereals and grains, <0.1 to >0.8; dairy products, <0.1 to 0.3; and fruits and vegetables, <0.1.[54] The primary factor affecting the selenium content of plant foods is the amount of selenium available in the soil for uptake by plants in a given area. For example, corn, rice, and soybeans collected in an area of China with human selenosis contained an average of 8.1, 4.0, and 11.9 μg/g, respectively, whereas the same foods taken from a Keshan disease area contained only 0.005, 0.007, and 0.010 μg/g.[55] Animal products also show some variation in selenium content. However, the extreme values are moderated somewhat because animals tend to conserve selenium under conditions of deficiency and excrete it under conditions of excessive exposure.

Data from nationwide food surveys analyzed by the U.S. Food and Drug Administration show that the average selenium intake by adults between 1974 and 1982 was 108 μg/d with annual values ranging between 83 and 129 μg/d.[56] Thus, the well-balanced North American diet appears to provide ample selenium to satisfy the RDA for this element. The national dietaries of countries with soils poor in selenium furnish lower quantities of selenium. For example, dietary selenium intakes in New Zealand and Finland were reported to be 28–32 and 30–50 μg/d, respectively.[54] The low dietary intakes of selenium in Finland convinced the authorities there to supplement the fertilizers used in that country with sodium selenate. As a result serum selenium levels among the Finns increased by >50% between 1984 and 1986 to approach typical North American values.[57]

High dietary selenium intakes occur in areas with naturally seleniferous soils. In one region of China where endemic human selenosis was seen, intakes as high as 6690 μg/d were reported.[55] The source of selenium in this food chain was a highly seleniferous coal that lost its selenium to the soil because of weathering.

Investigations into the nutritional bioavailability of selenium in foods have only begun, but animal models already have shown great variation in the availability of selenium in different foods. On the basis of increased hepatic glutathione peroxidase activity in selenium-depleted rats, selenium fed as mushrooms, tuna, wheat, beef kidney, and Brazil nuts had 5%, 57%, 83%, 97%, and 124% of the availability of sodium selenite, respectively.[58,59] A bioavailability trial carried out with men of low-selenium status in Finland showed that a number of variables had to be considered in such studies, including short-term increases in glutathione peroxidase activity, long-term tissue retention of selenium, and metabolic conversion of retained forms of selenium to biologically active forms.[60]

Toxicity

Human selenium poisoning from consumption of toxic foods containing high levels of selenium was reported in Enshi county, China, where chronically intoxicated individuals ingested an average of 4.99 mg selenium/d in a vegetable diet.[55] Signs of selenosis included loss of hair and nails, skin lesions, tooth decay, and abnormalities of the nervous system. Concomitant fluorosis may have been a complicating factor in the appearance of the latter two signs.[8] Acutely poisoned persons (loss of hair in 3–4 d) may have consumed as much as 38 mg selenium/d.[61]

Human selenium poisoning was reported in 13 persons in the United States who consumed a "health food" supplement that contained ~182 times more selenium than stated on the label.[62–64] The total amount of selenium thought to be ingested by the victims ranged between 27 and 2387 mg. The most common symptoms were nausea, vomiting, hair loss, nail changes, irritability, fatigue, and peripheral neuropathy.

The biochemical basis of selenium toxicity is not fully understood, but several possible reaction mechanisms have been suggested, such as interference with sulfur metabolism, catalytic oxidation of sulfhydryl groups, and inhibition of protein synthesis.[65]

Because there are no sensitive and specific biochemical indicators of dietary selenium overexposure at this time,[54] it is not possible to propose with certainty a safe dietary selenium intake. Recent field studies in Enshi county, China, suggest that 900 μg selenium/d can result in persistent clinical signs (fingernail changes) and 750 μg/d can lead to biochemical abnormalities (alterations in the ratio of plasma to red blood cell selenium).[66] Until better indices of selenium overexposure are developed, it would seem imprudent (and unnecessary from the nutritional point of view) to consume routinely more than the 200 μg upper limit of the Food and Nutrition Board's 1980 safe and adequate daily dietary intake.[48]

References

1. K. Schwarz and C.M. Foltz (1957) Selenium as an integral part of factor 3 against dietary necrotic liver degeneration. *J. Am. Chem. Soc.* 79:3292–3293.
2. Board on Agriculture, Committee on Animal Nutrition, National Research Council (1983) *Selenium in Nutrition*, revised ed., National Academy of Sciences, Washington, DC.
3. K.E.M. McCoy and P.H. Weswig (1969) Some selenium responses in the rat not related to vitamin E. *J. Nutr.* 98:383–389.
4. J.N. Thompson and M.L. Scott (1969) Role of selenium in the nutrition of the chick. *J. Nutr.* 97:335–342.
5. M.E. Whitacre, G.F. Combs, Jr., S.B. Combs, and R.S. Parker (1987) Influence of dietary vitamin E on nutritional pancreatic atrophy in selenium-deficient chicks. *J. Nutr.* 117:460–467.
6. G.F. Combs, Jr., C.H. Liu, Z.H. Lu, and Q. Su (1984) Uncomplicated selenium deficiency produced in chicks fed a corn-soy-based diet. *J. Nutr.* 114:964–976.
7. Y.C. Awasthi, E. Beutler, and S.K. Srivastava (1975) Purification and properties of human erythrocyte glutathione peroxidase. *J. Biol. Chem.* 250:5144–5149.
8. G. Yang, K. Ge, J. Chen, and X. Chen (1988) Selenium-related endemic diseases and the daily selenium requirement of humans. *World Rev. Nutr. Diet.* 55:98–152.
9. M.F. Robinson (1976) The moonstone: more about selenium. *J. Hum. Nutr.* 30:79–91.
10. K.E. Hill, R.F. Burk, and J.M. Lane (1987) Effect of selenium depletion and repletion on plasma glutathione and glutathione-dependent enzymes in the rat. *J. Nutr.* 117:99–104.
11. J.G. Yang, J. Morrison-Plummer, and R.F. Burk (1987) Purification and quantitation of a rat plasma selenoprotein distinct from glutathione peroxidase using monoclonal antibodies. *J. Biol. Chem.* 262:13372–13375.
12. O.E. Olson, E.J. Novacek, E.I. Whitehead, and I.S. Palmer (1970) Investigations on selenium in wheat. *Phytochemistry* 9:1181–1188.
13. W.C. Hawkes, E.C. Wilhelmsen, and A.L. Tappel (1985) Abundance and tissue distribution of selenocysteine-containing proteins in the rat. *J. Inorg. Biochem.* 23:77–92.
14. P.D. Whanger, N.D. Pedersen, J. Hatfield, and P.H. Weswig (1976) Absorption of selenite and selenomethionine from ligated digestive tract segments in rats. *Proc. Soc. Exp. Biol. Med.* 153:295–297.
15. D.G. Brown, R.F. Burk, R.J. Seely, and K.W. Kiker (1972) Effect of dietary selenium on the gastrointestinal absorption of $^{75}SeO_3^{2-}$ in the rat. *Int. J. Vitam. Nutr. Res.* 42:588–591.
16. I.H. Waschulewski and R.A. Sunde (1988) Effect of dietary methionine on utilization of tissue selenium from dietary selenomethionine for glutathione peroxidase in the rat. *J. Nutr.* 118:367–374.
17. W. Leinfelder, E. Zehelein, M.A. Mandrand-Berthelot, and A. Bock (1988) Gene for a novel tRNA species that accepts L-serine and cotranslationally inserts selenocysteine. *Nature* 331:723–725.
18. R.A. Sunde and J.K. Evenson (1987) Serine incorporation into the selenocysteine moiety of glutathione peroxidase. *J. Biol. Chem.* 262:933–937.
19. I. Chambers, J. Frampton, P. Goldfarb, N. Affara, W. McBain, and P.R. Harrison (1986) The structure of the mouse glutathione peroxidase gene: the selenocysteine in the active site is encoded by the 'termination' codon, TGA. *EMBO J.* 5:1221–1227.
20. N. Esaki, T. Nakamura, H. Tanaka, and K. Soda (1982) Selenocysteine lyase, a novel enzyme that specifically acts on selenocysteine. *J. Biol. Chem.* 257:4386–4391.
21. B.A. Bopp, R.C. Sonders, and J.W. Kesterson (1982) Metabolic fate of selected selenium compounds in laboratory animals and man. *Drug Metab. Rev.* 13:271–318.
22. I.S. Palmer, D.D. Fischer, A.W. Halverson, and O.E. Olson (1969) Identification of a major selenium excretory product in rat urine. *Biochim. Biophys. Acta* 177:336–342.

23. J.T. Rotruck, A.L. Pope, H.E. Ganther, A.B. Swanson, D.G. Hafeman, and W.G. Hoekstra (1973) Selenium: biochemical role as a component of glutathione peroxidase. *Science* 179:588–590.

24. F. Ursini, M. Maiorino and C. Gregolin (1985) The selenoenzyme phospholipid hydroperoxide glutathione peroxidase. *Biochim. Biophys. Acta* 839:62–70.

25. R.F. Burk, R.A. Lawrence, and J.M. Lane (1980) Liver necrosis and lipid peroxidation in the rat as a result of paraquat and diquat administration. *J. Clin. Invest.* 65:1024–1031.

26. R. Reiter and A. Wendel (1983) Selenium and drug metabolism I. Multiple modulations of mouse liver enzymes. *Biochem. Pharmacol.* 32:3063–3067.

27. R.F. Burk and J.M. Lane (1983) Modification of chemical toxicity by selenium deficiency. *Fundam. Appl. Toxicol.* 3:218–221.

28. R.F. Burk (1983) Biological activity of selenium. *Annu. Rev. Nutr.* 3:53–70.

29. T.C. Stadtman (1980) Selenium-dependent enzymes. *Annu. Rev. Biochem.* 49:93–110.

30. M.A. Motsenbocker and A.L. Tappel (1982) A selenocysteine-containing selenium-transport protein in rat plasma. *Biochim. Biophys. Acta* 719:147–153.

31. D. Behne, H. Hilmert, S. Scheid, H. Gessner, and W. Elger (1988) Evidence for specific selenium target tissues and new biologically important selenoproteins. *Biochim. Biophys. Acta* 966:12–21.

32. M.S. Saedi, C.G. Smith, J. Frampton, I. Chambers, P.R. Harrison, and R.A. Sunde (1988) Effect of selenium status on mRNA levels for glutathione peroxidase in rat liver. *Biochem. Biophys. Res. Commun.* 153:855–861.

33. S. Yoshimura, S. Takekoshi, K. Watanabe, and Y. Fujii-Kuriyama (1988) Determination of nucleotide sequence of cDNA coding rat glutathione peroxidase and diminished expression of the mRNA in selenium deficient rat liver. *Biochem. Biophys. Res. Commun.* 154:1024–1028.

34. G. Yang, J. Chen, Z. Wen, et al. (1984) The role of selenium in Keshan disease. *Adv. Nutr. Res.* 6:203–231.

35. J. Bai, S. Wu, K. Ge, X. Deng, and C. Su (1980) The combined effect of selenium deficiency and viral infection on the myocardium of mice. *Acta Acad. Med. Sin.* 2:29–31.

36. L. Sokoloff (1987) Kashin-Beck disease: historical and pathological perspectives. In: *AIN Symposium Proceedings. Nutrition '87* (O.A. Levander, ed.), pp. 61–63, American Institute of Nutrition, Bethesda, MD.

37. O.A. Levander (1987) Etiological hypotheses covering Kashin-Beck disease. In: *AIN Symposium Proceedings. Nutrition '87* (O.A. Levander, ed.), pp. 67–71, American Institute of Nutrition, Bethesda, MD.

38. O.A. Levander and R.F. Burk (1986) Report on the 1986 A.S.P.E.N. Research Workshop on Selenium in Clinical Nutrition. *JPEN* 10:545–549.

39. C.R. Fleming, J.T. McCull, J.F. O'Brien, R.W. Forsman, D.M. Ilstrup, and J. Petz (1984) Selenium status in patients receiving home parenteral nutrition. *JPEN* 8:258–262.

40. A.M. van Rij, C.D. Thomson, J.M. McKenzie, and M.F. Robinson (1979) Selenium deficiency in total parenteral nutrition. *Am. J. Clin. Nutr.* 32:2076–2085.

41. M.R. Brown, H.J. Cohen, J.M. Lyons, et al. (1986) Proximal muscle weakness and selenium deficiency associated with long-term parenteral nutrition. *Am. J. Clin. Nutr.* 43:549–554.

42. AMA Department of Foods and Nutrition (1979) Guidelines for essential trace element preparations for parenteral use. *JAMA* 241:2051–2054.

43. O.A. Levander (1987) A global view of human selenium nutrition. *Annu. Rev. Nutr.* 7:227–250.

44. G.F. Combs, Jr. and S.B. Combs (1986) *The Role of Selenium in Nutrition,* Academic Press, Orlando, FL.

45. D.F. Birt, A.D. Julius, C.E. Runice, L.T. White, T. Lawson, and P.M. Pour (1988) Enhancement of BOP-induced pancreatic carcinogenesis in selenium-fed Syrian golden hamsters under specific dietary conditions. *Nutr. Cancer* 11:21–33.

46. W.C. Willett and M.J. Stampfer (1988) Selenium and cancer. *Br. Med. J.* 297:573–574.

47. J.T. Salonen and J.K. Huttunen (1986) Selenium in cardiovascular disease. *Ann. Clin. Res.* 18:30–35.

48. National Research Council (1980) *Recommended Dietary Allowances,* 9th ed., National Academy Press, Washington, DC.

49. W.R. Meyer, D.C. Mahan, and A.L. Moxon (1981) Value of dietary selenium and vitamin E for weanling swine as measured by performance and tissue selenium and glutathione peroxidase activities. *J. Anim. Sci.* 52:302–311.

50. W. Mertz (1987) Use and misuse of balance studies. *J. Nutr.* 117:1811–1813.

51. O.A. Levander (1986) Selenium. In: *Trace Elements in Human and Animal Nutrition,* 5th ed. (W. Mertz, ed.), pp. 209–279, Academic Press, Orlando, FL.

52. G. Yang, L. Zhu, S. Liu, L. Gu, P. Qian, J. Huang, and M. Lu (1987) Human selenium requirements in China. In: *Selenium in Biology and Medicine, Part B* (G.F. Combs, Jr., J.E. Spallholz, O.A. Levander, and J.E. Oldfield, eds.), pp. 589–607, AVI Publishing Co., Westport, CT.

53. National Research Council (1989) *Recommended Dietary Allowances,* 10th ed., National Academy Press, Washington, DC.

54. International Programme of Chemical Safety (1987) *Selenium,* Environmental Health Criteria 58, World Health Organization, Geneva.

55. G.Q. Yang, S. Wang, R. Zhou, and S. Sun (1983) Endemic selenium intoxication of humans in China. *Am. J. Clin. Nutr.* 37:872–881.

56. J.A.T. Pennington, D.B. Wilson, R.F. Newell, B.F. Harland, R.D. Johnson, and J.E. Vanderveen (1984) Selected minerals in foods surveys, 1974 to 1981/82. *J. Am. Diet. Assoc.* 84:771–780.

57. P. Varo, G. Alfthan, A. Ekholm, A. Aro, and P. Koivistoinen (1988) Selenium intake and serum selenium in Finland: effects of soil fertilization with selenium. *Am. J. Clin. Nutr.* 48:324–329.

58. O.A. Levander (1983) Considerations in the design of selenium bioavailability studies. *Fed. Proc.* 42:1721–1725.

59. M.W. Chansler, M. Mutanen, V.C. Morris, and O.A. Levander (1986) Nutritional bioavailability to rats of selenium in Brazil nuts and mushrooms. *Nutr. Res.* 6:1419–1428.

60. O.A. Levander, G. Alfthan, H. Arvilommi, et al. (1983) Bioavailability of selenium to Finnish men as assessed by platelet glutathione peroxidase activity and other blood parameters. *Am. J. Clin. Nutr.* 37:887–897.

61. G.Q. Yang (1985) Keshan disease: an endemic selenium-related deficiency disease. In: *Trace Elements in Nutrition of Children* (R.K. Chandra, ed.), pp. 273–290, Raven Press, New York.

62. R. Jensen, W. Closson, and R. Rothenberg (1984) Selenium intoxication-New York. *MMWR* 33:157–158.

63. Anonymous (1984) Toxicity with superpotent selenium. *FDA Bull.* 14:19.

64. K. Helzlsouer, R. Jacobs, and S. Morris (1985) Acute selenium intoxication in the United States. *Fed. Proc.* 44:1670.

65. O.A. Levander (1982) Selenium: biochemical actions, interactions, and some human health implications. In: *Clinical, Biochemical, and Nutritional Aspects of Trace Elements* (A.S. Prasad, ed.), pp. 345–368, Alan R. Liss, New York.

66. G.Q. Yang, L. Gu, R. Zhou, and S. Yin (in press) Studies of human maximal and minimal safe intake and requirement of selenium. In: *Proceedings Fourth International Symposium on Selenium in Biology and Medicine* (A. Wendel, ed.), Springer-Verlag, Berlin.

Chapter 31

Robert H. Ophaug

Fluoride

The importance of fluoride in mammalian nutrition has been recognized since the late 1930s, when extensive epidemiological surveys established the relationship between the fluoride content of drinking water and the prevalence of dental caries and dental fluorosis, a form of enamel hypomineralization.[1,2] These studies demonstrated that lifelong consumption of optimally fluoridated drinking water (0.7–1.2 mg/L depending on the mean maximal daily temperature) reduced dental caries by 50–65% and produced only the mildest forms of dental fluorosis, which are not of esthetic concern, in ~10% of the population. Recently there has been an expanded nutritional interest in fluoride stimulated by an additional 30–50% decline in the prevalence of dental caries[3] and by reports that the prevalence of dental fluorosis, one of the earliest and most sensitive indicators of fluoride toxicity, is also increasing in both fluoridated and nonfluoridated areas.[4]

Essential Status and Dietary Requirements

According to Underwood and Mertz,[5] the essentiality of a trace element is established when a reduction in ingestion below the range of safe and adequate intake results in a consistent and reproducible impairment of a physiological function. These authors and the Committee on Dietary Allowances of the Food and Nutrition Board, National Research Council[6] consider fluoride to be an essential trace element ". . . on the basis of its proven beneficial effect on dental caries." Although there is insufficient data to establish a Recommended Dietary Allowance (RDA) for fluoride, the Committee on Dietary Allowances[6] established an "estimated safe and adequate daily dietary intake" of fluoride for seven age categories. The estimated safe and adequate daily dietary intakes range from 0.1–0.5 mg fluoride/d for infants 0–6 mo of age to 1.5–4.0 mg fluoride/d for adults.

Metabolism

The plasma fluoride concentration varies in predictable ways depending on the physiological balance between the quantity of fluoride ingested and absorbed and its clearance from plasma by renal and extrarenal mechanisms, mainly uptake by calcified tissues.[7] In humans the plasma fluoride level reflects the quantity of fluoride ingested[8] and tends to increase with age.[9–11] When fluoride is ingested in small multiple doses, as in the case of optimally fluoridated drinking water, the plasma fluoride levels remain in a narrow range of 0.01–0.04 mg/L.[12] Conversely, when a large fraction of the total daily fluoride intake is ingested as a single dose, such as fluoride supplements, transient spikes in the plasma fluoride levels are observed.[13]

Fluoride Transfer Across Biological Membranes. The transfer of fluoride across cell membranes and epithelia is critically important in the metabolism of ingested fluoride. In the past 10 y our knowledge of the fundamental mechanisms involved in the transfer process has increased significantly. Over 40 y ago Borei[14] noted that fluoride was more toxic to a variety of cells at low pH and speculated that fluoride crossed cell membranes only as the undissociated acid (HF) and that the membranes are essentially impermeable to ionic fluoride (F$^-$). In a classical series of investigations, Whitford and coworkers[15,16] showed that pH gradients across biological membranes promote the passive diffusion of HF from regions of low pH to regions of higher pH where the fluoride is trapped by dissociation to ionic fluoride. These investigations clearly demonstrated the importance of transmembrane and transepithelial pH gradients on the gastric absorption,[17] tissue distribution,[18] and renal excretion[19] of fluoride.

Gastrointestinal Absorption. The rapidity with which ingested fluoride is found in plasma[20] and studies with isolated stomachs of laboratory animals[21,22] support the conclusion that, in contrast to most substances, fluoride is rapidly absorbed from the stomach. The absorption of fluoride from the stomach is passive[22,23] and is promoted by conditions that increase gastric acidity.[17] This finding is consistent with the concept that fluoride is transferred across the gastric mucosa by passive diffusion of HF. Fluoride also is absorbed from the intestine[22,23] by mechanisms that are not pH dependent[24,25] and may involve the diffusion of hydrated fluoride ions through paracellular channels.[26] The absorption of fluoride from water or NaF tablets in fasting subjects is essentially 100%.[27] The concomitant intake of food and variations in the chemical composition of the food also influence the absorption of fluoride.[28–31] In human diets ~50–80% of the fluoride is absorbed.[32]

Distribution. Fluoride has a very high affinity for calcified tissues, and 95% of the fluoride present in the body is found in the bones and teeth.[33] The fluoride concentration in human bone increases with age and is proportional to the quantity of fluoride ingested over a wide range of fluoride intakes.[34] Animal studies showed that as bone ages, with or without exposure to fluoride, it exhibits a decreased capacity to incorporate fluoride.[35] However, there is disagreement as to whether human bone fluoride concentrations reach a plateau with age.[34] An age-related reduction in bone fluoride uptake is indirectly supported by the observation that individuals in the fifth and sixth decades of life excrete more fluoride via the urine than do younger age groups.[9] Although comparable data for humans are not available, animal studies showed that less fluoride is incorporated into bone with a protracted previous high fluoride exposure than into similarly aged bones with little previous fluoride exposure.[35]

The distribution of fluoride in soft tissues was studied by administering radioactive fluoride (^{18}F) to experimental animals and determining the tissue water to plasma water (T:P) concentration ratios of fluoride at equilibrium.[18,20] Typically, T:Ps of 0.3–1.0 are obtained and demonstrate that (1) fluoride can penetrate the intracellular fluid compartment of soft tissues, (2) the intracellular-extracellular distribution of fluoride varies among tissues, and (3) fluoride is not accumulated intracellularly.[18,20] Whitford[15,18] proposed that soft-tissue distribution of fluoride is determined by the diffusion equilibrium of HF, with F$^-$ considered to be essentially impermeable. Thus, fluoride is found in the highest concentration in the more alkaline (extracellular) compartment with the distribution of fluoride for each tissue dependent on the magnitude of the intracellular-extracellular pH gradient.

Excretion. Renal excretion represents the major route of removal of fluoride from the body. In an individual relatively unexposed to fluoride, ~50%

of an oral dose is excreted in the urine within 24 h,[36] with ≤30% excreted within 4 h.[20] The amount of fluoride excreted in urine increases with age[9] and, after prolonged periods of relatively constant fluoride intake, approximately equals the amount absorbed.[36] Renal clearance of fluoride is a pH-dependent process characterized by glomerular filtration followed by varying degrees of tubular reabsorption.[15,19] Because tubular epithelium is very permeable to the undissociated HF molecule (but not to fluoride ion), conditions leading to acidification of urine increase tubular reabsorption and decrease renal clearance of fluoride. Conversely, alkalinization of urine decreases tubular reabsorption and increases the clearance of fluoride.[15,19]

Sources of Ingested Fluoride

Although fluoride is ubiquitous in nature and is found in all foods, the fluoride content of drinking water is the major factor influencing the dietary fluoride intake of man. Because of its widespread use as a caries-prevention agent, young children also ingest significant quantities of fluoride from nondietary sources.

Dietary Fluoride Intake. The dietary (food, beverages, and water) fluoride intake of average 6-mo-old infants ranges from 0.42 mg/d in fluoridated (>0.7 mg/L) areas to 0.23 mg/d in areas where the drinking water contains <0.3 mg/L fluoride.[37,38] These estimates of average dietary fluoride intake, however, are influenced dramatically by the type of milk or milk formula that is fed.[38,39] Human milk and cow milk contain very low levels of fluoride (<0.10 mg/L) and, even though consumed in large quantities by infants, contribute only small amounts of fluoride to the dietary intake. Although commercial ready-to-feed formulas are now prepared with low-fluoride water and contain lower concentrations of fluoride than previously,[40] formulas prepared in the home by dilution of liquid concentrates or powders with fluoridated water may contain >1 mg/L fluoride. Therefore, some infants may have dietary fluoride intakes that exceed 0.10 mg/kg body weight.[38,39] Studies of the milk feeding patterns of infants indicate that the percentage of infants fed formula decreases rapidly from 62% at age 2 mo to 11% at age 1 y.[41] In addition, from 1971 to 1980 the percentage of newborn infants fed prepared formula decreased from 77.4% to 50.4%, with a corresponding increase in the percentage of newborn infants being breast-fed.[41] Thus, the high fluoride intake associated with the feeding of formula prepared with fluoridated water appears to be affecting fewer infants than previously and to be restricted, for the most part, to infants <1 y of age.

Average 2-y-old children have dietary fluoride intakes of 0.62 and 0.21 mg/d in fluoridated (>0.7 mg/L) and nonfluoridated (<0.3 mg/L) areas, respectively.[37] Approximately 70% of the dietary fluoride intake is derived from drinking water and beverages.

Singer et al.[42] estimated that male adults (15–19 y of age) consuming 2800 kcal/d and residing in a fluoridated (>0.7 mg/L) community ingest an average of 1.85 mg fluoride/d, with 0.37 mg being derived from foods and the remainder from beverages and water. On the basis of the analysis of 93 individual food items in a hospital diet, Taves[43] estimated the daily fluoride intake from foods to be 0.40 mg. When the fluoride content of drinking water is <0.3 mg/L, the dietary (foods, beverages, and water) fluoride intake of young, male adults was calculated to be 0.86 mg/d.[42]

From analysis of market-basket food collections, average 6-mo-old infants, regardless of the fluoride content of the drinking water, have dietary fluoride intakes that fall within the range of estimated safe and adequate daily dietary intakes established by the Committee on Dietary Allowances of the Food and Nutrition Board, National Research Council.[6] Conversely, the daily dietary fluoride intakes of average 2-y-old children[37] and 15–19-y-old male adults[42] fall within the estimated safe and adequate intakes only if the drinking water contains >0.7 mg/L of fluoride.

Nondietary Fluoride Intake. Depending on the age of the child and the fluoride content of the drinking water, supplemental fluoride may be prescribed for children from birth up to at least 13 y of age.[44,45] The American Academy of Pediatrics (AAP) and the American Dental Association (ADA) currently recommend fluoride supplements (0.25 mg/d) for children <2 y of age only if the drinking water contains <0.3 mg/L fluoride. From 2 to 3 y of age a daily fluoride supplement of 0.50 and 0.25 mg is recommended for children in areas where the drinking water contains <0.3 mg/L and 0.3–0.7 mg/L, respectively. From 3 to 13 (or 16) y of age fluoride supplements recommended for these areas are increased to 1.0 and 0.50 mg/d, respectively. No supplemental fluoride is recommended at any age if the drinking water contains >0.7 mg/L fluoride. The recommended doses of supplemental fluoride adjust the fluoride intakes of 6-mo-old and 2-y-old children residing in areas with suboptimal water fluoride levels to those that are safe and adequate[6] and similar to those of children in optimally fluoridated areas.[37]

Fluoride-containing dentifrice is a source of ingested fluoride that is particularly important for young children because of their relative inability to control their swallowing reflex and because the crowns of cosmetically important teeth are calcifying and are susceptable to the development of dental fluorosis. Children <5 y of age ingest 26–35% of the dentifrice used,[46–48] and it was reported that children 2–4 y of age ingest an average of 0.30 mg fluoride each time teeth are brushed.[46] Thus the daily fluoride intake of an average 2-y-old child in a fluoridated community would be approximately doubled by brushing twice daily with a fluoride-containing (0.1%) dentifrice. Because nearly 80% of the parents of 3-y-old children indicate that they start the brushing of teeth in their children by age 18 mo[49] and because by age 3 y 55% are brushing at least twice daily,[50] fluoride ingestion from dentifrice affects significant numbers of children at an early age.

Fluoride Toxicity

Acute Fluoride Toxicity. In the absence of treatment, the ingestion of a single dose of 32–64 mg fluoride/kg body weight (70–140 mg sodium fluoride/kg body weight) is a certainly lethal dose (CLD) in man.[51] A single dose of 8–16 mg fluoride/kg body weight is safely tolerated.[52] Accidental acute fluoride toxicity in man is relatively rare, although a single hospital accident resulted in 263 cases of acute fluoride poisoning and 43 deaths.[53] The addition of inappropriately high quantities of fluoride to the drinking water by school-water fluoridation systems produced symptoms in children of acute fluoride toxicity but no deaths.[54,55] The accidental overfluoridation of a community water supply was without severe effects on the general population but resulted in acute fluoride toxicity and one death in patients undergoing hemodialysis.[56] One fatality caused by the inappropriate use of fluoride in a dental clinic was reported.[57]

Chronic Fluoride Toxicity. Dental fluorosis is a hypomineralization of the enamel that varies in severity from small, parchment-white areas covering only a small part of the tooth surface to confluent staining and pitting of the enamel.[58] In humans the development of fluorosis in the permanent dentition (except third molars) is associated with excessive fluoride intake during the first 5 y of life when the crowns of the permanent teeth are undergoing calcification. Epidemiologic studies indicate that dental fluorosis becomes significant from a public health standpoint when the fluoride content of the drinking water exceeds 2 mg/L. A daily fluoride intake of 0.10 mg/kg body weight is associated with the development of dental fluorosis in animals and humans.[59,60] Data from animal studies indicate that the development and severity of dental fluorosis is dependent not only on an elevated fluoride intake but also on the duration of the elevated intake and on the pattern of elevated plasma fluoride levels that result. In rats, for example, enamel mineralization disturbances are produced by single daily (for 1 wk) peak plasma fluoride concentrations of 0.19 mg/L but not 0.10 ppm.[61] Relatively constant plasma fluoride levels of 0.06–0.09 mg/L for 1 wk,[61] or 0.03 ppm for 56 d[62] also resulted in microradiographic evidence of fluorotic changes in rat incisor enamel. Recent data indicate that the prevalence of dental fluorosis in the United States is increasing in both fluoridated and nonfluoridated cities.[4,63,64] Although a few cases of moderate-to-severe fluorosis were reported in optimally fluoridated communities,[58] the fluorosis reported in the recent studies is nearly all of the very mild forms that are not of esthetic concern.

Crippling skeletal fluorosis is an advanced stage of chronic fluoride intoxication resulting from the ingestion of 10–25 mg fluoride/d for 10–20 y.[65] Skeletal fluorosis is characterized by a progressive hypermineralization of the skeleton, particularly the spinal column and pelvis; calcification of the tendons and ligaments; and exostosis formation. In the United States crippling skeletal fluorosis is not seen in communities with water supplies containing ≤20 mg/L fluoride.[65]

Beneficial Effects of Fluoride in Man

The reduction of dental caries is clearly the major beneficial effect of fluoride in man and is the basis for its recognition as an essential trace element.[5,6] Several mechanisms were proposed for the anticaries activity of fluoride including (1) inhibition of enamel demineralization, (2) enhancement of enamel remineralization, (3) effects on plaque bacteria, and (4) effects on tooth morphology.[66] All of these factors are probably involved, to some extent, in the anticaries effectiveness of fluoride. Because of difficulty in establishing a clear relationship between surface enamel fluoride levels and caries, more emphasis is currently being placed on the topical effects of fluoride on plaque colonization, composition, and metabolic activity and on the remineralization-demineralization reactions of enamel.[67,68]

References

1. H.T. Dean (1946) Epidemiology of studies in the United States. In: *Dental Caries and Fluorine* (F.R. Moulton, ed.), pp. 5–31, Science Press Printing Company, Lancaster, PA.

2. H.T. Dean (1942) Investigation of physiological effects by the epidemiological method. In: *Fluorine and Dental Health*, Publication no. 19. (F.R. Moulton, ed.), pp. 23–31, Science Press Printing Company, Lancaster, PA.

3. C.E. Renson, P.J.A. Crielaers, S.A.J. Ikikunle, et al. (1985) Changing patterns of oral health: implications for oral health manpower. Part I. *Int. Dent. J.* 35:235–251.

4. S.M. Szpunar and B.A. Burt (1987) Trends in the prevalence of

5. E.J. Underwood and W. Mertz (1987) Introduction. In: *Trace Elements in Human and Animal Nutrition*, vol. 1, 5th ed. (W. Mertz, ed.), pp. 1–19, Academic Press, Inc., San Diego.

6. National Research Council (1989) *Recommended Dietary Allowances*, 10th ed., National Academy Press, Washington, DC.

7. D.R. Taves and W.S. Guy (1979) Distribution of fluoride among body compartments. In: *Continuing Evaluation of the Use of Fluorides*, AAAS Selected Symposium 11 (E. Johansen, D.R. Taves, and T.O. Olsen, eds.) pp. 159–185, Westview Press, Boulder, CO.

8. W.S. Guy, D.R. Taves, and W.S. Brey (1976) Organic fluorocarbons in human plasma: prevalence and characterization. In: *Biochemistry Involving Carbon-Fluorine Bonds*, American Chemical Society Symposium Series no. 28 (R. Filler, ed.), pp. 117–134, American Chemical Society, Washington, DC.

9. H.C. Kuo and J.W. Stamm (1975) The relationship of creatinine clearance to serum fluoride concentration and urinary fluoride excretion in man. *Arch. Oral Biol.* 20:235–238.

10. L. Singer and R.H. Ophaug (1979) Concentration of ionic, total and bound fluoride in plasma. *Clin. Chem.* 25:523–525.

11. H. Husdan, R. Vogl, D. Oreopoulos, C. Gryfe, and A. Rapoport (1976) Serum inorganic fluoride: normal range and relationship to age and sex. *Clin. Chem.* 22:1884–1888.

12. J. Ekstrand (1978) Relationship between fluoride in the drinking water and the plasma fluoride concentration in man. *Caries Res.* 12:123–127.

13. J. Ekstrand, G. Alvan, L.O. Boreus, and A. Norlin (1977) Pharmacokinetics of fluoride in man after single and multiple doses. *Europ. J. Clin. Pharmacol.* 12:311–317.

14. H. Borei (1945) Inhibition of cellular oxidation by fluoride. *Arkh. Kimi. Mineral Geol.* 20A:1–215.

15. G.M. Whitford (1983) Physiologic determinants of plasma fluoride concentrations. In: *Fluorides: Effects on Vegetation, Animals and Humans* (J.L. Shupe, H.B. Peterson, and N.C. Leone, eds.), pp. 167–182, Paragon Press, Inc., Salt Lake City.

16. G.M. Whitford and D.H. Pashley (1979) The effect of body fluid pH on fluoride distribution, toxicity, and renal clearance. In: *Continuing Evaluation of the Use of Fluorides*, AAAS Selected Symposium II (E. Johansen, D.R. Taves, and T.O. Olsen, eds.), pp. 187–221, Westview Press, Boulder, CO.

17. G.M. Whitford and D.H. Pashley (1984) Fluoride absorption: the influence of gastric acidity. *Calcif. Tissue Int.* 36:302–307.

18. G.M. Whitford, D.H. Pashley, and K.E. Reynolds (1979) Fluoride tissue distribution: short-term kinetics. *Am. J. Physiol.* 236:F141–F148.

19. G.M. Whitford, D.H. Pashley, and G.I. Stringer (1976) Fluoride renal clearance: a pH-dependent event. *Am. J. Physiol.* 230:527–532.

20. C.H. Carlson, W.D. Armstrong, and L. Singer (1960) Distribution and excretion of radiofluoride in the human. *Proc. Soc. Exp. Biol. Med.* 104:235–239.

21. G.K. Stookey, D.B. Crane, and J.C. Muhler (1962) Effect of molybdenum on fluoride absorption. *Proc. Soc. Exp. Biol. Med.* 109:580–583.

22. G.K. Stookey, E.L. Dellinger, and J.C. Muhler (1964) In vitro studies concerning fluoride absorption. *Proc. Soc. Exp. Biol. Med.* 115:298–301.

23. H.D. Cremer and W. Buttner (1970) Absorption of fluorides. In: *Fluorides and Human Health*, pp. 75–91, World Health Organization, Geneva.

24. G.M. Whitford and J.L. Williams (1986) Fluoride absorption: independence from plasma fluoride levels. *Proc. Soc. Exp. Biol. Med.* 181:550–554.

25. K. Quan, J. Nopakun, L. Harriman, and H.H. Messer (1987) Fluoride

dental fluorosis in the United States: a review. *J. Public Health Dent.* 47:71–79.

absorption from rat small intestine. *J. Dent. Res.* 66:318(abstr. 1688).

26. S.G. Schultz (1977) The role of paracellular pathways in isotonic fluid transport. *Yale J. Biol. Med.* 50:99–112.

27. J. Ekstrand, M. Ehrnebo, and L.O. Boreus (1978) Fluoride bioavailability after intravenous and oral administration: importance of renal clearance and urine flow. *Clin. Pharmacol. Ther.* 23:329–337.

28. G.K. Stookey, D.B. Crane, and J.C. Muhler (1964) Further studies on fluoride absorption. *Proc. Soc. Exp. Biol. Med.* 115:295–298.

29. K. Trautner and J. Einwag (1986) Bioavailability of fluoride from some health food products in man. *Caries Res.* 20:518–524.

30. K. Trautner and J. Einwag (1987) Factors influencing the bioavailability of fluoride from calcium-rich health food products and CaF_2 in man. *Arch. Oral Biol.* 32:401–406.

31. K. Trautner and G. Siebert (1986) An experimental study of bioavailability of fluoride from dietary sources in man. *Arch. Oral Biol.* 31:223–228.

32. H.C. Hodge and F.A. Smith (1965) Biological properties of inorganic fluoride. In: *Fluorine Chemistry,* vol. IV (J.H. Simons, ed.), p. 137, Academic Press, New York.

33. I. Zipkin (1973) Fluoride in the calcified structures. In: *Biological Mineralization* (I. Zipkin, ed.), pp. 487–505, John Wiley and Sons, New York.

34. S.M. Weidmann and J.A. Weatherell (1970) Distribution of fluorides. In: *Fluorides and Human Health,* pp. 93–139, World Health Organization, Geneva.

35. I. Zipkin and F.J. McClure (1952) Deposition of fluoride in the bones and teeth of the growing rat. *J. Nutr.* 47:611–620.

36. H.C. Hodge, F.A. Smith, and I. Gedalia (1970) Excretion of fluorides. In: *Fluorides and Human Health,* pp. 141–161, World Health Organization, Geneva.

37. R.H. Ophaug, L. Singer, and B.F. Harland (1985) Dietary fluoride intake of 6-month and 2-year-old children in four dietary regions of the United States. *Am. J. Clin. Nutr.* 42:701–707.

38. R.W. Dabeka, A.D. McKenzie, H.B.S. Conacher, and D.C. Kirkpatrick (1982) Determination of fluoride in Canadian infant foods and calculation of fluoride intake by infants. *Can. J. Public Health* 73:188–191.

39. L. Singer and R. Ophaug (1979) Total fluoride intake of infants. *Pediatrics* 63:460–465.

40. J. Johnson and J.W. Bawden (1986) Fluoride content of commercially available infant formulas. *J. Dent. Res.* 65:183(abstr. 124).

41. G.A. Martinez, D.A. Dodd, and J. Samartgedes (1981) Milk feeding patterns in the United States during the first 12 months of life. *Pediatrics* 68:863–868.

42. L. Singer, R.H. Ophaug, and B.F. Harland (1985) Dietary fluoride intake of 15–19-year-old male adults residing in the United States. *J. Dent. Res.* 64:1302–1305.

43. D.R. Taves (1983) Dietary intake of fluoride: ashed (total fluoride) v. unashed (inorganic fluoride) analysis of individual foods. *Br. J. Nutr.* 49:295–301.

44. Council on Dental Therapeutics, American Dental Association (1982) *Accepted Dental Therapeutics,* 39th ed., pp. 344–368, American Dental Association, Chicago.

45. American Academy of Pediatrics, Committee on Nutrition (1986) Fluoride supplementation. *Pediatrics* 77:758–761.

46. W.E. Barnhart, L.K. Hiller, G.J. Leonard, and S.E. Michaels (1974) Dentifrice usage and ingestion among four age groups. *J. Dent. Res.* 53:1317–1322.

47. J.A. Hargreaves, G.S. Ingram, and B.J. Wagg (1972) A gravimetric study of the ingestion of toothpaste by children. *Caries Res.* 6:237–243.

48. Y. Ericsson and B. Forsman (1969) Fluoride retained from mouthrinses and dentifrices in preschool children. *Caries Res.* 3:290–299.

49. T.B. Dowell (1981) The use of toothpaste in infancy. *Br. Dent. J.* 150:247–249.

50. J.D. Palmer and D.L. Prothero (1981) Young children and toothpaste. *Br. Dent. J.* 150:338–339.

51. H.C. Hodge and F.A. Smith (1965) Biological properties of inorganic fluorides. In: *Fluorine Chemistry,* vol. IV (J.H. Simons, ed.), pp. 2–365, Academic Press, New York.

52. S.B. Heifetz and H.S. Horowitz (1984) The amounts of fluoride in current fluoride therapies—safety considerations for children. *J. Dent. Child.* 51:257–269.

53. W.L. Lidbeck, I. Hill, and J.A. Beeman (1943) Acute sodium fluoride poisoning. *JAMA* 121:826–827.

54. Centers for Disease Control (1974) Acute fluoride poisoning—North Carolina. *MMWR* 23:199.

55. R. Hoffman, J. Mann, J. Calderone, J. Turnbull, and M. Burkhart (1980) Acute fluoride poisoning in a New Mexico elementary school. *Pediatrics* 65:897–900.

56. Centers for Disease Control (1980) Fluoride intoxication in a dialysis unit—Maryland. *MMWR* 29:134–136.

57. L.E. Church (1976) Fluoride—use with caution. *J. Maryland Dent. Assoc.* 19:106.

58. H.S. Horowitz, S.B. Heifetz, W.S. Driscoll, A. Kingman, and R.J. Meyers (1984) A new method for assessing the prevalence of dental fluorosis—the tooth surface index of fluorosis. *J. Am. Dent. Assoc.* 109:37–41.

59. B. Forsman (1977) Early supply of fluoride and enamel fluorosis. *Scand. J. Dent. Res.* 85:22–30.

60. J.W. Suttie, J.R. Carlsson, and E.C. Faltin (1972) Effects of alternating periods of high and low fluoride ingestion on dairy cattle. *J. Dairy Sci.* 55:790–804.

61. B. Angmar-Mansson and G.M. Whitford (1982) Plasma fluoride levels and enamel fluorosis in the rat. *Caries Res.* 16:334–339.

62. B. Angmar-Mansson and G.M. Whitford (1984) Enamel fluorosis related to plasma fluoride levels in the rat. *Caries Res.* 18:25–32.

63. S.M. Szpunar and B.A. Burt (1988) Dental caries, fluorosis and fluoride exposure in Michigan schoolchildren. *J. Dent. Res.* 67:802–806.

64. D.H. Leverett (1986) Prevalence of dental fluorosis in fluoridated and nonfluoridated communities—a preliminary investigation. *J. Public Health Dent.* 46:184–187.

65. H.C. Hodge (1979) The safety of fluoride tablets or drops. In: *Continuing Evaluation of the Use of Fluorides,* AAAS Selected Symposium 11 (E. Johansen, D.R. Taves, and T.O. Olsen, eds.), pp. 253–274, Westview Press, Boulder, CO.

66. P.F. DePaola and S. Kashket (1983) Prevention of dental caries. In: *Fluorides: Effects on Vegetation, Animals and Humans* (J.L. Shupe, H.B. Peterson, and N.C. Leone, eds.), pp. 199–211, Paragon Press, Inc., Salt Lake City.

67. E.A.M. Kidd, A. Thylstrup, O. Fejerskov, and C. Bruun (1980) Influence of fluoride in surface enamel and degree of dental fluorosis on caries development in vitro. *Caries Res.* 14:196–202.

68. D.H. Retief, B.E. Harris, and E.L. Bradley (1987) Relationship between enamel fluoride concentration and dental caries experience. *Caries Res.* 21:68–78.

Manganese

The essentiality of manganese was first reported in 1931 when Kemmerer et al.[1] and Orent and Mc-Collum[2] demonstrated poor growth in mice and impaired reproduction in rats fed diets devoid of manganese. Although it has long been appreciated that a deficiency of manganese can be a practical problem in the pig and poultry industry,[3] the idea that manganese deficiency may be a problem in human population subgroups is relatively recent. This chapter briefly summarizes some of the literature related to manganese nutrition, metabolism, and metabolic function. For additional information the reader is referred to more comprehensive reviews.[3-7] Because of space constraints, review articles rather than original sources are cited in many cases; the reader is directed to these reviews for the appropriate original citations.

Body Compartments

An average human contains between 200 and 400 μmol of manganese, which is fairly uniform in distribution throughout the body.[4] There is relatively little variation among species with regard to tissue manganese concentrations.[3] Manganese tends to be highest in tissues rich in mitochondria; its concentration in mitochondria is higher than in cytoplasm or other cell organelles. Hair can accumulate high concentrations of manganese, and it has been suggested that hair manganese concentrations may reflect manganese status. High concentrations of manganese are normally found in pigmented structures, such as retina, dark skin, and melanin granules. Bone, liver, pancreas, and kidney tend to have higher concentrations of manganese (20–50 μmol/g) than do other tissues. Concentrations of manganese in brain, heart, lung, and muscle are typically <20 nmol/g; blood and serum concentrations are ~200 and 20 nmol/L, respectively. Typical milk concentrations are on the order of 1 μmol/L. Bone can account for up to 25% of total body manganese because of its mass.

Bone manganese concentrations can be raised or lowered by substantially varying dietary manganese intake, but bone manganese is not thought to be a readily mobilizable pool.[3] In contrast to the situation for several other essential trace elements, the fetus does not accumulate liver manganese before birth, and fetal concentrations are significantly less than adult concentrations. This lack of fetal storage can be attributed to the apparent lack of manganese-storage proteins and the fact that most manganese enzymes are not expressed prenatally.[3,4]

Methods of Analysis

The most common analytical methods that can sensitively measure manganese (18 nmol/L) include neutron-activation analysis, x-ray fluorescence, proton-induced x-ray emission, inductively coupled plasma emission, electron paramagnetic resonance (EPR), and flameless atomic-absorption spectrophotometry (AAS). Currently the most common method employed is flameless AAS. All of these methods, with the exception of EPR, measure the total concentration of manganese in the sample. In contrast, the use of EPR allows the investigator to selectively measure bound vs. free manganese. Given the idea that changes in the intracellular free Mn^{2+} pool may be an important factor in cellular metabolic control,[8] use of this method to measure manganese will probably increase in the near future.

Absorption and Transport

Studies on the absorption and excretion of manganese were carried out primarily with the isotope ^{54}Mn, a γ emitter with a half-life of 312 d. Absorption of manganese is thought to occur throughout the small intestine. The efficiency of manganese absorption is relatively low and is not thought to be under homeostatic control.[4] For adults, manganese absorption was reported to range from 2% to 15% when [54]Mn-labeled test meals were used, whereas values >25% were reported from balance studies.[9,10] Manganese absorption and retention are higher in neonates than in adults, and it was suggested that, for this reason, neonates may be particularly susceptible to manganese toxicosis.[11]

The higher retention of manganese in young animals in relation to adults may reflect an absence of manganese excretion during the neonatal period. For example, in mice, rats, and kittens there is nearly a total absence of manganese excretion during the neonatal period, even though absorption and accumulation can be vigorous.[12] The avid retention of the small amount of manganese in milk and the postnatal changes in its excretory pattern underscore the important changes in manganese metabolism that take place during the neonatal period.

At present there are only limited data concerning the effects of individual dietary components on manganese absorption. In experimental animals, high amounts of dietary calcium, phosphorus, fiber, and phytate were reported to increase the requirements for manganese; such interactions presumably occur via the formation of insoluble manganese complexes in the intestinal tract with a concomitant reduction in the soluble fraction available for absorption.[3,13] The significance of these dietary factors with regard to human manganese requirements remains to be clarified. Using rats as a model system, Lee and Johnson[14] showed that the absorption/retention of manganese from soy protein can be higher than from casein protein. The mechanisms underlying this putative effect of soy protein on manganese absorption/retention have not been identified.

An interaction between iron and manganese was demonstrated in several species. Manganese absorption was shown to increase under conditions of iron deficiency in both experimental animals and humans, whereas high amounts of dietary iron were shown to accelerate the development of manganese deficiency in chickens. The mechanisms underlying the interactions between iron and manganese have not been identified; however, they likely involve either a transport site or a ligand.[3]

Metal-specific intestinal transport proteins for manganese have not been identified. Using isolated brush border membrane preparations, Bell et al.[15] reported that the mucosal transport of manganese occurs through a nonsaturable simple diffusion process when manganese is present in concentrations ranging from 1 to 90 μmol/L. However, using intestinal-perfusion techniques, Garcia-Aranda et al.[16] reported that the intestinal absorption of manganese is a rapidly saturable process involving a high-affinity, low-capacity active-transport mechanism. The discrepancy between these two reports may reflect the fact that in membrane vesicle studies the data reflect the initial uptake of manganese across the mucosal membrane, whereas in intestinal-perfusion studies the data reflect manganese uptake across the mucosal membrane and its subsequent serosal transfer. A high-affinity, low-capacity intestinal transfer system for manganese would be of value to the animal, because it would help ensure efficient uptake and retention of the element from diets low in manganese while simultaneously protecting the animal from absorbing excessive amounts of the element.

Manganese entering into the portal blood from the gastrointestinal tract may either remain free or rapidly become associated with α_2-macroglobulin before transversing to the liver, where it is almost completely removed. A small fraction enters the systemic circulation where it may become oxidized to Mn^{3+} and bound to transferrin.[4] Manganese uptake by the liver was reported to occur by a unidirectional, saturable process with the properties of passive mediated transport.[8] Once entering the liver, manganese enters at least five metabolic pools. One pool represents manganese taken up by the lysosomes, from which it is thought to be transferred subsequently to the bile canaliculus. The regulation of manganese is thought to be maintained in part through biliary excretion of the element; up to 50% of manganese injected intravenously can be recovered in the feces within 24 h. A second pool of manganese is associated with the mitochondria. Mitochondria have a large capacity for manganese uptake and it is thought that mitochondrial uptake and release of manganese and calcium may be related. A third pool of manganese is found in the nuclear fraction of the cell; the roles of nuclear manganese have not been delineated. A fourth manganese pool is incorporated into newly synthesized manganese proteins (*see* below); biological half-lives for these proteins have not been agreed upon. The fifth identified intracellular pool of manganese is free Mn^{2+}. It is thought that fluctuations in the free manganese pool may be an important regulator of cellular metabolic control in a manner analogous to free Ca^{2+} and Mg^{2+}.[4,8]

The mechanisms by which manganese is transported to and taken up by extrahepatic tissues have not been identified. Transferrin was reported to be the major manganese-binding protein in plasma; however, it is not known to what extent transferrin facilitates the uptake of manganese by extrahepatic tissue.[17] Manganese uptake by extrahepatic tissue does not appear to be increased under conditions of manganese deficiency, suggesting a lack of inducible manganese-transport proteins.[18]

Currently there is only limited information concerning the hormonal regulation of manganese metabolism. Fluxes in the concentrations of adrenal, pancreatic, and pituitary-gonadal axis hormones were shown to affect tissue manganese concentrations.[19] However, it is not clear to what extent hormone-induced changes in tissue manganese concentrations are due to alterations in cellular uptake of manganese or to changes in the expression of manganese metalloenzymes or manganese-activated enzymes.

Biochemical Functions

Manganese functions as a constituent of metalloenzymes and as an enzyme activator. Manganese-containing enzymes include arginase, pyruvate carboxylase, and manganese-superoxide dismutase (MnSOD). Arginase, the cytosolic enzyme responsible for urea formation, contains 4 mol Mn^{2+}/mol enzyme. The activity of arginase is affected by diet, with concentrations in Mn-deficient rats being <50% of controls. Despite this marked influence of manganese deficiency on arginase activity, the functional significance of this reduction has not been agreed upon.[3] With experimental diabetes, liver and kidney manganese concentrations can be elevated; this increase was associated with an increase in arginase activity.[19] Whether this finding implies an increased manganese requirement for diabetics has not been determined.

Pyruvate carboxylase, the enzyme that catalyzes the first step of carbohydrate synthesis from pyruvate, contains 4 mol Mn^{2+}/mol enzyme. Although the activity of this enzyme can be slightly lower in Mn-deficient animals than in controls, gluconeogenesis was not shown to be markedly inhibited in deficient animals.[20]

MnSOD catalyzes the disproportionation of O_2^- to H_2O_2 and O_2. The activity of MnSOD in tissues of manganese-deficient rats can be significantly lower than in controls. That this reduction is functionally significant is suggested by the observation of high levels of hepatic mitochondrial lipid peroxidation in deficient rats compared with controls.[21] Tissue MnSOD activity can be increased by environmental insults, such as ozone and alcohol, that increase the production of the superoxide radical. This increase can be attenuated in manganese-deficient animals, potentially increasing their sensitivity to these insults.[21]

For manganese-activated reactions, the metal can act by binding either to the substrate (such as ATP) or directly to the protein, resulting in conformational changes. In contrast to the relatively few manganese metalloenzymes, there are a large number of manganese-activated enzymes, including hydrolases, kinases, decarboxylases, and transferases.[4,5] Many of these metal activations are nonspecific in that other

metal ions, particularly Mg^{2+}, can replace Mn^{2+}. One exception to the nonspecific manganese activation of enzymes is the manganese-specific activation of glycosyltransferases. Several manganese-deficiency–induced pathologies have been attributed to a low activity of this enzyme class (see below). A second example of an enzyme that may be specifically activated by manganese is phosphoenolpyruvate carboxykinase (PEPCK); low activities of this enzyme were reported in manganese-deficient animals.[20]

A third example of a manganese-activated enzyme is glutamine synthetase. This enzyme, which is found in high concentrations in brain, catalyzes the reaction

$$NH_3 + glutamate + ATP \rightarrow$$

$$glutamine + ADP + pi$$

Although the influence of manganese deficiency on this enzyme has not been reported, it can be speculated that a manganese-deficiency–induced reduction in its activity could explain some of the behavioral defects associated with manganese deficiency. It should also be noted that this enzyme can be inactivated by oxygen radicals;[22] thus a manganese-deficiency–induced reduction in MnSOD activity theoretically could act to further depress the activity of this enzyme.

Deficiency Signs

Manganese deficiency was demonstrated in a number of species, including rats, mice, pigs, and cattle.[3] Signs of manganese deficiency include impaired growth, skeletal abnormalities, impaired reproductive performance, ataxia, and defects in lipid and carbohydrate metabolism.

The effects of manganese deficiency on bone development have been studied extensively, in part because the first abnormality to be recognized as resulting from inadequate intake of this element was perosis in chickens.[3] It is now recognized that in most species, manganese deficiency can result in shortened and thickened limbs, curvature of the spine, and swollen and enlarged joints.[3,6] The basic biochemical defect underlying the development of these bone defects is a reduction in proteoglycan synthesis secondary to a reduction in the activities of glycosyltransferases. These enzymes are needed for the synthesis of chondroitin sulfate side chains of proteoglycan molecules.[6] Strause and Saltman[23] reported that manganese deficiency in adult rats can result in an inhibition of both osteoblast and osteoclast activity. The implications of this observation in regard to human bone disease need to be ascertained.

One of the most striking effects of manganese deficiency occurs during pregnancy. When pregnant animals are deficient in manganese, their offspring exhibit a congenital, irreversible ataxia characterized by incoordination, lack of equilibrium, and retraction of the head. This condition is the result of impaired development of the otoliths, the calcified structures in the inner ear responsible for normal body righting reflexes. The otoliths are made up of otoconia, small crystalline structures embedded in an amorphous, proteoglycan-rich matrix. In the otolithic matrix and in both the cells and matrix of the otic cartilage of manganese-deficient animals there is a deficit of proteoglycans. Thus, it is thought that the block in otolith development is secondary to depressed proteoglycan synthesis because of low activity of manganese-requiring glycosyltransferases.[4]

Defects in carbohydrate metabolism, in addition to those described above, have been shown in manganese-deficient rats and guinea pigs. In the guinea pig, perinatal manganese deficiency results in severe pancreatic pathology, with animals exhibiting aplasia or marked hypoplasia of all cellular components. When manganese-deficient guinea pigs are given a glucose challenge, they respond with a diabetic-type glucose tolerance curve. Manganese supplementation completely reverses the pancreatic pathology and abnormal glucose tolerance observed in these animals.[4]

In addition to its effect on pancreatic tissue integrity, manganese deficiency can directly impair pancreatic insulin synthesis and secretion. In rats, manganese deficiency results in depressed pancreatic insulin synthesis and enhanced intracellular insulin degradation as well as a depression in the insulin secretory process.[24] The mechanisms underlying the effects of manganese on pancreatic insulin metabolism have not been delineated; however, they are thought to be multifactorial. For example, the flux of islet cell manganese from the cell surface to an intracellular pool may be a critical signal for insulin release.[25,26] Insulin mRNA concentrations are decreased ~10-fold in manganese-deficient rats compared with controls;[27] this finding is consistent with the observation of depressed insulin synthesis in these animals. Finally, the effect of manganese deficiency on insulin production also may be due to the destruction of pancreatic β cells. Diabetogenic agents such as streptozotocin were postulated to function via the production of high concentrations of superoxide radicals. The activity of MnSOD in pancreatic islet cells is low relative to other tissues; thus a manganese-deficiency–induced reduction in MnSOD activity could render the pancreas particularly susceptible to free radical damage.[4]

In addition to its effect on endocrine function, manganese deficiency was shown to affect pancreatic exocrine function. For example, manganese-deficient rats are characterized by an increase in pancreatic amylase content. The mechanism underlying this effect of manganese deficiency has not been delineated. However, it is thought to involve a shift in amylase synthesis or degradation, because secretagogue-stimulated acinar secretion is comparable in control and manganese-deficient rats.[28]

Although the influence of manganese deficiency on carbohydrate metabolism was demonstrated primarily in experimental animals, there is one report in the literature of an insulin-resistant diabetic patient who responded to oral doses of manganese chloride with decreasing blood glucose concentrations.[29] The rationale for testing the use of manganese in this patient was his reported use of an extract of lucerne, an old South African folk medicine, to treat his diabetes. Upon analysis the extract was found to contain high concentrations of manganese. Large-scale studies evaluating the therapeutic effect of manganese supplementation in treatment of diabetes have not been reported.

Abnormal lipid metabolism can result from manganese deficiency, and a lipotropic role for this element was suggested.[3] Manganese-deficient animals can be characterized by high liver fat concentrations. Manganese was reported to be a cofactor in steroid biosynthesis, and hypocholesterolemia was observed in deficient animals. Abnormal lipoprotein metabolism also was demonstrated in manganese-deficient animals, with deficient rats characterized by lower high-density-lipoprotein (HDL) concentrations than were controls. Deficient animals are also characterized by a shift to smaller plasma HDL particles, lower HDL apolipoprotein (apo E) concentrations, and higher apo C concentrations.[30]

Abnormal lipid metabolism was suggested as one of the factors contributing to the observation of ultrastructural abnormalities in the tissues of manganese-deficient animals. Reported ultrastructural changes include alterations in the integrity of cell membranes, swollen and irregular endoplasmic reticulum, and elongated mitochondria with stacked cristae. The effect of manganese deficiency on cell membrane integrity could be caused by either an effect of the deficiency on membrane lipid composition and/or an increased rate of membrane lipid peroxidation, because the activity of MnSOD is lower in deficient animals than in controls.[21] Given the above, it is interesting that the ob/ob mouse is characterized by low tissue manganese concentrations and MnSOD activity compared with those of controls.[31] It is not known if the low manganese status of the ob/ob mouse contributes to the pathological expression of this genotype.

It is evident that a deficiency of manganese can result in a number of biochemical and structural defects in experimental animals. That manganese deficiency could potentially be a problem in humans was first suggested by Doisy in 1972,[32] who described a male subject who developed manganese deficiency after its accidental omission from a purified diet that was being used to investigate the effects of vitamin K deficiency. Signs that were associated with the feeding of this diet that are not normally considered consequences of vitamin K deficiency included weight loss, reddening of the subject's black hair, dermatitis, reduced growth of hair and nails, and hypocholesterolemia. Unfortunately, it is not known which of these signs were due to the manganese deficiency per se, because the subject was switched to a hospital diet after it was recognized that manganese had been left out of the diet. Thus, the effect of selectively adding manganese back to the diet on the above signs was not determined.

The effect of chronic manganese deficiency in young men was investigated by Friedman et al.[33] As part of a manganese balance study, seven male subjects were fed manganese-deficient diets (0.11 mg Mn/d) for 39 d. During the depletion period all of the subjects were in negative manganese balance and five of the subjects developed a fleeting dermatitis (miliaria crystallina) that disappeared with manganese repletion. Serum calcium, phosphorus, and alkaline phosphatase concentrations increased significantly during the depletion period, consistent with the suggestion by Strause and Saltman[23] that manganese deficiency may affect bone remodeling.

Although the study of Friedman et al.[33] leaves many unanswered questions about the etiology of the metabolic defects observed during the depletion period, the study is significant because it indicates the ease with which manganese deficiency may occur. Although manganese deficiency has not been documented in humans consuming natural diets, several disease states have been linked to possible disturbances in manganese metabolism.[18] For example, some epileptics have been reported to have low blood manganese concentrations, and low tissue manganese concentrations were reported in children with maple syrup urine disease and phenylketonuria. Manganese deficiency was suggested as a potential underlying factor in the development of joint disease, hip abnormalities, osteoporosis, and congenital malformations.[18] Although it is evident from the above that the potential role of manganese deficiency in the etiology or promulgation of several human pathologies is an area of active research, it should be stressed that evidence for widespread manganese deficiency in human populations is lacking. Thus, given the recognized toxicity of manganese (see below), there is little support for manganese supplementation of the typical diet.

Genetic Disorders That Interact with Manganese

The importance of manganese during perinatal development is illustrated in several genetic mutants that possess errors of manganese metabolism. Interactions affecting development can be classified into two groups. The first type of interaction involves a single mutant gene with a phenotypic expression that can be reduced or prevented by prenatal, postnatal, or perinatal nutritional manipulation. The second type involves strain differences that produce differential responses to a dietary deficiency of the element.

An example of the first group of gene-nutrient interactions is the mutant gene *pallid* in mice. This gene is characterized by pale coat color and ataxia caused by missing or absent otoliths. In a classic study in the area of gene-nutrient interactions, Erway et al.[34] demonstrated that supplementing the diet with high amounts of manganese (2000 µg Mn/g diet) during pregnancy prevents abnormal otolith development and congenital ataxia. The mutant gene itself and the effect of the gene on pigmentation are unaltered by manganese supplementation. The biochemical lesion underlying the enhanced requirement of the pallid mouse for manganese has yet to be identified. It was reported that the concentration of manganese in bone and brain but not in liver or kidney is lower in pallid mice than in controls and that these mice have a reduced ability to synthesize brain serotinin from L-tryptophan compared with controls. The biochemical lesions underlying these phenomena have not been identified.[3]

A gene analogous to *pallid*, *screwneck*, was identified in mink. This mutant is characterized by a pale coat color, abnormal or missing otoliths in the inner ear, and ataxia. This genetic lesion was shown to be alleviated by dietary manganese supplementation.[3] Similar to the situation for *pallid*, the precise biochemical lesions caused by *screwneck* have not been identified, but the genes *pallid* and *screwneck* both provide excellent models in which to study manganese metabolism.

Representative of the second category of gene-nutrient interactions is the observation that when pregnant mice of several different strains are fed diets containing either a normal (45 µg Mn/g diet) or a low amount of manganese (3 µg Mn/g diet), the effects on otolith development of the fetuses are dependent upon the mother's genetic background. Most strains show normal otolith development when fed the normal amount of manganese; however, with the lower-manganese diet, some strains show up to 30% of normal otolith development in their fetuses, whereas others show only 5% of normal otolith development.[3] The biochemical differences underlying these strain variations are not known, but possible sites include differences in manganese absorption by the mother, maternal blood manganese transport, placental manganese transport, and fetal requirements for glycosyltransferase enzymes.

A second example of strain variation in response to manganese deficiency is the observation of Klimis-Tavantzis et al.[35] that Wistar rats differ from RICO rats in that manganese deficiency results in a reduction in hepatic fatty acid synthesis in the former but not the latter strain.

A final example of a rat strain that may be characterized by abnormal manganese metabolism is the genetically epilepsy-prone rat (GEPR). GEPR is characterized by low tissue manganese concentrations compared with those of control rats.[36] This observation is intriguing given the observations that manganese-deficient rats are more susceptible to convulsions than are normal rats and that whole-blood manganese concentrations are lower in subgroups of humans with epilepsy than in control subjects.[37] Although it is premature to suggest that manganese deficiency is a causative factor for epilepsy in either humans or GEPRs, this is an area that merits further investigation.

One human autosomal-recessive genetic disorder that was reported to be characterized by abnormal manganese metabolism is prolidase deficiency. Prolidase is a manganese-activated dipeptidase with absolute specificity for dipeptides with carboxy terminal amino acids. The clinical findings in prolidase deficiency include skin ulcers and recurrent infections, mild mental retardation, and bone abnormalities. Patients with this disorder have been reported to have elevated erythrocyte manganese concentrations; however, both erythrocyte prolidase and arginase activities are lower than in normal individuals.[38] The above observation suggests that there may be a block in the intracellular transfer of manganese in these individuals.

Requirements and Allowances

The 1989 Recommended Dietary Allowances state that the estimated safe and adequate daily dietary intakes (ESADDI) for manganese should be 0.3–1.0 mg/d for infants, 1.0–3.0 mg/d for children, and 2.0–5.0 mg/d for adults.[39] The lower range for the ESADDI figure for adults was based on the review of a number of balance studies in which equilibrium or accretion of manganese occurred whenever the intake was ≥2.5 mg/d. According to the results from the Food and Drug Administration's Total Diet Study (1982–1986),[40] manganese intakes were within the ESADDI range for young children, teenage boys, adult men, and older men. Intakes for infants tended

to exceed the ESADDI, whereas teenage, adult, and older women had intakes that were slightly lower than the appropriate ESADDI ranges. Although the results from the Total Diet Study are encouraging, it should be noted that on the basis of evaluation of several recent balance studies, it was argued that the recommended dietary intake of manganese for adults be increased to 3.5 mg/d.[10] If this recommendation were followed, a significant proportion of the female population would have intakes <50% of this value.

Food items considered high in manganese include nuts, whole cereals, dried fruits, and leafy vegetables. Tea has high concentrations of manganese; usual drinking water contributes little to the dietary intake. Meats, dairy products, poultry, and seafood are considered poor sources of manganese.[3,7]

Toxicity

In domestic animals the major reported biochemical lesion associated with dietary manganese toxicosis is an induction of iron deficiency that may result from an inhibitory effect of manganese on iron absorption.[3]

In humans manganese toxicity represents a serious health hazard. Toxic intakes of the element (either through the air or diet) result in severe pathologies particularly of the central nervous system.[7,41] It has been estimated that the incidence of manganese toxicity in workers in manganese mines in Chile is from 1% to 4%. In its more severe forms, manganese toxicity can result in a syndrome characterized by severe psychiatric symptoms, including hyperirritability, violent acts, and hallucinations. The toxicity results in a permanent crippling of the extrapyramidal system, the morphological lesions of which are similar to Parkinson's disease. Although the majority of reported cases of manganese toxicity have been in individuals exposed to excessive airborne amounts of the element (>5 mg/m^3), manganese toxicity was reported in an individual who consumed high amounts of manganese supplements over a period of years.[42] There have been a number of cases of manganese toxicity in individuals who consume water containing high manganese concentrations.[43] In addition to extensive neural damage, reproductive and immune system dysfunction, nephritis, testicular damage, pancreatitis, and hepatic damage can occur with manganese toxicity, but the frequency of these disorders is not known.[7] Manganese is known to be mutagenic in nonmammalian systems, but mutagenicity has not been reported in mammalian systems.[7]

There has been concern recently that the risk for manganese toxicity may be increasing in some areas because of the use of methylcyclopentadenyl manganese tricarbonyl in gasoline as an antiknock agent.

However, there is little evidence that air, water, or food manganese concentrations have markedly increased in geographical areas in which this fuel additive has been used.[7]

The mechanisms underlying the cellular toxicity of manganese have not been firmly identified, although there is evidence that it involves manganese-initiated catechol autooxidation and tissue lipid peroxidation.[41] Abnormal carbohydrate metabolism may also underlie some of the effects of manganese toxicosis, given the observation that insulin production can be impaired in animals subjected to high amounts of the element.[8]

Summary

The absorption of manganese is not well regulated and is influenced by several dietary factors. Homeostatic regulation is mainly through excretion of manganese into the intestinal tract via bile. Absorbed manganese is transported via α_2-macroglobulin and transferrin; retained manganese concentrates in mitochondria-rich tissues. Fluctuations in the intracellular concentration of free Mn^{2+}, like that of Mg^{2+} and Ca^{2+}, may be a mechanism of cellular metabolic control. Manganese functions both as an enzyme activator and as a constituent of metalloenzymes. It is the preferred metal cofactor for a number of glycosyltransferases, and many of the connective tissue defects seen with manganese deficiency may be explained by reduced activity of these enzymes. Manganese metalloenzymes affected by manganese status include arginase and superoxide dismutase. Some of the membrane abnormalities seen with manganese deficiency may be caused by low superoxide dismutase activity resulting in increased lipid peroxidation.

Manganese is involved in carbohydrate metabolism; a deficiency of the element can produce abnormal insulin metabolism and abnormal glucose tolerance. The relationship of manganese to lipid metabolism has not been defined, but it appears to have a lipotropic action and is involved in cholesterol and fatty acid synthesis.

Manganese is essential for normal brain function, partly via its role in the metabolism of biogenic amines. Manganese toxicity is a serious health hazard in some industries, resulting in a permanently crippling neurological disorder of the extrapyramidal system.

The adequacy of manganese nutrition in humans has not been well characterized, in part because of the lack of methods for detecting suboptimal manganese status. Future studies defining manganese status of various population groups at risk, coupled with a greater understanding of the element's func-tion in metabolism, will further delineate the role of manganese in biological systems.

References

1. A.R. Kemmerer, C.A. Elvehjem, and E.B. Hart (1931) Studies on the relation of manganese to the nutrition of the mouse. *J. Biol. Chem.* 92:623–630.
2. E.R. Orent and E.V. McCollum (1931) Effects of deprivation of manganese in the rat. *J. Biol. Chem.* 92:651–678.
3. L.S. Hurley and C.L. Keen (1987) Manganese. In: *Trace Elements in Human Health and Animal Nutrition* (E. Underwood and W. Mertz, eds.), pp. 185–223, Academic Press, New York.
4. C.L. Keen, B. Lönnerdal, and L.S. Hurley (1984) Manganese. In: *Biochemistry of the Essential Ultratrace Elements* (E. Frieden, ed.), pp. 89–132, Plenum Publishing Co., New York.
5. A.R. McEuen (1981) Manganese metalloproteins and manganese-activated enzymes. In: *Inorganic Biochemistry* (H.A.O. Hill, ed.), pp. 249–282, Royal Society of Chemistry, Burlington House, London.
6. R.M. Leach, Jr. (1986) Mn(II) and glycosyltransferases essential for skeletal development. In: *Manganese in Metabolism and Enzyme Function* (V.L. Schramm and F.C. Wedler, eds.), pp. 81–89, Academic Press, Orlando, FL.
7. C.L. Keen and R.M. Leach (1987) Manganese. In: *Handbook on Toxicity of Inorganic Compounds* (H.G. Seiler and H. Sigel, eds.), pp. 405–415, Marcel Dekker, New York.
8. V.L. Schramm and M. Brandt (1986) The manganese(II) economy of rat hepatocytes. *Fed. Proc.* 45:2817–2820.
9. L. Davidsson, Å. Cederblad, E. Hagebø, B. Lönnerdal, and B. Sandström (1988) Intrinsic and extrinsic labeling for studies of manganese absorption in humans. *J. Nutr.* 118:1517–1521.
10. J.H. Freeland-Graves, F. Behmardi, C.W. Bales, et al. (1988) Metabolic balance of manganese in young men consuming diets containing five levels of dietary manganese. *J. Nutr.* 118:764–773.
11. C.L. Keen, J.G. Bell, and B. Lönnerdal (1986) The effect of age on manganese uptake and retention from milk and infant formulas in rats. *J. Nutr.* 116:395–402.
12. G.C. Cotzias, S.T. Miller, P.S. Papavasiliou, and L.C. Tang (1976) Interactions between manganese and brain dopamine. *Med. Clin. North Am.* 60:729–738.
13. J.H. Freeland-Graves, C.W. Bales, and F. Behmardi (1987) Manganese requirements of humans. In: *Nutritional Bioavailability of Manganese* (C. Kies, ed.), pp. 90–104, American Chemical Society, Washington, DC.
14. D.-Y. Lee and P.E. Johnson (1989) ^{54}Mn absorption and excretion in rats fed soy protein and casein diets. *Proc. Soc. Exp. Biol. Med.* 190:211–216.
15. J.G. Bell, C.L. Keen, and B. Lönnerdal (1989) Higher retention of manganese in suckling than in adult rats is not due to maturational differences in manganese uptake by rat small intestine. *J. Toxicol. Environ. Health* 26:387–398.
16. J.A. Garcia-Aranda, R.A. Wapnir, and F. Lifshitz (1983) *In vivo* intestinal absorption of manganese in the rat. *J. Nutr.* 113:2601–2607.
17. L. Davidsson, B. Lönnerdal, B. Sandström, K. Kunz, and C.L. Keen (1989) Identification of transferrin as the major plasma carrier protein for manganese introduced orally or intravenously or after in vitro addition in the rat. *J. Nutr.* 119:1461–1464.
18. C.L. Keen, S. Zidenberg-Cherr, and B. Lönnerdal (1987) Dietary manganese toxicity and deficiency: effects on cellular manganese metabolism. In: *Nutritional Bioavailability of Manganese* (C. Kies, ed.), pp. 21–34, American Chemical Society, Washington, DC.
19. M.L. Failla (1986) Hormonal regulation of manganese metabolism.

In: *Manganese in Metabolism and Enzyme Function* (V.L. Schramm and F.C. Wedler, eds.), pp. 93–105, Academic Press, Orlando, FL.

20. D.L. Baly, C.L. Keen, and L.S. Hurley (1985) Pyruvate carboxylase and phosphoenolpyruvate carboxykinase activity in developing rats: effect of manganese deficiency. *J. Nutr.* 115:872–879.

21. S. Zidenberg-Cherr and C.L. Keen (1987) Enhanced tissue lipid peroxidation: a mechanism underlying pathologies associated with dietary manganese deficiency. In: *Nutritional Bioavailability of Manganese* (C. Kies, ed.), pp. 56–66, American Chemical Society, Washington, DC.

22. N.F. Schor (1988) Inactivation of mammalian brain glutamine synthetase by oxygen radicals. *Brain Res.* 456:17–21.

23. L. Strause and P. Saltman (1987) Role of manganese in bone metabolism. In: *Nutritional Bioavailability of Manganese* (C. Kies, ed.), pp. 46–55, American Chemical Society, Washington, DC.

24. D.L. Baly, D.L. Curry, C.L. Keen, and L.S. Hurley (1985) Dynamics of insulin and glucagon release in rats: influence of dietary manganese. *Endocrinology* 116:1734–1740.

25. P. Rorsman and B. Hellman (1983) The interaction between manganese and calcium fluxes in pancreatic β-cells. *Biochem. J.* 210:307–314.

26. M. Korc and M.H. Schöni (1988) Quin 2 and manganese define multiple alterations in cellular calcium homeostasis in diabetic rat pancreas. *Diabetes* 37:13–20.

27. D.L. Baly, I. Lee, and R. Doshi (1988) Mechanism of decreased insulinogenesis in manganese-deficient rats: decreased insulin mRNA levels. *FEBS Lett.* 239:55–58.

28. L. Werner, M. Korc, and P.M. Brannon (1987) Effects of manganese deficiency and dietary composition on rat pancreatic enzyme content. *J. Nutr.* 117:2079–2085.

29. A.H. Rubenstein, N.W. Levin, and G.A. Elliott (1962) Manganese-induced hypoglycemia. *Lancet* 2:1348–1351.

30. J. Kawano, D.N. Ney, C.L. Keen, and B.O. Schneeman (1987) Altered high density lipoprotein composition in manganese-deficient Sprague-Dawley and Wistar rats. *J. Nutr.* 117:902–906.

31. N. Bégin-Heick and J.R. Deeks (1987) Hypercorticism and manganese metabolism in brown adipose tissue of the obese mouse. *J. Nutr.* 117:1708–1714.

32. E. Doisy, Jr. (1972) Micronutrient controls of biosynthesis of clotting proteins and cholesterol. In: *Trace Substances in Environmental Health,* vol. VI (D. Hemphill, ed.), pp. 193–199, University of Missouri, Columbia.

33. B.J. Friedman, J.H. Freeland-Graves, C.W. Bales, et al. (1987) Manganese balance and clinical observations in young men fed a manganese-deficient diet. *J. Nutr.* 117:133–143.

34. L. Erway, L.S. Hurley, and A. Fraser (1966) Neurological defect: manganese in phenocopy and prevention of a genetic abnormality of the inner ear. *Science* 152:1766–1768.

35. D.J. Klimis-Tavantzis, R.M. Leach, and P.M. Kris-Etherton (1983) The effect of dietary manganese deficiency on cholesterol and lipid metabolism in the Wistar rat and in the genetically hypercholesterolemic RICO rat. *J. Nutr.* 113:328–338.

36. G.F. Carl, J.W. Critchfield, J.L. Thompson, G.L. Holmes, B.B. Gallagher, and C.L. Keen (in press) Genetically epilepsy prone rats are characterized by altered tissue trace element concentrations. *Epilepsia.*

37. G.F. Carl, C.L. Keen, B.B. Gallagher, and L.S. Hurley (1987) Manganese metabolism in epilepsy: normal or abnormal? In: *Nutritional Bioavailability of Manganese* (C. Kies, ed.), pp. 105–111, American Chemical Society, Washington, DC.

38. I. Lombeck, U. Wendel, J. Versieck, et al. (1986) Increased manganese content and reduced arginase activity in erythrocytes of a patient with prolidase deficiency (iminodipeptiduria). *Eur. J. Pediatr.* 144:571–573.

39. National Research Council (1989) *Recommended Dietary Allowances,* 10th ed., National Academy Press, Washington, DC.

40. J.A.T. Pennington, B.E. Young, and D.B. Wilson (1989) Nutritional elements in U.S. diets: results from the Total Diet Study, 1982 to 1986. *J. Am. Diet. Assoc.* 89:659–664.

41. J. Donaldson (1987) The physiopathologic significance of manganese in brain: its relation to schizophrenia and neurodegenerative disorders. *Neurotoxicology* 8:451–462.

42. G. Banta and W.R. Markesbery (1977) Elevated manganese levels associated with dementia and extrapyramidal signs. *Neurology* 27:213–216.

43. X.G. Kondakis, N. Makris, M. Leotsinidis, M. Prinou, and T. Papapetropoulos (1989) Possible health effects of high manganese concentration in drinking water. *Arch. Environ. Health* 44:175–178.

Chapter 33

Barbara J. Stoecker

Chromium

Chromium (Cr) is a transition element that occurs most commonly in oxidation states of 0, 2+, 3+, and 6+. The most stable valence state is the trivalent state. Chromium forms complexes and chelates that help to prevent formation of biologically inert chromium oxides and to retain solubility at the pH of intestinal contents. These chromium complexes have a slow rate of ligand exchange.[1]

History of Discovery of Essentiality

In 1957 Mertz and Schwarz[2] reported that a compound extracted from pork kidney, which they called glucose tolerance factor, restored impaired glucose tolerance in rats. Chromium was identified as the active component of the glucose tolerance factor.[3] Subsequently, malnourished children with impaired glucose tolerance were supplemented orally with 250 μg chromium as $CrCl_3 \cdot 6H_2O$, and improvements were noted in children presumed to be in poor chromium status.[4] Similar studies of impaired glucose tolerance were reviewed in more detail.[5–9] In these studies chromium supplementation usually improved glucose tolerance in a number of subjects. Improvement was greater in subjects who initially deviated more from optimal glucose tolerance.[8] However, impaired glucose tolerance clearly has multiple etiologies and is not always due to insufficient chromium intake.

More recently, chromium depletion, presumably uncomplicated by other nutrient deficiencies, was reported in patients receiving total parenteral nutrition (TPN).[10–12] In these cases chromium supplementation reversed symptoms including glucose intolerance and elevated insulin requirements.

Body Compartments

In rats intubated with $^{51}CrCl_3$, ^{51}Cr reached its highest peak in the blood by 1 h after administration

and decreased logarithmically to 20% of the peak value after 24 h.[13] Because chromium disappears from the blood very rapidly but remains in various organs much longer, the circulating chromium may not be in equilibrium with tissue chromium stores.[1]

Mertz and coworkers[14] injected rats intravenously with $^{51}CrCl_3$ and used whole-body counting to determine ^{51}Cr retention. On the basis of retention rates, they proposed at least three body chromium compartments with half-lives estimated at 0.5, 5.9, and 83.4 d. Onkelinx[15] also proposed a three-compartment model of chromium metabolism from data obtained in rats, whereas Jain and coworkers[16] suggested a rapidly exchanging chromium pool and an "inner" pool with "sink-like" characteristics.

In humans the distribution of intravenous $^{51}Cr(III)$ was observed with whole-body scanning and counting and plasma counting in three normal subjects. A model was proposed with a plasma pool in equilibrium with fast ($t\frac{1}{2}$ = 0.5–12 h), medium (1–14 d), and slow (3–12 mo) compartments.[17]

After injection of trivalent radiochromium in rats, generally there is accumulation of ^{51}Cr in spleen, bone, pancreas, kidney, and liver.[16,18] In rats with experimentally induced diabetes mellitus, there was a significant reduction in total body retention of ^{51}Cr that could be partially restored toward normal with insulin.[19]

Methods of Analysis

Reported chromium concentrations of serum, urine, and other tissues have declined markedly in recent years because of better instrumentation and more attention to contamination control. The inadequacy of conventional deuterium-background correction systems for determination of chromium in urine by atomic absorption spectrometry (AAS) with graphite furnace was illustrated in 1978;[20] the decreases in reported plasma or serum chromium concentrations and in urinary chromium excretion were summarized.[5,6] Utmost care in sample collection and handling and the use of Standard Reference Materials certified for chromium concentration by the National Institute of Standards and Technology are essential for studies involving tissue chromium analyses.[21,22]

Accepted concentrations for chromium in urine and serum or plasma are substantially <1 ppb. Most studies find serum chromium concentrations <2.9 nmol/L.[6,8] Plasma values are higher but are still <5.8 nmol/L.[9] Urinary chromium typically ranges from 1.0 to 20.0 nmol/L with group means of ~3.9 nmol/L.[5,6,23] Such low concentrations preclude the use of flame AAS, but graphite furnace AAS with an appropriate background correction system, neutron activation, and mass spectrometry are among the methods with adequate sensitivity. Graphite furnace AAS is most widely used; methods for analysis of chromium in urine and plasma have been thoroughly validated.[24,25]

Absorption

Intestinal absorption of trivalent chromium is low. Estimates of absorption in fasted rats range from 0.5% to 2–3%.[1] When $^{51}CrCl_3$ was administered intravenously to rats, small amounts of ^{51}Cr were recovered in the feces.[18] Thus, apparently there is some excretion of chromium into the gastrointestinal tract. Nevertheless, the amounts in the feces were small, and urinary chromium excretion is considered to be a reasonably accurate estimation of chromium absorption.

Several research groups have related chromium intake and urinary excretion. In a study in which normal subjects were given a dose of $^{51}CrCl_3$, a mean of 0.69% (range = 0.3–1.3%) of the dose was found in the urine within 72 h.[26] In a 12-d metabolic balance study, two men consuming an average of 36.8 μg chromium/d had a mean apparent net absorption of chromium of 1.8%.[27] In other studies, diet and urinary chromium excretion of 10 adult males and 22 females were measured. In adults consuming 60 or 260 μg chromium/d, minimum absorption (does not include losses through hair, sweat, etc.) was estimated at 0.4%.[23] When dietary chromium intake was 10 μg, ~2% of that amount was absorbed (estimated as urinary excretion) whereas at chromium intakes of 40 μg, only 0.4–0.5% of the chromium was recovered in the urine.[28] Absorption was similar from $CrCl_3$ supplements and from food chromium.[23] These studies did not provide evidence for higher absorption of dietary chromium sources than of chromium chloride. Urinary chromium excretion measured by recent techniques is also consistent with overall low absorption of dietary chromium.

Dietary Factors Affecting Chromium Absorption. Chelation of a mineral may increase or decrease its availability. When oxalate (0.1 mmol/L) and $^{51}CrCl_3$ were mixed together and administered as an oral dose, ^{51}Cr levels in the blood, whole body, and urine of rats were markedly increased at 24 h. The same concentration of phytate caused a much smaller but still significant decrease in ^{51}Cr levels.[29] However, a somewhat higher phytate-to-chromium molar ratio did not impair glucose tolerance, fasting plasma insulin, nor lipoprotein lipase activity of rats. The phytate in this study was 0.35% endogenous phytate in soy protein; it is possible that mixing chromium and phytate in a solution may produce a more pronounced effect than feeding a phytate-containing diet.[30]

A number of years ago a difference in the action of chromium in rats fed sucrose and starch diets was reported.[31] In obese and lean mice there was a significant effect of type of dietary carbohydrate on tissue chromium. Animals fed starch as the dietary carbohydrate generally had higher tissue chromium concentrations than did mice fed sucrose, fructose, or glucose. In addition, a carbohydrate load of starch generally increased the ^{51}Cr absorption from $^{51}CrCl_3$ compared with that from carbohydrate loads of sucrose, fructose, and glucose.[32] In humans, changing a diet from 35% of total calories as complex carbohydrates and 15% as simple sugars to a diet with 15% of total calories as complex carbohydrates and 35% as simple sugars for 6 wk significantly increased urinary chromium excretion.[33] Data from these three studies are consistent in suggesting that consumption of diets high in monosaccharides and disaccharides impair chromium status.

Other Factors Affecting Absorption. Diabetes mellitus appears to affect the urinary excretion and presumably the absorption of chromium. Insulin-requiring diabetic patients excreted a mean of 1.95% of an orally administered dose (0.9–3.2%) of $^{51}CrCl_3$; this excretion was two- to threefold higher than excretion from nondiabetic subjects.[26]

The very rapid passage of chromium through the gastrointestinal tract may impede its absorption. Eighty-five percent of rats intubated with $^{51}CrCl_3$ had ^{51}Cr below the cecum 4 h after intubation. In rats in which ligatures had been placed at various points in the intestine, ^{51}Cr seemed to accumulate with pools of water at each ligature, which may indicate that chromium is moving through the lumen with water.[34]

The percentage chromium absorbed may be increased by low chromium intakes. Earlier studies indicated no effect of chromium status or dose on percent absorption.[1] However, in guinea pigs depleted of chromium for 23 wk, ^{51}Cr concentrations in blood and liver were significantly higher than in chromium-supplemented animals 3 h after an oral dose of $^{51}CrCl_3$.[35] Similarly, in humans consuming <40 µg chromium/d, the percent absorption of chromium was inversely related to the amount of chromium in the diet.[28]

Transport

In rats gavaged with physiological levels of $^{51}CrCl_3$, <99% of the ^{51}Cr in blood was associated with the plasma or serum 24 h after ^{51}Cr administration. From paper electrophoresis ~90% of the ^{51}Cr on the protein fractions was attached to the β-globulin band whether the ^{51}Cr had been administered in vivo or added to the serum in vitro. Iron added to the serum before the addition of ^{51}Cr resulted in a dose-responsive reduction in ^{51}Cr bound to siderophilin (transferrin). Human serum labeled with ^{51}Cr, ^{55}Fe, or both showed these two labels to be bound to the same band. Chromium showed an affinity for transferrin that approached that of iron.[13]

Biochemical Functions

Chromium potentiates insulin action. Addition of chromium to epididymal fat tissue from chromium-deficient rats stimulated glucose uptake in the presence of added insulin.[1,36] Exogenous insulin stimulated significantly more uptake of amino acids by heart protein in chromium-supplemented rats than in chromium-depleted controls.[37] Mertz[36] hypothesized that chromium forms a complex between insulin and insulin receptors that facilitates the insulin-tissue interaction. Because trivalent chromium complexes have a very slow rate of ligand exchange, they are less likely to be the active sites of enzymes[1] and no chromium-dependent enzyme has been identified.

Glucose Tolerance Factor. A factor was extracted from brewer's yeast that improved glucose tolerance of chromium-deficient rats. This complex appeared to contain nicotinic acid, glutamic acid, glycine, and a sulfur-containing amino acid.[1] However, isolation or synthesis of glucose tolerance factor has been very difficult.[38] Controversy has continued about the precise structure of glucose tolerance factor. Some laboratories have prepared extracts that contain different ligands. A low-molecular-weight chromium-binding substance was recently isolated from bovine colostrum; it stimulated glucose oxidation and conversion into lipid in rat adipocytes.[39] This substance contained aspartic acid, glutamic acid, glycine, and cysteine. Nicotinic acid was not detected, but there was a constituent that had an absorption maximum at 260 nm, which is the peak for nicotinic acid. Further research is needed to resolve questions about structure and

function of glucose tolerance factor. However, it seems that chromium as found in brewer's yeast and in some other naturally occurring and synthetic complexes is more effective in stimulating glucose utilization than is chromium chloride or chromium found in torula yeast.[40,41]

Response to Glucose. Chromium was reported to increase in plasma after glucose administration in persons assumed to have adequate chromium status.[1,42] However, using a different subject population and improved methods of chromium analysis, Anderson and coworkers[43] found that serum chromium did not increase significantly after a glucose load in subjects previously given either 200 µg chromium/d as $CrCl_3$ or a placebo. Similarly, in elderly subjects Offenbacher and colleagues[44] found that plasma chromium did not increase in response to a glucose load. Thus, plasma or serum chromium response after a glucose challenge does not seem to be an appropriate indicator of chromium status.

Like serum chromium, urinary chromium excretion in response to a glucose load does not provide a reliable means for assessing Cr status. An increase in urinary chromium excretion in response to a glucose load was demonstrated for ~80% of subjects not supplemented with chromium, but results were variable and the effect disappeared when subjects were supplemented daily with 200 µg trivalent chromium.[45]

Both exercise and trauma increase glucose utilization and the subsequent appearance of chromium in the urine. After a 9.66-km run, urinary chromium and zinc were increased whereas no change was observed in urinary sodium, potassium, or calcium.[46] Severalfold increases in urinary chromium were measured in traumatized patients.[47]

Effects on Lipid Metabolism. Data on effects of chromium on serum cholesterol levels in experimental animals and humans are equivocal, with some studies showing decreased serum cholesterol and increased HDL cholesterol and others showing no effect of chromium supplementation.[1,6,8,9,31] Some of these discrepancies no doubt reflect the lack of an adequate measure of chromium status. Chromium supplementation would not be expected to be beneficial to subjects already consuming sufficient chromium.

Chromium reduced serum cholesterol and aortic plaque in rats,[1,31] whereas combined chromium and ascorbate deprivation increased serum cholesterol of guinea pigs.[48] However, inconsistent data make definitive conclusions from experimental animals very difficult.

Interactions with Nucleic Acids. Chromium in mouse liver was concentrated in the nuclei 48 h after intraperitoneal injection of 0.005–5 mg $CrCl_3$/kg body weight.[49] The chromium dose in this experiment was high, but results confirmed earlier studies noting association of chromium with nucleic acids.[8] The synthesis of DNA and protein in liver was not affected significantly by chromium administration; however, prior administration of chromium chloride enhanced RNA synthesis.[49] Using partially hepatectomized rats, this research group concluded that Cr in the nucleoli may participate in gene expression.[50]

Deficiency Symptoms

Identification of chromium as an essential element was based on its role in restoration of glucose tolerance in rats.[3] However, because of the ubiquitous nature of chromium in the environment, it is not easy to produce a clear chromium deficiency in laboratory animals. Imposed stress, such as exercise, illness, imbalanced diets, or hemorrhage, exacerbates the deficiency state.[1,6,8,46,51] In human beings there is not yet a good method for assessment of chromium status. Therefore, most studies that seek to reverse a possible chromium-deficiency symptom by supplementation are hampered by inadequate means to assess the initial chromium status of the subjects. Nonetheless, understanding of chromium deficiency symptoms is increasing.

Growth and Survival. Several studies cited by Mertz[1] reported an increase in growth and survival of chromium-supplemented rats and mice. Growth is also impaired in guinea pigs fed diets containing <60 ng chromium/g diet.[52] A significantly increased rate of growth was observed in malnourished children supplemented with chromium compared with a similar group who received no chromium supplementation.[53] Two patients receiving chromium-deficient TPN solutions showed weight loss that was restored with chromium supplementation.[10,11]

Impaired Glucose Tolerance, Hyperglycemia, and Elevated Circulating Insulin. Numerous reports through the years have noted that chromium depletion impairs glucose tolerance in experimental animals. These studies were extensively reviewed.[1,6,8,9]

In patients receiving no chromium or inadequate chromium supplementation in TPN solutions, chromium supplementation reduced insulin requirements and reversed glucose intolerance.[10–12] The Nutrition Advisory Group of the American Medical Association[54] recommended that 10–15 μg chromium/d be given to stable adults receiving TPN. This recommendation should be evaluated carefully. Assuming similar utilization of orally and intravenously administered chromium, an intravenous dose of 15 μg chromium/d is equivalent to a daily oral intake of 3000 or 1500 μg/d at absorption rates of 0.5% or 1%, respectively.

Supplementation of elderly subjects with 10.8 μg

chromium/d as a high-chromium yeast improved glucose tolerance, whereas supplementation with an equivalent amount of torula yeast (<0.45 μg chromium/d) did not.[55] Patients with noninsulin-dependent diabetes showed improvement in glucose tolerance in this study.[55] In eight hypoglycemic women, chromium supplementation (200 μg chromium/d for 3 mo) resulted in increased minimum serum glucose values 2–4 h after a glucose load, insulin binding to erythrocytes, and insulin receptor numbers.[56] In other studies chromium did not improve hyperglycemia in diabetic or elderly subjects.[44,57] The divergent results in these studies illustrate the complex etiology of diabetes mellitus and glucose intolerance, the possible effects of form of chromium on the prognosis for improvement with supplementation, and the uncertainty of initial chromium status of subjects.

Lipid Metabolism. In rats supplemented with trivalent chromium, lower serum cholesterol and aortic plaque incidence were reported.[31] In obese mice, hepatic lipid concentration decreased in chromium-supplemented animals.[58] Hepatic lipid was positively correlated with circulating insulin levels in these mice. However, further research is needed to explain inconsistencies in the lipid response of chromium-depleted animals.

In human subjects supplementation with a high-chromium brewer's yeast resulted in significantly lower serum cholesterol.[55] Both serum triglycerides and total lipids were reduced in subjects with initial serum cholesterol >7.76 mmol/L.[55] Chromium supplementation was reported to increase HDL cholesterol in men.[59] However, in other studies chromium supplementation did not affect serum lipids.[5,8,9,60]

Other Signs of Deficiency. Peripheral neuropathy was seen in one patient receiving TPN without chromium.[10] This neuropathy was reversed with chromium supplementation. Decreased fertility and sperm count were found in rats depleted of chromium.[61] Urinary creatinine and hydroxyproline excretion of chromium-depleted guinea pigs was significantly higher than that of supplemented animals.[52]

Requirements and Allowances

The first recommendation for dietary chromium was established in 1989 as an estimated safe and adequate intake of 50–200 μg/d.[62] Recent estimates of chromium intakes in the United States were quite low, with group means of 24.5–89 μg/d.[27,28,44,63] The safety of 200-μg intakes has been established but the long-term effects of dietary intakes <50 μg have not been evaluated adequately. Further, our pattern of relatively high consumption of simple sugars may increase urinary chromium excretion.[33]

Better indicators of chromium status in humans and more research are needed to establish whether many people consume diets that are inadequate to meet their need for chromium or whether the recommended intake range is somewhat higher than necessary for healthy people.

Pregnancy. Concern has been expressed about suboptimal chromium nutrition during gestation, and chromium deficiency was suggested as one potential etiological factor in the glucose intolerance of pregnancy.[64] Plasma immunoreactive insulin response to a glucose load was significantly greater in pregnant than in nonpregnant women.[65] Hair chromium was reported to be significantly lower in parous women than in nulliparous subjects.[64,66]

Exercise. In humans urinary chromium losses were increased twofold on the day of a 9.66-km run compared with a rest day.[46] Trained athletes had lower resting urinary chromium concentrations but greater urinary chromium losses because of exercise.[67] In experimental animals plasma ultrafiltrable chromium was excreted rapidly by glomerular filtration without significant tubular reabsorption.[68]

Age. It was suggested that chromium deficiency contributes to the impaired glucose tolerance in elderly subjects.[1] However, two recent studies of elderly subjects showed mean intakes of 25 and 37 μg chromium/d,[44,69] which are similar to intakes of younger adults. Both of these groups were healthy, apparently well-nourished volunteers. If elderly subjects are chromium deficient, their chromium intakes may be lower than noted in these studies or their need for chromium may be increased by various types of physiological stress. Age per se may not be a factor causing chromium deficiency.

Sources

Many self-selected diets are near or <50 μg chromium/d. Meats and whole-grain products are some of the best sources of chromium in the food supply;[70,71] however, there are considerable losses of chromium with milling.[72] Fruits, vegetables, and milk have very low chromium concentrations.[70] Mean chromium concentration of breast-milk samples from American mothers was 5.8 nmol/L, which would provide 0.2–0.3 μg chromium/d.[73] Data are not available on the absorption of chromium from formula compared with breast milk, but the current recommendation of 10–40 μg/d for the 0–6 mo-old infant seems disproportionately high.

There may also be a substantial amount of chromium added to the food supply during processing and preparation. Chromium can be leached from stainless steel containers particularly when acidic juices are heated in them.[74] Some beers contain significant quantities of chromium that can be absorbed by humans, but the chromium concentration among brands is quite variable.[75]

Toxicity

The therapeutic–toxic-dose ratio for chromium of ~1:10,000 means that intakes of trivalent chromium that will produce a physiological effect are quite safe.[1] Because trivalent chromium is poorly absorbed, very high oral intakes would be necessary to attain toxic levels.

Toxic effects of industrial exposure to chromium have been documented. Symptoms include allergic dermatitis, skin ulcers, and increased incidence of bronchogenic carcinoma.[76] Airborne hexavalent chromium has been assumed to be responsible for most of the toxicity problems because trivalent chromium is less well absorbed and less irritating. However, a recent study in which workers were chronically exposed to trivalent chromium showed clear indication of elevated body loads of chromium.[77] Median serum chromium was 9.4 nmol/L in tannery workers and 2.9 nmol/L in control subjects. Median urinary chromium was fourfold higher in tannery workers than in control subjects. Workers handling wet hides had significantly higher serum chromium levels and urinary chromium-creatinine ratios than did workers in other areas of the tannery. Hexavalent chromium in the air was below the detection limit, and the authors indicated that tannery compounds contain almost exclusively trivalent chromium.

Further studies on potential toxicity of chromium are needed. A low-molecular-weight compound has been found that binds chromium in the liver of mice.[78] This compound was hypothesized to have a role in chromium detoxification.[78]

In conclusion, the essentiality of chromium has been demonstrated, but further research is necessary to clarify physiological functions of chromium. Needed research is hampered by lack of satisfactory measures for chromium status and by problems of sample contamination. Many people in the United States consume <50 μg chromium/d. Long-term consequences of these dietary intakes and of the effects of various kinds of stress on chromium metabolism need to be evaluated.

References

1. W. Mertz (1969) Chromium occurrence and function in biological systems. *Physiol. Rev.* 49:163–239.
2. K. Schwarz and W. Mertz (1957) A glucose tolerance factor and its differentiation from factor 3. *Arch. Biochem. Biophys.* 72:515–518.
3. K. Schwarz and W. Mertz (1959) Chromium(III) and the glucose tolerance factor. *Arch. Biochem. Biophys.* 85:292–295.

4. L.L. Hopkins, Jr., O. Ransome-Kuti, and A.S. Majaj (1968) Improvement of impaired carbohydrate metabolism by chromium(III) in malnourished infants. *Am. J. Clin. Nutr.* 21:203–211.

5. R.A. Anderson (1981) Nutritional role of chromium. *Sci. Total Environ.* 17:13–29.

6. J.S. Borel and R.A. Anderson (1984) Chromium. In: *Biochemistry of the Essential Ultratrace Elements* (E. Frieden, ed.), pp. 175–199, Plenum Press, New York.

7. S. Wallach (1985) Clinical and biochemical aspects of chromium deficiency. *J. Am. Coll. Nutr.* 4:107–120.

8. R.A. Anderson (1987) Chromium. In: *Trace Elements in Human and Animal Nutrition* (W. Mertz, ed.), 5th ed., pp. 225–244, Academic Press, Inc., New York.

9. E.G. Offenbacher and F.X. Pi-Sunyer (1988) Chromium in human nutrition. In: *Annual Reviews of Nutrition* (R.E. Olson, ed.), 8th ed., pp. 543–563, Annual Reviews Inc., Palo Alto, CA.

10. K.N. Jeejeebhoy, R.C. Chu, E.B. Marliss, G.R. Greenberg, and A. Bruce-Robertson (1977) Chromium deficiency, glucose intolerance, and neuropathy reversed by chromium supplementation, in a patient receiving long-term total parenteral nutrition. *Am. J. Clin. Nutr.* 30:531–538.

11. H. Freund, S. Atamian, and J.E. Fischer (1979) Chromium deficiency during total parenteral nutrition. *JAMA* 241:496–498.

12. R.O. Brown, R. Forloines-Lynn, R.E. Cross, and W.D. Heizer (1986) Chromium deficiency after long-term total parenteral nutrition. *Dig. Dis. Sci.* 31:661–664.

13. L.L. Hopkins, Jr., and K. Schwarz (1964) Chromium (III) binding to serum proteins, specifically siderophilin. *Biochim. Biophys. Acta* 90:484–491.

14. W. Mertz, E.E. Roginski, and R.C. Reba (1965) Biological activity and fate of trace quantities of intravenous chromium(III) in the rat. *Am. J. Physiol.* 209:489–494.

15. C. Onkelinx (1977) Compartment analysis of metabolism of chromium in rats of various ages. *Am. J. Physiol.* 232:E478–E484.

16. R. Jain, R.L. Verch, S. Wallach, and R.A. Peabody (1981) Tissue chromium exchange in the rat. *Am. J. Clin. Nutr.* 34:2199–2204.

17. T.H. Lim, T. Sargent, III, and N. Kusubov (1983) Kinetics of trace element chromium(III) in the human body. *Am. J. Physiol.* 244: R445–R454.

18. L.L. Hopkins, Jr. (1965) Distribution in the rat of physiological amounts of injected Cr-51(III) with time. *Am. J. Physiol.* 209:731–735.

19. J.L. Kraszeski, S. Wallach, and R.L. Verch (1979) Effect of insulin on radiochromium distribution in diabetic rats. *Endocrinology* 104: 881–885.

20. B.E. Guthrie, W.R. Wolf, and C. Veillon (1978) Background correction and related problems in the determination of chromium in urine by graphite furnace atomic absorption spectrometry. *Anal. Chem.* 50:1900–1902.

21. J. Versieck, F. Barbier, R. Cornelis, and J. Hoste (1982) Sample contamination as a source of error in trace-element analysis of biological samples. *Talanta* 29:973–984.

22. C. Veillon (1988) Chromium. *Methods Enzymol.* 158:334–343.

23. R.A. Anderson, M.M. Polansky, N.A. Bryden, K.Y. Patterson, C. Veillon, and W.H. Glinsmann (1983) Effects of chromium supplementation of urinary Cr excretion of human subjects and correlation of Cr excretion with selected clinical parameters. *J. Nutr.* 113: 276–281.

24. C. Veillon, K.Y. Patterson, and N.A. Bryden (1982) Chromium in urine as measured by atomic absorption spectrometry. *Clin. Chem.* 28:2309–2311.

25. C. Veillon, K.Y. Patterson, and N.A. Bryden (1984) Determination of chromium in human serum by electrothermal atomic absorption spectrometry. *Anal. Chim. Acta* 164:67–76.

26. R.J. Doisy, D.H.P. Streeten, M.L. Souma, M.E. Kalafer, S.L. Rekant, and T.G. Dalakos (1971) Metabolism of chromium-51 in human subjects. In: *Newer Trace Elements in Nutrition* (W. Mertz and W.E. Cornatzer, eds.), pp. 155–168, Dekker, New York.

27. E.G. Offenbacher, H. Spencer, H.J. Dowling, and F.X. Pi-Sunyer (1986) Metabolic chromium balances in men. *Am. J. Clin. Nutr.* 44:77–82.

28. R.A. Anderson and A.S. Kozlovsky (1985) Chromium intake, absorption and excretion of subjects consuming self-selected diets. *Am. J. Clin. Nutr.* 41:1177–1183.

29. N.S.C. Chen, A. Tsai, and I.A. Dyer (1973) Effect of chelating agents on chromium absorption in rats. *J. Nutr.* 103:1182–1186.

30. K.S. Keim, B.J. Stoecker, and S. Henley (1987) Chromium status of the rat as affected by phytate. *Nutr. Res.* 7:253–263.

31. H.A. Schroeder (1968) The role of chromium in mammalian nutrition. *Am. J. Clin. Nutr.* 21:230–244.

32. C.D. Seaborn and B.J. Stoecker (1988) Effects of starch, sucrose, fructose, and glucose on chromium absorption and tissue concentrations in obese and lean mice. *FASEB J.* 2:A423(abstr.).

33. A.S. Kozlovsky, P.B. Moser, S. Reiser, and R.A. Anderson (1986) Effects of diets high in simple sugars on urinary chromium losses. *Metabolism* 35:515–518.

34. D. Oberleas, Y.C. Li, and B.J. Stoecker (1987) Intestinal transit of ^{51}-Cr in the rat. *Fed. Proc.* 64:904(abstr.).

35. B.J. Stoecker, C.D. Seaborn, H.C. Lin, X.X. Xu, and Y.C. Li (1988) Effects of chromium and ascorbate depletion on ^{51}chromium absorption and urinary excretion in guinea pigs. *FASEB J.* 2: A840(abstr.).

36. W. Mertz, E.W. Toepfer, E.E. Roginski, and M.M. Polansky (1974) Present knowledge of the role of chromium. *Fed. Proc.* 33:2275–2280.

37. E. Roginski and W. Mertz (1969) Effects of chromium(III) supplementation on glucose and amino acid metabolism in rats fed a low protein diet. *J. Nutr.* 97:525–530.

38. R.W. Tuman, J.T. Bilbo, and R.J. Doisy (1978) Comparison and effects of natural and synthetic glucose tolerance factor in normal and genetically diabetic mice. *Diabetes* 27:49–56.

39. A. Yamamoto, O. Wada, and H. Suzuki (1988) Purification and properties of biologically active chromium complex from bovine colostrum. *J. Nutr.* 118:39–45.

40. E.W. Toepfer, W. Mertz, M.M. Polansky, E.E. Roginski, and W.R. Wolf (1977) Preparation of chromium-containing material of glucose tolerance factor activity from brewer's yeast extracts and by synthesis. *J. Agric. Food Chem.* 25:162–166.

41. B.J. Stoecker, Y.-C. Li, D.B. Wester, and S.-B. Chan (1987) Effects of torula and brewer's yeast diets in obese and lean mice. *Biol. Trace Elem. Res.* 14:249–254.

42. V.J.K. Liu and J.S. Morris (1978) Relative chromium response as an indicator of chromium status. *Am. J. Clin. Nutr.* 31:972–976.

43. R.A. Anderson, N.A. Bryden, and M.M. Polansky (1985) Serum chromium of human subjects: effects of chromium supplementation and glucose. *Am. J. Clin. Nutr.* 41:571–577.

44. E. Offenbacher, C. Rinko, and F.X. Pi-Sunyer (1985) The effects of inorganic chromium and brewers yeast on glucose tolerance, plasma lipids, and plasma chromium in elderly subjects. *Am. J. Clin. Nutr.* 42:454–456.

45. R.A. Anderson, M.M. Polansky, N.A. Bryden, et al. (1982) Urinary chromium excretion of human subjects: effects of chromium supplementation and glucose loading. *Am. J. Clin. Nutr.* 36:1184–1193.

46. R.A. Anderson, M.M. Polansky, and N.A. Bryden (1984) Acute effects on chromium, copper, zinc, and selected clinical variables in urine and serum of male runners. *Biol. Trace Elem. Res.* 6:327–336.

47. J.S. Borel, T.C. Majerus, M.M. Polansky, P.B. Moser, and R.A. Anderson (1984) Chromium intake and urinary chromium excretion of trauma patients. *Biol. Trace Elem. Res.* 6:317–326.

48. B.J. Stoecker and W.K. Oladut (1985) Effects of chromium and

ascorbate deficiencies on glucose tolerance and serum cholesterol of guinea pigs. *Nutr. Rep. Int.* 32:399–405.

49. S. Okada, M. Suzuki, and H. Ohba (1983) Enhancement of ribonucleic acid synthesis by chromium(III) in mouse liver. *J. Inorg. Biochem.* 19:95–103.

50. S. Okada, H. Tsukada, and H. Ohba (1984) Enhancement of nucleolar RNA synthesis by chromium(III) in regenerating rat liver. *J. Inorg. Biochem.* 21:113–124.

51. F.H. Nielsen (1988) Nutritional significance of the ultratrace elements. *Nutr. Rev.* 46:337–341.

52. C.D. Seaborn, N.Z. Cheng, L.M. Campbell, and B.J. Stoecker (1989) Chromium and ascorbate effects on urinary excretion of hydroxyproline and creatinine in male guinea pigs. *FASEB J.* 3: A761(abstr.).

53. C.T. Gurson and G. Saner (1973) Effects of chromium supplementation on growth in marasmic protein-calorie malnutrition. *Am. J. Clin. Nutr.* 26:988–991.

54. Anonymous (1979) Guidelines for essential trace element preparations for parenteral use. *JAMA* 241:2051–2054.

55. E.G. Offenbacher and F.X. Pi-Sunyer (1980) Beneficial effect of chromium-rich yeast on glucose tolerance and blood lipids in elderly subjects. *Diabetes* 29:919–924.

56. R.A. Anderson, M.M. Polansky, N.A. Bryden, S.J. Bhathena, and J.J. Canary (1987) Effects of supplemental chromium on patients with symptoms of reactive hypoglycemia. *Metabolism* 36:351–355.

57. L. Sherman, J.A. Glennon, W.J. Brech, G.H. Klomberg, and E.S. Gordon (1968) Failure of trivalent chromium to improve hyperglycemia in diabetes mellitus. *Metabolism* 17:439–442.

58. Y.-C. Li and B.J. Stoecker (1986) Chromium and yogurt effects on hepatic lipid and plasma glucose and insulin of obese mice. *Biol. Trace Elem. Res.* 9:233–242.

59. R. Riales and M.J. Albrink (1981) Effect of chromium chloride supplementation on glucose tolerance and serum lipids including high-density lipoprotein of adult men. *Am. J. Clin. Nutr.* 34:2670–2678.

60. R.A. Anderson, M.M. Polansky, N.A. Bryden, E.E. Roginski, W. Mertz, and W. Glinsmann (1983) Chromium supplementation of human subjects: effects on glucose, insulin, and lipid variables. *Metabolism* 32:894–899.

61. R.A. Anderson and M.M. Polansky (1981) Dietary chromium deficiency: effect on sperm count and fertility in rats. *Biol. Trace Elem. Res.* 3:1–5.

62. National Research Council (1989) *Recommended Dietary Allowances,* 10th ed., National Academy Press, Washington, DC.

63. J.T. Kumpulainen, W.R. Wolf, C. Veillon, and W. Mertz (1979) Determination of chromium in selected United States diets. *J. Agric. Food Chem.* 27:490–494.

64. K.M. Hambidge and D.O. Rodgerson (1969) Comparison of hair chromium levels of nulliparous and parous women. *Am. J. Obstet. Gynecol.* 103:320–321.

65. I.W.F. Davidson and R.L. Burt (1973) Physiologic changes in plasma chromium of normal and pregnant women: effect of a glucose load. *Am. J. Obstet. Gynecol.* 116:601–608.

66. J.R. Mahalko and M. Bennion (1976) The effect of parity and time between pregnancies on maternal hair chromium concentration. *Am. J. Clin. Nutr.* 29:1069–1072.

67. W.W. Campbell and R.A. Anderson (1987) Effects of aerobic exercise and training on the trace minerals chromium, zinc and copper. *Sports Med.* 4:9–18.

68. D.L. Donaldson, C.C. Smith, and A.A. Yunice (1984) Renal excretion of chromium-51 chloride in the dog. *Am. J. Physiol.* 246: F870–F878.

69. V.W. Bunker, M.S. Lawson, H.T. Delves, and B. Clayton (1984) The uptake and excretion of chromium by the elderly. *Am. J. Clin. Nutr.* 39:797–802.

70. R.S. Gibson, A.C. Macdonald, and O.B. Martinez (1985) Dietary chromium and manganese intakes of a selected sample of Canadian elderly women. *Hum. Nutr. Appl. Nutr.* 39A:43–52.

71. E.W. Toepfer, W. Mertz, E.E. Roginski, and M.M. Polansky (1973) Chromium in foods in relation to biological activity. *J. Agric. Food Chem.* 21:69–73.

72. H.A. Schroeder (1971) Losses of vitamins and trace minerals resulting from processing and preservation of foods. *Am. J. Clin. Nutr.* 24:562–573.

73. C.E. Casey and K.M. Hambidge (1988) Chromium in human milk from American mothers. *Br. J. Nutr.* 52:73–77.

74. E.G. Offenbacher and F.X. Pi-Sunyer (1983) Temperature and pH effects on the release of chromium from stainless steel into water and fruit juices. *J. Agric. Food Chem.* 31:89–92.

75. R. Anderson and N.A. Bryden (1983) Concentration, insulin potentiation, and absorption of chromium in beer. *J. Agric. Food Chem.* 31:308–311.

76. L. Fishbein (1988) Perspectives of analysis of carcinogenic and mutagenic metals in biological samples. *Int. J. Environ. Anal. Chem.* 28:21–69.

77. J.A. Randall and R.S. Gibson (1987) Serum and urine chromium as indices of chromium status in tannery workers. *Proc. Soc. Exp. Biol. Med.* 185:16–23.

78. A. Yamamoto, O. Wada, and T. Ono (1984) Distribution and chromium-binding capacity of a low-molecular-weight, chromium-binding substance in mice. *J. Inorg. Biochem.* 22:91–102.

Other Trace Elements

All elements that have not been assigned separate chapters in this volume fit into the category of elements that have become known as the ultratrace elements. Ultratrace elements are those with estimated dietary requirements usually <1 μg/g and often <50 ng/g of diet for laboratory animals.[1] At least 14 elements have been suggested as ultratrace elements: arsenic, boron, bromine, cadmium, chromium, fluorine, lead, lithium, molybdenum, nickel, selenium, silicon, tin, and vanadium. The quality of the experimental evidence supporting the suggestion of nutritional essentiality varies widely among these elements. Here, an element is considered essential if a dietary deficiency of the element consistently results in a suboptimal biological function that is preventable or reversible by an intake of physiological amounts of that element. The evidence for the essentiality (initially appearing in 1950s) of chromium and selenium is substantial and noncontroversial. They are discussed in chapters 33 and 30, respectively. A critical review of the experimental evidence supporting the suggestion of nutritional essentiality of the other 12 ultratrace elements indicates that only arsenic, boron, molybdenum, nickel, and silicon meet the definition of essentiality. Thus, those five elements will be discussed here. Vanadium will also be discussed because recent findings lend credence to the suggestion of essentiality for vanadium. Other ultratrace elements will not be discussed because only weak or limited evidence supports them as essential.

Arsenic

History. The first conclusive evidence for arsenic essentiality was published in 1975–1976.[2] Arsenic deprivation signs were described for rats, pigs, and goats. Subsequently, signs also were described for chickens and hamsters. Thus, it is only recently that arsenic has been studied from the biochemical, nutritional, and physiological, and not only the toxicological or pharmacological, points of view.

Method of Analysis. One of the most precise and sensitive methods for the determination of arsenic in biological material involves measuring arsine generated from dry combusted samples by graphite-furnace atomic absorption spectrometry.[3,4]

Absorption, Transport, Retention, and Excretion. The metabolism of arsenic is markedly affected by the dose and form of arsenic.[5] Moreover, the metabolism of arsenic in some animal species is quite unusual. For example, rats, unlike other mammals, concentrate arsenic in their red blood cells.[6] The marmoset monkey is unable to methylate arsenite,[7,8] which is a major reaction in the elimination of arsenic from the body for most animals. Studies with rabbits, hamsters, and chicks seem to give findings on the metabolism of arsenic most applicable to humans.

Absorption of inorganic arsenic from the gastrointestinal tract correlates well with the solubility of the compounds ingested.[5,9] The form of organic arsenic also determines whether or not it is well absorbed. For example, >90% of an oral dose of arsenobetaine was found in the urine of hamsters;[10] 70–80% of an oral dose of arsenocholine was found in the urine of mice, rats, and rabbits;[11] and 45% of an oral dose of dimethylarsinic acid was found in the urine of hamsters.[12] On the other hand, when sodium-*p*-N-glycolylarsanilate was given orally to rats or humans, >90% was recovered in the feces within 3 d, and urinary excretion accounted for only 4–5% of the dose.[13]

Only a limited number of studies have examined the mechanisms involved in the intestinal absorption of arsenic. Contrary to an early suggestion, recent findings indicate that despite structural similarities arsenate and phosphate do not share a common transport pathway in the duodenum.[14] Apparently the absorption of arsenate involves a simple movement down a concentration gradient. In rats some forms of organic arsenic are absorbed at rates directly proportional to their intestinal concentration over a

100-fold range.[15] This suggests that organic arsenicals are absorbed mainly by simple diffusion through lipoid regions of the intestine.

Blood contains both inorganic (probably protein bound) and methylated forms of arsenic. Before arsenate is methylated, it is reduced to arsenite.[16] Methylation takes place in the liver with S-adenosylmethionine as the methyl donor.[17] In humans the final product, dimethylarsinic acid, results from the methylation of the monomethylarsenic acid precursor formed from arsenite.[18] The methylation of arsenic can be modified by changes in the glutathione,[19] methionine, and choline[20] status of the animal.

The fate of absorbed organic arsenic depends upon its form. Arsenobetaine passes through the body into the urine unchanged.[21] After oral administration of arsenocholine, arsenobetaine is the major urinary metabolite although some arsenocholine appears in the urine.[11] In addition, some arsenocholine is retained in the body and is incorporated into phospholipids in a manner similar to choline.[11] After the oral administration of dimethylarsinic acid, hamsters synthesize a trimethylarsenic compound of unknown structure. Approximately 16% of an administered dose of dimethylarsinic acid appeared in the urine as a trimethylated arsenic compound.[12]

If the ingestion of arsenic is low, no tissue significantly accumulates arsenic.[22] In unexposed humans, the highest amounts of arsenic are usually found in skin, hair, and nails.[5]

Ingested arsenic is excreted rapidly in urine. Minor amounts also are excreted through other routes, including sweat, hair and skin losses, and bile.[5] Following an oral dose of inorganic arsenic as arsenic acid, the proportions of arsenic compounds in human urine were reported to be 51% dimethylarsinic acid, 21% monomethylarsonic acid, and 27% inorganic arsenic.[23] However, if the arsenic had been in organic form, the amounts of the different forms of arsenic in urine would have been completely different. For example, an analysis of urine from 102 Japanese students, a population consuming luxuriant amounts of organic arsenic in seafood, revealed 9.4% inorganic arsenic, 3.0% monomethylarsonic acid, 28.9% dimethylarsinic acid, and 58.2% trimethylated arsenic compound.[24]

Biochemical Function. The evidence showing that arsenic is essential does not clearly define its biochemical function. Possibly, arsenic has a role related to or involved in phospholipid metabolism. Studies with hamsters suggest that significant amounts of dimethylarsinic acid[12] and small amounts of inorganic arsenic[25] can be converted into trimethylated arsenic compounds in vivo; perhaps some of this is arsenocholine. Arsenocholine administration results in the incorporation of arsenocholine into phospholipids in

the same way as choline.[11] In higher animals arsenocholine can replace choline in some of its functions.[26] Arsenocholine is antiperotic and growth promoting in the choline-deficient fowl.

In addition to phospholipids, choline is involved in labile methyl metabolism. Recent findings have shown that arsenic deprivation in the rat, chick, and hamster affects labile methyl metabolism.[27] Thus, it is possible that arsenic has a biochemical function as a methylated compound.

Deficiency Signs. Several reviews summarized the signs of arsenic deprivation in four animal species—chick, goat, miniature pig, and rat.[2,28,29] In the goat, miniature pig, and rat the most consistent signs of arsenic deprivation were depressed growth and abnormal reproduction characterized by impaired fertility and elevated perinatal mortality. Other signs of deprivation in goats were depressed serum triglycerides and death during lactation. Myocardial damage was present in lactating goats. The myocardial organelle most markedly affected was the mitochondrion membrane.[30] In advanced stages, the membrane ruptured allowing mitochondrial materials to lie free in the cytoplasm.

Other signs of arsenic deprivation have been reported. Studies with chicks, rats, and hamsters, however, have revealed that the nature and severity of the signs of arsenic deprivation are affected by variations in the dietary concentration of zinc, arginine, choline, methionine, taurine, and guanidoacetic acid, all of which can affect methyl metabolism.[27]

Requirements, Allowances, and Sources. Only data from animal studies are available for estimating the arsenic need of humans. An arsenic requirement of <50 ng/g and probably ~25 ng/g was suggested for growing chicks and rats fed an experimental diet containing 20% protein, 9% fat, 60% carbohydrate, 11% fiber, minerals, and vitamins.[28] Thus, the arsenic requirement is apparently between 6.25 and 12.5 μg/ 1000 kcal. From these data a possible arsenic requirement for humans eating 2000 kcal would be ~12–15 μg/d. The reported arsenic content of diets from various parts of the world indicates that the average daily intake of arsenic is in the range of 12–40 μg.[31-33] Fish, grain, and cereal products contribute most of the arsenic to the diet.

Toxicity. Because there are mechanisms for homeostatic regulation of arsenic, the toxicity of arsenic through oral intake is relatively low. It is much less toxic than selenium, a trace element of known nutritional value. Toxic quantities of inorganic arsenic generally are measured in milligrams and the ratio of the toxic to nutritional dose for rats apparently is ~1250. The organic forms of arsenic that occur naturally in foods are virtually nontoxic; a 10 g/kg body-weight dose of arsenobetaine depressed spontaneous motility and respiration in male mice, but these symptoms disappeared within an hour.[34]

Signs of subacute and chronic exposure of arsenic in humans include the development of dermatoses of various types (hyperpigmentation, hyperkeratosis, desquamation, and loss of hair), hematopoietic depression, liver damage characterized by jaundice, portal cirrhosis and ascites, sensory disturbances, peripheral neuritis, anorexia, and loss of weight.[35,36]

Numerous epidemiological studies have suggested an association between chronic arsenic overexposure and cancer. However, the role of arsenic in carcinogenesis remains controversial. Recent examinations of the evidence indicate that arsenic is not a primary carcinogen[37] and is either an inactive or extremely weak mutagen.[38]

Boron

History. Between 1939 and 1944 several attempts to induce a boron deficiency in rats were unsuccessful, although the diets used apparently contained only 155–163 ng boron/g.[39] In 1945 a report indicated that supplemental dietary boron enhanced survival and maintenance of body fat and elevated liver glycogen in potassium-deficient rats.[40] Those findings were not confirmed in a subsequent study in which rats were fed a different diet with an unknown boron content supplemented with different levels of boron.[41] Thereafter, boron was generally accepted as essential for plants (discovered in 1910, confirmed in 1923) but not for animals.[39] Since 1981, however, accumulating evidence indicates that boron is an essential element and is important in macromineral metabolism in humans.[42]

Method of Analysis. Analytical methods for the determination of boron in biological materials are still being established. One relatively precise and sensitive method involves low-temperature wet ashing of samples in Teflon® containers and measurement of boron in the resultant solution by inductively coupled plasma emission spectrometry.[43]

Absorption, Transport, Retention, and Excretion. Food boron, sodium borate, and boric acid are rapidly absorbed and are excreted largely in the urine. In 1941 Kent and McCance[44] did balance studies in humans given a 352 mg dose of boron as boric acid. At the end of 1 wk, >90% of the boron was recovered from the urine. Over 40 y later, Jansen et al.[45] fed six male volunteers a single dose of boric acid (750–1473 mg) as either a water solution or a 3% water-emulsifying ointment. After 96 h mean urinary recoveries for the two sources were 93.9% and 92.4%, respectively. More than 50% of the dose was eliminated during the first 24 h.

Very little is known about the mechanism by which boron is absorbed or transported in the body. Boron is distributed in tissues and organs of animals at concentrations mostly between 0.05 and 0.6 µg/g fresh weight. Several times these levels are found in bones.[46]

Biochemical Function. Many findings support the hypothesis that boron has a function that influences macromineral metabolism. Because boron affects steroid hormone metabolism in humans[42] and animals[47] and because the response to boron seems to be enhanced in nutritional disorders characterized by secondary hyperparathyroidism, i.e., magnesium deficiency[48] and aluminum toxicity,[49] it would not be surprising to find that boron affects mineral metabolism via a regulatory role involving a hormone. In plants boron is suspected of having a regulatory role involving such hormones as auxin, gibberellic acid, and cytokinin, perhaps through control of second messengers, such as calcium, at the cell-membrane level.[50]

The possibility that boron has a function at the cell membrane level is supported by a number of different findings. Some recent reviews[51–53] presented evidence consistent with the view that boron is directly associated with membranes and is involved in their functional efficiency in plants. Many symptoms of boron deficiency in plants appear to be secondary effects caused by changes in membrane permeability. In animals boron affects the response to magnesium[48,49] and potassium[54] deficiencies; these deficiencies affect membrane integrity.[55]

Boron stimulates RNA synthesis by rat liver.[56] RNA synthesis in plants is also stimulated by boron.[57] It has been hypothesized that boron has a fundamental role in pyrimidine metabolism because such a hypothesis unifies the seemingly separate roles of boron in plants.[58]

Deficiency Signs. The response to boron deprivation is affected by variables that affect macromineral metabolism. The reported signs of boron deficiency in animals vary in nature and severity as the diet is varied in content of calcium, phosphorus, magnesium, potassium, cholecalciferol, aluminum, and methionine.[1,27,28,39,47–49,54] The most consistent sign of deficiency is depressed growth. A recent study with postmenopausal women indicated that boron deprivation elevated urinary excretion of calcium and magnesium and depressed serum concentrations of 17β-estradiol and testosterone.[42]

Requirements, Allowances, and Sources. No boron requirement or allowance has been set for humans. A recent study with chicks indicated that this species requires ~1 µg boron/g diet,[59] and reports indicate that low dietary boron altered mineral metabolism in rats fed basal diets containing 0.3–0.4 µg boron/g.[47–49,54,59] Postmenopausal women responded to a boron supplement of 3 mg/d to a diet supplying 0.25 mg boron/d.[42] This suggests that humans might have a dietary boron requirement near 1 mg/d.

The daily intake of boron by humans can vary widely depending upon the proportions of various food groups in the diet.[39,60] Foods of plant origin, especially fruits, leafy vegetables, nuts, and legumes, are rich sources of boron. Wine, cider, and beer are also high in boron. Meat, fish, and dairy products are poor sources. A limited number of surveys indicate average daily intakes of boron of 0.5–3.1 mg/d.[60,61]

Toxicity. Boron has a low order of toxicity when administered orally. Excellent reviews of the toxicity of boron indicate that toxicity signs generally occur in animals only after the dietary boron concentration exceeds 100 μg/g.[62,63] In pigs weighing ~60 kg, 8 mg boron·kg^{-1}·d^{-1} detrimentally affected calcium metabolism.[64] The ~500 mg/d dose apparently resulted in osteoporosis associated with a reduction in parathyroid activity. In humans the signs of acute toxicity are well known and include nausea, vomiting, diarrhea, dermatitis, and lethargy.[63,65] In addition, high boron ingestion induces increased urinary excretion of riboflavin.[65]

Molybdenum

History. Evidence for the essentiality of molybdenum first appeared in 1953 when xanthine oxidase was identified as a molybdenum metalloenzyme. Subsequently, attempts to produce molybdenum deficiency in rats and chicks were successful only when the diet contained massive amounts of tungsten, an antagonist of molybdenum metabolism. These studies showed that the dietary requirement to maintain normal growth of animals was <1 μg molybdenum/g diet, a level substantially lower than requirements for other trace elements recognized as essential at the time. Thus, molybdenum was not considered to be of practical importance in animal and human nutrition. Consequently, relatively little effort has been devoted to the study of the metabolism and nutrition of molybdenum in monogastric animals or humans.

Method of Analysis. Inductively coupled plasma emission spectrometric methods have produced accurate measurements of molybdenum in biological material.[66]

Absorption, Transport, Retention, and Excretion. Molybdenum (except as MoS$_2$) in foods and in the form of soluble complexes is readily absorbed. In humans, between 25% and 80% of ingested molybdenum is absorbed. Studies with rats indicated that molybdenum absorption takes place in the stomach and small intestine, the rate of absorption being higher in the proximal than in the distal parts of the small intestine.[67] Whether an active or a passive

mechanism is more important in the absorption of molybdenum is uncertain. One study produced evidence indicating that at low concentrations of molybdenum, absorption was carrier-mediated and active.[68] Another study showed that in vivo absorption rates were essentially the same over a 10-fold range of molybdenum concentrations.[69] This finding and the finding that the rates of absorption in both stomach and small intestine were high suggest that molybdate is absorbed via diffusion. Winston[67] raised the possibility that molybdate is absorbed by diffusion and by active transport, but at high concentrations the relative intensity of the latter is small. The absorption and retention of molybdenum are influenced markedly by interactions between molybdenum and various dietary forms of sulfur.[70] Evidence suggests that molybdenum in blood and urine exists mainly as the molybdate ion (MoO$_4^{2-}$).[67] In blood much of the molybdate is loosely attached to the erythrocytes and tends to specifically bind to α_2-macroglobulin.[71] Molybdate in food and water apparently is not radically changed by absorption and transport in the blood.

The liver retains the highest amounts of molybdenum. Skeleton and kidney also retain significant amounts.[67,70–72] Unlike the situation in blood, it is unknown whether inorganic molybdenum is present to any extent in cells.[73] The molybdenum in liver was found to be entirely present in macromolecular association, part as known molybdoenzymes and the remainder as a pool of molybdenum cofactor.[74] Over 50% of the nonenzymatic form of molybdenum in the liver exists as the cofactor bound to the mitochondrial outer membrane. This cofactor can be transferred to an apoenzyme of xanthine oxidase or sulfite oxidase, transforming it into an active enzyme molecule. The molybdenum cofactor has been identified as di-(carboxamido-methyl) molybdopterin, which is a 5,6,7,8-tetrahydropterin.[75]

After absorption most molybdenum is rapidly turned over and eliminated as molybdate via the kidney, indicating that this, rather than regulated absorption, is the major homeostatic mechanism for this element. However, significant amounts of molybdenum also are excreted in bile.[71]

Biochemical Functions. Molybdenum functions as an enzyme cofactor.[73,74] Animal molybdoenzymes catalyze the hydroxylation of substrates using the elements of water.[76] Aldehyde oxidase oxidizes and detoxifies various pyrimidines, purines, pteridines, and related compounds. Xanthine oxidase (dehydrogenase) catalyzes the transformation of hypoxanthine to xanthine and xanthine to uric acid. Sulfite oxidase catalyzes the transformation of sulfite to sulfate.

In addition to an enzyme cofactor, evidence suggests that molybdenum as molybdate might have an important physiological function in stabilizing the steroid-binding ability of the unoccupied glucocorticoid receptor. During isolation procedures molybdate protects steroid hormone receptors, particularly the glucocorticoid receptor, against inactivation.[77] It is hypothesized, however, that molybdate affects the glucocorticoid receptor because it mimics an endogenous compound called modulator.[78]

Deficiency Signs. The signs of molybdenum deficiency have been reviewed by Mills and Bremner.[79] In rats and chickens molybdenum deficiency aggravated by excessive dietary tungsten results in the depression of molybdenum enzymes, disturbances in uric acid metabolism, and increased susceptibility to sulfite toxicity. Under field conditions a molybdenum-responsive syndrome was found in hatching chicks. This syndrome was characterized by a high incidence of late embryonic mortality, mandibular distortion, anophthalmia, and defects in leg bone development and feathering. Skeletal lesions, subsequently detected in older birds, included separation of the proximal epiphysis of the femur, osteolytic changes in the femoral shaft, and lesions in the overlying skin that were ultimately attributed to intense irritation in these areas. The incidence of this syndrome was particularly high in commercial flocks reared on diets containing high concentrations of copper (a molybdenum antagonist) as a growth stimulant. These apparently dissimilar pathologic changes were suggested to be caused by a defect in sulfur metabolism.

Deficiency uncomplicated by high dietary tungsten or copper was produced in goats and pigs fed diets containing <60 ng molybdenum/g.[80] Deficiency signs were depressed feed consumption and growth, impaired reproduction characterized by elevated mortality in both mothers and offspring, and elevated copper concentrations in liver and brain.

Evidence of the role of molybdenum as a component of sulfite oxidase and that sulfite oxidase deficiency markedly deranges cysteine metabolism resulted in the recognition of human disorders caused by the lack of functioning molybdenum. A genetic deficiency of sulfite oxidase was identified in humans; this deficiency is characterized by severe brain damage, mental retardation, and dislocation of ocular lenses, and results in increased urinary output of sulfite, S-sulfocysteine, and thiosulfate and a marked decrease in sulfate output.[73] A patient receiving prolonged total parenteral nutrition therapy acquired a syndrome described as acquired molybdenum deficiency.[81] This syndrome, exacerbated by methionine administration, was characterized by hypermethioninemia, hypouricemia, hyperoxypurinemia, hypouricosuria, and very low urinary sulfate excretion. In addition, the patient suffered mental disturbances

that progressed to coma. The symptoms were indicative of a defect in sulfur amino acid metabolism at the level of sulfite oxidation to sulfate (sulfite oxidase deficiency) and a defect in uric acid production at the level of xanthine and hypoxanthine transformation to uric acid (xanthine oxidase deficiency). Supplementation of the patient with ammonium molybdate improved the clinical condition, reversed the sulfur handling defect, and normalized uric acid production.

Low dietary molybdenum might also be detrimental to human health and well-being in the detoxification of xenobiotic compounds. Molybdenum deprivation depresses the activity of the molybdenum hydroxylases (see above) without any apparent overall detrimental effect in animals; perhaps the same phenomenon occurs in humans. It seems possible that low molybdenum hydroxylase activity would have undesirable consequences when a person or animal is stressed by high intakes of xenobiotics. This possibility does not seem to have been examined closely. The molybdenum hydroxylases apparently are as important as the microsomal monooxygenase system in the metabolism of drugs and foreign compounds.[76]

Requirements, Allowances, and Sources. Minimum dietary requirements for molybdenum to maintain optimal health and performance of animals and humans are unknown. Deficiency studies not utilizing molybdenum antagonists have not been helpful for determining dietary requirement of molybdenum because, although molybdoenzyme levels are affected, health and performance are not noticeably altered. Thus, human requirements can be estimated only from balance studies. The National Research Council[82] estimated that an adequate and safe intake of molybdenum is 75–250 μg/d. As with other elements, the daily intake of molybdenum varies depending upon the composition of the diet. Recent surveys indicate that the daily intake of molybdenum is 50–350 μg.[83–85] However, most diets apparently supply ~50–100 μg molybdenum/d; these levels barely meet the lowest suggested safe and adequate level of intake (75 μg/d). The richest food sources of molybdenum include milk and milk products, dried legumes, organ meats (liver and kidney), cereals, and baked goods. The poorest sources of molybdenum include vegetables other than legumes, fruits, sugars, oils, fat, and fish.

Toxicity. Large oral doses are necessary to overcome the homeostatic control of molybdenum. Thus, molybdenum is a relatively nontoxic element; in nonruminants an intake of 100–5000 mg/kg of food or water is required to produce clinical toxicity symptoms.[67,70] Ruminants are more susceptible to elevated dietary molybdenum. The mechanisms behind molybdenum toxicity need further clarification. However, many of the signs are similar or identical to those of copper deficiency or indicate abnormal sulfur metabolism.[67,70] Both occupational and high dietary exposure to molybdenum have been linked through epidemiologic methods to elevated uric acid in blood and increased incidence of gout.

Nickel

History. Although nickel was first suggested to be an essential element for animals in 1936, conclusive evidence for essentiality did not appear until 1970–1975.[1,28,86] However, early studies were conducted under conditions that produced suboptimal growth in experimental animals.[28,86] Since 1975, diets and environments that allow optimal growth and survival of experimental animals have been used in nickel nutrition and metabolism. Thus, most significant findings supporting the nutritional essentiality of nickel have appeared after 1975.

Method of Analysis. The determination of nickel in biological material after appropriate collection and preparation is most precisely done with great analytical sensitivity through the use of electrothermal atomic absorption spectrometry.[87]

Absorption, Transport, Retention, and Excretion. When ingested with diet, most nickel remains unabsorbed by the gastrointestinal tract. Limited studies suggest that <10% of nickel ingested with food is absorbed.[86,88,89] However, a much higher percentage, up to 50% of the dose, is absorbed when nickel is ingested in water after an overnight fast.[88,89] Nickel absorption apparently is also enhanced by iron deficiency,[90] gravidity,[91] and lactation.[92] For example, pigs absorbed >19% of nickel ingested from day 21 of gravidity until parturition.[91]

The mechanisms involved in the transport of nickel through the gut are not conclusively established. Becker et al.[93] reported that the transport of nickel across the mucosal epithelium apparently is an energy-driven process rather than simple diffusion and suggested that nickel ions use the iron transport system located in the proximal part of the small intestine. On the other hand, Foulkes and McMullen[94] presented evidence that indicates no existence of a specific nickel carrier mechanism at the brush border membrane; thus nickel absorption probably depends upon the efficiency of mucosal trapping through charge neutralization on the membrane. This suggests that nickel crosses the basolateral membrane through passive leakage or diffusion, perhaps in the form of an amino acid or other low-molecular-weight complex. The passage as a lipophilic complex is a possibility, because nickel affects the absorption of ferric ions, which probably traverse biomembranes as lipophilic complexes.[95] Oral intakes of lipophilic nickel-pyridinethione complexes markedly increased the concentrations of nickel in tissues of mice.[96]

The extracellular transport of nickel is probably through a variety of ligands; however, the principal ligand in blood apparently is serum albumin.[97] The remaining nickel in serum is associated with the amino acid L-histidine[97] and with α_2-macroglobulin.[98]

No tissue significantly accumulates orally administered physiological doses of nickel. Recently reported reference values for nickel concentrations in some human tissues are (mean μg/kg dry weight) lung, 173; thyroid, 141; adrenal, 132; kidney, 62; heart, 54; liver, 50; brain, 44; spleen, 37; and pancreas, 34.[99] The physiological significance of the relatively high nickel concentrations in thyroid and adrenal glands is unknown.

Although fecal nickel excretion (mostly unabsorbed nickel) is 10–100 times as great as urinary excretion, the small fraction of nickel absorbed from the intestine and transported to the plasma is rapidly excreted via the kidney as urinary low-molecular-weight complexes.[97,100] In human renal cytosol the low-molecular-weight fraction contains two nickel-binding components; these are anionic oligosaccharides that bind 70% of the nickel and an acidic peptide that binds the remaining 30%.[100] High-molecular-weight proteins ranging from 10 to 13 kDa were also fractionated from renal cytosol and microsomes.[101] The role of these proteins in the renal handling of nickel needs clarification.

Although urine is the major excretory route of nickel, significant amounts are lost through sweat and bile. The nickel content of sweat is high,[102] indicating active nickel secretion by the sweat glands. The loss of nickel through the bile has been estimated at 2–5 μg/d.[99]

Biochemical Function. No evidence clearly defines the biochemical function of nickel in higher animals. However, it seems possible that nickel functions as a cofactor or structural component in specific metalloenzymes. This hypothesis is supported by the discovery of nickel-containing enzymes in plants and microorganisms. Several reviews described the four kinds of nickel-containing enzymes, which are urease, hydrogenase, methylcoenzyme M reductase, and carbon monoxide dehydrogenase.[103–105] Walsh and Orme-Johnson[105] in their review stated that it is not clear why Ni^{2+} is used in place of Zn^{2+} in urease. However, there is no other biologically available metal that could replace nickel in the other three enzymes where nickel redox chemistry most likely is involved in biohydrogenation catalysis, reductive biodesulfurization catalysis, and biocarboxylation.

The finding of the 3^+ oxidation state of nickel, which apparently is essential for the biohydrogenation, biodesulfurization, and biocarboxylation reactions in mostly anaerobic microorganisms, does not seem very likely in aerobic organisms. However, some of the redox action of nickel might involve the 1^+ oxidation state of nickel, especially that of methyl-CoM reductase.[104,105] This oxidation state might occur more easily in aerobic organisms. Moreover, nickel acts in a structural manner in some of the studied enzymes[106] and possibly is required for the transcription of hydrogenase-related genes.[107] These three facts plus the need for Ni^{2+} for urease activity make the finding of some mammalian nickel-containing enzyme quite plausible. Other interesting possibilities for such a finding follow.

Ni^{2+} is a potent in vitro activator of calcineurin, a Ca^{2+} and calmodulin-dependent phosphoprotein phosphatase.[108] The high concentration of Ni^{2+} required for the activation of calcineurin suggests that activation may not occur in vivo. However, it is possible that the presence of certain factors and a high affinity of calcineurin for nickel could result in an important role for nickel in the action of calcineurin in vivo.

Fishelson et al.[109,110] found that Ni^{2+} could replace Mg^{2+} and was more efficient than Mg^{2+} in the formation of the two C3 convertases of the complement system—C3b, Bb of the alternative pathway, and C4b, 2a of the classical pathway. α_2-Macroglobulin, which contains nickel, complexes with C3 convertase.[98] Fixation of nickel in the C3b, Bb (Ni) complex and binding of the complex to serum α_2-macroglobulin were suggested as a possible explanation for the presence of nickel in a specific subclass of α_2-macroglobulin, i.e., nickeloplasmin.[98]

Recent reports indicate that vitamin B-12 status affects the signs of nickel deprivation in the rat or that vitamin B-12 must be present for optimal nickel function.[27,111] Thus, nickel may have a function in higher animals that involves a pathway utilizing vitamin B-12.

Deficiency Signs. The reported signs of nickel deprivation for six animal species—chick, cow, goat, pig, rat, and sheep—are extensive and have been listed in several reviews.[28,86,91,112,113] Unfortunately, the described signs probably will have to be redefined because recent studies indicate that many of the reported signs of nickel deprivation may be manifestations of pharmacological actions of nickel.[114,115] That is, a high dietary level of nickel was alleviating an abnormality caused by something other than a nutritional deficiency of nickel or was causing a change in a variable that was not necessarily subnormal. In many studies in which the nickel-deprived animals were compared with controls fed 5–20 μg Ni/g diet, the iron content of the diet was inadequate. This is of concern because nickel can partially alle-viate many manifestations of iron deficiency by pharmacological mechanisms.[114,115]

The suggestion that some of the reported signs of nickel deprivation are misinterpreted manifestations of a pharmacological action does not necessarily detract from the conclusion that nickel is an essential element. The following signs apparently are representative of nickel deficiency. If nickel deficiency is severe, growth and hematopoiesis are depressed especially in marginally iron-adequate or in methyl-depleted animals. Iron utilization is impaired. The trace element profiles of femur and liver change. In the femur the concentrations of calcium and manganese are depressed and the concentrations of copper and zinc are elevated. As with other elements, the extent and severity of nickel deprivation signs are markedly affected by diet composition.[115]

Requirements, Allowances, and Sources. No nickel requirement or allowance has been set for humans. However, because nickel is essential for several animal species, it seems reasonable that nickel is required by humans also. Moreover, the nickel requirement of animals may indicate the amount of nickel required by humans. The suggested requirements for various animal species have ranged from 50 to 1000 μg/kg diet.[39,112,116] Analysis of available information indicates that most monogastric animals have a dietary nickel requirement of <200 μg/kg diet. This suggests that the dietary nickel requirement of humans would be <150 μg/d. Any requirement for nickel probably could be modified by a number of factors, including iron status,[114,115] methionine status,[27,111] pregnancy,[91] and contraceptive drugs.[117] Thus, recent reports indicating that diets often provide <150 μg/d (some ≤60 μg/d) are not particularly comforting.[31,84,118–120] Diets based on foods of animal origin and fats may be low in nickel. Rich sources of nickel include chocolate, nuts, dried beans and peas, and grains.[84,118–120]

Toxicity. Life-threatening toxicity of nickel through oral intake is unlikely. Because of excellent homeostatic regulation, nickel salts exert their toxic action mainly by gastrointestinal irritation and not by inherent toxicity. Generally, ≥250 μg nickel/g diet are required to produce signs of nickel toxicity (such as depressed growth) in rats, mice, chickens, rabbits, and monkeys.[116,121] If animal data can be extrapolated to humans, a daily dose of 250 mg of soluble nickel would produce toxic symptoms in humans.

Some findings, however, suggest that oral intake of nickel in moderate doses could adversely affect health under certain conditions. Moderate amounts of dietary nickel exacerbate signs of severe iron deficiency and copper deficiency in rats.[86,113–115] Nickel may act similarly in humans. Some evidence suggests that the ingestion of small amounts of nickel may be of greater importance than external contacts in maintaining eczema caused by nickel allergy. An oral dose as low as 0.6 mg nickel as nickel sulfate given with water to fasting subjects (thus nickel was highly available, see preceding section) produced a positive reaction in some nickel-sensitive individuals.[122] This dose is only a few times higher than the human daily requirement postulated from animal studies.

Silicon

History. Until 1972, silicon was generally considered to be nonessential except in some lower classes of organisms (diatoms, radiolarians, and sponges) in which silica serves a structural role. In 1972 the first substantial evidence was published that indicated that silicon is an essential element for chickens and rats.[123] Most of the limited studies on the biochemical, nutritional, and physiological roles of silicon have been published since 1974.

Method of Analysis. Inductively coupled argon plasma emission and graphite-furnace atomic absorption spectrometric methods have been used to obtain apparently accurate measures of silicon in biological material.[123–125]

Absorption, Transport, Retention, and Excretion. Little is known about the metabolism of silicon.[39] Increasing silicon intake increases urinary excretion up to fairly well-defined limits in humans, rats, and guinea pigs. However, the upper limits of urinary silicon excretion apparently are not determined exclusively by the excretory ability of the kidney, because urinary excretion can be elevated above these limits by peritoneal injections of silicon. Thus, the upper limits apparently are set by the rate and extent of silicon absorption from the gastrointestinal tract.

The form of dietary silicon determines whether it is well absorbed. In one study, humans absorbed only ~10% of a large single dose of an alumino-silicate compound but absorbed >70% of a single dose of methylsilanetriol salicylate, a drug used in the treatment of circulatory ischemias and osteoporosis. Further evidence that some forms of silicon, including that in food, are well absorbed is that in rats and humans urinary excretion can be a high percentage (close to 50%) of daily silicon intake. Silicon absorption has been found to be affected in rats by age, sex, and the activity of various endocrine glands. The mechanisms involved in the intestinal absorption of silicon are unknown.

Silicon is not protein bound in plasma; it is believed to exist in plasma almost entirely in the undissociated monomeric silicic acid form, $Si(OH)_4$.[123,126] The elimination of absorbed silicon is mainly via the urine,[126] where it probably exists as magnesium orthosilicate.[123]

Connective tissues, including aorta, trachea, tendon, bone, and skin, and its appendages contain much of the silicon that is retained in the body.[127] The high silicon content of connective tissues apparently is the result of its presence as an integral component of the glycosaminoglycans and their protein complexes that contribute to structural framework. The bound form of silicon has never been clearly identified. Silicon may be present in biological material as a silanolate (an ether or ester-like derivative of silicic acid). R_1-O-Si-O-R_2 or R_1-O-Si-O-Si-O-R_2 may be the form of silicon in its structural roles.

Biochemical Function. The distribution of silicon and the effect of silicon deficiency on the form and composition of connective tissue support the view that silicon functions as a biological cross-linking agent and thus contributes to the architecture and resilience of connective tissue.

Silicon is apparently required for maximal bone prolylhydroxylase activity.[127] Silicon also increases the activities of prolyl 4-hydroxylase, galactosyl-hydroxyllysyl glucosyltransferase, and lysyl oxidase (three enzymes catalyzing posttranslational modifications of collagen) in lungs of rats.[128] These findings suggest that silicon has an important role in bone and cartilage collagen biosynthesis.

Silicon is apparently involved in bone calcification;[127] however, the mechanism of involvement remains unclear. Some findings suggest a catalytic function for silicon. The marked influence of silicon on collagen and mucopolysaccharide formation and structure may result in its indirect influence on bone calcification. In support of this latter view is the finding, in silicon-deficient animals, that the formation of organic matrix, whether cartilage or bone, is apparently more impaired than the mineralization process.[127]

Recently, it was found that silicon affects gene expression in some diatoms.[129] Perhaps this functional aspect should be examined in higher animals.

Deficiency Signs. Most of the signs of silicon deficiency in chickens and rats indicate aberrant metabolism of connective tissue and bone.[127] Chicks fed a semisynthetic, silicon-deficient diet exhibited skull-structure abnormalities associated with depressed collagen content in bone and long-bone abnormalities characterized by small, poorly formed joints and defective endochondral bone growth. Tibias of silicon-deficient chicks exhibit depressed contents of articular cartilage, water, hexosamine, and collagen. In optimally growing chickens, growth is not significantly retarded by silicon deficiency.

More work is needed to clarify the consequences of silicon deficiency in humans. This need has not prevented speculation that the lack of silicon is involved in the causation of several human disorders, including atherosclerosis, osteoarthritis, and hypertension, as well as the aging process.[39] Those speculations indicate the need for studying the importance of silicon in nutrition especially in aging humans.

Requirements, Allowances, and Sources. Although the essentiality of silicon was suggested almost 20 y ago, the form of silicon needed and the minimum requirement for it have not been ascertained for any animal; therefore little can be said about possible human requirements. Deficiency signs in chickens were prevented by 100–200 μg silicon as sodium silicate/g diet or ~26–52 mg/1000 kcal of an experimental diet.[1] However, other silicon compounds might be 5–10 times more effective, per atom of silicon, in preventing nutritional deficiency.[130] Thus, if humans have a requirement for silicon, it probably is in the range of 5–20 mg/d. This range is similar to the reported average daily intake of silicon.

Total dietary silicon intake of humans varies greatly with the amounts and proportions of foods of animal (silicon low) and plant (silicon high) origin consumed and with the amounts of refined and processed foods in the diet.[1] The richest sources of silicon are unrefined grains of high fiber content, cereal products, and root vegetables. The average British diet has been estimated to supply 31 mg silicon/d.[124] A human balance study[125] indicated that the oral intake of silicon could be ~21–46 mg/d.

Toxicity. Silicon is essentially nontoxic when taken orally. Evidence for its nontoxicity is the observation that magnesium trisilicate, an over-the-counter antacid, has been used by humans for >40 y without obvious deleterious effects. Other silicates are food additives used as anticaking or antifoaming agents.[131] However, ruminants consuming plants with a high silicon content may develop siliceous renal calculi. Renal calculi in humans may also contain silicates.[127]

Vanadium

History. The hypothesis that vanadium may be an essential element for higher animals has had a long and inconclusive history. In 1950 Bertrand[132] stated that "we are completely ignorant of the physiological role of vanadium in animals, where its presence is constant." In 1949 Rygh[133] reported that vanadium might be needed by animals because vanadium markedly stimulated the mineralization of bones and teeth and prevented caries formation in rats and guinea pigs. In 1963 Schroeder et al.[134] stated that although vanadium behaves like an essential trace metal, final proof of essentiality for mammals is still lacking. Between 1971 and 1974, a number of findings led many to conclude that vanadium is an essential nutrient.[1,28,135] Recently, however, a con-

vincing argument indicated that most evidence presented as proof for the essentiality of vanadium is nothing more than evidence showing the very active in vitro and pharmacologic properties of vanadium.[115,135] It seems that the statement of Schroeder et al.[134] that "no other trace metal has so long had so many supposed biological activities without having been proved to be essential" still holds true today. However, the recent discovery of vanadium-containing enzymes in plants and microorganisms supports the concept that vanadium is an essential nutrient for higher animals. Therefore, some of the nutritional and metabolic aspects of vanadium from the voluminous literature, mainly about the in vitro and pharmacological actions of vanadium, are presented here.

Method of Analysis. Both neutron activation analysis[136] and graphite furnace atomic absorption spectrometry[137] have been used to obtain apparently accurate measures of vanadium in biological material.

Absorption, Transport, Retention, and Excretion. Limited information exists about metabolism of physiological amounts of vanadium in animals. Nonetheless, it is apparent that most ingested vanadium is unabsorbed and is excreted via the feces.[39,138] On the basis of the estimated daily vanadium intake, the very low concentrations of vanadium normally found in urine, and the fecal level of vanadium, apparently <5% of vanadium ingested is absorbed. However, more evidence is needed to confirm this because two studies with rats indicated much greater vanadium absorption (>30%) from the intestine.[139,140] Dietary composition and the chemical form of vanadium probably affect the percentage of ingested vanadium absorbed from the intestine. Regardless, the rat studies suggest caution in assuming that ingested vanadium will always be poorly absorbed from the gastrointestinal tract.

The chemistry of vanadium is complex because the element can exist in oxidation states from 1^- to 5^+ and can form polymers. The tetravalent (VO^{2+}) and pentavalent (VO_2^+, $H_2VO_4^-$, or more simply VO_3^-) forms are the most important in biological systems.

Evidence suggests that the binding of the vanadyl ion (VO^{2+}) to iron-containing proteins is important in vanadium metabolism.[141–143] Regardless of the oxidation state administered to animals, vanadium apparently is converted into vanadyl-transferrin and vanadyl-ferritin complexes in plasma and body fluids.[141–143] If vanadate (VO_3^-) appears in the blood, it is quickly converted to vanadyl, most likely in the erythrocytes.[143] It remains to be determined whether ferritin is a storage vehicle for vanadium as well as for iron in the liver and whether vanadyl-transferrin can transfer vanadium through the transferrin receptor. A review of recent analyses using reliable techniques indicates that very little vanadium is retained in the body under normal conditions; most tissues contain <10 ng vanadium/g wet weight.[138] However, tissue vanadium is markedly elevated in animals fed high dietary vanadium. In rats, liver vanadium increased from 10 to 55 ng vanadium/g wet weight when dietary vanadium was increased from 0.1 to 25 μg/g.[139] In sheep, bone vanadium increased from 220 to 3320 ng/g dry weight when dietary vanadium was increased from 10 to 220 μg/g.[144] Bone apparently is a major sink for retained vanadium. Rat tissue vanadium is affected also by age. In rats aged 21–115 d the vanadium concentration decreased in kidney, liver, lung, and spleen and increased in fat and bone.[145]

Biochemical Function. Because vanadium is such an active element in vitro and pharmacologically, there have been numerous biochemical and physiological functions suggested for it. Recently, a number of reviews appeared that discussed the evidence behind the suggestions that vanadium might have a role in the regulation of Na^+, K^+-ATPase, phosphoryl transfer enzymes, adenylate cyclase, and protein kinase.[1,39,135,138,146,147] They also discuss the possible role of vanadium as an enzyme cofactor in the form of vanadyl in hormone metabolism, glucose metabolism, lipid metabolism, and bone and tooth metabolism. However, no specific biochemical function has been identified for vanadium in higher animals. The recent discovery in lower forms of life of two enzymes that require vanadium lends credence to the possibility that vanadium has a similar role in higher animals. These enzymes are nitrogenase in bacteria,[148,149] which reduce dinitrogen to ammonia and bromoperoxidase in algae,[150,151] and in lichens,[152] which catalyze the oxidation of halide ions by hydrogen peroxide, thus facilitating the formation of a carbon-halogen bond.

The findings that some haloperoxidases require vanadium for activity make one wonder if it acts in a similar manner in higher organisms. The best known haloperoxidase in animals is thyroid peroxidase. Recently it was shown that vanadium deprivation in rats elevated thyroid weight and thyroid weight–body weight ratio and affected the response of thyroid peroxidase to changing dietary iodine.[153] Another finding that suggests that vanadium affects halogen metabolism is that in chicks dietary chloride reduces the toxicity of vanadium, and increasing dietary vanadium reduces plasma chloride concentrations.[154]

Deficiency Signs. Most of the deficiency signs reported for vanadium are questionable.[115,135] Recent studies suggest that the reported differences between vanadium-deprived and vanadium-supplemented animals were the consequences of high-vanadium supplements (10–100 times the amount normally found in the diet) that resulted in pharmacologic changes in suboptimally performing animals fed imbalanced diets. The diets used in vanadium-deprivation studies have had widely varying contents of protein, sulfur amino acids, ascorbic acid, iron, copper, and perhaps other nutrients that affect or can be affected by vanadium.

Recently, Anke et al.[155] reported some deficiency signs for goats. More than 50% of kids from goats fed 10 ng vanadium/g diet died between days 7 and 91 of life; some deaths were preceded by convulsions. In addition, skeletal deformations were seen in the forelegs, and forefoot tarsal joints were thickened. Confirmation of these signs is needed because control diets contained high, probably pharmacologic, amounts of vanadium (2 μg/g).

Requirements, Allowances, and Sources. The failure to establish vanadium as an essential element prevents any suggestion of a vanadium requirement. If vanadium is essential, any human requirement likely would be very small. The diets used in animal deprivation studies contained only 4–25 ng vanadium/g; these often did not markedly affect the animals. Recent surveys indicate dietary intakes of vanadium between 6 and 20 μg/d.[83,84,136,156] Foods rich in vanadium include shellfish, mushrooms, parsley, dill seed, black pepper, and some prepared foods.[39,136,137] Beverages, fats and oils, and fresh fruits and vegetables contain the least vanadium, ranging from <1 to 5 μg/g.

Toxicity. Vanadium can be a relatively toxic element. The threshold level for toxicity apparently is near 10–20 mg/d or 10–20 μg/g of diet.[138] Recent reviews indicate that the concentration of dietary vanadium that is toxic can be affected by dietary composition.[115,138] A number of substances can ameliorate vanadium toxicity, including ascorbic acid, EDTA, chromium, protein, ferrous iron, chloride, and perhaps aluminum hydroxide. Age and animal species also influence vanadium toxicity. From their in-depth study of vanadium toxicity, Proescher et al.[157] concluded that vanadium was a neurotoxic and a hemorrhagic-endotheliotoxic poison with a nephrotoxic, hepatotoxic, and probably a leukocytotoxic and hematotoxic component. Thus, it is not surprising that a variety of signs of vanadium toxicity exist and that they can vary among species and with dosage. Some of the more consistent signs include depressed growth, elevated organ vanadium, diarrhea, depressed food intake, and death. Excessive in vivo vanadium was suggested as a factor in manic-depressive illness.[158,159]

References

1. F.H. Nielsen (1984) Ultratrace elements in nutrition. *Annu. Rev. Nutr.* 4:21–41.
2. F.H. Nielsen and E.O. Uthus (1984) Arsenic. In: *Biochemistry of the Essential Ultratrace Elements* (E. Frieden, ed.), pp. 319–340, Plenum, New York.
3. E.O. Uthus, M.E. Collings, W.E. Cornatzer, and F.H. Nielsen (1981) Determination of total arsenic in biological samples by arsine generation and atomic absorption spectrometry. *Anal. Chem.* 53:2221–2224.
4. W.J. Wang, S. Hanamura, and J.D. Winefordner (1986) Determination of arsenic by hydride generation with a long absorption cell for atomic absorption spectrometry. *Anal. Chim. Acta* 184:213–218.
5. M. Vahter (1983) Metabolism of arsenic. In: *Biological and Environmental Effect of Arsenic* (B.A. Fowler, ed.), pp. 171–198, Elsevier, Amsterdam.
6. H. Lanz, Jr., P.C. Wallace, and J.G. Hamilton (1950) The metabolism of arsenic in laboratory animals with As74 as a tracer. *Univ. Calif. Publ. Pharmacol.* 2:263–282.
7. M. Vahter, E. Marafante, A. Lindgren, and L. Dencker (1982) Tissue distribution and subcellular binding of arsenic in marmoset monkeys after injection of 74As-arsenite. *Arch. Toxicol.* 51:65–77.
8. M. Vahter and E. Marafante (1985) Reduction and binding of arsenate in marmoset monkeys. *Arch. Toxicol.* 57:119–124.
9. E. Marafante and M. Vahter (1987) Solubility, retention, and metabolism of intratracheally and orally administered inorganic arsenic compounds in the hamster. *Environ. Res.* 42:72–82.
10. H. Yamauchi, T. Kaise, and Y. Yamamura (1986) Metabolism and excretion of orally administered arsenobetaine in the hamster. *Bull. Environ. Contam. Toxicol.* 36:350–355.
11. E. Marafante, M. Vahter, and L. Dencker (1984) Metabolism of arsenocholine in mice, rats and rabbits. *Sci. Total Environ.* 34:223–240.
12. H. Yamauchi and Y. Yamamura (1984) Metabolism and excretion of orally administered dimethylarsinic acid in the hamster. *Toxicol. Appl. Pharmacol.* 74:134–140.
13. E.W. McChesney, J.O. Hoppe, P. McAuliff, and W.F. Banks, Jr. (1962) Toxicity and physiological disposition of sodium *p*-N-glycolylarsanilate. I. Observations in mouse, cat, rat and man. *Toxicol. Appl. Pharmacol.* 4:14–23.
14. C.S. Fullmer and R.H. Wasserman (1985) Intestinal absorption of arsenate in the chick. *Environ. Res.* 36:206–217.
15. S.W. Hwang and L.S. Schanker (1973) Absorption of organic arsenical compounds from the rat small intestine. *Xenobiotica* 3:351–355.
16. M. Vahter and J. Envall (1983) *In vivo* reduction of arsenate in mice and rabbits. *Environ. Res.* 32:14–24.
17. E. Marafante and M. Vahter (1984) The effect of methyltransferase inhibition on the metabolism of (74As) arsenite in mice and rabbits. *Chem. Biol. Interact.* 50:49–57.
18. J.P. Buchet and R. Lauwerys (1985) Study of inorganic arsenic methylation by rat liver in vitro: relevance for the interpretation of observations in man. *Arch. Toxicol.* 57:125–129.
19. J.P. Buchet and R. Lauwerys (1987) Study of factors influencing the *in vivo* methylation of inorganic arsenic in rats. *Toxicol. Appl. Pharmacol.* 91:65–74.
20. M. Vahter and E. Marafante (1987) Effects of low dietary intake of methionine, choline or proteins on the biotransformation of arsenite in the rabbit. *Toxicol. Lett.* 37:41–46.
21. M. Vahter, E. Marafante, and L. Dencker (1983) Metabolism of arsenobetaine in mice, rats and rabbits. *Sci. Total Environ.* 30:197–211.
22. H. Yamauchi and Y. Yamamura (1983) Concentration and chemical species of arsenic in human tissue. *Bull. Environ. Contam. Toxicol.* 31:267–270.
23. G.K.H. Tam, S.M. Charbonneau, F. Bryce, C. Pomroy, and E. Sandi (1979) Metabolism of inorganic arsenic (74As) in humans following oral ingestion. *Toxicol. Appl. Pharmacol.* 50:319–322.
24. N. Yamato (1988) Concentrations and chemical species of arsenic in human urine and hair. *Bull. Environ. Contam. Toxicol.* 40:633–640.
25. H. Yamauchi and Y. Yamamura (1985) Metabolism and excretion of orally administered arsenic trioxide in the hamster. *Toxicology* 34:113–121.
26. H.J. Almquist and C.R. Grau (1944) Interrelation of methionine, choline, betaine and arsenocholine in the chick. *J. Nutr.* 27:263–269.
27. F.H. Nielsen (1988) Possible future implications of ultratrace elements in human health and disease. In: *Essential and Toxic Trace Elements in Human Health and Disease, Current Topics in Nutrition and Disease,* vol. 18 (A.S. Prasad, ed.), pp. 277–292, Liss, New York.
28. F.H. Nielsen (1982) Possible future implications of nickel, arsenic, silicon, vanadium, and other ultratrace elements in human nutrition. In: *Clinical, Biochemical, and Nutritional Aspects of Trace Elements, Current Topics in Nutrition and Disease,* vol. 6 (A.S. Prasad, ed.), pp. 379–404, Liss, New York.
29. M. Anke (1986) Arsenic. In: *Trace Elements in Human and Animal Nutrition,* vol. 2 (W. Mertz, ed.), pp. 347–372, Academic Press, Orlando, FL.
30. A. Schmidt, M. Anke, B. Groppel, and H. Kronemann (1984) Effects of As-deficiency on skeletal muscle, myocardium and liver. A histochemical and ultrastructural study. *Exp. Pathol.* 25:195–197.
31. W.H. Evans and J.C. Sherlock (1987) Relationships between elemental intakes within the United Kingdom total diet study and other adult dietary studies. *Food Addit. Contam.* 4:1–8.
32. J.P. Buchet, R. Lauwerys, A. Vandevoorde, and J.P. Pycke (1983) Oral daily intake of cadmium, lead, manganese, copper, chromium, mercury, calcium, zinc and arsenic in Belgium: a duplicate meal study. *Food Chem. Toxicol.* 21:19–24.
33. H. Mykkänen, L. Räsänen, M. Ahola, and S. Kimppa (1986) Dietary intakes of mercury, lead, cadmium, and arsenic by Finnish children. *Hum. Nutr. Appl. Nutr.* 40A:32–39.
34. T. Kaise, S. Watanabe, and K. Itoh (1985) The acute toxicity of arsenobetaine. *Chemosphere* 14:1327–1332.
35. K.S. Squibb and B.A. Fowler (1983) The toxicity of arsenic and its compounds. In: *Biological and Environmental Effects of Arsenic* (B.A. Fowler, ed.), pp. 233–269, Elsevier, Amsterdam.
36. N. Ishinishi, K. Tsuchiya, M. Vahter, and B.A. Fowler (1986) Arsenic. In: *Handbook on the Toxicology of Metals,* 2nd ed., (L. Friberg, G.F. Nordberg, and V. Vouk, eds.)pp. 43–83, Elsevier, Amsterdam.
37. A. Furst (1983) A new look at arsenic carcinogenesis. In: *Arsenic: Industrial, Biomedical, Environmental Perspectives* (W.H. Lederer and R.J. Fensterheim, eds.), pp. 151–165, Van Nostrand Reinhold, New York.
38. D. Jacobson-Kram and D. Montalbano (1985) The reproductive effects assessment group's report on the mutagenicity of inorganic arsenic. *Environ. Mutagen.* 7:787–804.
39. F.H. Nielsen (1988) The ultratrace elements. In: *Trace Minerals in Foods* (K.T. Smith, ed.), pp. 357–428, Marcel Dekker, New York.
40. J.T. Skinner and J.S. McHargue (1945) Response of rats to boron supplements when fed rations low in potassium. *Am. J. Physiol.* 143:385–390.
41. R.H. Follis, Jr. (1947) The effect of adding boron to a potassium-deficient diet in the rats. *Am. J. Physiol.* 150:520–522.
42. F.H. Nielsen, C.D. Hunt, L.M. Mullen, and J.R. Hunt (1987) Effect

of dietary boron on mineral, estrogen, and testosterone metabolism in postmenopausal women. *FASEB J.* 1:394–397.

43. C.D. Hunt, E.S. Halas, and M.J. Eberhardt (1988) Long-term effects of lactational zinc deficiency on bone mineral composition in rats fed a commercially modified Luecke diet. *Biol. Trace Element Res.* 16:97–113.

44. N.L. Kent and R.A. McCance (1941) The absorption and excretion of "minor" elements by man. I. Silver, gold, lithium, boron, and vanadium. *Biochem. J.* 35:837–844.

45. J.A. Jansen, J.S. Schou, and B. Aggerbeck (1984) Gastro-intestinal absorption and *in vitro* release of boric acid from water-emulsifying ointments. *Food Chem. Toxicol.* 22:49–53.

46. F.H. Nielsen (1986) Other elements: Sb, Ba, B, Br, Cs, Ge, Rb, Ag, Sr, Sn, Ti, Zr, Be, Bi, Ga, Au, In, Nb, Sc, Te, Tl, W. In: *Trace Elements in Human and Animal Nutrition,* vol. 2 (W. Mertz, ed.), pp. 415–463, Academic Press, Orlando, FL.

47. C.D. Hunt and F.H. Nielsen (1981) Interaction between boron and cholecalciferol in the chick. In: *Trace Element Metabolism in Man and Animals,* vol. 4 (J.McC. Howell, J.M. Gawthorne, and C.L. White, eds.), pp. 597–600, Australian Academy of Science, Canberra.

48. F.H. Nielsen, T.R. Shuler, T.J. Zimmerman, and E.O. Uthus (1988) Magnesium and methionine deprivation affect the response of rats to boron deprivation. *Biol. Trace Element Res.* 17:91–107.

49. F.H. Nielsen, T.R. Shuler, T.J. Zimmerman, and E.O. Uthus (1988) Dietary magnesium, manganese and boron affect the response of rats to high dietary aluminum. *Magnesium* 7:133–147.

50. P.M. Tang and R.R. Dela Fuente (1986) Boron and calcium sites involved in indole-3-acetic acid transport in sunflower hypocotyl segments. *Plant Physiol.* 81:651–655.

51. D.J. Pilbeam and E.A. Kirkby (1983) The physiological role of boron in plants. *J. Plant Nutr.* 6:563–582.

52. A.J. Parr and B.C. Loughman (1983) Boron and membrane function in plants. *Annu. Proc. Phytochem. Soc. Eur.* 21:87–107.

53. H. Goldbach (1985) Influence of boron nutrition on net uptake and efflux of ^{32}P and ^{14}C-glucose in *Helianthus annuus* roots and cell cultures of *Daucus carota. J. Plant Physiol.* 118:431–438.

54. F.H. Nielsen, T.J. Zimmerman, and T.R. Shuler (1988) Dietary potassium affects the signs of boron and magnesium deficiency in the rat. *Proc. N.D. Acad. Sci.* 42:61.

55. M.P. Ryan and R. Whang (1983) Interrelationships between potassium and magnesium. In: *Potassium: Its Biologic Significance* (R. Whang and J.K. Aikawa, eds.), pp. 97–107, CRC Press, Boca Raton, FL.

56. U. Weser (1967) Stimulation of rat liver RNA synthesis by borate. *Proc. Soc. Exp. Biol. Med.* 126:669–671.

57. A.H.N. Ali and B.C. Jarvis (1988) Effects of auxin and boron on nucleic acid metabolism and cell division during adventitious root regeneration. *New Phytol.* 108:383–391.

58. C.J. Lovatt (1985) Evolution of xylem resulted in a requirement for boron in the apical meristems of vascular plants. *New Phytol.* 99:509–522.

59. C.D. Hunt (1988) Boron homeostasis in cholecalciferol-deficient chicks. *Proc. N.D. Acad. Sci.* 42:60.

60. D. Schlettwein-Gsell and S. Mommsen-Straub (1972) Übersicht Spurenelemente in Lebensmitteln. IX. Bor. *Int. Z. Vitam. Ernahrungsforsch.* [Beih.] 43:93–109.

61. P. Varo and P. Koivistoinen (1980) Mineral element composition of Finnish foods. XII. General discussion and nutritional evaluation. *Acta. Agricul. Scand.* 22(suppl.):165–171.

62. Anonymous (1980) Boron. In: *Mineral Tolerance of Domestic Animals,* pp. 71–83, National Academy Press, Washington, D.C.

63. Life Sciences Research Office (1980) *Evaluation of the Health Aspects of Borax and Boric Acid as Food Packaging Ingredients,* Federation of American Societies of Experimental Biology, Bethesda, MD.

64. J. Franke, H. Runge, R. Bech, et al. (1985) Boron as an antidote to fluorosis? Part I: Studies on the skeletal system. *Fluoride* 18:187–197.

65. J. Pinto, Y.P. Huang, R.J. McConnell, and R.S. Rivlin (1978) Increased urinary riboflavin excretion resulting from boric acid ingestion. *J. Lab. Clin. Med.* 92:126–134.

66. F.A. Ward, L.F. Marciello, L. Carrara, and V.J. Luciano (1980) Simultaneous determination of major, minor, and trace elements in agricultural and biological samples by inductively coupled argon plasma spectrometry. *Spect. Lett.* 13:803–831.

67. P.W. Winston (1981) Molybdenum. In: *Disorders of Mineral Metabolism* (F. Bronner and J.W. Coburn, eds.), vol. 1, pp. 295–315, Academic Press, New York.

68. C.J. Cardin and J. Mason (1976) Molybdate and tungstate transfer by rat ileum. Competitive inhibition by sulphate. *Biochim. Biophys. Acta* 455:937–946.

69. L.J. Kosarek and P.W. Winston (1977) Absorption of molybdenum-99 (Mo-99) as molybdate with various doses in the rat. *Fed. Proc.* 36:1106.

70. C.F. Mills and G.K. Davis (1987) Molybdenum. In: *Trace Elements in Human and Animal Nutrition* (W. Mertz, ed.), vol. 1, pp. 429–463, Academic Press, San Diego.

71. J. Lener and B. Bibr (1984) Effects of molybdenum on the organism (a review). *J. Hyg. Epidemiol. Microbiol. Immunol.* 28:405–419.

72. N.D. Grace and P.L. Martinson (1985) The distribution of Mo between the liver and other organs and tissues of sheep grazing a ryegrass white clover pasture. In: *Trace Elements in Man and Animals—TEMA 5* (C.F. Mills, I. Bremner, and J.K. Chesters, eds.), pp. 534–536, Commonwealth Agricultural Bureaux, Farnham Royal.

73. K.V. Rajagopalan (1988) Molybdenum: An essential trace element in human nutrition. *Annu. Rev. Nutr.* 8:401–427.

74. J.L. Johnson, H.P. Jones, and K.V. Rajagopalan (1977) In vitro reconstitution of demolybdosulfite oxidase by a molybdenum cofactor from rat liver and other sources. *J. Biol. Chem.* 252:4994–5003.

75. S.P. Kramer, J.L. Johnson, A.A. Ribeiro, D.S. Millington, and K.V. Rajagopalan (1987) The structure of the molybdenum cofactor. *J. Biol. Chem.* 262:16357–16363.

76. C. Beedham (1985) Molybdenum hydroxylases as drug-metabolizing enzymes. *Drug Metab. Rev.* 16:119–156.

77. P. Blanchardie, P. Lustenberger, J.L. Orsonneau, M. Denis, and S. Bernard (1984) Influence of molybdate, ionic strength and pH on ligand binding to the glucocorticoid receptor. *Steroids* 44:159–174.

78. P.V. Bodine and G. Litwack (1988) Evidence that the modulator of the glucocorticoid-receptor complex is the endogenous molybdate factor. *Proc. Natl. Acad. Sci. USA* 85:1462–1466.

79. C.F. Mills and I. Bremner (1980) Nutritional aspects of molybdenum in animals. In: *Molybdenum and Molybdenum-Containing Enzymes* (M.P. Coughlan, ed.), pp. 517–542, Pergamon, Oxford.

80. M. Anke, B. Groppel, and M. Grün (1985) Essentiality, toxicity, requirement and supply of molybdenum in human and animals. In: *Trace Elements in Man and Animals—TEMA 5* (C.F. Mills, I. Bremner, and J.K. Chesters, eds.), pp. 154–157, Commonwealth Agricultural Bureaux, Farnham Royal.

81. N.N. Abumrad, A.J. Schneider, D. Steel, and L.S. Rogers (1981) Amino acid intolerance during prolonged total parenteral nutrition reversed by molybdate therapy. *Am. J. Clin. Nutr.* 34:2551–2559.

82. National Research Council (1989) *Recommended Dietary Allowances,* 10th ed., National Academy Press, Washington, DC.

83. W.H. Evans, J.I. Read, and D. Caughlin (1985) Quantification of results for estimating elemental dietary intakes of lithium, rubidium, strontium, molybdenum, vanadium and silver. *Analyst* 110:873–877.

84. J.A.T. Pennington and J.W. Jones (1987) Molybdenum, nickel, cobalt, vanadium and strontium in total diets. *J. Am. Diet. Assoc.* 87:1644–1650.

85. K. Shiraishi, Y. Yamagami, K. Kameoka, and H. Kawamura (1988) Mineral contents in model diet samples for different age groups. *J. Nutr. Sci. Vitaminol. (Tokyo)* 34:55–65.

86. F.H. Nielsen (1984) Nickel. In: *Biochemistry of the Essential Ultratrace Elements* (E. Frieden, ed.), pp. 293–308, Plenum, New York.

87. F.W. Sunderman, Jr., S.M. Hopfer, and M.C. Crisostomo (1988) Nickel analysis by electrothermal atomic absorption spectrometry. *Methods Enzymol.* 158:382–391.

88. N.W. Solomons, F. Viteri, T.R. Shuler, and F.H. Nielsen (1982) Bioavailability of nickel in man. Effects of foods and chemically-defined dietary constituents on the absorption of inorganic nickel. *J. Nutr.* 112:39–50.

89. F.W. Sunderman, Jr., S.M. Hopfer, T. Swift, et al. (1988) Nickel absorption and elimination in human volunteers. In: *Trace Element Metabolism in Man and Animals-TEMA 6,* Plenum, New York.

90. F.H. Nielsen (1983) Studies on the interaction between nickel and iron during intestinal absorption. In: *4. Spurenelement-Symposium* (M. Anke, W. Bauman, H. Braünlich, and C. Brückner, eds.), pp. 11–18, Friedrich-Schiller-Universitat, Jena.

91. M. Kirchgessner, D.A. Roth-Maier, and A. Schnegg (1981) Progress of nickel metabolism and nutrition research. In: *Trace Element Metabolism in Man and Animals—TEMA 4* (J. McC. Howell, J.M. Gawthorne, and C.L. White, eds.), pp. 621–624, Australian Academy of Science, Canberra.

92. M. Kirchgessner, D.A. Roth-Maier, and R. Spörl (1983) Spurenelementbilanzen (Cu, Zn, Ni and Mn) laktierender Sauen. *Z. Tierphysiol. Tierernhr. Futtermittelkd.* 50:230–239.

93. G. Becker, U. Dörstelmann, U. Frommberger, and W. Forth (1980) On the absorption of cobalt (II)- and nickel (II)-ions by isolated intestinal segments in vitro of rats. In: *3. Spurenelement-Symposium, Nickel* (M. Anke, H.-J. Schneider, and C. Brückner, eds.), pp. 79–85, Friedrich-Schiller-Universitat, Jena.

94. E.C. Foulkes and D.M. McMullen (1986) On the mechanism of nickel absorption in the rat jejunum. *Toxicology* 38:35–42.

95. F.H. Nielsen (1980) Effect of form of iron on the interaction between nickel and iron in rats: growth and blood parameters. *J. Nutr.* 110:965–973.

96. S. Jasim and H. Tjälve (1986) Effect of sodium pyridinethione on the uptake and distribution of nickel, cadmium and zinc in pregnant and non-pregnant mice. *Toxicology* 38:327–350.

97. B. Sarkar (1985) Metal-protein interaction in transport, accumulation and excretory processes of metals. *Nutr. Res.* 1(suppl.): 489–498.

98. S. Nomoto and F.W. Sunderman, Jr. (1988) Presence of nickel in alpha-2 macroglobulin isolated from human serum by high performance liquid chromatography. *Ann. Clin. Lab. Sci.* 18:78–84.

99. W.N. Rezuke, J.A. Knight, and F.W. Sunderman, Jr. (1987) Reference values for nickel concentrations in human tissue and bile. *Am. J. Ind. Med.* 11:419–426.

100. D.M. Templeton and B. Sarkar (1986) Low molecular weight targets of metals in human kidney. *Acta. Pharmacol. Toxicol. (Copenh.)* 59(suppl.):416–423.

101. F.W. Sunderman, Jr., B.L.K. Mangold, S.H.Y. Wong, S.K. Shen, M.C. Reid, and I. Jansson (1983) High-performance size-exclusion chromatography of ^{63}Ni-constituents in renal cytosol and microsomes from ^{63}NiCl$_2$-treated rats. *Res. Commun. Chem. Pathol. Pharmacol.* 39:477–492.

102. J.R. Cohn and E.A. Emmett (1978) The excretion of trace metals in human sweat. *Ann. Clin. Lab. Sci.* 8:270–275.

103. R.K. Thauer (1985) Nickelenzyme in Stoffwechsel von methanogenen Bakterien. *Biol. Chem. Hoppe Seyler* 366:103–112.

104. R.P. Hausinger (1987) Nickel utilization by microorganisms. *Microbiol. Rev.* 51:22–42.

105. C.T. Walsh and W.H. Orme-Johnson (1987) Nickel enzymes. *Biochemistry* 26:4901–4906.

106. K. Schneider, R. Cammack, and H.G. Schlegel (1984) Content and localization of FMN, Fe-S clusters and nickel in the NAD-linked hydrogenase of *Nocardia opaca* 1b. *Eur. J. Biochem.* 142:75–84.

107. L.W. Stults, W.A. Sray, and R.J. Maier (1986) Regulation of hydrogenase biosynthesis by nickel in *Bradyrhizobium Japonicum.* *Arch. Microbiol.* 146:280–283.

108. C.J. Pallen and J.H. Wang (1986) Stoichiometry and dynamic interaction of metal ion activators with calcineurin phosphatase. *J. Biol. Chem.* 261:16115–16120.

109. Z. Fishelson and H.J. Müller-Eberhard (1982) C3 convertase of human complement: enhanced formation and stability of the enzyme generated with nickel instead of magnesium. *J. Immunol.* 129:2603–2607.

110. Z. Fishelson, M.K. Pangburn, and H.J. Müller-Eberhard (1983) C3 convertase of the alternative complement pathway. *J. Biol. Chem.* 258:7411–7415.

111. B. Brossart, T.J. Zimmerman, and F.H. Nielsen (1987) Interactions between nickel and vitamin B-12 in the methyl-depleted rat: effect on growth and blood indices. *Proc. N.D. Acad. Sci.* 41:87.

112. M. Anke, B. Groppel, H. Kronemann, and M. Grün (1984) Nickel—an essential element. In: *Nickel in the Human Environment* (F.W. Sunderman, ed.), pp. 339–365, International Agency for Research on Cancer, Lyon.

113. J.W. Spears (1984) Nickel as a "newer trace element" in the nutrition of domestic animals. *J. Anim. Sci.* 59:823–835.

114. F.H. Nielsen, T.R. Shuler, T.G. McLeod, and T.J. Zimmerman (1984) Nickel influences iron metabolism through physiologic, pharmacologic and toxicologic mechanisms in the rat. *J. Nutr.* 114:1280–1288.

115. F.H. Nielsen (1985) The importance of diet composition in ultratrace element research. *J. Nutr.* 115:1239–1247.

116. M. Kirchgessner, A. Reichlmayr-Lais, and R. Maier (1985) Ni retention and concentrations of Fe and Mn in tissues resulting from different Ni supply. In: *Trace Elements in Man and Animals—TEMA 5* (C.F. Mills, I. Bremner, and J.K. Chesters, eds.), pp. 147–151, Commonwealth Agricultural Bureaux, Farnham Royal.

117. S. Nayel, M. Zahran, A.A. Gawad, A. Mokhtar, S. Gawish, and G. El-Tabbakh (1986) Serum nickel concentration in normal menstrual cycle and after combined contraceptive pill. *Contraception* 34:395–401.

118. M.-A. Flyvholm, G.D. Nielsen, and A. Andersen (1984) Nickel content of food and estimation of dietary intake. *Z. Lebensm. Unters Forsch.* 179:427–431.

119. N.K. Veien and M.R. Andersen (1986) Nickel in Danish food. *Acta. Derm. Venereol. (Stockh.)* 66:502–509.

120. G.A. Smart and J.C. Sherlock (1987) Nickel in foods and the diet. *Food Addit. Contam.* 4:61–71.

121. F.H. Nielsen (1977) Nickel toxicity. In: *Advances in Modern Toxicology: Toxicology of Trace Elements*, vol. 2, (R.A. Goyer and M.A. Mehlman, eds.) pp. 129–146, Wiley, New York.

122. E. Cronin, A.D. Di Michiel, and S.S. Brown (1980) Oral challenges in nickel-sensitive women with hand eczema. In: *Nickel Toxicology* (S.S. Brown and F.W. Sunderman, Jr., eds.), pp. 149–152, Academic Press, New York.

123. E.M. Carlisle (1984) Silicon. In: *Biochemistry of the Essential Ultratrace Elements* (E. Frieden, ed.), pp. 257–291, Plenum, New York.

124. G.M. Berlyne, A.J. Adler, N. Ferran, S. Bennett, and J. Holt (1986) Silicon metabolism. I. Some aspects of renal silicon handling in normal men. *Nephron* 43:5–9.

125. H.J.M. Bowen and A. Peggs (1984) Determination of the silicon content of food. *J. Sci. Food Agric.* 35:1225–1229.

126. J.L. Kelsay, K.M. Behall, and E. Prather (1979) Effect of fiber from fruits and vegetables on metabolic responses of human subjects. II. Calcium, magnesium, iron and silicon balances. *Am. J. Clin. Nutr.* 32:1876–1880.

127. A.J. Adler, Z. Etzion, and G.M. Berlyne (1986) Uptake, distribution, and excretion of ^{31}silicon in normal rats. *Am. J. Physiol.* 251:E670–E673.

128. A. Poole, R. Myllyla, J.C. Wagner, and R.C. Brown (1985) Collagen biosynthesis enzymes in lung tissue and serum of rats with experimental silicosis. *Br. J. Exp. Pathol.* 66:567–575.

129. C.D. Reeves and B.E. Volcani (1985) Role of silicon in diatom metabolism. Messenger RNA and polypeptide accumulation patterns in synchronized cultures of *Cylindrotheca fusiformis*. *J. Gen. Microbiol.* 131:1735–1744.

130. K. Schwarz (1974) Recent dietary trace element research, exemplified by tin, fluorine, and silicon. *Fed. Proc.* 33:1748–1757.

131. R. Villota and J.G. Hawkes (1986) Food applications and the toxicological and nutritional implications of amorphous silicon dioxide. *CRC Crit. Rev. Food Sci. Nutr.* 23:289–321.

132. D. Bertrand (1950) Survey of contemporary knowledge of biogeochemistry. 2. The biogeochemistry of vanadium. *Bull. Am. Mus. Nat. Hist.* 94:403–456.

133. O. Rygh (1949) Recherches sur les oligo-éléments. II. De l'importance du thallium et du vanadium, du silicium et du fluor. *Bull. Soc. Chim. Biol. (Paris)* 31:1403–1407.

134. H.A. Schroeder, J.J. Balassa, and I.H. Tipton (1963) Abnormal trace metals in man-vanadium. *J. Chronic Dis.* 16:1047–1071.

135. B.R. Nechay, L.B. Nenninga, P.S.E. Nechay, et al. (1986) Role of vanadium in biology. *Fed. Proc.* 45:123–132.

136. A.R. Byrne and L. Kosta (1978) Vanadium in foods and in human body fluids and tissues. *Sci. Total Environ.* 10:17–30.

137. D.R. Myron, S.H. Givand, and F.H. Nielsen (1977) Vanadium content of selected foods as determined by flameless atomic absorption spectroscopy. *J. Agric. Food Chem.* 25:297–300.

138. F.H. Nielsen (1987) Vanadium. In: *Trace Elements in Human and Animal Nutrition*, 5th ed. (W. Mertz, ed.), pp. 275–300, Academic Press, San Diego.

139. J.D. Bodgen, H. Higashino, M.A. Lavenhar, J.W. Bauman, Jr., F.W. Kemp, and A. Aviv (1982) Balance and tissue distribution of vanadium after short-term ingestion of vanadate. *J. Nutr.* 112:2279–2285.

140. T.B. Wiegmann, H.D. Day, and R.V. Patak (1982) Intestinal absorption and secretion of radioactive vanadium ($^{48}VO_3^-$) in rats and effect of Al(OH)$_3$. *J. Toxicol. Environ. Health* 10:233–245.

141. E. Sabbioni and E. Marafante (1978) Metabolic patterns of vanadium in the rat. *Bioinorg. Chem.* 9:389–407.

142. E. Sabbioni and E. Marafante (1981) Relations between iron and vanadium metabolism: *in vivo* incorporation of vanadium into iron proteins of the rat. *J. Toxicol. Environ. Health* 8:419–429.

143. W.R. Harris, S.B. Friedman, and D. Silberman (1984) Behavior of vanadate and vanadyl ion in canine blood. *J. Inorg. Biochem.* 20:157–169.

144. S.L. Hansard, II, C.B. Ammerman, K.R. Fick, and S.M. Miller (1978) Performance and vanadium content of tissues in sheep as influenced by dietary vanadium. *J. Anim. Sci.* 46:1091–1095.

145. J. Edel, R. Pietra, E. Sabbioni, E. Marafante, A. Springer, and L. Ubertalli (1984) Disposition of vanadium in rat tissues at different ages. *Chemosphere* 13:87–93.

146. D.W. Boyd and K. Kustin (1984) Vanadium: a versatile biochemical effector with an elusive biological function. *Adv. Inorg. Biochem.* 6:311–365.

147. B.R. Nechay (1984) Mechanisms of action of vanadium. *Annu. Rev. Pharmacol. Toxicol.* 24:501–524.

148. B.J. Hales, E.E. Case, J.E. Morningstar, M.F. Dzeda, and L.A. Mauterer (1986) Isolation of a new vanadium-containing nitrogenase from *Azotobacter vinelandii*. *Biochemistry* 25:7251–7255.

149. B.E. Smith, F. Campbell, R.R. Eady, et al. (1987) Biochemistry of nitrogenase and the physiology of related metabolism. *Philos. Trans. R. Soc. Lond. [Biol.]* 317:131–146.

150. E. de Boer, M.G.M. Tromp, H. Plat, G.E. Krenn, and R. Wever (1986) Vanadium (V) as an essential element for haloperoxidase activity in marine brown algae: purification, and characterization of a vanadium (V)-containing bromoperoxidase from *Laminaria saccharina*. *Biochim. Biophys. Acta.* 872:104–115.

151. B.E. Krenn, H. Plat, and R. Wever (1987) The bromoperoxidase from the red alga *Ceramium rubrum* also contains vanadium as a prosthetic group. *Biochim. Biophys. Acta* 912:287–291.

152. H. Plat, B.E. Krenn, and R. Wever (1987) The bromoperoxidase from the lichen *Xanthoria parietina* is a novel vanadium enzyme. *Biochem. J.* 248:277–279.

153. E.O. Uthus and F.H. Nielsen (1988) The effect of vanadium, iodine and their interaction on thyroid status indices. *FASEB J.* 2:A841.

154. C.H. Hill (1985) Interaction of vanadate with chloride in the chick. *Nutr. Res. [Suppl.]* 1:555–559.

155. M. Anke, B. Groppel, K. Gruhn, T. Kośla, and M. Szilágyi (1986) New research on vanadium deficiency in ruminants. In: *5. Spurenelement-Symposium: New Trace Elements* (M. Anke, W. Baumann, H. Bräunlich, C. Brückner, and B. Groppel, eds.), pp. 1266–1275, Friedrich-Schiller-Universitat, Jena.

156. D.R. Myron, T.J. Zimmerman, T.R. Shuler, L.M. Klevay, D.E. Lee, and F.H. Nielsen (1978) Intake of nickel and vanadium by humans. A survey of selected diets. *Am. J. Clin. Nutr.* 31:527–531.

157. F. Proescher, H.A. Seil, and A.W. Stillians (1917) A contribution to the action of vanadium with particular reference to syphilis. *Am. J. Syph.* 1:347–405.

158. G.J. Naylor (1984) Vanadium and manic depressive psychosis. *Nutr. Health* 3:79–85.

159. G.J. Naylor, F.M. Corrigan, A.H.W. Smith, P. Connelly, and N.I. Ward (1987) Further studies of vanadium in depressive psychosis. *Br. J. Psychiatry* 150:656–661.

Iodine Deficiency: An International Public Health Problem

Iodine is an essential constituent of the thyroid hormones, 3,5,3'5'-tetraiodothyronine (thyroxine, T_4) and 3,5,3'-triiodothyronine (T_3). The major role of iodine in nutrition arises from the importance of thyroid hormones to the growth and development of humans and animals.

The daily requirement of iodine in adults is 1–2 μg/kg body weight. A daily iodine intake between 50 and 1000 μg is considered safe. The 1989 Recommended Dietary Allowance (RDA) is in the range of 40–120 μg for children up to the age of 10 y and 150 μg for older children and adults. An additional 25 and 50 μg are recommended during pregnancy and lactation, respectively.[1]

The effects of iodine deficiency on growth and development are now denoted by the term *iodine deficiency disorders* (IDD). The term *goiter* has been used for many years to describe the effect of iodine deficiency. Goiter is indeed the most obvious and familiar feature of iodine deficiency. However, knowledge has greatly expanded in the last 25 y so that it is not surprising that a new term (i.e., IDD) is needed.[2] Strategies for preventing IDD were reviewed extensively.[3–5]

Iodine-deficiency Disorders

Goiter. Iodine deficiency causes depletion of thyroid iodine stores with reduced production of T_4. A decrease in the blood concentration of T_4 triggers the secretion of increased amounts of pituitary thyroid-stimulating hormone, which increases thyroid activity and results in hyperplasia of the thyroid gland. An increased efficiency of the thyroid iodide pump occurs with faster turnover of thyroid iodine, which can be demonstrated by an increased thyroidal uptake of radioactive isotopes ^{131}I and ^{125}I. This increase in iodine uptake was first demonstrated in the field

in the classical observations of Stanbury et al.[6] in the Andes in Argentina.

Recent research showed that staple foods from the Third World, such as cassava, maize, bamboo shoots, sweet potatoes, lima beans, and millets, contain cyanogenic glucosides that are capable of liberating large quantities of cyanide by hydrolysis.[7] Not only is the cyanide itself toxic, but the metabolite formed in the body from cyanide is predominantly thiocyanate, which is a goitrogen. With the exception of cassava, these glycosides are located in the inedible portions of plants. If located in the edible portion, they are present in such small quantities that they do not cause a major problem. Cassava, on the other hand, is cultivated extensively in developing countries and represents an essential source of energy for more than 200 million people living in the tropics.[7] The role of cassava along with iodine deficiency in the etiology of endemic goiter and endemic cretinism was demonstrated by Delange et al.[7] from their studies in nonmountainous Zaire. These observations also were confirmed by Maberly et al.[8] in Sarawak, Malaysia.

The Fetus. Iodine deficiency of the fetus is the result of iodine deficiency in the mother. The condition is associated with a greater incidence of stillbirths, abortions, and congenital abnormalities, which can be reduced by iodine supplementation during pregnancy. The effects are similar to those observed with maternal hypothyroidism, which can be reduced by thyroid hormone replacement therapy.[9] Iodine supplementation of iodine-deficient pregnant women also results in a significant reduction in fetal and neonatal deaths. This finding is consistent with evidence from studies in experimental animals indicating the effect of iodine deficiency on fetal survival.[10–12]

Further data from Papua New Guinea indicate a

relationship between the level of maternal T_4 and the outcome of current and recent past pregnancies, including mortality and the occurrence of cretinism. The rate of perinatal deaths was twice as high among mothers with very low serum concentrations of total T_4 (TT_4) <30 nmol/L (36.0%) compared with women with levels >30 nmol/L (16.4%); the same results were evident for free T_4 (FT_4).[13]

A major effect of fetal iodine deficiency is the condition of endemic cretinism, which is quite distinct from the condition of sporadic cretinism.[11] This condition, which occurs with an iodine intake of <25 µg/d in contrast to a normal intake of 80–150 µg/d, is still widely prevalent, affecting up to 10% of populations living in severely iodine-deficient areas in India,[11] Indonesia,[11] and China.[14] In its most common form, it is characterized by mental deficiency, deaf mutism, and spastic diplegia. This condition is referred to as the *nervous* or *neurological* type of cretinism in contrast to the less common *myxedematous* type characterized by hypothyroidism with dwarfism.

Apart from its prevalence in Asia and Oceania (Papua New Guinea), cretinism also occurs in Africa (Zaire) and in South America in the Andean region (Ecuador, Peru, Bolivia, and Argentina).[11] In all these situations, with the exception of Zaire, neurological features are predominant.[11] In Zaire the myxedematous form is more common, probably because of the high intake of cassava.[7] However, there is considerable variation in the clinical manifestations of neurological cretinism, which include isolated deaf mutism and mental defect of varying degrees. In China the term *cretinoid* is used to describe such individuals.

The common form of endemic cretinism is not usually associated with severe clinical hypothyroidism as in the case of the so-called sporadic cretinism, although mixed forms with both the neurological and myxedematous features do occur. Unlike the situation for hypothyroidism, however, the neurological features of cretinism are not reversed by the administration of thyroid hormones.[15]

The apparent spontaneous disappearance of endemic cretinism in southern Europe raised considerable doubt as to the relation of iodine deficiency to the condition. Such a spontaneous disappearance without iodization was noted by Costa et al.[16] in northern Italy and by Konig and Veraguth[17] in Switzerland. The apparent spontaneous disappearance of the condition is now attributed to increase in iodine intake because of dietary diversification as a result of social and economic development affecting more remote rural areas.

A controlled trial in the western highlands of Papua New Guinea revealed that endemic cretinism could be prevented by correction of iodine deficiency with the injection of iodized oil before pregnancy.[18,19] The value of iodized-oil injection in the prevention of endemic cretinism was confirmed in Zaire[12] and in South America.[20] Mass injection programs were carried out in New Guinea, Zaire, Indonesia, and China. Evaluations of these mass programs in Indonesia and China indicate that endemic cretinism was prevented when correction of iodine deficiency was achieved.[14,21]

The Neonate. An increased perinatal mortality because of iodine deficiency was demonstrated in Zaire.[12] The injection of iodized oil in the latter half of pregnancy resulted in a substantial decrease in perinatal and infant mortality and improved birth weight.

Apart from the question of mortality, the importance of the state of thyroid function in the neonate relates to the fact that at birth the brain of the human infant has only reached about one-third of its full size and continues to grow rapidly until the end of the second year.[22] Thyroid hormone, dependent on an adequate supply of iodine, is essential for normal brain development, as was confirmed by animal studies.[23,24]

Data on iodine nutrition and neonatal thyroid function in Europe confirm the continuing presence of severe iodine deficiency affecting neonatal thyroid function and hence threatening early brain development.[25] Similar observations were made in Zaire, where rates of 10% of chemical hypothyroidism among neonates were found.[26] This hypothyroidism persists into infancy and childhood if the deficiency is not corrected and results in retardation of physical and mental development.

These observations indicate a much greater risk of mental defect in severely iodine-deficient populations than is indicated by the presence of classical cretinism.

The Child. Iodine deficiency in children is characteristically associated with goiter. The classification of goiter that was standardized by the World Health Organization is discussed elsewhere.[5] The goiter rate increases with age and reaches a maximum during adolescence. The prevalence is higher among girls than among boys. Observations of goiter rates in schoolchildren 8–14 y of age provide a convenient indication of the presence of iodine deficiency in a community.

Recent studies in schoolchildren living in iodine-deficient areas from a number of countries indicate impaired school performance and lower intelligence quotients (IQs) in comparison with matched groups from areas that are not iodine deficient. These studies are difficult to design and interpret because of the problem of an adequate control group. There are many possible causes for impaired school performance and impaired performance on an IQ test that may be operating. For example, the iodine-deficient areas are likely to be more remote and to suffer more social deprivation with a disadvantage in school facilities, a lower socioeconomic status, and poorer general nutrition. All such factors have to be taken into account apart from the problem of adapting tests developed in Western countries for use in Third World countries.

Initially, studies of psychomotor development, as indicated by tests of motor coordination, revealed differences that could be regarded as largely independent of educational status. However, more recent critical studies by Bleichrodt et al.[27] in Indonesia and in an iodine-deficient area in Spain, which used a wide range of psychological tests, showed that the mental development of children from iodine-deficient areas lags behind that of children from areas that are not iodine deficient. The differences in psychomotor development became apparent from age 2.5 y.

The obvious question is whether these differences can be affected by correction of the iodine deficiency. In a pioneering study initiated in Ecuador in 1966, Fierro-Benitez et al.[28] reported the long-term effects of iodized-oil injections by comparison of two highland villages—one (Tocachi) treated and the other (La Esperanza) untreated and acting as a control. The results indicate a significant role of iodine deficiency. However, other factors such as social deprivation and other nutritional factors were considered to be important in the school performance of these Ecuadorean children.[28]

A controlled trial carried out with oral iodized oil in a small Bolivian village (Tiquipaya) 2645 m above sea level revealed significant benefits to schoolchildren's mental performance associated with reduction of goiter.[29]

The Adult. Iodine administration in the form of iodized salt, iodized bread, or iodized oil was demonstrated to be effective in increasing circulating T_4 and in preventing goiter in adults. Iodine administration may also reduce existing goiter in adults. This effect is particularly true of iodized-oil injections and leads to ready acceptance of the intervention measure by people living in iodine-deficient communities.[3]

The major determinant of brain (and pituitary) T_3 is serum T_4 rather than T_3 as is true of liver, kidney, and muscle.[30] Low levels of brain T_3 were demonstrated in the iodine-deficient rat in association with reduced levels of serum T_4. These levels return to normal with correction of iodine deficiency.[31] This finding provides a rationale for suboptimal brain function in subjects with endemic goiter and lowered serum T_4 levels and its improvement after correction of iodine deficiency.

In northern India a high degree of apathy has been noted in populations living in iodine-deficient areas. This effect is also observed in domestic animals such as dogs. It is apparent that reduced mental function is widely prevalent in iodine-deficient communities with effects on their capacity for initiative and decision making. This observation suggests that iodine deficiency is a major block to the human and social development of communities living in an iodine-deficient environment. Correction of the iodine deficiency is indicated as a major contribution to development.

An instructive and broad example of such possibilities is provided by observations of the effect of an iodized-salt program dating only from 1978 in the Northern Chinese village of Jixian in Heilongjiang Province.[32] In 1978 there were 1313 people with a goiter rate of 65% with 11.4% cretins. The cretins included many severe cases which caused the village to be known locally as "the village of idiots." The economic development of the village was retarded—for example, no truck driver or teacher was available. Girls from other villages did not want to marry and live in the village. The intelligence of the student population was known to be low; children aged 10 y had a mental development equivalent to those aged 7 y.

After the introduction of iodized salt in 1978, the goiter rate dropped to 4% by 1982. No cretins were born during that period. The attitude of the people changed greatly; they were much more positive in their approach to life in contrast to the previous listless attitude. The economy improved accompanied by changes in the lives of the villagers. Average income increased from 43 yuan per head in 1981 to 223 yuan in 1982 and 414 yuan in 1984 and was higher than the average per capita income in the district. In 1983 cereals were exported for the first time. Before iodization no family had a radio. Now 55 families have been able to obtain a television set. Girls now come from other villages to marry young men in Jixian. Seven men joined the People's Liberation Army, whereas previously they had been rejected because of goiter. These effects are largely due to the correction of hypothyroidism by iodized salt.

Correction of Iodine Deficiency

Iodized Salt. Iodized salt has been the major method for combatting iodine deficiency since the 1920s, when it was first successfully used in Switzerland. Since then successful programs have been reported from a number of countries including Central and South America (e.g., Guatemala and Colombia), Finland in Europe, and China and Taiwan in Asia.[5]

The difficulties in the production and maintenance

of quality of iodized salt, especially in Asia, are vividly demonstrated in India where there has been a breakdown in supply. The difficulties have led to the adoption of universal salt iodation for India to be achieved by 1992.

In Asia, the cost of iodized-salt production and distribution at present is of the order of 3–5 cents per person per year.[3] This amount must be considered cheap in relation to the health and social benefits to be obtained.

However, there is still the problem of the salt reaching the iodine-deficient person. There may be problems with distribution or preservation of the iodine content of salt (i.e., the salt may be left uncovered or exposed to heat). Iodized salt also should be added after cooking to reduce the loss of iodine.

Finally, there is the difficulty of actual consumption of the salt. Although the addition of iodine makes no difference to the taste of salt, the introduction of a new variety of salt to an area where a salt source is already available and familiar is likely to be resisted. For example, in the Chinese provinces of Sinjiang and Inner Mongolia, the strong preference of the people for desert salt of very low iodine content led to a mass iodized-oil injection program to prevent cretinism.[14]

Iodized Oil by Injection. The value of iodized-oil injection in the prevention of endemic goiter and endemic cretinism was first established in New Guinea with controlled trials involving the use of saline injection as a control.[19] These trials established the value of the oil in the prevention of goiter and the prevention of cretinism. Experience in South America confirmed the value of the measure.[21] Correction of severe iodine deficiency by a single intramuscular injection (2–4 mL) was demonstrated for a period of over 4 y.[33]

The injection of iodized oil can be administered through local health services (where they exist) or by special teams. In New Guinea the injection of a population in excess of 100,000 was carried out by public health teams along with the injection of triple antigen. In Nepal 2 million injections have now been given by the immunization teams. The obvious disappearance of goiter ensured ready acceptance.[3,4]

Iodized oil is especially appropriate for isolated village communities characteristic of mountainous endemic goiter areas. The oil should be administered to all females up to the age of 40 y and males up to the age of 20 y. A repeat of the injection is required in 3–5 y depending on the dose given and the age of the individual. In children the need is greater than in adults, and the recommended dose should be repeated in 3 y if severe iodine deficiency persists.[3] Iodized walnut oil and iodized soya bean oil are new preparations developed in China since 1980.[34]

It is now clear that iodized oil (Lipiodol, a poppy seed oil with 480 mg iodine/mL; Guerbet, Paris, France) is suitable for use in a mass program. In Indonesia >1 million injections were given between 1974 and 1978 along with the massive distribution of iodized salt. A further 4.9 million were given by specially trained paramedical personnel during the period 1979–83. In China in Sinjiang, 707,000 injections were given by barefoot doctors between 1978 and 1981; a further 3–4 million were given in 1982.[14]

A major advantage of iodized-oil injections is the association of injections with the successful eradication of smallpox. One disadvantage is the immediate discomfort produced and the risk of transmission of infection such as Hepatitis B and AIDS. Sensitivity phenomena were not reported.[3–5,34] However, the major disadvantage of injections has been cost. Currently cost has been reduced by mass packaging and now is of a similar order of magnitude to that of iodized salt especially if the population to be injected is restricted to women of reproductive age and children and if a primary health-care team is available.[3,5,34]

Iodized Oil by Mouth. The effectiveness of a single oral administration of iodized oil for 1–2 y was demonstrated in South America and in Burma.[4] More recent studies in India and China revealed that oral iodized oil is effective for at least 1 y, only one-fourth as long as a similar dose given by injection.[34] The main hazard of such iodization is transient hyperthyroidism, which is seen mainly in persons over the age of 40 y. It is caused by autonomous thyroid function resulting from long-standing iodine deficiency and can be reduced by minimizing iodization in those over the age of 40.[3–5]

Indications for Different Methods of Iodine Supplementation. There are three grades of severity of IDD in a population on the basis of urinary iodine excretion.[3]

1. Mild IDD with goiter prevalence in the range 5–20% (schoolchildren) and with median urine iodine concentrations > 43.5 nmol/nmol creatinine. Mild IDD can be controlled with iodinated salt at a concentration of 10–25 mg/kg.

2. Moderate IDD with goiter prevalence up to 30% along with some hypothyroidism and median urine iodine concentrations in the range 21.8–43.5 nmol/nmol creatinine. Moderate IDD may be controlled with iodinated salt (25–40 mg/kg) or iodized oil, either orally or by injection, administered through the primary health-care system.

3. Severe IDD indicated by a high prevalence of goiter (≥30%), endemic cretinism (prevalence 1–10%), and median urine iodine <21.8 nmol/nmol creatinine. Severe IDD requires iodized oil either

orally or by injection for complete prevention of central nervous system defects.

Prevention and Control of IDD

Many populations are at risk of iodine deficiency because they live in an iodine-deficient environment characterized by soil from which iodine has been leached by glaciation, high rainfall, or flood. This situation occurs most often in mountainous areas such as the Himalayan region, the Andean region, and the vast mountain ranges of China.

However, low-lying areas subject to flooding, as in the Ganges Valley in India and Bangladesh, are also severely iodine deficient. This problem will continue until there is dietary diversification such as that which occurred in Europe late in the 19th century and in the early decades of this century or, alternatively, until some form of iodine supplement is given.

An estimated 800 million persons are at risk of iodine deficiency; of these, 190 million are suffering from goiter, >3 million are overt cretins (Table 1), and millions more suffer from some intellectual or motor deficit.[3] The major concentrations of population are in Asia where there has been a major escalation of IDD control programs in the last 5 y in India, Indonesia, Nepal, Burma, and Bhutan.

In Latin America earlier efforts have produced a large measure of control in such countries as Argentina, Brazil, Colombia, and Guatemala. However, there is evidence of recurrence of the problem of iodine deficiency in Colombia and Guatemala that is associated with political and social unrest. Major IDD problems have persisted in Ecuador, Peru, and Bolivia, but significant progress has been made in the last 3 y with the combination of national government initiative and support from international agencies.

In Africa there has been a lag in the development of IDD control programs by comparison with the other continents. However, new initiatives began after a Joint WHO/UNICEF/ICCIDD Regional Seminar held in Yaounde, Cameroon, in March 1987.[33] This seminar set up a Joint IDD Task Force that initiated comprehensive planning for the prevention and control of IDD in Africa.

China has also made rapid progress since the passing of the Cultural Revolution in 1976. One-third of the population of China (370 million) is at risk of IDD because of the extensive mountainous areas in that country.[14]

The gap between our new knowledge of IDD and the application of this knowledge in national IDD-control programs (particularly in developing countries) led to the formation of the International Council for the Control of Iodine Deficiency Disorders (ICCIDD). The inaugural meeting of this multidisciplin-

Table 1. Prevalence of iodine-deficiency disorders in developing countries and numbers of persons at risk*

	At risk	Goiter	Overt cretinism
		$\times 10^6$	
Southeast Asia	280	100	1.5
Asia (other countries)	400	30	0.9
Africa	60	30	0.5
Latin America	60	30	0.25
Total	800	190	3.15

* From Hetzel et al.[3] (Used with permission.)

ary group of epidemiologists, nutritionists, endocrinologists, chemists, health planners, and economists was held in Kathmandu, Nepal, in March 1986. Papers covering all aspects of IDD control programs presented in Kathmandu were published as a monograph.[3] The ICCIDD established a global multidisciplinary network of some 300 persons with expertise relevant to IDD and IDD control programs and works closely with WHO, UNICEF, and national governments within the United Nations in the development of national programs.[3,33]

The feasibility of substantial progress in the prevention and control of IDD in the next 5–10 y was endorsed in a World Health Assembly Resolution in 1986, and a global strategy for a 10-y program was adopted by the UN agencies.[3]

These developments encourage the hope that significant progress can be made in the prevention and control of IDD within the next decade with great benefits to the quality of life of the many millions of people affected.[35]

References

1. National Research Council (1989) *Recommended Dietary Allowances*, 10th ed., National Academy Press, Washington, DC.
2. B.S. Hetzel (1983) Iodine deficiency disorders (IDD) and their eradication. *Lancet* 2:1126–1129.
3. B.S. Hetzel, J.T. Dunn, and J.B. Stanbury, eds. (1987) *The Prevention and Control of Iodine Deficiency Disorders*, Elsevier, Amsterdam.
4. J.B. Stanbury and B.S. Hetzel, eds. (1980) *Endemic Goiter and Endemic Cretinism: Iodine Nutrition in Health and Disease*, Wiley, New York.
5. J.T. Dunn, E.A. Pretell, C.H. Daza, and F.E. Viteri, eds. (1986) *Towards the Eradication of Endemic Goiter, Cretinism, and Iodine Deficiency*, Pan American Health Organization, Washington, DC.
6. J.B. Stanbury, G.L. Brownell, D.S. Riggs, H. Perinetti, J. Itoiz, and E.B. DelCastillo (1954) *The Adaptation of Man to Iodine Deficiency*, Harvard University Press, Cambridge.
7. F. Delange, F.B. Iteke, and A.M. Ermans (1982) *Nutritional Factors Involved in the Goitrogenic Action of Cassava.* Canada 1, International Development Research Center, Ottawa.
8. G.F. Maberly, C. Eastman, K.V. Waite, J. Corcoran, and V. Rashford (1983) The role of Cassava. In: *Current Problems in Thyroid*

Research (N. Ui, K. Torizuka, S. Nagataki, and K. Miyai, eds.) pp. 341–344, Excerpta Medica, Amsterdam.

9. A.J. McMichael, J.D. Potter, and B.S. Hetzel (1980) Iodine deficiency, thyroid function, and reproductive failure. In: *Endemic Goiter and Endemic Cretinism* (J.B. Stanbury and B.S. Hetzel, eds.), pp. 445–460, Wiley, New York.

10. B.S. Hetzel, B.J. Potter, and E.M. Dulberg (in press) The iodine deficiency disorders: nature, pathogenesis and epidemiology. *World Rev. Nutr. and Diet.*

11. P.O.D. Pharoah, F. Delange, R. Fierro Benitez, and J.B. Stanbury (1980) Endemic cretinism. In *Endemic Goiter and Endemic Cretinism* (J.B. Stanbury and B.S. Hetzel, eds.), pp. 395–421, Wiley, New York.

12. C.H. Thilly (1981) Goitre et cretinisme endemiques: role etiologique de la consommation de manioc et strategie d'eradication. *Bull. Belg. Acad. Med.* 136:389–412.

13. P.O.D. Pharoah, S.M.N. Ellis, R.P. Ekins, and E.S. Williams (1976) Maternal thyroid function, iodine deficiency and fetal development. *Clin. Endocrinol.* (Oxf.) 5:159–166.

14. T. Ma, T. Lu, U. Tan, B. Chen, and H.I. Zhu (1982) The present status of endemic goiter and endemic cretinism in China. *Food Nutr. Bull.* 4:13–19.

15. R. Fierro-Benitez, J.B. Stanbury, A. Querido, L. De Groot, R. Alban, and J. Endova (1970) Endemic cretinism in the Andean region of Ecuador. *J. Clin. Endocrinol. Metab.* 30:228–236.

16. A. Costa, F. Cottino, M. Mortara, and U. Vogliazzo (1964) Endemic cretinism in Piedmont. *Panminerva Med.* 6:250–259.

17. M.P. Konig and P. Veraguth (1961) Studies of thyroid function in endemic cretins. In: *Advances in Thyroid Research* (R. Pitt-Rivers, ed.), pp. 294–298, Pergamon, London.

18. P.O.D. Pharoah, I.H. Buttfield, and B.S. Hetzel (1971) Neurological damage to the fetus resulting from severe iodine deficiency during pregnancy. *Lancet* 1:308–310.

19. P.O.D. Pharoah and K.J. Connolly (1987) A controlled trial of iodinated oil for the prevention of endemic cretinism: a long term follow up. *Int. J. Epidemiol.* 16:68–73.

20. E.A. Pretell, T. Torres, V. Zenten, and M. Comejo (1972) Prophylaxis of endemic goiter with iodized oil in rural Peru. In: *Human Development and the Thyroid Gland—Relation to Endemic Cretinism* (J.B. Stanbury and R. Kroc, eds.), *Advances in Experimental Medicine and Biology,* vol. 30, pp. 249–265, Plenum, New York.

21. E.M. Dulberg, K. Widjaja, R. Djokomoeljanto, B.S. Hetzel, and L. Belmont (1983) Evaluation of the iodization program in Central Java with reference to the prevention of endemic cretinism and motor coordination defects. In: *Current Problems in Thyroid Research* (N. Ui, K. Torizuka, S. Nagataki, and K. Miyai, eds.), pp. 19–22, Excerpta Medica, Amsterdam.

22. J. Dobbing (1974) The later development of the brain and its vulnerability. In: *Scientific Foundations of Paediatrics* (J. Davis and J. Dobbing, eds.), pp. 565–577, Heinemann Medical, London.

23. B.S. Hetzel and B.J. Potter (1983) Iodine deficiency and the role of thyroid hormones in brain development. In: *Neurobiology of the Trace Elements* (I. Dreosti and R.M. Smith, eds.), pp. 83–133, Humana Press, New Jersey.

24. B.S. Hetzel, J. Chavadej, and B.J. Potter (1988) The brain in iodine deficiency. *Neuropathol. Appl. Neurobiol.* 14:93–104.

25. F. Delange, P. Heidemann, P. Bourdoux, et al. (1986) Regional variations of iodine nutrition and thyroid function during the neonatal period in Europe. *Biol. Neonate* 49:322–330.

26. A.M. Ermans, N.M. Moulameko, F. Delange, and R. Alhuwalia, eds. (1980) *Role of Cassava in the Aetiology of Endemic Goiter and Cretinism,* International Development Research Center, Ottawa.

27. N. Bleichrodt, I. Garcia, C. Rubio, G. Morreale de Escobar, and F. Escobar Del Rey (1987) Developmental disorders associated with severe iodine deficiency. In: *The Prevention and Control of Iodine Deficiency Disorders* (B.S. Hetzel, J.T. Dunn, and J.B. Stanbury, eds.), pp. 65–84, Elsevier, Amsterdam.

28. R. Fierro-Benitez, R. Cazar, J.B. Stanbury, et al. (1986) Long-term effect of correction of iodine deficiency on psychomotor and intellectual development. In: *Towards the Eradication of Endemic Goiter, Cretinism, and Iodine Deficiency* (J.T. Dunn, E.A. Pretell, C.H. Daza, and F.E. Viteri, eds.), pp. 182–200, Pan American Health Organization, Washington, DC.

29. A. Bautista, P.A. Barker, J.T. Dunn, M. Sanchez, and D.L. Kaiser (1982) The effects of oral iodized oil on intelligence, thyroid status, and somatic growth in school-age children from an area of endemic goiter. *Am. J. Clin. Nutr.* 35:127–134.

30. F.R. Crantz and P.R. Larsen (1980) Rapid thyroxine to 3,5,3'-triiodothyronine conversion binding in rat cerebral cortex and cerebellum. *J. Clin. Invest.* 65:935–938.

31. M.J. Obregon, P. Santisteban, A. Rodriguez-Pena, et al. (1984) Cerebral hypothyroidism in rats with adult-onset iodine deficiency. *Endocrinology* 115:614–624.

32. J. Li and X. Wang (1987) Jixian: a success story in IDD control. *IDD Newslett.* 3:4–5.

33. B.S. Hetzel (1987) Progress in the prevention and control of iodine deficiency disorders. *Lancet* 2:266.

34. J.T. Dunn (1987) Iodized oil in the treatment and prophylaxis of IDD. In: *The Prevention and Control of Iodine Deficiency Disorders* (B.S. Hetzel, J.T. Dunn, and J.B. Stanbury, eds.), pp. 127–134, Elsevier, Amsterdam.

35. B.S. Hetzel (1989) *The Story of Iodine Deficiency. An International Challenge in Nutrition,* Oxford University Press, Oxford.

Chapter 36

Janet C. King and Jean Weininger

Pregnancy and Lactation

Fetal growth during pregnancy and milk secretion during lactation are nutrient-requiring processes. In well-nourished women normal physiologic and metabolic adjustments in nutrient utilization probably provide the additional nutrients needed for fetal growth and milk secretion. In poorly nourished women the additional demand for nutrients during these processes may lead to maternal and/or fetal nutrient deficiencies. The extensive physiologic and metabolic adjustments occurring during pregnancy lead to an increased risk of maternal clinical problems, such as toxemia. The nutrient requirements for pregnancy and lactation and the consequences of insufficient intakes are reviewed in this chapter.

Physiological Adjustments in Nutrient Utilization in Pregnancy

Weight Gain. Healthy women eating an unrestricted diet generally gain 10–12 kg during the course of pregnancy.[1] There is usually little weight gain during the first trimester, followed by a steady gain of ~350–400 g/wk during the second and third trimesters.[1] Maternal tissue stores (including fat, blood, and uterine and breast tissue) accumulate primarily in the second trimester and account for ~6 kg of an average 11-kg total gain. The remaining 5 kg is accounted for by the fetus, placenta, and amniotic fluid. An 11-kg gain contains on average ~7 kg water, 3 kg fat, and 1 kg protein.[2] About 5–6 kg of the 7-kg water gain is in the extracellular fluid of the mother. Considerably more water may be retained by pregnant women with edema.

Metabolic Changes. Changes in maternal hormone secretions from the placenta and other maternal endocrine glands lead to alterations in carbohydrate, fat, and protein utilization during pregnancy. Glucose, the main fuel used by the fetus, is transported across the placenta by facilitated diffusion, amino acids are transported by active transport, and fatty acids are transported by simple diffusion. Near term, the fetus uses ~35 g glucose/d, 7 g amino acids/d, and 1.7 g fatty acids/d for energy.[3] When maternal glucose concentrations drop, as during fasting, fatty acids and ketones are more readily used by the fetus.

In the first trimester increased serum concentrations of estrogen and progesterone and the accompanying increased maternal-tissue insulin sensitivity result in an anabolic state whereby glycogen and fat are stored by the mother.[4] This fat storage comprises most of the extra dietary energy required in the first and second trimesters. During the third trimester maternal glucose is spared for fetal use primarily because of increased maternal tissue insulin resistance as a result of the placental secretion of human chorionic somatomammotropin (hCS; formerly known as placental lactogen, hPL) and accompanying maternal fat mobilization.[5]

Reductions in urea production and excretion late in pregnancy contribute to nitrogen retention for tissue synthesis. Elevated concentrations of plasma insulin may increase the uptake of some amino acids, especially the branched-chain amino acids, which seem to provide a large proportion of the amino acid fuel needed by the fetus.[3]

Blood Volume and Hemodynamic Changes. The plasma volume increases ~40% above the nonpregnancy value of 2.6 L, and accounts for just over 1 kg of the total water gain.[6] Larger plasma volumes tend to correspond to larger fetuses. The erythrocyte volume increases ~18% without iron supplementation and ~30% with iron supplementation from a nonpregnancy volume of 1.4 L. Both erythrocyte and plasma volumes begin to increase after about the 10th week of pregnancy; the erythrocyte volume continues to expand until term, whereas the plasma volume reaches a plateau and levels off at ~30–34 wk.

The total serum protein concentration decreases (primarily reflecting a decrease in albumin) by the end of the first trimester of pregnancy because of expanded plasma volume and altered rates of protein synthesis. Serum protein concentration remains at ~10 g/L nonpregnancy values for the second half of pregnancy.[6] Alpha 1-globulin and α,2-globulin increase by ~1 g/L, β-globulin increases by ~3 g/L, and γ-globulin decreases slightly during the course of pregnancy. Altered amounts of transport proteins affect the serum concentrations of minerals such as calcium, iron, and zinc.

Nutrient Requirements of Pregnant Women

Energy. The total energy requirement for pregnancy—covering the energy equivalents of protein and fat synthesis and increased metabolism—has been estimated to be ~85,000 kcal.[7] About 36,000 kcal are needed for metabolism, 41,000 kcal are deposited as fat and lean tissue, and 8,000 kcal are used to convert dietary energy to metabolizable energy.

A number of investigators reported an increase in the resting metabolic rate—the rate of energy expenditure for metabolism—during pregnancy. The amount of increase by term varies with the population studied, ranging from 7,000 to 46,500 kcal.[8] The nutritional state of the mother may affect metabolic energy needs. Work in The Gambia showed that underfed pregnant women have less of an increase in resting metabolism than do pregnant women receiving nutritional supplementation.[9,10] The metabolic needs of pregnancy may be significantly lower than Hytten's estimates of 36,000 kcal.[8,11]

In developing countries where women regularly perform heavy physical work, studies have shown some decrease in the intensity of work late in pregnancy. For those with limited energy intakes, heavy physical work in late pregnancy tends to reduce birth weight, possibly because the energy demand for physical activity diverts energy from tissue synthesis.[8]

Contrary to popular assumption there is little evidence that women in industrialized societies become more sedentary during pregnancy, although they may reduce work intensity.[11–13] In addition, increasing numbers of such women perform recreational exercise throughout pregnancy. Those pregnant women who spend a significant amount of time in weight-bearing activity, such as walking, will need additional energy in proportion to their gain in weight.[8]

Because so many factors—prepregnancy weight and body composition, composition and amount of weight gain, stage of pregnancy, and level of activity—affect energy needs, there is no single value for energy requirements that would apply to all pregnant women.[8] On the basis of Hytten's figure of 85,000

kcal, divided by the 280 d of gestation, an additional energy intake of 300 kcal/d is suggested during pregnancy.[14] The Food and Agriculture Organization[15] recommends an extra 285 kcal/d for those pregnant women who maintain their prepregnancy level of physical activity and 200 kcal/d for those who reduce their activity.

Protein. Maternal, placental, and fetal needs increase protein requirements during pregnancy. Protein comprises ~0.9 kg of an average pregnancy weight gain of 12.5 kg.[2] About 50% of this extra protein is deposited in the fetus, 25% in the uterus and breasts, 10% in the placenta, and 15% in blood and amniotic fluid. Fetal protein deposition is greatest during the last quarter of gestation, which corresponds to the period of maximum fetal growth.[8]

Nitrogen balance studies fail to show that nitrogen is retained as maternal lean tissue during the first half of pregnancy (D.D. Marino, unpublished observation, 1982), but indicate that ~6–8 g protein/d is retained in the last half of pregnancy. In addition, the fetus is estimated to use ~2.8 g protein $\cdot$ kg^{-1} $\cdot$ d^{-1} in the last trimester for tissue synthesis and fuel.[3] Reduced urinary nitrogen excretion during pregnancy and other metabolic adaptations that improve nitrogen utilization probably make it possible for most pregnant women to provide the additional protein need with only small adjustments in their intakes.[8]

Vitamins. The circulating concentrations of many vitamins are reduced during pregnancy, but it is difficult to evaluate how much of these reductions are due to normal physiological adjustments of pregnancy and how much to true increases in need. As discussed above, the plasma volume expands ~50% as pregnancy progresses, thereby diluting the concentrations of many of the vitamins and their carrier proteins. The resting metabolic rate increases to varying degrees in different populations studied. The glomerular filtration rate also increases early in pregnancy and increases to ~50% higher than nonpregnancy rates. In addition, changing enzyme activities responding to the new hormone concentrations of pregnancy may alter the apparent status of various vitamins, although this change may not represent a true deficiency. All of these factors contribute to the notion that the decrease in many vitamin (and mineral) concentrations is a normal adjustment to pregnancy and not necessarily reflective of significantly increased needs.[8] Those vitamins of particular concern during pregnancy are vitamins A, D, and B-6 and folate.

Although plasma retinol concentrations tend to decrease during pregnancy, vitamin A deficiency is not considered a particular hazard for pregnant women except in those populations where vitamin A deficiency is common. Rather, the main concern is with the possible hazards from excess, particularly of vitamin A analogues used pharmacologically. In the early 1980s major congenital defects were seen in more than a dozen infants whose mothers had taken isotretinoid during pregnancy for treatment of severe cystic acne.[16,17] Product labels and warnings to physicians were instituted as protective measures. Vitamin A supplementation should be done very cautiously because of the teratogenic potential.

Vitamin D deficiency during pregnancy is associated with disorders of calcium metabolism in the newborn, although deficiency is not likely unless the mother also has a low intake of calcium and insufficient exposure to sunlight.[18] If the mother is only marginally deficient in vitamin D, there may be a slight reduction in bone calcification or reduced bone density in the fetus. This syndrome has been seen in infants of low-income women in India, and it can be prevented by giving calcium supplements during pregnancy.[19] Vitamin D deficiency during pregnancy can also contribute to neonatal hypocalcemia[20] as well as defects in tooth formation.[21] Classical signs of rickets in a newborn are rare and are seen only with the most severe cases of vitamin D deficiency. Because of the potential for toxicity with this fat-soluble vitamin, supplementation should be done very cautiously.

Significantly lower blood concentrations of vitamin B-6 and its active form, pyridoxal 5'-phosphate, as well as reduced activity of the vitamin as evidenced by various functional tests were reported in pregnant women.[14] Despite reports of morning sickness, depression, and other symptoms that responded to vitamin B-6 supplementation, the clinical significance of altered vitamin B-6 metabolism during pregnancy is unclear, and there is no association with poor birth outcomes.[8] Dietary allowance committees of various countries recommend roughly an additional 0.5 mg vitamin B-6 during pregnancy—related to the increased protein allowance, although studies show that it would take several more milligrams per day to maintain normal vitamin B-6 status during pregnancy.[22,23]

It is understandable that during pregnancy there would be a great demand for folate for DNA synthesis in rapidly growing fetal, placental, and maternal tissues as well as for increased erythropoiesis. Even in well-nourished women there is a predictable decrease in serum and red cell folate during pregnancy, an increased urinary excretion of folate, and alterations in other laboratory findings indicative of folic acid deficiency—although megaloblastic anemia is not common. Severe malformations result when women take folate antagonists early in pregnancy, but it is controversial whether folate deficiency in pregnancy contributes to abortion, stillbirth, pre-

maturity, abruptio placentae, or low birth weight.[24] Some reports indicate that folate supplementation around the time of conception may help prevent a recurrence of neural-tube defects in the offspring of women who have already had one child with neural tube defects,[24,25] but this finding still needs confirmation. The World Health Organization[24] recommends 400 μg additional folate intake during pregnancy. This amount is double the nonpregnancy recommendation. Recommendations vary from an additional 100 to 400 μg/d.

Minerals. As with vitamins the physiological changes of pregnancy—including increased plasma volume and increased glomerular filtration rate—result in generally lowered circulating concentrations of various minerals. Alterations in protein metabolism lead to changes in some of the carrier proteins for minerals. These changes result in lowered circulating concentrations of minerals and are not necessarily indicative of altered mineral status.[8] Of particular concern are three minerals that might be lacking in the diets of pregnant women: calcium, iron, and zinc.

A complex series of hormonal and physiological adjustments allows for increased calcium retention beginning early in pregnancy. Most of the ~30 g calcium gained during pregnancy goes into the fetal skeleton.[26] Calcium absorption doubles by 20 wk gestation and remains high throughout pregnancy.[27] Extra calcium early in pregnancy is thought to be stored in maternal bone and is available for the fetus in the third trimester when the needs are greatest.[8] Calcium losses in the urine are increased probably as a result of the increased glomerular filtration rate.[28] Additional calcium is recommended throughout pregnancy to ensure that the maternal skeleton is not depleted, but the specific quantity varies from country to country.

Iron-deficiency anemia is a common problem among nonpregnant women, and many women start their pregnancies with diminished iron stores. A total of ~1,200 mg iron covers both fetal and maternal needs during the course of pregnancy and at delivery.[8,29] Hemoglobin and serum iron concentrations tend to decrease during pregnancy and the percent transferrin saturation increases, but these changes are not necessarily indicative of iron deficiency. The total oxygen-carrying capacity of the blood actually increases with the expansion of blood volume. Iron absorption increases significantly, and maternal iron stores are mobilized to satisfy the fetal demand for iron that comes late in pregnancy. The amount of iron absorbed, the degree of maternal red blood cell expansion, and the amount of iron stores in the newborn are influenced by maternal iron status.[8,29] Many dietary allowance committees recommend supplemental iron during pregnancy, because the increased need cannot be met by usual diets even among well-nourished populations.

Although fetal needs for zinc are highest in late pregnancy, zinc is critically important in very early pregnancy organogenesis. Zinc concentration in human embryos was reported to be seven times greater on the 35th day of gestation than on the 31st day.[30] Zinc appears to be conserved in early pregnancy by a decrease in urinary excretion as compared with nonpregnant control subjects.[31] Increases in urinary zinc excretion late in pregnancy are consistent with increased losses of calcium, water-soluble vitamins, and other substances through increased glomerular filtration rate.[32] Increased absorption and possible release of bone and muscle zinc may help meet the fetal zinc needs of 0.5–0.75 mg/d during the last trimester.[8] The circulating zinc mass actually increases in late pregnancy along with the expanded plasma volume[33] even though serum zinc concentrations decline, possibly reflecting lowered concentrations of serum albumin to which much of zinc is bound.[34] An additional 3–5 mg zinc is suggested during pregnancy.

Problems During Pregnancy

Insufficient Weight Gain. Insufficient weight gain during pregnancy has been associated with small-for-gestational-age (SFGA) infants, that is, infants weighing ≤2,500 g at birth.[8] SFGA infants are also at greater risk for neonatal death and various defects and disabilities.[8]

Underweight or Overweight at Conception. The incidence of delivering SFGA infants is greater in women who are underweight before pregnancy—below 90% of the standard weight for height. Ideally, such underweight women should gain weight before they become pregnant or, if not, they should try to compensate by gaining more weight during pregnancy. In one study the perinatal mortality rate was lowest in underweight women who gained ~14 kg during pregnancy.[35]

Improving the nutritional status of women before they become pregnant has a positive effect on subsequent birth outcome. In one study women who received food supplementation for 5–7 mo after the birth of the first child had a better pregnancy outcome with the second child than did women who received supplementation for only ≤2 mo. Infants of women whose diets were supplemented for the longer period of time had a higher mean birth weight and birth length and a lower risk of being SFGA.[36]

Obese women—those ≥ 135% of the standard weight for height—have an increased risk of complications during pregnancy, including hypertension, gestational diabetes, induced and assisted labor,

postpartum hemorrhage, and cesarean section.[37–39] Such a pregnancy is also more likely to result in a large-for-gestational-age (LFGA) or macrosomatic infant—one weighing >4,000 g. These infants have a higher rate of neonatal morbidity and mortality.[40,41] Although pregnancy is not the time to lose weight, even for obese women, many obese women have good outcomes with lower weight gains.

Alcohol and Other Drugs. Roughly half the infants born to alcoholic women have fetal alcohol syndrome, a life-threatening condition characterized by intrauterine growth retardation, facial and other anomalies, and mental retardation.[42] Significant alcohol intake during pregnancy, if not resulting in full-blown fetal alcohol syndrome, may be associated with increased risk of low-birth-weight infants, abruptio placenta, and spontaneous abortion in the first and second trimester as well as learning disorders in the offspring.[43] Pregnant women are advised to avoid alcohol completely, if possible, because no safe intake has been established.

The Food and Drug Administration has advised pregnant women to avoid unnecessary consumption of caffeine because of animal studies suggesting that it causes birth defects.[42] Although studies in humans are inconsistent and generally have failed to demonstrate a negative effect of caffeine on birth outcome, pregnant women who choose to use caffeine should do so in moderation.[42,43] Caffeine is found in tea, cocoa, certain soft drinks, and some over-the-counter drugs as well as in coffee.

The adverse effects of smoking during pregnancy on fetal growth are well documented.[43] Pregnant women would be wise to avoid other commonly used "recreational" drugs, such as marijuana and cocaine, as well as any other drug not specifically prescribed by their physician.

Toxemia. Toxemia—the hypertensive disorders of pregnancy—includes preeclampsia (hypertension with proteinuria and/or edema) and the convulsive end state, eclampsia. Fluid retention alone, which is quite common in pregnant women, is not sufficient to diagnose preeclampsia.

There has been much controversy over the role of salt intake, inadequate protein intake, excessive weight gain, and calcium deficiency in the etiology of toxemia. It is likely that improved nutrition has contributed to the decline in incidence and mortality rate of toxemia, but the cause of toxemia is still unknown. The former practice of restricting salt and prescribing diuretics for edema during pregnancy is not recommended, and pregnant women are advised to use salt to taste.[43]

Lactation

Physiology of Lactation. Lactation is established during the first week after birth. Milk secretion is a two-stage process: (*1*) the synthesis and secretion of milk components by the mammary alveolar cells and (*2*) the passage of milk along the duct system. Milk synthesis is the most active during infant suckling. The stimulus for milk secretion is derived largely from the hormone prolactin, but other anterior pituitary hormones are required for maintenance of milk secretion. If suckling stops, release of these hormones ceases and milk secretion usually stops in a few days.

Milk Volume and Composition. A milk volume of ~750 mL/d is generally accepted as standard during the first 6 mo of lactation,[14] although milk volumes vary considerably even among well-nourished populations.[44] In developing societies where women often breast-feed longer than in industrialized societies, breast-milk volumes range from ~300 to 900 mL/d in the second 6 mo and from 200 to 600 mL/d in the second year of life.[45]

The overall composition of human milk is quite constant even among women whose nutritional status varies. Human milk, compared with other mammalian milk, is high in lactose and relatively low in protein and minerals. Protein in human milk (~8–9 g/L) has a relatively low casein content (20% of the total protein) and a large whey protein fraction that includes α-lactalbumin, lactoferrin, and immunoglobulin IgA—the latter two of which help protect against gastrointestinal infections in the young infant.[46] Human milk also contains a relatively high content (25% of total nitrogen) of nonprotein nitrogen (urea, free amino acids, and other compounds).

The fat content of human milk is ~3.8%, although it varies considerably throughout the day and within a particular feeding. The higher fat content at the end of a feeding may have some bearing on appetite control in the infant. The fatty acid content of human milk is influenced by the maternal diet but generally tends toward a substantial amount of unsaturated fatty acids (including oleic and linoleic) and a lower saturated fatty acid content than cow milk. The cholesterol content of human milk is relatively high and may be important in the infant's development of mechanisms to handle cholesterol later in life.[46]

The vitamin content of human milk varies to some extent with maternal dietary intake and, for the most part, is well suited for the infant. Vitamin D levels are low but are adequate for the normal term infant. The relatively low mineral content of human milk (2 g/L) compared with cow milk is physiologically important because it provides a lower renal solute load for the immature kidney of the human infant. The iron content of human milk is also low (0.3–0.5 mmol/L), but its very high availability (≥75% is absorbed in the gut) combined with the infant's own iron stores of ~1.34 mmol/kg seems adequate to protect the infant from iron deficiency during the first 4–6 mo of life.[46,47]

Maternal Nutrient Requirements. The energy content of human milk depends on its carbohydrate, fat, and protein content and ranges from ~670 to 770 kcal/L.[14] About 5% of the energy comes from protein, 38% from lactose, and >50% from fat.[46] The efficiency of conversion of maternal energy to milk energy is 80–90%. Thus, to produce 850 mL milk/d requires ~750 kcal/d.[14] Women who gain 11–12.5 kg during pregnancy will store ~2–4 kg fat. These fat stores can be drawn on during lactation.

Maternal Nutritional Status and Lactation. Poor maternal nutritional status, as indicated by low weight-for-height values, is associated with lower milk production.[48] For example, the milk volumes of underweight women in India ranged from 450 to 560 mL/d in comparison to the usual volume of 750 mL/d among well-nourished women. The effect of maternal nutritional status on milk composition is more variable. Only protein concentration is consistently reduced in women of poor nutritional status. These changes in milk volume and composition in poorly nourished women are likely to have a negative effect on infant growth and development.

References

1. R.M. Pitkin and W.N. Spellacy (1978) Physiologic adjustments in general. In: *Laboratory Indices of Nutritional Status in Pregnancy* (Committee on Nutrition of the Mother and Preschool Child, Food and Nutrition Board, National Research Council), pp. 1–8, National Academy of Sciences, Washington, DC.
2. F.E. Hytten (1980) Weight gain in pregnancy. In: *Clinical Physiology in Obstetrics* (F.E. Hytten and G. Chamberlain, eds.), pp. 193–233, Blackwell, Oxford.
3. P. Rosso (1983) Nutritional needs of the human fetus. *Clin. Nutr.* 2:4–8.
4. D.R. Hollingsworth (1985) Maternal metabolism in normal pregnancy and pregnancy complicated by diabetes mellitus. *Clin. Obstet. Gynecol.* 28:457–472.
5. R. Osathanondh and D. Tulchinsky (1980) Placental polypeptide hormones. In: *Maternal-fetal Endocrinology* (D. Tulchinsky and K.J. Ryan, eds.), pp. 17–44, Saunders, Philadelphia.
6. F.E. Hytten and T. Lind (1973) *Diagnostic Indices in Pregnancy*, Ciba-Geigy, Basel.
7. F.E. Hytten (1980) Nutrition. In: *Clinical Physiology in Obstetrics* (F.E. Hytten and G. Chamberlain, eds.), pp. 163–192, Blackwell, Oxford.
8. J.C. King, M.N. Bronstein, W.L. Fitch, and J. Weininger (1987) Nutrient utilization during pregnancy. *World Rev. Nutr. Diet.* 52: 71–142.
9. M. Lawrence, F. Lawrence, W.H. Lamb, and R.G. Whitehead (1984) Maintenance energy cost of pregnancy in rural Gambian women and influence of dietary status. *Lancet* 2:363–365.
10. A.M. Prentice, R.G. Whitehead, M. Watkinson, W.H. Lamb, and T.J. Cole (1983) Prenatal dietary supplementation of African women and birth weight. *Lancet* 1:489–492.
11. J.V.G.A. Durnin, F.M. McKillop, S. Grant, and G. Fitzgerald (1985) Is nutritional status endangered by virtually no extra intake during pregnancy? *Lancet* 2:823–825.

12. M.L. Blackburn and D.H. Calloway (1974) Energy expenditure of pregnant adolescents. *J. Am. Diet. Assoc.* 65:24–30.

13. M.L. Blackburn and D.H. Calloway (1976) Basal metabolic rate and work energy expenditure of mature, pregnant women. *J. Am. Diet. Assoc.* 69:24–28.

14. National Research Council (1989) *Recommended Dietary Allowances,* 10th ed., National Academy Press, Washington, DC.

15. Joint FAO/WHO/UNU Expert Consultation (1985) *Energy and Protein Requirements.* Technical Report Series 724, World Health Organization, Geneva.

16. P.M. Fernhoff and E.J. Lammer (1984) Craniofacial features of isotretinoin embryopathy. *Pediatrics* 105:595–597.

17. I.T. Lott, M. Bocian, H.W. Pribram, and M. Leitner (1984) Fetal hydrocephalus and ear anomalies associated with maternal use of isotretinoin. *J. Pediatr.* 105:597–600.

18. P. Rosso and S.A. Lederman (1985) Nutrition and fetal growth. In: *Advances in Perinatal Medicine,* vol. 4 (A. Milunsky, E.A. Friedman, and L. Gluck, eds.), pp. 1–61, Plenum, New York.

19. C.A. Smith (1947) The effect of wartime starvation in Holland upon pregnancy and its product. *Am. J. Obstet. Gynecol.* 53:599–606.

20. S.A. Roberts, M.D. Cohen, and J.O. Forfar (1973) Antenatal factors associated with neonatal hypocalcaemic convulsions. *Lancet* 2:809–811.

21. R.J. Purvis, W.J. McK. Barrie, G.S. MacKay, E.M. Wilkinson, F. Cockburn, and N.R. Belton (1973) Enamel hypoplasia of the teeth associated with neonatal tetany: a manifestation of maternal vitamin-D deficiency. *Lancet* 2:811–814.

22. K. Schuster, L.B. Bailey, and C.S. Mahan (1984) Effect of maternal pyridoxine-HCl supplementation on the vitamin B_6 status of mother and infant and on pregnancy outcome. *J. Nutr.* 114:977–988.

23. L. Lumeng, R.E. Cleary, R. Wagner, P.-L. Yu, and T.-K. Li (1976) Adequacy of vitamin B_6 supplementation during pregnancy: a prospective study. *Am. J. Clin. Nutr.* 29:1376–1383.

24. A.M. Shojania (1984) Folic acid and vitamin B_{12} deficiency in pregnancy and in the neonatal period. *Clin. Perinatol.* 11:433–459.

25. K.M. Laurence, N. James, M.H. Miller, G.B. Tennant, and H. Campbell (1981) Double-blind randomised controlled trial of folate treatment before conception to prevent recurrence of neural-tube defects. *Br. Med. J.* 282:1509–1511.

26. J. Villar and J.M. Belizan (1986) Calcium during pregnancy. *Clin. Nutr.* 5:55–62.

27. I.S. Shenolikar (1970) Absorption of dietary calcium in pregnancy. *Am. J. Clin. Nutr.* 23:63–67.

28. A.T. Howarth, D.B. Morgan, and R.B. Payne (1977) Urinary excretion of calcium in late pregnancy and its relation to creatinine clearance. *Am. J. Obstet. Gynecol.* 129:499–502.

29. T.H. Bothwell, R.W. Charlton, J.D. Cook, and C.A. Finch (1979) *Iron Metabolism in Man,* Blackwell, Oxford.

30. S. Chaube, H. Nishimura, and C.A. Swinyard (1973) Zinc and cadmium in normal human embryos and fetuses. *Arch. Environ. Health* 26:237–240.

31. K.M. Hambidge, N.F. Krebs, M.A. Jacobs, A. Favier, L. Guyette, and D. Ikle (1983) Zinc nutritional status during pregnancy: a longitudinal study. *Am. J. Clin. Nutr.* 37:429–442.

32. J.M. Davison (1980) The urinary system. In: *Clinical Physiology in Obstetrics* (F.E. Hytten and G. Chamberlain, eds.), pp. 289–327, Blackwell, Oxford.

33. S. Tuttle, P.J. Aggett, D. Cambell, and I. MacGillivray (1985) Zinc and copper nutrition in human pregnancy: a longitudinal study in normal primigravidae and in primigravidae at risk of delivering a growth retarded baby. *Am. J. Clin. Nutr.* 42:1032–1041.

34. C.A. Swanson and J.C. King (1983) Reduced serum zinc concentration during pregnancy. *Obstet. Gynecol. N.Y.* 62:313–318.

35. R.L. Naeye (1979) Weight gain and the outcome of pregnancy. *Am. J. Obstet. Gynec.* 135:3–9.

36. B. Caan, D.M. Horgen, S. Margen, J.C. King, and J.P. Jewell (1987) Benefits associated with WIC supplemental feeding during the interpregnancy interval. *Am. J. Clin. Nutr.* 45:29–41.

37. C. Calandra, D.A. Abell, and N.A. Beischer (1981) Maternal obesity in pregnancy. *Obstet. Gynecol. N.Y.* 567:8–11.

38. L.E. Edwards, W.F. Dickes, I.R. Alton, and E.Y. Hakanson (1978) Pregnancy in the massively obese: course, outcome, and obesity prognosis of the infant. *Am. J. Obstet. Gynecol.* 131:479–483.

39. T. Gross, R.J. Sokol, and K.C. King (1980) Obesity in pregnancy: risks and outcome. *Obstet. Gynecol. N.Y.* 56:446–450.

40. H.D. Modanlon, W.L. Dorchester, A. Thorisian, and R.K. Freeman (1980) Macrosomia—maternal, fetal, and neonatal implications. *Obstet. Gynecol. N.Y.* 55:420–424.

41. D.K. Stevenson, A.O. Hopper, R.S. Cohen, L.R. Bucalo, J.A. Kerner, and P. Sunshine (1982) Macrosomia: causes and consequences. *J. Pediatr.* 100:515–520.

42. B. Worthington-Roberts (1987) Nutritional support of successful reproduction: an update. *J. Nutr. Ed.* 19:1–10.

43. K.K. Shy and Z.A. Brown (1984) Maternal and fetal well-being. *West. J. Med.* 141:807–815.

44. D.B. Jelliffe and E.F.P. Jelliffe (1978) The volume and composition of human milk in poorly nourished communities: a review. *Am. J. Clin. Nutr.* 31:492–515.

45. K.G. Dewey, D.A. Finley, and B. Lonnerdal (1984) Breast milk volume and composition during late lactation (7–20 months). *J. Pediatr. Gastroenterol.* 3:713–720.

46. L. Hambraeus (1984) Human milk composition. *Nutr. Abstr. Rev.* 54:219–236.

47. Committee on Nutrition, American Academy of Pediatrics (1981) Nutrition and lactation. *Pediatrics* 68:435–443.

48. K.M. Rasmussen (1988) Maternal nutritional status and lactational performance. *Clin. Nutr.* 7:147–155.

Chapter 37

Infancy

Recent investigations in infant nutrition have focused increasingly on relationships between food consumption and the enhancement of health rather than on the avoidance of frank nutrient deficiencies. The major exception to this generality in the United States is iron deficiency among selected socioeconomic groups.[1] In the economically developing world, deficiencies of vitamin A, iron, and iodine and protein-energy malnutrition continue to be major public health concerns.[2] Nutrient requirements for the prevention of deficiency diseases are published by national and international agencies.[3]

Food and Maturational Development

Studies of the constituents of human milk illustrate one type of interrelationship between diet and functional competencies.[4] Foods usually are viewed solely as a source of amino acids, carbohydrates, lipids, and other nutrients needed in the synthesis of functional and structural constituents of all tissues. Recent investigations of the nutrient needs of infants suggest that foods may have wider roles.[4] Human milk appears to deliver a significant proportion of basic nutrients as complex molecules with diverse yet complementary activities that are expressed before digestion and absorption. These activities complement maturation and, thereby, enhance specific functional competencies in the young infant. Examples of this functional relationship are noted between human milk constituents and the infant's immune and digestive systems.[4] Secretory immunoglobulin A (SIgA) in human milk provides passive mucosal protection to the infant by neutralizing specific antigens harmful to mucosal functions. This supplementary protection is provided when the infant's capacity for SIgA production is most limited. Recent data also suggest that human milk may stimulate the enhancement of the infant's production of mucosal immune factors.[4] A second example is the bile-salt–stimulated lipase in human milk. This enzyme enhances the infant's capacity for fat digestion and also may help protect the infant against parasitic infestation, e.g., *Giardia lamblia*.

Energy Intake and Growth

Most pediatric texts indicate that infants require ~100–120 kcal/kg in the first year of life. This represents significantly higher intakes than are consumed ad libitum by healthy breast-fed infants. Recent estimates of intake indicate that 1–2-mo-old infants consume 100–120 kcal/kg but that their energy intakes decrease to ~70–85 kcal/kg by age 4 mo.[5,6] These lower intakes persist after the ad libitum addition of solid foods to the infant's diet.[6,7]

Growth has been used as the principal criterion for the assessment of dietary adequacy in infancy. This criterion is difficult to assess, because growth patterns observed over the last 30–50 y among presumably normal infants demonstrate a plasticity that apparently is diet dependent.[8] The common expectation is that body weights and lengths of infants generally track birth percentiles. Sustained negative trends in anthropometric percentiles often trigger advice for increased feeding. Breast-fed infants studied in this country, however, exhibit negative trends in National Center for Health Statistics weight-for-age and length-for-age percentiles during the latter phase of exclusive breast-feeding, i.e., after the third month, and sustain those trends during the ensuing period of ad libitum mixed feedings of human milk and solid foods after the fourth or fifth month.[7,9] The magnitude of those negative trends is seldom sufficiently pronounced to be labeled frank growth failure, and its functional significance is not clear. Identification of an optimal growth pattern between the extremes of maximal growth and clear stunting represents a challenge. Maximal growth may not be desirable over the long term, and the health risks associated with stunting have been well documented.

Preliminary evidence is available that functional differences may be associated with distinct patterns of growth that fall within normal ranges. Recent studies indicate that breast-fed infants maintain lower minimal rates of energy expenditure, body temperature, and heart rates than do formula-fed infants who consume greater quantities of energy under ad libitum feeding conditions.[10] It is not clear whether those functional differences represent adaptations to inadequately low energy intakes among breast-fed infants or a response to excessive energy consumption by those fed artificial formulas. Applications of the doubly labeled water technique to measure energy expenditure and body composition are expected to be useful in the understanding of relationships among nutrient intake, growth, body composition, and functional capacities.

Recent observations of energy intake and growth of breast-fed infants also suggest a need to reassess concepts of growth monitoring and the expected tracking of anthropometric characteristics measured at birth and early infancy. A clearer assessment of desirable growth patterns is of most acute significance to infants who live in environments with high endemic levels of enteric disease. Sustained negative trends in weight or length percentiles often lead to the recommendation of supplementary foods. The introduction of supplementary foods in those environments is associated commonly with increased morbidity from gastrointestinal disease.[11] A premature introduction of solid foods therefore increases unnecessarily the risk to enteric disease. The inappropriate delay of supplementary foods commonly results in wasting and stunting.

Issues of Nutrition and Acute Morbidity

Diarrhea. From an international perspective, gastroenteritis continues to be a major cause of unacceptably high morbidity and mortality in infants. Low nutrient intakes, contaminated foods, and unsafe feeding practices account for an excessive proportion of that morbidity and mortality. Although oral rehydration therapy is efficacious in the treatment of the more acute effects of gastroenteritis, it is not sufficient. The initiation of feeding immediately after rehydration is an essential component of optimal management. Recent data demonstrate that nutrient balances are improved significantly when feeding is initiated early.[7] Improvements in net nutrient retentions early in the treatment phase ameliorate the deterioration of nutritional status caused by diarrheal diseases.

Field studies suggest an inverse relationship between the severity of diarrheal illnesses and nutritional status.[11] A relationship between nutritional status and the incidence of diarrhea is less clear, but the evidence suggests a higher incidence of diarrhea with declines in nutritional status.[11] The weakness of the relationship between nutritional status and diarrheal incidence is unexpected because of anticipated adverse affects of malnutrition on immune function. These findings suggest a need to investigate relationships between the mucosal immune system and nutritional states, particularly the role of micronutrients in normal mucosal immune function.

Vitamin A. The role of subclinical nutrient deficiencies in the predisposition to infectious illnesses is of current interest. Recent studies in Aceh, Indonesia, are particularly relevant to this discussion. Annual mortality of children aged 60–71 mo was reported to decrease from 8.0/1000 to 6.0/1000, i.e., a 25% reduction, in children to whom two doses of 200,000 IU vitamin A were administered orally at 6-mo intervals.[12] Children with any evidence of xerophthalmia were excluded from the analyses. If a reduction in mortality after the supplementation of the diet with vitamin A is replicable at other sites and the expected associated decrease in morbidity is documented in younger age groups, the impact of this intervention on nutritional strategies to improve infant health will be significant.

Biologically plausible mechanisms that may account for these putative effects on mortality and morbidity are suggested by the adverse effects of vitamin A deficiency on immunocompetence[13] and mucosal integrity.[14] In the absence of vitamin A, cultured hamster tracheal epithelial cells fail to develop into mature columnar mucous cells.[14] A squamous cell type is observed in their place. This response is similar to that seen in vivo in vitamin A–deficient animals. In the small intestine, vitamin A deficiency is not associated with squamous metaplasia but instead with the reduced production of mucin.[14] Reduced mucus production by the small intestine may reduce the effectiveness of an important protective barrier against the attachment or invasion of pathogens.

Breast-feeding. Breast-feeding is the most effective single nutritional strategy that has been identified for the prevention of diarrheal disease in infants.[4] This protection has been demonstrated in economically developed and developing nations. Protective effects of breast-feeding on otitis media and respiratory infections are less well established. Specific protective mechanisms remain unclear. Passive protection via human milk's immune components, active protection by unidentified inductive factors in human milk that are capable of stimulating the infant's immune system, and the decreased likelihood of consuming contaminated foods when an infant is breast-fed are possible explanations for the lower morbidities associated with breast-feeding.

Nutrition and Chronic Disease

Increased attention in nutrition is focused on the prevention of chronic diseases that become clinically significant in adult life. Genetically related disorders that become evident in infancy and childhood (e.g., allergy, asthma, insulin-dependent diabetes, and celiac disease), early adult life (e.g., inflammatory bowel disease and duodenal ulcer), and late adulthood (e.g., atherosclerosis, noninsulin-dependent diabetes, hypertension, and colon cancer) have been identified.[15] The expression of many of those disorders possibly is modulated by diet. Of the 10 leading causes of death in the United States, 5 (i.e., coronary heart disease, some cancers, stroke, diabetes mellitus, and atherosclerosis) have been associated with diet. There is no direct evidence, however, that any of the conditions with onset after childhood are significantly influenced by the diet in infancy. A clear demonstration that the diet during infancy influences the occurrence or severity of chronic diseases during adult life is difficult, because intervening events, exposures, and behaviors are likely to diminish the consistency, strength, and specificity of putative interrelationships among diet, genetic endowment, environmental factors, and disease outcomes in later stages of life. Evidence that the diet in infancy modulates a genetic predisposition to chronic diseases therefore focuses on extrapolated associations noted in epidemiologic investigations, short-term clinical studies, or animal experiments and on the biological plausibility of hypothetical relationships.

Breast-feeding vs. Formula Feeding. Breast-feeding was suggested to prevent or ameliorate allergies, asthma, insulin-dependent diabetes, and some forms of childhood cancers, but the evidence is not conclusive. Most work that has led to these suggestions has been epidemiologic in nature and is difficult to evaluate because of problems with study design and data analysis. These problems stem from difficulties in the control of pertinent behavioral and socioeconomic variables. The types of difficulties that usually are encountered were summarized by Kramer.[16] Evaluations of feeding studies often place excessive reliance on prolonged maternal recalls, there often is not blind ascertainment of infant-feeding history, and the duration and exclusivity of breast-feeding commonly are not sufficient to ascribe an outcome to a particular feeding mode. In the assessments of outcomes associated with feeding mode, strict diagnostic criteria of target outcomes often are not applied, outcome is not ascertained blindly, the severity of outcomes is not graded, and the age of onset is not identified

clearly. Finally, statistical analyses are difficult to interpret because controls for confounding variables commonly are not sufficient, dose-effect responses are not assessed, and statistical power often is inadequate.

Atherosclerosis. The prevention of atherosclerosis through nutritional strategies also has been discussed because of the concern that this condition may originate in early childhood.[17,18] Blood cholesterol measured at 6 mo is found to correlate with levels measured at 7 y, and by age 1 y blood cholesterol correlates with the dietary intake of saturated fatty acids and cholesterol.[17] Genetic aspects are relevant, because children whose parents have high levels of blood cholesterol are two to three times more likely to have cholesterol levels >95% compared with children whose parents have low cholesterol levels. Most expert groups however recommend no changes in the amounts of fat normally included in the infant's diet because of (1) the lack of evidence that 40–50% fat in the diets of infants exacerbates a genetic predisposition to atherosclerosis or that a reduction in dietary fat ameliorates it and (2) the possibility that lowered amounts of fat may dilute the energy content of the diet sufficiently to interfere with normal development.

There is less consensus regarding the optimal fat composition of the infant's diet. Generally, saturated fatty acids increase plasma cholesterol; the cholesterolemic effect of saturated fatty acids is lessened by increases in carbon-chain length. The relative effects of the diet's fatty acid composition is illustrated by a recent investigation that demonstrates a lowering of plasma cholesterol when stearic acid is substituted for dietary palmitic acid.[19] Polyunsaturated fatty acids tend to lower plasma cholesterol more than monounsaturated fatty acids do. High levels of polyunsaturated fatty acids, however, may increase the risk for certain cancers and adversely affect immune function.[20,21] The incompletely understood role of longer-chain (>20 carbons) polyunsaturated fatty acids in the development of membrane structures in the central nervous system and other organs also complicates evaluations of fatty acid mixtures in infant diets.[22]

Obesity. The prevention and control of obesity during infancy are of concern to the prevention of morbidity in childhood and in later life stages. Although it is clear that not all obese infants become obese adults, obesity in infancy increases the risk of long-term obesity. Secular trends demonstrate an increasing prevalence of obesity in early life.[23] The persistence of juvenile onset obesity is significant, and it increases with the severity of obesity.[24]

Although there is no basis for recommending hypocaloric diets for the treatment, control, or prevention of infantile obesity, it is advisable to avoid its development because of excess energy consumption or inappropriately low levels of activity. Obesity predisposes children to psychological dysfunction, orthopedic problems, abnormal glucose tolerance, respiratory disease, and hypertension.[25] Increases in childhood obesity also are associated with increasingly atherogenic lipoprotein profiles.[26]

Dental Caries. The prevalence of dental caries in children appears to be declining but remains a significant cause of morbidity in this age group. The role of sugars, particularly sucrose, in the promotion of tooth decay is well established. Fluoridation of the water supply and a decrease in the frequency and quantity of foods rich in sugar remain mainstays of sound oral hygiene programs, which should have their origin in infancy. Fluoride supplements are not indicated for young infants who live in areas without fluoridation. Fluoride supplements, however, are appropriate for infants older than age 6 mo. The desired supplemental amount is dependent upon fluoride concentrations in the water supply.

Feeding Considerations

The increased emphasis on health promotion has underscored the recommendation that infants be exclusively breast-fed for the first 4–6 mo of life. Although it is not unusual for some cultures to support the breast-feeding of children through the second year, in this country it is unusual after the 9th–12th month. When complementary foods are introduced, single foods should be added to the diet at intervals that permit the assessment of the infant's tolerance to the new foods. The recommended interval between the introduction of new foods is ~4 d. The introduction of whole cow milk should be delayed until after the first year, and its intake should be limited to <900 mL/d. Greater amounts of milk often limit the intake of other foods and result in an imbalanced diet, e.g., resulting in inadequately low levels of iron and vitamin C. The infant's total diet should provide ~10–15% of calories as protein, ~40–50% as carbohydrate, and the remainder as fat.

During the period of exclusive breast-feeding, supplementation with vitamin D may be suggested in climates that limit sun exposure. Fluoride supplements also may be necessary in areas without fluoridation in infants aged ≥6 mo. During the period of mixed feeding, the need for other supplemental micronutrients is dependent upon specific diets. If human milk or synthetic formulas make up ≥80% of the diet, it is unlikely that the infant will require any supplements except for iron. As the proportion of milk in the diet decreases, the need for supplemental nutrients will depend increasingly on the composition of the remaining part of the diet. Nutrient allowances published by the National Research Council[3] provide useful guidelines for the assessment of the micronutrient composition of the diet. The assessment of an infant's nutritional status should include an evaluation of anthropometric indicators, dietary intake, activity pattern, and selected biochemical indices as indicated.

Summary

In this country the major emphasis in infant nutrition is the relationship between diet and health rather than a focus on the prevention of deficiency diseases. The complementarity between human milk composition and the infant's developmental competencies is an example of this interest. From an international perspective, iron, iodine, and vitamin A deficiency and protein-energy malnutrition continue to be of major public health importance. Nutritional strategies remain a mainstay of efforts targeted at the prevention of diarrheal disease and the amelioration of its adverse effects. Breast-feeding is the best single nutritional approach for the prevention of infectious diseases in young infants. No change in the usual fat content (~40% of energy) of the infant's diet is recommended as a means of lessening a genetic predisposition to diet-related adult-onset diseases. A similar consensus is not available regarding the optimal composition of dietary fats. Although hypocaloric diets have no place in the treatment or control of infantile obesity, it is prudent to prevent this condition by discouraging excessive intakes of energy and inactivity. The frequent and excessive intake of refined carbohydrates increases the risk for dental caries.

This work was funded in part by grant no. 5R01 HD21049 from the National Institute of Child Health and Human Development and in part by Hatch Project no. 199408.

References

1. Nutrition Policy Board, U.S. Department of Health and Human Services (1988) *The Surgeon General's Report on Nutrition and Health.* DHHS (PHS) Publication No. 88-50210, U.S. Government Printing Office, Washington, DC.

2. United Nations Administrative Committee on Coordination, Subcommittee on Nutrition (1987) *First Report on the World Nutrition Situation,* ACC/SCN, FAO, Rome, Italy.

3. National Research Council (1989) *Recommended Dietary Allowances,* 10th ed., National Academy Press, Washington, DC.

4. C. Garza, R.J. Schanler, N.F. Butte, and K.J. Motil (1987) Special properties of human milk. *Clin. Perinatol.* 14:104–128.

5. N.F. Butte, C. Garza, E.O. Smith, and B.L. Nichols (1984) Human milk intake and growth performance of exclusively breast-fed infants. *J. Pediatr.* 104:187–195.

6. K.G. Dewey, M.J. Heinig, L.A. Nommsen, and B. Lönnerdal (1989) Low energy intake and growth velocity of breast-fed infants at 6–

12 mo: are there functional consequences? *FASEB J.* 3:4813 (abstracts, part II).

7. C. Garza, J. Stuff, and N. Butte (1988) Growth of the breast-fed infant. In: *The Effects of Human Milk upon the Recipient Infant* (A.S. Goldman, S.A. Atkinson, and L.A. Hanson, eds.), pp. 109–122, Plenum Press, New York.

8. R.G. Whitehead and A.A. Paul (1985) Human lactation, infant feeding, and growth: secular trends. In: *Nutritional Needs and Assessment of Normal Growth* (M. Gracey and F. Falkner, eds.), Raven Press, New York.

9. M.J. Heinig, L.A. Nommsen, B. Lönnerdal, and K.G. Dewey (1989) Growth patterns of breast-fed infants during the weaning period: 6–18 mo. *FASEB J.* 3:4806 (abstracts, part II).

10. N.F. Butte, W.W. Wong, C. Garza, and P.D. Klein (in press) Adequacy of human milk for meeting energy requirements during early infancy. In: *Proceedings of the Fourth International Symposium on Human Lactation* (S. Atkinson, R. Chandra, and L. Hanson, eds.), ARTS Biomedical, St. Johns, Newfoundland.

11. J. Sepulveda, W. Willett, and A. Munoz (1988) Malnutrition and diarrhea. A longitudinal study among urban Mexican children. *Am. J. Epidemiol.* 127:365–376.

12. A.I. Sommer, I. Tarwotjo, E. Djunaedi, et al. (1986) Impact of vitamin A supplementation on childhood mortality. A randomised controlled community trial. *Lancet* 1:1169–1173.

13. W.R. Beisel (1982) Single nutrients and immunity. *Am. J. Clin. Nutr.* 35:417–468.

14. L. De Luca and G. Wolf (1970) Vitamin A and mucus secretion, a brief review of the effect of vitamin A on the biosynthesis of glycoproteins. *Int. Z. Vitaminforsch.* 40:284–290.

15. J.L. Rotter (1987) Genetic predisposition to common adult disease. In: *Frontiers in Genetic Medicine* (M.M. Kaback and L.J. Shapairo, eds.), pp. 35–43, Ross Laboratories, Columbus, OH.

16. M.S. Kramer (1988) Does breast feeding help protect against atopic disease? Biology, methodology, and a golden jubilee of controversy. *J. Pediatr.* 112:181–190.

17. D.S. Freedman, S.R. Srinivasen, J.L. Cresanta, L.S. Webber, and G.S. Berenson (1987) Cardiovascular risk factors from birth to seven years of age: the Bogalusa Heart Study. Serum lipids and lipoproteins. *Pediatrics* 80(suppl.):789–796.

18. G.S. Berenson, S.R. Srinivasen, R.R. Frerichs, and L.S. Webber (1979) Serum high density lipoprotein and its relationship to cardiovascular disease risk factor variables in children—the Bogalusa Heart Study. *Lipids* 14:91–98.

19. A. Bonanome and S.M. Grundy (1988) Effect of dietary stearic acid on plasma cholesterol and lipoprotein levels. *N. Engl. J. Med.* 318:1244–1248.

20. P.C. Chan, K.A. Ferguson, and T.L. Dao (1983). Effects of different dietary fats on mammary carcinogenesis. *Cancer Res.* 43:1079–1083.

21. J. Mertin and R. Hunt (1976) Influence of polyunsaturated fatty acids on survival of skin allografts and tumor incidence in mice. *Proc. Natl. Acad. Sci. USA* 73:928–931.

22. M.T. Clandinin, J.E. Chappell, S. Leong, F. Heim, P.R. Swyer, and G.W. Chance (1980) Extrauterine fatty acid accretion in infant brain: implications for fatty acid requirements. *Early Hum. Dev.* 4:131–138.

23. C.L. Shea, D.S. Freedman, G.L. Burke, D.W. Harsha, L.S. Webber, and G.S. Berenson (1988) Secular trends of obesity in early life: the Bogalusa Heart Study. *Am. J. Public Health* 78:75–77.

24. D.S. Freedman, C.L. Shear, G.L. Burke, et al. (1987) Persistence of juvenile-onset obesity over eight years: the Bogalusa Heart Study. *Am. J. Public Health* 77:588–592.

25. S.L. Gortmaker, W.H. Dietz, A.M. Sobol, and C.A. Wehler (1987) Increasing pediatric obesity in the United States. *Am. J. Dis. Child.* 141:535–540.

26. D.S. Freedman, G.L. Burke, D.W. Harsha, et al. (1985) Relationship of changes in obesity to serum lipid and lipoprotein changes in childhood and adolescence. *JAMA* 254:515–520.

Chapter 38

Betty Ruth Carruth

Adolescence

The biological variation among individuals during periods of rapid growth such as adolescence is most evident from the contrast between chronological age and markers of maturation, e.g., stature and secondary sex characteristics. Although individuals progress through the teenage years within a relatively short period, the diversity at any age is remarkable, often to the chagrin of adolescents who wish to fit society's expectations for ideal body image and physical attractiveness.

The major influences on nutrient needs during adolescence relate to genetic potential; to normal patterns of growth and development in the absence of trauma, stress, injury, or other environmental and health factors; and to physical activities that increase energy and nutrient needs.

Factors Influencing Nutrient Needs: Genetics and Environment

Increases in linear height reflect genetic potential, and the rate of growth is used as a reference point for predicting adult height in growing adolescents. In animal and human studies, measurements correlated between body weight and genetic potential are less clear and are further confounded by energy imbalance problems in adolescence.[1] In serial measurements of height change and growth velocities of adolescents, individual patterns of development evolve that correlate with inheritable traits. Rates of growth can be influenced by environmental factors, e.g., food availability, family systems and food distribution, abuse of substances, and accidents, injuries, and traumas resulting from risk-taking behavior that is characteristic of the adolescent years. Because many of these environmental factors are present in the lifestyles of adolescents, nutrient intake, utilization, and metabolism are negatively influenced and result in less than optimal nutrition during the adolescent years.

Assessing Growth and Development

Changes in Linear-height and Peak-height Velocity Rates. Tanner and Davies[2] published longitudinally based weight and height velocity charts for North American children. The percentiles described early, middle, and late maturers by age according to velocity of height growth in centimeters. These charts provide a means of comparing children and adolescents of the same chronological age at different heights according to their rate of growth (J.M. Tanner, unpublished observations, 1986). The average age at peak-height velocity (PHV) is 13.5 y for males and 11.5 for females. For those who mature late, PHV occurs at 15.4 y in males and at 13.5 y in females. During a year of PHV, females may grow 8.3 cm and males 9.5 cm, resulting in an average height difference of 13.0 cm.[2] By describing the velocity of growth and relating this to other indicators of physiological maturation, e.g., pubic hair, testes weight, or breast development, adolescents may be compared with their cohort age group in terms of individual development and progression—changes that often are misunderstood by adolescents and parents.

Menarche. The onset of menses begins about 1 y after PHV. Thereafter, increases in height are minimal. According to Garn and Wagner[3] any changes in stature after menarche are in the magnitude of 0.5 cm, and Rosenfeld[4] estimated that 98% of adult height has been reached. Menarche is followed by a deceleration in rate of growth with an increase in the deposition of adipose tissue as indicated by increasing triceps skinfold measurements and decreasing lean body mass as a percent of total body weight. In contrast, males continue to grow linearly post-PHV at a decelerated rate. For both sexes, major changes in body composition occur, resulting in increased nutrient and energy needs to accommodate the rapid gain in skeletal and body mass.

In children endocrine function and gender differences are not statistically significant. Consequently dietary adequacy and nutrient allowances for both sexes are treated similarly.[5] However, when neuroendocrine systems initiate the pubertal phase, estimates of nutrient needs should be based on gender differences in the amount of lean body mass, physical activity, rate of velocity, and changes in body composition that influence the amount of nutrients required during this period of rapid growth.

Developmental Issues and Nutrient Needs of Adolescents

Height-weight Ratios. Charts from the National Center for Health Statistics (NCHS) are the most frequently cited norm for comparing heights and weights of individuals by age and sex for ages 12–17 y.[6] These charts provide percentiles based on height, weight, sex, and chronological age and were derived from a large cross-sectional, national probability sample. Their limitations have been discussed and acknowledged as suitable for group comparisons. They are not suitable, however, for individual adolescents. For those who mature late and early, the discrepancy between longitudinal and cross-sectional norms for height attained are even more pronounced than for adolescents with a mean growth rate, i.e., 50th percentile for age and sex. The growth charts do not address changes in body composition when energy intakes exceed activity and growth needs other than by classifying an individual by weight percentile. For example, the 90th percentile indicates obesity for height, age, and sex.

In the prepubertal years a tendency toward overweight may occur in both males and females. The accompanying gynecomastia in males may initiate restrictive food practices and weight loss during a period of preparation for the rapid linear growth associated with the onset of puberty. Normal teens can expect to gain ~50% of their adult weight and approximately 15% of adult height.[4] Lean body mass increases significantly in males, almost doubling in the prepubertal and pubertal years (ages 10–17 y). Estrogen and progesterone promote greater fat deposition in females, whereas testosterone and the adrenal androgens alter body composition in males, resulting in more lean body mass than fat, a greater skeletal mass, and a larger blood cell mass than in females.[7] Thus, proportional gains in weight as increments in height occur are desirable; however, the variations in rate of growth among individuals can result in height-weight ratios that are diverse from the NCHS charts based on age, sex, and height indices. In our present society the percent of body fat and gains in lean muscle mass for both males and females are of greater concern to the adolescent's self-image than are dietary adequacy of nutrients, such as iron, calcium, and zinc, that directly affect

biochemical and metabolic systems promoting normal growth patterns.

Several researchers reported on the efficacy of the body mass index (BMI, wt/ht^2) and triceps skinfold measurement as indicators of percent of body fat.[8–10] Johnston[11] concluded that both relative weight and triceps skinfold measurement can falsely categorize adolescents as having normal amounts of body fat. For example, triceps skinfold measurement was more highly correlated with body fatness in males, and wt/ht^2 was more indicative of body fatness in females. Thus, the distribution of fat in females vs. males and total amount of fat as percent of body weight must be considered in periods of rapid growth. It was suggested that in preadolescent children, weight-height ratios may not correlate with skinfold measurements and other indicators of body fat.[12] Thus, for an individual, serial data represent the best basis for determining nutrient needs, including energy requirements for growth and physical activity.

McKeag[13] reviewed current knowledge about the effect of exercise on growth and development and the potential negative impact of excessive exercise. Although skills may be built by repetitive exercise, the onset of puberty must occur before muscle building and endurance capacity increase as a result of training activities. If exercise is not continued, muscle development of adolescents will regress to their prepubertal or untrained status.

For teenage girls the national profiles for physical fitness are discouraging. According to the President's Council on Physical Fitness and Sports,[14] fitness test scores in 1975 and 1984 indicated that girls plateaued at 13–14 y of age, and over the decade no gains were observed. Girls had better scores on upper-body flexibility than did boys. Boys demonstrated greater cardiovascular capacity and endurance than did girls; however, a large percentage of both groups scored lower than the 50th and 25th percentiles compared with the same tests in 1975.

Changes in body composition are exceedingly important in recommending nutrients and food patterns that promote health in the adolescent population. Energy requirements increase with rapid growth, a greater proportion of lean body mass, a lesser proportion of body fat as percent of total weight, increased physical activity that promotes cardiovascular fitness, and large muscle development and skeletal maturation. When these conditions exist to a lesser degree, energy needs may be reduced, but the requirements for micronutrients, such as zinc, folic acid, pyridoxine, vitamin B-12, etc. do not decrease proportionately to the calorie reductions reported by females in NHANES II data.[15,16]

In summary, nutrient needs during adolescence are influenced by elevated amounts of estrogen and progesterone in females and testosterone in males as well as by the anabolic adrenal androgens that increase with the onset of puberty and trigger the subsequent changes in linear height, body weight, and body composition.[17] Overall increased energy needs during the adolescent years and the genetic expression as reflected by early, normal, or late maturation necessitate individualizing dietary recommendations and approaches for promoting better nutritional practices and healthier lifestyles.

Dietary and Nutrient Standards. The 1989 Recommended Dietary Allowances currently are used to assess the nutrient intakes of adolescents.[5] Nutrient allowances are increased overall from the prepubertal years with the exception of energy per unit of weight. The allowances are considered adequate for the nutritional needs of practically all healthy people and do not represent requirements. Requirements for adolescents have received limited study.

For protein, values represent calculations from body composition and growth rates and are based on the assumption that protein utilization is comparable with adult maintenance requirements. Energy allowances for adolescents represent average needs by age and at an assumed amount of activity. For children and adolescents, energy allowances reflect the median calorie intake of children followed in longitudinal growth studies. Nutrient allowances for adolescents are mostly extrapolated from nutrient recommendations for infants and adults; only a few are based on studies of nutrient requirements of adolescents. However, frequently dietary data for individuals are compared with these dietary standards, and nutrient adequacy is judged by percent of the standard present in the diet.

Woteki[18] described data from national surveys available to the public and indicated their proper uses and limitations. The National Health and Nutrition Examination Surveys I (NHANES I, 1971–1974) and II (NHANES II, 1976–1980) involved a representative sample of the civilian population (noninstitutionalized). These surveys included health histories, physical examinations, and selected laboratory assessments. Hematological assessments and serum indicators of vitamins and some minerals as well as anthropometric measurements are available for comparing health and dietary data about adolescents. The cross-sectional data are categorized by chronological age with standard deviations given for sample variations.[15,16]

Another source used as a standard to compare dietary data is the Nationwide Food Consumption Survey (NFCS), 1977–1978, conducted by the Human Nutrition Information Service (HNIS), Department of Agriculture (USDA).[19] Members of the household recalled 1 d of food intake and a diary was kept for 2 additional days. Adolescents did not meet the standard for calcium, iron, pyridoxine, magnesium, and energy when expressed as percent of RDA. However, when the data are expressed as nutrients per 1000 kcal, dietary deficiencies are not as apparent. As the energy intake decreases per day, it becomes important to consume nutrient-dense foods. However, the current most-favored snacks and many meals consumed by adolescents are more likely to provide calories without providing essential vitamins and minerals.[20]

Energy and Nutrient Intakes of Adolescents

Energy. Data from the NHANES I survey indicate that 12–14-y-old girls consumed 1,932 kcal/d; the amount decreased to 1,739 kcal/d for 18–19-y-olds. For males ages 12–14 y, the average intake was 2,519 kcal/d compared with 2,949 kcal/day for 18–19-y-olds. With increments in lean body mass and linear height and increased activities with sponsored sports for many males, the larger energy intake with increasing age is appropriate. In addition, most males met or exceeded two-thirds of the RDA for minerals, such as iron, calcium, and zinc, that tend to be deficient in the diets of girls.[15,16,19]

Wait et al.[21] compared energy intakes of girls at the prepubescent, rapidly growing, and postpubescent stages of development. Energy intakes were not related to chronological ages but were related to physiological indices. The researchers proposed that calories per unit of height and age was a better estimate of energy need, a suggestion that has been recommended by practitioners in the field.[22]

Protein. Protein needs are increased during adolescence because of the increased lean body mass, erythrocyte and myoglobin requirements, and hormonal changes. Males increase muscle mass into adulthood, whereas females increase in adipose tissue postmenarche and have almost twice the amount that males[7] have, i.e., 22–24% compared with 12–14%, respectively. To meet expanding protein requirements for growth and tissue development, it was recommended that males consume 0.3 g protein/cm height, with a range of 0.29–0.32 g/cm height.[22] For girls, the protein recommendation is 0.27–0.29 g/cm height. These recommendations, thus, link increments in height to nutrient requirements rather than to chronological age.

Overall, protein intake was not a dietary problem in the most recent surveys of adolescents' reported diets.[15,16] Protein intake for males ages 9–11 y was 205% and for 15–18 y was 190% of the standard. Protein intake for females ages 9–11 y was 181% and for ages 15–18 y was 152% of the standard.[19] For females who reduce caloric intake to achieve weight loss, protein may be used for gluconeogenesis. In addition, other nutrients, such as iron, calcium, and zinc, may be adversely affected by dietary restriction of protein.

Carbohydrate and Fat. Current recommendations for these energy sources relate to the percent of calories derived from carbohydrate and fat and the types of foods chosen. The recommendations are aimed at the food habits of the adult population in the United States and are as follows: <30–35% of calories from total fat, with 10% from saturated sources, 10% of calories from polyunsaturated fats, and ≥50% of the total calories from carbohydrates with emphasis on foods rich in fiber and other complex carbohydrates.[23]

In general, diets of adolescents are characterized by a fat intake >35% of calories, more foods providing simple sugars, and a diet that is essentially low in vegetable and plant sources that would provide fiber and complex carbohydrates. Although the recommendations were not developed for youth, it is likely that diets of adolescents will be modified as part of the family's changes in dietary habits. The effects of reducing these nutrients on growth and development are unknown, and prospective studies are needed to determine the effect of altering fat intake and its distribution among food sources.

Vitamins. In general, water-soluble vitamins and some of the fat-soluble vitamins are not of concern except in subgroups of adolescents where a dietary deficiency is secondary to other factors. NHANES and NFCS data indicated that both males and females exceeded the standard of 100% of the RDA for vitamin A, thiamin, riboflavin, preformed niacin, vitamin B-12, and vitamin C.

Pyridoxine. The role of vitamin B-6 in protein and amino acid metabolism is well recognized during periods of rapid growth, both as a cofactor and in providing plasma pyridoxal phosphate (PLP) for catabolism of excess amino acids. Driskell et al.[24] reported on vitamin B-6 status of 112 black and white adolescent girls, using the coenzyme stimulation of erythrocyte alanine aminotransferase and dietary intake to estimate vitamin B-6 status. About half the subjects reported 0.02 mg vitamin B-6/g of protein in 1981 and 1983, and >40% were judged as having inadequate vitamin B-6 status. In vitamin B-6 requirements studies in young adults and animals, growth retardation improved and urinary excretion of vitamin B-6 metabolites decreased when supplements were given after a deficient diet and/or higher protein meals were provided.[25]

Folate. Folic acid's primary role as a methyl donor is essential to protein metabolism and erythropoiesis during periods of rapid growth. Unlike the situation for other water-soluble vitamins, such as vitamin C,[26] dietary deficiencies were reported for adolescent groups. Reiter et al.[27] found that 97% of black adolescent females consumed less than two-thirds of the RDA for folate and 74% had marginal plasma concentrations.

Herbert[28] proposed intakes for adolescent males and females, ages 11–18 y, of 6.8 nmol folate/kg (3 μg/kg), providing a range of 249–385 nmol/d for males and 295 nmol/d for females. The 1989 RDA[5] are somewhat higher. Although the North American diet may provide two-thirds or more of 300 μg/d proposed by Sauberlich et al.[29] for nonpregnant adult women, folate is labile to heat, storage, and cooking losses that further reduce its availability from the diet. In addition, the better sources of folate, i.e., liver and leafy vegetables, are not consumed in appreciable amounts by adolescents although fortified breakfast cereals may contribute to folate intake.

Vitamin C. Vitamin C performs as an antioxidant and as an electron donor in multiple, complex biological processes. For adolescents the reported intakes in most recent surveys were 175% of the RDA for males and 132–186% of the RDA for females.[19] Olson and Hodges[26] proposed 30 mg vitamin C for males and 40 mg for females during the adolescent years. These recommendations are lower than the 1989 RDA, e.g., 50–60 mg vitamin C/d for both adolescent males and females. Given the reportedly low dietary intake of iron, the larger consumption of vitamin C may enhance the bioavailability of dietary iron. A recommendation of 40 mg provides a 40% safety factor and is four to seven times the therapeutic dose required to cure scurvy.

Minerals

Iron. Iron is one of three minerals (calcium, iron, and zinc) frequently reported as deficient in adolescents' diets; the incidence of anemia, indicated by a plasma ferritin concentration of <10 μg/L, was reported as 10% in females and 3% in males.[30] The most recent reports of iron status (NHANES II) showed a prevalence of impaired iron status in 4–12% of males aged 11–14 y and 5–14% of females aged 15–44 y.[31]

Iron is essential for the formation of hemoglobin and myoglobin and as a cofactor in a number of enzyme systems. The degree of iron storage depletion is evaluated by decreases in plasma-ferritin concentrations; subsequent stages include iron-deficient erythropoiesis, and iron-deficiency anemia as characterized by microcytic-hypochromic changes in erythrocytes.[32] Because of assay ease and tissue availability, hemoglobin and hematocrit values are most frequently reported as indicators of iron-deficiency anemia in the adolescent population. Racial differences in hemoglobin values that were independent of nutrient intake and maturational changes have been reported.

Iron absorption increases when iron deficiency occurs, enabling the body to maintain a close regulation of body iron content. In recent years interests in dietary composition of foods consumed together and of other nutrients that may enhance absorption have changed dietary recommendations for absolute amounts of dietary iron. Monsen and Balintfy[33] proposed that heme and nonheme forms of iron could be calculated in any particular meal because of the difference in absorption of the two forms and because of their availability when other constituents of the diet were considered. For calculation purposes the average amount of heme iron in all animal tissue is estimated at 40%; the remaining 60% of dietary iron in plant products and animal tissue is treated as nonheme iron. On the basis current knowledge, the 60% nonheme iron may be enhanced by the presence of organic acid, such as ascorbic acid, and the quantity of animal tissue (enhancing factor) present in the meal.

For adolescents the consumption of protein exceeds the RDA threefold and vitamin C intakes are in the range of 130–186% of the dietary standard. Although Herbert[32] does not specifically discuss the iron stores of adolescents and rates of absorption, he reported that mean absorption rates of adult women with 500-mg iron stores are 5–10% and could increase to 15–20% when stores are <100 mg. If those extrapolations can be made to the adolescent population, then the low incidence of reported iron-deficiency anemia may reflect the positive synergistic interaction of higher protein intake from animal tissue and adequate ascorbic acid intakes in this age group.

The 1989 RDA for iron are similar to intakes proposed by Herbert,[32] i.e., 12 mg for males aged 10–17.9 y and 15 mg for females aged 10–17.9 y. An allowance of 10 mg/d was recommended for children, with an additional 2 mg to support the pubertal growth spurt in males and an additional 5 mg for the growth spurt and menses in females. These recommendations are based on the average omnivorous U.S. diet eaten by an individual with adequate iron stores, on the premise that an average of 10% of the total dietary iron is absorbed.[32] However, the iron bioavailability was less in a study reported by Viglietti and Skinner.[34] They calculated total iron availability to be <10% of that assumed in the RDA, and neither boys nor girls met the amount of 1.8 mg iron bioavailability as reported in the Nationwide Food Consumption Survey.

Dietary supplements are used by adolescents to offset the effect of a poor diet, to augment physical strength, to impart a specific result such as virility, and for emotional reasons that have little to do with sound nutrition science. Sobal and Muncie[35] reported on 17 studies involving vitamin-mineral supplementation by adolescents and concluded that the range

of use was 1–57% compared with a prevalence of ≥40% in the adult population. Use of dietary supplements by adolescents is not supported by professional groups other than in cases of pregnancy, trauma, and disease that impair nutrient absorption, utilization, and metabolism.[36]

Calcium. Approximately 99% of the body calcium is in the skeletal structure and 1% is ionized. During adolescence long bones and vertebrae increase by intramembranous ossification and by endochondral ossification. In x rays, the epiphyseal plate shows up as a dense shadow with a translucent zone interstitial with the shaft. Both ends of the long bones have epiphyseal plates and are subject to trauma or injury during periods of rapid growth. The wrist site is a more active growth site than the lower limbs and is used to assess biological maturity (vs. chronological age).[3]

Although no control studies on calcium balance in adolescents were found in the literature, Nordin et al.'s study[37] of premenopausal and postmenopausal women showed a requirement of 500–700 mg/d of calcium to provide for the obligatory urinary losses of filtered calcium (3 mmol/d) and to achieve positive calcium balance. In adolescents, increases in estrogen, growth hormone, testosterone, and other anabolic hormones favor osteoblastic activity. However, the low dietary intake of calcium among girls represents a potential health problem for osteoporosis in the postmenopausal years because peak skeletal mass is formed during the adolescent years before growth ceases.[38] In addition, protein intakes in the United States are well above estimated needs and may compromise utilization of dietary calcium.[39]

Intense physical activity can also cause increased urinary loss of calcium. Because the RDA assume moderate amounts of activity, adolescents involved in intensive sports and dance may represent an at-risk group for calcium deficiency. If dietary supplements and/or food sources of protein are self-administered, e.g., 2–3 g/kg weight in an attempt to enhance athletic performance through anabolic and morphological changes of protein within muscle fibers, the interaction of nutrients may negatively influence patterns of growth and development during adolescence.

Zinc. Zinc is now known to be involved with some 70 enzyme systems and is of particular importance in adolescence. Zinc is required for synthesis of nucleic acids and protein, and zinc deficiency may be manifested by weight loss, intercurrent infections, hypogonadism in males, growth retardation, poor appetite, lethargy, delayed wound healing, and other symptoms depending upon the severity of the deficiency. Zinc deficiencies may occur secondary to hypercatabolic states, such as multiple injuries, major fractures, and other types of injuries that can be associated with the risk-taking behavior of adolescents. Prasad[40] described the difficulty in diagnosing zinc deficiency, because reduced plasma or urine zinc are not necessarily indicators of low-body-zinc status and plasma zinc concentration may remain normal in cases of mild zinc deficiency. However, diminished growth rates in height and body weight were corrected with zinc supplements in patients with sickle cell anemia in studies using zinc-supplemented and placebo groups.[40]

Controlled studies on zinc requirements during adolescence have not been conducted. The RDA are extrapolated from adult requirements, and limited data on zinc nutriture are reported in the literature.[41] In a biracial study of 14- and 16-y-old girls, Sloane et al.[42] found mean plasma zinc concentrations to be significantly higher for white (0.0133 ± 0.005 mmol/L) than for black (0.0121 ± 0.005 mmol/L) subjects. Although dietary fiber did not influence zinc status, it was negatively related to copper plasma concentrations. Height in both groups was positively related to dietary zinc intake. It appears that mild deficiency may influence growth patterns without evidence of severe deficiency as described by Prasad.[40]

As with iron, over a range of zinc intakes, the absorption rate is regulated, and other dietary components, such as cadmium, copper, calcium, and ferrous irons, function as inhibitors of zinc absorption. The presence of dietary phytates, hemicellulose, and lignin also negatively influence zinc absorption.

Sandstead and Evans[41] reported that ~30% of ingested dietary zinc is absorbed and only ~5% is excreted in the urine. The best sources of zinc are seafood, poultry, and meats, although nuts, seeds, beans, and lentils are important plant sources. With the exception of those consuming vegetarian diets, teenagers do not usually choose foods high in complex carbohydrates and vegetables that contain fiber and phytate. The amount of phosphorus in the diet influences zinc requirements and increases zinc need when phosphorus and protein intakes are high.[41] Because adolescent diets are likely to be high in protein and phosphorus, zinc requirements for normal growth and development may be increased.[42] Other behaviors, such as alcohol consumption, can cause overall dietary deficiencies and may be associated with zinc deficiencies.[40]

Very little information is available on requirements of adolescents. Consequently many recommendations for adolescents are based on maintenance requirements of adults. The recently suggested recommended dietary intakes for zinc, calcium, and iron[32] represent extrapolated values that involve approximated absorption rates, body stores, and increments for rapid growth and development characteristics of adolescents in addition to adult maintenance requirements. These recommendations also recognized the significance of nutritional differences resulting from differences in biological maturation. Indeed, chronological age alone is a poor indicator for the individual adolescent's nutritional needs.

Eating Disorders

The prevalence of eating disorders in the adolescent population is unknown, and results of studies done with selected groups vary with the health-care setting, gender of the clients, and intensity of reported physical activity.[43,44] The published incidences range from <4% to >40% of the school-age children studied who reported some type of binging, vomiting, or other types of maladaptive behavior.

The revised Diagnostic and Statistical Manual of Mental Disorders (DSM III-R) supports expanded diagnostic criteria in regard to a weight loss of 15% compared with the former 25% below expected or original body weight and amenorrhea for a minimum of 3 consecutive months in anorexia nervosa.[45] Bulimia nervosa criteria include a minimum average of two binge-eating episodes a week for at least 3 mo. Other behaviors associated with body image and excessive concern with body shape and weight were unchanged.

A review by Lucas[44] provides a historical perspective and describes biopsychosocial determinants that are relevant to practitioners working with both female and male anorectics. The importance of recognizing anorexia nervosa as an entity separate from other forms of psychogenic undernutrition and changes in hormones that represent physiological adaptations to semistarvation is stressed. The perpetuating mechanism in both anorexia nervosa and bulimia as evidenced by abnormalities of norepinephrine and serotonin metabolism, endorphinergic activity, and sympathetic alterations lessens the adolescent's sense of control. The person increases dysfunctional behavior to gain control, thus perpetuating both mental and physiological symptoms of the disorder.[46]

In addition to the perpetuating nature of starvation, eating disorders are sustained by dysfunctional familial influences and interactions.[47] Most research findings support the model of a family environment that hampers identity development, attaining autonomy and self-sufficiency, and skill development in conflict resolution. Familial transmission of eating disorders was suggested because of their occurrence in biological relatives of patients along with severe depressive symptoms in both male and female relatives.

Adams and Shafer[48] compiled a list of characteristics of adolescents with and without eating disorders derived from a variety of studies and published literature. By assessment of eating and related behaviors, body image and body satisfaction, health status, personal functioning at home and at school, and environmental influences, responses could be categorized as warning signals that an adolescent was a potential candidate for anorexia nervosa and bulimia nervosa. Although most adolescents practice food-related behaviors that could be considered dysfunctional at times as part of their quest for autonomy, those with eating disorders manifest identifiable patterns of behavior.

An assessment of nutritional status should include collection and correlation of anthropometric, biochemical, clinical, and dietary information.[49] With the overall goal of restoring nutritional status, refeeding to achieve body weight and normal endocrine function, and establishing an adequate nutrient intake, treatment necessarily must be individualized and guided by the severity of the disease and the motivation of the individual. Kilbourne[49] suggested an initial calorie intake at basal metabolic rate (BMR) and added increments to 1.5 times BMR as BMR becomes normal. As weight increases, 100 kcal for each 2.3 kg is added. A daily protein intake of 1.5–2.0 g/kg weight along with vitamin and minerals is considered adequate to support the anabolic processes, and a supplement to provide for micronutrients comparable to the Recommended Dietary Allowances should be adequate. Controlled exercise also is recommended to prevent osteoporotic changes that occur with immobility. Although severe cases may require nasogastric or parenteral feeding, these interventions are not without serious physical and emotional risks to the patient.

In our Western society females are more likely than males to develop eating disorders. With the emphasis on physical fitness and sports, males are susceptible to weight configurations that enhance their athletic ability, and they may manifest the same obsessional behavior seen in females with eating disorders. It has been postulated that eating disorders occur in adolescents from non-Westernized societies who are exposed to the Western culture for even brief periods of time.[50]

Summary

Present knowledge in nutrition of adolescents lacks an experimental database that addresses the diversity of growth acceleration and endocrine changes and their impact upon food choices of adolescents. Indicators of inadequate nutriture may reflect a complex interaction among nutrient needs, environmental factors, and societal values about food consumption. In the majority of the adolescent population, consumption practices that influence total food intake as well as nutrient interactions should be of increasing concern, e.g., vitamin-mineral supplementation, lack of diversity in choosing a variety of foods, and high sodium intakes.[51]

In addition, addictive behaviors (i.e., eating disorders and alcoholism) that decrease food intake and/or increase maladaptive behaviors (e.g., excessive exercising) may place otherwise normal adolescents at greater risk than their counterparts who practice moderation in eating and physical activities. Although the relationships between reported food intakes and subsequent clinical diagnoses of nutrient deficiencies in adolescents are poorly correlated, food-related practices that result in marginal deficiencies may in turn interrupt the normal sequence of growth and development and severely impair health status during the teenage years.

References

1. C. Susanne (1980) Developmental genetics of man. In: *Human Physical Growth and Maturation* (F.E. Johnston, A.F. Roche, and C. Susanne, eds.), pp. 221–242, Plenum Press, New York.
2. J.M. Tanner and P.S.W. Davies (1985) Clinical longitudinal standards for height and height velocity for North American children. *J. Pediatr.* 107:317–329.
3. S.M. Garn and B. Wagner (1969) The adolescent growth of the skeletal mass and its implication to mineral requirements. In: *Adolescent Nutrition and Growth* (F.P. Heald, ed.), pp. 139–161, Appleton-Century-Crofts, New York.
4. R.G. Rosenfeld (1982) Evaluation of growth and maturation in adolescence. *Pediatr. Rev.* 4:175–183.
5. National Research Council (1989) *Recommended Dietary Allowances,* 10th ed., National Academy Press, Washington, DC.
6. National Center for Health Statistics (1973) *Height and Weight of Youths 12–17 Years, United States.* Vital and Health Statistics, series 11, no. 124, U.S. Government Printing Office, Washington, DC.
7. D.B. Cheek (1974) Body composition, hormones, nutrition and adolescent growth. In: *Control of the Onset of Puberty* (M.M. Grumbach, G.D. Grave, and F.E. Mayer, eds.), pp. 426–447, John Wiley and Sons, New York.
8. S.M. Garn and S.D. Pesick (1982) Comparison of the Benn index and other body mass indices in nutritional assessment. *Am. J. Clin. Nutr.* 36:573–575.
9. F.E. Johnston (1985) Validity of triceps skinfold and relative weight as measures of adolescent obesity. *J. Adolesc. Health Care* 6:185–190.
10. A.R. Frisancho and P.N. Flegel (1982) Relative merits of old and new indices of body mass with reference to skinfold thickness. *Am. J. Clin. Nutr.* 36:697–699.
11. F.E. Johnston, A.N. Paolone, H.L. Taylor, and L.M. Schell (1982) The relationship of body fat weight, determined densitometrically, to relative weight and triceps skinfold in American youths, 12–17 years of age. *Am. J. Phys. Anthropol.* 57:1–6.
12. R. Michielutte, R.A. Diseker, W.T. Corbett, H.M. Schey, and J.R. Ureda (1984) The relationship between weight-height indices and the triceps skinfold measure among children age 5 to 12. *Am. J. Public Health* 74:604–606.
13. D.B. McKeag (1986) Adolescents and exercise. *J. Adolesc. Health Care* 7(suppl.)121–129.
14. G.G. Reiff, W.R. Dixon, D. Jacoby, G.X. Ye, C.G. Spain, and P.A. Hunsicker (1986) *The President's Council on Physical Fitness and Sports 1985. National School Population Fitness Survey.* HHS Office of the Assistant Secretary for Health, Research Project 282-84-0086. University of Michigan.
15. National Center for Health Statistics (1979) *Caloric and Selected*

Nutrient Values for Persons 1–74 Years of Age. First Health and Nutrition Examination Survey, 1971–1974. DHEW Publication no. (PHS) 79-1657, series 11, no. 209, U.S. Department of Health, Education and Welfare, Hyattsville, MD.

16. U.S. Department of Health, Education and Welfare (1977) *Dietary Intake Findings. United States, 1971–1974.* DHEW Publication no. (HRA) 77-1647, series 11, no. 202. National Center for Health Statistics, Hyattsville, MD.

17. E.D. Nottelmann, E.J. Susman, L.D. Dorn, et al. (1987) Developmental processes in early adolescence. Relations among chronological age, pubertal stage, height, weight, and serum levels of gonadotropins, sex steroids, and adrenal androgens. *J. Adolesc. Health Care* 8:246–260.

18. C.E. Woteki (1986) Dietary survey data: source and limits to interpretation. *Nutr. Rev.* 40(suppl.):204–212.

19. Human Nutrition Information Service, U.S. Department of Agriculture (1985) *Nutrient Intake: Individuals in 48 States, Year 1977–1978 Nationwide Food Consumption Survey, 1977–1978* (1985) HNIS Report no. 1-2, U.S. Government Printing Office, Washington, DC.

20. R.J. Kuczmarski, E.R. Brewer, F.J. Cronin, B. Dennis, K. Graves, and S. Haynes. (1986) Food choices among white adolescents: the Lipid Research Clinics prevalence study. *Pediatr. Res.* 20: 309–315.

21. B. Wait, R. Blair and L.J. Roberts (1969) Energy intake of well-nourished children and adolescents. *Am. J. Clin. Nutr.* 22:1383–1396.

22. E.J. Gong and F.P. Heald (1988) Diet, nutrition, and adolescence. In: *Modern Nutrition and Health* (M.E. Shils and V.R. Young, eds.), pp. 969–981, Lea and Febiger, Philadelphia.

23. Nutrition Committee, American Heart Association (1988) Dietary guidelines for healthy American adults. A statement for physicians and health professionals. *Circulation* 77:721A–724A.

24. J.A. Driskell, A.J. Clark, and S.W. Moak (1987) Longitudinal assessment of vitamin B-6 status in southern adolescent girls. *J. Am. Diet. Assoc.* 87:307–310.

25. Anonymous (1987) Dietary protein and vitamin B-6 requirements. *Nutr. Rev.* 45:23–25.

26. J.A. Olson and R.E. Hodges (1987) Recommended dietary intakes (RDI) of vitamin C in humans. *Am. J. Clin. Nutr.* 45:693–703.

27. L.A. Reiter, L.M. Boylan, J. Driskell, and S. Moak (1987) Vitamin B-12 and folate intakes and plasma levels of black adolescent females. *J. Am. Diet. Assoc.* 87:1065–1067.

28. V. Herbert (1987) Recommended dietary intakes (RDI) of folate in humans. *Am. J. Clin. Nutr.* 45:661–670.

29. H.E. Sauberlich, M.J. Kretsch, J.H. Skala, H.L. Johnson, and P.C. Taylor (1987) Folate requirements and metabolism in nonpregnant women. *Am. J. Clin. Nutr.* 46:1016–1028.

30. L. Bailey, J. Ginsburg, P. Wagner, W. Noyes, G. Christakis, and J. Denning (1982) Serum ferritin as a measure of iron stores in adolescents. *J. Pediatr.* 101:774–776.

31. Life Sciences Research Office (1984) *Assessment of the Iron Nutritional Status of the United States Population Based on Data Collected in the Second NHANES Survey, 1976–1980.* Federation of American Societies for Experimental Biology, Bethesda, MD.

32. V. Herbert (1987) Recommended dietary intakes (RDI) of iron in humans. *Am. J. Clin. Nutr.* 45:679–686.

33. E.R. Monsen and J.L. Balintfy (1982) Calculating dietary iron bioavailability: refinement and computerization. *J. Am. Diet. Assoc.* 80:307–311.

34. G.C. Viglietti and J.D. Skinner (1987) Estimation of iron bioavailability in adolescents' meals and snacks. *J. Am. Diet. Assoc.* 87: 903–908.

35. J. Sobal and H.L. Muncie (1988) Vitamin/mineral supplement use among adolescents. *J. Nutr. Educ.* 20:314–318.

36. American Academy of Pediatrics, Committee on Nutrition (1980) Vitamin and mineral supplement needs in normal children in the United States. *Pediatrics* 66:1015–1021.

37. B.E.C. Nordin, K.J. Polley, A.G. Need, H.A. Morris, and D. Marshall (1987) The problem of calcium requirement. *Am. J. Clin. Nutr.* 45:1295–1304.

38. R.B. Sandler, C.W. Slemenda, R.E. LaPorte, et al. (1985) Postmenopausal bone density and milk consumption in childhood and adolescence. *Am. J. Clin. Nutr.* 42:270–274.

39. V.R. Young and P.L. Pellett (1987) Protein intake and requirements with reference to diet and health. *Am. J. Clin. Nutr.* 45:1323–1343.

40. A.S. Prasad (1988) Zinc in growth and development and spectrum of human zinc deficiency. *J. Am. Coll. Nutr.* 7:377–384.

41. H.H. Sandstead and G.W. Evans (1984) Zinc. In: *Present Knowledge in Nutrition,* 5th ed. (R.E. Olson, H.P. Broquist, C.O. Chichester, W.J. Darby, A.C. Kolbye, Jr., and R.M. Stalvey, eds.), pp. 479–505, Nutrition Foundation, Inc., Washington, DC.

42. B.A. Sloane, C.C. Gibbons, and M. Hegsted (1985) Evaluation of zinc and copper, nutritional status and effects upon growth of southern adolescent females. *Am. J. Clin. Nutr.* 42:235–241.

43. J.R. Braisted, L. Mellin, E. Gong, and C.E. Irwin (1985) The adolescent ballet dancer. Nutritional practices and characteristics associated with anorexia nervosa. *J. Adolesc. Health Care* 6:365–371.

A.R. Lucas (1986) Anorexia nervosa: historical background and biopsychosocial determinants. *Semin. Adolesc. Med.* 2:1–9.

45. American Psychiatric Association (1987) *Diagnostic and Statistical Manual of Mental Disorders,* 3d ed., American Psychiatric Association, Washington, DC.

46. P. Garfinkel and A.S. Kaplan (1985) Starvation based perpetuating mechanism in anorexia nervosa and bulimia. *Int. J. Eating Dis.* 4: 651–665.

47. M. Strober and L.L. Humphrey (1987) Familial contributions to the etiology and course of anorexia nervosa and bulimia. *J. Consult. Clin. Psychol.* 55:654–659.

48. L.B. Adams and M.B. Shafer (1988) Early manifestations of eating disorders in adolescents: defining those at risk. *J. Nutr. Educ.* 20: 307–313.

49. K.A. Kilbourne (1986) Nutritional evaluation and management of anorexic and bulimic patients. *Semin. Adolesc. Med.* 2:47–55.

50. H.L. Holden and P.H. Robinson (1988) Anorexia nervosa and bulimia nervosa in British blacks. *Br. J. Psychiatry* 152:544–549.

51. G.C. Frank, L.S. Webber, T.A. Nicklas, and G.S. Berenson (1988) Sodium, potassium, calcium, magnesium and phosphorus intakes of infants and children: Bogalusa Heart Study. *J. Am. Diet. Assoc.* 88:801–807.

Chapter **39**

Helen Smiciklas-Wright

Aging

The world's elderly population is growing at a rate of 2.4%/y.[1] Older Americans are increasing in absolute numbers, comprising a steadily increasing proportion of the total population, and are living longer.[2] The percentage of the U.S. population that is ≥65 y is projected to increase from 12.4% to 13.9% by the year 2010. Presently, 9.6% of those in the ≥65 y age category are ≥85 y. This proportion is expected to increase steadily to 15.5% in 2010. If present trends continue, within the next 10–20 y almost half of deaths will occur after age 80.[3]

Detailed reviews of biomedical conditions among elderly persons appear in *Principles of Geriatric Medicine* by Andres et al.[4] The leading causes of death have changed little in recent years. Cardiovascular diseases, cancers, pneumonia, and diabetes mellitus continue to be the dominant causes of death.[3] The most frequently reported chronic conditions include arthritis, hypertension, and heart disease. The coexistence of chronic diseases, i.e., comorbidity, increases with age and is higher for women than men.[5]

Many elderly persons are healthier than most stereotypes suggest; many rate their health as good to excellent despite chronic conditions and are not constrained by their illnesses. However, some elderly persons, particularly those with comorbidity and those who are older, have physical disabilities that limit their independence in food shopping and preparation. Approximately 4% of noninstitutionalized Americans ≥ 65 y and 17% of those ≥ 85 y reported that they could not prepare their own meals because of a health or a physical problem.[6] More than 30% of a group of homebound older persons reported difficulty in preparing meals (V. Bernardo, H. Smiciklas-Wright, D. J. Lago, et al., unpublished observations, 1990).

Chronic conditions may compromise nutrition in ways other than through impaired physical functioning. Some elderly persons have restrictive dietary practices.[7] Many take drugs prescribed by physicians for chronic illnesses. Many also take nonprescription drugs for conditions such as dizziness, weakness, and constipation and nutrient supplements and tonics to improve appetite and well-being.[8] Excellent reviews on the effects of drugs on appetite, nutrient absorption, metabolism, and excretion are available.[8,9] Drug-induced fatigue, weakness, or depression may further compromise food intake. The potential for adverse drug reactions is not exaggerated given that some elderly persons, particularly those in nursing homes, may be taking ≥20 drugs/d.

Many older Americans live in families usually consisting of an elderly married couple.[3] Over 60% of men live with their wives but only ~30% of women live with their husbands. Older people are also more apt to live alone at least until they are in their 90s; urban and rural nonfarm elderly persons, too, are more likely to be alone.[10,11] Davis et al.[12] used National Health and Nutrition Examination Survey (NHANESII) data to compare living arrangements and eating behaviors of older adults. Those who lived alone, particularly men, were more likely to have practices, e.g., skipping meals, that placed them at higher nutritional risk.

Older Americans generally have experienced economic gains. Poverty among noninstitutionalized elderly persons fell from 35% in 1959 to ~12% in the 1980s.[13] However, poverty rates are much higher among minority elderly persons and women, particularly widows.[14] There are mixed findings on the relationship between income and nutrition.[15] Fanelli and Woteki[16] reported that median intakes of energy and some nutrients were notably lower for 65–74-y-old NHANESII participants who were below the poverty level. Other studies showed no association between income and nutrition.[17] The mixed findings on the relationship between income and diet may reflect the failure to consider other variables, such as education and nutrition knowledge.[15]

Biomedical Changes

Changes in body structure and function occur with age but do so with different rates in different persons. The grosser manifestations of aging have been described, but there is relatively limited understanding of the inevitability of changes or of molecular mechanisms responsible for the changes. There is also insufficient information on biological and environmental factors that moderate change.

Body Composition. Lean body mass decreases and fatness increases with aging. Most of the data describing these changes come from cross-sectional studies.[18] Flynn et al.[19] documented cross-sectional observations in their longitudinal measurements of total body potassium. Women of reproductive age showed a lower rate of potassium loss than did males of the same age but a greater rate of loss than did males after age 60 y. Not only does body fatness increase, there is also a redistribution of body fat. Brozek[20] described a centralization or shift of subcutaneous fat from limbs to trunk in elderly persons. More information is needed on this aspect of body composition relative to metabolic complications and consequent health outcomes, e.g., hypertension, hyperlipidemia, and gallbladder disease.[18]

Peak bone mass is achieved at 30–35 y. Females experience a precipitous decline in bone mass during postmenopausal years. Changes in bone mass in women and elderly men result in various degrees of osteoporosis and susceptibility to bone fractures.[18] Bone fractures in older persons occur not only because of decreased bone mass but also because of fatigue damage and reduced trabecular connectivity.[21] The complexity of bone health complicates our understanding of the role that nutritional factors play in bone strength.[21]

Total body water is decreased in older persons and it is decreased even more in very old persons.[22] Cross-sectional studies suggest that the major decrease is in intracellular water. Because most intracellular water is associated with fat-free mass, its loss could be concurrent with the loss of lean body mass. The average hydration of fat-free mass appears to remain relatively constant in healthy persons.[22] Longitudinal studies, however, demonstrate that the loss of body water is due to changes in extracellular water.[23] There may be several explanations for the differences in cross-sectional and longitudinal studies, e.g., differences in survival characteristics, or in early or late nutrition.[22] The changes in body water are significant for the disposition of water-soluble drugs, for the administration of diuretics, and for thermal regulation.

More longitudinal data are needed to describe body composition changes. More work is also necessary to understand the modulating effects of ethnic-genetic, nutritional, physical activity, and other determinants.

Physiological Changes. Age-related changes have been reported at all levels of biological organization. Reviews of cellular- and organ-level changes have appeared in many papers and books and will not be described here.[24–27]

There is certainly evidence of adaptive responses with aging. For example, it has generally been assumed that there is neuronal loss with age. However, Terry et al.[28] showed that although large neurons decrease in number during normal aging, there is a compensatory increase in medium-sized neurons.

It is generally assumed that physiological functions continue to be appropriate in the absence of disease but the reserve capacity, or the ability to respond to stress, diminishes over time. An example is the work of Odio and Brodish,[29] who studied the effect of age in rats on the capacity to mobilize glucose and free fatty acids during the stress of electric shock. They found an age-dependent loss of plasticity of response mechanisms associated with energy metabolism during stress and speculated that age-associated deficits might force the older animal to mobilize more of its physiological resources than would a younger animal when dealing with environmental stress. The work of Carrillo et al.[30] is another example of reduced reserve capacity with age. Young, middle-aged, and old mice had similar control values of hepatic glutathione (GSH) and glutathione-5-transferase (GST) activity, but there were marked age differences when animals were stressed with protein-free diets.

Any overview of age-related changes must conclude that there is considerable heterogeneity from the cellular level to the total organism. Cellular-level studies suggest that heterogeneity may be expressed within a single cell population; e.g., whereas overall amounts of glucose-6-phosphatase are decreased in hepatocytes from old animals, some cells contain apparently normal amounts.[27] Biochemical and physiological indices show increased variation with age.[31] Longitudinal studies show that many individuals follow patterns of aging that could not be predicted from cross-sectional data.[32] Many older men in the Baltimore Longitudinal Study of Aging experienced 5–10 y during which their kidney function was unchanged, and a few showed improved kidney function whereas the average curve showed a decline in function.[33]

Nutrient Requirements

Energy. The current (10th) edition of the Recommended Dietary Allowances (RDA) divides adults in two age categories: 25–50 y and ≥51 y.[34] This is similar to the previous edition except for the energy recommendation.[35] In the ninth edition, older adults were divided into two age categories, 51–75 y and ≥75 y. The committee responsible for the current RDA recognized that there was no rational basis to support the assertion that all people >51 y are sufficiently similar to warrant grouping them together but concluded that there were not sufficient data available to make differential recommendations.

A decreased caloric intake is recommended for older persons to adjust for age-associated decreases in resting energy expenditure and physical activity. The recommended average energy allowance for 21–50-y-old males and females is 2900 kcal and 2200 kcal, respectively. The allowance for persons above age 50 is 2300 kcal for males and 1900 kcal for females, with a normal variation of ±20% accepted for both age categories. The RDA do not assume that marked decline in activity is either inevitable or desirable.

Schneider et al.[36] questioned whether energy allowances should be based on observed changes in body composition, resting energy expenditure, and physical activity and argued that age-related morbidity and mortality might be decreased if lean body mass and physical activity were maintained rather than diminished with age. Several studies show that basal metabolic rates will be only negligibly lower in elderly persons who do not have marked changes in lean body mass.[37,38] Buskirk's review of data on health maintenance and exercise supports the assumption that regular exercise blunts many of the physiological declines associated with aging.[39]

Nutrients. Estimates for nutrient requirements for older persons have been based largely on extrapolation of data from studies on young adults.[40] A number of recent papers reviewed available data on nutrient requirements.[25,40–44]

There is considerable literature showing protein changes at the molecular and tissue levels and changes in turnover of body proteins.[45] It is not clear how these changes affect protein requirements. There are data to show similar, lower, and higher requirements for healthy older persons compared with younger subjects.[46–49] Some of the contradictions may be due to study designs as well as variations in activity level and disease prevalence. At present, the RDA for reference protein (0.75 g/kg) is the same for elderly adults as for young adults.[34] Munro et al.[50] reported that a group of free-living healthy elderly persons had average protein intakes well above the recommendation and that there was no relationship between protein intakes and plasma protein concentrations or selected body measurements. Protein requirements for the older person experiencing disease and other traumas may be higher than for healthy elderly persons.[46]

For other nutrients, the RDA for adults aged 21–50 y and ≥51 y are essentially the same except for thiamin and riboflavin, which are expressed in terms of total caloric intake, and for iron. RDA for iron are 15 and 10 mg for females in the two age categories, respectively. Suter and Russell,[42] in their review of vitamin requirements of elderly persons, confirm that data for many vitamins are limited. They concluded that some subgroups of older persons may require higher amounts of some vitamins, including vitamins D and B-12. They cite several age-related changes in vitamin D production and metabolism and lack of sun exposure as influencing vitamin D requirements and atrophic gastritis as impairing vitamin B-12 absorption.

Schneider et al.[36] proposed that RDA based on age alone may be misleading and that formulas for calculating allowances should include coefficients for specific diseases and laboratory test results. The data for such an approach are insufficient but the recommendation serves as a reminder that RDA are not intended to cover special nutritional needs arising from chronic diseases, other medical conditions, and drug therapies.[34]

Nutritional Status of Older Americans

Assessment of Status. The importance of assessment and the problems in determining nutritional status of older persons were the focus of a recent conference sponsored by the National Institute on Aging (NIA).[51] A major theme of the conference was the need for appropriate reference standards. Chumlea and Baumgartner[52] noted that for Americans older than age 80 y, reference data for stature, weight, and other body measurements are limited to small samples primarily of white ambulatory individuals.

Reference intervals for many laboratory tests are calculated by using tissue samples from young adults. Longitudinal studies are beginning to provide clinical-chemistry reference intervals for healthy elderly subjects.[53] However, the interpretation of clinical indicators can be confounded in less-healthy persons. An example is the association of anemia with chronic inflammatory disease and even with acute infections that can lead to overestimation of iron deficiency in elderly persons.[54]

A second theme of the NIA conference was the need for adjustments in measuring techniques, particularly for anthropometry.[52] Recumbent measures were developed for persons who cannot assume an erect position. Several alternatives to height measurement are available, e.g., knee height.[52,55] More data are needed about the reliability of these measures across diverse samples of elderly individuals.[56]

A comprehensive evaluation of nutritional status is usually based on anthropometric, dietary, clinical, and biochemical information. Valuable data also may be derived from indirect indicators of nutritional risk, e.g., information about the number of meals missed per week or about perceived need for assistance with food-related activities.[57] Wolinsky et al.[58] showed that older individuals assessed to be at nutritional risk, on the basis of simple questionnaires, were more likely to have restricted activities, bed-disability days, more physicians' visits, and hospital episodes.

Nutritional Status. Nutritional status data are available from national surveys, i.e., the Nationwide Food Consumption Survey (NFCS)[59] and the National Health and Nutrition Examination Survey (NHANES). NHANESIII, which will be in the field from 1988 to 1994, will be the first NHANES to include a sample older than 74 y.[60] Most of the data on nutritional status of older Americans come from cross-sectional studies of relatively small selected samples.[25,40,41]

Many studies report that older persons consume smaller amounts of food and, hence, energy than do younger persons. Reasonably healthy, institutionalized elderly persons have intakes comparable with those of free-living populations,[61] whereas sedentary homebound persons have lower intakes.[7] There are some longitudinal data to support cross-sectional observations. Elahi et al.[62] reported that energy intake decreased with age over a period of 15 y for men participating in the Baltimore Longitudinal Study of Aging, whereas Garry et al.[63] found that energy intake remained relatively constant for healthy elderly males and females over a 6-y period.

Average energy intakes in most studies are comparable to average recommended allowances but a proportion of the older population reports low energy intakes. The proportion may be exaggerated when data are collected by 24-h recall. Nevertheless, many older persons may have such low energy intakes that appropriate nutrient densities would be hard to achieve.[64,65]

Nutritional state of older persons is associated with health or frailty. Protein-calorie malnutrition is a major problem that has been documented in geriatric patients in various acute and extended-care facilities.[66,67] Nutritional variables such as serum albumin[68] and weight loss[69] may predict mortality for institutional patients. Routine assessment of patients could provide early identification of older people at increased risk of death.[68]

The possibility of malnutrition also exists for moderately frail elderly persons.[70] Limited mobility and drug use are only two of many contributing factors. Lips et al.[71] studied elderly subjects with hip fractures and control subjects. Vitamin D status as assessed by serum concentrations of 25-hydroxyvitamin D and 1,25-dihydroxyvitamin D was poor in patients with hip fracture; the status was mainly due to low exposure to sunshine.

Even healthy elderly persons may experience undesirable nutritional changes at times of stress. Willis et al.[72] reported that major life crises were associated with significant decreases in lymphocyte counts, caloric intake, and body weight in a group of healthy older persons.

There is a great need for studies that examine factors that may affect nutritional status.[73,74] Gibbs and Turner[75] called for new theoretical paradigms that account for social, health, and demographic variables as determinants of nutritional status. There is also a great need for information about the health consequences of minor nutritional problems. Many health outcomes are associated with overt malnutrition, including delayed wound healing and decubitus ulcers in patients with protein-calorie malnutrition.[67] Goodwin et al.[76] found an association between nutritional status measures and cognition in a healthy noninstitutionalized population with no clinical evidence of impaired nutritional status. Their work suggests that very subtle nutritional changes may have adverse affects on functional status.

Nutrition as a Modulator of Aging

Restricting calories while administering essential nutrients was shown in many studies to have a reproducible impact on aging in rodents.[77,78] The first evidence is found in the work of McKay et al.[79] who restricted caloric intakes of weanling rats. Animals who survived the first year of the regimen had reduced skeletal growth, delayed sexual maturation, and markedly longer lives. Other investigators have shown that moderate as well as severe restrictions may influence both life expectancy and life span in laboratory rodents.[80] The increase in longevity appears to be the result of caloric restriction, because restriction of protein,[80] fat, or minerals[81] has little or no effect.

Caloric restriction delays some but not all age-related physiologic processes.[82] Increased concentrations of plasma lipids and diminished ability of adipocytes to respond to lipolytic action of glucagon are delayed, but systolic blood pressure decreases are unaffected. There are also changes in the onset of disease processes common to many laboratory rodents, e.g., progressive chronic nephropathy. The breadth of processes affected suggests that caloric restriction influences primary aging processes.[82]

The mechanisms underlying the effects of caloric restriction have not been determined. Food restriction may exert its effect through protection from free radicals.[83] It may inhibit an age-related increase in membrane 22:5 fatty acid and, thus, a reduction of peroxidation of membrane lipids.

Harmon[84] believes that the free radical theory of aging suggests practical means of increasing healthy life span in humans. He proposes that judicious selection of diets and antioxidant supplements, e.g., vitamins E and C, can be reasonably expected to increase active life span by 5–10 y. Other investigators advise caution before considering large doses of selective vitamins and minerals.[78] Certainly more work is necessary to define judicious antiaging nutrient intakes.

Nutritional Care for Elderly Persons

Noninstitutionalized Elderly Persons. The family is the primary provider of long-term care, including food assistance, for elderly persons who live at home. However, demographic and social trends indicate that the family's ability to provide support will be strained.[85] Nutrition programs for both ambulatory and homebound elderly persons represent an important area of support. Balsam and Osteraas[86] recommend that the framework for nutrition programs should be a continuum of community nutrition needs ranging from services for independent and healthy elderly persons to those who are frail and needy of considerable back-up support.

Home-delivered meals have been available for many years under the sponsorship of voluntary agencies.[87] Government's commitment to food assistance developed out of the Older American's Act of 1965.[88] The Nutrition Program for Older Americans was originally established under Title VII of the act to provide meals in a social setting for persons ≥ 60 y with special emphasis on low-income and minority elderly persons. The program was reorganized under Title III-C in 1978 with separate funding for home-delivered and congregate meals.[89] The home-delivered meals feature of the program has grown rapidly to >94 million meals in 1988.

Many investigators noted the program's successes in improving food intake, nutritional status, and social activities of participants.[90–92] There are concerns, however, about groups of elderly persons who are underserved, such as ethnic and linguistic minorities and the homeless.[92] There are also concerns about declining support at a time when the elderly population is growing rapidly. Some programs have become innovative in the face of fiscal austerity, with practices such as buyer consortiums.[93]

Title III-C nutrition programs are mandated to target persons who are in the greatest social and economic need, but there is no means of testing for participation. Many insightful papers recently focused on the dilemma of age or need as a basis for public policy for older Americans and specifically for nutrition programs.[94–97]

Institutionalized Elderly Persons. About 5% of older Americans live in institutions, mostly in nursing homes. Although only a small percentage of people ≥ 65 y live in nursing homes at any one time, a much higher proportion will spend some time in such facilities.[98] Furthermore, the proportion of institutionalized elderly persons is much higher (~20%) for those who are ≥85 y.

Nursing home residents are becoming older and are more likely to be acutely ill because of earlier hospital discharges.[99] These characteristics, as well as environments in many nursing homes, increase residents' dependency. Rodin[100] showed relationships between residents' dependency and health outcomes, which may be mediated through such physiological mechanisms as increased catecholamine and corticosteroid concentrations.

There are a number of approaches to enhancing residents' self-control. Some strategies, such as better positioning of subjects, adaptive equipment, and providing adequate time for eating, enhance the ability of individuals to feed themselves.[101] Some residents need more direct nutrition support, ranging from provision of food supplements[102,103] to more aggressive support, such as tube and parenteral feedings. Sullivan et al.[99] and Maslow[104] reviewed both the nutrition and ethics related to decisions about nutrition support.

Conclusion

The aging of the American population is one of the most compelling issues on the nation's health-policy agenda. There are various projections about the morbidity and quality of life for older persons. The optimistic projection is that morbidity will be compressed and disabilities will occupy a smaller portion of the typical lifespan;[105] the less-optimistic projection is that periods of disability and need for care will increase.[3] Both of these projections may be partially correct in that differences in subgroups of elderly persons may become more pronounced, ranging from independent and reasonably healthy individuals to even frailer elderly persons with multiple disabilities.

An important question concerns what distinguishes the healthy older population, those experiencing what has been termed "successful aging," from the severely disabled elderly persons.[106] Nathan Shock, one of the most distinguished scientists in gerontology, was quoted as saying, "Aging is not a disease!"[107] Rowe and Kahn[106] argued that the modifying effects of psychosocial factors, exercise, and diet have been underestimated in aging research.

Considerable work needs to be done in order to understand the reciprocity between nutrition and aging—work on nutrition needs and on norms for the healthy population. Work is also required in describing the role of nutrition in both successful and adverse health outcomes and in understanding how much diet can be expected to contribute to active life expectancy.

References

1. U.S. Department of Commerce, Bureau of the Census (1987) *An Aging World.* International Population Reports, Series P-95, no. 78. U.S. Government Printing Office, Washington, DC.

2. J.A. Brody, D.B. Brock, and T.F. Williams (1987) Trends in the health of the elderly population. *Annu. Rev. Public Health* 8:211–234.

3. J.A. Brody and D.B. Brock (1985) Epidemiologic and statistical characteristics of the United States elderly population. In: *Handbook of the Biology of Aging* (C.E. Finch and E. Schneider, eds.), pp. 3–26, Van Nostrand Reinhold, New York.

4. R. Andres, E.L. Bierman, and W.R. Hazzard (1985) *Principles of Geriatric Medicine,* McGraw-Hill, New York.

5. J.M. Guralnik, A.Z. LaCroix, D.F. Everett, and M.G. Kovar (1989) Aging in the eighties: the prevalence of comorbidity and its association with disability. *Adv. Data* 170:1–8.

6. U.S. Department of Health and Human Services, Public Health Service, Centers for Disease Control (1989) *Physical Functioning of the Aged United States, 1984.* DHHS Publication no. (PHS)89-1595, DHHS, Hyattsville, MD.

7. E. Schlenker (1984) *Nutrition in Aging,* Times Mirror/Mosby, St. Louis, MO.

8. D. Roe (1987) *Geriatric Nutrition,* Prentice-Hall, Englewood Cliffs, NJ.

9. J.N. Hathcock (1987) Nutrient-drug interactions. *Clin. Geriatr. Med.* 3:297–307.

10. R.T. Coward, S.J. Cutler, and F.E. Schmidt (1989) Differences in the household composition of elders by age, gender and area of residence. *Gerontologist* 29:814–821.

11. W.J. McAuley, M.D. Jacobs, and C.S. Carr (1984) Older couples: patterns of assistance and support. *J. Gerontol. Soc. Work* 6:35–48.

12. M.A. Davis, S.P. Murphy, and J.M. Neuhaus (1988) Living arrangements and eating behaviors of older adults in the United States. *J. Gerontol.* 43:S96–S98.

13. K.C. Holden (1988) Poverty and living arrangements among older women: are changes in economic well-being underestimated? *J. Gerontol.* 43:S22–S27.

14. M.D. Hurd (1989) The economic status of the elderly. *Science* 244:659–664.

15. J. Hendricks and T.M. Calasanti (1986) Social-psychological aspects of nutrition among the elderly. Part I. Social dimensions of nutrition. In: *Nutritional Aspects of Aging,* vol. 1 (L.H. Chen, ed.), pp. 77–97, CRC Press, Boca Raton, FL.

16. M.T. Fanelli and C.E. Woteki (1989) Nutrient intakes and health status of older Americans: data from the NHANESII. *Ann. N.Y. Acad. Sci.* 561:94–103.

17. D.P. Slesinger, M. McDivitt, and F.M. O'Donnell (1980) Food patterns in an urban population: age and sociodemographic correlates. *J. Gerontol.* 35:432–438.

18. R.J. Kuczmarski (1989) Need for body composition information in elderly subjects. *Am. J. Clin. Nutr.* 50(suppl.):1150–1157.

19. M.A. Flynn, G.B. Nolph, A.S. Baker, W.M. Martin, and G. Krause (1989) Total body potassium in aging humans: a longitudinal study. *Am. J. Clin. Nutr.* 50:713–717.

20. J. Brozek (1952) Changes of body composition in man during maturity and their nutritional implications. *Fed. Proc.* 11:784–793.

21. R.P. Heaney (1989) Nutritional factors in bone health in elderly subjects: methodological and contextual problems. *Am. J. Clin. Nutr.* 50:1182–1189.

22. D.A. Schoeller (1989) Changes in total body water with age. *Am. J. Clin. Nutr.* 50:1176–1181.

23. G.T. Lesser, S. Deutsch, and J. Mankofsky (1980) Fat-free mass, total body water, and intracellular water in the aged rat. *Am. J. Physiol.* 238:R82–R90.

24. D.A. Roe (1987) *Geriatric Nutrition,* Prentice-Hall, Englewood Cliffs, NJ.

25. W.R. Bidlack and C.H. Smith (1988) Nutritional requirements of the aged. *CRC Crit. Rev. Food Sci. Nutr.* 27(3):189–218.

26. J.W. Roe and K.L. Minaker (1985) Geriatric medicine. In: *Handbook of Biology and Aging* (C.E. Finch and E.L. Schneider, eds.), pp. 932–959, Van Nostrand Reinhold, New York.

27. P. Wilson (1983) The histochemistry of aging. *Histochem. J.* 15:393–410.

28. R.D. Terry, R. DeTeresa, and L.A. Hansen (1987) Neocortical cell counts in normal human adult aging. *Ann. Neurol.* 21:530–539.

29. M.R. Odio and A. Brodish (1988) Effects of age on metabolic responses to acute and chronic stress. *Am. J. Physiol.* 254:E617–E624.

30. M.-C. Carrillo, K. Kitani, S. Kanai, et al. (1989) Differences in the influence of diet on hepatic glutathione S-transferase activity and glutathione content between young and old C57 black female mice. *Mech. Ageing Dev.* 47:1–15.

31. G.T. Baker and R.L. Sprott (1988) Biomarkers of aging. *Exp. Gerontol.* 23:223–239.

32. E.W. Campion, L.O. deLabry, and R.J. Glynn (1988) The effect of age on serum albumin in healthy males: report from the normative aging study. *J. Gerontol.* 43:M18–M20.

33. N.W. Shock (1985) Longitudinal studies of aging in humans. In: *Handbook on the Biology of Aging* (C.E. Finch and E.L. Schneider, eds.), pp. 721–743, Van Nostrand Reinhold, New York.

34. National Research Council (1989) *Recommended Dietary Allowances,* 10th ed., National Academy Press, Washington, DC.

35. National Research Council (1980) *Recommended Dietary Allowances,* 9th ed., National Academy Press, Washington, DC.

36. E.L. Schneider, E.M. Vining, E.C. Hadley, and S.A. Farnham (1986) Recommended dietary allowance and the health of the elderly. *N. Engl. J. Med.* 314:157–160.

37. A. Keys, H.L. Taylor, and F. Grande (1973) Basal metabolism and age of adult men. *Metabolism* 22:579–587.

38. S.P. Tzankoff and A.H. Norris (1978) Longitudinal changes in basal metabolism in man. *J. Appl. Physiol.* 45:536–539.

39. E.R. Buskirk (1985) Health maintenance and longevity: exercise. In: *The Handbook of Biology and Aging* (C.E. Finch and E.L. Schneider, eds.), pp. 894–931, Van Nostrand Reinhold, New York.

40. H.A. Guthrie (1988) Nutrient requirements of the elderly. In: *Health Promotion and Disease Prevention in the Elderly* (R. Chernoff and D. Lipschitz, eds.), pp. 33–43, Raven Press, New York.

41. J.E. Morley (1986) Nutritional status of the elderly. *Am. J. Med.* 81:679–695.

42. P.M. Suter and R.M. Russell (1987) Vitamin requirements of the elderly. *Am. J. Clin. Nutr.* 45:501–512.

43. R. Chernoff and D. Lipschitz (1985) Aging and nutrition. *Compr. Ther.* 11(8):29–34.

44. E.A. Young (1983) Nutrition, aging and the aged. *Med. Clin. North Am.* 67:295–313.

45. M.J. McKay and J. Bond (1986) Protein and amino acids. In:

Nutritional Aspects of Aging, vol. I (L.H. Chen, ed.), pp. 173–194, CRC Press, Boca Raton, FL.

46. M. Gersovitz, K. Motil, H.N. Munro, and V.R. Young (1982) Human protein requirements: assessment of the adequacy of the current recommended dietary allowance for dietary protein in elderly men and women. *Am. J. Clin. Nutr.* 35:6–14.

47. E. Zanni, D.H. Calloway, and A.Y. Zezulka (1979) Protein requirements of elderly men. *J. Nutr.* 109:513–524.

48. A.H.R. Cheng, A. Gomez, J.G. Gergan, T.C. Lee, F. Monckberg, and C.O. Chicester (1978) Comparative nitrogen balance study between young and aged adults using three levels of protein intake from a combination of wheat-soy-milk mixture. *Am. J. Clin. Nutr.* 31:12–22.

49. R. Uauy, N.S. Scrimshaw, and V.R. Young (1978) Human protein requirements: nitrogen balance response to graded levels of egg protein in elderly men and women. *Am. J. Clin. Nutr.* 31:779–785.

50. H.N. Munro, R.B. McGandy, S. Hartz, R.M. Russell, R.A. Jacob, and C.L. Otradovec (1987) Protein nutriture of a group of free-living elderly. *Am. J. Clin. Nutr.* 46:568–592.

51. A.W. Sorensen (1989) Epidemiologic and methodologic problems in determining nutritional status of older persons: introduction. *Am. J. Clin. Nutr.* 50(suppl.):xi–xii.

52. W.C. Chumlea and R.N. Baumgartner (1989) Status of anthropometry and body composition data in elderly subjects. *Am. J. Clin. Nutr.* 50(suppl.):1158–1166.

53. P.J. Garry, W.C. Hunt, D.J. Vanderjagt, and R.L. Rhyne (1989) Clinical chemistry reference intervals for healthy elderly subjects. *Am. J. Clin. Nutr.* 50(suppl.):1219–1230.

54. R. Yip and P.R. Dallman (1988) The roles of inflammation and iron deficiency as causes of anemia. *Am. J. Clin. Nutr.* 48:1295–1300.

55. H.L. Muncie, J. Sobal, J.M. Hoopes, J.H. Tenney, and J.W. Warren (1987) A practical method of estimating stature of bedridden female nursing home patients. *J. Am. Geriatr. Soc.* 35:285–289.

56. M.T. Fanelli (1987) The ABCs of nutritional assessment in older adults. *J. Nutr. Elderly* 6(3):33–40.

57. D.A. Roe (1989) Nutritional surveillance of the elderly: methods to determine program impact and unmet need. *Nutr. Today* 24(5):24–29.

58. F.D. Wolinsky, R.M. Coe, D.K. Miller, J.M. Prendergast, M.J. Greel, and M. Chavez (1983) Health services utilization among the non-institutionalized elderly. *J. Health Soc. Behav.* 24:325–337.

59. E.M. Pao, S.J. Mickle, and M.C. Burk (1985) One-day and 3-day nutrient intakes by individuals—Nationwide Food Consumption Survey findings, spring 1977. *J. Am. Diet. Assoc.* 85:313–324.

60. T. Harris, C. Woteki, R.R. Briefel, and J.C. Kleinman (1989) NHANESIII for older persons: nutrition content and methodological considerations. *Am. J. Clin. Nutr.* 50(suppl.):1145–1149.

61. N.R. Sahyoun, C.L. Otradovec, S.C. Hartz, et al. (1988) Dietary intakes and biochemical indicators of nutritional status in an elderly, institutionalized population. *Am. J. Clin. Nutr.* 47:524–533.

62. V. Elahi, D. Elahi, R. Andres, J. Tobin, M. Butler, and A.A. Norris (1983) A longitudinal study of nutritional intake in men. *J. Gerontol.* 38:162–182.

63. P.J. Garry, R.L. Rhyne, L. Halioua, and C. Nicholson (1989) Changes in dietary patterns over a 6-year period in an elderly population. *Ann. N.Y. Acad. Sci.* 561:104–112.

64. M.B. Kohrs (1982) A rational diet for the elderly. *Am. J. Clin. Nutr.* 36:735–736.

65. B. Shannon and H. Smiciklas-Wright (1979) Nutrition education in relation to the needs of the elderly. *J. Nutr. Educ.* 11:85–89.

66. H.L. Muncie and C. Carbonetto (1982) Prevalence of protein-calorie malnutrition in an extended care facility. *J. Fam. Pract.* 14:1061–1064.

67. T. Welch (1989) Nutrition-related problems in the institutionalized elderly. *Diet. Curr.* 16:1–4.

68. N. Agarwal, F. Acewedo, L.S. Leighton, C.G. Cayten, and C.S. Pitchumoni (1988) Predictive ability of various nutritional variables for mortality in elderly people. *Am. J. Clin. Nutr.* 48:1173–1178.

69. J.T. Dwyer, K.A. Coleman, E. Krall, et al. (1987) Changes in relative weight among institutionalized elderly adults. *J. Gerontol.* 42:246–251.

70. A.A. Spindler and M.A. Renvall (1989) Nutritional status and psychometric test scores in cognitively impaired elders. *Ann. N.Y. Acad. Sci.* 561:167–177.

71. P. Lips, F.C. van Ginkel, M.J.M. Jongen, F. Rubertus, W.J.F. van der Vijgh, and J.C. Netelenbos (1987) Determinants of vitamin D status in patients with hip fracture and in elderly control subjects. *Am. J. Clin. Nutr.* 46:1005–1010.

72. L. Willis, P. Thomas, P.J. Garry, and J.S. Goodwin (1987) A prospective study of response to stressful life events in initially healthy elders. *J. Gerontol.* 42:627–630.

73. J.S. Goodwin (1989) Social, psychological, and physical factors affecting the nutritional status of elderly subjects: separating cause and effect. *Am. J. Clin. Nutr.* 50(suppl.):1201–1209.

74. A.M. Ferris and V.B. Duffy (1989) Effect of olfactory deficits on nutritional status: does age predict persons at risk? *Ann. N.Y. Acad. Sci.* 561:113–123.

75. S.E. Gibbs and H.B. Turner (1986) Social-psychological aspects of nutrition among the elderly. Part II. Psychological dimensions of nutrition. In: *Nutritional Aspects of Aging,* vol. I (L.H. Chen, ed.), pp. 98–115, CRC Press, Baco Raton, FL.

76. J.S. Goodwin, J.M. Goodwin, and P.J. Garry (1983) Association between nutritional status and cognitive functioning in a healthy elderly population. *JAMA* 249:21917–21921.

77. A.M. Holeman and B.J. Merry (1986) The experimental manipulations of aging by diet. *Biol. Rev.* 61:329–368.

78. E.L. Schneider and J.D. Reed (1985) Life extension. *N. Engl. J. Med.* 312:213–222.

79. C. McKay, M. Crowell, and L. Maynard (1935) The effect of retarded growth upon the length of life and upon ultimate size. *J. Nutr.* 10:63–79.

80. B.P. Yu, E.J. Masoro, and C.A. McMahan (1985) Nutritional influences on aging or Fischer 344 Rats: I. physical, metabolic, and longevity characteristics. *J. Gerontol.* 40:657–670.

81. K. Iwasaki, C.A. Gleiser, E.J. Masoro, C.A. McMahan, E.-J. Seo, and B.P. Yu (1988) The influence of dietary protein source on longevity and age-related disease processes of Fischer rats. *J. Gerontol.* 43:B5–B12.

82. E.J. Masoro (1988) Minireview: food restriction in rodents: an evaluation of its role in the study of aging. *J. Gerontol.* 43:B59–B64.

83. F.S. Langaniere and B.P. Yu (1987) Anti-lipoperoxidation action of food restriction. *Biochem. Biophys. Res. Commun.* 145:1185–1191.

84. D. Harmon (1988) Free radicals in aging. *Mol. Cell. Biochem.* 84:155–161.

85. Select Committee on Aging, House of Representatives, Ninety-Eighth Congress (1984) *Tomorrow's Elderly.* Committee Publication no. 98-457, U.S. Government Printing Office, Washington, DC.

86. A. Balsam and G. Osteraas (1987) Developing a continuum of community nutrition services: Massachusetts Elderly Nutrition Programs. *J. Nutr. Elder.* 6(4):51–67.

87. G.M. Piper, B. Frank, and R.M. Thorner (1965) Survey of home-delivered meals programs. *Public Health Rep.* 80:432–436.

88. Older American's Act of 1965. Public law 89-73. 1965.

89. Older American's Act Amendments of 1978. Public law 95-478. 1978.

90. J.P. McNaughton and L.T. Kilgore (1985/86) Impact of Title III funded feeding program on nutrient intake and blood profiles of elderly in Mississippi. *J. Nutr. Elder.* 5(2):35–47.

91. M.B. Kohrs, J. Nordstrom, E.L. Plowman, et al. (1980) Association

of participation in a nutritional program for the elderly with nutritional status. *Am. J. Clin. Nutr.* 33:2643–2656.

92. Kirschner Associates, Inc. (1983) *An Evaluation of the Nutrition Services for the Elderly.* DHHS Publication no. (OHDS)83-20917. U.S. Government Printing Office, Washington, DC.

93. A.L. Balsam and B.L. Rogers (1988) *Service Innovations in the Elderly Nutrition Program: Strategies for Meeting Unmet Needs.* A Report prepared for the American Association of Retired Persons. Andrus Foundation, Washington, DC.

94. B.L. Neugarten (1982) Policy for the 1980s: age or need entitlement. In: *Age or Need? Public Policies for Older People* (B.L. Neugarten, ed.), pp. 19–32, Sage, Beverly Hills, CA.

95. M.A. Smyer (1984) Aging and social policy: contrasting Western Europe and the United States. *J. Fam. Iss.* 5:239–253.

96. C.L. Estes, S. Fox, and C.W. Mahoney (1986) Health care and social policy: health promotion and the elderly. In: *Wellness and Health Promotion for the Elderly* (K. Dychtwald and J. Macheam, eds.), pp. 55–69, Aspen, Rockville, MD.

97. H. Smiciklas-Wright and G.J. Fosmire (1895) Government nutrition programs for the aged. In: *Handbook of Nutrition and Aging* (R. Watson, ed.), pp. 323–334, CRC Press, Boca Raton, FL.

98. Kastenbaugh (1983) The 4% fallacy: R.I.P. *Int. J. Aging Hum. Dev.* 17:71–74.

99. D. Sullivan, R. Chernoff, and D.A. Lipschitz (1987) Nutritional support in long-term care facilities. *Nutr. Clin. Prac.* 2:6–13.

100. J. Rodin (1986) Aging and health: effects of the sense of control. *Science* 233:1271–1276.

101. J.C. Rogers and T. Snow (1982) An assessment of the feeding behavior of the institutionalized elderly. *Am. J. Occup. Ther.* 36:375–380.

102. L.E. Mathews (1988) Use of supplemental feeding for nursing home residents. *J. Nutr. Elder.* 7(4):35–41.

103. M. Katakity, J.F. Webb, and J.W.T. Dickerson (1983) Some effects of a food supplement in elderly hospital patients: a longitudinal study. *Hum. Nutr. Appl. Nutr.* 37A:85–93.

104. K. Maslow (1988) Total parenteral nutrition and tube feeding for elderly patients: findings of an OTA study. *JPEN* 12:425–432.

105. J.F. Fries (1980) Aging, natural death, and the compression of morbidity. *N. Engl. J. Med.* 303:133–140.

106. R.W. Rowe and R.L. Kahn (1987) Human aging: usual and successful. *Science* 237:143–149.

107. V.J. Cristofalo and G.T. Baker (1990) In memoriam Nathan W. Shock 1906–1989. *J. Gerontol.* 45:B1–B2.

Chapter 40

Elsworth R. Buskirk

Exercise

The coverage here of perspectives and special physiological needs is not all encompassing with respect to diet, physical fitness, and exercise. Rather, a broad view of our understanding in certain relevant areas is presented as are questions and problems for research. Thus, the desired implication is to convey that we still have much to learn even though the Greeks presumably initiated the learning process centuries ago.

The interaction of nutrition, regular exercise, and physical fitness has received considerable attention in recent years. The research relative to these interactions has considered a variety of factors including appropriate methods for nutritional and fitness assessment, nutritional factors that ostensibly contribute to fitness, nutrition and endurance capacity, substrate utilization during performance of various types of exercise, nutritional and exercise-induced adaptations, the impact of genetic endowment, relationship to risk factors associated with the development of chronic disease, and the development of a healthy lifestyle.

History

Perspectives with respect to diet and exercise have an extensive history that was recently reviewed by Simopoulos.[1] It is reputed that trainers of athletes occupied an important place in Greek society, for in addition to teaching athletic skills, they supervised training and diet. Porridge, cheese, figs, and meal cakes constituted their dietary regimen; meat was eaten only occasionally. A meat diet did appear about the middle of the fifth century B.C. and perhaps reached a peak through the example set by Milo of Croton, who won numerous wrestling matches from 536 to 520 B.C. Milo ostensibly ate 9 kg of meat, 9 kg of bread, plus 8.5 L of wine in a day. Even by today's dietary excesses undertaken by some of the huge men engaged in athletics, Milo's dietary indulgence remains impressive.

Among the Greeks, scientific medicine began to take shape and dietary management, i.e., nutrition together with exercise, formed part of the training regimen. The concept of positive health was regarded by the Greeks as important, and many trusted their health management to professional trainers. Hippocrates in his regimen I emphasized that if there is any deficiency in food or exercise, the body will fall sick. The concept that special physiques needed special diets was adhered to, thus bringing genetic endowment into the picture. Simopoulos[1] in summarizing nutrition and fitness from the first Olympiad in 776 B.C. to 393 A.D. offers the following view:

"In the near future, research will enable us to write prescriptions specifying the type and quantity of exercise and the type of food on the basis of the genetic profile, the physique, and the type of work of the individual and environment and season of the year." An ambitious forecast to say the least, but a perspective to motivate investigators.

General Considerations

Exercise capacity and physical performance are improved and/or sustained with appropriate nutrition but can deteriorate with nutritional deficiencies. Essential to appropriate nutrition are the energy-supply nutrients, i.e., carbohydrates, fats, and to some extent protein, vitamins for their role in metabolic and other reactions, plus minerals and water. The latter are of considerable consequence when exercise is intense, sustained, or performed in warm or hot environments. Of primary concern is the provision of adequate energy to support the active person's needs. Of secondary concern is the provision of sufficient carbohydrate to provide for adequate glycogen stores and for glucose metabolism. Similarly, the provision of adequate amounts of vitamins and minerals is necessary to sustain the enzymatic-metabolic interactions. An appropriate diet would contain sufficient protein, but our usual diets contain more than the protein necessary to sustain growth, development, and the turnover process in skeletal muscle and other body protein reservoirs.

On the basis of present evidence, there appears little reason for the physically active person's diet to deviate in major ways from that of other healthy persons, with the possible exception that more complex carbohydrates and less fat would be desirable. A recognizable exception would involve athletes in training who require ≥3,500 kcal/d, and the problems of nutrient bulk and caloric density are of concern. A moderate increase in fat intake reduces bulk and enables the athlete to obtain sufficient energy to support the high rate of energy turnover. Adaptation to a higher-fat diet that continues well beyond the training period undertaken at a young age may facilitate atherogenesis. The former athlete should be made aware of this possibility.

The major impetus for an increase in physical activity among population groups at large is the belief, fostered by numerous articles in the popular literature (including newspapers and TV), that good nutrition and physical activity facilitate wellness and help prevent chronic diseases such as coronary heart disease, maturity-onset or non-insulin-dependent diabetes, osteoporosis, and obesity. It is important to acknowledge that a considerable number of investigations have added to our current understanding of the health-related consequences of physical activity and the importance of a physically active lifestyle that is maintained for as long as possible.

General Nutrient Needs for Physically Active Persons

The nutrient needs for active individuals are generally provided by a nutritionally balanced diet that supplies sufficient energy to meet energy demands. Thus, the nutrient needs of active and sedentary individuals are similar but differ in quantity, with the active person requiring more food-derived energy. A diet containing ~10% protein, 30% fat, and 60% carbohydrate with a large proportion of the latter comprising complex carbohydrates is recommended.[2] Physical activity is the major variable that affects energy expenditure and energy needs. Under most circumstances the responsiveness of the appetite and satiety mechanisms compensate for changes in physical activity so that body weight and composition remain relatively constant.[3] An exception would be the response to intense training regimens during which both body weight and fat are lost. The effect is more pronounced in physically untrained individuals initially. As training continues they may respond similarly to those who are well trained.[4]

Other modifiers of nutrient needs include periods of rapid growth, maturation, gender, and aging. More nutrients are needed to sustain growth and development; girls generally need fewer calories than boys need and women need fewer than men; as we age beyond the achievement of adulthood, our energy needs decrease because of both a gradual reduction in fat-free body weight associated with a lower resting metabolic rate and the lesser physical activity that is undertaken.[5]

Participation in regular physical exercise of sufficient intensity is characterized by an increase in fat-free body mass and perhaps some reduction in body fat stores. The circulating lipid and lipoprotein profiles are modified, generally with an increase in high-density-lipoprotein concentration and a decrease in triglyceride, total cholesterol, and low-density-lipoprotein concentrations. There is a tendency toward lower blood pressure. Carbohydrate metabolism is modified, reflecting an increased insulin sensitivity in muscle and a greater propensity for glucose uptake as well as greater mobilization of free fatty acids from adipose tissue and more extensive capacity to oxidize free fatty acids within muscle. These changes are all influenced by the type, frequency, intensity, and duration of exercise with the general trends mentioned associated with regular weight-bearing exercise that exceeds ~60% of the person's aerobic power.[2]

When glycogen stores are lowered through intensive exercise in a person consuming a low-fat and limited-energy diet, the reservoir of fat in adipose tissue is tapped for fuel.[6,7] Thus, body fat stores are reduced by the combination of relatively intense exercise undertaken for a prolonged period under conditions of caloric restriction with little dietary fat. Under these circumstances, progress can be made in achievement and ultimate maintenance of a more ideal body weight.[8] An argument can be made that food intake is more precisely regulated in the person engaged in relatively high amounts of regular physical activity, at least with respect to the maintenance of a more ideal body weight.

In postabsorptive persons engaged in prolonged moderate-intensity exercise, glucose production increases primarily from hepatic glycogenolysis and secondarily from hepatic gluconeogenesis. Plasma free fatty acid (FFA) and glycerol concentrations also increase. A decrease in the respiratory quotient occurs, indicating a shift in substrate metabolism from carbohydrate to fat oxidation.[9] The relative increase in availability of FFA during exercise was shown to reduce the rate of muscle glycogen utilization effectively delaying the onset of exhaustion.[10–12] With the consumption of a diet high in fat, FFA oxidation increases[12,13] as does gluconeogenesis.[14,15] A high-protein diet increases amino acid oxidation and hepatic gluconeogenesis, at least on a relatively short-term basis.[16] On the basis of a variety of substrate feeding studies, it appears reasonable that with exercise, hepatic cyclic AMP is involved in the control of the pathways for glycogenolysis, glycolysis, and gluconeogenesis.[17–19]

Food Selection and Exercise

Studies of food selection among physically active people including athletes have not been comprehensive and have failed to take into account seasonal changes in appetite, food-item availability and cost, changes in housing or occupation, etc.[4] Brotherhood[20] put together a compendium of energy intake and gross dietary composition of men and women athletes compared with control subjects. The compendium revealed that more energy was consumed by the athletes than by the control subjects and that athletes in training consumed more energy than when not training. There was essentially no difference in the percentage of energy derived from carbohydrate (40–50%), fat (31–41%), or protein (11–17%). In other words, the athletes did not consume diets high in carbohydrates.

Hartung et al.[21] compared the dietary habits of three groups of men: marathoners, joggers, and relatively sedentary men. They reported that the marathoners and joggers ate less meat and fewer meat items than did the inactive men. Interestingly, the joggers ate fewer sweets, including candy, than the inactive men. There were no differences in the consumption of high-fat foods other than meat, but the exercising men had slightly lower fat intakes. Similarly, Blair et al.[22] compared middle-aged men and women runners with control subjects. The runners consumed ~600 kcal/d more than did the nonrunners when running 55–65 km/wk. The percentage consumption of the major nutrients was essentially the same.

Despite these general findings of little change in food-item selection, the dietary pattern of many health-conscious exercisers suggests that most are careful with their diets and tend to eat fewer meat items, less fat, and more vegetables and other sources of complex carbohydrates. For those interested in the food selection of exercisers, the brief review by Titchenal[4] is recommended. It is fair to conclude that longitudinal studies covering seasonal changes in dietary and exercise habits as well as the effects of gender and stage of life are necessary to provide a more comprehensive picture of what the active person eats under various circumstances.

Special Physiological Needs: Substrates

When exercise begins, energy turnover increases rapidly with rapid mobilization of carbohydrate and lipid stored within the contracting muscle. In addition, there is a gradual increase in the uptake of glucose and FFA from the circulation supplying the contracting muscle. If the exercise is of high intensity, the major source of energy is glycogen, but with longer periods of exercise that are less intense, the substrates supplied by the perfusing blood account for up to 90% of the energy turnover. In terms of multiples of resting utilization, glucose uptake by contracting muscle may increase up to 40-fold with glucose turnover in the whole body increasing up to fourfold.[23]

With many types of exercise, blood glucose concentration remains relatively constant as exercise continues because hepatic glycogenolysis and gluconeogenesis provide sufficient glucose to match peripheral glucose utilization. With prolonged relatively high-intensity exercise beyond 90 min–2 h, glucose utilization decreases, and FFA supplies the majority of the energy needs. In terms of a controlling system, the sympathetic nervous system releases norepinephrine, and blood insulin concentrations decline. The counterregulatory hormones involved with glucose control are released in greater quantities, i.e., epinephrine, glucagon, cortisol, and growth hormone.[24] Two major balancing situations exist with respect to substrate control: (1) the opposing effects of norepinephrine and insulin on adipose tissue lipolysis and release of FFA and (2) the roles of insulin and glucagon with respect to hepatic glucose production.

During recovery after exercise, the restoration processes begin with the recouping of muscle and liver glycogen and lipid stores within muscle and adipose tissue as well as the resynthesis of some muscle. The restoration process is aided by rest and the consumption of nutrients. During the first few hours after intense exercise, FFA continue to be utilized accompanied by a relative sparing of carbohydrate. Glucose utilization proceeds at a rate usually associated with rest. In recovery, the nonexercised muscles and the exercised muscles react differently. Glucose is taken up by the exercised muscles for resynthesis of glycogen whereas the nonexercised muscles display insulin resistance—and perhaps even release alanine for gluconeogenesis. The net effect is a relatively low total rate of glucose utilization.[23]

The eating of a carbohydrate-rich diet after glycogen depletion increases the glycogen stores in both muscle and liver. In fact, larger than normal amounts of glycogen can be stored—a phenomenon that has been labeled *super compensation*. Endurance has been found to increase during exercise that follows super compensation.

During exercise glucose ingestion may enhance endurance by maintaining blood glucose concentration when glycogen stores are low. This is particularly true for the continued high-intensity effort.

The breakdown and utilization of glycogen in muscle is influenced by several factors. A calcium-induced transient increase in phosphorylase a activity (transformation from phosphorylase b) and increases in intramuscular inorganic phosphate (P_i) are associated with the increased glycogenolysis induced by muscular contractions. Increases in AMP and IMP concentrations may well increase phosphorylase activity. The rate of glycogen breakdown is related to the initial glycogen concentration plus the combined effects of insulin (inhibits) and epinephrine (enhances). Epinephrine increases cyclic AMP production, which, in turn, increases phosphorylase activity in contracting muscle. In addition, the availability of substrates from the blood may influence muscle glycogenolysis and physical performance, particularly endurance.[25] In patients suffering from glycogen phosphorylase deficiency or McArdle's disease, exercise capacity is reduced by at least one-third from expected normal values because of inadequate glycogenolysis.[26]

A question remains as to how muscle glycogen can be preserved during exercise of low to moderately high intensity. An increase in plasma FFA concentration presumably results in a slower rate of glycogen utilization,[27] and a decrease in FFA availability increases glycogen utilization.[28] A citrate-mediated inhibition of phosphofructokinase that results from increased FFA utilization may well be responsible for the reduced glycogenolysis.[29]

Glucose-6-phosphate accumulates and activates glycogen synthase and inhibits phosphorylase. Because caffeine ingestion increases FFA availability in some subjects, it has been suggested that it could modify the interrelation between carbohydrate and fat metabolism and improve performance.[30] However, the results are not consistent[31] and perhaps are modified by prior nutrition, e.g., a high-carbohydrate diet.[32] At this time there is no substantial evidence that caffeine utilization decreases glycogen usage during relatively intense endurance exercise. The side effects of caffeine and interindividual differences in tolerance may well preclude any small advantage its use might convey.

The elevation in blood glucose by carbohydrate ingestion within an hour before exercise often increases muscle glycogen use during exercise,[25] whereas feeding carbohydrate much earlier may not have this effect. Hyperinsulinemia is presumably produced by carbohydrate ingestion and it, along with muscular contraction, produces an early decrease in blood glucose during exercise and more dependence on muscle glycogen. Insulin also has an antilipolytic action that results in lower circulating

concentrations of FFA which, in turn, favors greater glycogen utilization.[33] There are large interindividual differences in the response to preexercise glucose ingestion. However, the general advice to the competitive athlete might well be to consume the carbohydrate >1 h before the endurance event to facilitate performance by avoiding the insulin-induced decrease in blood glucose during the early stages of exercise. Even so, it is not clear at present that such practices have an effect on the rate of muscle glycogen depletion during exercise.

Oral carbohydrate administration during exercise has produced mixed results. For example, Hargreaves et al.[34] found a glycogen-sparing effect whereas Coyle et al.[35] did not. These two studies utilized different types of exercise. Hargreaves et al. used an intermittent exercise that may have permitted some glycogen repletion during the rest period, whereas Coyle et al. used continuous exercise. It is possible that glycogenolytic rate is not affected much by carbohydrate feeding during high-intensity exercise. Muscle glucose uptake may be impaired under these conditions.[36,37] Hargreaves and Richter[25] hypothesized that during intense exercise glucose disposal rather than membrane transport may limit glucose uptake in the contracting muscle. Therefore, increased blood glucose concentrations may not result in increased glucose metabolism. A membrane-limiting effect has not been ruled out, however. Nevertheless, there is reasonably good evidence that when muscle glycogen is depleted, the availability of blood glucose will facilitate continuation of exercise.[35]

A perspective generated by the extraordinary improvement that women have made in long-distance running, including the marathon, is that this improvement is related not only to the larger number of women now engaged in the requisite training to run these distances but also to the distinct possibility that they can derive energy from their body fat stores more readily than men can. This latter possibility perhaps is related to their relatively greater fat stores and to the gender-associated differences in circulating hormones. Thus, in women, transition from depletion of carbohydrate reserves (glycogen stores) to utilization of fatty acids is smooth and efficient and protects them from the phenomenon that runners call "hitting the wall." Investigation of this gender-associated distinction is well worth pursuing and should include the effects of gender vs. training frequency, intensity, and duration, and muscle fiber type and distribution as well as running mechanics.

Fat metabolism has been thought to be stimulated by cold exposure both acutely and over the long term.[38–40] Exercise of long duration and low to moderately high intensity also is associated with enhanced lipid metabolism, which presumably is associated with catecholamine-mediated mobilization of FFA from adipose tissue.[41] Nevertheless, when the supposed two stimuli for increased fat metabolism were combined, the results were variable. O'Hara et al.[40] observed large losses of body fat with 1–2 wk of intermittent exercise in a cold environment. Similarly, Timmons et al.[42] found a 35% greater energy expenditure with exercise at −10 °C than at 22 °C. In contrast, Patton and Vogel[43] found that the respiratory exchange ratio was unaltered during intermittent high-intensity exercise in a −20 vs. a 20 °C environment. Sink et al.[44] came to similar conclusions when they had moderately fit men exercise at 50 or 60% of aerobic power in environments of 0 or 22 °C. They concluded that cold exposure does not act synergistically with exercise to further stimulate lipid metabolism. Nevertheless, with continuing hard work in a natural environment in which the terrain and environmental conditions are rugged and the food supply is marginal, lipid metabolism no doubt is enhanced.

Special Issues

Weight Loss and Chronic Disease. Wood et al.[45] conducted a randomized trial involving overweight men who either dieted or exercised for 1 y. Both the dieters and exercisers lost body weight and body fat. However, the exercisers preserved their fat-free mass whereas the dieters did not. Although plasma concentrations of total cholesterol and low-density lipoproteins did not differ, the exercisers had a greater increase in high-density lipoproteins and a greater decrease in their triglycerides than did the dieters. In general, conventional wisdom suggests that either an increased energy expenditure, a decreased energy intake, or a combination of the two results in metabolic changes that favorably modify risk factors associated with the development of chronic diseases such as coronary heart disease and maturity-onset diabetes.

For those participating in regimens designed to enhance weight loss, the combination of diet plus exercise has many positive features and few negative ones. Fat-free mass tends to be preserved despite a transient negative nitrogen balance.

Another issue is the possibility of an effect of regular exercise in protecting against the development of chronic disease, e.g., coronary heart disease. It appears clear that physical inactivity is a significant risk factor, at least for a significant number of men.[46] We need to know the rate of development of the increased risk, how early in life the process starts, if risk can be lessened to a greater extent by regular exercise at certain stages of life, how much exercise is needed, and whether the answers are the same irrespective of gender?

Starvation. With fasting or complete starvation, substrate availability for the performance of physical exercise is altered. Within 2–3 d hepatic glycogen stores and circulating blood glucose concentrations are significantly reduced, hypoinsulinemia and hyperglucagonemia stimulate lipolysis with the release of FFA from adipose tissue, and ketogenesis occurs. Some gluconeogenesis may occur but in insufficient amounts to preserve normoglycemia. Although there is some evidence that ketone bodies can be utilized for fuel in the brain, there is no evidence that they are metabolized in exercising muscle. In any event, the capacity for exercise is reduced and as starvation continues, malaise characterizes the starved individual.

Diabetes. In diabetic children insulin therapy is required, but muscular activity can be performed and many insulin-dependent diabetics have gone on to become successful athletes. Nevertheless, exercise can provoke severe hypoglycemia among those with inadequate metabolic control and can lead to ketoacidosis and, in some instances, hyperglycemia. Several recommendations have been made to facilitate the performance of physical activity by the insulin-dependent diabetic: (1) self-measurement of blood glucose concentration, (2) programmed ingestion of carbohydrates, (3) reduction of insulin dose with appropriate timing relative to the exercise session, and (4) choosing a noninvolved-muscle injection site. Each regimen related to diet, exercise, and insulin therapy needs to be managed individually. Consistency is essential.[47]

Elderly People. A special problem exists among elderly people. Because of progressive loss of function (or dysfunction) of organs beyond middle age, elderly people have lower physical capacities.[48] These functional losses are not unlike the cardiovascular or musculoskeletal decrements that occur with physical inactivity or bed rest. Exercise programs can blunt such losses or even reverse them. Obesity is all too common and in elderly people is associated with physical inactivity with a resultant increase in cardiac morbidity, cerebral and peripheral vascular disease, and maturity-onset diabetes. In contrast, undernutrition is also common among elderly people, particularly among those who are physically compromised. Nutrient deficiencies result from poor appetites and low food intakes. Physical inactivity prevails along with depression, dementia, cognitive losses, and dependence. The possible role of regular exercise in counteracting such debilitation deserves further attention.[5]

Iron

Physiological function and physical performance can be influenced by iron status, and it is well known that iron-deficiency anemia impairs oxygen transport and, thereby, aerobic power and performance capacity.[49,50] If the anemia is only marginal but there are lower than normal iron stores, circulating maximal lactate concentrations are increased and subsequently decreased with iron repletion.[50]

A number of studies indicate that between 2% and 5% of exceptional athletes have iron deficiency or relatively low body iron stores.[51-54] The percentage is higher for women athletes than for male athletes. Hematocrits and hemoglobins may be low or relatively normal but tend to be lower among women athletes.

An important problem that has surfaced for those athletes susceptible to iron-deficiency anemia is gastrointestinal bleeding. A survey of 110 participants in a 1985 Canadian triathalon revealed that three (2.7%) of the participants had subsequent bloody bowel movements in either competition or training.[55] Other young distance runners have displayed similar problems[56,57] as have cyclists.[58] Although gastrointestinal bleeding is more frequent the higher the intensity of exercise, the specific cause is unknown. The following have been implicated as a cause for bloody stools: hemorrhagic gastritis predisposing iron-deficiency anemia, compromised gastrointestinal blood flow, melena perhaps associated with peptic ulcer disease, increased circulating epinephrine and cortisol, and therapeutic use of aspirin. To help with the problem, a gastrointestinal workup is necessary along with, perhaps, avoidance of the following: prerace aspirin use, antacid therapy, use of hydrogen ion blockers, and extra dietary iron.[57]

Hematuria has been observed for years in distance runners, particularly in those running on hard surfaces. Heel strike, rapid perfusion through small blood vessels with rupturing of red blood cells, along with mechanical shaking of the kidney have been commonly referred to as causes of hematuria.

The mechanisms proposed for iron deficiency include inadequate iron intake,[59] inadequate iron absorption,[60] losses in sweat,[61] gastrointestinal blood loss,[62] and red cell hemolysis with hematuria.[63]

Copper

Among athletes and physically active people there is little evidence that copper metabolism is altered. Haralambie and Keul[64] found no essential difference in serum copper between trained and sedentary men. Similarly, Lukaski et al.[65] reported similar plasma copper concentrations for collegiate athletes and control subjects as did Dressendorfer and Sockolov,[66] who measured runners and nonrunners. In contrast, Dowdy and Burt[67] observed swimmers during a 6-mo training period and reported a decrease in ceru-

loplasmin from 370 to 250 mg/L during the first month; no change was found thereafter. Serum copper concentration declined from 10.1 to 7.9 μmol/L at the end of the training period. The results from this training study have not been confirmed, and there is no reason at present to suspect a significant impact of regular exercise on copper metabolism. Nevertheless, the right questions may not have been asked, the right variables measured, or copper turnover assessed.

Zinc

Low concentrations of serum zinc were found in long distance runners compared with sedentary men (e.g., 11.6 vs 14.4 μmol/L).[66] The more the daily running distance, the lower the serum zinc concentration. Among athletes Haralambie[68] found that 23% of men and 43% of women had serum zinc concentrations <11.5 μmol/L. Similarly, Deuster et al.[54] found that 25% of the women runners whom they studied had serum zinc values <12.2 μmol/L. In contrast, Lukaski et al.[65] found no difference in plasma zinc values between athletes and control subjects.

Unfortunately, data on iron, copper, and zinc intakes seldom have been incorporated in studies of the circulating concentrations of these elements. Thus, a more complete physiological interpretation of the results found in blood is not possible. More complete studies of trace element metabolism in relation to physical activity would be welcome.

Questions

There are many questions concerning the regulation and utilization of metabolic substrates under different environmental, nutritional, and exercise conditions, e.g., can one adapt over time to a relatively high-fat diet and maintain at least moderate exercise capacity? The sequence of substrate replacement during recovery is not well understood nor is it clear what anabolic events occur. The role of the counter-regulatory hormones under different nutritional and exercise conditions needs to be better understood, particularly in relation to the development and management of maturity-onset diabetes. For example, is there an improvement in insulin sensitivity? In addition, studies are needed to define the role of exercise in relation to dietary restriction for purposes of weight loss or maintenance for those with a propensity for obesity. In addition, the role that trace elements play in support of metabolism during physical activity needs considerably more research.

References

1. A.P. Simopoulos (1989) Opening address: nutrition and fitness from the first Olympiad in 776 BC to 393 AD and the concept of positive health. *Am. J. Clin. Nutr.* 49:921–926.

2. E.R. Buskirk (1981) Some nutritional considerations in the conditioning of athletes. *Annu. Rev. Nutr.* 1:319–350.

3. J.H. Wilmore (1983) Appetite and body composition consequent to physical activity. *Res. Q. Exerc. Sport* 54:415–425.

4. C.A. Titchenal (1988) Exercise and food intake: what is the relationship? *Sports Med.* 6:135–145.

5. E.R. Buskirk (1985) Health maintenance and longevity: exercise. In: *Handbook of the Biology of Aging* (C.E. Finch and E.L. Schneider, eds.), pp. 894–931, Van Nostrand Reinhold, New York.

6. K.J. Acheson, A. Thelin, E. Ravussin, M.J. Arnaud, and E. Jequier (1985) Contribution of 500 g naturally labeled ^{13}C dextrin maltose to total carbohydrate utilization and the effect of the antecedent diet, in man. *Am. J. Clin. Nutr.* 41:881–890.

7. R. Bielinski, Y. Schutz, and E. Jequier (1985) Energy metabolism during the postexercise recovery in man. *Am. J. Clin. Nutr.* 42:69–82.

8. K.D. Brownell, G.A. Marlott, E. Lichtenstein, and G.T. Wilson (1986) Understanding and preventing relapse. *Am. Psychol.* 41:765–782.

9. J. Wahren (1979) Metabolic adaptation to physical exercise in man. In: *Endocrinology* (L.J. DeGroot, ed.), pp. 1911–1926, Grune and Stratton, New York.

10. M.S. Rennie, W.W. Winder, and J.O. Holloszy (1976) A sparing effect of increased plasma fatty acids on muscle and liver glycogen content in the exercising rat. *Biochem. J.* 156:647–655.

11. R.C. Hickson, M.J. Rennie, R.K. Conlee, W.W. Winder, and J.O. Holloszy (1977) Effects of increased plasma fatty acids on glycogen utilization and endurance. *J. Appl. Physiol.* 43:829–833.

12. W.C. Miller, G.R. Bryce, and R.H. Conlee (1984) Adaptations to a high-fat diet that increase exercise endurance in male rats. *J. Appl. Physiol.* 56:78–83.

13. E.W. Askew, G.L. Dohm, and R.L. Huston (1975) Fatty acid and ketone body metabolism in the rat: response to diet and exercise. *J. Nutr.* 105:1422–1432.

14. B. Friedman, E.W. Goodman, and S. Weinhouse (1967) Effects of fatty acids on gluconeogenesis in the rat. *J. Biol. Chem.* 242:3620–3627.

15. A.B. Eisenstein, I. Strack, and A. Steiner (1974) Increased hepatic gluconeogenesis without a rise of glucagon secretion in rats fed a high fat diet. *Diabetes* 23:869–875.

16. M. Tiedgen and H.J. Seitz (1980) Dietary control of circadian variations in serum insulin, glucagon and hepatic cyclic AMP. *J. Nutr.* 110:876–882.

17. H. Galbo (1983) *Hormonal and Metabolic Adaptation to Exercise*, Thieme, Stuttgart.

18. G.L. Dohm, J. Kasperec, and J. Barakat (1985) Time course of changes in gluconeogenic enzyme activities during exercise and recovery. *Am. J. Physiol.* 249:E6–E11.

19. P. Satabin, B. Bois-Joyeux, M. Chanez, C.Y. Guezennec, and J. Peret (1989) Effects of long-term feeding of high-protein or high-fat diets on the response to exercise in the rat. *Eur. J. Appl. Physiol.* 58:568–576.

20. J.R. Brotherhood (1984) Nutrition and sports performance. *Sports Med.* 1:350–389.

21. G.H. Hartung, J.P. Foreyt, R.E. Mitchell, I. Wlasek, and A.M. Gotto (1980) Relation of diet to high-density-lipoprotein cholesterol in middle-aged marathon runners, joggers and inactive men. *N. Engl. J. Med.* 302:357–361.

22. S.N. Blair, N.M. Ellsworth, W.L. Haskell, M.P. Stern, J.W. Farquhar, and P.D. Wood (1981) Comparison of nutrient intake in middle aged men and women runners and controls. *Med. Sci. Sports Exerc.* 13:310–315.

23. E.S. Horton (1989) Metabolic fuels, utilization and exercise. *Am. J. Clin. Nutr.* 49:931–932.

24. M. Kjaer (1989) Epinephrine and some other hormonal responses to exercise in man: with special reference to physical training. *Int. J. Sports Med.* 10:2–15.

25. M. Hargreaves and E.A. Richter (1988) Regulation of skeletal muscle glycogenolysis during exercise. *Can. J. Sports Sci.* 13:197–203.

26. S.F. Lewis and R.G. Haller (1986). The pathophysiology of McArdle's disease: clues to regulation in exercise and fatigue. *J. Appl. Physiol.* 61:391–401.

27. D.L. Costill, E. Coyle, G. Dalsky, W. Evans, W. Fink, and D. Hoopes (1977) Effects of elevated plasma FFA and insulin on muscle glycogen usage during exercise. *J. Appl. Physiol.* 43:695–699.

28. A.C. Juhlin-Dannfelt, S.E. Terblanche, R.D. Fell, J.C. Young, and J.O. Holloszy (1982) Effects of β-adrenergic receptor blockade on glycogenolysis during exercise. *J. Appl. Physiol.* 53:549–554.

29. M.J. Rennie and J.O. Holloszy (1977) Inhibition of glucose uptake and glycogenolysis by availability of oleate in well-oxygenated perfused skeletal muscle. *Biochem. J.* 168:161–170.

30. D.L. Costill, G.P. Dalsky, and W.J. Fink (1978) Effects of caffeine ingestion on metabolism and exercise performance. *Med. Sci. Sports* 10:155–158.

31. D.C. Casal and A.S. Leon (1985) Failure of caffeine to affect substrate utilization during prolonged running. *Med. Sci. Sports Exerc.* 17:174–179.

32. J. Weir, T.D. Noakes, K. Myburgh, and B. Adams (1987) A high carbohydrate diet negates the metabolic effects of caffeine during exercise. *Med. Sci. Sports Exerc.* 19:100–105.

33. V. Koivisto, S. Karonen, and E.A. Nikkila (1981) Carbohydrate ingestion before exercise: comparison of glucose, fructose and sweet placebo. *J. Appl. Physiol.* 51:783–787.

34. M. Hargreaves, D.L. Costill, A. Coggan, W.J. Fink, and I. Nishibata (1984) Effect of carbohydrate feedings on muscle glycogen utilization and exercise performance. *Med. Sci. Sports Exerc.* 16:219–222.

35. E.F. Coyle, A.R. Coggan, M.K. Hemmert, and J.L. Ivy (1986) Muscle glycogen utilization during prolonged strenuous exercise when fed carbohydrate. *J. Appl. Physiol.* 61:165–172.

36. P.D. Gollnick, B. Pernow, B. Essen, E. Jansson, and B. Saltin (1981) Availability of glycogen and plasma FFA for substrate utilization in leg muscle of man during exercise. *Clin. Physiol.* 1:27–42.

37. E.A. Richter and H. Galbo (1986) High glycogen levels enhance glycogen breakdown in isolated contracting skeletal muscle. *J. Appl. Physiol.* 61:827–831.

38. P.G. Hanson and R.E. Johnson (1965) Variation of plasma ketones and free fatty acids during acute cold exposure in man. *J. Appl. Physiol.* 20:56–60.

39. E.J. Masaro (1966) Effects of cold on metabolic use of lipids. *Physiol. Rev.* 46:67–101.

40. W.J. O'Hara, C. Allen, R.J. Shephard, and J. Allen (1979) Fat loss in the cold: a controlled study. *J. Appl. Physiol.* 46:872–877.

41. B. Saltin and J. Karlsson (1971) Muscle glycogen utilization during work of different intensities. In: *Muscle Metabolism During Exercise* (B. Pernow and B. Saltin, eds.), pp. 289–299, Plenum Press, New York.

42. B.A. Timmons, J. Araujo, and T.R. Thomas (1985) Fat utilization enhanced by exercise in a cold environment. *Med. Sci. Sports Exerc.* 17:673–678.

43. J.F. Patton and J.A. Vogel (1984) Effects of acute cold exposure on submaximal endurance performance. *Med. Sci. Sports Exerc.* 16:494–497.

44. K.R. Sink, T.R. Thomas, J. Araujo, and S.F. Hill (1989) Fat energy use and plasma lipid changes associated with exercise intensity and temperature. *Eur. J. Appl. Physiol.* 58:508–513.

45. P.D. Wood, M.I. Stefanik, D.M. Dreon, et al. (1988) Changes in plasma lipids and lipoproteins in overweight men during weight loss through dieting as compared with exercise. *N. Engl. J. Med.* 319:1173–1179.

46. R.S. Paffenbarger and R.T. Hyde (1984) Exercise as a protection against coronary heart disease. *N. Engl. J. Med.* 302:726–1027.

47. H. Dorchy and J. Poortmans (1989) Sport and the diabetic child. *Sports Med.* 7:248–262.

48. E.R. Buskirk and S.S. Segal (1988) The aging motor system. In: *Physical Activity and Aging* (W.W. Spirduso and H.M. Eckert, eds.), American Academy of Physical Education Papers no. 22, pp. 19–36, Human Kinetics Books, Champaign, IL.

49. O.D. Vellar and L. Hermansen (1971) Physical performance and hematological parameters, with special reference to hemoglobin and maximal oxygen uptake. *Acta Med. Scand.* 190(Suppl. 522): 1–40.

50. R.B. Schoene, P. Escourrou, H.T. Robertson, K.L. Nelson, J.R. Parsons, and N.J. Smith (1983) Iron repletion decreases maximal exercise lactate concentrations in female athletes with minimal iron deficiency anemia. *J. Lab. Clin. Med.* 102:306–312.

51. J.F. DeWijn, J.L. DeLongste, W. Mosterd, and D. Willebrand (1971) Haemoglobin packed cell volume, serum iron and iron binding capacity of selected athletes during training. *J. Sports Med.* 11: 42–51.

52. E.M. Haymes (1980) Iron supplementation. In: *Encyclopedia of Physical Education, Fitness and Sports: Training, Environment, Nutrition and Fitness,* pp. 335–344, Brighton, Salt Lake City.

53. S.A. Plowman and P.C. McSwegin (1981) The effects of iron supplementation on female cross-country runners. *J. Sports Med.* 21: 407–416.

54. P.A. Deuster, S.B. Kyle, P.B. Moser, R.A. Vigersky, A. Sing, and E.B. Schoomaker (1986) Nutritional survey of highly trained women. *Am. J. Clin. Nutr.* 44:954–962.

55. S.N. Sullivan (1987) Exercise-associated symptoms in triathletes. *Phys. Sportsmed.* 15:105–110.

56. G. Selby, D. Frame, and E.R. Eichner (1988) Effort-related gastrointestinal blood loss in young distance runners during a competitive season. *Med. Sci. Sports Exerc.* 20:S79(abstr.).

57. E.R. Eichner (1989) Gastrointestinal bleeding in athletes. *Phys. Sportsmed.* 17:128–140.

58. T.W. Dobbs, M. Atkins, and R. Ratliff (1988) Gastrointestinal bleeding in competitive cyclists. *Med. Sci. Sports Exerc.* 20: 578(abstr.).

59. D.B. Clement and R.C. Asmundson (1982) Nutritional intake and hematological parameters in endurance runners. *Phys. Sportsmed.* 10:7–41.

60. L. Ehn, B. Carlmark, and S. Hoglund (1980) Iron status in athletes involved in intense physical activity. *Med. Sci. Sports Exerc.* 12: 61–64.

61. J.M.C. Gutteridge, D.A. Rowley, B. Halliwell, D.F. Cooper, and D.M. Heeley (1985) Copper and iron complexes catalytic for oxygen radical reactions in sweat from human athletes. *Clin. Chim. Acta* 145:267–273.

62. L.F. McMahon, M.J. Ryan, D.L. Larson, and R.L. Fisher (1984) Occult gastrointestinal blood loss in marathon runners. *Ann. Intern. Med.* 100:846–847.

63. A. Hunding, R. Jordal, and P.E. Paulev (1981) Runners anemia and iron deficiency. *Acta Med. Scand.* 209:315–318.

64. G. Haralambie and J. Keul (1970) Das verhalten von serum ceruloplasmin und kupfer bei langdavernder korperbulastrung. *Arztl. Forsch.* 24:112–115.

65. H.C. Lukaski, W.W. Bolonchuk, L.M. Klevay, D.B. Milne, and H.H. Sandstead (1983) Maximal oxygen consumption as related to magnesium, copper, and zinc nutriture. *Am. J. Clin. Nutr.* 37: 407–415.

66. R.H. Dressendorfer and R. Sockolov (1980) Hypozincemia in runners. *Phys. Sportsmed.* 8:97–100.

67. R.P. Dowdy and J. Burt (1980) Effect of intensive, long-term training on copper and iron nutriture in man. *Fed. Proc.* 39:786(abstr.).

68. G. Haralambie (1981) Serum zinc in athletes in training. *Int. J. Sports Med.* 2:131–138.

Chapter **41**

Donald J. McNamara

Coronary Heart Disease

Cardiovascular diseases accounted for 48% of all deaths in the United States in 1985 with over 900,000 Americans dying from heart attacks, strokes, and other blood-vessel diseases. It was estimated that 65 million Americans have some form of heart or blood-vessel disease and that the cost of cardiovascular disease in 1985 approached $84 billion. Although these data clearly document the impact of cardiovascular diseases on the health and well-being of the American public, it is encouraging to note that there has been a significant reduction in cardiovascular disease morbidity and mortality rates through advances in medical care and lifestyle changes. Since 1964, coronary heart disease (CHD) mortality has declined steadily with a 42% decrease between 1964 and 1985. Even with these dramatic and encouraging results from medical care and lifestyle changes, CHD remains the leading cause of mortality in the United States.

Epidemiological studies indicate that CHD is a disease of multiple etiologies and results from a variety of risk factors, some amenable to reduction and others impervious to intervention. Heredity no doubt plays a significant role in CHD risk and a family history of premature CHD is considered a major risk factor. Other risk factors that cannot be altered are male sex and increasing age. Lifestyle risk factors that are modifiable include cigarette smoking, high blood pressure, high blood cholesterol concentrations, glucose intolerance, obesity, and physical inactivity. On the basis of epidemiological evidence, cigarette smoking is considered the most significant of the major risk factors followed by hypertension and hypercholesterolemia.[1] These risk factors are known to be interactive and any combinations of risk factors have a greater impact on CHD risk than the sum of their independent effects.

A number of dietary factors can have a significant impact on CHD risk factors that involve hyperlipidemia, hypertension, obesity, and glucose intoler-ance. Dietary recommendations from various health agencies are to reduce total fat and saturated fatty acids, cholesterol, and salt in the diet and to maintain an ideal body weight.[2-4] These recommendations are based on the best available evidence relating dietary factors to CHD morbidity and mortality risk.

Diet-related Risk Factors for CHD

Hyperlipidemia. An elevated plasma cholesterol concentration has been shown to be a major risk factor for CHD. Risk is positively related to an elevated plasma low-density-lipoprotein (LDL) cholesterol concentration. LDL was identified as the major atherogenic plasma lipoprotein by a variety of epidemiologic, clinical, metabolic, and animal studies. Variations in LDL-cholesterol concentrations account for a large part of the variance in CHD incidence within populations at high risk. The National Cholesterol Education Program classified CHD risk as being average for individuals with a plasma total cholesterol concentration of <5.2 mmol/L, moderate at 5.2–6.2 mmol/L, and high at >6.2 mmol/L.[3] The extent of CHD risk in the moderate-risk group depends on the presence or absence of other risk factors, such as hypertension, cigarette smoking, obesity, and male sex.

Although elevated concentrations of LDL cholesterol were shown to increase CHD risk, studies also showed that low plasma high-density-lipoprotein (HDL) cholesterol is a risk factor for CHD and that one of the strongest determinants of CHD risk is the LDL-HDL ratio.[5] There are a number of factors related to a low plasma HDL-cholesterol concentration, including cigarette smoking, obesity, lack of exercise, androgenic steroids, β-adrenergic blocking agents, hypertriglyceridemia, and genetics. Although there is some debate regarding the advisability of measuring HDL cholesterol in all patients, it would seem reasonable that the LDL-HDL ratio be determined in

349

moderate-risk individuals as part of an overall risk evaluation. An intervention program should include analysis of the patient's LDL-HDL ratio, and if it is >3.5 (or a total cholesterol-to-HDL ratio of >5.0), then diet therapy to reduce CHD risk is indicated. At this time, however, the primary emphasis of diet therapy is to reduce an elevated plasma LDL cholesterol.[6]

Calories and Obesity. There has been a continuing controversy over whether obesity is a primary or secondary risk factor in the development of CHD. Data from the Framingham Heart Study showed that increased relative body weight is an independent risk factor for CHD in addition to its contribution to hypertension, low concentrations of HDL, decreased glucose tolerance, and elevated plasma triglyceride and cholesterol concentrations.[7] Recent data provide evidence that androgenic obesity (increased waist-to-hip circumference ratio) represents a greater CHD risk than lower body obesity.[8] The extent of a patient's obesity can be determined most readily from the body mass index (body weight in kilograms divided by the height in meters squared, kg/m^2), with a mean value of 23 representing normal body weight. Overweight is defined as a value >27, and severely overweight is characterized by a body mass index value >31.[4]

Metabolic studies showed that obesity is associated with a number of abnormalities of both cholesterol and lipoprotein metabolism that are related to hyperlipidemia. For every excess kilogram of body weight, endogenous cholesterol synthesis is increased by 20 mg/d; in other words, being 10 kg overweight results in an additional cholesterol input of 200 mg/d that must be catabolized, excreted, or stored in tissues.[9] In a similar manner obese subjects have increased hepatic synthesis of very-low-density lipoproteins (VLDL), which is associated with hypertriglyceridemia, decreased plasma HDL-cholesterol concentration, and increased production of LDL.[10]

Hypertension. The relationship between hypertension and increased cardiovascular disease risk is established, and the benefit of reducing an elevated blood pressure in reducing risk of cardiovascular diseases and strokes is generally recognized. The incidence of hypertension was shown to be related to obesity, high sodium intakes, excess alcohol consumption, and low dietary calcium. Hypertension is defined as a diastolic pressure of >90 mm Hg and a systolic pressure >140 mm Hg and can take various forms (mild, moderate, or severe) depending upon the extent of the increase in diastolic pressure or the extent of an increase in systolic pressure alone (isolated systolic hypertension).[4]

Recommended Dietary Changes: Rationale

Caloric Intake. Obesity is associated with increased rates of cholesterol, VLDL triglyceride, and apolipoprotein B synthesis, which often result in hyperlipidemia. Obesity is also associated with low concentrations of plasma HDL cholesterol, hypertension, and glucose intolerance. Weight reduction often effectively reduces these CHD risk factors and represents an effective treatment modality for a number of significant diet-related CHD risk factors. In terms of plasma lipoprotein synthesis, weight reduction results in a corresponding decrease in the elevated rates of cholesterol and VLDL synthesis.[9] Obese patients with fasting hypertriglyceridemia have both an overproduction of VLDL triglyceride and a reduced fractional catabolism of plasma VLDL. Reduction of the plasma VLDL-triglyceride concentration by weight reduction results in an increase in plasma HDL-cholesterol concentration and a less-atherogenic plasma lipoprotein profile. Because obesity is associated with a number of clearly defined CVD risk factors (hypertension, low concentrations of HDL, elevated plasma glucose concentrations, high blood cholesterol concentrations, and hypertriglyceridemia), any effective dietary intervention to lower CHD risk must include a weight-reduction component to increase its effectiveness. A primary objective should be to attain and maintain ideal body weight through both decreased caloric intake and increased energy expenditure. The finding that male-type obesity is an independent risk factor for CHD, along with the other risk factors that develop secondary to obesity, clearly stresses the importance of obesity as a prevalent CHD risk factor and emphasizes the importance of weight reduction in a CHD risk-reduction program.

Dietary Fat. It is generally thought that the current American diet contains an excess amount of saturated fatty acids that should be reduced so that the polyunsaturated-to-saturated fatty acids ratio (P:S) is increased from 0.45 to 1.0. The plasma cholesterol-lowering response to a change in dietary fat quality from a low to a high P:S is documented extensively.[2] The evidence indicates that the hypocholesterolemic effects of an increased dietary fat P:S do not result from changes in endogenous cholesterol synthesis or catabolism but rather from changes in the synthesis and catabolism of plasma lipoproteins.[9] Kinetic studies indicate that shifting dietary fat quality from a low to high P:S results in decreased production of VLDL and LDL apolipoprotein B (the apolipoprotein associated with LDL) and that this decreased production reduces the plasma cholesterol concentration.[9] Another mechanism involved in lower plasma cholesterol concentrations that result from an increase in the P:S of the diet is an induction of hepatic LDL (apolipoproteins B and E) receptors[11] that, in turn, results in increased LDL fractional catabolic rate and reduced plasma LDL-cholesterol concentrations. It should be noted that intake of diets containing dietary fat with very high P:S not only lowers plasma concentrations of atherogenic LDL cholesterol but also lowers the protective HDL cholesterol concentration. There are some concerns regarding long-term consequences of such changes, and for that reason it is not advisable to increase the P:S of dietary fat >1.0.[12]

Dietary Fat Quantity. There is some debate regarding the rationale for reducing the percent of calories from fat from 37% to 30% as part of a plasma cholesterol-lowering diet, because such a reduction can result in lowering of plasma HDL-cholesterol concentrations.[12] Most of the evidence indicates that a 30%-fat diet with a P-S ratio of 1.0 effectively reduces plasma total and LDL-cholesterol concentrations in most hypercholesterolemic patients.[2] However, further reductions in total fat calories were shown to reduce HDL-cholesterol concentrations and to increase plasma triglyceride concentrations in some patients.[13] As discussed below, current theories for lowering plasma LDL-cholesterol concentrations of hypercholesterolemic patients support maintenance of a 30% fat intake, with replacement of saturated fatty acids with monounsaturated fatty acids. This approach can provide additional LDL-cholesterol lowering without an increase in plasma triglyceride concentrations and a decrease in HDL concentrations.[12]

Dietary Cholesterol. Dietary recommendations advise a dietary cholesterol intake of <300 mg/d as compared with the current average intake of 450 mg/d. Because dietary cholesterol is derived solely from animal products, this recommendation is usually associated with a decreased consumption of saturated animal fatty acids in the diet. Of all the dietary changes recommended, reducing dietary cholesterol probably has the least effect on plasma cholesterol concentrations for most people. Considering that absorption of dietary cholesterol averages 60% and the rate of endogenous cholesterol synthesis is 11–13 mg/kg body weight per day, a reduction in dietary cholesterol intake of 150 mg/d results in a decrease of absorbed cholesterol of 90 mg/d, an amount that is <10% of the total daily input of absorbed dietary and endogenously synthesized cholesterol.[9]

Analysis of the effect of dietary cholesterol on plasma cholesterol concentrations from 68 studies in 1,490 subjects demonstrated that the average effect of a 100 mg/d increment in dietary cholesterol is a 0.06 mmol/L change in plasma cholesterol concentrations. On the basis of these data, a 150 mg/d reduction in dietary cholesterol intake would reduce the population mean plasma cholesterol value by 0.08 mmol/L, a 1.4% reduction (assuming an average cholesterol concentration of 5.4 mmol/L). The analysis of these studies also indicated that the response to a dietary cholesterol challenge is independent of dietary fat quality and quantity, initial and final dietary cholesterol intakes, and initial plasma cholesterol concentrations. There was no evidence of a threshold level of dietary cholesterol, of an interactive effect between fat quality and cholesterol quantity, or of an increased sensitivity to dietary cholesterol in hypercholesterolemic patients.[14]

Approximately one-third of the population is sensitive to dietary cholesterol, and reducing dietary cholesterol intake results in some reduction of plasma cholesterol concentration in these dietary-cholesterol-sensitive individuals.[15] This sensitivity to dietary cholesterol appears to be related to an inability to suppress endogenous cholesterol synthesis when dietary cholesterol intake is increased, i.e., the individual lacks appropriate feedback mechanisms to regulate endogenous cholesterol synthesis. Data suggest that under such conditions the resulting increase in plasma cholesterol concentrations may be related not only to a steady endogenous synthesis and to an increased dietary intake but also to a suppression of LDL receptors that decreases LDL catabolism and results in a further expansion of the plasma LDL cholesterol pool because of a decreased LDL fractional catabolic rate.[16]

Efficacy and Safety of Dietary Changes

Heterogeneous Responses. A number of recent studies addressed the question of heterogeneity in the population of plasma cholesterol responses to dietary interventions. Although mean population reductions in plasma cholesterol in response to dietary changes are significant, a large degree of variability exists within the population. The heterogeneity of responses to changes in dietary fat quality can be quite pronounced and can range from little or no effect to as much as a 30% reduction in LDL-cholesterol concentrations.[17,18] Although there is significant heterogeneity of responses to changes in dietary fat quality, there is even more pronounced heterogeneity of responses to changes in dietary cholesterol intake. When dietary cholesterol intake is varied over a physiological intake range (0–1000 mg/d), a small percentage of patients exhibit a variable increase in plasma cholesterol concentrations, whereas the majority of study subjects have no detectable change in plasma cholesterol concentrations.[15,19] The existence of precise feedback mechanisms balancing exogenous dietary cholesterol and endogenous synthesis of cholesterol in the majority of individuals is a primary reason that a reduction in dietary cholesterol intake has relatively little effect on plasma cholesterol concentrations in most patients.

Public Perceptions and Misperceptions. The hypercholesterolemic patient is faced with a constant barrage of messages on how to lower the risk for CHD. Some such messages are rendered purely on a commercial basis; many are from well-meaning promoters of wellness. Because many of these messages are confusing and contradictory, the hypercholesterolemic patient is faced with a constant challenge of trying to separate scientifically based information from the marketing and advertising messages regarding the latest hypocholesterolemic product or fad available. Unfortunately for many patients, this steady stream of information results in reliance on an overly simplistic approach of excluding what are perceived as bad foods from the diet in the hope of reducing CHD risk. Often such decisions are made on the basis of the cholesterol content of a food item with little awareness of the importance of the type or amount of fat in the food. Patients making food choices based on a pocket-size cholesterol counter are not always making the most effective dietary decisions. Many patients are able to reduce total fat and cholesterol intake yet fail to achieve a suitable dietary fat P-S ratio, which has the major effect on plasma LDL-cholesterol concentrations. Effective dietary interventions to reduce plasma cholesterol concentrations rely primarily on the reduction of saturated fatty acid intake and the substitution of unsaturated fatty acids in the diet to achieve a P-S ratio of 1.0.[2-4]

Population vs. Individual Therapy. There are two approaches to the diet-CHD relationship: the population-based approach and the high-risk approach. The population-based approach is based on the rationale that because a large percentage of the population is at increased risk for CHD because of elevated plasma LDL-cholesterol concentrations, it is reasonable to reduce that risk factor by mass intervention. The high-risk approach, on the other hand, recommends detection of hypercholesterolemia and individualized treatment of the high-risk patient to reduce the CHD risk profile. These are not mutually exclusive approaches and indeed, if properly executed, can be complementary. If this is the case, why is there considerable debate regarding the approach to be taken in reducing CHD incidence in the American population?

There are a number of concerns regarding the population-based approach to dietary intervention, not the least of which is the limited scientifically based nutrition knowledge of the population as a whole. An additional potential problem with a major emphasis on a population approach deals with the

diagnosis and determination of severe hypercholesterolemia requiring pharmacologic intervention to reduce CHD risk. Measurement of plasma cholesterol concentrations and education in how to incorporate effective dietary changes while maintaining overall nutritional balance must be essential components of any population-wide CHD risk-reduction program.[2-4]

Benefit-risk Considerations. The best available evidence indicates that lowering an elevated plasma cholesterol concentration reduces CHD risk. However, there is little evidence to indicate that the associated reduction in CHD mortality results in decreased total mortality.[20,21] Neither the long-term benefits of lowering an elevated plasma cholesterol concentration nor the health consequences of a low-fat, high-carbohydrate diet when applied to the American population are clearly defined. Drastic changes in dietary patterns may not be totally without risk, especially for the very young and the very old.[22] Although the widely recommended dietary reduction in total fat and saturated fatty acid intake does not appear to present any known health problems, dietary extremes to lower fat and cholesterol intake and to increase fiber consumption may have deleterious effects for some segments of the population.

New Areas of Research

Fiber. Numerous studies have demonstrated that an increased dietary fiber intake, primarily water-soluble fiber, lowers plasma cholesterol concentrations. Most studies indicate that a significant plasma cholesterol lowering response can be achieved when total and soluble fiber intakes are increased to 50 and 20 g/d, respectively.[23]

Tropical Oils. The finding that dietary intake of palmitic acid results in increased plasma LDL-cholesterol concentrations has been widely publicized.[24] The hypercholesterolemic effect of palmitic acid led to a movement to remove palm and coconut oils, the so-called tropical oils, from products in the market place. Many companies responded by altering the oils added to their products. It should be kept in mind that palm oil contributes a very small percentage to the overall fat intake in the diet (~2%), and its removal from the diet will have little impact on the average plasma cholesterol concentration.

Fish Oils. Epidemiological evidence relating increased intake of fish rich in n−3 fatty acids with reduced incidence of CHD resulted in intense investigation of the effects of n−3 fatty acids on plasma cholesterol concentrations and CHD risk. The majority of studies indicate that moderate intake of fish oils can effectively lower plasma triglyceride concentrations in hypertriglyceridemic individuals, whereas intake of n−3 fatty acids have a relatively modest, if any, plasma LDL-cholesterol–lowering activity.[25] One concern regarding the intake of large amounts of fish oils is the increased fat intake associated with commercially prepared products. Addition of fish to the diet may have benefits by other modalities including decreased intake of animal protein and saturated fatty acids and potential antithrombic activity associated with n−3 fatty acids. As a supplement to a low-saturated fatty acids, low-cholesterol diet, fish oil capsules are not recommended for the hypercholesterolemic patient.

Monounsaturated Fatty Acids. Studies by Grundy and co-workers[12,13] demonstrated that monounsaturated dietary fatty acids, previously considered to be neutral with respect to changes in plasma cholesterol concentrations, effectively lower plasma LDL-cholesterol concentrations without an associated reduction in HDL-cholesterol concentrations. In addition, studies indicated that an olive-oil–rich diet more favorably affected plasma lipoprotein profiles than did a high-carbohydrate diet[26] (in terms of reducing plasma concentrations of VLDL triglyceride and LDL cholesterol while maintaining HDL cholesterol and apolipoprotein A-I concentrations). These data raise the possibility that a 30%-fat diet may not necessarily be the most effective diet for reducing elevated concentrations of plasma lipoproteins. Substitution of saturated fatty acids in the diet with monounsaturated fatty acids not only lowers plasma LDL concentrations but may also provide a more palatable diet, which could enhance compliance with dietary guidelines. These studies raised the question of whether the traditional low-fat Asian diet is preferable to a Mediterranean diet that is higher in total fat and rich in monounsaturated fatty acids for lowering CHD risk in the population.[12]

Stearic Acid. Dietary saturated fatty acids are usually considered to be hypercholesterolemic, and dietary guidelines recommend reduction in the dietary saturated fat intake to 10% of total calories. Recent studies by Bonanome and Grundy[24] demonstrated that intake of stearic acid (18:0) does not result in elevated plasma cholesterol concentrations but, as compared with dietary palm oil (16:0), reduces cholesterol concentrations. This finding has a significant impact on the plasma-cholesterol-elevating potential of foods, such as beef fat and cocoa butter, that have a high stearic acid content and on the role of hydrogenated vegetable oils in a plasma-cholesterol-lowering diet. Because hydrogenation saturates the polyunsaturated fatty acids found in vegetable oils (primarily linoleic acid, 18:2, to stearic acid, 18:0), the recommendation that hydrogenated vegetable oils be limited in a plasma-cholesterol-lowering diet may not be necessary.

Alcohol. There is an increasing evidence from international studies that moderate alcohol consumption is protective against CHD as judged by the observation of negative correlations between total alcohol consumption and CHD mortality.[27] Although the negative effects of excess alcohol consumption are well documented, including the implication that excess alcohol consumption is related to hypertension and hypertriglyceridemia, these data suggest that moderate alcohol intake, at the level of one to two drinks a day, may have an important CHD risk-reduction effect.

Summary

There is little debate regarding the advisability of lowering an elevated plasma LDL-cholesterol concentration to reduce the associated CHD risk. In the case of a patient with a plasma total cholesterol value >6.2 mmol/L or a patient with a cholesterol value between 5.2 and 6.2 mmol/L with CHD or with two additional primary risk factors, the initial approach to risk reduction is dietary modification to lower saturated fatty acid intake to <10% of total calories and cholesterol intake to <300 mg/d. If this initial dietary intervention fails to lower plasma cholesterol concentrations sufficiently, it is recommended that dietary intake of saturated fatty acids be further restricted to <7% of total calories and dietary cholesterol to <200 mg/d.[3] Unfortunately, for many patients with severely elevated plasma LDL-cholesterol concentrations, dietary modification alone may not be sufficient to lower the levels below 5.2-mmol/L, and pharmacological interventions probably will be necessary.

Effective dietary intervention does not rely on a "good food, bad food" approach to the problem but rather to a modification of the eating habits of the high-risk patient to attain ideal body weight and to reduce saturated fatty acids in the diet. There are multiple approaches to this goal that can fit most lifestyles and that will greatly enhance compliance to this life-long dietary change. The previous overemphasis given to dietary cholesterol as a factor in elevated plasma cholesterol concentrations will make it much more difficult to communicate the message that dietary fat and, primarily, saturated fatty acids are the major dietary factors targeted for intervention in any plasma-cholesterol-lowering diet.

The most important dietary factor involved in CHD risk may be total calories and incidence of obesity in the population. Obesity is not only an independent risk factor for CHD but is also related to a number of other risk factors for heart disease. Weight loss to attain ideal body weight corrects a number of abnormalities of lipid metabolism associated with obesity and can be an effective modality for lowering elevated plasma lipid concentrations. The importance of maintaining an ideal body weight as part of an overall CHD risk-reduction program requires that any dietary intervention program include a weight-loss component if the patient is overweight and maintenance of ideal body weight by balancing caloric intake with energy expenditure.[4]

References

1. J. Stamler, D. Wentforth, and J.D. Neaton (1986) Is relationship between serum cholesterol and risk of premature death from coronary heart disease continuous and graded? Findings in 356,222 primary screenees of the Multiple Risk Factor Intervention Trial (MRFIT). *JAMA* 256:2823–2828.

2. Nutrition Committee and the Council on Arteriosclerosis (1984) Recommendations for treatment of hyperlipidemia in adults. *Circulation* 69:1065A–1090A.

3. National Cholesterol Education Program Expert Panel (1988) Detection, evaluation, and treatment of high blood cholesterol in adults. *Arch. Intern. Med.* 148:36–69.

4. U.S. Department of Health and Human Services (1988) *The Surgeon General's Report on Nutrition and Health.* DHHS (PHS) Publication no. 88-50210, U.S. Government Printing Office, Washington, DC.

5. D.J. Gordon, J.L. Probstfield, R.J. Garrison, et al. (1989) High-density lipoprotein cholesterol and cardiovascular disease. Four prospective American studies. *Circulation* 79:8–15.

6. S.M. Grundy, DeW.S. Goodman, B.M. Rifkind, and J.I. Cleeman (1989) The place of HDL in cholesterol management. A perspective from the National Cholesterol Education Program. *Arch. Intern. Med.* 149:505–510.

7. H.B. Hubert, M. Feinleib, P.M. McNamara, and W.P. Castelli (1983) Obesity as an independent risk factor for cardiovascular disease: a 26-year follow-up of participants in the Framingham Heart Study. *Circulation* 67:968–977.

8. P. Bjorntorp (1988) The associations between obesity, adipose tissue distribution and disease. *Acta Med. Scand.* [*Suppl.*] 723: 121–134.

9. D.J. McNamara (1987) Effects of fat-modified diets on cholesterol and lipoprotein metabolism. *Annu. Rev. Nutr.* 7:273–290.

10. Y.A. Kesaniemi and S.M. Grundy (1983) Increased low density lipoprotein production associated with obesity. *Arteriosclerosis* 3: 170–177.

11. D.K. Spady and J.M. Dietschy (1988) Interaction of dietary cholesterol and triglycerides in the regulation of hepatic low density lipoprotein transport in the hamster. *J. Clin. Invest.* 81:300–309.

12. S.M. Grundy (1989) Monounsaturated fatty acids and cholesterol metabolism: implications for dietary recommendations. *J. Nutr.* 119:529–533.

13. S.M. Grundy (1986) Comparison of monounsaturated fatty acids and carbohydrates for lowering plasma cholesterol. *N. Engl. J. Med.* 314:745–748.

14. D.J. McNamara (in press) Relationship between blood and dietary cholesterol. *Adv. Meat Sci.*

15. D.J. McNamara, R. Kolb, T.S. Parker, et al. (1987) Heterogeneity of cholesterol homeostasis in man: response to changes in dietary fat quality and cholesterol quantity. *J. Clin. Invest.* 79:1729–1739.

16. P. Mistry, N.E. Miller, M. Laker, W.R. Hazzard, and B. Lewis (1981) Individual variation in the effects of dietary cholesterol on plasma lipoproteins and cellular cholesterol homeostasis in man. *J. Clin. Invest.* 67:493–502.

17. R.N. Wolf and S.M. Grundy (1983) Influence of exchanging carbohydrate for saturated fatty acids on plasma lipids and lipoproteins in men. *J. Nutr.* 113:1521–1528.

18. M.B. Katan, A.C. van Gastel, C.M. de Rover, M.A.J. van Montfort, and J.T. Knuiman (1988) Differences in individual responsiveness of serum cholesterol to fat-modified diets in man. *Eur. J. Clin. Invest.* 18:644–647.

19. M.B. Katan and A.C. Beynen (1987) Characteristics of human hypo- and hyperresponders to dietary cholesterol. *Am. J. Epidemiol.* 125:387–399.

20. J. McCormick and P. Skrabanek (1988) Coronary heart disease is not preventable by population interventions. *Lancet* 2:839–841.

21. A.M. Garber, H.C. Sox, and B. Littenberg (1989) Screening asymptomatic adults for cardiac risk factors: the serum cholesterol level. *Ann. Intern. Med.* 110:622–639.

22. G.M. Reaven (1986) Looking at the world through LDL-cholesterol colored glasses. *J. Nutr.* 116:1143–1147.

23. J.W. Anderson and N.J. Gustafson (1988) Hypocholesterolemic effects of oat and bean products. *Am. J. Clin. Nutr.* 48:749–753.

24. A. Bonanome and S.M. Grundy (1988) Effect of dietary stearic acid on plasma cholesterol and lipoprotein levels. *N. Engl. J. Med.* 318:1244–1248.

25. A. Leaf and P.C. Weber (1988) Cardiovascular effects of n-3 fatty acids. *N. Engl. J. Med.* 318:549–557.

26. R.P. Mensink, M.J.M. de Groot, L.T. van den Broeke, A.P. Severijnen- Nobels, P.N.M. Demacker, and M.B. Katan (1989) Effect of monounsaturated fatty acid v. complex carbohydrates on serum lipoproteins and apoproteins in healthy men and women. *Metabolism* 38:172–178.

27. D.M. Hegsted and L.M. Ausman (1988) Diet, alcohol and coronary heart disease in men. *J. Nutr.* 118:1184–1189.

Hypertension

Considerable evidence has accumulated that suggests that dietary factors in combination with genetics play a major role in the development of hypertension in humans. Rather than attempting to critically assess all of the controversies in the area, this summary will focus upon presenting an overview in which most literature references will be to recent reviews. The aim will be to present a summary of the controversial points and to discuss the limitations of the epidemiological and experimental data that confuse the interpretation of the literature. It is hoped that, by this means, the reader will become better equipped to evaluate both existing work and the many papers that will be devoted to this expanding subject in the near future.

There is an increasing appreciation that the majority of hypertensive patients, i.e., those with mild blood pressure elevations, have not been demonstrated to derive a cardiac benefit from drug therapy.[1,2] In fact, the health risk of some drugs used to treat mild hypertension probably outweighs the marginal benefit that many patients in this group (who may not actually have hypertension) would obtain. Dietary and other nonpharmacological therapies, therefore, are being avidly sought with the hope of increased benefit for this large number of patients along with decreased risk and cost.[3,4] Prior to a discussion of the studies relating diet and blood pressure, a general description of hypertension study design and methods will make it easier to understand how misleading results can be generated.

Dietary Experiments on Volunteers

Studying blood pressure in outpatients in a meaningful way requires careful attention to study design, subject selection, and observer bias. Similar issues arise in studies performed in metabolic wards but, in addition, one is faced with the issue of how applicable the findings are to the blood pressures of patients in

the real world performing their normal daily tasks. The recent advent of ambulatory blood pressure monitors revealed considerable difference between subjects' blood pressures obtained in the clinic, at work, and at home.[5] This discrepancy can be in either direction, depending upon the circumstances. For example, about one-third of patients believed to have mild hypertension on the basis of blood pressure measurement in clinics are found to be normotensive away from the doctor's office. On the other hand, patients believed to be receiving adequate antihypertensive therapy, on the basis of supine blood pressure readings obtained after 5 min of rest, may be found to lack significant blood pressure control when assessed with ambulatory monitors during a routine stressful day. Obviously, the latter values are more pertinent in predicting end-organ damage and morbidity from elevated blood pressure, and it was shown that blood pressure values obtained with ambulatory monitors correlate with left ventricular hypertrophy much better than do blood pressures obtained in clinics.[6]

Although ambulatory monitors can provide useful data if one is practiced in evaluating their performance, it is possible to use random-zero sphygmomanometers to at least eliminate observer bias in pressure measurement. Blood pressure is highly variable in both normotensive and hypertensive subjects, and it is essential to take into account a number of well-known problems in assessing changes. The blood pressures of most subjects entering studies will fall as they become accustomed to having their pressures measured. Because blood pressure changes continuously during the day, subjects selected for inclusion in a study on the basis of a high (for them) pressure measurement will exhibit a better picture of their true (lower) mean pressure with repeated measurement. These effects of habituation and regression upon the mean require that diet–blood pressure studies have pretreatment pe-

Table 1. Problems in studying hypertension

Problem	Solution
Measurement errors and bias	Ambulatory monitors Random-zero sphygmomanometer
Marked variability of blood pressure	Multiple measurements
Effects of multiple dietary changes	Adequate controls, careful dietary-change assessment
Habituation and regression-on-the-mean effects	Pretreatment and recovery periods
Seasonal and environmental effects	Parallel, randomized controls

riods that are long enough (≤6 wk) and have enough measurements so that the subjects' true mean pressures are revealed. For example, in a randomized crossover study, several weeks of placebo treatment resulted in actual decreases in urinary catecholamine excretion and decreases of 10 mm Hg in blood pressure.[7] This degree of blood pressure reduction is larger than that reported in most dietary-intervention studies. Such observations also raise the issue of needing appropriate placebo control groups in these types of studies.

Another study design feature almost never employed in dietary-intervention studies of blood pressure is the posttreatment recovery period. If the true baseline pressures are achieved before the dietary intervention and a diet-related change is observed, one would expect the blood pressures to return to baseline after the patients return to their usual diet. When such measurements are taken, it is sometimes obvious that the subjects' blood pressures never go back up toward the presumed baseline and that the observed reduction was only a habituation effect occurring during the treatment period, i.e., the pretreatment period was inadequate. Other issues not usually addressed by studies in this area include blinding of subjects to the dietary intervention when possible and actually assessing the subjects' diets during the study to see whether the intended dietary change has provoked unanticipated alterations in the subjects' eating patterns because of gastrointestinal intolerance of the trial diet. Such evaluation of personal habits should also include documenting the use of alcohol and other drugs that may affect blood pressure or other variables (e.g., prostaglandins, plasma lipids, etc.) being measured. In addition, it should be appreciated how difficult it is to change one dietary component in isolation and that eating more of one type of food means that less of some-

thing else must be consumed to avoid weight changes, which also can alter blood pressure.[8,9]

Finally, study design issues that are routine in clinical pharmacology often seem to be unappreciated or ignored in dietary-intervention trials. These issues include randomization of subjects in both treated and control groups and matched parallel control groups to account for environmental or seasonal changes and to avoid crossover effects. Statistical power calculations are notably rare as well and would give some assurance that experiments include enough subjects to allow for a reasonable chance of detecting a biologically meaningful change in blood pressure. A summary of some problems encountered in studying outpatient blood pressure is presented in Table 1.

Epidemiological Studies

There are a number of problems in the interpretation of data relating diet and blood pressure in populations. It is rare to find two groups of people eating diets that differ in only one dietary component. Most groups eating diets with a high fish content, for example, also have a high intake of salt, which could obscure any hypotensive influence of fish. The consumption of an unusual type of food over many generations may result in genetic adaptation to some components that would therefore have different effects in different population groups. It is possible, for example, that a high intake of n−3 fatty acids by Eskimos on a marine diet may have fewer or different long-term effects for them than would the same amounts of these compounds consumed as dietary supplements by American volunteers.

Many nutrients have a high degree of association in foodstuffs, and it is important to remember that people eat food, not specific nutrients. It is, therefore, very difficult to isolate the health effects of particular dietary components. Many dietary habits that are believed to influence blood pressure directly also are related to other personal characteristics that are known to have an effect, such as alcohol intake, body size, physical activity, and obesity. It has been noted that total energy intake is intimately related to the consumption of all major nutrients and is driven by physical activity level. Schoolchildren found to have lower blood pressures also were found to have a higher intake of all nutrients, primarily because of their being more active.[4] As a result it would be difficult to interpret any inverse associations found between particular nutrients and blood pressure. An additional problem in population studies is estimating nutrient intake accurately and being sure that standardized methods of blood pressure measurement are used in the different groups being compared. Because of these numerous difficulties in interpretation, epidemiological studies are useful in finding associations and generating hypotheses, but these hypotheses must be tested in carefully controlled dietary-intervention studies. Some of the issues confounding epidemiological studies of diet–blood pressure relationships are summarized in Table 2.

Alcohol and Vascular Function

Although an entire chapter of this volume is devoted to the nutritional aspects of alcohol, it must be mentioned as a confounding variable in population studies on vascular disease and blood pressure. Mediterranean populations have a lower incidence of vascular disease than do Northern European populations, which is frequently ascribed to differences in the amount and type of lipid in their diets.[10] The dietary component that correlated most strongly with a healthy vasculature in the famous Seven Countries Study, however, was red wine intake.[11] The percent of total calories that populations consume as alcohol is highly variable and seems to be frequently overlooked in studies of hypertension and atherosclerosis. In the United States it was estimated that excess alcohol intake is responsible for ~10% of hypertension especially in middle-aged males.[3,12] As a result it is the leading cause of secondary hypertension in this group. Statistically, individuals who regularly consume >60 mL ethanol daily have a higher prevalence of hypertension,[12] and a reduced consumption is recommended for hypertensive patients. Because the hypertensive effects of even small doses of alcohol have been well documented,[3] it is difficult to see how dietary-intervention studies on blood pressure could be conducted without taking this factor into account.

Obesity and Weight Loss

The effect of obesity on blood pressure appears to be independent of dietary components other than alcohol, with which it has an additive effect.[3,4] It is now appreciated that a male obesity pattern, predominately upper body and abdominal, is more strongly correlated with hypertension than is the female pattern, where excess weight is distributed mainly in the buttocks and thighs.[13] In the United States there has been a strong and consistent association between obesity and hypertension, especially in men < 45 y.[14] This influence must be appreciated when comparing data across populations as well as between different subgroups within a country. It has long been considered that an increase in blood pressure with age was a hallmark of populations eating a diet high in salt.[15] There is some evidence, however, that this phenomenon is actually related to the in-

Table 2. Problems in diet–blood pressure epidemiology

- Lack of standardized blood pressure measurements.
- Inaccuracy of nutrient intake estimates.
- Confounding effects of environmental and social factors.
- Possible genetic differences in response to nutrients.
- Comparisons of noncontemporaneous populations with different levels of public health measures, infections.

crease in weight with age in most acculturated societies; it is rarely seen in populations without such a weight increase. In addition, the responses of obese hypertensive subjects to dietary manipulations may not be the same as those of lean subjects, so it is important that the subjects' weights be taken into account in study design. This would include setting study inclusion criteria for body mass index (height/weight^2) as well as being sure that the randomization process produces comparable numbers of similar patients in the different study groups.

The effects of weight loss on blood pressure have been studied extensively but with controversial results.[8,16] Calorie-restricted diets are usually low in sodium as well, but a number of well-designed trials indicated a significant lowering of blood pressure in hypertensive subjects that was attributable to weight loss.[16] It is important that dietary interventions be designed with such effects in mind and that the subjects' weights be measured during the study. Because achieving ideal body weight will nearly normalize the blood pressures of many obese male (and some female) hypertensive patients, weight reduction is a first step in blood pressure management.

Sodium

There have been a number of observations that hypertension is virtually nonexistent in primitive societies that consume diets low in salt.[15] This topic has been the subject of much controversy, but there is some consensus that a diet high in calories, fat, and sodium and low in potassium is associated with the development of hypertension.[3,4] People in primitive societies are for the most part physically active throughout life and are lean vegetarians who are not exposed to alcohol. Therefore, it is not clear which dietary component is actually responsible for the development of hypertension.[4] The role of sodium in causing hypertension is difficult to study within a population, because there may not be a sufficiently diverse intake of sodium, i.e., the dose-response relationship between sodium and blood pressure may be flat over the range of intake in a population. Studies of migrations and recruitment of primitive people into modern armies, however, lend support to the importance of chronically high sodium intake in increased blood pressure. Major criticisms of the available epidemiological data include the difficulty in measuring sodium intake and the lack of standardization of blood pressure measurement.[3,4,17]

Clinical trials of sodium restriction in hypertensive subjects were reviewed,[18] and there is reasonable evidence that low sodium diets will lower blood pressure in many patients and reduce their need for antihypertensive drugs. Although the blood pressure response to sodium restriction is quite heterogeneous, there is no known hazard to a moderate sodium restriction and it will benefit the salt-sensitive subset of patients. From a practical standpoint reducing sodium intake in the American diet would most likely also lead to a reduction in dietary fat content, which is considered desirable from several health standpoints.[10] If dietary sodium were a major factor in the development of hypertension in industrialized countries, however, one would expect that increased intake would increase blood pressure in normotensive subjects, especially those with strong family histories of hypertension and who are at increased risk of developing it themselves. This has not been found to be the case. In addition, the fact that strict vegetarians or thin nondrinkers can have a low prevalence of hypertension and a high sodium intake suggested that sodium intake alone has a minor role in the development of hypertension.[4]

Potassium

It has been proposed that primitive societies lack hypertension because of their high potassium rather than low sodium intake.[19] As is the case with sodium, the epidemiological data have many limitations. A number of workers, however, believe that the dietary potassium-sodium ratio is an important predictor of the tendency to blood pressure elevation, and studies found an inverse correlation between blood pressure and the ratio of these electrolytes in urine but no correlation with the excretion of either electrolyte alone.[3,4]

Trials of dietary potassium supplementation all have involved small numbers of patients for a short duration, and these data have been summarized.[3,4,20] Such supplements have no effect upon the blood pressures of normotensive subjects, although it has been shown recently that potassium depletion of normal individuals causes sodium retention and increased blood pressure both at baseline and in response to a saline infusion.[21] The effects of potassium supplements on hypertensive individuals also appear

to involve a natriuresis that is dependent upon the subjects' sodium status. If the patients have low potassium intake and have not had sodium restricted, then additional potassium seems to have a moderate hypotensive effect.[20]

Calcium, Magnesium, and Trace Elements

During the last few years there has been considerable discussion of the role of dietary calcium in the prevention and management of hypertension. On the basis of an extensive population survey, it was suggested that calcium intake had a potent blood pressure–lowering effect, and some small clinical trials have reported positive results.[22] After the epidemiological data were reanalyzed to account for the confounding effects of age, income, alcohol consumption, and obesity, the effects of calcium were less clear-cut.[4,23] In addition, several well-designed intervention trials performed more recently were negative,[4] and it has been appreciated that the intake of calcium, mainly derived from dairy products, is strongly associated with intakes of potassium and protein. Some bias in the population survey data may also have been introduced because social class and activity level strongly influence both dairy-product consumption and blood pressure. Not only have intervention trials given conflicting results, but even those that are considered by the authors to show a hypotensive effect of calcium supplements reveal a very heterogeneous response with substantial increases in blood pressure in some subjects. This, plus the reports of increased urinary calcium[24] or altered calcium metabolism[25] in hypertensive patients, makes for a confusing picture and suggests that recommending changes in dietary calcium for the purpose of lowering blood pressure may be premature.

Although magnesium sulfate has effective hypotensive properties when rapidly infused, there is little evidence for its role in blood pressure regulation. In properly designed clinical trials no effect of dietary magnesium supplements on blood pressure of hypertensive patients was found[26] except in those who were taking diuretics and were potassium depleted.[27] There have been a number of observations that correlate lower urinary or erythrocyte magnesium with higher blood pressure in population groups, but this finding has not been corroborated by other workers.[28] Much of these data suffer from the disadvantage of small numbers of subjects and the fact that negative findings are less likely to be published. Perhaps future work will clarify the interrelations of dietary magnesium, other cations, blood pressure, and renin as has been speculated.[29]

A major portion of trace element intake is via drinking water. Although blood pressure elevation can be demonstrated in studies of animals given toxic amounts of cadmium and in humans poisoned chronically with cadmium, lead, mercury, and thallium,[30] there is no epidemiological evidence relating the intake of these elements to hypertension in the general population.[31] Work in this area is continuing, however.[32] A direct involvement of selenium, copper, zinc, and other essential trace elements in blood pressure regulation in man has not been suggested by clinical or animal studies thus far.

Lipids

The association of obesity and a high-fat diet with hypertension in population studies[8] was made more clinically plausible by the reported correlation between dietary saturated fatty acids, plasma cholesterol, and atherosclerotic vascular disease.[10] Because dietary polyunsaturated fatty acids (at the expense of saturated fatty acids) have been determined to benefit atherosclerotic vascular disease, it seemed reasonable to hypothesize that the ratio of dietary polyunsaturated to saturated fatty acids (P:S) would influence blood pressure regulation. More recently, it has been appreciated that the two biochemical classes of polyunsaturated fatty acids have different metabolic effects in humans. Therefore, the concept of P:S as an important dietary index requires some modification.

Briefly, nature constructs fatty acids from the noncarboxyl (ω) end, and mammals are not able to produce long-chain fatty acids with unsaturated bonds beyond the ninth carbon from the omega end. Such acids are referred to as being in the n−9 (or ω-9) class, and the monounsaturate oleic acid is one example. Humans must obtain polyunsaturated fatty acids via the diet, and there are two major classes of these, which we cannot interconvert. These are the n−6 class, long regarded as essential for mammals, and the more recently studied n−3 class. The former are present in large amounts in the vegetable oils most widely used in the United States (e.g., corn, sunflower, and safflower) whereas the latter primarily are found in marine oils. Some terrestrial sources of 18-carbon n−3 fatty acids exist (e.g., linseed and canola), but there is controversy as to whether these acids are metabolically equivalent in humans to the longer-chain acids (20 and 22 carbons) from marine oils. The epidemiological data relating either of these polyunsaturate classes to human blood pressure are confounded by the many variables discussed above.[33,34]

Unlike many dietary lipid components, a small fraction of the polyunsaturated fatty acids ingested each day is converted in the body to local hormone-like compounds that exert a wide variety of very potent biological activities.[34] Because the precursor acids for these substances (e.g., prostaglandins, thromboxanes, prostacyclin, leukotrienes, etc.) have 20 carbons (eicosanoic acids), these autocoids are often called eicosanoids, and they are known to be involved in numerous processes regulating blood pressure in humans. As a result any physiological changes taking place during supplementation studies of polyunsaturates were ascribed to alterations in the types or amounts of eicosanoids produced in vivo. Very few studies have directly addressed this hypothesis, however, and the many problems in this field were recently reviewed.[34]

Intervention studies have been carried out with both n−6 and n−3 fatty acid supplements in both normotensive and hypertensive subjects. The literature on dietary n−6 fatty acids and blood pressure recently was summarized.[33] In a number of the studies in which a lowering of blood pressure was observed with increased dietary n−6 fatty acids, several dietary components were changed simultaneously (e.g., total fat and sodium), making it difficult to ascribe the hypotensive effect to an altered dietary P:S alone. In fact, more recent work that carefully controlled total dietary fat, calories, and other components found no effect of greatly increased n−6 fatty acid intake.[35] The opposite experiment, practically eliminating saturated fat from the diet of normotensive subjects to increase P:S, also failed to show any change in blood pressure.[36]

There has been a great enthusiasm in recent years for exploring the vascular benefits of n − 3 fatty acids from marine oils. Epidemiological data, however, do not reveal lower blood pressures in populations with a high fish consumption. In fact, Eskimos have the same age-related increase in blood pressure as do Europeans, and Oriental groups with a large intake of fish also have some of the highest prevalences of hypertension in the world, perhaps because of their high amounts of dietary salt.[34] Numerous intervention trials have claimed that fish oils have a hypotensive effect, whereas several negative studies have been published. Generally poor study design and a lack of attention to basic principles of hypertension research make much of this literature uninterpretable. Despite this it now appears likely that large doses of n−3 fatty acids have hypotensive effects in humans and that the mechanism is not simply one of altered eicosanoid formation.[37] The amount of n−3 fatty acids needed to achieve the effect in a short time, however, would be essentially impossible to obtain by dietary means (~1 kg oily fish/d). This area also was recently reviewed.[34]

Currently, studies with highly enriched (>80%) n−3 fatty acid preparations (as opposed to fish oils containing <30% n−3 acids) are in progress to de-

Table 3. Status of dietary factors in hypertension management

Achieving ideal body weight	Always recommended
Reducing alcohol intake (<60 mL/d)	Always recommended
Reduced sodium intake (<2 g/d)	Usually recommended
Increased potassium intake	Appears worthwhile
Increased calcium	Not clearly indicated
Increased magnesium	Not clearly indicated
Increased n−6 polyunsaturates	Not beneficial
Increased n−3 polyunsaturates	Benefit under study

termine the mechanisms and dose-response relationship of their hypotensive effect. Such preparations avoid the large caloric load of chronic, high-dose fish-oil supplements. Because the duration of the effect, necessary dose, and possible complications of long-term n−3 fatty acid supplements have not yet been explored, it is not possible at this time to make a recommendation for fish oil or n−3 fatty acids as a therapy for hypertension.[37] This area is one of very active research, so the data necessary to define the therapeutic role (if any) of these compounds should be available shortly. An important consideration would be just how such supplements would fit into the American diet and whether other dietary modification (e.g., lower total fat and salt restriction) would allow a hypotensive effect to be revealed at a more easily achievable dose of n−3 acids.

Summary

It seems clear that much of the hypertension in acculturated societies is related to dietary habits. The majority of hypertensive patients have only mild blood pressure elevations and can benefit significantly from dietary management alone.[38] A summary of possible dietary changes benefitting blood pressure is presented in Table 3. Unfortunately, many patients are not able to modify their dietary habits, and so drug therapy will continue to be necessary for subjects with moderately elevated blood pressure (diastolic pressure >100 mm Hg). Achieving ideal body weight and reducing excess consumption of salt and alcohol can be recommended to lower blood pressure. From a practical standpoint this regimen also means lowering dietary fat and increasing potassium, which are likely to be beneficial dietary changes. Increased dietary n−6 fatty acid intake does not appear to lower blood pressure, whereas n−3 fatty acids do have hypotensive properties. The nutritional or therapeutic role of the latter group remains to be defined.

This work was supported in part by a grant from the National Institutes of Health (HL-35380). Dr. Knapp is an Established Investigator of the American Heart Association.

References

1. E.D. Freis (1982) Should mild hypertension be treated? *N. Engl. J. Med.* 307:306–309.
2. Medical Research Council Working Party (1985) MRC trial of treatment of mild hypertension: principal results. *Br. Med. J.* 291:97–104.
3. Subcommittee on Nonpharmacological Therapy of High Blood Pressure (1986) Nonpharmacological approaches to the control of high blood pressure. *Hypertension* 8:444–467.
4. L.J. Beilin (1987) Diet and hypertension: critical concepts and controversies. *J. Hypertens.* 5(suppl 5):S447–S457.
5. T.G. Pickering, G.A. Harshfield, R.B. Devereux, and J.H. Laragh (1985) What is the role of ambulatory blood pressure monitoring in the management of hypertensive patients? *Hypertension* 7:171–177.
6. R.B. Devereux, T.G. Pickering, G.A. Harshfield, et al. (1983) Left ventricular hypertrophy in patients with hypertension: importance of blood pressure response to regularly recurring stress. *Circulation* 68:470–476.
7. V. Hossman, G.A. FitzGerald, and C.T. Dollery (1981) Influence of hospitalization and placebo therapy on blood pressure and sympathetic function in essential hypertension. *Hypertension* 3:113–118.
8. M.F. Hovell (1982) The experimental evidence for weight-loss treatment of essential hypertension: a critical review. *Am. J. Public Health* 72:359–368.
9. M.L. Tuck, J. Sowers, L. Dornfield, G. Kledzik, and M. Maxwell (1981) The effect of weight reduction on blood pressure, plasma renin activity, and plasma aldosterone levels in obese patients. *N. Engl. J. Med.* 304:930–933.
10. R.A. Stallones (1983) Ischemic heart disease and lipids in blood and diet. *Annu. Rev. Nutr.* 3:155–185.
11. A.S. St. Leger, A.L. Cochrane, and F. Moore (1979) Factors associated with cardiac mortality in developed countries, with particular reference to the consumption of wine. *Lancet* 1:1017–1020.
12. G.D. Friedman, A.L. Klatsky, and A.B. Siegelaub (1983) Alcohol intake and hypertension. *Ann. Intern. Med.* 98:846–849.
13. R.L. Weisner, D.J. Norris, R. Birch, et al. (1985) The relative contribution of body fat and fat pattern to blood pressure level. *Hypertension* 7:578–585.
14. B.N. Chiang, L.V. Perlamn, and F.H. Epstein (1969) Overweight and hypertension: a review. *Circulation* 39:403–421.
15. L.K. Dahl (1958) Salt intake and salt need. *N. Engl. J. Med.* 258:1152–1157.
16. R.R. Wing, A.W. Caggiula, M.P. Norwalk, R. Koeske, S. Lee, and H. Langford (1984) Dietary approaches to the reduction of blood pressure: the independence of weight and sodium/potassium interventions. *Prev. Med.* 13:233–244.
17. F.C. Luft (1989) Salt and hypertension: recent advances and perspectives. *J. Lab. Clin. Med.* 114:215–221.
18. R.J. Prineas and H. Blackburn (1985) Clinical and epidemiologic relationships between electrolytes and hypertension. In: *NIH Workshop on Nutrition and Hypertension: Proceedings from a Symposium* (M.J. Horan, M. Blaustein, J.B. Dunbar, W. Kachadorian, N.M. Kaplan, and A.P. Simopoulos, eds.), pp. 63–85, Biomedical Information Corp., New York.
19. L. Tobian (1988) Potassium and hypertension. *Nutr. Rev.* 46:273–282.
20. W.N. Suki (1988) Dietary potassium and blood pressure. *Kidney Int.* 34(suppl. 25):S175–S176.
21. G.G. Krishna, E. Miller, and S. Kapoor (1989) Increased blood pressure during potassium depletion in normotensive men. *N. Engl. J. Med.* 320:1177–1182.
22. D.A. McCarron, C.D. Morris, H.J. Henry, and J.L. Stanton (1984) Blood pressure and nutrient intake in the United States. *Science* 224:1392–1398.

23. E.T. Zawada and N. Brautbar (1985) Calcium supplement therapy of hypertension—has the time come? *Nephron* 41:129–131.

24. H. Kestleloot, J. Geboers, and R. Van Hoof (1983) Epidemiological study of the relationship between calcium and blood pressure. *Hypertension* 5(suppl. II): 52–56.

25. L.M. Resnick (1989) Calcium metabolism in the pathophysiology and treatment of clinical hypertension. *Am. J. Hypertens.* 2:179S–185S.

26. F.P. Cappuccio, N.D. Markandu, G.W. Beynon, A.C. Shore, B. Sampson, and G.A. MacGregor. (1985) Lack of effect of oral magnesium on high blood pressure: a double-blind study. *Br. Med. J.* 291:235–238.

27. T. Dyckner and P.O. Wester (1983) Effect of magnesium on blood pressure. *Br. Med. J.* 286:1847–1849.

28. P.K. Whelton and M.J. Klag (1989) Magnesium and blood pressure: review of the epidemiologic and clinical trial experience. *Am. J. Cardiol.* 63:26G–30G.

29. L.M. Resnick, J.H. Laragh, J.E. Sealley, and M.H. Alderman (1983) Divalent cations in essential hypertension: relations between serum ionized calcium, magnesium, and plasma renin activity. *N. Engl. J. Med.* 309:888–891.

30. P. Saltman (1983) Trace elements and blood pressure. *Ann. Intern. Med.* 98:823–827.

31. D. Sparrow, A.R. Sharrett, A.J. Garvey, G.F. Craun, and J.E. Silbert (1984) Trace metals in drinking water: lack of influence on blood pressure. *J. Chronic Dis.* 371:59–65.

32. W. Mertz (1985) Trace metals and hypertension. In: *NIH Workshop on Nutrition and Hypertension: Proceedings from a Symposium* (M. Horan, M. Blaustein, J.B. Dunbar, W. Kachadorian, N.M. Kaplan, and A.P. Simopoulos, eds.), pp. 271–276, Biomedical Information Corp., New York.

33. F.M. Sacks (1989) Dietary fats and blood pressure: a critical review of the evidence. *Nutr. Rev.* 47:291–300.

34. H.R. Knapp (1989) Omega-3 fatty acids, endogenous prostaglandins, and blood pressure regulation in humans. *Nutr. Rev.* 47: 301–313.

35. B.M. Margetts, L.J. Beilin, B.K. Armstrong, et al. (1985) Blood pressure and dietary polyunsaturated and saturated fats: a controlled trial. *Clin. Sci.* 69:165–177.

36. F.M. Sacks, P.G. Wood, and E.H. Kass (1984) Stability of blood pressure in vegetarians receiving dietary protein supplements. *Hypertension* 6:199–201.

37. H.R. Knapp and G.A. FitzGerald (1989) The antihypertensive effects of fish oil: a controlled study of polyunsaturated fatty acid supplements in essential hypertension. *N. Engl. J. Med.* 320:1037–1043.

38. J. Stamler, E. Farinaro, L.M. Mojonnier, Y. Hall, D. Moss, and R. Stamler (1980) Prevention and control of hypertension by nutritional-hygienic means: long-term experience of the Chicago coronary prevention evaluation program. *JAMA* 243:1819–1823.

Clarie B. Hollenbeck and Ann M. Coulston

Chapter 43

Diabetes Mellitus

Diabetes mellitus is a chronic condition characterized primarily by an elevation of plasma glucose, although abnormalities in lipoprotein and amino acid metabolism also are a common finding. The prevalence of diabetes in the United States is estimated at 11 million.[1] There are two major types of diabetes mellitus: Type I, or insulin-dependent diabetes mellitus (IDDM), and Type II, or non-insulin-dependent diabetes mellitus (NIDDM). The National Diabetes Data Group has defined specific criteria for the classification of IDDM and NIDDM as well as for the diagnosis of gestational diabetes (GDM).[2]

IDDM accounts for ~10% of individuals with diabetes. It usually occurs as a primary diagnosis in individuals under the age of 30 y and, thus, is the predominate form of diabetes in children, adolescents, and young adults. Onset of symptoms tend to be abrupt and symptoms are characterized by a lack of insulin. IDDM may be acutely life threatening, and these individuals are dependent on daily injections of insulin to sustain life. Although the cause of IDDM is not known, both viral and cytotoxic factors that cause pancreatic beta cell destruction are thought to play a role in the etiology of IDDM. Despite the fact that the etiology of IDDM is currently a very active area of research, there is no known means of preventing the development of this form of diabetes.

NIDDM accounts for the great majority of individuals with diabetes. It appears most commonly in midlife and is frequently associated with obesity. NIDDM has a more insidious onset and may exist with few or no symptoms for many years before diagnosis. In fact, there are estimates that approximately half the individuals in the United States with NIDDM are not yet diagnosed. Although decreased insulin secretion in response to a glucose stimulus can be seen in individuals with NIDDM, most individuals maintain normal or greater than normal levels of circulating insulin in response to meals. Thus, the primary cause of ambient hyperglycemia in these individuals appears to be reduced insulin sensitivity of peripheral tissue rather than reduced insulin secretion.

GDM occurs in ~2% of pregnancies. Onset of glucose intolerance occurs during pregnancy and glucose tolerance generally reverts to normal after parturition. If unrecognized or untreated, GDM may increase the risk of perinatal morbidity and mortality. GDM, like NIDDM, is associated with reduced insulin sensitivity of peripheral tissue rather than insulin deficiency.

Introduction to Nutritional Management

In this chapter we will discuss dietary strategies for the nutritional management of individuals with diabetes. In our evaluation of these strategies we will focus on the dietary factors that have the greatest impact on the regulation of carbohydrate and lipoprotein metabolism. In addition, we will emphasize data from studies of dietary strategies likely to gain long-term patient compliance.

Although diabetes is usually categorized as a disease of carbohydrate metabolism, it has been apparent for some time that abnormalities of lipoprotein metabolism also are common in patients with this syndrome. These abnormalities are particularly important given the accelerated atherogenesis frequently associated with diabetes. Concern for the increased morbidity and mortality from vascular disease has resulted in dietary recommendations for these individuals designed to reduce the risk of developing coronary artery disease (CAD). Specifically, dietary recommendations were made to reduce the total amount of fat and increase carbohydrate.[3,4] The rationale for this approach is based on the premise that a decrease in total dietary fat will lead to a reduction in plasma low-density-lipoprotein (LDL) cholesterol concentrations with a concomitant reduction in morbidity and mortality from CAD. Although elevated concentrations of LDL cholesterol predispose individuals to increased risk of developing vascular disease, LDL-cholesterol concentrations generally are not increased in individuals with diabetes when compared with the general population.[5] On the other hand, risk factors for CAD present in individuals with diabetes include increased plasma glucose, insulin, and total plasma triglyceride and very-low-density-lipoprotein (VLDL) triglyceride and decreased high-density-lipoprotein (HDL) cholesterol. Of even greater importance is evidence that high-carbohydrate, low-fat diets accentuate plasma glucose, insulin, total triglyceride, and VLDL-triglyceride concentrations while lowering plasma HDL-cholesterol concentrations.[6–10]

Because the goal of reducing the risk of cardiovascular complications in patients with diabetes is important, it is essential that dietary strategies address the metabolic abnormalities of carbohydrate and lipid metabolism present in individuals with diabetes. Moreover, the primary abnormality of carbohydrate metabolism, i.e., hyperglycemia, may also predispose these individuals to complications of peripheral and cerebral vascular disease, retinopathy, nephropathy, and neuropathy. Thus, although normalization of blood glucose concentration may be the primary goal of treatment for all types of diabetes, therapy must be directed toward preventing or reducing the progression of all metabolic complications associated with this condition.

Weight Reduction

As mentioned earlier, the majority of patients with diabetes have NIDDM. Many of these individuals are overweight or obese. It has been evident for more than 40 y that glucose tolerance can be returned toward normal with a reduction in body weight.[11] Evidence also demonstrates that many of the defects in lipoprotein metabolism improve with attainment of glycemic control. It is not surprising, then, that weight reduction is an effective tool in improving abnormalities in both carbohydrate and lipid metabolism present in overweight individuals with diabetes. Several studies demonstrated significant beneficial effects on carbohydrate and lipid metabolism without the necessity of obtaining ideal body weight.[12–15] Indeed, weight loss in the range of 6–10 kg in individuals with NIDDM who remain obese after weight loss was associated with improvement in glycemic control and the disappearance of glucosuria. These studies also showed significant reductions of total triglyceride and VLDL-triglyceride, apoprotein B, and total plasma cholesterol concentrations. The fact that beneficial metabolic effects occur even though individuals remain substantially obese emphasizes the

therapeutic benefit of modest weight reduction and should provide encouragement for obese individuals to undergo relatively short periods of weight reduction.

Although there is little disagreement that weight reduction should be the primary nutritional intervention in obese patients with diabetes, the exact nature of these diets is more controversial. The optimal method of producing sustained weight loss has yet to be identified. Moderate caloric restriction of 500–1000 kcal/d less than weight-maintenance calories is useful to produce a gradual sustained weight loss. Such a caloric level is sufficient to allow for a nutritionally balanced diet using ordinary foods.

Because modest caloric restriction results in very slow weight loss, the possibility of using more marked caloric restriction for shorter periods of time was studied. Such very-low-calorie diets were originally designed for the severely obese but otherwise healthy individual. These diets have been studied in individuals with NIDDM and are reported to be effective for weight loss and to be safe in short-term applications.[16,17]

Very-low-calorie diets generally provide 500–800 kcal/d in a liquid formula drink of high-quality protein, low in carbohydrate and fat, and supplemented with vitamins and minerals. They may contain either a high proportion of protein or may have a more balanced caloric distribution, containing protein, carbohydrate, and fat in varying ratios.

Both types of diets will result in weight loss, but it is unclear whether there are advantages or disadvantages to differing proportions of macronutrients. Carbohydrate-containing diets reduce the level of ketosis and may provide maintenance of muscle glycogen and sustained exercise tolerance. Higher protein diets, on the other hand, may provide for better nitrogen balance,[18] although not all studies support this finding.[19] Other studies indicate that the distribution of macronutrients has no measurable effect on either appetite or mood.[20,21] In any case, maintenance of weight loss for patients with NIDDM is as difficult as for the normal individual. The exact composition of a weight loss diet should be individually tailored and based upon considerations such as metabolic abnormalities present, individual dietary preference, and ability to achieve compliance.

Effects of Variations in Amount of Dietary Carbohydrate and Fat

The major focus of dietary advice for patients with diabetes over the past several years has been the emphasis on high-carbohydrate, low-fat diets. The rationale for this approach was discussed earlier.

However, replacing dietary fat with carbohydrate may not be the most appropriate means of reducing cardiovascular risk factors in individuals with diabetes. Currently, there are conflicting reports on the metabolic effects of high-carbohydrate, low-fat diets in individuals with diabetes. Much of the confusion exists to a large degree because of the inability and/or unwillingness on the part of investigators to divorce the changes in relative amount of fat and carbohydrate from those due to variations in either the kind of fat or the amount of dietary cholesterol. An example of this approach is a study published by Simpson et al.[22] These investigators reported that the consumption of a high-carbohydrate, low-fat diet leads to a decline in total plasma cholesterol concentrations and improved overall diabetic control. However, in addition to the changes in the amount of carbohydrate and fat in the diet, the diets differed in the ratio of polyunsaturated to saturated fatty acids (P:S, 0.3 vs. 1.1), amount of dietary cholesterol (700 vs. 100 mg/d), and the amount of dietary fiber (18 vs. 97 g/d). Because all of these dietary changes have been shown to influence plasma glucose and lipoprotein concentrations, it is difficult to attribute the observed changes solely to the effects of the high-carbohydrate, low-fat nature of the diets. Indeed, in a subsequent study by the same group[10] in which P:S, dietary cholesterol, and fiber were held constant, high-carbohydrate, low-fat diets resulted in significantly higher total and 2-h postprandial glucose concentrations as well as significant reductions in HDL-cholesterol concentrations with no significant decrease in total cholesterol or LDL-cholesterol concentrations. The comparison of these two studies serves to emphasize the importance of controlling dietary variables that may alter carbohydrate and lipoprotein metabolism independently of the amount of dietary carbohydrate and fat per se.

Isocaloric Substitution of Carbohydrate for Fat. Studies conducted by our group[6,7] and others[8-10] have indicated consistently that the isocaloric substitution of carbohydrate for fat in the diet of individuals with diabetes results in an increase in plasma glucose, insulin, total triglyceride, and VLDL-triglyceride concentrations and a reduction in HDL-cholesterol levels without appreciably affecting total plasma cholesterol concentrations. For example, Sestoft et al.[8] demonstrated that increasing complex carbohydrate from 40% to 50% of the total calories in individuals with diabetes resulted in a significant increase in postprandial plasma glucose and insulin concentrations. In addition, total plasma triglyceride and VLDL-triglyceride concentrations were significantly increased, total plasma cholesterol concentrations were unchanged, and LDL- and HDL-cholesterol concentrations were decreased. A recent study by our group

revealed similar results in patients with NIDDM.[6] Postprandial plasma glucose and insulin as well as fasting total triglyceride and VLDL-triglyceride concentrations were significantly increased and HDL-cholesterol concentrations were significantly decreased as a result of increasing dietary carbohydrate from 40% to 60% of total daily calories. Moreover, these deleterious effects persisted throughout a 6-wk period.

Not all studies have reported similar deleterious effects. However, data indicating that high-carbohydrate, low-fat diets lead to beneficial effects on carbohydrate or lipid metabolism are confounded either by the lack of suitable dietary control,[22-25] or by the fact that the diets also differed in type of dietary fat[22-25] and amount of dietary cholesterol[22-24] or were enriched with dietary fiber.[22-24] When these factors are taken into consideration, there appears to be little evidence in support of the view that substituting carbohydrate for fat in the diet of individuals with diabetes results in any measurable beneficial effect on either carbohydrate or lipoprotein metabolism. Indeed, it could be argued that the available evidence supports the conclusion that the most characteristic defects in carbohydrate and lipoprotein metabolism in patients with diabetes (that is, increased glucose, insulin, total plasma triglyceride, and VLDL-triglyceride concentrations and decreased HDL-cholesterol concentrations) have a marked tendency to deteriorate in response to high-carbohydrate, low-fat diets.

Modified-fat, Cholesterol-restricted Diets. Several studies assessing the metabolic effects of an isocaloric substitution of carbohydrate for fat in the diet illustrate the deleterious effects of the high-carbohydrate nature of the diets.[6-8,10] However, this finding should not divert attention from the fact that these studies also have a positive interpretation. That is, they clearly demonstrate that diets containing conventional quantities of fat (35-40% of total calories) in which a portion of the saturated fatty acids is replaced with unsaturated fatty acids will reduce total cholesterol and LDL cholesterol to the same extent as replacement of saturated fatty acids with complex carbohydrate without increasing fasting or day-long plasma glucose, insulin, and triglyceride concentrations or decreasing HDL-cholesterol concentrations. These observations are consistent with studies conducted in individuals with normal glucose tolerance that demonstrated that diets containing 40-45% carbohydrate with an increased P:S and decreased dietary cholesterol content resulted in lower VLDL triglyceride and higher HDL cholesterol concentrations than did 60%-carbohydrate, modified-fat, cholesterol-restricted diets.[26,27] Thus, the beneficial effects of modifying fat appear to be independent of whether total fat is reduced. These data suggest that a modification of fat and reduction of cholesterol content of conventional diets might prove to be more beneficial in correcting abnormalities in carbohydrate and lipoprotein metabolism of individuals with diabetes than low-fat diets would be.

The beneficial effects of replacing saturated fatty acids with unsaturated fatty acids in the diet may not be limited solely to the effects generally attributed to polyunsaturated fatty acids. Recently Garg et al.[9] demonstrated beneficial effects on lipid metabolism with the substitution of monounsaturated fatty acids for saturated fatty acids. Specifically, they assessed the metabolic effects of replacing saturated fatty acids in the diet with either complex carbohydrate (high-carbohydrate, low-fat diet) or monounsaturated fatty acids in diets of diabetic individuals treated with insulin. They reported an increase in 24-h urinary excretion, postprandial plasma glucose and insulin, and fasting and postprandial triglyceride concentrations and a decrease in fasting HDL-cholesterol concentrations during the high-carbohydrate phase. In addition, insulin requirements were significantly higher when dietary carbohydrate was increased. Thus, these data are consistent with data previously discussed in regard to the deleterious effects of increasing dietary carbohydrate in individuals with diabetes, and they suggest that the beneficial effects of reducing saturated fatty acids also can be achieved with the use of monounsaturated fatty acids.

Following the report of Kromhout et al.[28] that the consumption of fish and other marine mammals may confer special benefits in decreasing CAD, there has been an increased interest in the role of these fatty acids and the development of CAD in patients with diabetes. The long-chain, polyunsaturated fatty acids found primarily in marine mammals belong to the n−3 series fatty acids, and this difference in chemical structure affects several metabolic processes related to blood platelet function, thrombosis, and lipoprotein metabolism that may relate to CAD seen in individuals with diabetes.

Clinical studies in normoglycemic individuals demonstrated that fish oils were at least as effective as polyunsaturated vegetable oils (n−6 series fatty acids) in reducing serum cholesterol levels. Studies of the effect of these fatty acids on lipoprotein metabolism also showed a marked reduction in total plasma triglyceride and VLDL-triglyceride concentrations, unlike other dietary fatty acids.[29] Because elevated total plasma triglyceride and VLDL-triglyceride concentrations are a common finding in patients with diabetes, there has been widespread interest in the use of n−3 fatty acids or fish oils. Two recent studies in patients with NIDDM demonstrated a significant decrease in total plasma triglyceride and VLDL-triglyceride concentrations with fish-oil sup-

plements of ~5 g/d with no change in LDL or HDL cholesterol concentrations.[30,31] However, in both studies a deterioration in plasma glucose control was noted at higher doses of fish-oil supplements. There was less deterioration in plasma glucose control in treated patients with a mean fasting plasma glucose of 7.8 mmol/L[31] than in untreated patients with a mean fasting plasma glucose of 12.8 mmol/L.[30] Whether these differences were due to differences in treatment, degree of glycemic control, or study populations is not clear. At this point there does not appear to be sufficient data to make any definitive statement on the efficacy and safety of fish-oil supplementations in patients with diabetes.

Effects of Variations in Type of Dietary Carbohydrate

The potential deleterious effects of high-carbohydrate diets have not gone unrecognized by their adherents, but it has been argued that these dangers can be avoided by changes in the type of carbohydrate ingested. It is generally recommended that patients with diabetes should (1) decrease intake of simple carbohydrate in favor of complex carbohydrate, (2) select foods with low rather than high glycemic-index values, and (3) increase intake of dietary fiber. Thus, it seems important to examine available information as to the impact of these changes on carbohydrate and lipoprotein metabolism in individuals with diabetes.

Simple vs. Complex Carbohydrate. It is generally recommended that the ingestion of simple carbohydrates (monosaccharides and disaccharides) should be discouraged and ingestion of complex (polysaccharide) carbohydrates encouraged in patients with diabetes. This recommendation appears to be based on the belief that simple carbohydrate foods will be absorbed readily and, therefore, will cause marked increases in plasma glucose response. Thus, restriction of simple carbohydrate foods would be necessary to avoid wide excursions in plasma glucose concentration. Despite the popular acceptance of this notion, it is not based on a large body of scientific evidence. Indeed, there appears to be only one study that addresses the specific issue of the metabolic effects of simple and complex carbohydrates in the diets of individuals with diabetes.[32] In this study postprandial glycemia and glucosuria were significantly increased when diets containing 80% complex carbohydrate and 20% simple carbohydrate were compared with diets containing 80% simple carbohydrate and 20% complex carbohydrate. It should be emphasized that changes in the percentage of simple and complex carbohydrate in this study were accomplished by varying the relative quantities of naturally occurring carbohydrate foods. For example, all of the carbohydrate in fruits and dairy products and from 50% to 100% of the carbohydrate in vegetables is present as simple carbohydrate. Thus, the proportion of simple carbohydrate in the diet was increased by incorporating more fruits and vegetables into the menu, not by adding refined sugars to the meals.

The result of this study suggests that instructing individuals with diabetes to decrease their consumption of fruits, vegetables, or dairy products in favor of complex carbohydrate is not likely to be of benefit to plasma glucose control. It is essential that the results of this study not be misinterpreted; these data may be applicable only to situations involving naturally occurring carbohydrate-rich foods. However, the distinction between naturally occurring and refined simple sugars is rarely made in general dietary recommendations. Although these data appear to be in conflict with the traditional concept of the metabolic effects of simple and complex carbohydrate, they are quite consistent with data demonstrating that plasma glucose and insulin responses to dietary carbohydrate vary widely as a function of the source of dietary carbohydrate.[33,34]

Glycemic Index. The *glycemic index* is a classification of foods based on the plasma glucose response of single foods compared with the response to a reference standard food or oral glucose challenge. Evidence indicates that plasma glucose response to equivalent amounts of dietary carbohydrate varies as a function of the specific carbohydrate-rich food consumed.[33,34] It has been suggested that meals containing foods with a low glycemic response or glycemic index will result in lower postprandial glucose responses in diabetic patients than will meals containing foods with a high glycemic index.[34] As attractive as this notion may be, many factors besides the total carbohydrate of a food or meal alter plasma glucose response. It remains to be seen whether this observation will lead to a clinically useful reduction in postprandial hyperglycemia when used to plan meals for individuals with diabetes. To date, studies designed to evaluate the clinical utility of the glycemic index in the context of mixed meals for individuals with diabetes have not been successful. In fact, the results of these studies generally have failed to show any significant difference among test meals varying widely in their predicted glycemic response.[35,36] Thus, it would appear that the use of the glycemic index in its present form would provide little clinical assistance in designing meals for individuals with diabetes.

Dietary Fiber. Over the past several decades there has been an increased interest in the role of dietary fiber in human health and disease. This interest has heightened as a result of several studies that reported hypoglycemic and/or hypolipemic effects of increased dietary fiber. However, the results of these studies are difficult to assess. They are either acute studies that lack suitable controls[23,24,37,38] or use enormous amounts of dietary fiber.[22,24] Moreover, both carbohydrate and fiber content are often increased in parallel, making it difficult to address the independent effects of increased carbohydrate from those of increased fiber.[22–25]

Studies that have shown the greatest effects on carbohydrate or lipoprotein metabolism have relied on fiber levels between 70 and 100 g/d.[22–24] Although it is entirely possible that beneficial effects on carbohydrate and lipoprotein metabolism may occur at these levels of dietary fiber intake, one must also acknowledge that these levels of dietary fiber intake may be impossible to achieve consistently in a large segment of the population. Several well-controlled metabolic studies using levels of 45–50 g/d showed little or no significant benefits to either carbohydrate or lipid metabolism in patients with diabetes.[39–42] A complete discussion of the clinical relevance of these studies can be found in a recent review of the dietary management of hyperlipidemia in individuals with diabetes.[43]

It appears that increasing dietary fiber within practical and acceptable limits will have at best marginal beneficial effects on plasma glucose and lipoprotein concentrations in patients with diabetes. This conclusion, however, should not be taken to mean that dietary fiber is unimportant in individuals with diabetes. Indeed, there are several general nutritional considerations for which individuals with diabetes should be encouraged to increase dietary fiber intake. These considerations include the beneficial effects of dietary fiber on gastrointestinal motility and diverticular disease. It would seem reasonable, therefore, to advise individuals with diabetes to increase their intake of fiber-rich foods such as fruits and vegetables and whole-grain breads and cereals for these reasons without any undue expectations of correcting abnormalities in carbohydrate or lipoprotein metabolism.

Refined Carbohydrates. Traditionally, individuals with diabetes have been instructed to avoid foods containing refined sugars. The rationale for this dietary advice is similar to that used for simple carbohydrates. That is, refined simple sugars would be readily absorbed, leading to large swings in plasma glucose response. However, it was demonstrated that the replacement of sucrose for a portion of carbohydrate in a single meal for individuals with diabetes did not lead to an exaggerated increase in postprandial glucose or insulin concentrations.[44,45] These data suggest that the addition of moderate amounts of sucrose to a single meal would not result in exaggerated plasma glucose or insulin response. However, caution should be exercised in expanding these findings to a more chronic situation. The effects of continued sucrose intake in individuals with diabetes over days, weeks, or even months remain controversial. Substantial evidence from a number of well-controlled prospective studies demonstrates that the consumption of moderate amounts of sucrose results in postprandial hyperglycemia, hyperinsulinemia, and hypertriglyceridemia in addition to increased fasting hypertriglyceridemia, hypercholesterolemia, and decreased HDL-cholesterol concentrations.[7,46–49] We have published two studies in which the effects of increased dietary sucrose on carbohydrate and lipoprotein metabolism in diabetes were evaluated. In one study the only variable was the amount of total calories present as sucrose.[46] After 15 d of diets containing 16% of the total calories as added sucrose, we documented a significant increase in day-long glucose and triglyceride concentrations. In addition, there were significant elevations in fasting total plasma triglyceride, VLDL-triglyceride, and total plasma cholesterol concentrations when compared with a sucrose-free diet. Twenty-four–hour urinary glucose excretion was also significantly greater when sucrose was present in the diet despite no change in the total carbohydrate content. In a second study lasting 4 wk, we evaluated the effects of increased dietary sucrose and carbohydrate in individuals with diabetes.[7] The combination of these two dietary manipulations appeared to exacerbate the metabolic changes seen with increased dietary sucrose alone.

The results of longer-term studies in nondiabetic individuals also raise questions about the safety of increasing sucrose in the diets of individuals with diabetes. The findings are particularly true for individuals without diabetes but who share some of the same metabolic abnormalities as individuals with diabetes. For example, Reiser et al.[47,48] demonstrated in normoglycemic, hyperinsulinemic individuals that the isocaloric addition of sucrose for 6 wk increased fasting plasma glucose, insulin, total triglyceride, and VLDL-triglyceride concentrations. Moreover, these increases were proportional to the amount of sucrose added. Similarly, Liu et al.[49] demonstrated that the magnitude of the increase in fasting total triglyceride and VLDL-triglyceride concentrations in patients with endogenous hypertriglyceridemia varied as a function of the sucrose content of the diet.

In contrast to these studies, there are several reports in which the authors concluded that increased sucrose consumption did not lead to adverse metabolic effects. In perhaps the best-controlled of these studies, Bantle et al.[50] reported no significant differences

in metabolic control in individuals with diabetes after 8 d of increased sucrose consumption. However, fasting, 1- and 2-h postprandial, and overall mean plasma glucose concentrations were higher after the sucrose diet. In addition, fasting and postprandial peak triglyceride concentrations also were elevated after the sucrose diet. The fact that the differences reported did not reach levels of significance may be the result of the statistical analyses or the length of time of the study. This study lasted only 8 d, and the magnitude of these metabolic changes may well have reached levels of significance with increased duration of the diet.

The fact that all studies do not show deleterious effects does not negate the positive data. There should be no doubt that sucrose can and does have deleterious effects on metabolic control in individuals with diabetes. It is likely that the magnitude of the deleterious effects will vary based on such factors as plasma glucose and lipid concentrations, amount of sucrose ingested, and other dietary constituents. Because current information does not permit prediction of individuals who may be adversely affected or at what sucrose levels adverse effects will occur, perhaps the best approach is to limit sucrose consumption, be aware of the potential deleterious effects, monitor patients closely, and modify sucrose intake appropriately in accordance with any change in the individual's metabolic status.

Sugar Substitutes. Alternative sweeteners, such as the sugar alcohols, aspartame, and saccharin, have been advocated as substitutes for sucrose to provide sweetness without hyperglycemia or increased calories for persons with diabetes. The risk, benefits, and effects of different sweeteners in individuals with diabetes have not been fully tested. Because individuals with diabetes are likely to ingest greater quantities of these sweeteners than the general population, the use of these substances is an important issue. In 1977 it was estimated that as many as 91% of all individuals with diabetes used sugar substitutes.[51] However, few studies have addressed whether the use of sweeteners either increases adherence to prescribed diets or facilitates weight reduction in obese individuals with diabetes. Thus, there seems to be a need for such studies before we can assess the importance of sweeteners in the dietary management of diabetes. Because the role of sugar substitutes in the treatment of individuals with diabetes has been the focus of several recent reviews, we will comment only briefly here.[52,53]

Sorbitol, a sugar alcohol, has been used as an alternative sweetener because it is absorbed more slowly from the gastrointestinal tract and, thus, reduces the prompt increase in plasma glucose characteristic of dietary carbohydrate.[54] Sorbitol has the same caloric equivalent as that of its parent carbohydrate and is about half as sweet as sucrose. The slow passive absorption of sorbitol can cause osmotic diarrhea and abdominal discomfort even with relatively low doses (30–50 g). The sugar alcohols do not cause any increase in plasma glucose, glucosuria, or insulin requirement in patients with diabetes.[55]

Aspartame, which is produced commercially from phenylalanine and aspartic acid, has been in use since 1981. It is ~200 times sweeter than sucrose and, thus, is used in quantities that provide insignificant amounts of amino acids or calories.[56] Aspartame has a chemical structure that breaks down with heating, resulting in the loss of sweetening ability. Thus, aspartame is used only in foods that will not be subjected to high temperatures. Although there have been scattered reports of toxic effects from aspartame ingestion, these reports have been difficult to substantiate. The Food and Drug Administration (FDA) and other regulatory agencies found it to be safe for human consumption and set the acceptable daily intake at 50 mg/kg body weight.[57] This amount represents about 17 354-mL cans of aspartame-sweetened beverage for a 70-kg individual. Consumption levels, in general, are well below the acceptable daily intake.

Saccharin was the first man-made sugar substitute and gained widespread use during the sugar shortages of World Wars I and II. Saccharin is ~300–400 times sweeter than sucrose, although it leaves a bitter aftertaste that has diminished its widespread acceptability. Bans on the use of saccharin were proposed as a result of findings indicating that sodium saccharin produced bladder cancer in experimental animals (FDA, unpublished observations, 1980). However, additional evidence in humans failed to define any association between bladder cancer risk and consumption of saccharin.[58] Although the FDA has not defined acceptable intakes, the acceptable daily intake suggested by the Food and Agriculture Organization/World Health Organization is <2.5 $mg \cdot kg^{-1} \cdot d^{-1}$.[52] One teaspoon or packet of saccharine contains 14–20 mg saccharin.

Conclusion

Because the major cause of morbidity and mortality in patients with diabetes is vascular disease, a major goal of nutritional management must be to decrease the incidence of these complications. The amount of carbohydrate and fat that should be incorporated into the diet of individuals with diabetes remains controversial. However, data presented in this review suggest that diets containing conventional quantities of fat (35–40% of total calories), in which the composition of fat has been modified to reduce saturated fatty acids and dietary cholesterol, appear to offer the best overall control of carbohydrate and lipoprotein metabolism in individuals with diabetes. The popular recommendation to substitute carbohydrate for saturated fatty acids in the diet results in increased postprandial plasma glucose, insulin, and total triglyceride concentrations; increased fasting triglyceride total and VLDL-triglyceride concentrations; and decreased HDL-cholesterol concentrations. Furthermore, it does not appear that the deleterious effects of increasing dietary carbohydrate can be prevented by substituting complex for simple carbohydrate, by selecting low-glycemic-index foods, or by increasing dietary fiber content to within acceptable limits. Consequently, we believe that the current available information does not support the view that patients with diabetes should be encouraged to follow high-carbohydrate, low-fat diets. This statement should not be taken to indicate that dietary fat is unimportant. Indeed, we have tried to point out that the type of dietary fat and amount of dietary cholesterol appear to be two important constituents in the regulation of lipoprotein metabolism in individuals with diabetes. On the basis of the above considerations, we believe that individuals with diabetes should be encouraged to reduce intake of saturated fatty acids, cholesterol, and refined sugars and individuals who are overweight should be encouraged to lose weight.

References

1. M.I. Harris, W.C. Hadden, W.C. Knowler, and P.H. Bennet (1987) Prevalence of diabetes and impaired glucose tolerance and plasma glucose levels in U.S. population aged 20–74 years. *Diabetes* 36: 523–534.
2. National Diabetes Data Group International Work Group (1979) Classification and diagnosis of diabetes and other categories of glucose intolerance. *Diabetes* 28:1039–1057.
3. American Diabetes Association (1987) Nutritional recommendations and principles for individuals with diabetes mellitus: 1986. *Diabetes Care* 10:126–132.
4. Canadian Diabetes Association (1981) Special report committee guidelines for the nutritional management of diabetes mellitus: a special report from the Canadian Diabetes Association. *J. Can. Diet. Assoc.* 42:110–118.
5. E.A. Nikkila (1981) Plasma lipid and lipoprotein abnormalities in diabetes. In: *Diabetes and Heart Disease* (R.J. Jarett, ed.), pp. 133–167, Elsevier Science, New York.
6. A.M. Coulston, C.B. Hollenbeck, A.L.M. Swislocki, and G.M. Reaven (1989) Persistence of the hypertriglyceridemic effect of high-carbohydrate, low-fat diets in patients with type 2 diabetes mellitus. *Diabetes Care* 12:94–101.
7. A.M. Coulston, C.B. Hollenbeck, A.L.M. Swislocki, Y.-D.I. Chen, and G.M. Reaven (1987) Deleterious metabolic effects of high carbohydrate, sucrose containing diets in patients with NIDDM. *Am. J. Med.* 82:213–220.
8. L. Sestoft, T. Krarup, and B. Palmvig (1985) High carbohydrate, low-fat diet: effect on lipid and carbohydrate metabolism, GIP and insulin secretion in diabetics. *Dan. Med. Bull.* 32:64–69.
9. A. Garg, A. Bonanone, S.M. Grundy, Z.-J. Zhang, and R.H. Unger

(1988) Comparison of a high-carbohydrate diet with high-mono-unsaturated fat diet in patients with non-insulin-dependent diabetes mellitus. *N. Engl. J. Med.* 319:829–834.

10. H.C.R. Simpson, R.W. Simpson, S. Lousley, and J. Mann (1982) Digestible carbohydrate—an independent effect on diabetic control in type 2 (non-insulin-dependent) diabetic patient? *Diabetologia* 23:235–239.

11. L.H. Newburgh, J.W. Conn, and M.W. Johnston (1938) A new interpretation of diabetes mellitus in obese, middle-aged persons: recovery through reduction of weight. *Trans. Assoc. Am. Physicians* 53:245–257.

12. G. Liu, A.M. Coulston, C.K. Lardinois, C.B. Hollenbeck, J. Moore, and G.M. Reaven (1985) Moderate weight loss and sulfonylurea treatment on non-insulin-dependent diabetes mellitus. *Arch. Intern. Med.* 145:665–669.

13. R.R. Wing, R. Koeske, L.H. Epstein, M.P. Nowalk, W. Gooding, and D. Becker (1987) Long-term effects of modest weight loss in type II diabetic patients. *Arch. Intern. Med.* 147:1749–1753.

14. P. Weisweiler, M. Drosner, and P. Schwandt (1982) Dietary effects of very low density lipoproteins in type 2 (non-insulin-dependent) diabetes mellitus. *Diabetologia* 23:101–103.

15. J.K. Wales (1982) Treatment of type 2 (non-insulin-dependent) diabetes mellitus. *Diabetologia* 23:240–245.

16. R.R. Henry, T.A. Wiest-Kent, and L. Scheaffer, O.G. Kolterman, and J.M. Olefsky (1986) Metabolic consequences of very-low-calorie diet therapy in non-insulin-dependent diabetic and non-diabetic subjects. *Diabetes* 35:155–164.

17. T.A. Hughes, J.T. Gwynne, B.R. Switzer, C. Herbst, and G. White (1984) Effects of caloric restriction and weight loss on glycemic control, insulin release and resistance, and atherosclerotic risk in obese patients with type II diabetes mellitus. *Am. J. Med.* 77:7–17.

18. L.J. Hoffer, B.R. Bistrian, V.R. Young, G.L. Blackburn, and D.E. Mathews (1984) Metabolic effects of very low calorie weight diets. *J. Clin. Invest.* 73:750–758.

19. M.U. Yang and T.B. Van Itallie (1984) Variability in body protein loss during protracted, severe caloric restriction: role of triiodothyronine and other possible determinants, *Am. J. Clin. Nutr.* 40:611–622.

20. J.C. Rosen, D.A. Hunt, E.A.H. Sims, and C. Bogardus (1982) Comparison of carbohydrate containing and carbohydrate-restricted hypocaloric diets in the treatment of obesity: effects on appetite and mood. *Am. J. Clin. Nutr.* 36:464–469.

21. J.C. Rosen, J. Gross, D. Loew, and E.A.H. Sims (1985) Mood and appetite during minimal carbohydrate and carbohydrate-supplemented hypocaloric diets. *Am. J. Clin. Nutr.* 42:371–379.

22. H.C.R. Simpson, R.W. Simpson, S. Lousley, and J. Mann (1981) High carbohydrate leguminous fibre diet improves all aspects of dietary control. *Lancet* 1:1–5.

23. J.W. Anderson, W.J.L. Chen, and B. Sieling (1980) Hypolipemic effects of high-carbohydrate, high-fiber diets. *Metabolism* 29:551–558.

24. R.W. Simpson, J.I. Mann, and J. Eaton (1979) Improved glucose control in maturity-onset diabetes treated with high-carbohydrate-modified fat diets. *Br. J. Med.* 1:1753–1756.

25. T.G. Kiehm, J.W. Anderson, and K. Ward (1976) Beneficial effects of a high-carbohydrate, high-fiber diet on hyperglycemic diabetic men. *Am. J. Clin. Nutr.* 29:895–899.

26. B. Lewis, F. Hammett, and M. Katan (1981) Toward an improved lipid-lowering diet: additive effects of changes in nutrient intake. *Lancet* 2:1310–1313.

27. J.H. Brussard, G. Dallinga-Thie, P.H.E. Groot, and M.B. Datan (1980) Effects of amount and type of dietary fat on serum lipids, lipoproteins, and apoproteins in man. *Atherosclerosis* 36:515–527.

28. D. Kromhout, E.B. Bosschieter, and C.D. Coulander (1985) The inverse relation between fish consumption and 20 year mortality from coronary heart disease, *N. Engl. J. Med.* 312:1205–1224.

29. P.J. Nestel, W.E. Connor, M.F. Reardon, S. Connor, S. Wong, and R. Boston (1984) Suppression by diets rich in fish oil of very low density lipoprotein production in man. *J. Clin. Invest.* 74:82–89.

30. H. Glauber, P. Wallace, K. Griver, and G. Brechtel (1988) Adverse metabolic effects of omega-3 fatty acids in non-insulindependent diabetes mellitus, *Ann. Intern. Med.* 108:663–668.

31. G. Schectman, K. Sushma, and A.H. Kissebah (1988) Effect of fish oil concentrate on lipoprotein composition in NIDDM. *Diabetes* 37:1567–1573.

32. C.B. Hollenbeck, A.M. Coulston, C.C. Donnor, R.A. Williams, and G.M. Reaven (1985) The effects of variations in percent of naturally occurring complex and simple carbohydrates on plasma glucose and insulin response in individuals with non-insulin-dependent diabetes mellitus. *Diabetes* 34:151–155.

33. P.A. Crapo, G.M. Reaven, and J.M. Olefsky (1977) Postprandial glucose and insulin response to different complex carbohydrates. *Diabetes* 26:1178–1183.

34. D.J.A. Jenkins, T.M.S. Wolever, R.H. Taylor, et al. (1981) Glycemic index of foods: a physiological basis for carbohydrate exchange. *Am. J. Clin. Nutr.* 34:184–190.

35. C.B. Hollenbeck, A.M. Coulston, and G.M. Reaven (1988) Comparison of plasma glucose and insulin responses to mixed meals of high-, intermediate-, and low-glycemic potential. *Diabetes Care* 11:323–329.

36. D.C. Laine, W. Thomas, M.D. Levitt, and J.P. Bantle (1987) Comparison of the predictive capabilities of the diabetic exchange list and the glycemic index of foods. *Diabetes Care* 10:387–394.

37. D.J.A. Jenkins, T.M.S. Wolever, and T.D.R. Hockaday (1977) Treatment of diabetes with guar gum. *Lancet* 2:779–780.

38. D.J.A. Jenkins, T.M.S. Wolever, and R. Nineham (1978) Guar crisp breads in the diabetic diet. *Br. J. Med.* 2:1744–1746.

39. C.B. Hollenbeck, A.M. Coulston, and G.M. Reaven (1986) To what extent does increased dietary fiber improve glucose and lipid metabolism in patients with noninsulin-dependent diabetes mellitus (NIDDM)? *Am. J. Clin. Nutr.* 43:16–24.

40. G. Riccardi, A. Rivellese, and D. Pacioni (1984) Separate influences of dietary carbohydrate and fiber on metabolic control of diabetes. *Diabetologia* 26:116–121.

41. B. Karlstom, B. Vessby, and N.-G. Asp (1984) Effects of an increased content of cereal fiber in the diet of type 2 (non-insulin-dependent) diabetic patient. *Diabetologia* 26:272–277.

42. M. Uusitupa, O. Siitonen, K. Savolainen, M. Silvasti, and I. Penttila (1989) Metabolic and nutritional effects of long-term use of guar gum in the treatment of noninsulin-dependent diabetes of poor metabolic control. *Am. J. Clin. Nutr.* 49:345–351.

43. C.B. Hollenbeck and A.M. Coulston (1987) Effect of variation in diet on lipoprotein metabolism in patients with diabetes mellitus. *Diabetes Metab. Rev.* 3:669–689.

44. J.P. Bantle, D.C. Laine, G.W. Castle, J.W. Thomas, B.J. Hoogwerf, and F.C. Goetz (1983) Postprandial glucose and insulin responses to meals containing different carbohydrates in normal and diabetic subjects. *N. Engl. J. Med.* 309:7–12.

45. G. Slama, P. Jean-Joseph, I. Giogolea, et al. (1984) Sucrose taken during a mixed meal had no additional hyperglycaemic action over isocaloric amounts of starch in well controlled diabetics. *Lancet* 2:122–125.

46. A.M. Coulston, C.B. Hollenbeck, C.C. Donnor, R.A. Williams, Y.-A.M. Chiou, and G.M. Reaven (1985) Metabolic effects of added dietary sucrose in individuals with non-insulin-dependent diabetes mellitus (NIDDM). *Metabolism* 34:962–966.

47. S. Reiser, E. Bohn, J. Hallfrisch, O.E. Michaelis, M. Keeney, and E.S. Prather (1981) Serum glucose and insulin in hyperinsulinemic

subjects fed three different levels of sucrose. *Am. J. Clin. Nutr.* 34:2348–2358.

48. S. Reiser, M.C. Bickard, J. Hallfrisch, O.E. Michaelis, and E.S. Prather (1981) Blood lipids and their distribution in lipoproteins in hyperinsulinemic subjects fed three different levels of sucrose. *J. Nutr.* 111:1045–1057.

49. G. Liu, A.M. Coulston, C.B. Hollenbeck, and G.M. Reaven (1984) The effects of sucrose content in high and low carbohydrate diets on plasma glucose, insulin, and lipid responses in hypertriglyceridemic humans. *J. Clin. Endocrinol. Metab.* 59:636–641.

50. J.P. Bantle, D.C. Laine, and J.W. Thomas (1986) Metabolic effects of dietary fructose and sucrose in type I and type II diabetic subjects. *JAMA* 256:3241–3246.

51. Committee on Saccharin and Food Safety Policy, National Research Council, National Academy of Sciences (1978) *Saccharin: Technical Assessment of Risk and Benefits,* National Academy Press, Washington, DC.

52. P.A. Crapo (1988) Use of alternative sweeteners in diabetic diet. *Diabetes Care* 11:174–182.

53. American Dietetic Association (1987) Position of the American Dietetic Association: appropriate use of nutritive and non-nutritive sweeteners. *J. Am. Diet. Assoc.* 87:1687–1694.

54. L.H. Adock and C.H. Gray (1957) The metabolism of sorbitol in the human subject. *Biochem. J.* 65:554–560.

55. J. Steinke, F.C. Wood, L. Domenque, A. Marble, and A.E. Renol (1961) Evaluation of sorbitol in the diet of diabetic children at camp. *Diabetes* 10:218–227.

56. D.L. Horwitz (1984) Aspartame use by persons with diabetes. In: *Aspartame: Physiology and Metabolism* (L.D. Stegink and L.J. Filer, Jr., eds.), pp. 633–640, Dekker, New York.

57. Food and Drug Administration (1981) Aspartame: commissioner's final decision. *Fed. Regist.* 46:38285–38308.

58. A.S. Morrison and J.E. Buring (1980) Artificial sweeteners and cancer of the lower urinary tract. *N. Engl. J. Med.* 302:537–541.

Osteoporosis and Osteomalacia

There are at least two nutritionally related skeletal diseases that are important in adulthood: osteoporosis and osteomalacia. Osteoporosis is defined as a decrease in the amount of bone leading to fractures after minimal trauma. In osteoporosis, matrix of bone mineral and protein is lost, resulting in less overall bone. Composition of the remaining bone, however, is normal. Osteomalacia is characterized also by inadequate bone mineralization. In contrast to osteoporosis, persons with osteomalacia have normal protein matrix that is not fully mineralized. These two diseases may coexist in the same individual.

Nutritional studies of skeletal diseases have been hampered by at least three factors. Until ~10 y ago, sensitive methodologies to study bone were usually highly invasive. Although less-invasive technology is now more available, the widely used measures of bone mass, including photon densitometry, describe only the mineral content. They do not characterize the protein matrix or bone architecture. More indepth and invasive studies, both biochemical and radiographical, are required to generate differential diagnoses of these diseases. Because the less-invasive measures of bone mass do not discriminate between osteoporosis and osteomalacia, studies of diet and bone mass may lack sensitivity in describing true relationships. A second impediment to studies of diet and bone is that even the osteoporotic process may have three different phases (maximal bone mass, postmenopausal bone loss, and senile bone loss), with a differential response to nutritional factors. Finally, observation of the individual for clinically important bone loss may require a time period exceeding 4–5 y given the metabolic processes associated with skeletal loss and the error associated with bone-mass measurement. In spite of these limitations, investigation of the role of diet in adult skeletal bone maintenance has continued and will be described in this chapter.

Calcium

Because ~99% of the calcium in the body is stored in the skeleton, a net loss of calcium from the body must be accompanied by a net loss from the skeleton. Questions remain as to whether consistent loss of skeletal bone arises from inadequate calcium intake, inadequate calcium absorption, or excessive excretory loss.

Inadequate Intake—Maximal Bone Mineralization. Bone mass is believed to accrue in young adult women as a result of increased bone formation relative to bone resorption. After menopause the balance between formation and resorption apparently is altered in favor of increased bone resorption, at least in some women.[1] It has been suggested that promoting greater bone mass in young adult women may be the most effective method of sustaining sufficient bone mass as aging progresses. Conceptually, maximal bone will establish a *track* that will characterize the relative bone mass of the individual during aging. Young women with a higher track will be more likely to maintain that position in relation to peers and may have lower risk of osteoporosis and fracture in later years.[2]

There is some consistent evidence that increased dietary calcium intake may be influential in promoting greater maximal bone mass. This consistency is observed in both human and animal studies using a variety of study designs. Sowers et al.[3] found that higher calcium intake was associated with greater bone mass (measured by single-photon densitometry) in a geographically defined population of women aged 20–35 y after considering the effect of age, body size, lifestyle habits, and reproductive events. Sandler et al.[4] found that postmenopausal women who had consumed milk during childhood and adolescence were more likely to have greater bone mass than those women whose milk consumption ceased during childhood. A Yugoslav study indicated that differences in bone mass observed in persons from a dairying region vs. a nondairying region were evident from age 30 y (maximal bone accumulation).[5] A recent study by Sinha et al.[6] suggests that dietary calcium intake does not affect the bone dynamics observed in aged female rats but does increase bone formation in younger rats. Potentially, dietary calcium intake and exercise may have a synergistic effect on maximal bone mass as suggested in a recent paper by Kanders et al.[7]

Calcium Intake—Postmenopausal and Senile Osteoporosis. Although the pathogenesis of osteoporosis remains unclear, investigators have suggested that there may be two processes within the syndrome. Type I, or postmenopausal osteoporosis, is suggested as occurring within 15–20 y of menopause and is clinically observed as the vertebral crush fracture or Colles fracture. Type II, or senile osteoporosis, reflects changes in bone status with aging and is not as likely to be associated with hypersensitivity associated with estrogen loss after cessation of the menses. Clinically, this stage is suggested by the increased hip fracture rate after age 70.[8] Whether two separate processes underlie bone loss of aging is not established. Moreover, the response to dietary or supplemental calcium intake may be different if two processes are operational.

Several lines of evidence were initially proposed to suggest that calcium deficiency was responsible for bone loss with aging. The statement from the Consensus Development Conference on Osteoporosis[9] cited national food consumption surveys indicating that the average daily intake of calcium for American women was 450–550 mg, an amount substantially lower than the Recommended Dietary Allowance (RDA) of 800 mg. The statement also drew upon the balance studies reported by Heaney et al.,[10,11] which suggested that estrogen-treated and premenopausal women could come into calcium balance with an intake of 1000 mg calcium/d whereas nontreated postmenopausal women could come into balance with an intake of 1500 mg calcium/d.

Equally notable was the Yugoslav study[5] that described greater bone mass and significantly fewer fractures in a population residing in a dairying region as compared with a nondairying region. In 1982 Heaney et al.[12] pointed out that although regional differences in bone mass and fracture were observed, the difference was associated with an effect during maximal bone mineralization; high calcium consumption did not appear to generate an additional effect in the postmenopausal period. In attempting to replicate the concept of the Yugoslav study, Sowers et al.[13] observed that postmenopausal women living in a community with a mean content of 350 mg calcium/L in the community water supply had no different bone mass than those living in a community whose water supply provided <60 mg calcium/L. When total calcium intake, including water, supplements, and food, were considered, calcium was not observed to have an independent effect on bone mass. Only when postmenopausal women had sufficient calcium and vitamin D, as determined by

comparison with the RDA, was a greater bone mass observed.

The issue of dietary calcium deficiency as a factor in bone loss was addressed in several clinical trials (Table 1). The results were inconclusive and plagued by deficiencies in study design. Notable among the design deficiencies are the failure to determine total calcium intake, which includes food and water as well as supplements; lack of adequate sample size to detect a difference if it existed; and failure to randomize or to use matched treated and control groups. Study populations may not be homogeneous with regard to age of individuals, time since onset of menopause, and potential type of osteoporotic process. These factors make the issue of effective randomization or matching even more critical.

The lack of consistency of findings from the clinical trials suggests that calcium supplementation as an effective intervention agent for bone loss in postmenopausal women is suspect. However, there has been very little investigation of potential synergistic effects of calcium supplementation along with other therapeutic modalities. For example, Ettinger et al.[23] reported an additive effect on prevention of bone loss when calcium supplementation was given to women receiving hormone replacement therapy following natural menopause. Although another investigation did not replicate this work, this approach may be a fruitful avenue of exploration.[24]

Inadequate Dietary Calcium Absorption. Although calcium status is certainly influenced by dietary intake, calcium absorption is equally critical. Absorption is determined by the interaction of calcium with other substances in the intestine, the chemical configuration of the calcium product relative to the stomach and intestinal environment, and the level of both passive and active transport across the gut wall. Because change in bone status is a relatively inefficient way to assess calcium absorption, we will not address this issue in detail in this chapter but refer the reader to Chapter 24.

Some investigators suggest that bone loss is a reflection of both marginal calcium intake and impaired calcium absorption with aging. It has been observed that the body can adapt to a wide range of calcium intakes by adjusting the amount of calcium absorbed; however, there appears to be increasing compromise in calcium absorption with aging.[25,26] The adaptive process is accomplished by increasing the fraction of calcium available for absorption when intake is low and reducing active transport when consumption is high.[27] Thus, the absolute amount of calcium absorbed is a function of both intake and rate of absorption. Although absorption may be decreased with greater intakes, the absolute amount of calcium crossing the gut wall may be higher in those consuming a high-calcium diet.

Table 1. Some trials of calcium supplementation

Reference	Date	Subjects	Dose	Duration (y)	Bone mass measurement	Significant improvement	Randomized	Blinded
14	1975	17 Controls 12 Cases Postmenopausal women	750 mg +400 IU vit D	3	X-ray density	No	No	No
15	1977	20 Controls 20 Cases Postmenopausal women	1000 mg	2	Single photon	No	Yes	No
16	1977	18 Controls 24 Cases Postmenopausal women	800 mg	1–2 1/2	Single photon	No	No	No
17	1978	20 Controls 20 Cases Postmenopausal women	800 mg	1	X ray	No	Yes	No
18	1980	41 Controls 20 Cases Postmenopausal women with vertebral fractures	1200 mg	Variable	X ray	No	No	No
19	1981	18 Controls 10 Treated 80–82 y	750 mg	3	Single	Yes	Yes	Yes
20	1982	46 Controls 27 Treated	575–1000 mg (some vit D)	Variable	Vertebral compression	Yes	No	Yes
21	1984	103 Treated in three groups Young postmeno-pausal women	500 mg + food	2	Single photon	No	No	No
22	1987	52 Controls 158 Cases Postmenopausal women	1000–1250 mg	9 mo	Single photon	Yes	No	No

Excretory Loss of Calcium. The primary excretion routes for calcium are through the feces and urine. Renal regulation of urinary calcium excretion has been of substantial interest because excess urinary loss has been associated with lower bone mass and increased hip fractures. Increasing the level of protein in the diet appears to increase the amount of urinary calcium excretion. Hegsted[28] suggested a positive association between protein intake and hip fracture incidence. The mechanism for calcium loss resulting from high protein intakes is still under investigation. Work by Tshope and Ritz[29] suggests that by reducing the amount of dietary sulfur-containing amino acids, calcium excretion can be reduced. The potentially adverse effects of high-protein diets have been suggested as a mechanism to support the observations of differential bone mass levels in vegetarian and nonvegetarian populations.[30]

The importance of urinary calcium excretion is also supported by recent studies in men and women using thiazide medications. Renal calcium retention promoted by thiazide-based antihypertensive medications is associated with greater bone mass.[13,31]

Vitamin D

Potentially, vitamin D may be associated with both major skeletal diseases, osteoporosis and osteomalacia. As discussed in Chapter 12, vitamin D precursors from skin epithelial tissue and food are hydroxylated in the liver to the 25-hydroxyvitamin D; this product then is hydroxylated in the kidney to the hormonally active form, 1,25-dihydroxyvitamin D. The active form interacts with a receptor in the cytosol of the intestinal epithelial cell and is transferred to the nucleus, promoting the synthesis of RNA for calcium-binding protein. The net effect is increased intestinal absorption of calcium.

Reports on levels of the hormonally active 1,25-dihydroxyvitamin D in persons with greater age, persons with lower bone mass, persons with osteoporosis, or persons with fracture are ambiguous. Both abnormal[32–34] and normal levels[35–37] of 1,25-dihydroxyvitamin D associated with aging and bone loss were reported. For example, Christiansen and Rodbro[37] report no difference in 1,25-dihydroxyvitamin D levels among population-based groups of early postmenopausal women (postmenopausal women losing bone rapidly) and older women with and without fracture. In contrast, Tsai et al.[38] reported a substantial contrast in 1,25-dihydroxyvitamin D values when younger women were compared with women older than 70 y. The differences observed between age groups appear to be related to menopause rather than age per se.

It was suggested that an age-related decline in quantity or efficiency of 1,25-dihydroxyvitamin D is of sufficient magnitude to contribute to negative calcium balance and potentially to promote osteoporosis (M.F.R. Sowers, R.B. Wallace, B.W. Hollis, and J.H. Lemke, unpublished observations, 1989).[31,39] Kidney function declines with age[40] and may be related to the observed impairment of intestinal calcium absorption with age.[1,41–43] One mechanism for lowered calcium absorption might be impaired 1-alpha hydroxylation of 25-dihydroxyvitamin D in the kidney to its hormonally active form, substantially impeding production of a calcium-binding protein. Other mechanisms might include alteration in secondary factors related to the 1,25-dihydroxyvitamin D response to serum calcium.[44]

There is speculation that mild to moderate vitamin D deficiency leading to occult osteomalacia may contribute significantly to the excess bone loss and fracture observed in Caucasian women.[45] This speculation is supported, in part, by the observation that vitamin D intake was lower in patients with femoral neck fracture than in control subjects.[46] It was observed that in countries where vitamin D deficiency and osteomalacia are widespread, hip fractures are commonly reported.[47,48] Parfitt et al.[45] observed that approximately one-third of patients in a nursing home have serum 25-hydroxyvitamin D levels characteristic of osteomalacia. However, a population-based study indicated that 2% of postmenopausal women had serum vitamin D and alkaline phosphatase levels indicative of osteomalacia.[49] These data suggest that the effects of vitamin D deficiency resulting in osteomalacia may be observed in populations identified as having low bone mass and fracture. Studies of low bone mass and fracture fail to discriminate whether low bone mass is attributable to osteoporosis, osteomalacia, or both.

Fluoride

Fluoride has also been associated with both the promotion and prevention of skeletal diseases.

Chronic ingestion of fluoride leads to its accumulation in skeletal tissue, with the fluoride ion substituting for the hydroxyl ion. This substitution results in conversion of hydroxyapatite to fluorapatite.[50,51]

A positive influence of fluoride on bone mass was suggested by studies of the 1950s and 1960s, when radiography was the primary technology for studying bone mass. Leone et al.[52] examined a limited number of residents (age 45+) twice in 10 y in two communities in which the water supplies contained either 0.4 or 8 mg fluoride/L. Fewer cases of osteoporosis were reported from the higher-fluoride area than from the lower-fluoride area. These same investigators observed a much higher incidence of osteoporosis in Framingham, MA, where the water had only trace amounts of fluoride, than in several west Texas communities where water fluoride concentrations were much higher.[53] Unfortunately, the study populations were poorly described, and there was no adjustment for confounding factors such as exposure to sunlight, race, ethnicity, and dietary pattern.

Bernstein et al.[54] contrasted lumbar roentgenograms from 300 male and female volunteers living in areas of southwest North Dakota, where water fluoride ranged from 4 to 5.8 mg/L, with roentgenograms from 715 men and women from northeast North Dakota living in areas with water fluoride <0.3 mg/L. The percent with decreased radiographic bone density and with one or more collapsed vertebrae was greater in women aged ≥55 y who lived in the low-fluoride area ($p < 0.01$). Men had more collapsed vertebrae than women, but frequency in men was not associated with type of water consumed.

Recent work suggests that the level of fluoride required to produce an increase in bone mass vs. fluorosis is ill defined. It appears that bone generated by excess fluoride may be architecturally unsound and susceptible to increased fracture. Leone et al.[53] found that 10% of lifelong residents of a community in which the fluoride content of the water supply was 8 mg/L developed osteosclerosis. A more recent study found significantly increased numbers of fractures in a community in which the fluoride content of the water supply was 4 mg/L as compared with communities where the fluoride content of the water supply was 1 mg/L.[55] Some investigators using sodium fluoride therapy for treatment of osteoporosis report defective mineralized bone.[56,57]

Appropriate levels of fluoride to promote osteoblastic activity without producing osteosclerosis are complicated by individual response. Riggs et al.[20] reported that almost 40% of osteoporotic patients treated with sodium fluoride were nonresponsive. This differential response was not explained by variations in the severity of the osteoporosis or the fluoride dose. Other nutrients from diet and/or diet supplements may contribute to the variability of fluoride response. Fluoride is cleared via the kidney, fecal excretion, and bone uptake. Greater calcium intake partially blocks the intestinal absorption of fluoride, promotes fecal excretion, and results in lessened bone uptake.[58] Inadequate calcium intake secondary to greater fluoride intake resulted in defective mineralized bone in kittens.[59]

Summary

Studies of food and water intake as a source of nutrients including calcium, vitamin D, and fluoride suggest important roles for these nutrients in relation to bone mass. The relationship between these nutrients and specific diseases including osteoporosis and osteomalacia may be difficult to ascertain when either the nutrient exposure is not well characterized or when the disease outcome is not well characterized. Much additional work is needed to describe the relative influence of nutrient intake at different stages of the life cycle as well as the interactive nature between each of the three nutrients and bone. Investigators also need to determine whether they are evaluating impact of nutritional status on osteoporosis, osteomalacia, or other metabolic bone diseases. Future investigations also appear promising in the area of other minerals, such as aluminum[60] and boron,[61] and other vitamins, including vitamin A and vitamin C.

References

1. L.V. Avioli and S.M. Krane (1977) *Metabolic Bone Disease,* vol. 1, Academic Press, New York.
2. H.F. Newton-John and D.B. Morgan (1968) Osteoporosis: disease of senescence? *Lancet* 1:323–333.
3. M.F.R. Sowers, R.B. Wallace, and J.H. Lemke (1985) Correlates of forearm bone mass among women during maximal bone mineralization. *Prev. Med.* 14:585–596.
4. R.B. Sandler, C.W. Slemenda, R.E. LaPorte, et al. (1985) Postmenopausal bone density and milk consumption in childhood and adolescence. *Am. J. Clin. Nutr.* 42:270–274.
5. V. Matkovic, K. Kostial, I. Simonovic, R. Buzina, A. Brodarec, and B.E.C. Nordin (1979) Bone statues and fracture rates in two regions of Yugoslavia. *Am. J. Clin. Nutr.* 32:540–549.
6. R. Sinha, J.C. Smith, and J.H. Soares (1988) The effect of dietary calcium on bone metabolism in young and aged female rats using a short-term in vivo model. *J. Nutr.* 118:1217–1222.
7. B. Kanders, D.W. Dempster, and R. Lindsay (1988) Interaction of calcium nutrition and physical activity on bone mass in young women. *J. Bone Min. Res.* 3:145–149.
8. B.L. Riggs and L.J. Melton (1983) Evidence for two distinct syndromes of involutional osteoporosis. *Am. J. Med.* 75:899–901.
9. National Institutes of Health (1984) *Statement of the Consensus Development Conference on Osteoporosis.* DHHS Publication no. (PHS) 421-132, vol. 5, no. 3, U.S. Government Printing Office, Washington, DC.
10. R.P. Heaney, R.R. Recker, and P.D. Saville (1978) Menopausal changes in calcium balanced performance. *J. Lab. Clin. Med.* 92:953–963.
11. R.P. Heaney, R.R. Recker, and P.D. Saville (1977) Calcium balance and calcium requirements in middle-age women. *Am. J. Clin. Nutr.* 30:1603–1611.
12. R.P. Heaney, J.C. Gallagher, C.C. Johnston, et al. (1982) Calcium nutrition and bone health in the elderly. *Am. J. Clin. Nutr.* 36:986–1013.
13. M.F.R. Sowers, R.B. Wallace, and J.H. Lemke (1985) Correlates of mid-radius bone density among postmenopausal women: a community study. *Am. J. Clin. Nutr.* 41:1045–1053.
14. A.A. Albanese, A.H. Edelson, E.J. Lorenze, et al. (1975) Problems of bone health in the elderly. *N.Y. State Med. J.* 75:326–336.
15. R.R. Recker, P.D. Daville, and R.P. Heany (1977) Effect of estrogens and calcium carbonate on bone loss in postmenopausal women. *Ann. Intern. Med.* 87:649–655.
16. A. Horsman, J.C. Gallagher, M. Simpson, et al. (1977) Prospective trial of oestrogen and calcium in postmenopausal women. *Br. Med. J.* 2:789–792.
17. B. Lamke, H.E. Sjoberg, and M. Sylven (1978) Bone mineral content in women in Colles' fracture: effect of calcium supplementation. *Acta. Orthop. Scand.* 49:143–149.
18. B. Nordin, A. Horsman, R. Crilly, et al. (1980) Treatment of spinal osteoporosis in postmenopausal women. *Br. Med. J.* 280:451–454.
19. E.L. Smith, W. Reddan, and P.E. Smith (1981) Physical activity and calcium modalities for bone mineral increase in aged women. *Med. Sci. Sports Exerc.* 13:60–64.
20. B. Riggs, E. Seeman, S. Hodgson, et al. (1982) Effect of the fluoride/calcium regimen on vertebral fracture occurrence in postmenopausal osteoporosis. *N. Engl. J. Med.* 306:446–450.
21. L. Nilas, C. Christiansen, and P. Rodbro (1984) Calcium supplementation and postmenopausal bone loss. *Br. Med. J.* 289:1103–1106.
22. K.J. Polley, B.E.C. Nordin, P.A. Baghurst, C.J. Walker, and B.E. Chatterton (1987) Effect of calcium supplementation on forearm bone mineral content in postmenopausal women: a prospective, sequential controlled trial. *J. Nutr.* 117:1929–1935.
23. B. Ettinger, H.K. Genant, and C.E. Cann (1987) Post menopausal bone loss prevented by treatment with low dose estrogen and calcium. *Ann. Intern. Med.* 106:40–45.
24. J.C. Stevenson, M.I. Whitehead, M. Padwick, et al. (1988) Dietary intake of calcium and postmenopausal bone loss. *Br. Med. J.* 297:15–17.
25. R.P. Heaney and R.R. Recker (1986) Distribution of calcium absorption in middle aged women. *Am. J. Clin. Nutr.* 43:299–305.
26. M. Horowitz, J. Wishart, L. Mundy, and C. Nordine (1987) Lactose in calcium absorption in post-menopausal osteoporosis. *Arch. Intern. Med.* 147:534–536.
27. H. Spencer and L. Kramer (1986) Factors contributing to osteoporosis. *J. Nutr.* 116:316–319.
28. D.M. Hegsted (1986) Calcium and osteoporosis. *J. Nutr.* 116:2316–2319.
29. W. Tshope and E. Ritz (1985) Sulfur containing amino acids are a major determinate of urinary calcium. *Min. Electrol. Metab.* 11:137–139.
30. J.J.B. Anderson and R.A. Tylavsky (1984) Diet and osteopinia in elderly caucasian women. In: *Osteoporosis 1. Copenhagen International Symposium on Osteoporosis* (C. Christiansen, C.D. Arnaud, B.E.C. Nordin, A.M. Parfitt, W.A. Peck, and B.L. Riggs, eds.), pp. 299–303, Department Clinical Chemistry, Glostrup Hospital, Copenhagen.
31. R.D. Wasnich, R.J. Benfante, K. Yano, L. Heilbrun, and J.M. Vogel (1983) Thiazide effect on the mineral content of bone. *N. Engl. J. Med.* 309:344–347.
32. J.C. Gallagher, B.L. Riggs, J. Eisman, A. Hamstra, S.B. Arnaud, and H.F. DeLuca (1979) Intestinal calcium absorption and serum vitamin D metabolites in normal subjects and osteoporotic patients. *J. Clin. Invest.* 69:729–736.
33. S. Lawoyin, J.E. Zerwekh, K. Glass, and C.Y.C. Pak (1980) Ability of 25-dihydroxyvitamin D_3 therapy to augment serum 1,25- and

24,25-dihydroxyvitamin D in postmenopausal women. *J. Clin. Endocrinol. Metab.* 50:593–596.

34. D.M. Slovik, J.S. Adams, R.M. Neer, M.F. Holick, and J.T. Potts (1981) Deficient production of 1,25-dihydroxyvitamin D in elderly osteoporotic patients. *N. Engl. J. Med.* 304:372–374.

35. M.R. Haussler, M.K. Drezner, J.W. Pike, J.S. Chandler, and L.A. Hagan (1979) Assay of 1,25-dihydroxyvitamin D and other active vitamin D metabolites in serum: application to animals and humans. In: *Vitamin D: Basic Research and Its Clinical Application* (A.W. Norman, K. Schaefer, D.V. Herrath, et al., eds.), pp. 189–196, de Gruyter, Berlin.

36. B.E.C. Nordin, M. Peacock, R.G. Crilly, G. Taylor, and D.H. Marshall (1986) Plasma 25-hydroxy and 1,25-dihydroxyvitamin D levels and calcium absorption in post-menopausal women. In: *Molecular Endocrinology* (I. MacIntyre and M. Szelke, eds.), pp. 63–94, Elsevier/North Holland, Amsterdam.

37. C. Christiansen and P. Rodbro (1984) Serum vitamin D metabolites in younger and elderly postmenopausal women. *Calcif. Tissue Int.* 36:19–24.

38. K.S. Tsai, H. Heath, R. Kumar, and B.L. Riggs (1984) Impaired vitamin D metabolism with aging in women: possible role in pathogenesis of senile osteoporosis. *J. Clin. Invest.* 73:1668–1672.

39. O.H. Sorenson, B. Lumholtz, B. Lund, et al. (1982) Acute effects of parathyroid hormone on vitamin D metabolism in patients with bone loss of aging. *J. Clin. Endocrinol. Metab.* 54:1258–1261.

40. D.F. Davies and N.W. Shock (1950) Age changes in glomerular filtration rate (ERPS) and tubular resorption capacity in adult males. *J. Clin. Invest.* 29:491–507.

41. L.V. Avioli, J.E. McDonald, and S.W. Lee (1965) The influence of age on the intestinal absorption of ^{47}Ca in women and its relation of ^{47}Ca absorption in postmenopausal osteoporosis. *J. Clin. Invest.* 44:1960–1967.

42. D.D. Alevizaki, D. Ikkos, and P. Singhelakis (1973) Progressive decrease of true intestinal calcium absorption with age in normal man. *J. Nucl. Med.* 14:760–762.

43. J.R. Bullamore, J.C. Gallagher, R. Wilkinson, B.E.C. Nordin, and D.H. Marshall (1970) Effects of age on calcium absorption. *Lancet* 2:535–537.

44. B.L. Riggs, A. Hanstra, and H.F. DeLuca (1981) Assessment of 25-dihydroxyvitamin D 1-alpha hydroxylase reserve in postmenopausal osteoporosis by administration of parathyroid extract. *J. Clin. Endocrinol. Metab.* 53:833–835.

45. A.M. Parfitt, B. Chir, J.C. Gallagher, et al. (1982) Vitamin D and bone health in the elderly. *Am. J. Clin. Nutr.* 36:1014–1031.

46. M.R. Baker, H. McDonnell, M. Peacock, and B.E.C. Nordin (1979) Plasma 25-hydroxy vitamin D concentration in patients with fractures of the femoral neck. *Lancet* 1:589–590.

47. J. Chalmers, W.D.H. Conacher, D.L. Gardner, and P.J. Scott (1967) Osteomalacia—a common disease in elderly women. *J. Bone Joint Surg.* [Am] 49B:403–423.

48. H. Vaishnava and S.N.A. Rizvi (1974) Frequency of osteomalacia and osteoporosis in fractures of proximal femur. *Lancet* 1:676–677.

49. M.F.R. Sowers, R.B. Wallace, B.W. Hollis, and J.H. Lemke (1986) Parameters related to 20-OH-D levels in a population-based study of women. *Am. J. Clin. Nutr.* 43:621–628.

50. H.C. Hodge and F.A. Smith (1965) Biological effects of inorganic fluorides. In: *Fluorine Chemistry* (J.H. Simmons, ed.), pp. 155–171, Academic Press, New York.

51. E.D. Eanes, I. Zipkin, and R.A. Harper (1965) Small-angle x-ray diffraction analysis of the effect of fluoride on human bone apatite. *Arch. Oral Biol.* 10:161–173.

52. N.C. Leone, C.A. Stevenson, T.F. Hilbish, and M.C. Sosman (1955) Roentgenologic study of a human population exposed to high-fluoride domestic water: a ten year study. *Am. J. Roentgenol. Radium Ther. Nucl. Med.* 74:874–875.

53. N.C. Leone, C.A. Stevenson, B. Besse, L.E. Hawes, and T.R. Dawber (1960) The effects of the absorption of fluoride. *Arch. Ind. Health* 21:326–327.

54. D.S. Bernstein, N. Sadowsky, D.M. Hegsted, G.D. Guri, and F.J. Stare (1966) Prevalence of osteoporosis in high- and low-fluoride areas in North Dakota. *JAMA* 198:499–504.

55. M.F.R. Sowers, R.B. Wallace, and J.H. Lemke (1986) Bone mass in three communities: a study of calcium and fluoride intake. *Am. J. Clin. Nutr.* 44:889–898.

56. V.H. Vigorita, J.M. Lane, and E. Schwartz (1984) Is fluoride bone osteomalacic: a histomorphometric analysis. In: *Osteoporosis. Proceedings of Copenhagen International Symposium on Osteoporosis* (C. Christiansen, C.D. Arnaud, B.E.C. Nordin, A.M. Parfitt, W.A. Peck, B.L. Riggs, eds.), pp. 635–638, Glostrup Hospital, Copenhagen.

57. E.F. Eriksen, L. Mosekilde, and F. Melsen (1984) Effect of sodium fluoride, calcium phosphate and vitamin D_2 for 5 years on bone balance and remodeling in osteoporosis. In: *Osteoporosis. Proceedings of the Copenhagen International Symposium on Osteoporosis* (C. Christiansen, C.D. Arnaud, B.E.C. Nordin, A.M. Parfitt, W.A. Peck, and B.L. Riggs, eds), pp. 659–663, Glostrup Hospital, Copenhagen.

58. B.L. Riggs (1978) Effect of concurrent calcium ingestion on intestinal absorption of fluoride. *Metabolism* 27:971–974.

59. J.M. Burkhart and J. Jowsey (1968) Effect of variations in calcium intake on the skeleton of fluoride-fed kittens. *J. Lab. Clin. Med.* 72:943–950.

60. S.M. Ott, N.A. Maloney, G.L. Klein, et al. (1983) Aluminum is associated with low bone formation in patients receiving chronic parenteral nutrition. *Ann. Intern. Med.* 98:910–914.

61. F.H. Nielsen, C.D. Hunt, L.M. Mullen, and J.R. Hunt (1987) Effect of dietary boron on mineral, estrogen, and testosterone metabolism in postmenopausal women. *FASEB J.* 1:394–397.

Chapter 45

Saulo Klahr

Renal Disease

The hallmark of chronic renal disease is a decrease in glomerular filtration rate (GFR). This decrease may occur through three major mechanisms: (1) a decrease in single-nephron filtration rate (the filtration rate per nephron in humans is 60 nL/min for a total GFR of 120 mL/min, assuming 1 million nephrons in each of the two kidneys); (2) a decrease in the number of functional nephrons; or (3) most likely a combination of these two events. The progressive loss of nephrons affects most of the functions of the kidney summarized in Table 1. As GFR falls solutes that are excreted by the kidney preferentially by filtration (urea, creatinine) accumulate in body fluids and concentrations in plasma increase.[1] Indeed, the plasma concentration of urea and creatinine provides a crude measurement of the decrease in GFR. As GFR falls to values <25% of normal ($\sim$ 30 mL/min), other solutes that are either filtered and reabsorbed or secreted by the renal tubules may also accumulate in body fluids.[1,2] These solutes include phosphate, sulfate, uric acid, magnesium, and hydrogen and result in the development of metabolic acidosis. Finally, a number of other compounds are retained in body fluids when renal disease is far advanced. These compounds include phenols, guanidines, organic acids, indoles, a number of metabolic products, and certain peptides. Some of these solutes may be toxic at certain concentrations and could contribute to the symptoms and signs of advanced chronic renal insufficiency (uremia).

As renal function decreases, the ability of the patients to respond rapidly to changes in dietary intake, particularly of sodium, potassium, and water, is markedly restricted.[1,2] Although the excretion of solute and water per nephron increases as renal function decreases, the fewer the number of functional nephrons, the smaller is the range of solute or water excretion achievable by the composite nephron population. Thus, the upper limit of excretion for many solutes and for water is less in patients with renal insufficiency than that achieved in normal subjects.

There is also a restriction on the minimum amount of sodium and water that may be excreted. As renal disease progresses there is decreased flexibility in response to changes in the intakes of sodium, other solutes, and water.[1,2] Therefore, the volume and composition of the extracellular fluid compartment may change as renal function decreases.

A decrease in renal function also imposes restrictions on the dose and frequency of administration of certain drugs, particularly those in which metabolism is greatly dependent on renal excretion. Drug interactions also may be modified in patients with uremia. Two reviews were published regarding appropriate dosage for numerous drugs in patients with different levels of renal functional impairment.[3,4]

The loss of synthetic functions of the kidney also may contribute to the abnormalities seen in renal insufficiency. For example, decreased production of erythropoietin, a hormone synthesized in the kidney that plays a key role in the maturation of red blood cell precursors in bone marrow, is a major cause of the anemia seen in patients with renal disease.[5,6] Decreased synthesis of 1,25-dihydroxycholecalciferol [1,25(OH)$_2$D3], the active metabolite of cholecalciferol, by the diseased kidney results in decreased serum concentrations of this compound and may lead to decreased calcium absorption from the gastrointestinal tract.[7] Decreased concentrations of 1,25(OH)$_2$D3 also may contribute to the development of hyperparathyroidism (high concentrations of circulating parathyroid hormone) in patients with renal disease.[8]

The kidney is the main site of degradations of several peptides (β_2 microglobulin, light chains), proteins, and peptide hormones including insulin, glucagon, growth hormone, and parathyroid hormone.[9] The kidney also is involved in gluconeogenesis, the synthesis of glucose from noncarbohydrate precursors, and in lipid metabolism.[9] Failure of the kidneys, therefore, leads to multiple abnormalities that may

Table 1. Principal functions of the kidney

1. Excretion of metabolic waste products, i.e., urea, creatinine, uric acid
2. Maintenance of volume and ionic composition of body fluids
3. Elimination and detoxification of drugs and toxins
4. Regulation of systemic blood pressure
5. Production of erythropoietin
6. Endocrine control of mineral metabolism: synthesis of 1,25-dihydroxycholecalciferol and 24,25-dihydroxycholecalciferol
7. Degradation and catabolism of peptide hormones insulin, glucagon, parathyroid hormone, etc. and of small–molecular-weight proteins β_2 microglobulin and light chains
8. Metabolic interconversions: gluconeogenesis, lipid metabolism

have a marked impact on intermediary metabolism, levels of circulating hormones, and absorption of certain nutrients. In addition, as renal failure progresses anorexia, nausea, and vomiting may develop, which may further compromise adequate nutrient and energy intake. Specific abnormalities affecting nutritional status and changes requiring modifications of the diet of patients with progressive renal disease are outlined below.

Phosphate and Calcium

Phosphate excretion changes little as GFR falls, because there is a progressive decrease in tubular reabsorption of phosphate, which is mediated mainly by increased plasma concentrations of parathyroid hormone.[10] However, when GFR falls below 30 mL/min, even a marked decrease in tubular reabsorption of phosphate is not enough to overcome the substantial decrease in the filtered load. Thus, phosphate accumulates. Hyperphosphatemia, therefore, is seen commonly in patients with GFRs of ≤ 25 mL/min unless dietary phosphate is restricted.[10] It is also at this level of GFR that changes in serum calcium occur. These changes in calcium concentration presumably are related to several factors. An increase in serum phosphate produces a reciprocal decrease in serum ionized calcium. There is also evidence that the levels of 1,25(OH)$_2$D3 decrease at GFR values <30 mL/min because of decreased production of 1,25(OH)$_2$D3. The latter effect decreases absorption of calcium from the gastrointestinal tract, a phenomenon that has been documented in patients with this level of GFR.[11] The ability of parathyroid hormone to remove calcium from bone may be impaired, and this "skeletal resistance" to the action of this hormone may also contribute to the development of hypocalcemia.[12] It should be remembered that acidosis tends

to increase the fraction of plasma calcium that is in the ionized form and, thus, prevents some of the clinical consequences of hypocalcemia. Rapid correction of acidosis may decrease the concentrations of ionized calcium and cause acute manifestations of hypocalcemia, including tetany and convulsions in patients with chronic renal disease.

Evidence has accumulated to indicate that a reduction in phosphorus intake in patients with mild renal insufficiency reduces the levels of parathyroid hormone (PTH) and improves the skeletal response to the hormone.[13] Phosphorus absorption from the gastrointestinal tract can be decreased by the use of phosphate binders. Until the last few years aluminum salts (hydroxide, carbonate) were used as phosphate binders. However, it is now known that aluminum can be absorbed and may accumulate in plasma and tissues.[14] Because aluminum accumulation is toxic,[14] other phosphate-binding agents such as calcium carbonate have been introduced.[15] When prescribed as a phosphate binder, calcium carbonate should be administered with meals. Because the major sources of dietary phosphorus are mainly dairy products (milk, cheese) and meat, restriction of these foods in the diet will decrease the amount of phosphorus ingested. Dietary phosphorus can be decreased to 600–900 mg/d by reducing the protein intake, particularly by avoiding meats and dairy products.

Such protein-restricted diets often restrict calcium intake, resulting in negative calcium balance in patients with renal insufficiency. Therefore, calcium supplements of 500–1500 mg/d are recommended in such patients. When calcium supplements are given, they should be administered between meals to increase calcium absorption. The amount of the calcium supplement required depends on the size of the individual, the concentrations of serum calcium, and the gastrointestinal absorption of calcium. Several calcium salts (carbonate, gluconate, lactate, citrate, or chloride) have been used as calcium supplements. In hypocalcemic patients with GFR values <30 mL/min, administration of small doses of 1,25(OH)$_2$D3 may be necessary to increase serum calcium. Administration of 1,25(OH)$_2$D3 may reduce the circulating concentrations of PTH in patients with renal insufficiency by increasing serum calcium and by inhibiting the synthesis of PTH in the parathyroid gland.[11]

In summary, the goals of calcium and phosphorus therapy in patients with renal insufficiency are (1) to maintain plasma concentrations of phosphorus and ionized calcium within normal limits, (2) to prevent the development of secondary hyperparathyroidism or to decrease the concentrations of PTH when hyperparathyroidism is already established, and (3) to prevent or reverse skeletal disease, soft tissue calcification, pruritus, and other manifestations of abnormal calcium-phosphorus homeostasis.

Magnesium

Clinically significant hypermagnesemia is rare in patients with chronic renal insufficiency. Although the kidney is the major route of magnesium excretion, decreased magnesium reabsorption per nephron as renal failure progresses prevents marked increases in plasma concentrations of magnesium.[16] In far-advanced renal insufficiency, mild hypermagnesemia is common. Protein-restricted diets may decrease the total amount of magnesium ingested to ~200 mg/ d. Clinically important hypermagnesemia (serum magnesium concentrations >1.7–2.1 mmol/L) does not occur unless additional magnesium is taken in because of the use of antacids, enemas, or laxatives with a high magnesium content.[17] Such magnesium-containing preparations should be avoided in patients with marked renal insufficiency.

Water Excretion

Renal disease causes a progressive impairment in the urinary concentrating capacity.[18] In health the urine osmolality may be as high as 1200 mmol/kg of water, but in renal insufficiency the maximum urine osmolality approaches that of plasma (300 mmol/kg). If total solute excretion in uremic subjects remains at 600 mmol/d and maximal urine osmolality is ≤300 mmol/kg water, an obligatory water excretion of 2 L/d is necessary to eliminate the osmolar load. This obligatory excretion restricts the capacity of patients with renal insufficiency to decrease water excretion to the levels seen in normal individuals.

The upper limit of water excretion is also decreased in patients with renal insufficiency.[19] Although the ability to dilute the urine is well preserved in patients with renal disease (free water generation calculated per 100 mL of GFR is preserved), the total amount of free water that can be excreted decreases as GFR falls. For example, if water diuresis is induced in a normal person and a uremic patient and both excrete 10 mL free water/100 mL GFR, urine volume will increase in both. However, the increments will be quite different. The normal person (GFR = 120 mL/ min) can increase urine volume from 2 L isosmotic urine/d to 19.3 L dilute urine/d, whereas the uremic patient (GFR = 4 mL/min) can increase urine volume from 2 to only 2.6 L/d.

The obligatory increase in water excretion in the patient with chronic renal disease may lead to polyuria and result in the development of nocturia, a manifestation of late renal insufficiency. Occasionally, particularly when extra fluids containing dextrose and water are administered in an effort to flush the kidneys, hyponatremia can occur because of the inability of the patient with chronic renal failure to increase appropriately the excretion of water.

Sodium Excretion

As renal disease progresses fractional sodium excretion increases in a manner that is adequate to maintain external balance (Figure 1). This adaptation occurs until very late in the course of renal disease so that normal extracellular fluid volume is preserved. However, when sodium intake changes, the fractional excretion of sodium must change substantially to maintain sodium balance in the patient with chronic renal failure.[1] For example, in a normal individual, doubling sodium intake from 3.5 to 7 g/d necessitates a change in fractional excretion of sodium from 0.25% to 0.5%. The same increment in salt intake requires a change in fractional sodium excretion from 8% to 16% in a patient with a GFR of 4 mL/min. Hence, the patient with chronic renal disease can vary sodium excretion only over a rather restricted range, and this range narrows as GFR declines.[1,20] With chronic renal disease an upper and a lower limit of sodium excretion develop. The lower limit, or floor, is important because it limits the ability of patients with chronic renal disease to conserve sodium maximally, and a low-salt diet can result in a negative sodium balance with loss of a corresponding volume of water. Extracellular fluid (ECF) volume, plasma volume, and GFR all fall.

Patients with advanced renal insufficiency also cannot tolerate high intakes of sodium. If excessive

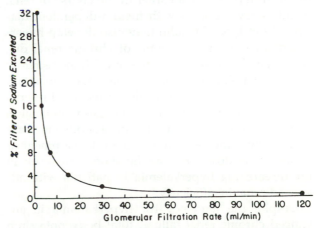

Figure 1. The patterns of sodium excretion, expressed as the percentage of filtered sodium excreted, are shown at different levels of glomerular filtration rate (from 2 to 120 mL/min) in subjects with normal renal function or chronic renal disease ingesting 7.0 g sodium chloride/d. (Reproduced with permission from reference 1.)

sodium is ingested, sodium retention with expansion of the extracellular fluid may occur and may produce or aggravate preexisting hypertension, edema, fluid overload, congestive heart failure, and pulmonary edema. Thus, the loss of flexibility for both sodium and water excretion must be carefully considered in the dietary management of patients with renal insufficiency.

Potassium

Normally, ~90–95% of ingested potassium is excreted in the urine; the remainder is excreted in the stool.[21] In chronic renal failure a greater fraction of ingested potassium is excreted in the stool with 20–50% of the ingested amount appearing in the stool when the GFR falls below 5 mL/min.[22] Potassium excretion per nephron also increases, and potassium excretion approaches and may even surpass the filtered load of potassium. In chronic renal failure, aldosterone and other factors, such as increased flow of fluid through the distal nephron, are the major mediators of increased potassium secretion in the distal tubule. Therefore, adjustments in renal mechanisms that increase potassium excretion in addition to increased stool excretion are sufficient to maintain a normal plasma and potassium balance until the GFR reaches <10 mL/min, even when the intake of potassium is normal (100 mmol/d).

Plasma potassium may increase in chronic renal disease as acidosis develops because of redistribution of potassium between intracellular and extracellular compartments.[23] Intracellular potassium leaves the cells and is replaced by hydrogen and sodium. In addition, hormonal deficiencies such as low aldosterone concentrations in hyporeninemic patients may result in hyperkalemia earlier in the course of renal insufficiency. Patients with insulin-dependent diabetes from lack of insulin may also develop hyperkalemia earlier in the course of chronic renal disease.[24] Finally, at very low rates of GFR, the secretory rate of potassium may be near maximal to maintain the steady state. Thus, very little functional reserve remains to respond to sudden changes in potassium intake. Conditions such as oliguria, a sudden increase in potassium intake, and a sudden development of metabolic acidosis or catabolic states can result in life-threatening hyperkalemia in patients with advanced renal insufficiency.

Despite the tendency for hyperkalemia in advanced chronic renal failure, total body potassium may in fact be decreased. This apparent paradox is related to the fact that the vast majority of potassium in the body is located intracellularly. Decreased intake, increased catabolism, and decreased extrusion of sodium from cells in advanced uremia can lead to decreased intracellular potassium, leading to some degree of potassium depletion despite an elevation in ECF potassium.

Emergency therapy of life-threatening hyperkalemia includes stimulation of cellular uptake of potassium by the administration of glucose and insulin or sodium bicarbonate and removal of potassium by the use of intestinal cation-exchange resins (kayexalate) or dialysis. Patients with advanced chronic renal failure should be advised to restrict the intake of foods rich in potassium, such as citrus fruits, avocados, beans, figs, and bananas. It should be kept in mind that patients on low-sodium diets and using salt substitutes may develop hyperkalemia from the high potassium content of some salt substitutes.

Acid-base Balance

The contribution of the kidneys to the preservation of acid-base balance in normal persons requires the reabsorption of the daily filtered load of ~4000 mmol of bicarbonate and the excretion of 50–100 mmol of hydrogen ions in the form of ammonium and titratable acid (H$^+$ bound to phosphate and other buffer ions).[25] In acid-base regulations as with many other nephron functions, there are remarkable compensatory responses by the residual functioning kidney mass as overall renal function declines. Except for a small group of patients with hyperchloremic acidosis, most subjects with renal disease do not show significant acidemia attributable to renal disease per se until the GFR falls below roughly 20% of normal.[25] Although plasma bicarbonate concentration may be depressed at higher levels of GFR, blood pH remains normal or is only barely depressed because of ventilatory compensation. Even when GFR falls below 20 mL/min, the extent of acidosis is highly variable. Causes of this variability include the nature of the renal disease, diet, intake of acidic ion salts, extracellular volume status, potassium balance, and efficiency of respiratory compensation.[25]

Because metabolism of proteins is the major source of hydrogen, dietary protein restriction or efforts to decrease endogenous catabolism, if present, will markedly decrease the generation of hydrogen.[26] Phospholipids contribute to a smaller degree to the generation of hydrogen. Bicarbonate salts may be administered orally to correct the metabolic acidosis of renal insufficiency. It should be remembered that low plasma levels of phosphate may lead to decreased titratable acid excretion and aggravation of the metabolic acidosis of uremia.

Nitrogen Metabolism and Protein Intake

In the early 1900s it was noted that ingestion of protein aggravated the clinical symptoms of patients with renal failure. Ambard[27] observed that uremic individuals were often wasted and did poorly particularly after ingestion of a meal containing meat. These initial clinical correlations suggested that uremic toxicity could be ameliorated by reducing the amount of protein in the diet. Volhard[28] noticed that "in patients with chronic renal insufficiency a reduction in nitrogen intake to levels of 3–5 grams per day (about 20–30 grams of protein) prevents the rise in blood urea for long periods of time; . . . considerably elevated urea, indican and xanthoprotein values decrease and initial signs of uremic intoxication disappear." These and subsequent observations clearly established that restriction of dietary protein in patients with advanced renal insufficiency improves many of the uremic symptoms. In the last decade or so there has also been a great deal of interest in the potential effect of low-protein diets on renal function and on the progression of renal disease in humans.[29] However, definitive evidence that dietary protein restriction ameliorates or halts the progression of renal disease in humans is still lacking.

Blood urea levels and particularly urea production (usually measured as the total excretion of urea nitrogen in a 24-h urine collection) have been used to estimate protein intake. However, increased tissue catabolism and degradation of endogenous protein may also increase urea production. Inadequate energy intake, acidosis, intercurrent infections, sodium depletion, or excess glucocorticoid secretion may result in increased urea nitrogen in patients with renal insufficiency. Metabolic acidosis may be responsible for the abnormal metabolism of branched-chain amino acids in uremia.[30,31] Metabolic acidosis significantly decreased the levels of branched-chain amino acids in plasma and muscle and increased the oxidation of valine and leucine. Correction of the acidosis by sodium bicarbonate administration diminishes protein catabolism and the altered metabolism of branched-chain amino acids observed in uremia.[31,32]

It has not been clearly established at what point in the course of progressive renal insufficiency protein restriction should be initiated. It seems prudent to restrict protein to prevent an elevation of blood urea nitrogen (BUN) > 35.7 mmol/L, and perhaps BUN values < 25 mmol/L should be the goal.[33] Certainly in patients with GFR values < 20–25 mL/min, some degree of protein restriction is recommended to ameliorate symptoms of uremia. Protein intake should be restricted to ~0.6 g protein/kg standard body weight. However, in patients with GFR values < 10 mL/min some clinicians have utilized diets providing ~0.3 g protein/kg body weight supplemented with keto acids or amino acids. Protein restriction alone may not prevent uremic symptoms in patients with

GFR values < 5 mL/min. The potential problem of inducing malnutrition by prolonged protein restriction should be considered, and the nutritional status of patients should be carefully evaluated at periodic intervals.[34]

Protein malnutrition of severe degree is less common today than two decades ago when dialysis facilities were in short supply. A combination of inadequate energy intake because of anorexia and rigid reduction of protein intake over many months yielded patients with marked wasting. Patients were often 15–30% below customary weight during the early phase of dialysis after edema fluid had been removed. The nutritional status of patients with end-stage renal disease and those treated by dialysis no doubt has been greatly improved in recent years because of early initiation of dialysis and better application of nutritional knowledge. However, a number of observations indicate that a lesser but still significant degree of protein malnutrition still may be prevalent.[35] Extravascular pools of albumin may be reduced even though serum albumin concentration remains normal. Serum concentration of transferrin, possibly a more sensitive indicator of protein malnutrition, has been found to be low in many patients with moderate-to-advanced renal failure and was also subnormal in a group of patients on chronic dialysis despite ingestion of 1 g protein$\cdot$kg$^{-1}\cdot$d^{-1}.[36] Although inadequate protein or energy intake or both may be the major cause of malnutrition in chronic renal failure, the possibility that one or more steps in the complex process of protein synthesis are disturbed by renal failure per se has not received sufficient study. This possibility is supported by the finding of reduced alkali-soluble protein in muscle from patients with only moderate renal failure.

Energy Turnover

A gradual onset of anorexia in chronic renal failure leads to inadequate energy intake.[36,37] In adults this change leads to loss of adipose tissue, utilization of body proteins, and diversion of dietary protein for use as fuel. In children an energy deficit contributes to impaired growth. Although few measurements have been made, it is a general clinical observation that both mental and physical activity progressively decline in advancing uremia and remain impaired in some patients on dialysis. There has been some success in improving energy intake, especially by patients on long-term hemodialysis. There is, unfortunately, little information on energy turnover at the cellular level in chronic renal failure. Adenosine triphosphate (ATP) levels are elevated in erythrocytes, whereas phosphorylating activity and ATPase activity may be reduced, suggesting decreased energy turnover.

The protein and energy requirements of patients with end-stage renal disease undergoing maintenance dialysis are somewhat different.[38,39] It has been suggested that patients on maintenance hemodialysis should receive 1.2 g protein/kg body weight. Patients on continuous ambulatory peritoneal dialysis who have protein and amino acid losses into the dialysate should receive diets containing ~1.5 g protein/kg body weight. Energy requirements in these individuals are usually adequate because glucose dialysate solutions are used, and enough glucose is absorbed from the peritoneal cavity. In general, hemodialysis patients as well as predialysis patients with chronic renal failure[40] should receive 35 kcal/kg standard body weight.

Lipid Metabolism

Lipid abnormalities are common in patients with chronic renal disease, particularly those with the nephrotic syndrome.[41] This syndrome is characterized by heavy proteinuria (mainly albuminuria), hypoalbuminemia, high levels of serum cholesterol, and variable degrees of edema. Hyperlipidemia type IV, with low levels of high-density lipoproteins (HDLs), is common in patients with chronic uremia and in patients undergoing maintenance hemodialysis.[42–44] Cardiovascular disease is a major cause of death in long-term hemodialysis patients. Many of the known risk factors for the development of atherosclerosis and coronary artery disease are present in these patients, including hypertension, cigarette smoking, reduced levels of HDL cholesterol, hypertriglyceridemia, hyperinsulinemia, glucose intolerance, stress, and a sedentary lifestyle.

Hypertriglyceridemia is the most common lipid abnormality in patients with chronic renal failure.[44,45] Patients exhibit increased very-low-density-lipoprotein (VLDL) triglyceride, reduced HDL cholesterol, and an increased ratio of low-density-lipoprotein (LDL) cholesterol to HDL cholesterol. The primary defect is a reduction in the removal of triglyceride-rich lipoproteins caused by reductions in lipoprotein lipase and hepatic lipase activities. Reduction in dietary carbohydrate and increase in the ratio of polyunsaturated to saturated fatty acids are effective in lowering plasma triglyceride levels.[43] However, lipid-lowering drugs such as clofibrate or carnitine may be required. In patients with the nephrotic syndrome and hypercholesterolemia, lovastatin administration effectively reduces the levels of serum cholesterol.[46] Exercise training also was shown to ameliorate hyperlipidemia in patients with chronic renal insufficiency, whereas sedentary control subjects during the same period showed a deterioration in serum lipid profile.[47]

Disorders of Carbohydrate Metabolism

Carbohydrate tolerance is impaired in uremia. This is evident after oral or intravenous glucose loads. The abnormal glucose metabolism of chronic renal failure is characterized by fasting euglycemia, abnormal glucose tolerance, delayed glucose response to insulin, hyperinsulinemia, and hyperglucagonemia.[48,49] Although some studies suggest that the abnormal glucose tolerance is caused by resistance of peripheral tissues to insulin,[50,51] the presence of insulin resistance in skeletal muscle has not been clearly established;[52,53] there may be a circulating factor that induces insulin resistance in muscle.[54] Increased growth hormone concentrations in uremia also may contribute to the resistance of peripheral tissues to insulin.

Of interest is the fact that diabetic patients who develop progressive renal disease require diminishing doses of insulin as the disease progresses. Reduced energy intake and weight loss plus a reduced degradation of insulin probably play a role in this decreased insulin requirement of diabetics with progressive renal disease.

Vitamins

There is only limited information concerning vitamin nutrition in end-stage renal disease.[55–57] Evaluation of published reports is complicated by the frequent omission of information on dietary intake of protein, use of vitamin supplements, time of sampling in relation to dialysis treatment, and intake of drugs that potentially may affect vitamin metabolism. Reduced concentrations of a number of water-soluble vitamins in serum and/or in erythrocytes and leukocytes have been reported. Hematologic evidence of folate deficiency has been found at several centers but not at others.[55,56] These differences probably reflect variations in dietary intake and use of vitamin supplements. In one report patients who were not receiving vitamin supplements had low plasma and leukocyte concentrations of vitamin C, and a few patients had signs suggestive of mild scurvy. The plasma concentrations of other water-soluble vitamins were normal in most reports. Because the kidney is one route of elimination of water-soluble vitamins and their metabolites, decreased elimination by the kidney may be a protective mechanism, especially for patients on hemodialysis in whom removal of water-soluble vitamins may occur during the procedure. Different from water-soluble vitamins, the serum concentrations of retinol (vitamin A) and retinol-binding protein are increased in patients with renal failure.[57–59]

Trace Elements

The possible existence of deficiency of essential trace elements and of toxic accumulation of essential or nonessential trace elements was suggested in end-stage renal disease.[60–63] Highly protein-bound elements such as copper and zinc are lost in excessive amounts with increased proteinuria. Current available information on trace element metabolism comes from only a few geographical areas and is fragmentary. Most of the work on trace elements has been done in patients on dialysis, and the information is even more limited for patients with end-stage renal disease before initiation of dialysis.

References

1. N.S. Bricker, S. Klahr, H. Lubowitz, and E. Slatopolsky (1971) The pathophysiology of renal insufficiency: on the functional transformation in the residual nephrons with advancing disease. Symposium on Pediatric Nephrology. *Pediatr. Clin. North Am.* 18:595–611.

2. N.S. Bricker and L.G. Fine (1980) The pathophysiology of chronic renal failure. In: *Clinical Disorders of Fluid and Electrolyte Metabolism* (M.H. Maxwell and C.R. Kleeman, eds.), pp. 799–825, McGraw Hill, New York.

3. W.M. Bennett, R.S. Muther, R.A. Parker, et al. (1980) Drug therapy in renal failure: dosing guidelines for adults. I. *Ann. Intern. Med.* 93:62–89.

4. W.M. Bennett, R.S. Muther, R.A. Parker, et al. (1980) Drug therapy in renal failure: dosing guidelines for adults. II. *Ann. Intern. Med.* 93:286–325.

5. J.W. Eschbach and J.W. Adamson (1985) Anemia of end-stage renal disease (ESRD). *Kidney Int.* 28:1–5.

6. J.W. Eschbach, J.C. Egrie, M.R. Downing, J.K. Browne, and J.W. Adamson (1987) Correction of the anemia of end-stage renal disease with recombinant human erythropoietin: results of a combined phase I and II clinical trial. *N. Engl. J. Med.* 316:73–78.

7. L. Wilson, A. Felsenfeld, M.K. Drezner, and F. Llach (1985) Altered divalent ion metabolism in early renal failure: role of 1,25(OH)$_2$D. *Kidney Int.* 27:565–573.

8. S. Madsen, K. Olgaard, and J. Ladefoged (1981) Suppressive effect of 1,25-dihydroxyvitamin D$_3$ on circulating parathyroid hormone in renal failure. *J. Clin. Endocrinol. Metab.* 53:823–827.

9. S. Klahr (1983) Nonexcretory functions of the kidney. In: *The Kidney and Body Fluids in Health and Disease* (S. Klahr, ed.), pp. 65–90, Plenum Medical Publishing Co., New York.

10. R. Goldman and S. Basset (1954) Phosphorus excretion in renal failure. *J. Clin. Invest.* 33:1623–1628.

11. D.A. Feinfeld and L.M. Sherwood (1988) Parathyroid hormone and 1,25(OH)$_2$D$_3$ in chronic renal failure. *Kidney Int.* 33:1049–1058.

12. F. Llach, S.F. Massry, F.R. Singer, K. Kurokawa, J.H. Kaye, and J.W. Coburn (1975) Skeletal resistance to endogenous parathyroid hormone in patients with early renal failure. *J. Clin. Endocrinol. Metab.* 41:339–345.

13. P.J. Somerville and M. Kaye (1979) Evidence that resistance to the calcemic action of parathyroid hormone in rats is caused by phosphate retention. *Kidney Int.* 16:552–560.

14. A.C. Alfrey (1984) Trace metals. In: *The Systemic Consequences of Renal Disease* (G. Eknoyan and J.P. Knochel, eds.), pp. 443–460, Grune and Stratton, Orlando, FL.

15. E. Slatopolsky, C. Weerts, S. Lopez-Hilker, et al. (1986) Calcium carbonate as a phosphate binder in patients with chronic renal failure undergoing dialysis. *N. Engl. J. Med.* 315:157–161.

16. T.H. Steele, S.F. Wen, M.A. Evenson, and R.E. Rieselbach (1968) The contribution of the chronically diseased kidney to magnesium homeostasis in man. *J. Lab. Clin. Med.* 71:455–463.

17. R.E. Randall, M.D. Cohen, C.C. Spray, and E.C. Rossmeisl (1964) Hypermagnesemia in renal failure. Etiology and toxic manifestations. *Ann. Intern. Med.* 61:73–88.

18. D.J. Baldwin, J.H. Berman, H.O. Heinemann, and H.W. Smith (1955) The elaboration of osmotically concentrated urine in renal disease. *J. Clin. Invest.* 34:800–807.

19. C.R. Kleeman, D.A. Adams, and M.H. Maxwell (1961) An evaluation of maximal water diuresis in chronic renal disease. *J. Lab. Clin. Med.* 58:169–184.

20. S. Klahr and E. Slatopolsky (1973) Renal regulation of sodium excretion. *Arch. Intern. Med.* 131:780–791.

21. F.S. Wright and G. Giebisch (1985) Regulation of potassium excretion. In: *The Kidney: Physiology and Pathophysiology* (D.W. Seldin and G. Giebisch, eds.), pp. 1223–1249, Raven Press, New York.

22. R.G. Schultze (1973) Recent advances in the physiology and pathophysiology of potassium excretion. *Arch. Intern. Med.* 131:885–897.

23. H.J. Adrogue and N.E. Madias (1981) Changes in plasma potassium concentrations during acute acid-base disturbances. *Am. J. Med.* 71:456–467.

24. M.J. Bia and R.T. DeFronzo (1981) Extrarenal potassium homeostasis. *Am. J. Physiol.* 240:F257–F268.

25. L.L. Hamm and S. Klahr (1984) Alterations of acid-base balance. In: *Differential Diagnosis in Renal and Electrolyte Disorders*, 2nd ed. (S. Klahr, ed.), pp. 231–250, Appleton-Century-Crofts, Norwalk, CT.

26. A. Relman, E.J. Lennon, and J. Lemman, Jr. (1961) Endogenous production of fixed acid and the measurement of the net balance of acid in normal subjects. *J. Clin. Invest.* 40:1621–1630.

27. L. Ambard (1920) *Physiologie Normale et Pathologique des Reins.* Masson et Cie, Paris.

28. F. Volhard (1918) Die doppelseitigen hämatogenen Nierenkrankungen (Bright'sche Krankheit). In: *Handbuch der Inneren Medizin* (Mohr, Stachelin, eds.), pp. 1149–1172, Springer; Berlin.

29. S. Klahr and M.L. Purkerson (1988) Effects of dietary protein on renal function and on the progression of renal disease. *Am. J. Clin. Nutr.* 47:146–152.

30. R.C. May, Y. Hara, R.A. Kelly, K.P. Block, M.G. Buse, and W.E. Mitch (1987) Branched-chain amino acid metabolism in rat muscle: abnormal regulation in acidosis. *Am. J. Physiol.* 252:E712–E718.

31. Y. Hara, R.C. May, R.A. Kelly, and W.E. Mitch (1987) Acidosis, not azotemia, stimulates branched-chain, amino acid catabolism in uremic rats. *Kidney Int.* 32:808–814.

32. N.J. Papadoyannakis, C.S. Stefanidis, and M. McGeown (1984) The effect of the correction of metabolic acidosis on nitrogen and potassium balance of patients with chronic renal failure. *Am. J. Clin. Nutr.* 40:623–627.

33. J.D. Kopple and J.W. Coburn (1974) Evaluation of chronic uremia: importance of serum urea nitrogen, serum creatinine and their ratio. *JAMA* 227:41–44.

34. M.J. Blumenkrantz, J.D. Kopple, R.A. Gutman, et al. (1980) Methods for assessing nutritional status of patients with renal failure. *Am. J. Clin. Nutr.* 33:1567–1585.

35. G. Eknoyan (1988) Effects of renal insufficiency on nutrient metabolism and endocrine function. In: *Nutrition and the Kidney* (W.E. Mitch and S. Klahr, eds.), pp. 29–58, Little Brown Co., Boston.

36. B.S. Ooi, A.F. Darocy, and V.E. Pollak (1972) Serum transferrin levels in chronic renal failure. *Nephron* 9:200–208.

37. J.D. Kopple (1978) Abnormal amino acid and protein metabolism in uremia. *Kidney Int.* 14:340–348.

38. A. Alverstrand (1988) Nutritional requirements of hemodialysis patients. In: *Nutrition and the Kidney* (W.E. Mitch and S. Klahr, eds.), pp. 180–197, Little, Brown Co., Boston.

39. S.M. Diamond and W.L. Heinrich (1988) Nutrition and peritoneal dialysis. In: *Nutrition and the Kidney* (W.E. Mitch and S. Klahr, eds.), pp. 198–223, Little, Brown Co., Boston.

40. R.R. Hirshberg and J.D. Kopple (1988) Requirements for protein, calories and fat in the predialysis patient. In: *Nutrition and the Kidney* (W.E. Mitch and S. Klahr, eds.), pp. 131–153, Little, Brown Co., Boston.

41. C.H. Coggins and B.F. Cornell (1988) Nutritional management of the nephrotic syndrome. In: *Nutrition and the Kidney* (W.E. Mitch and S. Klahr, eds.), pp. 239–249, Little, Brown Co., Boston.

42. H.E. Norbeck and L.A. Carlson (1981) The uremic dyslipoproteinemia: its characteristics and relations to clinical factors. *Acta Med. Scand.* 209:489–503.

43. M. Okubo, Y. Tsukamoto, T. Yoneda, Y. Homma, H. Nakamura, and F. Marumo (1980) Deranged fat metabolism and the lowering effect of carbohydrate-poor diet on serum triglycerides in patients with chronic renal failure. *Nephron* 25:8–14.

44. G. Reaven, R.S. Swenson, and M.L. Sanfelippo (1980) An inquiry into the mechanism of hypertriglyceridemia in patients with chronic renal failure. *Am. J. Clin. Nutr.* 33:1476–1484.

45. M.L. Sanfelippo, R.S. Swenson, and G.M. Reaven (1977) Reduction of plasma triglyceride by diet in subjects with chronic renal failure. *Kidney Int.* 11:54–61.

46. G.L. Vega and S.M. Grundy (1988) Lovastatin therapy in nephrotic hyperlipidemia: effects on lipoprotein metabolism. *Kidney Int.* 33:1160–1168.

47. A.P. Goldberg (1984) A potential role for exercise training in modulating coronary risk factors in uremia. *Am. J. Nephrol.* 4:132–133.

48. R.A. DeFronzo, R. Andres, P. Edgar, and W.G. Walker (1973) Carbohydrate metabolism in uremia: a review. *Medicine* 52:469–497.

49. E.S. Horton, C. Johnson, and A.E. Lebovitz (1968) Carbohydrate metabolism in uremia. *Ann. Intern. Med.* 68:63–74.

50. R.A. DeFronzo, A. Alvestrand, D. Smith, R. Hendler, E. Hendler, and J. Wahren (1981) Insulin resistance in uremia. *J. Clin. Invest.* 67:563–568.

51. F.B. Westervelt (1969) Insulin effect in uremia. *J. Lab. Clin. Med.* 74:79–84.

52. T.A. Davis, S. Klahr, and I.E. Karl (1987) Glucose metabolism in muscle of sedentary and exercised rats with chronic uremia. *Am. J. Physiol.* 252:F138–F145.

53. A.J. Garber (1970) Skeletal muscle protein and amino acid metabolism in experimental chronic uremia in the rat: accelerated alanine and glutamine formation and release. *J. Clin. Invest.* 62:623–632.

54. M.L. McCaleb, M.S. Izzo, and D.H. Lockwood (1985) Characterization and partial purification of a factor from uremia serum that induces insulin resistance. *J. Clin. Invest.* 75:391–396.

55. H. Dobbelstein, W.F. Korner, W. Mempel, H. Grosse-Wilde, and H.H. Edel (1974) Vitamin B6 deficiency in uremia and its implications for the depression of immune responses. *Kidney Int.* 5:233–239.

56. N. Lasker, A. Harvey, and H. Baker (1963) Vitamin levels in hemodialysis and intermittent dialysis. *Trans. Am. Soc. Artif. Intern. Organs* 9:51–56.

57. J.D. Kopple (1981) Nutritional therapy in kidney failure. *Nutr. Rev.* 39:193–206.

58. F.R. Smith and D.S. Goodman (1971) The effects of diseases of the liver, thyroid and kidney on transport of vitamin in human plasma. *J. Clin. Invest.* 50:2426–2436.

59. A. Vahlquist, P.A. Peterson, and L. Wibell (1973) Metabolism of the vitamin A transporting protein complex. I. Turnover studies in normal persons and in patients with chronic renal failure. *Eur. J. Clin. Invest.* 3:352–362.

60. H. Zumkley, H.P. Bertram, A. Lison, O. Knoll, and H. Losse (1979) Aluminum, zinc and copper concentrations in plasma in chronic renal insufficiency. *Clin. Nephrol.* 12:18–21.

61. A.C. Alfrey, G.R. Legendre, and W.D. Kaehny (1976) The dialysis encephalopathy syndrome—possible aluminum intoxication. *N. Engl. J. Med.* 294:184–189.

62. G.A. Kaysen and P.Y. Schoenfeld (1984) Aluminum homeostasis in patients undergoing continuous ambulatory peritoneal dialysis. *Kidney Int.* 25:107–114.

63. R.J. McGonigle and V. Parsons (1985) Aluminum-induced anemia in haemodialysis patients. *Nephron* 39:1–9.

Daniel Rudman and Axel G. Feller

Chapter **46**

Liver Disease

The structure and function of the liver are profoundly affected by the state of nutrition. Liver abnormalities can be produced by deficiencies of carbohydrate, protein, lipids, vitamins, or minerals whether from diet or malabsorption.[1-17] In turn, established liver disease disturbs the normal metabolism of many nutrients, both organic and inorganic. This chapter focuses on protein and amino acid nutrition and metabolism in relation to liver disease. Three topics will be considered: how protein undernutrition contributes to the pathogenesis of liver disease, how liver disease perturbs the intermediary metabolism of the amino acids, and how dietary protein and supplementary amino acids are used in the treatment of various types and stages of liver disease.

Protein Undernutrition as a Cause of Liver Disease

Amino acid (protein) malnutrition as a cause of prolonged liver disease can be illustrated by a common human disorder, pediatric kwashiorkor, and by a widely studied rat model, the fatty liver–cirrhosis complex produced by protein deficiency during the period of rapid growth. Pediatric kwashiorkor is a chronic disorder of children with onset shortly after weaning from breast-feeding.[18-28] The clinical features are growth retardation (but with a relatively normal weight for height and with preservation of subcutaneous adipose tissue), fatigue and lethargy, anemia, hepatomegaly, and hypoalbuminemia leading to dependent edema. The leading pathologic features are an enlarged fatty liver and atrophy of the skeletal muscles. Untreated, these features persist to a fatal outcome for the majority of patients. The immediate cause of death usually is an infection. There is, however, no evidence of progression to cirrhosis of the liver. Kwashiorkor has a high prevalence in the nonindustrialized populations of the Third World (up to 30% of children) but is rarely seen in Western societies.

The evidence for a role of protein deficiency in kwashiorkor is as follows: (1) The presenting features of hypoalbuminemia and muscle atrophy are characteristic of protein undernutrition.[26-28] (2) Dietary histories confirm that protein intake is inadequate. The condition is precipitated by the transition from breast-feeding, adequate in protein and calories, to a starchy calorie-sufficient but protein-poor vegetarian diet. (3) Treatment with a diet adequate in protein and calories rapidly cures the syndrome.[19,22,26] (4) Epidemiologically, the incidence of kwashiorkor is correlated with the frequency of a low protein intake.[20] (5) In healthy subjects an experimental diet with protein intake below the minimal daily requirement but with adequate energy intake can cause fatty liver.[23]

When both dietary energy and dietary protein are inadequate, growth is more severely restricted and is associated with wasting of adipose as well as muscle tissue.[28,29] Under these conditions, liver histology and albumin concentration may remain normal. It is proposed that when the energy intake as well as the protein intake are deficient, the body adapts by curtailing the secretion of insulin and by augmenting the production of glucagon, cortisol, and growth hormone. These endocrine reactions mobilize muscle amino acids and glucose-sparing adipose fatty acids, thereby promoting the availability of amino acids for the liver. When energy intake is adequate, however, these liver-sparing adaptations to protein deprivation are less likely to occur.

Thus, protein undernutrition with adequate energy intake in early childhood appears to lead directly to a severe and potentially lethal form of fatty liver. Nevertheless, progression to necrosis and scarring, i.e., cirrhosis, does not occur.

Another illustration of the adverse effects of protein undernutrition on hepatic structure and function is provided by protein-restricted growing rats. The historic origin of this line of work was the observation that pancreatectomized, insulin-treated diabetic dogs developed a fatty liver followed by cirrhosis; this type of experimental liver disease could be prevented by supplementing the diet with protein or methionine.[30] In growing rats, inadequate protein with adequate calories was found to cause fatty liver progressing to cirrhosis.[31,32] If the rat's protein-deficient diet was supplemented with methionine or choline, which provide methyl groups, liver disease was prevented. Folate and vitamin B-12 enhanced the protective effect of these lipotrophic, methyl-group-generating nutrients. Similar results were produced by protein-deficient, energy-adequate diets, although in less severe form, in dogs[33] and in nonhuman primates.[34,35]

Dietary Protein and the Pathogenesis of Alcoholic Liver Disease

The sections above demonstrate how protein deprivation leads directly to fatty liver in children and to both fatty liver and cirrhosis in experimental animals. In adult humans the most common forms of fatty liver and cirrhosis occur in association with chronic alcoholism and therefore are termed alcoholic liver disease. The role of protein deficiency in the etiology and pathogenesis of this family of liver disorders has been studied extensively but still remains controversial. The main points of view are summarized below.

Alcoholic liver disease proceeds through a series of stages.[36,37] First is the stage of chronic alcoholism. If ethanol intake exceeds ~160 g/d (1136 kcal) for ~15 y, a substantial proportion of individuals will develop structural abnormalities in the liver. The most common form of alcoholic liver disease is fatty liver. This condition may be asymptomatic or it may be associated with weakness, fatigue, anemia, and hypoalbuminemia. Sometimes the steatosis is accompanied by accumulation of intracellular hyaline, necrosis of hepatocytes, infiltration by polymorphonuclear leukocytes, and perivenular and perisinusoidal fibrosis accompanied by intensified malaise and biochemical changes of liver injury and dysfunction. This condition is termed alcoholic hepatitis. In alcoholic hepatitis, especially in the face of continuous alcohol intake, the liver histology may evolve to micronodular cirrhosis by the continuing death of hepatocytes, the laying down of connective tissue, and the appearance of regenerating nodules. The eventual clinical manifestations are fatigue and weakness, jaundice, and ascites. Common complications are upper gastrointestinal bleeding caused by portal hypertension and recurrent episodes of delirium or coma (hepatic encephalopathy).

In the United States, the prevalence of chronic al-

coholism is ~10% in males and 4% in females.[38] Of these individuals, ~25% eventually develop alcoholic liver disease, and ~10% develop cirrhosis.[39,40] Alcoholic liver disease is now the fifth leading cause of death in the United States.[41-43]

Several types of evidence suggest a close connection between protein malnutrition and alcoholic liver disease: (1) On initial presentation, the majority of individuals with alcoholic hepatitis or cirrhosis have physical or laboratory evidence of protein undernutrition.[44] (2) Cirrhosis of the liver was reported in several populations in which there is no alcohol intake but in which protein deficiency is common.[45-47] (3) Before about 1940, clinicians managing cirrhosis were prone to prognostic pessimism and therapeutic nihilism. Nevertheless, experimental animal research on liver disease led Connors[48] in 1939 and Patek and Post[49] in 1941 to treat cirrhotic patients with a nutritious diet and abstinence from alcohol. This regimen resulted in improved outcomes. Subsequent work showed that even when alcohol intake continued, a well-balanced diet led to clinical improvement in patients with cirrhosis.[50-52] Consequently, the theory became popular from about 1940 to 1965 that the alcoholic fatty liver–cirrhosis complex is primarily a nutritional disease, resulting from the sequence ethanol and socioeconomic factors to protein undernutrition to alcoholic liver disease.[53-55]

However, since 1965, the following counterarguments to the nutritional hypothesis for alcoholic liver disease have been brought forward: (1) The fatty liver of pediatric kwashiorkor does not evolve into cirrhosis.[56] (2) The epidemiologic evidence of a nearly universal association of protein undernutrition with alcoholic liver disease was questioned. According to Sherlock,[57] the conclusion that virtually all patients presenting with untreated alcoholic liver disease have protein undernutrition was based on the study of derelict alcoholics who were existing under severely compromised socioeconomic conditions. In middle-class cirrhotic patients protein intake and body weight often appeared to be normal.[57] Although detailed measurements of protein nutrition were lacking, these observations raised the suspicion that protein deficiency perhaps was more often the result than the cause of alcoholic liver disease. (3) An apparently direct hepatotoxic effect of ethanol despite an apparently adequate diet was demonstrated in monkeys, in humans, and in rats. Using a special liquid formula diet, Lieber and coworkers[58-63] showed that if carbohydrate calories in an adequate diet were replaced by ethanol amounting to 50% of total calories, fatty liver developed in 1–2 mo, alcoholic hepatitis in 9–12 mo, and (in one-third of the animals) cirrhosis in 2–5 y. The same diet given to healthy young men for as little as 2 d caused abnormalities in sensitive biochemical and histologic liver tests. These observations led Lieber and colleagues to propose the sequence ethanol to alcoholic liver disease to protein-calorie malnutrition. The last step could result from several causes: displacement of dietary nutrients by alcohol's empty calories (energy unaccompanied by protein or other essential nutrients), anorexia caused by alcoholic disease of the stomach and liver, or impaired absorption of ingested nutrients because of abnormalities in pancreatic, biliary, and small intestine functions.[64-73]

In rebuttal to the alcohol hepatotoxin hypothesis, several arguments were presented by defenders of the nutritional theory of alcoholic liver disease.[74-77] (1) Quantitative information is still lacking on the dietary intakes of alcoholics during the many years that precede the onset of clinical liver disease. Patek et al.,[76] however, studied the consumption of food and alcohol in 304 alcoholics (both cirrhotic and noncirrhotic) for a period of 2 y. Protein intake in both subgroups was low but was lower in the cirrhotic alcoholics by ~15%. (2) The experimental effect of adding ethanol to a protein-adequate diet may be different from that of substituting ethanol for carbohydrate in such a diet. The second maneuver used by Lieber and coworkers[58-63] creates a low-carbohydrate, calorie-rich regimen.[75-77] The loss of the protein-sparing effect of carbohydrate may increase the requirement for protein thereby creating a relatively protein-deficient diet or a conditioned protein deficiency. Thus, the data on protein, calorie, and ethanol intake in middle-class English cirrhotic patients,[57] although not suggestive of absolute protein deficiency, may be compatible with an excessive alcohol-protein ratio, a suboptimal carbohydrate-protein ratio, or a relative protein deficiency. (3) The same theme was developed by Hartroft and colleagues[78-80] in their experiments with rats. This group showed that even when rats consume 32-46% of dietary calories as ethanol, fatty liver and cirrhosis can be prevented by abundant simultaneous intake of high-quality protein. As in the original development of liver disease in growing rats by means of alcohol-free imbalanced diets, the main hepatoprotective factor appeared to be the protein's content of methionine, which in part could be replaced in this role by choline. The protective action of both methionine and choline could be enhanced by vitamin B-12 and folate. With each increment in the level of ethanol intake, the requirement for protein, methionine, or choline in the prevention of liver damage was raised. Moreover, if the ethanol in the diet was replaced by another type of empty calorie, such as glucose or fat, the same results occurred. These experiments led Hartroft[77] to conclude that ethanol is not a direct hepatotoxic agent like carbon tetrachlo-

ride. He suggested instead that an ethanol-rich diet is damaging to the liver only if the ratio of calories to protein or surrogate hepatoprotector exceeds a critical threshold value. Hartroft concluded, ". . . in the growing rat, the hepatic damage produced by ethanol is determined by the daily intake of ethanol, by the duration of this intake, and by the nature of the accompanying diet."

In summary, the debate on the relative importance of malnutrition and alcohol in the liver disease of the chronic alcoholic continues. The available information is compatible with the dual role of protein deprivation and ethanol hepatotoxicity. This view is consistent with the earlier evidence that a low-protein diet predisposes to liver damage by known hepatotoxic agents such as halogenated hydrocarbons and inorganic phosphorus.[81-84]

Hepatic Encephalopathy

A new dimension has been added to the dietary protein–cirrhosis interaction since 1970 by the rising prevalence of hepatic encephalopathy as a complication of cirrhosis.[85-88] This condition rarely was mentioned in textbooks before 1960 and can be considered a disorder of medical progress. Now cirrhotic patients have a longer survival because of diuretics, antibiotics, better access to medical care, use of aggressive nutritional support, and improved management of esophagovariceal hemorrhages by shunt operations and endoscopic sclerosis. These varices result from the sequence hepatic fibrosis to portal hypertension to development of venous collaterals around the liver, which establish spontaneous portasystemic anastomoses. The variceal hemorrhages were the cause of death in up to one-third of cirrhotic patients until the portacaval and related types of shunt were introduced in the 1960s. These operations create a larger shunt around the liver by a new anastomosis between the portal venous and inferior caval systems thereby decompressing the varices.[89,90] The result is protection from further bleeding but at the expense of a more extensive venous bypass around the liver, which in turn predisposes to frequent attacks of hepatic encephalopathy.

This type of encephalopathy presents as recurrent episodes of tremor with altered mental status that may progress to coma.[85-88] It can occur in acute liver failure caused, for example, by acute viral hepatitis. However, the common setting is as a recurrent problem in cirrhotic patients. The two sine qua nons appear to be hepatic venous bypass and an excessive protein load. The risk of severe attacks of hepatic encephalopathy is proportional to the degree to which portal venous blood bypasses the liver, and it is sharply increased by portasystemic shunt operations. In addition, the most common precipitating factors are ingestion of substantial dietary protein or the introduction of a protein load into the upper gastrointestinal tract by a bleeding event.[91] Consequently, temporary removal of protein from the diet is the major treatment. Sterilization of the colon by nonabsorbable antibiotics or surgical removal of the colon reduces the occurrence of encephalopathy in high-risk patients. It is suspected that the bacterial flora in the colon produce cerebrotoxic nitrogenous factors from dietary amino acids. After absorption these factors apparently bypass the liver (where they would normally be removed) through the portasystemic shunt to reach the brain and cause encephalopathy. What are the cerebrototoxic substances? Ammonia, bioactive amines such as tyramine or tryptamine, and mercaptans all have been suggested.[85-88] The general parallelism of hyperammonemia to the occurrence of hepatic encephalopathy supports a role for ammonia, but the strength of the correlation has varied considerably in the hands of different investigators.[85-88,92-95]

Fischer and colleagues[96,97] introduced an alternate and influential hypothesis about the mechanism of hepatic encephalopathy. In this condition the plasma aminogram shows characteristic deviations from normal. The aromatic amino acids (AAs) phenylalanine and tyrosine and the sulfur-containing methionine are elevated whereas the branched-chain amino acids (BCAAs) are depressed. AAs and BCAAs must compete for entry into the brain at a shared transport site in the blood-brain barrier. Phenylalanine and tyrosine, moreover, once across the blood-brain barrier, are precursors of the neurotransmitter norepinephrine and of related molecules (tyramine, octopamine) that in a state of accumulation may act as false neurotransmitters by displacing norepinephrine from its receptor or storage sites. Fischer et al.[96,97] proposed, therefore, that the abnormally high plasma AA-BCAA ratio predisposes to, or causes, hepatic encephalopathy. This hypothesis led to the design of enteral and parenteral products with reduced AA and increased BCAA contents and their clinical trial, as described below.

Abnormalities of Amino Acid Metabolism in Patients with Cirrhosis

The narration above shows how protein deprivation predisposes to chronic liver disease with a loss of hepatocytes and a decrease of portal venous blood flow. In this section, we will consider how chronic liver disease, once established, proceeds to disturb amino acid metabolism within this organ.

Impairment of Hepatic Urea Synthesis. The original observation was a falling blood urea concentration in advanced liver disease, which suggested a curtailed ability of the organ to synthesize urea. This conclusion was amply confirmed during the period 1973–1980.[98-104] Administration of a load of protein in normal individuals caused a marked, prompt acceleration of urea excretion. In cirrhotic patients the rise was significantly blunted, suggesting impairment in the urea cycle.[98,99] When the nitrogenous load was given in the form of intravenous amino acids, a similar curtailment of urea production was observed.[100] Supporting data were provided by in vitro perfusion studies with amino acids.[101,102] Perfused cirrhotic rat liver incorporated labeled ammonia into urea at a significantly slower rate than did normal rat liver. The final proof of a reduced capacity for urea synthesis came from enzyme assays of normal vs. cirrhotic human livers.[103-105] The specific activities of all five enzymes in the cycle were only 40–60% as great (per milligram DNA or per milligram noncollagen nitrogen) as in a normal liver.

Impaired Metabolism of Phenylalanine and Tyrosine. The initial research in this field can be traced again to blood chemistry. The plasma concentrations of phenylalanine and tyrosine are generally elevated in advanced cirrhosis.[92,106] This abnormality suggested a restriction in the largely hepatic main pathway for tyrosine biosynthesis and for phenylalanine and tyrosine catabolism: phenylalanine to tyrosine to p-hydroxyphenylpyruvic acid (PHPA) to homogentisic acid (HGA) to CO_2. This problem has been researched since 1960 by numerous investigators. Levine and Conn[107] administered an oral load of phenylalanine to cirrhotic and normal individuals. In cirrhotic patients the load was followed by a greater rise in plasma phenylalanine and by a slower return to baseline than in normal subjects. Conversely, the rise in plasma tyrosine that followed the phenylalanine load was smaller in cirrhotic patients than in normal subjects. Levine and Conn concluded that the hydroxylation of phenylalanine to tyrosine, a largely hepatic process, was impaired by cirrhosis. Confirmatory results were reported by Heberer et al.[107] Using the intravenous rather than the oral route, Jagenburg and coworkers[108] confirmed the delayed plasma clearance of a load of phenylalanine in cirrhotic patients versus normal subjects. Hehir et al.[110] studied the hydroxylation of phenylalanine in a patient with end-stage hepatic disease by using a tracer dose of the amino acid. They infused labeled phenylalanine and showed its rate of clearance to be only 12% of normal and its rate of conversion to tyrosine to be only 60% of normal. Finally, Heberer et al.[108] measured the specific activity of phenylalanine hydroxylase in normal and cirrhotic human-liver biopsies; the values in the cirrhotic samples averaged only 20% of normal expressed per unit DNA or per unit wet weight.

The next segment in the pathway concerns the degradation of tyrosine via PHPA and HGA to CO_2. A slowing of this segment was shown by excessive accumulation of plasma tyrosine after an oral load of this amino acid[107-111] and by delayed clearance and delayed oxidation to CO_2 of an intravenous tracer dose of tyrosine in end-stage liver disease.[112,113] Nordlinger et al.[111] gave an oral load of tyrosine, PHPA, or HGA to cirrhotic and normal individuals and measured the basal and postload concentrations of tyrosine in plasma and of PHPA and HGA in urine. Delayed clearance was found for all three substances in the majority of cirrhotic patients, suggesting partial defects at the steps catalyzed by tyrosine transaminase, PHPA oxidase, and HGA oxidase. The first step appeared to be rate limiting. Nevertheless, when Henderson et al.[114] compared the specific activity of tyrosine transaminase in cirrhotic and normal livers, they found no difference. Apparently, cirrhotic patients' delay in converting tyrosine to PHPA resulted from shrunken hepatic mass, reduced hepatic blood flow, or deficiency of the enzyme's supply of pyridoxal pyrophosphate or α-ketoglutarate rather than from lower content of the apoenzyme within the surviving hepatocytes. A disorder in the hepatic metabolism and plasma concentrations of pyridoxine vitamers has, in fact, been found in alcoholic cirrhosis.[115-118]

Blocks in the Transsulfuration Pathway. Early researchers on this subject concluded that most patients with advanced cirrhosis have abnormally high plasma methionine concentrations.[92,106] The plasma clearance of this amino acid after an intravenous or oral load moreover was delayed.[119-121] These observations suggested a problem in the mainly hepatic principal pathway (transsulfuration pathway) for methionine degradation, which also serves to synthesize cyst(e)ine and taurine, and via S-adenosyl methionine (SAM) provides methyl groups for other vital biosyntheses: methionine to SAM to homocystine to cystathionine to cyst(e)ine to sulfate and taurine. Horowitz et al.[122] administered an oral load of methionine to cirrhotic and normal individuals and then measured in plasma or urine, as appropriate, the above-mentioned intermediates and end products of the transsulfuration pathway.[122] In cirrhosis the postload accumulation of plasma methionine was abnormally high and the urinary excretion of sulfate was abnormally low. Homocystine, homoserine, cystathionine, and cystine did not accumulate to an abnormal degree in cirrhotic patients during the delayed clearance of the plasma load, suggesting that the block was at SAM synthetase. This conclusion was verified later by Cabrero et al.[123,124] who dem-

onstrated a significantly reduced specific activity of this enzyme in cirrhotic liver. Because SAM plays a central role in the methylation reactions for proteins, hormones, and nucleic acids, a deficiency in hepatic SAM production could have far-reaching adverse effects on the health of cirrhotic patients. Another consequence of the block at SAM would be impaired biosynthesis of cyst(e)ine. This prediction was confirmed by the observation that some cirrhotic patients, unlike normal individuals, develop profound hypocyst(e)inemia when nourished exclusively by intravenous fluids providing methionine as the only sulfur-containing amino acid.[125]

Although cystine did not increase after the plasma load of methionine in cirrhotic patients, Horowitz et al.[122] observed a basal hypercystinemia in these patients. This finding was confirmed by Tribble et al.,[126] who administered an oral load of cystine to cirrhotic patients and normal individuals and showed, in the former, an excessively large accumulation of plasma cyst(e)ine and an abnormally delayed excretion of sulfate and taurine. They concluded that the hepatic degradation of cyst(e)ine to the latter two end products was delayed. This metabolic block may explain the accumulation in plasma of cirrhotic patients of methylmercaptan,[127,128] which is formed from cyst(e)ine by an alternative pathway to the transsulfuration sequence.

The studies reviewed in this section show that cirrhosis disrupts intermediary amino acid metabolism in at least three pathways: urea synthesis, phenylalanine and tyrosine synthesis and degradation, and transsulfuration. Unlike the situation for the genetic disorders of these pathways, blocks exist at multiple points because of apoenzyme deficiency, curtailed blood flow, reduced hepatic mass, or cofactor deficiency. The consequences of this complex acquired disorder of amino acid metabolism could include amino acid imbalance syndromes causing food aversion and cachexia, accumulation of cerebrotoxic amines, and altered nutritional requirements and tolerances for protein as a whole and for phenylalanine, tyrosine, methionine, or cyst(e)ine individually.

Amino Acids in the Treatment of Liver Disease

Nutritional treatment with protein or amino acid mixtures is an important modality in the management of liver-disease patients.

Pediatric Kwashiorkor. Adequate intake of protein and calories provides specific, generally successful therapy both for curative and preventive purposes.[19,22,24,26-28] Before the nutritional origin of this syndrome was recognized, the mortality rate was 30–90%. In recent years, treatment with 2–3 g protein $\cdot$ kg^{-1} $\cdot$ d^{-1} and 150 kcal $\cdot$ kg^{-1} $\cdot$ d^{-1} lowered the mortality rate to 10–20%. Moreover, raising the protein intake for children after breast-feeding through nutritional education and food supplements in some at-risk communities reduced the incidence of kwashiorkor substantially.[24]

Alcoholic Liver Disease. In the absence of encephalopathy, the use of dietary protein to correct protein undernutrition is universally accepted. Hepatitic and cirrhotic alcoholic patients usually present some degree of protein deficiency.[44,74] The etiology appears to be a combination of primary and secondary factors. As demonstrated by Connors[48] in 1939 and by Patek and Post[49] in 1941, a nutritious diet accelerates the clinical improvement of cirrhotic patients who are able to take nourishment by mouth. Nevertheless, in today's hospitals the severely ill hepatitic or cirrhotic alcoholic patient is often so anorectic that force-feeding, either by the enteral or, less commonly, by the parenteral route, is required. Both methods have been shown to be successful in accelerating nutritional repletion and improvement in liver biochemical tests, but whether the mortality rate improves is still being debated.[129–136] Researchers, once again, are left with the unanswered question as to whether protein malnutrition is a partial cause of alcoholic liver disease or whether it is merely a consequence, that is, either

Ethanol → liver disease → high mortality rate
                    ↓
           protein deficiency

or

Protein deficiency & ethanol → liver disease →
        ↑ ——————————————————————— ↑

high mortality rate

When alcoholic liver disease is associated with encephalopathy, the physician confronts the dilemma of the narrowed nutritional window. Patients with alcoholic liver disease plus hepatic encephalopathy usually have concomitant protein undernutrition.[137–139] On the other hand, the Recommended Dietary Allowance of protein in these individuals often will precipitate hepatic encephalopathy. To maintain a clear sensorium, it may be necessary to keep protein intake at a deliberately inadequate level (20 or 30 g/d).[86–87] In keeping with the amino acid imbalance theory of Fischer et al.,[97] a strategy was developed to provide by mouth or by vein a mixture of amino acids designed to correct the abnormal plasma aminogram, that is, enteral[140,141] and parenteral[142] formulas enriched in BCAAs and de-

pleted in AAs. Such mixtures when administered at ~60–80 g amino acids/d tend to reduce the plasma AAs and to increase the plasma BCAAs.[143–146] Thereby, the abnormally high AA-BCAA ratio postulated by Fischer's group to be a major cause of hepatic encephalopathy can be restored to normal. In many cases, moreover, nitrogen balance becomes positive.[145,147] However, a benefit on the encephalopathy by this normalization of the AA-BCAA ratio has not been observed regularly,[147–152] thereby casting doubt on Fischer's theory. An unanticipated side effect of the intravenous amino acid mixture designed for hepatic encephalopathy, moreover, was a profound depression of plasma tyrosine and cyst(e)ine concentrations.[125] The reason appears to be as follows: The intravenous formula contains no tyrosine or cystine because of the insolubility of these two compounds in water. Normally, the metabolic production of tyrosine from phenylalanine and of cyst(e)ine from methionine would be sufficient. However, as described above, the impairments in phenylalanine hydroxylase and in SAM synthetase in cirrhotic liver apparently compromise these conversions in cirrhotic patients. Thus, these individuals may have new conditional requirements for tyrosine and cystine.[153]

Summary

Protein deficiency with adequate calorie intake causes a fatty liver in rats and in humans. In rats the process progresses spontaneously to cirrhosis; in humans an additional hepatotoxic insult probably is necessary. On a wide scale, ethanol provides this insult. It seems likely that the protein deficiency so common in the alcoholic-liver-disease population represents both a contributory cause and a consequence of liver disease.

Once established, liver disease then impairs the intrahepatic intermediary metabolism of amino acids at multiple points. Three impaired pathways so far have been analyzed in detail: the urea cycle, the phenylalanine-hydroxylase pathway, and the transsulfuration pathway. Multiple defects in the metabolic sequence were identified in each case.

Protein and amino acid mixtures are commonly used to treat liver disease. The preventive or curative results in pediatric kwashiorkor are excellent. Similarly, in alcoholic liver disease without encephalopathy, nutritional and clinical improvement usually are promoted. In alcoholic liver disease complicated by hepatic encephalopathy, however, the conventional approach to the protein undernutrition is hazardous, and treatment with BCAA-enriched, AA-poor synthetic mixtures is of doubtful efficacy; a solution to this problem has not yet been found.

Supported by grants from the Department of Veterans Affairs and the USPHS (grant ID31PE95008-01).

References

1. M. Adler and F. Schaffner (1979) Fatty liver hepatitis and cirrhosis in obese patients. *Am. J. Med.* 67:811–816.

2. Z.T. Cossack and J. Bouquet (1986) The treatment of Wilson's disease in paediatrics: oral zinc therapy versus penicillamine. *Acta Pharmacol. Toxicol.* (Copenh.) 59:514–517.

3. E. Drenick, F. Simons, and J.F. Murphy (1970) Effect on hepatic morphology of treatment of obesity by fasting, reducing diets and small-bowel bypass. *N. Engl. J. Med.* 282:829–834.

4. V.R. Gordeuk, B.R. Bacon, and G.M. Brittenham (1987) Iron overload: causes and consequences. *Annu. Rev. Nutr.* 7:485–508.

5. J.P. Grant, C.E. Cox, L.M. Kleiman, et al. (1977) Serum hepatic enzyme and bilirubin elevations during parenteral nutrition. *Surg. Gynecol. Obstet.* 145:573–580.

6. N.L. Keim and J.A. Mares-Perlman (1984) Development of hepatic steatosis and essential fatty acid deficiency in rats with hypercaloric, fat-free parenteral nutrition. *J. Nutr.* 114:1807–1815.

7. W.H. Kern, A.H. Heger, J.H. Payne, et al. (1973) Fatty metamorphosis of the liver in morbid obesity. *Arch. Pathol.* 96:342–346.

8. H.E. Kosterlitz (1947) The effects of changes in dietary protein on the composition and structure of the liver cell. *J. Physiol.* 106:194–210.

9. C.M. Leevy, A. Thomson, and H. Baker (1970) Vitamins and liver injury. *Am. J. Clin. Nutr.* 23:493–498.

10. R.L. Peters, T. Gay, and T.B. Reynolds (1975) Post-jejunoileal bypass hepatic disease: its similarity to alcoholic hepatic disease. *Am. J. Clin. Pathol.* 63:318–331.

11. D.A. Peura, F.W. Stromeyer, and L.F. Johnson (1980) Liver injury with alcoholic hyaline after intestinal resection. *Gastroenterology* 79:128–130.

12. P. Rozenthal, C. Biava, H. Spencer, and H.J. Zimmerman (1967) Liver morphology and function tests in obesity and during total starvation. *Am. J. Dig. Dis.* 12:198–208.

13. S. Sherlock and V. Walske (1948) Effect of under-nutrition in man on hepatic structure and function. *Nature* 161:604.

14. M.T. Soyer, R. Ceballas, and J.S. Aldrete (1976) Reversibility of severe hepatic damage caused by jejunoileal bypass after re-establishment of normal intestinal continuity. *Surgery* 79:601–604.

15. J.O. Westwater and D. Fainte (1958) Liver impairment in the obese. *Gastroenterology* 34:686–693.

16. F.C. Ames, E.M. Copeland, D.C. Leeb, et al. (1976) Liver dysfunction following small-bowel bypass for obesity: nonoperative treatment of fatty metamorphosis with parenteral hyperalimentation. *JAMA* 235:1249–1252.

17. A.L. Baker, C.O. Elson, J. Jaspan, and J.L. Boyer (1979) Liver failure with steatonecrosis after jejunoileal bypass: recovery with parenteral nutrition and reanastomosis. *Arch. Intern. Med.* 139:289–292.

18. J.F. Annegers (1973) The protein-calorie ratio of West African diets and their relationship to protein calorie malnutrition. *Ecol. Food Nutr.* 2:225–235.

19. M. Behar, F. Viteri, and N.S. Scrimshaw (1957) Treatment of severe protein deficiency in children (kwashiorkor). *Am. J. Clin. Nutr.* 5:506–515.

20. J.M. Bengoa, D.B. Jelliffe, and C. Perez (1959) Some indicator for the broad assessment of the magnitude of protein-calorie malnutrition in young children in population groups. *Am. J. Clin. Nutr.* 7:714–720.

21. A.K. Bhattacharyya (1986) Protein-energy malnutrition (kwashiorkor-marasmus syndrome): terminology, classification and evolution. *World Rev. Nutr. Diet.* 47:80–133.

22. J.F. Brock, J.D.L. Hansen, P.J. Pretorius, R.G. Hendricske, and J. Davel (1955) Kwashiorkor and protein malnutrition. A dietary therapeutic trial. *Lancet* 2:355–360.

23. M.G. Deo, S.K. Sood, and V. Ramalingaswami (1965) Experimental protein deficiency. *Arch. Pathol.* 80:14–23.

24. J.D.L. Hansen (1961) Protein malnutrition and its prevention and treatment with special reference to kwashiorkor and in marasmus. In: *Recent Advances in Human Nutrition, with Special Reference to Clinical Medicine* (J.F. Brock, ed.), pp. 267–281, Churchill, London.

25. A. Kattachaudhuri, A.K. Bhattacharyya, and A.M. Mukherjee (1972) The liver in pre-kwashiorkor and kwashiorkor-marasmus syndromes. *Trans. R. Soc. Trop. Med. Hyg.* 66:258–263.

26. S.M. Pereira and A. Begum (1974) The manifestations and management of severe protein-calorie malnutrition (kwashiorkor). *World Rev. Nutr. Diet.* 19:1–50.

27. H.C. Trowell, J.N.P. Davies, and R.F.A. Dean (1954) *Kwashiorkor,* Arnold, London.

28. G.A.O. Alleyn, et al. (1977) *Protein-Energy Malnutrition.* Butler & Tanner, London.

29. D.J. Becker (1983) The endocrine responses to protein calorie malnutrition. *Annu. Rev. Nutr.* 3:187–212.

30. C.H. Best, W.S. Hartroft, C.C. Lucas, and J.H. Ridout (1949) Liver damage produced by feeding alcohol or sugar and its prevention by choline. *Br. Med. J.* 2:1001–1006.

31. W.S. Hartroft (1954) The sequence of pathologic events in the development of experimental fatty liver and cirrhosis. *Ann. N.Y. Acad. Sci.* 57:633–645.

32. H.P. Himsworth (1950) Lectures on the liver and its diseases. Harvard University Press, Cambridge, MA.

33. I.L. Chaikoff and C.L. Connor (1940) Production of cirrhosis of liver of normal dog by high fat diets. *Proc. Soc. Exp. Biol. Med.* 43:638–641.

34. A.J. Patek, Jr., S. Bowry, and K.C. Hayes (1975) Cirrhosis of choline deficiency in the rhesus monkey. Possible role of dietary cholesterol. *Proc. Soc. Exp. Biol. Med.* 148:370–374.

35. G.F. Wilgram (1959) Experimental Laennec type of cirrhosis in monkeys. *Ann. Int. Med.* 51:1134–1158.

36. W.S. Hislop, I.A. Bouchier, J.G. Allan, et al. (1983) Alcoholic liver disease in Scotland and northeastern England: presenting features in 510 patients. *O. J. Med.* 52:232–243.

37. C.M. Leevy. (1962) Fatty liver: A study of 270 patients with biopsy proven fatty liver and a review of the literature. *Medicine* 41:249–278.

38. E.P. Nace (1986) Alcoholism: epidemiology, diagnosis, and biological aspects. *Alcohol* 3:83–87.

39. W.K. Lelbach (1976) Epidemiology of alcoholic liver disease. In: *Progress in Liver Disease,* vol. 5. (H. Popper and F. Schafner, eds.), pp. 494–515, Grune & Stratton, New York.

40. D. Wilkenson, J.N. Santanavia, and J.G. Rankin (1969) Epidemiology of alcoholic cirrhosis. *Aust. Ann. Med.* 18:222–226.

41. B.F. Grant, M.C. Dufour, and T.C. Harford (1988) Epidemiology of alcoholic liver disease. *Semin. Liver Dis.* 8:12–25.

42. M. Terris (1967) Epidemiology of cirrhosis of the liver: national mortality data. *Am. J. Public Health* 57:2076–2088.

43. U.S. Bureau of the Census (1979) *Statistical Abstract of the United States,* 100th ed., U.S. Government Printing Office, Washington, DC.

44. C.L. Mendenhall, S. Anderson, R.E. Weesner, S.J. Goldberg, and K.A. Crolic (1984) Protein-calorie malnutrition associated with alcoholic hepatitis. Veterans Administration Cooperative Study Group on Alcoholic Hepatitis. *Am. J. Med.* 76:211–222.

45. S. Tyagaraja (1937) Early pathological changes in the liver with special reference to cirrhosis. *Ceylon J. Sci. D* 4(3):119–146.

46. C.S. Yang (1928) Cirrhosis of the liver. Report of 84 cases. *Natl. Med. J. China* 14:195–210.

47. H.A. Yenikomshian (1934) Non-alcoholic cirrhosis of the liver in Lebanon and Syria. *JAMA* 103:660–661.

48. C.L. Connor (1939) The etiology and pathogenesis of alcoholic cirrhosis of the liver. *JAMA* 112:387–390.

49. A.J. Patek, Jr., and J. Post (1941) Treatment of cirrhosis of the liver by a nutritious diet and supplement rich in vitamin B complex. *J. Clin. Invest.* 20:481–505.

50. T.B. Reynolds, A.G. Redeker, and O.T. Kuzma (1965) Role of alcohol in pathogenesis of alcoholic cirrhosis. In: *Symposium on Therapeutic Agents and the Liver,* pp. 131–42, Blackwell Scientific Publications, London.

51. W.H. Summerskill, S.J. Wolfe, and C.S. Davidson (1957) Response to alcohol in chronic alcoholics with liver disease. *Lancet* 1:335–340.

52. W.C. Volwiller, C.M. Jones, and T.B. Mallory (1948) Criteria for the measurement of results of treatment in fatty cirrhosis. *Gastroenterology* 11:164–182.

53. C.S. Davidson (1986) Changing concepts in the pathogenesis of alcoholic liver disease. *Alcoholism Clin. Exp. Res.* 10:3S–4S.

54. R.M. Jacobs and M.F. Sorrell (1981) The role of nutrition in the pathogenesis of alcoholic liver disease. *Semin. Liver Dis.* 1:224–253.

55. A.J. Patek, J. Post, O.D. Ratnoff, et al. (1948) Dietary treatment of cirrhosis of the liver. Results in 124 patients observed during a 10 year period. *JAMA* 138:543–549.

56. G.C. Cook and M.S.R. Hutt (1967) The liver after kwashiorkor. *Br. Med. J.* 3:454–457.

57. S. Sherlock (1984) Nutrition and the alcoholic. *Lancet* 1:436–439.

58. C.S. Lieber, L.M. DeCarli, and E. Rubin (1975) Sequential production of fatty liver, hepatitis, and cirrhosis in subhuman primates fed ethanol with adequate diets. *Proc. Natl. Acad. Sci. USA* 72:437–441.

59. C.S. Lieber and L.M. DeCarli (1974) An experimental model of alcohol feeding and liver injury in the baboon. *J. Med. Primatol.* 3:153–163.

60. C.S. Lieber and L. M. DeCarli (1976) Animal models of ethanol dependence and liver injury in rats and baboons. *Fed. Proc.* 35:1232–1236.

61. C.S. Lieber, D.P. Jones, and L.M. DeCarli (1965) Effects of prolonged ethanol intake: production of fatty liver despite adequate diets. *J. Clin. Invest.* 44:1009–1021.

62. E. Rubin and C.S. Lieber (1968) Alcohol-induced hepatic injury in non-alcoholic volunteers. *N. Engl. J. Med.* 278:869–876.

63. E. Rubin and C.S. Lieber (1974) Fatty liver, alcoholic hepatitis and cirrhosis produced by alcohol in primates. *N. Engl. J. Med.* 290:128–135.

64. E. Baraona, H. Orrego, O. Fernandez, et al. (1962) Absorptive function of the small intestine in liver cirrhosis. *Am. J. Dig. Dis.* 7:318–330.

65. E. Baraona, R.C. Pirola, and C.S. Lieber (1974) Small intestinal damage and changes in cell population produced by ethanol ingestion in the rat. *Gastroenterology* 66:226–234.

66. E. Gottfried, M.A. Korsten, and C.S. Lieber (1978) Alcohol-induced gastric and duodenal lesions in man. *Am. J. Gastroenterol.* 70:587–592.

67. C.H. Halsted, E.A. Robles, and E. Mezey (1971) Decreased jejunal uptake of labeled folic acid (3H-PGA) in alcoholic patients: Roles of alcohol and nutrition. *N. Engl. J. Med.* 285:701–706.

68. C.H. Halsted, E.A. Robles, and E. Mezey (1973) Intestinal malabsorption in folate-deficient alcoholics. *Gastroenterology* 64:526–532.

69. Y. Israel, I. Salazar, and E. Rosenmann (1968) Inhibitory effects of alcohol on intestinal amino acid transport in vivo and in vitro. *J. Nutr.* 96:499–504.

70. W.G. Linscheer (1970) Malabsorption in cirrhosis. *Am. J. Clin. Nutr.* 23:488–492.

71. E. Mezey and J.J. Potter (1976) Changes in endocrine pancreatic function produced by altered dietary protein intake in drinking alcoholics. *John Hopkins Med. J.* 138:7–12.

72. E. Mezey (1975) Intestinal function in chronic alcoholism. *Ann. N.Y. Acad. Sci.* 252:215–227.

73. Z.R. Vlahcevic, P. Juttijudata, C.C. Bell, and L. Sewell (1972) Bile salt metabolism in patients with cirrhosis. II. Cholic and chenodeoxycholic acid metabolism. *Gastroenterology* 62:1174–1190.

74. A.J. Patek, Jr. (1979) Alcohol, malnutrition, and alcoholic cirrhosis. *Am. J. Clin. Nutr.* 32:1304–1312.

75. A.J. Patek, Jr., S.C. Bowry, and S.M. Sabesin (1976) Minimal hepatic changes in rats fed alcohol and a high casein diet. *Arch. Pathol. Lab. Med.* 100:19–24.

76. A.J. Patek, Jr., I.M. Toth, M.G. Saunders, G.A.M. Castro, and J.J. Engel (1975) Alcohol and dietary factors in cirrhosis. *Arch. Intern. Med.* 135:1053–1057.

77. W.S. Hartroft (1975) On the etiology of alcoholic liver cirrhosis. In: *Alcoholic Liver Pathology* (J.M. Khanna, Y. Israel, and H. Kalant, eds.), pp. 1989–197, Addiction Research Foundation, Toronto.

78. E.A. Porta, O.R. Koch, and W.S. Hartroft (1970) Recent advances in molecular pathology: a review on the effects of alcohol on the liver. *Exp. Mol. Pathol.* 12:104–132.

79. E.A. Porta, O.R. Koch, and W.S. Hartroft (1972) Recovery from chronic hepatic lesions in rats fed alcohol and a solid super diet. *Am. J. Clin. Nutr.* 25:881–896.

80. A. Takada, E.A. Porta, and W.S. Hartroft (1967) Regression of dietary cirrhosis in rats fed alcohol and a "super diet." *Am. J. Clin. Nutr.* 20:213–225.

81. S. Bulusu and I. Chakravarty (1984) Augmented hepatic susceptibility to malathion toxicity in rats on low-protein diets. *Environ. Res.* 35:53–65.

82. D.S. Sachan (1975) Effects of low and high protein diets on the induction of microsomal drug-metabolizing enzymes in rat liver. *J. Nutr.* 105:1631–1639.

83. G.O. Korsrud, T. Kuiper-Goodman, E. Hasselager, H.C. Grice, and J.M. McLaughlan (1976) Effects of dietary protein level on carbon tetrachloride-induced liver damage in rats. *Toxicol. Appl. Pharmacol.* 37:1–12.

84. P. Temcharoen, T. Anukarahanonta, and N. Bhamarapravati (1978) Influence of dietary protein and vitamin B_{12} on the toxicity and carcinogenicity of aflatoxins in rat liver. *Cancer Res.* 38:2185–2190.

85. I.R. Crossley, E.N. Wardle, and R. Williams (1983) Biochemical mechanisms of hepatic encephalopathy. *Clin. Sci.* 64:247–252.

86. S.H. Gammal and E.A. Jones (1989) Hepatic encephalopathy. *Med. Clin. North Am.* 73:793–813.

87. S. Sherlock (1987) Chronic portal systemic encephalopathy: update 1987. *Gut* 28:1043–1048.

88. L. Zieve (1987) Pathogenesis of hepatic encephalopathy. *Metab. Brain Dis.* 2:147–165.

89. J.T. Galambos, W.D. Waren, D. Rudman, et al. (1976) Selective and total shunts in the treatment of bleeding varices. A randomized controlled trial. *N. Engl. J. Med.,* 295:1089–1095.

90. L.S. Eriksso (1988) Hepatic encephalopathy and treatment of esophageal varices. *Scand. J. Gastroenterol.* 23:641–649.

91. R. Schwartz, G.B. Phillips, J.E. Seemiller, and G.J. Gabuzda (1954) Dietary protein in the genesis of hepatic coma. *N. Engl. J. Med.* 251:685–691.

92. J.D. Ansley, J.W. Isaacs, L.F. Rikkers, M.H. Kutner, B.M. Nordlinger, and D. Rudman (1978) Quantitative tests of nitrogen metabolism in cirrhosis: relation to other manifestations of liver disease. *Gastroenterology* 75:570–579.

93. G.G. Gerron, J.D. Ansley, J.W. Isaacs, et al. (1976) Technical

pitfalls in measurement of venous plasma HN_3 concentration. *Clin. Chem.* 22:663–666.

94. L. Rikkers, P. Jenko, D. Rudman, and D. Freides (1978) Subclinical hepatic encephalopathy: detection, prevalence, and relationship to nitrogen metabolism. *Gastroenterology* 75:462–469.

95. W.J.H. Summerskill, S.J. Wolfe, and C.S. Davidson (1957) The metabolism of ammonia and a-keto-acids in liver disease and hepatic coma. *J. Clin. Invest.* 36:361–372.

96. J.E. Fischer and R. Baldessarini (1971) False neurotransmitters and hepatic failure. *Lancet* 2:75–79.

97. J.E. Fischer, J.M. Funovics, A. Aguirre, et al. (1975) The role of plasma amino acids in hepatic encephalopathy. *Surgery* 78:276–290.

98. D. Rudman, T.J. DiFulco, J.T. Galambos, R.B. Smith III, A.A. Salam, and W.D. Warren (1973) Maximal rates of excretion and synthesis of urea in normal and cirrhotic subjects. *J. Clin. Invest.* 52:2241–2249.

99. R.J. Rafoth and G.R. Onstad (1974) Urea synthesis after oral protein ingestion in man. *J. Clin. Invest.* 56:1170–1174.

100. E.B. Rypins, J.M. Henderson, T.J. Fulenwider, et al. (1980) A tracer method for measuring rate of urea synthesis in normal and cirrhotic subjects. *Gastroenterology* 78:1419–1424.

101. M. Kekomaki, A.L. Schwartz, and P. Petikainen (1970) Rate of urea synthesis in normal and cirrhotic rat liver with reference to the arginine synthetase system. *Scand. J. Gastroenterol.* 5:375–380.

102. G.O. Perez, B. Rietberg, B. Owens, T. Parker, H. Obaya, and E.R. Schiff (1979) Urea synthesis by perfused rat liver—study of CCl_4-induced cirrhosis. *Biochem. Pharmacol.* 28:485–488.

103. B.S. Khatra, R.B. Smith, III, W.J. Millikan, C.W. Sewell, W.D. Warren, and D. Rudman (1974) Activities of Krebs-Henseleit enzymes in normal and cirrhotic human liver. *J. Lab. Clin. Med.* 84:708–715.

104. K.P. Maier, B. Volk, G. Hoppe-Seyler, and W. Gerok (1974) Urea-cycle enzymes in normal liver and in patients with alcoholic hepatitis. *Eur. J. Clin. Invest.* 4:193–195.

105. K.P. Maier, H. Talke, and W. Gerok (1979) Activities of urea-cycle enzymes in chronic liver disease. *Klin. Wochenschr.* 57:661–665.

106. M.Y. Morgan, J.P. Milsom, and S. Sherlock (1978) Plasma ratio of valine, leucine and isoleucine to phenylalanine and tyrosine in liver disease. *Gut* 19:1068–1073.

107. R.J. Levine and H.O. Conn (1967) Tyrosine metabolism in patients with liver disease. *J. Clin. Invest.* 46:2012–2020.

108. M. Heberer, H. Talke, K.P. Maier, and W. Gerok (1980) Metabolism of phenylalanine in liver disease. *Klin. Wochenschr.* 58:1189–1196.

109. R. Jagenburg, R. Olsson, C.G. Regardh, and S. Rodjer (1977) Kinetics of intravenous administered L-phenylalanine in patients with cirrhosis of the liver. *Clin. Chim. Acta* 78:453–463.

110. D.J. Hehir, R.L. Jenkins, B.R. Bistrian, et al. (1985) Abnormal phenylalanine hydroxylation and tyrosine oxidation in a patient with acute fulminant liver disease with correction by liver transplantation. *Gastroenterology* 89:659–663.

111. M. Nordlinger Bernard, T. Fulenwider, G.L. Ivey, et al. (1979) Tyrosine metabolism in cirrhosis. *J. Lab. Clin. Med.* 94:832–840.

112. S.J.D. O'Keefe, R. Abraham, A. El-Zayadi, W. Marshall, M. Davis, and R. Williams (1981) Increased plasma tyrosine concentrations in patients with cirrhosis and fulminant hepatic failure associated with increased plasma tyrosine flux and reduced hepatic oxidation capacity. *Gastroenterology* 81:1024–1057.

113. R.L.K. Shanbhogue, B.R. Bistrian, K. Lakshman, et al. (1987) Whole body leucine, phenylalanine, and tyrosine kinetics in end-stage liver disease before and after hepatic transplantation. *Metabolism* 36:1047–1053.

114. J.M. Henderson, B.A. Faraj, F.M. Ali, and D. Rudman (1981)

115. D. Labadarios, J.E. Rossouw, J.B. McDonnell, et al. (1977) Vitamin B6 deficiency in chronic liver diseases—evidence for increased degradation of pyridoxal-5' phosphate. *Gut* 18:23–27.

116. A.H. Merrill, Jr., J.M. Henderson, E. Wang, M.A. Codner, B. Hollins, and W.J. Millikan (1986) Activities of the hepatic enzymes of vitamin B-6 metabolism for patients with cirrhosis. *Am. J. Clin. Nutr.* 44:461–467.

117. L. Lumeng (1978) The role of acetaldehyde in mediating the deleterious effects of ethanol on pyridoxal 5' phosphate metabolism. *J. Clin. Invest.* 62:286–293.

118. D. Mitchell, C. Wagner, W.J. Stone, et al. (1976) Abnormal regulation of plasma pyridoxal 5'-phosphate in patients with liver disease. *Gastroenterology* 71:1043–1049.

119. H.A. Harper, L.W. Kinsell, and H.C. Barton (1947) Plasma l-methionine levels following intravenous administration in humans. *Science* 106:319–320.

120. L. Kinsell, H.A. Harper, H.C. Barton, et al. (1947) Rate of disappearance from plasma of intravenously administered methionine in patients with liver damage. *Science* 106:589–590.

121. L.W. Kinsell, H.A. Harper, and H.C. Barton (1948) Studies in methionine and sulfur metabolism. 1. The fate of intravenously administered methionine, in normal individuals and in patients with liver damage. *J. Clin. Invest.* 27:677–688.

122. J.H. Horowitz, E.B. Rypins, J.M. Henderson, et al. (1981) Evidence of impairment of transsulfuration pathway in cirrhosis. *Gastroenterology* 8:668–675.

123. C. Cabrero, A.M. Duce, P. Ortiz, S. Alemany, and J.M. Mato (1988) Specific loss of the high-molecular-weight form of S-adenosyl-l-methionine synthetase in human liver cirrhosis. *Hepatology* 6:1530–1534.

124. A.M. Duce, P. Ortiz, C. Cabrero, and J.M. Mato (1988) S-adenosyl-l-methionine synthetase and phospholipid methyltransferase are inhibited in human cirrhosis. *Hepatology* 8:65–68.

125. D. Rudman, M. Kutner, J. Ansley, et al. (1981) Hypotyrosinemia, hypocystinemia and failure to retain nitrogen during total parenteral nutrition of cirrhotic patients. *Gastroenterology* 81:1025–1035.

126. D.L. Tribble, D.P. Jones, A. Ardehali, R.M. Feeley, and D. Rudman (in press) Hypercysteinemia and delayed sulfur excretion in cirrhotics following oral cysteine loads. *Am. J. Clin. Nutr.*

127. L. Zieve, W.M. Doizaki, and F.J. Zieve (1974) Synergism between mercaptans and ammonia or fatty acids in the production of coma: a possible role for mercaptans in the pathogenesis of hepatic coma. *J. Lab. Clin. Med.* 83:16–28.

128. L. Zieve, W.M. Doizaki, and F.J. Zieve (1969) Pulmonary excretion of mercaptans and dimethyl sulfide in liver cirrhosis before and after ingestion of methionine. *J. Lab. Clin. Med.* 74:861.

129. J.L. Achord (1987) A randomized controlled clinical trial of peripheral amino acid-glucose infusion in acute alcoholic hepatitis. *Am. J. Gastroenterol.* 82:871–875.

130. H. Calvey, M. Davis, and R. Williams (1985) Controlled trial of nutritional supplementation with and without branched amino acid enrichment in the treatment of acute alcoholic hepatitis. *J. Hepatol.* 1:141–151.

131. A.M. Diehl, J. Boitnott, G. Herlong, et al. (1985) Effect of parenteral amino acid supplementation in alcoholic hepatitis. *Hepatology* 5:57–63.

132. J.T. Galambos, T. Hersh, J.T. Fulenwider, et al. (1979) Hyperalimentation in alcoholic hepatitis. *Am. J. Gastroenterol.* 72:535–541.

133. C. Mendenhall, G. Bongiovanni, S. Goldberg, et al. (1985) VA cooperative study on alcoholic hepatitis. III: Changes in protein-calorie malnutrition associated with 30 days of hospitalization with and without enteral nutrition therapy. *IPEN* 9:590–596.

134. S.M. Nasrallah and J.T. Galambos (1980) Aminoacid therapy of alcoholic hepatitis. *Lancet* 2:1276–1277.

Tyrosine transaminase activity in normal and cirrhotic liver. *Dig. Dis. Sci.* 26:124–129.

135. S. Naveau, G. Pelletier, T. Poynard, et al. (1986) A randomized clinical trial of supplementary parenteral nutrition in jaundiced alcoholic cirrhotic patients. *Hepatology* 6:270–274.

136. J. Smith, J. Horowitz, J.M. Henderson, et al. (1982) Enteral hyperalimentation in undernourished patients with cirrhosis and ascites. *Am. J. Clin. Nutr.* 35:56–72.

137. J.L. Achord (1988) Nutrition, alcohol and the liver. *Am. J. Gastroenterol.* 83:244–248.

138. C.L. Mendenhall, T. Tosch, R.E. Weesner, et al. (1986) VA cooperative study on alcoholic hepatitis II: prognostic significance of protein-calorie malnutrition. *Am. J. Clin. Nutr.* 43:213–218.

139. M.Y. Morgan (1981) Enteral nutrition in chronic liver disease. *Acta. Chir. Scand.* [Suppl.] 507:81–90.

140. D. Horst, N.D. Grace, H.O. Conn, et al. (1984) Comparison of dietary protein with an oral, branched chain-enriched amino acid supplement in chronic portal-systemic encephalopathy: a randomized controlled trial. *Hepatology* 4:279–287.

141. A. Sieg, S. Walker, P. Czygan, et al. (1983) Branched-chain amino acid-enriched elemental diet in patients with cirrhosis of the liver. A double blind crossover trial. *Z. Gastroenterol.* 21:644–650.

142. H. Freund, J. Dienstag, J. Lehrich, et al. (1982) Infusion of branched-chain enriched amino acid solution in patients with hepatic encephalopathy. *Ann. Surg.* 196:209–220.

143. J.E. Fischer, N. Yoshimura, A. Aguirre, et al. (1974) Plasma amino acids in patients with hepatic encephalopathy. Effects of amino acid infusions. *Am. J. Surg.* 127:40–47.

144. P.P. Keohane, H. Attrill, G. Grimble, R. Spiller, P. Frost, and D.B.A. Silk (1983) Enteral nutrition in malnourished patients with hepatic cirrhosis and acute encephalopathy. *IPEN* 7:346–350.

145. A. McGhee, M. Henderson, W.J. Millikan, et al. (1983) Comparison of the effects of hepatic-aid and a casein modular diet on encephalopathy, plasma amino acids, and nitrogen balance in cirrhotic patients. *Ann. Surg.* 197:288–293.

146. A. Watanabe, A. Takesue, T. Higashi, and N. Nagashima (1979) Serum amino acids in hepatic encephalopathy. Effects of branched chain amino acid infusion on serum aminogram. *Acta Hepatogastroenterol. (Stuttg.)* 26:346–357.

147. W.J. Millikan, Jr., J.M. Henderson, W.D. Warren, et al. (1983) Total parenteral nutrition with F080 in cirrhotics with subclinical encephalopathy. *Ann. Surg.* 197:292–304.

148. W.F. Alexander, E. Spindel, R.F. Harty, and J.J. Cerda (1989) The usefulness of branched chain amino acids in patients with acute or chronic hepatic encephalopathy. *Am. J. Gastroenterol.* 84:91–96.

149. L.S. Eriksson, A. Persson, and J. Wahren (1982) Branched chain amino acids in the treatment of chronic hepatic encephalopathy. *Gut* 23:801–806.

150. J.E. Fischer, H.M. Rosen, A.M. Eberd, et al. (1976) The effect of normalization of plasma amino acids on hepatic encephalopathy in man. *Surgery* 80:77–91.

151. H. Freund, N. Yoshimura, and J.E. Fischer (1979) Chronic hepatic encephalopathy. Long-term therapy with branched chain amino acid-enriched elemental diet. *JAMA* 242:347–349.

152. K. Schafer, M.B. Winther, M. Ukida, H. Leweling, H.J. Reiter, and J.C. Bode (1981) Influence of an orally administered protein mixture enriched in branched-chain amino acids on the chronic hepatic encephalopathy of patients with liver cirrhosis. *Z. Gastroenterol.* 19:356–362.

153. J.X. Chipponi, J.C. Bleier, M.T. Santi, and D. Rudman (1982) Deficiencies of essential and conditionally essential nutrients. *Am. J. Clin. Nutr.* 35:1112–1116.

Chapter 47

David Kritchevsky

Cancer

Although there has been a long-standing interest in nutrition, diet, and cancer in the United States, it is fair to say that current interest was stimulated by a paper by Doll and Peto[1] that attributed 10–70% of cancer deaths in the United States to diet but admitted that the attribution was ". . . highly speculative and chiefly refers to dietary factors which are not yet reliably identified." A more-recent estimate by one of the authors[2] modified the 10–70% downward drastically. A National Academy of Sciences review panel[3] considered in depth all aspects of the diet-cancer relationship. The only specific recommendation from this group was to reduce amounts of dietary fat.

Data relating to diet and cancer in humans are available from epidemiological studies. Such data are obtained by comparing cancer incidence in populations that are exposed or unexposed to total diet or specific components of the diet. These studies are designated as follow-up studies. In case-control studies, dietary histories of comparable diseased and nondiseased individuals are reviewed. It is also common to calculate correlations between and among diverse geographical populations. These correlations often provide striking differences, but they are flawed because the populations under study usually differ in many aspects of lifestyle and many confounding variables are introduced. Geographical correlations give rise to hypotheses, but these hypotheses must be validated by more stringent observations. In addition to the vagaries of the epidemiological input, the problems inherent in nutrition assessment also introduce problems for data accrual and interpretation. For example, total caloric intake may be relatively constant, but contributions of individual macronutrients may vary. Willett and Stampfer[4] suggested that the proportion of total calories provided by individual macronutrients should be assessed. Stavraky[5] described epidemiological findings as "hypothesis generating data," and so they are. However, efforts to validate or disprove the hypotheses either through further, more finely tuned epidemiological studies or animal studies are the wheels upon which this field advances. Such studies must be continued in order to approach an understanding of the disease.

Animal studies are relatively easy to carry out, but they yield data that should be extrapolated to man with great caution. Most animal studies are carried out in rodents, use defined diets that are easy to manipulate, most often require use of a chemical carcinogen, and are usually terminated at a specific time. The following discussion will consider data from both human and animal studies, and the inherent drawbacks that have been mentioned should be kept in mind.

Macronutrients

Carbohydrate. There are very few data relating to dietary carbohydrate and the risk of cancer in man. A review by Armstrong and Doll[6] suggested a possible connection between liver cancer and intake of potatoes, but the same authors cautioned that the correlations derived in their review were not to be taken as evidence of causation but rather as suggestions for further research. Intake of starch was related to gastric cancer.[7] However, dietary sucrose has no effect on spontaneous tumors in mice[8] or rats.[9]

Protein. In Western diets intakes of protein and fat are correlated closely. Therefore, care must be taken to disassociate one from the other. A relatively weak positive association between protein intake and meat intake with breast cancer was adduced in studies that did not control for caloric intake.[10,11] When protein intake was adjusted for total caloric intake, no correlation with breast cancer was found.[12] An excellent review by Rogers and Longnecker[13] listed 15 references in which protein or meat intake could not be correlated with colorectal cancer. Meat intake may be related to risk of pancreatic cancer,[14] but the additional roles of fat and caloric intake also should be assessed.

Most animal studies show that dietary protein does not affect carcinogenesis when fed at amounts required for optimum growth. A diet containing 31% casein fed to female rats before and after mating and then fed to their female pups increased incidence of dimethylbenzanthracene (DMBA)-induced mammary tumors.[15] A diet severely restricted in protein inhibited growth and reduced aflatoxin-induced liver tumors.[16]

Fat and Energy. Data from many geographic correlation studies support the hypothesis that a high-fat diet is a risk factor for cancers prevalent in developed countries, i.e., breast, colon, and prostate cancers. Berg[17] suggested that these cancers are the result of affluence and may be caused by overnutrition in general rather than by a surplus of any specific macronutrient.

A look at nutritional intake data and cancer mortality might be in order. In 1957 fat provided ~40% of food energy for Americans; this level decreased only recently to ~37%.[18] Between 1949–1951 and 1979–1981 the age-adjusted cancer death rates for all sites increased by 29% in men and decreased by 8% in women.[19] Breast cancer mortality increased by 2% in women whereas mortality from colorectal cancer decreased by 27% in women and 3% in men. During those 30 y, lung cancer mortality increased in women by 331% and in men by 224%.

Rogers and Longnecker[13] reviewed 14 case-control and follow-up studies of diet and breast cancer and found risk to be, at best, related weakly to intake of fat or fat-rich foods. The data that they reviewed included 6233 cancer cases and 265,683 controls. Miller,[20] in discussing the epidemiology of fat and breast cancer, stated that firmer evidence was needed to justify major changes in diet. Data from the National Health and Nutrition Examination Survey (NHANES) studies show no correlation between fat intake and breast cancer.[21] The report on diet, nutrition, and cancer of the National Academy of Sciences[3] suggested that fat intake be reduced to ~30% of calories but stated also that the available data (in 1982) did not provide a strong basis for the recommendation.

The correlation between fat intake and colon cancer is also fraught with inconsistency. The best recent review can be found in the work of Rogers and Longnecker.[13] In the 24 studies cited (19 case-control and 5 follow-up), there was no consistent trend. The authors took the liberty of assessing relative risks for colorectal cancer when none were given, and this author has taken the further liberty of calculating an average relative risk (±SD) for 21 studies to be 1.43 ± 0.84. Kolonel and LeMarchand[22] stated, ". . . at the present time, one cannot firmly conclude that dietary fat either promotes or has no effect on colon carcinogenesis in humans."

There are relatively few studies on the relation of fat intake to cancers other than colorectal or mammary. In a review of world data, MacLennan[23] found no relationship between fat intake and either prostate or gastrointestinal cancer. In no case are there data that consistently link fat intake with risk of a specific cancer.

Some data suggested that low concentrations of blood cholesterol may be associated with increased risk of cancer in man. In 1984 McMichael and his colleagues[24] reviewed the evidence linking exogenous (dietary) or endogenous cholesterol with cancer risk. They found a slightly increased risk for colon and breast cancer with increased cholesterol intake but stated that the close correlation with other nutrients precluded inference of causation. Insofar as blood cholesterol was concerned, they found that preclinical cancer results in a lowering of blood cholesterol but also found evidence that naturally low blood cholesterol placed males at increased risk for colon cancer.

Diets high in fat have been shown repeatedly to enhance chemically induced tumors in rats and mice. Because fat-rich diets are calorically dense, that property, rather than fat per se, may represent the link between fat intake and risk of cancer. In 1909 underfeeding was shown to reduce significantly the growth of transplanted tumors in mice.[25] Tannenbaum[26] showed that caloric restriction inhibits the growth of both induced and spontaneous tumors in mice. Caloric restriction inhibits tumor growth in rats even when the restricted animals ingest five times more fat daily than do controls.[27] In a review of 82 studies involving caloric restriction and carcinogenesis in mice, Albanes[28] found tumor incidence in 18 experiments in which the diets were high in calories but low in fat to be 52.4% ± 4.7%, whereas in 19 experiments in which diets were low in calories but high in fat, tumor incidence was 23.1% ± 4.7%.

A role for caloric intake in human carcinogenesis was suggested.[29,30] One of those studies concluded, "total energy intake must be evaluated before attempting to assign a causal role to any food or nutrient postulated to play a role in colon cancer."[30]

Fiber. Interest in the effects of dietary fiber on colon cancer stems from Burkitt's[31] suggestion of a correlation between incidence of colon cancer and diets low in fiber. As with the fat-fiber relationship, the connection between fiber or fiber-rich foods and colon cancer is probed via ecological or case-control studies. A recent review of physiological effects of dietary fiber compiled available data from both types of studies.[32] In the ecological area there were 15 negative and 1 positive correlations and 6 showed no effect; case-control data revealed 8 studies showing a negative correlation, 6 showing a positive correlation, and 8 finding no effect.[30]

The first epidemiological study of diet and colon cancer was carried out by Stocks and Karn[33] in England in 1933. They found breads, vegetables, and milk to be negatively correlated with colon cancer risk. Comparison of Finns and Danes shows the former to have a considerably lower incidence of colon cancer despite a diet high in meat, fat, and protein.[34] Dietary carbohydrate, fiber, and saturated fatty acids were found to be among negative risk factors. Comparison of colon cancer incidence and intakes of nonstarch polysaccharides in Japan, Finland, Denmark, and the United Kingdom indicates that all the populations have rather low intakes, but these data do not correlate with colon cancer incidence. The intakes of nonstarch polysaccharides in Japan and the United Kingdom are 10.9 and 12.4 g/d, respectively, and colon cancer incidence per 100,000 males per year is 7.8 in Japan and 21.3 in the United Kingdom.[35] Walker et al.[36] found the intake of fiber among South African rural or urban blacks, coloreds, Indians, and whites to be roughly similar whereas colon cancer incidence is very different.

One problem with all the data is that correlations are made with fiber-rich foods rather than with specific fibers. Therefore, these assessments may include effects of minerals or vitamins as well as those of fiber. A recent American study indicated that crude fiber but not neutral detergent fiber was negatively correlated with colon cancer risk.[37] Fruit and vegetable intake was correlated with decreased risk, but a high intake of grains was not protective.

Despite the lack of any clear-cut connection between fiber intake and colon cancer risk, the available data are intriguing and mandate further exploration of this phenomenon.

Micronutrients

Vitamin A and β-Carotene. Byers[38] reviewed six studies relating carotene intake to risk of lung cancer and found a consistent negative correlation between high intakes of carotene and relative risk. There may be an inverse correlation between dietary β-carotene and colon cancer risk.[39] However, the findings are inconsistent.[29] There seems to be no correlation between vitamin A intake and colon cancer risk,[29] and an inverse correlation exists between vitamin A intake and risk of breast cancer.[12,40] Data on vitamin A intake and risk of prostatic cancer are inconsistent, and there are negative correlations between intake of vegetables and fruits and pancreatic cancer.[41,42]

Vitamins C and E. The relationship of vitamin C intake to risk of colon cancer is either nonexistent or shows a slight inverse correlation.[13] There seems to be no connection between vitamin C intake and lung cancer, prostate cancer, or ovarian cancer.[13]

A review by Rogers and Longnecker[13] indicates no evidence of a correlation between vitamin E and risk of breast, lung, or prostate cancer. Insofar as colorectal cancer is concerned, a review of five studies suggests a small inverse association or none at all.

Selenium. Low selenium intake may be associated with the risk of gastrointestinal cancer,[43] but a relationship of selenium intake to breast or lung cancer is not remarkable.[44]

Calcium. Some recent data suggest an inverse association between calcium intake and risk of colorectal cancer.[39,45,46]

Alcohol. The effects of alcohol consumption on risk of breast cancer were reviewed.[13,38] Overall there appears to be a modest positive association. However, there is disagreement on the level of intake at which risk may become evident and at least one thorough study found no risk at all.[47] The wide range of correlations, ranging from no effect in light drinkers to heavy drinkers, suggests a possible bias in reporting of intake. Byers[38] suggested that subgroups in our population may be particularly susceptible to alcohol, and efforts to identify such groups should be made.

There is a moderate risk of large-bowel cancer associated with alcohol intake, and this risk is especially true for the susceptibility of male beer drinkers to rectal cancer.[3] Heavy drinking is associated with risk of cancer of the mouth, pharynx, larynx, esophagus, and liver.[3]

Summary

The recommendations related to diet and risk of cancer generally include maintenance of ideal weight, increased intake of cereals, vegetables and fruits, and some decrease in fat consumption. For the U.S. population these recommendations suggest moderation in food intake. For future assessment of a diet-cancer relationship, we need uniform experimental protocols, and we need especially to know more about nutrient interactions. For example, the study of Slattery et al.[37] indicated greater relative risk in the first and fourth quartiles of starch and grain consumption than in the second and third quartiles. Could it be that at the highest and lowest levels of starch intake there is a displacement of some other beneficial dietary component? More data on dietary interactions could provide an answer.

Sir Richard Doll[48] wrote about recent developments in the area of epidemiology and cancer prevention. With regard to diet, he encouraged action on current knowledge, i.e., increased intakes of fruits, vegetables, and fiber. He went on to say that such suggestions are justifiable only so long as we distinguish between recommendations based on established knowledge and those based on best guesses.

Most reviews of the subject of nutrition and cancer come to similar conclusions, because the available data are inconclusive. Investigation into the reasons for the dichotomies should be productive. Until then, the best advice is prudence, not panic.

References

1. R. Doll and R. Peto (1981) The causes of cancer: quantitative estimates of avoidable risks of cancer in the United States today. *JNCI* 66:1191–1308.

2. R. Peto (1984) Cancer around the world: evidence of avoidability. In: *Diet and Prevention of Coronary Heart Disease and Cancer* (B. Hallgren, O. Levine, S. Rossner, and B. Vessby, eds.), pp. 1–16, Raven Press, New York.

3. Committee on Diet, Nutrition and Cancer (1982) *Diet, Nutrition and Cancer*, National Academy Press, Washington, DC.

4. W.C. Willett and M.J. Stampfer (1986) Total energy intake: implication for epidemiologic analyses. *Am. J. Epidemiol.* 124:17–27.

5. K.M. Stavraky (1976) The role of ecological analysis in the etiology of disease. A discussion with reference to large bowel cancer. *J. Chronic Dis.* 29:435–445.

6. B. Armstrong and R. Doll (1975) Environmental factors and cancer incidence and mortality in different countries with special reference to dietary practices. *Int. J. Cancer* 15:617–631.

7. B. Modan, F. Lubin, V. Barell, R.A. Greenberg, M. Modan, and S. Graham (1974) The roles of starches in the etiology of gastric cancer. *Cancer* 34:2087–2092.

8. F.J.C. Roe, L.S. Levy, and R.L. Carter (1970) Feeding studies on sodium cyclamate, saccharin and sucrose for carcinogenic and tumor promoting activity. *Food Cosmet. Toxicol.* 8:135–145.

9. L. Friedman, H.L. Richardson, M.E. Richardson, E.J. Lethes, W.C. Wallace, and F.M. Sauro (1972) Toxic response of rats to cyclamates in chow and semi-synthetic diets. *J. Natl. Cancer Inst.* 49:751–764.

10. T. Hirayama (1978) Epidemiology of breast cancer with special reference to the role of diet. *Prev. Med.* 7:173–195.

11. R. Talamini, C. LaVecchia, A. Decarli, et al. (1984) Social factors, diet and breast cancer in a Northern Italian population. *Br. J. Cancer* 49:723–727.

12. K. Katsouyanni, W. Willett, D. Trichopoulos, et al. (1988) Risk of breast cancer among Greek women in relation to nutrient intake. *Cancer* 61:181–185.

13. A.E. Rogers and M.P. Longnecker (1988) Biology of disease. Dietary and nutritional influences on cancer: a review of epidemiologic and experimental data. *Lab. Invest.* 59:729–759.

14. S.E. Norell, A. Ahlbom, R. Erwald, et al. (1986) Diet and pancreatic cancer: a case-control study. *Am. J. Epidemiol.* 124:894–902.

15. E.J. Hawrylewicz (1986) Fat-protein interaction, defined 2-generation studies. *Prog. Clin. Biol. Res.* 222:403–433.

16. T.V. Madhavan and C. Gopolan (1968) The effect of dietary protein on carcinogenesis of aflatoxin. *Arch. Pathol.* 85:133–137.

17. J.W. Berg (1975) Can nutrition explain the pattern of international epidemiology of hormone-dependent cancer? *Cancer Res.* 35:3345–3350.

18. R.L. Rizek, S.O. Walsh, R.M. Marston, and E.M. Jackson (1983) Levels and sources of fat in the U.S. food supply and in diets of individuals. In: *Dietary Fats and Health* (E.D. Perkins and W.K. Visek, eds.), American Oil Chemists Society, Champaign, IL.

19. American Cancer Society (1988) *Cancer Facts and Figures*, American Cancer Society, New York.

20. A.B. Miller (1986) Dietary fat and the epidemiology of breast cancer. *Prog. Clin. Biol. Res.* 222:17–32.

21. D.Y. Jones, A. Schatzkin, S.B. Green, et al. (1987) Dietary fat and breast cancer in the National Health and Nutrition Examination Survey I epidemiologic follow-up study. *JNCI* 79:465–471.

22. L.N. Kolonel and L. LeMarchand (1986) The epidemiology of colon cancer and dietary fat. *Prog. Clin. Biol. Res.* 222:69–91.

23. R. MacLennan (1985) Fat intake and cancer of the gastrointestinal tract and prostate. *Med. Oncol. Tumor Pharmacother.* 2:137–142.

24. A.J. McMichael, O.M. Jensen, D.M. Parkin, and D.G. Zaridze (1984) Dietary and endogenous cholesterol and human cancer. *Epidemiol. Rev.* 6:192–216.

25. C. Moreschi (1909) Relationship between nutrition and tumor growth. *Z. Immunitatsforsch.* 2:651–675 (in German).

26. A. Tannenbaum (1945) The dependence of tumor formation on the degree of caloric restriction. *Cancer Res.* 5:609–615.

27. D. Kritchevsky and D.M. Klurfeld (1987) Caloric effects in experimental mammary tumorigenesis. *Am. J. Clin. Nutr.* 45:236–242.

28. D. Albanes (1987) Total calories, body weight and tumor incidence in mice. *Cancer Res.* 47:1987–1992.

29. J.D. Potter and A.J. McMichael (1986) Diet and cancer of the colon and rectum: a case-control study. *JNCI* 76:557–569.

30. J.L. Lyon, A.W. Mahoney, D.W. West, et al. (1987) Energy intake: its relation to colon cancer risk. *JNCI* 78:853–861.

31. D.P. Burkitt (1971) Epidemiology of cancer of the colon and rectum. *Cancer* 28:3–13.

32. S.M. Pilch, ed. (1987) *Physiological Effects and Health Consequences of Dietary Fiber,* Federation of American Societies for Experimental Biology, Bethesda, MD.

33. P. Stocks and M.K. Karn (1933) A cooperative study of the habits, homelife, dietary and family histories of 450 cancer patients and an equal number of control patients. *Ann. Eugen. (London)* 5:237–280.

34. O.M. Jensen, R. MacLennan, and J. Wahrendorf (1982) Diet, bowel function, fecal characteristics and large bowel cancer in Denmark and Finland. *Nutr. Cancer* 4:5–19.

35. J.H. Cummings and S.A. Bingham (1987) Dietary fibre, fermentation and large bowel cancer. *Cancer Surv.* 6:601–621.

36. A.R.P. Walker, B.F. Walker, and A.J. Walker (1986) Faecal pH, dietary fiber intake and proneness to colon cancer in four South African populations. *Br. J. Cancer* 53:489–495.

37. M.L. Slattery, A.W. Sorenson, A.W. Mahoney, T.K. French, D. Kritchevsky, and J.C. Street (1988) Diet and colon cancer: Assessment of risk by fiber type and food source. *JNCI* 80:1474–1480.

38. T. Byers (1988) Diet and cancer: any progress in the "interim"? *Cancer* 62:1713–1724.

39. S. Kune, G.A. Kune, and L.F. Watson (1987) Case-control study of dietary etiological factors: the Melbourne colorectal cancer study. *Nutr. Cancer* 9:21–42.

40. S. Graham, J. Marshall, C. Mettlin, T. Rzepka, T. Nemoto, and T. Byers (1982) Diet in the epidemiology of breast cancer. *Am. J. Epidemiol.* 116:68–75.

41. E.B. Gold, L. Gordis, M.D. Diener, et al. (1985) Diet and other risk factors for cancer in the pancreas. *Cancer* 55:460–467.

42. T.M. Mack, M.C. Yu, R. Hamsch, and B.E. Henderson (1986) Pancreas cancer and smoking, beverage consumption and past medical history. *JNCI* 76:49–60.

43. R.J. Shamberger and C.E. Willis (1971) Selenium distribution and human cancer mortality. *CRC Crit. Rev. Clin. Lab. Sci.* 2:211–221.

44. W.C. Willett, B.F. Polk, J.S. Morris, et al. (1983) Pre-diagnostic serum selenium and risk of cancer. *Lancet* 2:130–133.

45. G. Macquart-Moulin, E. Riboli, J. Cornee, B. Charmay, P. Berthezene, and N. Day (1986) Case-control study on colorectal cancer and diet in Marseilles. *Int. J. Cancer* 38:183–191.

46. C. Garland, R.B. Shekelle, E. Barrett-Connor, M.H. Criqui, A.H. Rossof, and P. Ogelsby (1985) Dietary vitamin D and calcium and risk of colorectal cancer: a 19-year prospective study in men. *Lancet* 1:307–309.

47. L.A. Webster, P.M. Layde, P.A. Wingo, H.W. Ory, and the Cancer and Steroid Hormone Study Group (1983) Alcohol consumption and risk of breast cancer. *Lancet* 2:724–726.

48. R. Doll (1988) Epidemiology and the prevention of cancer: some recent developments. *J. Cancer Res. Clin. Oncol.* 114:447–458.

Eleanor M. Pao and Yasmin S. Cypel

Chapter **48**

Estimation of Dietary Intake

Dietary intake estimation involves the collection of information on foods eaten by individuals and computation of the energy and nutrient contents of these foods by using values from food composition tables. The food intakes may be current or from the immediate, recent, or distant past. Factors to be considered in the selection of an appropriate method for estimating dietary intake are purpose of the study, population or group studied, precision of measurement required, costs, and length of time to be covered. This chapter describes methods for obtaining food intake information, processing the information, and deriving qualitative and quantitative estimates of dietary intake. This chapter also briefly reviews the strengths and weaknesses of these methods, their reliability and validity, and some implications for interpretation of dietary intake estimates.

Dietary intake estimates serve many purposes. Government, academia, industry, and numerous other groups have vital interests in the dietary status of both the overall population and particular subgroups. Dietary surveys are the principal means for obtaining descriptions of dietary patterns of population groups for use in making policy and program decisions. Four expert committees have provided helpful recommendations concerning appropriate assessment of food consumption patterns,[1] uses of national food-consumption-survey data,[2] assessment of nutrient adequacy using food-consumption-survey data,[3] and guidelines for interpreting dietary intake data.[4] Health professionals and clinicians need information relating diet to health or physical status; such information often requires consideration of usual dietary intake.

Data Collection Methods

Although four data-collection methods are identified and described here, researchers vary considerably in how they categorize and define each method. The food record or diary, for which foods are weighed or estimated by use of household measures, obtains current intake information; the dietary recall, food frequency method, and dietary history are used to measure past intake. Anderson[4] noted that the 1-d record and 1-d recall both measure quantitative daily consumption pertaining to food intake in a specified time period. To reflect total intake, foods eaten both at home and away from home must be reported. Supplements are sometimes included, but problems have been encountered with quantification because of the extremely large variety of dietary supplements available, the content change in their formulas, and the absence of reliable information about the content of many over-the-counter supplements. Survey questionnaires also collect demographic and personal information about individuals (for example, sex, age, race, income, and region and urbanization of residence) in order to characterize and compare dietary intakes by different groups. Several informative reviews of dietary intake methods are available.[5-8]

Food Record. The food record (also called food diary) is kept by the subject or by a designated surrogate (for example, a mother for her child) for a specified time period, usually 1–7 d. Longer periods of ≤1 y have been reported.[9] Although there is no true measure of dietary intake with which data from a study procedure can be compared, a weighed food record is often considered the most accurate method. Therefore, the weighed record is viewed by some as the standard for comparing the accuracy of other methods. In this method food is weighed before eating. For convenience, the subject may use a gram scale that can be set back to zero after a plate is placed on the scale and after each serving of food is added to the plate and the weight is recorded.[10] Leftovers are weighed and deducted. Foods eaten away from home are usually estimated in household measures. Few large-scale studies or surveys have used the weighed food record because of high costs, burden on the participants, and difficulty in maintaining a representative sample of the population. Further, studies showed that habitual eating patterns can be disrupted by the task of weighing, resulting in lower reported intakes.[9]

More often used than the weighed record is the less-burdensome estimated food record. Respondents are asked to describe foods and amounts as eaten. Descriptions of food include kind, preparation, brand name (if brand differences are significant), and main ingredients in mixtures. Several types of measurement varying in accuracy may appear on the estimated record. Standard measuring cups and spoons may be used to report volume of liquids, semisolids, and foods in small pieces. Solid foods may be measured with a ruler and described by shape (square, rectangle, cylinder, wedge) and dimensions (length, width, height, diameter). Count, such as one egg, and relative size, such as small, medium, or large, may be sufficient. Weight or volume measures on labels may be used for foods such as candy bars and beverages in containers. For items such as pies and cakes of which a portion of the whole is eaten, weight or dimensions of the whole and the proportion eaten are appropriate. Reports for meats must indicate whether amounts are for raw or cooked forms, with or without bone, and with or without skin or fat. In reporting volume, measures should be level, not rounded or heaping.

In the Nationwide Food Consumption Surveys (NFCSs) conducted by the U.S. Department of Agriculture (USDA), a set of measuring cups and spoons and a ruler are given to participating households for members to use in keeping 2-d food records. A food instruction booklet also is provided to help respondents describe kinds and amounts of food ingested.[11]

Interviewers or health professionals working with respondents, clients, or patients provide individuals with food record forms and verbal as well as written instructions for their completion. Use of measuring devices must be demonstrated, and the individual should have an opportunity to practice. Arrangements are made for the interviewer's return to collect and review completed records.

Validity refers to whether the method measures what it is supposed to measure. The validity of dietary intakes estimated by food records is especially important because food records are often used as the reference against which others are compared. Krall and Dwyer[12] assessed the validity of food diaries by comparing diary reports with weighed portions of food served in a metabolic research unit and found that ~9% of all food items were omitted. However, another study found that the burden of having to weigh foods eaten resulted in a 13% decrease in ca-

loric intakes, on average, compared with intakes from weekly diary records.[9] The possibility of systematic error is indicated by findings that in studies covering multiple days of food records, mean food intakes for the first few days often exceed those of later days.[13] Gersovitz et al.[13] found that the first 2 d yielded valid estimates of all nutrients studied except protein. Studies have shown significant correlation between some nutrients calculated from food records and biochemical measurements.[14] The studies described here indicate some pitfalls in use of the food record and some precautions that may help reduce errors in reporting.

Reliability often refers to repeatability or reproducibility of results using a particular method. Consumption in two time periods or as obtained by two different methods can be compared to appraise reliability. Todd et al.[15] found no significant differences in mean energy or protein intakes derived from data collected by two methods—weighed intakes recorded on tape and estimated food records. Similarly, in another study, four sets of 7-d records kept by 173 female nurses during 1 y showed little tendency to change over that time period; intraclass coefficients ranged from 0.41 for vitamin A to 0.72 for carbohydrate.[16]

Table 1 provides a list of the principal strengths and weaknesses of the food record. Comparison of this list with those for the other procedures can yield useful insights.

Twenty-four–hour Food Recall. The method most commonly selected for obtaining food intake information is the 24-h food recall. Large national dietary intake surveys,[11,17] diet-health studies,[18] as well as smaller studies[19] used this method to estimate dietary intakes by individuals. However, few studies using the 24-h recall follow identical procedures. Essentially, the individual is asked to recall and describe the kinds and amounts of all foods (including beverages) ingested during a 24-h period. Usually, the 24-h and 1-d recall are synonymous, referring to the preceding full day.[11,17] Occasionally, the 24-h period starts with the last eating event and moves backwards for 24 h.[10,19] Dietary recalls have covered shorter periods such as a few hours[20] or longer periods such as 7 d.[21] To obtain an indication of usual intake, six bimonthly 1-d food recalls were obtained from the same individuals during a 1-y panel survey.[11]

Dietary recall questionnaires may be administered by in-person or telephone interview[11] or they may be self-administered. The 24-h food recall takes 15–30 min to complete. Interviews may be conducted in the home,[11] in a clinic setting,[17] or at some other convenient site. The location should provide privacy to minimize distractions.

Because individuals vary in their ability and will-

Table 1. Strengths and weaknesses of food record methods

Strengths	Weaknesses
1. Respondent does not rely on memory.	1. Respondents must be literate.
2. Time period is defined.	2. Respondents must be highly cooperative.
3. Portions can be measured to increase accuracy.	3. Food consumed away from home may be less accurately reported.
4. Omission of foods is minimal.	4. Habitual eating pattern may be influenced or changed by the recording process.
5. For elderly people, records may be more accurate than recalls.	5. Requirement for literate respondents may introduce bias as a result of overrepresentation of more highly educated individuals.
6. Food intakes are quantified so nutrient contents can be calculated.	6. Record keeping increases respondent burden.
7. Multiple days may yield a measure of usual intake for a group.	7. Increased respondent burden may adversely affect response rates.
8. Multiple days provide reliable information about less frequently eaten foods.	8. Self-administered records require more callbacks and editing than interviewer-administered reports.
9. Two or more days provide data on intra- and interindividual variation in dietary intakes.	9. One-day records provide an inadequate indication of usual intake for groups or individuals.
10. One-day records kept intermittently over the year may provide an estimate of usual intake by an individual.	10. Validity of records may decrease as number of days increases.

ingness to recall, describe, and quantify foods eaten, interviewers are trained to ask probing questions that encourage and help organize the individuals' memories about eating events. Probes to clarify or check information must be neutral and vary with the kind of food. To obtain adequate descriptions of foods, interviewers usually ask about type (e.g., whole or skim milk), preparation (e.g., broiled or fried chicken), brand name (e.g., for ready-to-eat cereal), main ingredients in mixtures, and other special features (such as low calorie or low sodium). In automated interviews probing questions appear on the computer screen, reminding interviewers of essential information to be reported.[22] As a consequence, interviewer bias is reduced.

Usually some type of measurement aid is selected as a common reference to help individuals estimate portion sizes more precisely. Measurement aids include food models and geometric shapes,[18] household measuring utensils,[11] a product-identification notebook,[19] food-model drawings,[23] and other such means. Accuracy of portion size estimates using the different approaches has not been adequately tested.

Validity of the 24-h food recall was assessed in numerous studies by comparing recalled intakes with observed intakes or with intakes obtained by other methods. In a metabolic study in which foods were weighed before being served, actual and recalled intakes by adolescent girls were not significantly different on either of two nonconsecutive weekdays for energy, protein, calcium, and zinc content, but intakes were underestimated for five vitamins and iron on day 1 and overestimated for two vitamins and iron on day 2.[24] A study of older adults enrolled in a congregate meals program revealed that mean nutrient content of recalled intakes for a noon meal tended to be higher than mean content of observed intakes for all nutrients studied except vitamin A. However, differences were significant only for protein.[13] Other investigators found that recalled intakes compared with weighed intakes tended to be overestimated when intakes were low and underestimated when intakes were high.[25,26] Mean nutrient intakes estimated from 24-h recalls and 3-d food records were highly correlated and not statistically different (as measured by t test) in a study of vegetarians and nonvegetarians.[10] These studies provide evidence that reporting errors occur, but indications of their direction or extent are not consistent from study to study or from nutrient to nutrient.

Reliability of the 24-h dietary recall was studied by examining intra- and interindividual variation.[27] Sources of error that affect reliability of this survey method are discussed in enlightening detail by these researchers. Strengths and weaknesses of the 24-h food recall are outlined in Table 2.

Food Frequency Methods. In the last decade, use of food frequency methods in epidemiological studies of diet and disease relationships increased remarkably. As noted by Sampson,[28] usual dietary intake over an extended period is more pertinent in assessing the relationship of nutrition to chronic disease than is diet on a recent specific day or week. The method often is used to rank individuals by food or nutrient intakes and also by group intakes into categories so that high and low intakes may be studied. The questionnaires vary as to the number of foods listed, the length of time covered by the reference period, the response intervals for specifying frequency, and the procedure for estimating portion size.

Qualitative food frequency methods generally obtain only the usual number of times each food on a checklist is eaten during a specified period.[29] Information on portion size is necessary for calculations of nutrient intakes. Sometimes an average portion

Table 2. Strengths and weaknesses
of 24-h food recall methods

Strengths	Weaknesses
1. Respondent burden is small.	1. Repondent recall depends on memory.
2. Administration time is short.	2. Portion size is difficult to estimate accurately.
3. Reliance on memory is minimal.	3. Intakes tend to be underreported compared with other methods.
4. Time period is defined.	4. Dietary adequacy of an individual's intake cannot be assessed from one day's intake.
5. Food intake can be quantified.	
6. Procedure does not alter individual's habitual dietary patterns.	5. Trained interviewers are required.
7. Interviewer administration allows probing for omitted foods on incomplete information and fewer callbacks.	6. One-day intakes do not represent usual intake for groups or individuals.
8. Response rates are relatively high.	
9. A single contact is required.	
10. Procedure is often used to evaluate dietary intakes of large groups.	
11. Two or more days provide data on intra- and interindividual variation in dietary intakes.	
12. Multiple days are necessary to provide reliable data on less frequently eaten foods.	
13. Multiple days may yield a measure of usual intake.	
14. Repeated recalls over a year may provide an estimate of usual intake by an individual.	

size is estimated for the qualitative food frequency to allow for nutrient intakes to be calculated.[30] Quantitative methods require that the usual amount eaten be given; when this is combined with the frequency and nutrient content information, estimates of usual intake of a nutrient can be derived.[31] Semiquantitative methods also may allow estimation of a standard (or medium) portion by the researcher or ask respondents to indicate how often, on average, they consumed a specified common amount.[16] Estimation of portion size may be assisted by use of food models[32] or measuring utensils. The food lists may include only items high in a specified nutrient, such as vitamin A,[33] or may vary widely in the number of items, from as few as 18 food groups[17] to >100 foods and food groups.[31] To derive nutrient intakes, these methods require assignment of a nutrient value for

each group of foods. The value may be based on the predominant food in the group, on weighting each food in the group by usage, or on some other similar system.

Reference time periods vary from as short as a few days, 1 wk, 1 m, or 3 m to ≥1 y. For example, in an instrument with 61 food items designed by Willett et al.,[16] respondents indicated how often during the past year, on average, they ate a commonly used portion size. Nine response categories ranged from never to six or more times per day. Food frequency instruments may be administered by in-person or telephone interview or be self-administered by using mailed questionnaires.[16] A standardized food frequency method with wide acceptance has not yet appeared.

Validity of the food frequency procedure was evaluated by comparing results with those from alternative methods and by correlations of biochemical data with food frequency data. Willett et al.[16] compared results obtained with a 61-item food frequency questionnaire with data from four 1-wk food records for calorie-adjusted intakes of nine nutrients. They found that 49% of the 173 female nurses in the highest quintile for diet records were also in the highest quintile of data from food frequencies. They concluded that the food frequency method was useful in measuring intakes for a variety of nutrients. Pietinen et al.[30] found some nutrient values derived from a 44-item qualitative food frequency questionnaire and from diet records for 12 2-d periods were generally comparable. Axelson and Csernus[29] compared results from a 62-item qualitative instrument, completed by 89 university students, with NFCS 1965 and 1977–78 data for the same age cohort and concluded that their questionnaire provided similar data. Roidt et al.[34] found weak but significant correlations of 0.18–0.26 between serum indicators of vitamin A status and estimated nutrient intakes based on 302 mailed 71-item food frequency questionnaires. However, Sorenson et al.[32] determined that the food frequency procedure overestimated intakes compared with the 2-d record, 24-h dietary recall, and diet history methods. Krall and Dwyer[12] administered a food frequency questionnaire to volunteers in a metabolic study using weighed portions and found that the food frequency method significantly underestimated values for energy and nutrients. Flegal et al.[31] found poor agreement and poor relative validity between a 113-item food frequency procedure and 16 recalls and records.

Reliability of the food frequency method was assessed in terms of the correlation between two administrations of the instrument. Axelson and Csernus[29] found a significant correlation of 0.89 between two tests, 6 mo apart, involving 15 university

Table 3. Strengths and weaknesses of food frequency methods

Strengths	Weaknesses
1. An indication of usual dietary intake may be obtained.	1. Memory of food patterns in the past is required.
2. Highly trained interviewers are not required.	2. Recall period may be imprecise.
3. Method can be interviewer administered or self-administered.	3. Quantification of food intake may be imprecise because of poor estimation of recall of portions or use of standard sizes.
4. Administration may be simple.	4. Respondent burden is governed by number and complexity of foods listed and quantification procedure.
5. Customary eating patterns are not affected.	5. Recall of past diets may be biased by current diets.
6. Individuals may be ranked or classified by food intake.	6. Heterogeneity of populations influences the reliability of the method.
7. Response rates are high.	7. Suitability is questionable for certain segments of the population, such as individuals consuming atypical diets or foods not on the list.
8. Respondent burden is usually light.	8. Intakes tend to be overestimated compared with some other methods.
9. Relationship between diet and disease may be examined in epidemiological studies.	9. Validation of the method is difficult.

students. Pietinen et al.[30] demonstrated good reproducibility (correlations of 0.48–0.86) for nutrients in three administrations of a food frequency questionnaire to a fairly homogeneous group of Finnish middle-aged men. Strengths and weaknesses of the food frequency methods are listed in Table 3.

Diet History Method. The diet history method was developed originally to measure usual diets over a period of time in the past for use in longitudinal studies of human growth and development. As it evolved the method incorporated a combination of three methods—24-h dietary recall, food record, and food frequency.[35] More recently, modifications of the diet history were designed by epidemiologists to study associations between diet and onset of such chronic illnesses as cancer and heart disease.[6,36–38] The diet history generally obtains usual intake of foods in terms of frequencies and quantities ingested and is similar to quantitative food frequency methods. Diet histories, however, tend to focus on the more distant past than do food frequency questionnaires although there are exceptions. Diet histories may focus on foods in the total diet or on selected foods rich in a specific nutrient, such as vitamin A.[36]

Although highly trained interviewers with nutrition backgrounds most often are required, lay persons can be trained as procedures become more standardized.[39] Hankin[39] collected frequency and quantitative data on foods consumed by a population group as a basis for developing a suitable diet history questionnaire. To increase accuracy of reported portion sizes, she showed photographs of small, medium, and large servings of each food to respondents. Byers et al.[36] also used pictures of food, whereas others have used models.[40] Jain[40] described in detail a method used by an epidemiology unit in Canada.

In assessing validity of diet histories, Byers et al.[36] found some evidence that recall of past diets may be biased by current diets. However, the recall of past diets still provided more information about the past than recall of current intake did. Some researchers found that diet histories produce higher estimates of intakes than did food records.[36,38,41] Hankin et al.[37] and Howe et al.[42] found reproducibility of repeated administrations acceptable. Strengths and weaknesses of the diet history method are listed in Table 4.

Combination of Methods. Sometimes a combination of two or more methods can provide greater accuracy by counterbalancing the shortcomings of one method with strengths of another.[5,7] For example, the NFCSs conducted by the USDA use a combination of a 1-d food recall and a 2-d food record.[43]

Interviewers

The performance of interviewers is crucial for obtaining reliable and valid data in surveys as well as

Table 4. Strengths and weaknesses of diet history methods

Strengths	Weaknesses
1. Method yields a more representative pattern of intakes in the distant past than other methods.	1. Highly trained interviewers are usually required.
2. Measurement of past diet is useful in epidemiological studies of disease states that develop slowly over time.	2. Recall period is difficult to visualize accurately.
3. Respondent literacy is not required if interviewer administered.	3. Respondents must be highly cooperative.
4. Method may be designed to assess total diet or only selected food items.	4. Respondent and interviewer burden may be heavy.
	5. Method may require considerable time.
	6. The method tends to overestimate intakes compared with other methods.
	7. Recall of diets in the past may be biased by current diets.
	8. A commonly accepted method is not yet available.

in special studies. Consequently, interviewers' qualifications, training, and supervision must be given careful attention. Ideally, interviewers should have skill in interviewing techniques and knowledge of food preparation. Training courses provide standardized preparation and practice. Use of reference manuals promotes consistency in performance across time and among interviewers. Computer-assisted interviews may require additional training time. Field work is monitored to ensure that procedures are followed uniformly and problems are handled promptly. Telephone interviewers usually work in a central location, which simplifies supervision.

Data Processing

Plans for data processing and analysis are made as the survey or study is planned in order to ensure that required information is collected in usable form. After food intake information has been collected, it must be processed to provide variables and data for analyses that fulfill the objectives of the study. Questionnaires from large surveys are generally processed in a central office. They are reviewed, edited, and coded immediately upon arrival in case additional information is necessary. Coding is the assignment of numbers to responses for the purpose of data reduction and categorization either by hand tally or by computer. Food codes are used to organize food groups according to the system design.

In the USDA dietary intake surveys the coding scheme (available upon request) contains seven-digit food codes in which the first digit identifies one of nine major food groups. Subcategories within the nine major food groups form hierarchies that permit regrouping and extracting of information. Sometimes respondents supply inadequate descriptions or amounts of items and a default code or value is assigned; new food codes are created as needed. Amounts of food reported in common measures are converted to weights (in grams) by computer.

The amount of each nutrient in each food reported is calculated by using the weight in grams of the food and the nutritive value of 100 g of the food from an appropriate nutrient data base.[44] The food intake report and the nutrient database are linked by the food codes. Data are checked by computer for consistency and reasonableness.

A number of nutrient data bases are available for use in calculating nutrient content of food intakes by computer. Most of them are based on food composition values from the USDA National Nutrient Data Bank or revised sections of the standard reference Agriculture Handbook No. 8 (*Composition of Foods: Raw, Processed, Prepared*).[44] Values in food tables are not accurate enough for metabolic studies, which may require chemical analyses of specific food samples for particular nutrients. Accuracy of food composition tables and implications for energy and nutrient analysis of diets are discussed elsewhere.[2,5]

Data Analysis

A major use of dietary intake surveys is estimating the food and nutrient intakes of population groups categorized by sex, age, income, region, and other characteristics. Mean food and nutrient intakes among population subgroups are compared to determine the most commonly eaten foods and variations in eating patterns. Mean intakes by specific sex-age categories are compared with the latest Recommended Dietary Allowances (RDA)[45] to discern which nutrients are consumed in less than recommended amounts. Food intakes from the different food groups also may be evaluated.[46]

A variety of statistical procedures are applied in analysis of survey or study data. Descriptive statistics—frequency distributions, means, standard errors or standard deviations, and cross tabulations—are basic to understanding the data. Krebs-Smith et al.[47] illustrated the importance of properly stating the question to get the proper answer. Because not all sample households participate in a particular survey, weighting factors are usually derived to adjust for nonresponse. More complex relationships and variations may be examined using regression and other multivariate techniques.

Issues with Implications for Interpretation

Large national surveys provide baseline information for public decision making and for understanding trends or changes in dietary status of the population and its subgroups. However, users of dietary intake data should be cognizant of certain limitations in interpreting results. USDA has sponsored a number of methodologic studies to improve procedures for estimating dietary intake of individuals.[48]

Assessment of Diet Quality. The RDA[45] are standards commonly used to evaluate the quality of diets of population groups. Differences between mean nutrient intakes of sex-age groups and the appropriate RDAs should be interpreted with awareness that RDA provide margins of safety and are for a healthy reference individual. Therefore, an individual whose usual intake approximates or exceeds the RDA for a nutrient is unlikely to be deficient for this nutrient. An expert committee studied criteria for evaluating nutrient intake data derived from surveys and recommended that an approach be taken based on the probability that a specific nutrient intake would be inadequate to meet an individual's need.[3] However, lack of knowledge concerning mean nutrient requirements and their variations in the population precludes general use of the probability approach at this time.

Number of Days. The number of intake days obtained by food recall or record contributes to how the dietary intake estimates can be used.[4,49] One-day dietary intakes from a large sample provide reliable estimates of mean intakes for the group but not for an individual in the group. Intraindividual variation is greater in 1-d dietary data and may conceal relationships between diet and disease.[27] An expert committee considered 1-d data to be less preferable for such studies.[4]

Collection of multiple days of dietary information by using either the recall or record method decreases intraindividual variation and increases precision of intake estimates.[4] Beaton et al.[27] demonstrated that the width of a confidence interval for mean of the group was decreased by increasing sample size or number of intake days. Each additional day of intake information provides an increasingly smaller increment of independent information.[4] Intraindividual variation differs among nutrients. For data from a year-long study, the number of days needed to estimate adequately the usual intake for the group varied from 3 d for food energy to 41 d for vitamin A.[50] The number of days required depends on study purpose, desired precision, the particular nutrient, and the amount of intra- and interindividual variation.[4]

Measurement Error. Dietary intake measures can have both random and systematic errors. Food intakes are based on reports by respondents who describe the kinds and amounts of foods with an unknown degree of precision. Food composition tables consist of values representative of foods across the nation and across the seasons, but the values are not specific to the food items eaten by an individual. Impact of these and other errors on estimation of food and nutrient intakes is discussed in a Food and Nutrition Board report.[3]

Conclusions

Many factors are considered when a procedure for estimating dietary intake is chosen. No one method is suitable for all purposes, and all methods have strengths and weaknesses that require tradeoffs. Although four categories of data collection methods were described, numerous variations of each method can accommodate special circumstances of particular studies. However, each change in method can affect its validity and reliability. Short-term daily quantitative measures or estimates of intake obtained with food recalls or food records differ substantially in concept from longer-term usual measures or estimates of intake obtained with food frequencies or diet histories. Equally important to achievement of study goals is the processing of data, usually with computer assistance, from the food intake questionnaires—the review, editing, and coding as well as careful analysis and interpretation of results. Moreover, researchers and users of study results must recognize the limitations of the data and the implications for interpretation.

References

1. Food and Nutrition Board, National Research Council (1981) *Assessing Changing Food Consumption Patterns.* National Academy Press, Washington, DC.
2. Food and Nutrition Board, National Research Council (1984) *National Survey Data on Food Consumption: Uses and Recommendations.* National Academy Press, Washington, DC.
3. Food and Nutrition Board, National Research Council (1986) *Nutrient Adequacy: Assessment Using Food Consumption Surveys.* National Academy Press, Washington, DC.
4. S.A. Anderson, ed. (1986) *Guidelines for Use of Dietary Intake Data.* Life Sciences Research Office, Federation of American Societies for Experimental Biology, Bethesda, MD.
5. J.T. Dwyer (1988) Assessment of dietary intake. In: *Modern Nutrition in Health and Disease* (M.E. Shils and V.R. Young, eds.), pp. 887–905, Lea & Febiger, Philadelphia.
6. G. Block (1982) A review of validations of dietary assessment methods. *Am. J. Epidemiol.* 115:492–505.
7. M.C. Burk and E.M. Pao (1976) *Methodology for Large-Scale Surveys of Household and Individual Diets.* Home Economic Research Report no. 40, U.S. Government Printing Office, Washington, DC.
8. J.W. Marr (1971) Individual dietary surveys: purposes and methods. *World Rev. Nutr. Diet.* 13:105–164.
9. W.W. Kim, W. Mertz, J.T. Judd, M.W. Marshall, J.L. Kelsay, and E.S. Prather (1984) Effect of making duplicate food collections on nutrient intakes calculated from diet records. *Am. J. Clin. Nutr.* 40:1333–1337.
10. B.M. Calkins, D.J. Whittaker, P.P. Nair, A.A. Rider, and N. Turjman (1984) Diet, nutrition intake, and metabolism in populations at high and low risk for colon cancer. *Am. J. Clin. Nutr.* 40:896–905.
11. U.S. Department of Agriculture (1987) *Continuing Survey of Food Intakes by Individuals: Women 19–50 Years and Their Children 1–5 years, 4 days, 1985.* NFCS, CSFII Report no. 85-4, U.S. Government Printing Office, Washington, DC.
12. E.A. Krall and J.T. Dwyer (1987) Validity of a food frequency questionnaire and a food diary in a short-term recall situation. *J. Am. Diet. Assoc.* 87:1374–1377.
13. M. Gersovitz, J.R. Madden, and H. Smiciklas-Wright (1978) Validity of the 24-hr. dietary recall and seven-day record for group comparisons. *J. Am. Diet. Assoc.* 73:48–55.
14. A.W. Caggiula, R.R. Wing, M.P. Nowalk, N.C. Milas, S. Lee, and H. Langford (1985) The measurement of sodium and potassium intake. *Am. J. Clin. Nutr.* 42:391–398.
15. K.S. Todd, M. Hudes, and D.H. Calloway (1983) Food intake measurement: problems and approaches. *Am. J. Clin. Nutr.* 37:139–146.
16. W.C. Willett, L. Sampson, M.J. Stampfer, et al. (1985) Reproducibility and validity of a semiquantitative food frequency questionnaire. *Am. J. Epidemiol.* 122:51–65.
17. U.S. Department of Health and Human Services (1981) *Plan and Operation of the Second National Health and Nutrition Examination Survey 1976–80.* DHHS Publication no. (PHS) 81-1317, U.S. Government Printing Office, Washington, DC.

18. B.H. Dennis, S.G. Haynes, J.J.B. Anderson, S.B.L. Liu-Chi, J.D. Hosking, and B.M. Rifkind (1985) Nutrient intakes among selected North American populations in the Lipid Research Clinics Prevalence Study: composition of energy intake. *Am. J. Clin. Nutr.* 41: 312–329.

19. G.C. Frank, G.S. Berenson, P.E. Schilling, and M.C. Moore (1977) Adapting the 24-hr. recall for epidemiologic studies of school children. *J. Am. Diet. Assoc.* 71:26–31.

20. N.J. Krantzler, B.J. Mullen, H.G. Schutz, L.E. Grivetti, C.A. Holden, and H.L. Meiselman (1982) Validity of telephoned diet recalls and records for assessment of individual food intake. *Am. J. Clin. Nutr.* 36:1234–1242.

21. R. Karvetti and L. Knuts (1981) Agreement between dietary interviews. *J. Am. Diet. Assoc.* 79:654–660.

22. D. Feskanich, M. Buzzard, B.T. Welch, et al. (1988) Comparison of a computerized and a manual method of food coding for nutrient intake studies. *J. Am. Diet. Assoc.* 88:1263–1267.

23. M. Kirkcaldy-Hargreaves, G.W. Lynch, and C. Santor (1980) Assessment of the validity of four food models. *J. Can. Diet. Assoc.* 41:102–110.

24. J.L. Greger and G.M. Etnyre (1978) Validity of 24-hour dietary recalls by adolescent females. *Am. J. Public Health* 68:70–72.

25. J.P. Madden, S.J. Goodman, and H.A. Guthrie (1976) Validity of the 24-hr. recall. *J. Am. Diet. Assoc.* 68:143–147.

26. E.E.I. Linusson, D. Sanjur, and E.C. Erickson (1974) Validating the 24-hour recall method as a dietary survey tool. *Arch. Latinoam. Nutr.* 24:277–294.

27. G.H. Beaton, J. Milner, P. Corey, et al. (1979) Sources of variance in 24-hour dietary recall data: implications for nutrition study design and interpretation. *Am. J. Clin. Nutr.* 32:2546–2559.

28. L. Sampson (1985) Food frequency questionnaires as a research instrument. *Clin. Nutr.* 4:171–178.

29. J.M. Axelson and M.M. Csernus (1983) Reliability and validity of a food frequency checklist. *J. Am. Diet. Assoc.* 83:152–155.

30. P. Pietinen, A.M. Hartman, E. Haapa, et al. (1988) Reproducibility and validity of dietary assessment instruments. II. A qualitative food frequency questionnaire. *Am. J. Epidemiol.* 128:667–676.

31. K.M. Flegal, F.A. Larkin, H.L. Metzner, F.E. Thompson, and K.E. Guire (1988) Counting calories: partitioning energy intake estimates from a food frequency questionnaire. *Am. J. Epidemiol.* 128:749–760.

32. A.W. Sorenson, B.M. Calkins, M.A. Connolly, and E. Diamond (1985) Comparison of nutrient intake determined by four dietary intake instruments. *J. Nutr. Educ.* 17:92–99.

33. R. Russell-Briefel, A.W. Caggiula, and L.H. Kuller (1985) A comparison of three dietary methods for estimating vitamin A intake. *Am. J. Epidemiol.* 122:628–636.

34. L. Roidt, E. White, G.E. Goodman, et al. (1988) Association of food frequency questionnaire estimates of vitamin A intake with serum vitamin A levels. *Am. J. Epidemiol.* 128:645–654.

35. B.S. Burke (1947) The dietary history as a tool in research. *J. Am. Diet. Assoc.* 23:1041–1046.

36. T.E. Byers, J.R. Marshall, E. Anthony, R. Fiedler, and M. Zielezny (1987) The reliability of dietary history from the distant past. *Am. J. Epidemiol.* 125:999–1011.

37. J.H. Hankin, A.M.Y. Nomura, J. Lee, T. Hirohata, and L.N. Kolonel (1983) Reproducibility of a diet history questionnaire in a case-control study of breast cancer. *Am. J. Clin. Nutr.* 37:981–985.

38. M. Jain, G.R. Howe, K.C. Johnson, and A.B. Miller (1980) Evaluation of a diet history questionnaire for epidemiologic studies. *Am. J. Epidemiol.* 111:212–219.

39. J.H. Hankin (1986) 23rd Lenna Frances Cooper Memorial Lecture: a diet history method for research, clinical, and community use. *J. Am. Diet. Assoc.* 86:868–875.

40. M. Jain (1989) Diet history: questionnaire and interview techniques used in some retrospective studies of cancer. *J. Am. Diet. Assoc.* 89:1647–1652.

41. C.M. Young, G.C. Hagan, R.E. Tucker, and W.D. Foster (1952) A comparison of dietary study methods. II. Dietary history vs. seven-day record vs. 24-hr. recall. *J. Am. Diet. Assoc.* 28:218–221.

42. G.R. Howe, L. Harrison, and M. Jain (1986) A short diet history for assessing dietary exposure to n-nitrosamines in epidemiologic studies. *Am. J. Epidemiol.* 124:595–601.

43. B.B. Peterkin, R.L. Rizek, and K.S. Tippett (1988) Nationwide Food Consumption Survey, 1987. *Nutr. Today* 23:18–24.

44. B.P. Perloff (1989) Analysis of dietary data. *Am. J. Clin. Nutr.* 50: 11–15.

45. National Research Council (1989) *Recommended Dietary Allowances,* 10th ed., National Academy Press, Washington, DC.

46. U.S. Department of Agriculture (1986) *Nutrition and Your Health. Dietary Guidelines for Americans; Eat a Variety of Foods.* Home and Garden Bulletin no. 232-1, U.S. Government Printing Office, Washington, DC.

47. S.M. Krebs-Smith, P.S. Kott, and P.M. Guenther (1989) Mean proportion and population proportion: two answers to the same question? *J. Am. Diet. Assoc.* 89:671–676.

48. E.M. Pao, K.E. Sykes, and Y.S. Cypel (1990) *USDA Methodological Research for Large-Scale Dietary Intake Surveys.* Home Economics Research Report no. 49, U.S. Government Printing Office, Washington, DC.

49. G.H. Beaton, J. Milner, V. McGuire, T.E. Feather, and J.A. Little (1983) Source of variance in 24-hour dietary recall data: implications for nutrition study design and interpretation. Carbohydrate sources, vitamins, and minerals. *Am. J. Clin. Nutr.* 37:986–995.

50. P.P. Basiotis, S.O. Welsh, F.J. Cronin, J.L. Kelsay, and W. Mertz (1987) Number of days of food intake records required to estimate individual and group nutrient intakes with defined confidence. *J. Nutr.* 117:1638–1641.

Chapter **49**   Philip J. Garry and Kathleen M. Koehler

Problems in Interpretation of Dietary and Biochemical Data from Population Studies

The concept of nutritional assessment forms a bridge between the basic science of nutrient function and metabolism and the applied science of human nutrition. Nutritional assessment is the determination of nutritional status, i.e., the health condition of individuals or groups as influenced by the intake and utilization of nutrients. Nutritional assessment involves three basic types of examinations: a history and physical exam along with anthropometric measurements, assessment of past and/or recent dietary and supplement intakes, and biochemical measurements. In the past decade there have been considerable improvements in the categories of dietary intake and biochemical methodology.

The primary purpose of this chapter is to review some of the limitations of the dietary and biochemical methodology used to assess the nutritional status of populations in regional and national epidemiologic studies. In addition, we want to emphasize the difficulty in comparing results obtained in various studies designed to examine specific population subjects, as, for example, elderly subjects.

Both dietary analysis and biochemical measures have been used to assess the nutritional status of populations. However, because dietary assessment does not require specialized laboratory facilities, dietary intake information has been a primary source of nutritional data in epidemiologic studies assessing nutritional status of various populations. Dietary analysis has limitations that in large part are due to the difficulty in obtaining accurate estimates of intake. In addition, the analysis of diet alone cannot account for variations in the absorption of nutrients. Biochemical measures can corroborate the information obtained through dietary assessment and can take into account potential absorption problems. This aspect of biochemical assessment is generally most useful in evaluating specific nutrients, such as vitamins and minerals.

Interpretation of Dietary Intake Measurements

Dietary intakes have been estimated by a number of different methodologies that are designed to determine usual or habitual intakes of individuals. These include dietary histories, food records, and 24-h dietary recalls. Dietary history methods are primarily designed to estimate the habitual food intake over a long period of time ranging from 1 wk to several months and in some instances up to 1 y. The subjectivity involved in describing a usual eating pattern makes the dietary history method vulnerable to memory lapses and psychological tendencies to exaggerate or minimize self-described behavior.[1] Food record methodology requires an individual to record all foods eaten over a specified period of time, generally from a few days to 1 wk. Unlike dietary history methodology, which requires a trained interviewer, the burden is placed on the subject to provide accurate intake information. Thus, the individual must be highly motivated especially if required to keep records beyond several days. There also may be a tendency to alter eating behavior during the record-keeping period to make the task easier.[2] Thus, the dietary data may not reflect usual intakes. The 24-h dietary recall methodology also requires a trained interviewer and has been used with varying degrees of success in large population surveys such as the National Health and Nutrition Examination

Surveys (NHANES I and II). The major advantage of this methodology is the minimum amount of time required of the interviewer and subject to collect the dietary intake data. A major disadvantage of this technique, especially when used with elderly individuals, is the subjects' ability to remember with accuracy the food items and amounts eaten the previous day.

The difficulty in obtaining accurate estimates of dietary intake is a major limitation of dietary analysis. An understanding of the consequences of this error in measurement is essential to the interpretation of results. When estimating the usual or typical diet from the dietary intakes of a sample of daily observations, either by food record or recall, there are two sources of error. The first source of error is inaccuracy in the measurement of dietary intake for a particular day that is due to error in estimating quantities of foods eaten or the omission (or inclusion) of food items. This error is increased by incomplete or inaccurate knowledge of the nutrient content of the foods consumed. A second source of error arises because a small sample of daily observations is used to estimate the usual or typical intake. In theory this error can be minimized or eliminated by taking a sufficiently large sample of days. However, practical considerations make this alternative impossible in large studies, and error from this source can be considerable.

The practical effects of error in estimating dietary intake differ according to whether the error is biased or unbiased. If the error is biased, that is, not centered about zero, the distributions of nutrient intake will be shifted and will suggest intakes that are either too large or too small. Even if there is no bias, any amount of error will increase the observed variance of nutrient intake in the population above the true variance and will lead to overestimates of the proportions of the population in the extremes of the distribution. These extremes quite frequently are the areas of primary interest. Additionally, even unbiased measurement error will cause observed statistical associations of nutrient intake with other factors to be lower than the true associations, with a subsequent loss in power for statistical tests.[3]

It may be reasonable to assume that the error is unbiased from some sources, such as estimating quantities, but for other sources there is almost certainly bias. For example, incomplete information on the nutrient composition of foods must bias the estimates of intake toward quantities less than those consumed. If the sample of days from which the usual intake is estimated is not random, the error from this source also may be biased. For example, intakes on weekends may be higher than on weekdays, and the failure to include weekend days can lead to underestimation of usual intake. Finally, the

magnitude and bias of the error may differ for each nutrient.

Despite these problems, dietary information can be reasonably accurate for some macronutrients. For example, the approximate energy content of foods is generally known, and underestimation of daily energy intake is not a problem as long as accurate food records or recalls are obtained. The error of measurement, which is less than that of most other nutrients, has a variance that is about equal in magnitude to the true population variance in usual energy intake.[4] Therefore, the observed population variance in energy intake for a 1-d diet record is twice the true variance. Similarly, for a 3-d record the observed variance is only one and one-third times the true variance in energy intake. In this case, the standard deviation is inflated by ~15%, leading to only modest overestimations of the proportions of individuals in the extremes of the distribution. Similarly, correlations of energy intake with other factors are diminished only slightly. For some nutrients, however, the variance of the error may be three or four times the true variance of the nutrient intake in the population, and the consequences of estimating usual intake from a 3-d record may be much worse. Cholesterol intake and dietary vitamin B-12 are examples of nutrients for which the error of measurement appears to be large.

In summary, it is probably necessary to view most estimates of the proportion of the population with intakes below (or above) a critical value in the extremes of the distribution as being somewhat exaggerated especially when based on only a few days of diet records or recall. Similarly, observed correlations of dietary intake with biochemical measures are probably smaller than true correlations are.

Example of Dietary Intake of Populations

In the following example data from two different studies examining the intakes of elderly females are used to demonstrate the potential consequences of error in measurement of dietary intake. The studies illustrated are the NHANES II[5] and a regional survey, the New Mexico Aging Study (NMAS).[6] NHANES II examined 1,416 women aged 65–74 y. Dietary information was obtained by 24-h recall. In NMAS 79 women aged 65–84 y provided one 3-d diet record per year in five different years beginning in 1980.

Figure 1 shows the cumulative percent of daily energy intakes for the NMAS sample and for the 1,080 women in the NHANES II sample whose income was above the poverty level. In the NMAS, all 79 subjects had above-poverty incomes. As shown in Figure 1, the median intake of the NHANES II females was 264 kcal/d less than that of the NMAS

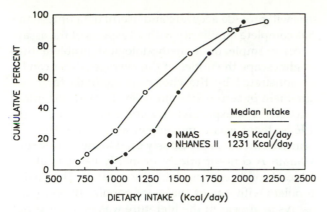

Figure 1. Cumulative percent of daily energy intakes for females in NMAS and NHANES II. For NMAS, n = 79 subjects; for NHANES II, n = 1,080 white and black women above poverty level.

females. Comparison of body weights of women in the two studies suggests that difference in weight is not a likely explanation for the difference in reported energy intake.

Figure 2 shows the cumulative percent of body weight for the NMAS women and for the 1,245 NHANES II women who were white (both above and below poverty level).[7] All of the 79 NMAS women were white. As shown in Figure 2, the median weight of the NHANES II women was 4.4 kg greater than that of the NMAS women.

Although the NHANES II subsamples in Figures 1 and 2 are not identical, white women above the poverty level predominate in both. (The total sample of 1,416 elderly women included 76% above the poverty level and 88% white.) Thus, the higher median body weight of the NHANES II women (Figure 2) does not provide an explanation for the lower median energy intake as compared with that of the NMAS women (Figure 1).

Because body weight does not support a true difference in energy intake between the NHANES II and NMAS women, the observed difference may represent bias in dietary intake measurement in one or both studies. Both surveys collected dietary intake information for weekdays only, so that different treatment of weekends is not a source of bias in comparing the two studies. The existence of bias can be investigated by comparing these results with the findings of other dietary surveys of elderly women. Two recent studies in Arizona[8] and Boston[9] collected 3-d diet records on elderly females, whereas a third study monitored dietary intake for 4 d at the Massachusetts Institute of Technology Clinical Research Center (MIT).[10] Table 1 shows that the mean energy intakes of elderly women in the Arizona, Boston, and MIT studies are very similar to that found in NMAS.

All four regional studies report mean energy intakes $\sim$ 200 kcal/d higher than that reported in NHANES II. This finding suggests that the NHANES II data are biased toward lower intakes than those usually consumed by elderly females.

Table 1 also shows that the standard deviation of energy intake in the four regional studies ranges from 294 to 388 kcal/d, whereas that for NHANES II is 624 kcal/d. This finding reflects not only differences in dietary methodology but also the decreased error associated with more days of dietary intake information. Thus, the variance for the 1-d recall in NHANES II is the largest followed by the 3-d records in the NMAS, Arizona, and Boston studies and lastly by the 4-d observation of the MIT study.

As stated previously, an inflated variance over the true variance results in an overestimation of the proportion of individuals in the extremes of the distribution. This effect can be demonstrated by considering the range of ascorbic acid intakes of elderly women in NMAS[6] and NHANES II[5] (above poverty). Figure 3 shows that the median intakes for both studies are similar and are well above the Recommended Dietary Allowance (RDA) of 60 mg/d.[11] However, the increased variance in NHANES II as compared with NMAS results in an overestimation of the number of individuals in the extremes of the distribution because of differences in the number of days of recorded intake. This variance can have serious consequences for proper interpretation of the data. For example, Figure 3 shows that $\sim$35% of the elderly females in NHANES II had intakes below the RDA whereas only 10% NMAS were below the RDA. Thus, the number of individuals with intakes below the RDA or even two-thirds of the RDA for ascorbic acid would appear to be inflated.

In summary, these examples demonstrate that possible bias and error in dietary information need

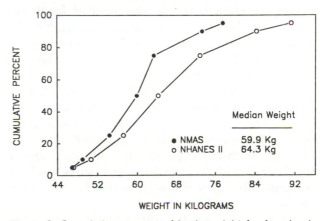

Figure 2. Cumulative percent of body weight for females in NMAS and NHANES II. For NMAS, n = 79 subjects; for NHANES II, n = 1,245 white women both above and below poverty level.

Table 1. Summary of five separate studies examining energy intakes in elderly women

Study	n	Age range	Energy intake (kcal/d)	Dietary methodology
NMAS[6]	79	65–84	1,515 ± 333	3-d diet records
Arizona[8]	138	60–96	1,536 ± 388	3-d diet records
Boston[9]	452	60–98	1,491 ± 376	3-d diet records
MIT[10]	24	65–85	1,485 ± 294	4-d diet records
NHANES II[5]	1,080	65–74	1,312 ± 624	24-h recall

to be evaluated and explained on the basis of differences in methodology and possibly other factors. NMAS as well as the Arizona, Boston, and MIT studies were regional studies with selected populations of elderly females, whereas NHANES II was a national sampling of a natural population of elderly females. Whether these dissimilarities in study design alone can explain the difference in dietary intakes is controversial and beyond the scope of this chapter. However, the example presented points out the need to be extremely cautious in interpreting and comparing various data sets examining dietary intake information in selected populations.

Sources of Error in Biochemical Assessment

The use of analytical and biochemical techniques to assess vitamin status of individuals and populations has undergone dramatic changes in the past 20 y. Most of these changes are related to improved instrumentation such as high-performance liquid chromatography, which is used to measure plasma retinol, α-tocopherol, and β-carotene. Another area of improvement is the development of functional enzyme assays of vitamin status. An example of a functional enzyme assay is the glutathione reductase assay (NADPH: oxidized glutathione oxidoreductase) for assessment of riboflavin status. Glutathione reductase is one of two erythrocyte enzymes that require flavin adenine dinucleotide (FAD) as a coenzyme. The ratio of enzyme activity (with FAD: without FAD) is termed the activity coefficient (AC), and the erythrocyte glutathione reductase activity coefficient (EGR-AC) has been used successfully to measure riboflavin status in a number of recent studies.

For most analyses there are usually a number of possible procedures and types of instrumentation from which to choose. It is not always apparent whether a published procedure for a particular anal-

ysis will provide accurate and useful data unless one has complete familiarity with all aspects of the assay.

An example of a methodological problem that might escape the notice of the average reader can be demonstrated by the choice of methods for measurement of serum vitamin A levels. With the introduction of inexpensive fluorometers in the early 1960s, there was a movement away from the colorimetric methods previously used to measure serum vitamin A concentrations, primarily because of the toxic chromogens used in the assay.[12] The major problem with one of the more popular fluorometric assays to appear in the literature was that it was not specific for vitamin A.[13] This procedure required only that the serum be extracted with an organic solvent, the extract be excited at a specific wavelength, and the fluorometric emission be measured at a longer wavelength. The upper range of normal by this fluorometric procedure was ~6.98 μmol/L as compared with 2.44 μmol/L by the standard Carr-Price colorimetric assay.[14] These differences in normal ranges led to considerable confusion when investigators tried to compare results between studies and to interpret results within a single study.[15] Thompson et al.[16] later found that serum contained variable amounts of phytofluene that had fluorescence characteristics very similar to retinol. Phytofluene is a conjugated long-chain hydrocarbon ($C_{40}H_{62}$) and is widely found in the vegetable kingdom, especially in tomatoes. Thus, even very slight contamination of serum by phytofluene will give biased results for serum vitamin A levels when measured with a nonspecific fluorometric assay.[13]

Similarly, the lack of standardized methodology, especially for the functional enzyme assays, can lead to inappropriate comparison of results obtained with different procedures. For example, the EGR-AC assay requires oxidized glutathione and NADPH as substrates in addition to the coenzyme FAD in the re-

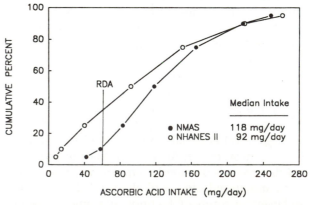

Figure 3. Cumulative percent of ascorbic acid intake for females in NMAS and NHANES II. For NMAS, n = 79 subjects; for NHANES II, n = 1,080 white and black women above poverty level.

action mixture. The activity of this enzyme is dependent not only on the sequence of substrate and coenzyme additions to the erythrocyte hemolysate[17] but also on the concentration of FAD required to activate the apoenzyme.[18] In published procedures, concentrations of FAD used to stimulate EGR range from 1.0 to 10 μmol/L.[17,19,20] However, final concentrations of FAD in the EGR reaction >5.0 μmol/L were shown to inhibit the reaction if very little apoenzyme is present. As a consequence, EGR-AC values of <1.0 often are found in studies in which riboflavin nutriture is adequate. In other words, a concentration of 10.0 μmol FAD/L may be needed to activate unsaturated enzyme to the maximum in vitro, but this concentration of FAD inhibits enzyme that is already saturated by FAD and results in an AC of <1.0. This inhibitory effect of FAD is negated in an automated procedure by preincubating the erythrocyte hemolysates with high concentrations of FAD followed by the subsequent reduction of FAD concentration to ~1.0 μmol/L during the assay.[18]

Because of the lack of a standardized methodology, it is not surprising that there has been some disagreement in regard to normal values for EGR-AC. Tillotson and Baker[21] suggested that a normal AC range should extend from 0.90 to 1.30, whereas Glatzle et al.[22] and Vo-Khactu et al.[20] suggested a normal range for human adults between 0.90 and 1.20. In the automated procedure mentioned above, the normal range was determined to be between 1.00 and 1.35.[18] Frequently, readers and sometimes investigators as well are not aware of the existence of such variations in procedures, which can result in improper comparison of data from different studies examining vitamin status in populations. For example, a study[1] on riboflavin status in a group of healthy elderly individuals used an AC of 1.2 as the upper range of normal and stated that a similar study of riboflavin status in healthy elderly subjects[23] found a substantial number of elderly subjects with AC values > 1.20. This comparison is not valid and is misleading to readers because of differences in normal ranges between the manual and automated methods used in these two separate studies.

An important aspect of biochemical assessment of populations is the establishment of reference intervals for vitamins and other clinical indices. It is easy to overlook the fact that reference intervals not only are dependent on the methodology chosen but also are influenced by preanalytical as well as analytical sources of variation. Preanalytical sources of variation evolve from secular, clinical, and intrinsic differences within the population being examined and from blood sample collection and handling techniques. Analytical sources of error relate primarily to the accuracy and the precision performance of the laboratory.

Secular sources of variation result from differences in lifestyle and dietary practices within the study population, such as alcohol consumption, smoking habits, and physical activity. Clinical sources of variation include those resulting from use of medications by subjects and from metabolic states altered by acute or chronic illness. For the most part, these secular and clinical sources of variation can be diminished by setting specific entrance criteria for the selection of the reference population. Intrinsic sources of variation arise from gender, age, and genetic differences in the sample population. Differences in the body size of the subjects may also contribute to the variance of the measurements obtained.

Blood sampling and handling techniques, such as posture during sample collection, differences in capillary-venous samples, use of anticoagulants, and fasting state of subjects, all should be controlled as much as possible to reduce variation from these sources. Sample storage conditions also must be carefully monitored if analyses are delayed for any period of time. For example, accurate lipid analyses require that serum or plasma samples be stored at −50 to −70 °C if analyses are to be delayed for an extended period.[24]

Finally, analytical sources of variation depend on the accuracy and precision performance of the laboratory. Poor accuracy and precision may result from the absence of an acceptable quality-assurance program. One factor affecting analytical error is the nature of the substance being analyzed. For example, if serum ascorbic acid levels are to be measured by the dichlorophenolindophenol method, the sample must be treated soon after collection.[25] Ascorbic acid is very labile and is easily oxidized to dehydroascorbic acid when plasma is separated from whole blood. If the plasma is not treated within 10 min with m-phosphoric acid, the results obtained will be biased on the low side. It is also imperative that individuals be in a fasting state ($\geq$12 h) in order for serum ascorbic acid levels to be free of influence from recent intakes of vitamin C. After a meal containing ascorbic acid, blood levels of ascorbic acid peak at ~3 h and can remain elevated $\leq$12 h before returning to a steady-state level.[25] If this tendency is not realized, values from analyses may be spuriously high and, therefore, misleading.

The total of these preanalytical and analytical sources of variation accounts for the range of laboratory results observed in any population study. The total variance can be separated into within- and between-subject variance components. Within-subject variance is a measure of the variability of an individual's test results around his or her own mean value as determined by repeat analyses over a specified time interval. Between-subject variance describes the variability of an individual's mean value about the population mean.

Recently Cooper et al.[26] discussed intraperson (within-subject) and interperson (between-subject) sources of variation for total cholesterol, high-density-lipoprotein (HDL) cholesterol, and triglycerides. The total intraperson source of variation, reported as the coefficient of variation (CV_p), was shown to be significant within a day and to increase within a month or year. CV_p measured on blood specimens collected once a month from adult males was ~6.1% for total cholesterol, 8.4% for HDL cholesterol, and 25.9% for triglycerides. In NMAS the corresponding CV_p values determined from samples collected 1 y apart were 8.2%, 11.9%, and 27.5%, respectively.[27] The slightly higher CV_p values found in the NMAS no doubt are related to the longer time interval between successive samplings. The within-subject variation is extremely helpful in understanding the amount of variation that can be expected in laboratory results if an individual is reexamined after a certain period of time. For example, with 90% confidence, one can expect the total cholesterol to vary as much as 1.09 mmol/L in an elderly male from year to year when it is determined also that the population mean cholesterol is ~5.75 mmol/L and the CV_p is 8.2%.

Cooper et al.[26] also reported interperson ranges of differences, i.e., the difference between the 5th and 95th percentiles. These values were ~2.84 mmol/L for cholesterol and low-density-lipoprotein (LDL) cholesterol for men and women, 0.90 mmol/L for HDL cholesterol for men and 1.29 mmol/L for women, and ~2.82 mmol/L for triglycerides (as triolein) for men and 1.69 mmol/L for women. In NMAS, values of 3.05 mmol/L for cholesterol and 2.76 mmol/L for LDL cholesterol for men and women were reported. These values are in agreement with those reported by Cooper et al. However, NMAS also reported HDL-cholesterol values of 0.80 mmol/L for men and 1.01 mmol/L for women and triglyceride values of 3.27 mmol/L for men and 2.37 mmol/L for women. These results are slightly different from those of Cooper et al. The overall comparisons between these two studies show the similarities in reported values even though the population size, age range, and methodology used (analytical and study design) are different.

The emphasis placed on lipid measurements in this chapter also reflects the national concern for identifying people at risk for developing coronary heart disease (CHD) by measuring total cholesterol and other lipid levels in blood. Because of the large within-subject variation found in total cholesterol

levels, it has been recommended that individuals have at least three successive cholesterol measurements 2 wk apart to minimize the error in misinterpreting a single measurement. Understanding the within-subject variation in total cholesterol also becomes an important factor when assessing certain dietary or drug therapies designed to lower total cholesterol levels.

To correctly identify individuals or populations at true risk for developing CHD because of elevated blood lipids, the National Cholesterol Education Program[28] recently stressed the need to improve the precision and accuracy of lipid measurements. Currently, 5% limits of imprecision and 5% of bias (accuracy) vs. a nationally accepted Abell-Kendall[29] reference method are recommended, with a goal of reducing these limits to 3% by 1992.[26] The emphasis on accurate and precise lipid measurements in individuals and populations is a recent development resulting from a need for clinical evaluation of elevated total and LDL-cholesterol levels in relation to risk for CHD.

Summary and Prospects for the Future

This chapter dealt with some problems associated with obtaining accurate and precise dietary intake and biochemical information in epidemiologic studies. Error associated with these measurements not only limits the ability to interpret properly the data obtained in such studies but also makes it difficult to compare published results from studies with similar design or purpose.

Major advances have been realized in the past decade to improve the quality of data collected in population surveys, especially in the biochemical area. The establishment of the National Cholesterol Education Program (NCEP)[30] is the result of an almost unprecedented movement in this country to improve the accuracy and precision of cholesterol measurements. Basic to this effort is the acceptance of a reference method, the Abell-Kendall cholesterol procedure,[29] that can be used to standardize and monitor the performance of laboratories using various methods for cholesterol analysis. In the future, investigators may have to present evidence that their cholesterol data meet the proposed NCEP requirements for accuracy and precision. This practice not only would validate published data but also would enable investigators to compare results among laboratories with confidence.

There are also initiatives to improve the accuracy and precision of vitamin measurements. In 1984 the National Institute of Standards and Technology (NIST), formerly known as the National Bureau of Standards, set up a quality-assurance program in support of clinical research funded by the National Cancer Institute. This program serves laboratories assaying vitamins A, C, E, and β-carotene in serum for epidemiological studies of treated and control populations.[31] The primary goal of the NIST quality-assurance program is to aid laboratories performing these assays to meet certain accuracy and precision criteria. Laboratories are provided with primary standards and then participate in a NIST study in which serum-based "spiked" samples are sent to each laboratory on a regular basis for vitamin A, C, E, and β-carotene analysis. Results are sent back to NIST for evaluation and reviewed in an annual NIST-sponsored workshop. The NIST personnel also make recommendations concerning technical problems such as sample storage, extraction, and separation techniques. Approximately 35 laboratories participate in the NIST program, and the performance quality of these laboratories has improved vastly since the introduction of the program. Although the NIST program is limited to selected vitamins, its success clearly indicates that a similar program is needed for the remaining water- and fat-soluble vitamins as well as for minerals.

The NIST and NCEP efforts are the beginnings of a much-needed movement to assure that biochemical assays conducted in various population studies are validated by some standardized reference material and/or by laboratory participation in a recognized quality-assurance program.

Similarly, the field of dietary assessment has emphasized critical evaluations of the validity of different methods for estimation of dietary intake. Strengths and weaknesses of the various methods were reviewed.[32] In the past decade, progress in obtaining accurate and precise dietary intake information included developments in the technology and completeness of computerized nutrient databases.[33] Continued progress is anticipated in computerized nutrient databases and in the methodology of national surveys. For epidemiological surveys, the further development of short-cut methods, such as quantitative food frequency instruments, may provide a measure of the usual diet not obtainable when food intake data are collected for a limited number of days.

There is little doubt that continued improvement and standardization of dietary and biochemical methodologies will enhance the effectiveness of epidemiologic studies in correctly assessing the nutritional problems of populations.

References

1. J.R. Mahalko, L.K. Johnson, S.K. Gallagher, and D.B. Milne (1985) Comparison of dietary histories and seven-day food records in a nutritional assessment of older adults. *Am. J. Clin. Nutr.* 42:542–553.

2. P.J. Garry, W.C. Hunt, and J.S. Goodwin (1985) Changes in dietary patterns over a four year period in an elderly population. In: *Proceedings of the XIII International Nutrition Congress* (T.G. Taylor and N.K. Jenkins, eds.), pp. 713–715, John Libbey, London.

3. K. Liu, J. Stamler, A. Dyer, J. McKeever, and P. McKeever (1978) Statistical methods to assess and minimize the role of intraindividual variability in obscuring the relationship between dietary lipids and serum cholesterol. *J. Chronic Dis.* 31:399–418.

4. W.C. Hunt, A.G. Leonard, P.J. Garry, and J.S. Goodwin (1983) Components of variance in dietary data for an elderly population. *Nutr. Res.* 3:433–444.

5. United States Department of Health and Human Services (1983) *Dietary Intake Source Data: United States, 1976–80.* DHHS Publication no. (PHS) 83-1681, U.S. Government Printing Office, Washington, DC.

6. P.J. Garry, R.L. Rhyne, L. Halious, and C. Nicholson (in press) Changes in dietary patterns over a 6-year period in an elderly population. *Ann. N.Y. Acad. Sci.*

7. United States Department of Health and Human Services (1987) *Anthropometric Reference Data and Prevalence of Overweight: United States, 1976–80.* DHHS Publication no. (PHS) 87-1688, U.S. Government Printing Office, Washington, DC.

8. L.A. Vaughan and M.M. Manore (1988) Dietary patterns and nutritional status of low income, free-living elderly. *Food Nutr. News* 60:27–30.

9. R.B. McGandy, R.M. Russell, S.C. Hartz, et al. (1986) Nutritional status survey of healthy noninstitutionalized elderly: energy and nutrient intakes from three-day diet records and nutrient supplements. *Nutr. Res.* 6:785–798.

10. J.J. Wurtman, H. Lieberman, R. Tsay, T. Nader, and B. Chew (1988) Calorie and nutrient intakes of elderly and young subjects measured under identical conditions. *J. Gerontol.* 43:B174–B180.

11. National Research Council (1989) *Recommended Dietary Allowances,* 10th ed., National Academy Press, Washington, DC.

12. P.J. Garry (1981) Vitamin A. In: *Clinics in Laboratory Medicine, Symposium on Laboratory Assessment of Nutritional Status* (Robert Labbe, ed.), pp. 699–711, Saunders Co., Philadelphia.

13. L.G. Hansen and W.J. Warwick (1968) A fluorometric micromethod for serum vitamin A. *Am. J. Clin. Pathol.* 50:525–528.

14. T.H. Carr and E.A. Price (1926) Color reactions attributed to vitamin A. *Biochem. J.* 20:497–501.

15. P.J. Garry (1975) Why such high serum levels of Vitamin A? *Pediatrics* 55:899(letter).

16. J.N. Thompson, P. Erdody, R. Brien, and T.K. Murray (1971) Fluorometric determination of vitamin A in human blood and liver. *Biochem. Med.* 5:67–89.

17. E. Beutler (1969) Effect of flavin compounds on glutathione reductase activity: in vivo and in vitro studies. *J. Clin. Invest.* 48:1957–1966.

18. P.J. Garry and G.M. Owen (1976) An automated flavin adenine dinucleotide dependent glutathione reductase assay for assessing riboflavin nutriture. *Am. J. Clin. Nutr.* 29:663–674.

19. G.E. Nicholads (1974) Assessment of status of riboflavin nutriture by assay of erythrocyte glutathione reductase activity. *Clin. Chem.* 20:624–627.

20. K.P. Vo-Khactu, R.L. Sims, R.H. Clayburgh, and H.H. Sandstead (1976) Effect of simultaneous thiamin and riboflavin deficiencies on the determination of transketolase and glutathione reductase. *J. Lab. Clin. Med.* 87:741–748.

21. J.A. Tillotson and E.M. Baker (1972) An enzymatic measurement of riboflavin status in man. *Am. J. Clin. Nutr.* 25:425–431.

22. D. Glatzle, W.F. Korner, S. Christeller, and O. Wiss (1970) Method for the detection of biochemical riboflavin deficiency. Stimulation of $NADPH_2$-dependent glutathione reductase from human erythrocytes by FAD in vitro. Investigation of the vitamin B_2 status in

healthy people and geriatric patients. *Int. J. Vitam. Res.* 40:166–183.

23. P.J. Garry, J.S. Goodwin, and W.C. Hunt (1982) Nutritional status in a healthy elderly population: riboflavin. *Am. J. Clin. Nutr.* 36:902–909.

24. A. Hainline, Jr., J. Karon, and K. Lippel, eds. (1982) *Lipid Research Clinics Program Manual of Laboratory Operations, Lipid and Lipoprotein Analysis,* 2nd ed. HEW Publication no. (NIH) 75-628 (revised), U.S. Government Printing Office, Washington, DC.

25. P.J. Garry, G.M. Owen, D.W. Lashley, and P.C. Ford (1974) Automated analysis of plasma and whole blood ascorbic acid. *Clin. Biochem.* 7:131–145.

26. G.R. Cooper, G.L. Myers, S.J. Smith, and E.J. Sampson (1988) Standardization of lipid, lipoprotein, and apolipoprotein measurements. *Clin. Chem.* 34:B95–B105.

27. P.J. Garry, W.C. Hunt, D.J. VanderJagt, and R.L. Rhyne (1989) Clinical chemistry reference intervals for healthy elderly people. *Am. J. Clin. Nutr.* 50(suppl.):1219–1230.

28. Laboratory Standardization Panel; National Cholesterol Education Program; National Heart, Lung, and Blood Institute. (1988) A report on current status of blood cholesterol measurement in clinical laboratories in the United States. *Clin. Chem.* 34:193–201.

29. L.L. Abell, B.B. Levy, B.B. Brodie, and F.E. Kendall (1952) Simplified methods for the estimation of total cholesterol in serum and demonstration of its specificity. *J. Biol. Chem.* 195:357–366.

30. National Cholesterol Education Program, National Heart, Lung, and Blood Institute (1988) Report of the Expert Panel on Detection, Evaluation and Treatment of High Blood Cholesterol in Adults. *Arch. Intern. Med.* 148:36–69.

31. W.A. MacCrehan and E. Schonberger (1987) Determination of retinol, alpha-tocopherol, and beta-carotene in serum by liquid chromatography with absorbance and electrochemical detection. *Clin. Chem.* 33:1585–1592.

32. G. Block (1982) A review of validations of dietary assessment methods. *Am. J. Epidemiol.* 115:492–505.

33. B.P. Perloff (1989) Analysis of dietary data. *Am. J. Clin. Nutr.* (suppl.) 50.

Chapter **50** Catherine E. Woteki and Marie T. Fanelli-Kuczmarski

The National Nutrition Monitoring System

Nutrition monitoring is defined as "an on-going description of nutrition conditions in the population, with particular attention to subgroups defined in socioeconomic terms, for the purposes of planning, analyzing the effects of policies and programs on nutrition problems and predicting future trends."[1] Nutrition monitoring is characterized by regular data collection and by linkages with policymaking and research (Figure 1). The data collected can be categorized into five areas—information about the food supply, food composition, food consumption patterns, dietary knowledge and attitudes, and the health and nutritional status of the population. As shown in Figure 1, monitoring provides a database for public policy decisions related to such issues as intervention programs, food fortification, and food safety. It also assists in the identification of nutrition research priorities of public health significance, thereby strengthening the research base for monitoring and policy making.

The National Nutrition Monitoring System (NNMS), as defined in the Joint Operational Plan, is an assortment of interrelated activities that provide regular information about the contributions that diet and nutritional status make to the health of the United States population and about the factors affecting diet and nutritional status (Figure 2). Knowledge about the relationships of food to nutritional and health status and of nutritional status to health is acquired from data gathered from either national surveys or surveillance activities. A survey implies the assessment of nutritional status on a one-time basis to identify problem areas and high-risk population groups, whereas a surveillance activity implies the frequent and continuous watching over of nutritional status usually using readily available data to identify and to quickly respond to problems. Two surveys—the National Health and Nutrition Examination Survey (NHANES) and the Nationwide Food Consumption Survey (NFCS)—form the core of the NNMS.

The coordination of the monitoring system is the responsibility of the Interagency Committee on Nutrition Monitoring.[2] The Committee is cochaired by the Assistant Secretary for Health, U.S. Department of Health and Human Services (DHHS), and the Assistant Secretary for Food and Consumer Services, U.S. Department of Agriculture (USDA). The purpose of this committee is to increase the effectiveness and productivity of federal nutrition monitoring efforts by improving planning, coordination, and communication among the agencies engaged in nutrition monitoring. The membership includes representatives from four Public Health Service (in DHHS) agencies, four USDA agencies, the Agency for International Development, the Bureau of Labor Statistics, the Census Bureau, the Department of Defense, and the Veterans Administration.

As indicated in Figure 1, the NNMS maintains formal linkages with federal nutrition policy makers through representation on the DHHS Nutrition Policy Board and the Subcommittee for Human Nutrition of the USDA Committee on Research and Education. It also maintains formal linkages with the federal nutrition research community through the Interagency Committee on Human Nutrition Research.

The purpose of this chapter is twofold: to present a history of nutrition monitoring activities in the United States and to critically evaluate the current NNMS.

Historical Development

The surveys and surveillance activities that now constitute the NNMS have evolved in response to

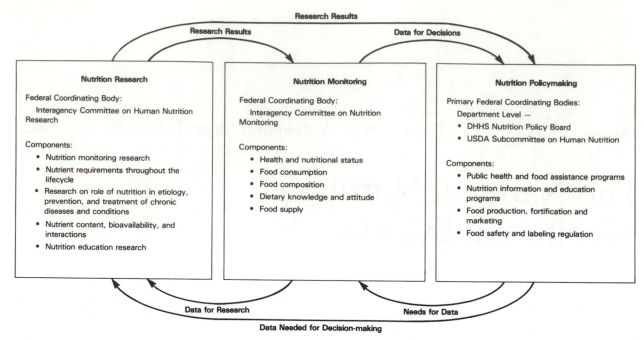

Figure 1. Relationships among nutrition research, monitoring, and policy making. Adapted from the Operational Plan for the National Nutrition Monitoring System (August 1987).

the information needs of federal agencies (Tables 1, 2). The earliest surveys were conducted by USDA and concentrated on food use by households. Later, as essential nutrients were identified, it became possible to assess the nutritional quality of the diet. In addition, hematological and biochemical tests were developed to assess nutritional status and were incorporated into national surveys.

The overall purpose for collecting this information has always been to provide information for planning and policy decisions. The underlying objectives for collecting information on food consumption from World War I to the mid-1940s were primarily to meet the needs of food production and marketing and distribution programs, both public and private. Since World War II, strong demands for much more in-

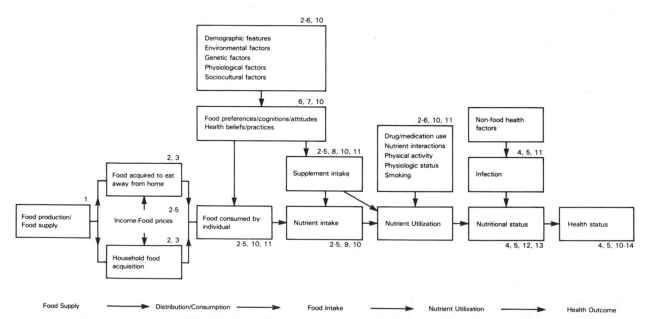

Figure 2. A conceptual model of the relationships of food to health: identification of data sources from the National Nutrition Monitoring System. Data source: 1 = U.S. Food Supply; 2 = NFCS; 3 = CSFII; 4 = NHANES; 5 = HHANES; 6 = BRFSS; 7 = HDS; 8 = VMSIS; 9 = TDS; 10 = NHIS; 11 = NEFS; 12 = PedNSS; 13 = PregNSS; 14 = Vital Statistics. Adapted from the Second National Nutritional Monitoring Report of the Expert Panel (July 1989).

formation especially about nutritional status, individual intakes, and their relationship to health have come from public and private agencies faced with making planning and policy decisions on food-assistance programs, health-services delivery programs, food fortification, and food safety. Secondarily, the surveys provide a rich database for epidemiologists, economists, and other researchers.

In the United States national policy makers have evidenced a growing interest in the role of nutrition in promoting health since the late 1940s.[3] The first national survey of household food consumption and dietary levels was in 1936–1937 as part of the Consumer Purchases Study conducted jointly by several federal agencies.[4] Between 1942 and 1965 four nationwide studies on household food consumption were conducted. During that time ~250 nutritional status and dietary evaluation studies of individuals also were conducted.[5,6] Unfortunately, data for selected age groups and populations were lacking because of the sampling design of these local studies. Thus, it was difficult, if not impossible, to characterize the nutritional health of the United States population. The first nationwide survey that provided a description of food intakes of individuals was conducted by the USDA in 1965.

The first comprehensive survey to evaluate the nutritional status of a large segment of the United States population was the Ten State Nutrition Survey (1968–70). In Section 14 of the Partnership for Health Amendments of 1967 (42 U.S.C. section 242C), Congress mandated that the Secretary of Health, Education and Welfare in collaboration with other federal government and state officials conduct a survey to assess the incidence and location of serious hunger, malnutrition, and health problems. To meet this mandate, a random selection of families was made from 1960 Census Bureau enumeration districts where the highest percent of families had incomes below the Orshansky Poverty Index in each of the 10 states selected. The sample population included middle- and upper-income persons who, because of changes in residential patterns subsequent to 1960, were living in the selected enumeration districts. Nutritional status was assessed on the basis of dietary intakes and food patterns, dental examinations, and anthropometric and biochemical measurements. Information on nonnutritional factors that affect food intake, such as socioeconomic characteristics, health status, and income, was also gathered. The findings of the Ten State Nutrition Survey indicated nutritional problems in selected age and income groups.[7]

After the Ten State Nutrition Survey, nutritional assessment was added to the National Health Examination Survey conducted by the National Center for Health Statistics (NCHS) to create the first NHANES. Conducted in 1971–74, this was the first survey to assess both the dietary intake and nutritional status of a representative sample of the civilian, noninstitutionalized population in the United States.

In the mid-1970s Congress recognized serious deficiencies in the federal nutrition monitoring program and sought to remedy them by legislative action.[8] The Food and Agriculture Act of 1977 (7 U.S.C. section 3178) required the Secretary of Agriculture and the Secretary of Health, Education and Welfare to "formulate and submit to Congress . . . a proposal for a comprehensive nutritional status monitoring system to include: (1) an assessment of a system consisting of periodic surveys and continuous monitoring to determine: the extent of risk of nutrition-related health problems in the United States; which population groups or areas of the country face greatest risk; and the likely causes of risk and changes in the above risk factors over time; (2) a surveillance system to identify remediable nutrition-related health risks to individuals or for local areas, in such a manner as to tie detection to direct intervention and treatment . . . ; and (3) program evaluations to determine the adequacy, efficiency, effectiveness, and side effects of nutrition-related programs in reducing health risks to individuals and populations."

A proposal for a comprehensive national nutrition monitoring system was submitted to Congress in 1978. It acknowledged the deficiencies in existing nutritional and dietary assessment methods, recognized delays in data analysis and the publication of results, pointed out the inadequate coverage of certain target groups and geographic areas, and admitted to the inadequate evaluation of nutrition intervention programs. The proposal also contained a series of recommendations for improving and expanding the scope of federal nutrition monitoring activities.

The proposal was reviewed by the General Accounting Office, which recommended that the departments develop an implementation plan for a national nutrition monitoring system. The Joint Implementation Plan for a Comprehensive National Monitoring System, submitted to Congress in 1981, identified and described the current efforts in nutrition monitoring conducted by USDA and DHHS and proposed major goals for the system. The implementation plan also established the Assistant Secretary for Food and Consumer Services, USDA, and the Assistant Secretary for Health, DHHS, as the people responsible for implementing compatible survey plans. Through their continuing efforts, the plans for nutrition monitoring were recently reviewed and updated, and an operational plan for the NNMS was completed in 1987.

Table 1. Dietary and nutrition status surveys and surveillance activities of National Nutrition Monitoring System

Date	Agency*	Survey	Target U.S. population	Sample selected	Number interviewed (response rate)	Number examined (response rate)
1909—annual	USDA	U.S. Food Supply Series	NA†	≈350 foods currently NR‡	NA	NA
1936-37	USDA	Household Food Consumption Survey—Household Food Use	Housekeeping households, with husband and wife, native born, nonrelief		20,466 households	NA
1942	USDA	Household Food Consumption Survey—Household Food Use	Housekeeping households	3,060 households	2,748 households	NA
1948	USDA	Household Food Consumption Survey—Household Food Use	Urban housekeeping households	5,681 households	4,489 households	NA
1955	USDA	Household Food Consumption Survey—Household Food Use	Civilian, housekeeping households	6,792 households	6,060 households	NA
1965-66	USDA	Household Food Consumption Survey—Household Food Use	Civilian, housekeeping households	18,890 households	15,112 households	NA
1965	USDA	Nationwide Food Consumption Survey—Individual Intakes	Eligible individuals residing in eligible households (all except half of persons 20-64 y)	NR	14,519 persons	NA
1968-70	DHEW	Ten State Nutrition Survey	Low-income families in 10 states	29,935 families	23,846 (80%) families	
1971-74	NCHS	First National Health and Nutrition Examination Survey	Civilian, noninstitutionalized individuals, 1-74 y	28,043 persons	86,352 persons (99%) / 27,753 (99%)	40,847 (47%) / 20,749 (74%)
1974-75	NCHS	NHANES I Augmentation Sample	Civilian, noninstitutionalized persons, 25-74 y	4,300 persons	4,288 (94%)	3,053 (71%)
1973—continuous	CDC	Pediatric Nutrition Surveillance System	Low-income, high-risk children, 0–17 y	5 states (in 1987, 36 states plus District of Columbia and Puerto Rico)	NA	NA
1976-80	NCHS	Second National Health and Nutrition Examination Survey	Civilian, noninstitutionalized individuals, 0.5-74 y	27,801 persons	25,286 (91%)	20,322 (73%)
1977-78	USDA	Nationwide Food Consumption Survey—Household Food Use	Civilian households	24,408 households	14,964 households	NA
1977-78	USDA	Nationwide Food Consumption Survey—Individual Intakes	Eligible individuals residing in eligible households (All except half of persons over 18 y in summer, fall, and winter)	44,169 persons	30,770 persons	NA
1977-78	USDA	Supplemental Nationwide Food Consumption Survey—Household Food Use	Civilian households in Puerto Rico, Alaska, Hawaii. Elderly adults in 48 states.	18,162 households	10,341 households	NA

Year	Agency	Survey	Population			
1977–78	USDA	Supplemental Nationwide Food Consumption Survey—Individual Intakes	Individuals residing in eligible households	28,984 persons	21,465 persons	NA
1977–78	USDA	Low-Income Nationwide Food Consumption Survey—Household Food Use	Low-income civilian households in 48 states	NR	4,623 households	NA
1977–78	USDA	Low-Income Nationwide Food Consumption Survey—Individual Intakes	Individuals residing in eligible households	16,208 persons	12,847 persons	NA
1979—continuous	CDC	Pregnancy Nutrition Surveillance System	Low-income, high-risk pregnant women	13 states (in 1986, 12 states plus District of Columbia)	NA	NA
1979–80	USDA	Low-Income Nationwide Food Consumption Survey—Household Food Use	Low-income civilian households	NR	3,002 households	NA
1979–80	USDA	Low-Income Nationwide Food Consumption Survey—Individual Intakes	Individuals in eligible households	NR	8,492 persons	NA
1982–84	NCHS	Hispanic Health and Nutrition Examination Survey	Civilian, noninstitutionalized individuals, 0.5–74 y			
			Mexican-American (AZ, CA, CO, NM, TX)	9,894 persons	8,554 (87%)	7,462 (75%)
			Cuban (FL)	2,244 persons	1,766 (79%)	1,357 (61%)
			Puerto Rican (CT, NJ, NY)	3,786 persons	3,369 (89%)	2,834 (75%)
1985–86	USDA	Continuing Survey of Food Intakes by Individuals	Women and men, 19–50 y; Children, 1–5 y	4,359 households	3,224 households; 4,618 persons	NA
1985–86	USDA	Continuing Survey of Food Intakes by Individuals in Low-Income Households	Low-income, women and men, 19–50 y, children 1–5 y	3,711 households	3,239 households; 5,619 persons	NA
1987	CDC	Surveillance of Severe Pediatric Undernutrition	Low-income, high-risk children, 0–5 y	4 states	NA	
1987–88	USDA	Nationwide Food Consumption Survey—Household Food Use	Civilian households	NR		NA
1987–88	USDA	Nationwide Food Consumption Survey—Individual Intakes	Individuals residing in eligible households	NR		NA
1988–94	NCHS	Third National Health and Nutrition Examination Survey	Civilian, noninstitutionalized individuals, 2 mo+	~40,000 persons		
1989–96	USDA	Continuing Survey of Food Intakes by Individuals	Individuals of all ages residing in eligible households			
			All income	1,500 each year		
			Low income	750 each year		

* USDA, U.S. Department of Agriculture; DHEW, Department of Health, Education and Welfare; NCHS, National Center for Health Statistics; CDC, Centers for Disease Control.
† Not applicable.
‡ Not reported.

Table 2. Specialized activities contributing to National Nutrition Monitoring System

Date	Agency*	Survey	Target U.S. population	Sample interviewed	Objective
1957—annual	NCHS	National Health Interview Survey	Civilian, noninstitutionalized individuals	~50,000 households	To collect data on personal and demographic features, incidence of acute illness and injuries, prevalence of chronic conditions and impairments, and utilization of health resources and other current health issues
		Supplemental topics:			
1984	NCHS	Aging	Persons, 55+ y	16,148 persons	To assess health status and care of elderly people
1985	NCHS	Health Promotion/Disease Prevention	Persons, 18+ y	33,630 persons	To measure progress towards 1990 Health Objectives for the Nation
1986	NCHS	Vitamin/Mineral Supplements	Children, 2–6 y Persons, 18+ y	1,877 children 1,775 persons	To determine supplement usage and intake levels
1987	NCHS	Cancer Epidemiology and Control	Persons, 18+ y	~45,000 persons	To assess cancer risk factors
1961—annual	FDA	Total Diet Study	Specific age-sex groups	NA†	To assess levels of a variety of nutritional components and contaminants in food supply and representative diets of target population
1980	FDA	Vitamin/Mineral Supplement Intake Survey	Civilian, noninstitutionalized persons, 16+ y	2,991 persons	To assess nutrient intakes from supplements and to examine characteristics of supplement users
1981–83, 1984—continuous	CDC	Behavioral Risk Factor Surveillance System	Persons, 18+ y, residing in participation states in households with telephones	23,113 persons (30,730 persons in 1986)	To assess prevalence of personal health practices related to leading causes of death
1982–84, 1986	NCHS	NHANES I Epidemiologic Followup Study	Persons examined in NHANES I, 25–75 y at baseline	12,220 persons (1982)	To examine relationship of baseline clinical, nutritional, and behavioral factors assessed in NHANES I to subsequent morbidity and mortality
1982, 1984, 1986, 1988	FDA	Health and Diet Study	Civilian, noninstitutionalized persons, 18+ y	4,000 persons response rate of 70–75%	To assess public knowledge, attitudes, and practices about diet and health and public's use of information on food labels
1988–90	NCHS	National Maternal and Infant Health Survey	Reproductive-age women	20,000 vital records, 60,000 persons linked with sampled vital records	To examine factors associated with low birth weight and fetal and infant deaths

* NCHS, National Center for Health Statistics; CDC, Centers for Disease Control; FDA, Food and Drug Administration.
† Not applicable.

NNMS Activities

Surveillance of the Food Supply. NNMS, as indicated in Figure 2, begins with the surveillance of the food supply. Since 1909 the Economic Research Service of the USDA has generated data on the per capita availability of all major food commodities. The estimates are conceptually similar to a balance sheet on which food that is exported or in stock or procured by the military is subtracted from the amount of food produced and imported to yield an estimate of the amount of food that is available for consumption by the civilian population. Because of the complexity of the food distribution system, use of all foods is not measured at the same point. Some foods are measured in the raw or primary state, whereas others are measured as retail product.[9] Because food procured by the military is also subtracted and the civilian population is used in the denominator, the data represent food disappearing into marketing channels for consumption by the civilian population. The U.S. Food Supply series provides estimates for approximately 350 foods. By use of tables of food composition, the nutrients available per capita can also be calculated. These data are used to assess the potential of the food supply to satisfy the nutritional needs of the population, to analyze trends in nutrient levels, and to provide insight into changes in overall food consumption patterns. The data are updated and published annually.[9]

The marketplace surveillance conducted by the Food and Drug Administration (FDA) provides supplementary information about the quality of the food supply. The Total Diet Study (TDS) program was first conducted by FDA in 1961. This annual study involves the purchase of approximately 200 foods from grocery stores across the United States and the analysis of these foods four times each year for 11 essential minerals and over 120 chemical contaminants.[10] The overall objective of the program is to monitor on a yearly basis the mineral and contaminant content of the food supply and to observe trends over time. Representative diets of specific age-sex groups derived from aggregated NFCS and NHANES dietary data are used to estimate average daily intake levels of these nutrients and contaminants. The target population groups include infants (6–11 mo), young children (2 y), male and female teenagers (14–16 y), male and female adults (25–30 y), and male and female older adults (60–65 y).

Household Food Acquisition. Progressing from the food supply to food acquired by households is the next step in monitoring, as indicated in Figure 1. Beginning in 1936–37 USDA has conducted seven national surveys of food use by households. Authority for nutrition research came originally from the general mission mandated by Congress when the department was established in 1862. The Research and Marketing Act of 1946 (7 U.S.C. sections 1621–1624) explicitly authorized research into problems of human nutrition and the nutritive value of agricultural commodities. More recently, the surveys and related activities have been carried out under broad legislative authority and the National Agricultural Research, Extension and Teaching Policy Act of 1977 (U.S.C. 3178 section 1428). The USDA data on per capita food availability and household food use represent the longest historical series related to nutrition that is maintained by the federal government.

The objective of the USDA surveys is to provide information on food used at home by *housekeeping households.* For these surveys a housekeeping household is defined as one in which at least one member ate 10 meals from the home food supplies. Since 1955 the design of the surveys has been a stratified probability sample of the 48 conterminous states, and since 1965 data have been collected over a 12-mo period to capture seasonal differences in food use.[11] Special surveys have included low-income households and households in Alaska, Hawaii, and Puerto Rico. In interviews with the person in the household most responsible for food purchasing and preparation, information is obtained about the quantity, form, source, and cost of food used during the previous 7 d. Detailed questions are also asked about income and participation in the food stamp program and other food assistance programs administered by USDA.[12,13]

Attitudes, Beliefs, and Practices. Information describing nutrition- and health-related attitudes, knowledge, and practices held by the United States population is obtained from a variety of federal monitoring activities. The National Health Interview Survey (NHIS) conducted by the NCHS is the principal source of national data on health characteristics of the population, specifically the incidence of acute illness and injuries, prevalence of chronic conditions and impairments known to or perceived by the individual, extent of disability, and utilization of health-care services. This survey was initiated in July 1957 as a response to the National Health Survey Act of 1956 (42 U.S.C. sections 242c–243h), which provided for a continuing survey and special studies to secure current and accurate information on the amount, distribution, and effects of illness and disability as well as the health services rendered. NHIS is a cross-sectional household interview survey of all adult household members ≥ 17 y of age who are present at the time of the interview. There are two parts to the interview questionnaire. The first section consists of a set of basic health and demographic items; the second consists of one or more sets of questions on special health topics in response to current interest and/or the need for data. The first section includes such items as disability days, physician visits, short-stay-hospitalization data, and long-term limitation of physical activity resulting from chronic conditions. These items are repeated each year, providing continuous information on basic health variables and permitting trend analyses. As shown in Table 2, the questions for the second section of the questionnaire range from health promotion to vitamin-mineral supplementation to cancer risk factors.[14,15] A random subsample of the adult household members is selected to answer the questions on current health topics. The combination of interview questions provides NHIS with a unique national health database as well as baseline data on current topics that are used by other federal agencies to design surveys.

FDA, created by the Pure Food and Drugs Act of 1906 (21 U.S.C. sections 1–15), has a major research effort aimed at measuring public knowledge, beliefs, and practices concerning diet and health, particularly such health problems as hypertension, heart disease, and cancer. In 1982, 1984, 1986, and again in 1988, FDA conducted the Health and Diet Survey, a consumer monitoring activity. The National Heart, Lung and Blood Institute, National Institutes of Health, collaborated on the 1982 and 1986 surveys whereas the Food Safety and Inspection Service, USDA, collaborated on the 1988 survey. The latter surveys included tracking questions designed to measure changes in the public's knowledge and concerns about nutrition and food safety since the 1982 and 1984 surveys. The Health and Diet Survey is conducted to assess the public's perceptions about diet-health relationships, health status, and preventive health behaviors and their use of information on food labels including the use of ingredients lists to avoid or limit food substances.[16,17]

In 1989 FDA plans to conduct a survey of weight-loss practices and of infant-feeding practices. The former survey will gather detailed information via telephone interviews about the types and combinations of practices being used by approximately 1200 individuals ≥ 18 y who are trying to lose weight. The latter survey will obtain time-specific information about feeding practices during the first 12 mo of life, such as transitions between breast-feeding and bottle feeding and the type and time of introduction of solid foods. Data will be collected by a series of mail questionnaires and a telephone interview from women who were first contacted when they were 3–7 mo pregnant.

In 1989 USDA will conduct a survey on consumer knowledge and attitudes on diet and health issues as a telephone follow-up to the Continuing Survey of Food Intakes by Individuals (CSFII). This project is a cooperative effort among two USDA agencies and FDA. It represents the first time that a nationwide sample will be used to study the relationship between individuals' dietary intakes and attitudes about dietary behavior.

At the state level the Behavioral Risk Factor Surveillance System (BRFSS), a surveillance activity of the Centers for Disease Control (CDC), is designed to assess the prevalence of personal health practices related to the leading causes of death and to prevention measures.[18,19] More specifically, questions concerning cigarette smoking, seat-belt use, alcohol use, drinking and driving, physical exercise, weight control, hypertension, and screening for breast cancer and cholesterol are asked of respondents. BRFSS uses a multistage cluster telephone survey design based on the Waksberg method.[20] Participants are selected randomly from adult civilian residents aged ≥ 18 y who have telephones. CDC collaborated with health departments in 28 states and the District of Columbia to conduct a one-time random-digit telephone survey between 1981 and 1983. Beginning in 1984 data were collected continuously throughout the year, during a specified 1-wk period every month. By 1987, 35 states were collecting information, many using computer-assisted telephone interviewing. The information generated by this surveillance system is used by state health departments to plan, initiate, and guide state health promotion and disease prevention programs and to monitor the progress of these programs over time.[21,22]

Supplement Intake. As shown in the conceptual model (Figure 1), health beliefs and practices can affect use of supplements, which in turn can influence total nutrient intake and utilization. In 1980 FDA conducted the Vitamin/Mineral Supplement Intake Survey (VMSIS). This survey was designed to determine prevalence and quantitative levels of selected nutrient supplementation among civilian, noninstitutionalized persons ≥ 16 y of age in the United States (Table 2).[23,24] It served as the model for the section on supplementation included in the 1986 NHIS. Data from these two surveys may be useful to determine trends in supplement usage.

Nutrient Intakes. Since 1965 USDA has collected information from individual household members about the food they have eaten. The major purpose of these surveys is to determine the adequacy of food and nutrient intake by the U.S. population by region and urbanization. Two series of surveys have been done—interviews with members of households selected for NFCSs in 1965–66, 1977–78, and 1987–88 and CSFII initiated in 1985. Special samples of low-income households were included in the recent NFCS and the CSFII. Dietary intake is obtained by personal interview using a 1-d recall technique in all the surveys. Since 1977 NFCS has also obtained an additional 2 d of dietary intake information by requesting that respondents complete a diary.[25] The 1985 and the 1986 CSFIIs attempted to obtain an additional 5 d of dietary intake through follow-up telephone interviews. Detailed descriptions were obtained of all foods and beverages consumed including food purchased and consumed away from home. Additional questions were asked about individual dietary practices and self-reported health characteristics.[26]

Beginning in 1989 CSFII will collect information on food and nutrient intakes by individuals annually and the data will be published with use of a moving-average approach. Dietary intakes will be obtained for 3 consecutive days using a 1-d recall and a 2-d record.

Current knowledge of the energy and nutrient composition of foods is essential for the analysis of data from NNMS surveys. The USDA nutrient data bank is the major mechanism for collecting, evaluating, and managing nutrient composition data for individual food items.[27] This bank is continually updated from sources that include federal government laboratories, such as USDA's Nutrient Composition Laboratory; FDA, university research, and commercial laboratories under government sponsorship; and industry laboratories. Approximately 65 nutrients currently receive priority at USDA for laboratory analysis and data collection, but information on all food components can be stored in the data bank.

Nutritional Status. The importance of a reliable assessment of nutritional status, particularly the extent of malnutrition and hunger, of the population in the United States was recognized at the 1969 White House Conference on Food, Nutrition and Health. Subsequently, the NHANES program, a core component of the NNMS, was undertaken by NCHS in response to a directive from the Secretary of Health, Education and Welfare under the authority of the National Health Survey Act of 1956. The objective of NHANES is the periodic assessment of the health and nutritional status of the United States population and the monitoring of changes in status over time. The first national survey, NHANES I, was conducted in 1971–74[28,29] and was followed by NHANES II in 1976–80[30] and NHANES III in 1988.[31] In addition, the NHANES I Augmentation Survey of Adults aged 25–74 y was conducted in 1974–75[32] and a special survey of three Hispanic groups—Mexican American, Cuban, and Puerto Rican—called Hispanic HANES (HHANES) was conducted in 1982–84.[33] The third national survey, NHANES III, is being conducted in 1988–94.

Each of the NHANES surveys has used multistage probability sampling to select a representative sample of the civilian noninstitutionalized population. Nutritional status is evaluated from data generated through interviews and physical examinations. The interviews include one or more 24-h dietary recalls; a food frequency questionnaire; questions related to eating habits, lifestyle, and other nutrition-related practices; and medical history. The NHANES III also will include a quantitative measure of intake of vitamins and minerals from supplements. Physical examinations include such components as anthropometric measurements, hematological and biochemical assessments, and medical and dental examinations. The results of these surveys have multiple uses that include the evaluation of dietary intake; the measurement conditions such as the prevalence of overweight, hypertension, growth retardation, and nutrition-related abnormalities; and the reassessment of fortification policies.[34,35]

Health Outcome. The conceptual model of the NNMS ends with health status (Figure 2). The NHANES I Epidemiologic Followup Study (NHEFS) was designed to examine the relationship of baseline nutritional, clinical, and behavioral factors assessed in NHANES I (1971–75) to subsequent morbidity and mortality from specific medical conditions. This study is a collaborative endeavor by NCHS, the National Institutes of Health, and other Public Health Service agencies. The initial follow-up was performed between 1982 and 1984 for those persons ≥ 25 y of age at baseline (NHANES I), whereas the follow-up for elderly adults, defined as persons ≥ 55 y of age at baseline, began in 1986. In-depth personal interviews with surviving NHANES I participants or with proxy respondents for individuals who were deceased or incapacitated were conducted. The data collected include a food frequency questionnaire, medical history, medications usage, smoking and alcohol histories, measurements of functional status, blood pressure, pulse and body weight, records of hospitalizations and nursing home stays, and death certificates.[36] The results provide a description of (*1*) mortality, morbidity, and institutionalization associated with suspected risk factors; (*2*) changes in the participant's characteristics between NHANES I and the follow-up study; and (*3*) the progression of chronic disease and functional impairments. Selected findings have been published,[37] but many analyses of the data collected are in progress. From the longitudinal data collected, better insight into the relationship of prior status to health in later years will be gained.

Information about breast-feeding practices and relationship of maternal weight gain to pregnancy outcome are also contributed to NNMS from the National Maternal and Infant Health Survey.[38] This survey, which is a combination of the former National Natality, National Fetal Mortality, and National Infant Mortality Surveys, is designed to collect nationally representative data on natality and fetal and infant mortality from vital records and from mothers and providers of prenatal care linked with the sampled vital records. NCHS in collaboration with 13 other government agencies fielded this survey in 1988. All data collection will be completed by 1990. Information on maternal weight gain; hematocrit, hemoglobin, and blood pressure; use of vitamin-mineral supplements by mothers and infants; infant-feeding practices; alcohol consumption; participation in food assistance programs; and nutrition-related health problems, such as nausea, diarrhea, and constipation, are being collected. These data will be used to investigate issues such as the causes of low birth weights and infant deaths, the effects of maternal alcohol consumption, and the use of public programs by women and infants.

Infant mortality data and rates for selected causes of death are critical for nutrition monitoring purposes. The Vital Statistics Program at NCHS is responsible for the coordination, reporting, and transmission of data on births and deaths from all 50 states, the District of Columbia, Puerto Rico, Guam, and the Virgin Islands. National vital statistics data are summarized each year in *Health, United States*.[39]

In summary, the surveys conducted by federal agencies as described in this section cover many aspects of the conceptual model for nutrition monitoring depicted in Figure 2. Data are produced annually on the per capita availability of foods and nutrients, decennially on food consumption by households, annually on food intakes by individuals, and periodically on nutritional status and morbidity. Vital statistics data published annually permit the tracking of infant-mortality rates and death rates for diseases with nutritional risk factors, including hunger. Special studies and targeted population surveys are also conducted to meet the information needs of the sponsoring agencies that cannot be met by the large population surveys.

Critical Analysis of the National Nutrition Monitoring System

It is widely recognized that the nutrition monitoring activities conducted in the United States are the most comprehensive in the world; it is also recognized that there is substantial room for improvement.[40,41] Criticisms of the system have tended to fall into six categories: the correct information is not collected, better population coverage is needed, needs are not being met for small-area data, agencies are slow in reporting the data, policy needs are not met, and better integration of the information is needed.

Types of Information Collected. NNMS must provide a broad spectrum of information from food availability through food distribution and consumption, food intake, and nutrient utilization (as reflected in nutritional status) to, ultimately, health status (Figure 2). At each step in this model, there are many factors that affect the outcome. For example, contraceptive agents, estrogen replacement drugs, cigarettes, aspirin, and other over-the-counter drugs can affect the levels of biochemical indicators of nutritional status. When nutritional status assessments are made, information on current and recent usage of these products is necessary for interpreting the data.

A careful review of Figure 2 along with Tables 1 and 2 will reveal that some areas appear to have been more intensely studied than others, indicating some gaps in the monitoring system. Probably the most apparent is nutrient utilization. Unfortunately, the research base is not sufficiently developed to permit field surveys to assess the level of nutrient utilization within the population. Only the outcome—nutritional status—can be measured. Other areas with rather limited coverage are food preferences, cognition, and attitudes and health beliefs and practices. It is widely recognized that these factors affect the food consumed by individuals. More comprehensive coverage and research in this area are recommended to further our understanding of the contribution of these factors to health. The 1989 CSFII will provide some information on consumer knowledge and attitudes toward diet and health that can be linked to dietary practices. Identification of current behaviors and beliefs seems essential to the development of effective public health policies and intervention programs for enhancing nutritional status. A third gap in the NNMS is estimates of total nutrient intake, that is, nutrient intake from food, supplements, and water. To date, no national survey has produced estimates of total nutrient intake because quantitative estimates of nutrients contributed by supplements and water have not been obtained.

Population Coverage. A second criticism of the NNMS is that the coverage of the population is poor with respect to timing of surveys and that some groups in the population suspected to be at higher risk of malnutrition are not covered by the surveys. Both criticisms have some merit but are difficult to remedy within the context of large federal surveys.

The issue of the timing of surveys is a complicated one. It is true that the timing of surveys has been rather haphazard as evidenced by the delays in fielding the 1977–78 NFCS and the NHANES III. During the 1970s, coverage was very good, with NHANES I and II in the field almost continuously, the NFCS in 1977–78, and the low-income NFCS in 1979–80. No national nutrition surveys were conducted during the early 1980s when dramatic changes were occurring in poverty rates among children and elderly persons in the United States.[42] This deficit is attributable more to the vagaries of the federal budget process than to any malign intent. Because surveys are costly, it is easy to postpone them when budgets are tight and to make do with information that may be slightly out of date. With the Interagency Committee on Nutrition Monitoring in place and an operational plan widely accepted, it is unlikely that this gap in coverage will occur again. A national survey or surveillance activity has been planned for every year between 1985 and 1996. These activities will result in a mechanism for continuous evaluation of the dietary and nutritional status of the U.S. population.

Coverage of populations at nutritional risk poses problems of different types. The national surveys are designed to be representative of the civilian, noninstitutionalized population in the United States. This definition and the method of sampling either eliminates or limits the size of some subgroups in the survey samples. Table 3 indicates groups in the population that are frequently identified as not covered adequately by NNMS. Both NFCS and NHANES exclude nursing homes, so the estimates of food and nutrient intake among older people is probably not representative of that age group.

Some subgroups (such as racial or ethnic minority groups and pregnant or lactating women) do not occur in the population in sufficient numbers to appear in the survey samples with sufficient representation to make reliable estimates of their health and nutrition status. For example, in the NHANES II only a few hundred Hispanics can be identified from the 20,322 people examined, and this sample represents

people with origins in Mexico, Puerto Rico, Cuba, and Central and South American countries. Each of these groups may have distinct dietary patterns and nutritional and health conditions influenced by their cultural and genetic inheritance. Therefore, a special survey of the three largest Hispanic groups in the conterminous United States was conducted by the NCHS in 1982–84.

Separate surveys of only low-income populations were done in the CSFII and NFCS. However, conducting special surveys of subgroups not covered adequately in national surveys may not always be feasible given fiscal constraints. Oversampling is a technique used to boost sample sizes so that one can improve the precision of estimates about health and nutritional status in selected subgroups. For example, in 1985 NHIS increased the number of black persons in the sample by ~75%, resulting in a >20% increase in the precision of statistics. However, this approach can also be very costly—to oversample the Asian population in the NHANES III, it was estimated that the total survey costs would be increased by ~27–45% depending upon the method of oversampling.[47] NHANES III is designed to oversample black and Hispanic persons, young children (<6 y of age), and old adults (>74 y of age).

By definition some groups are excluded from the core NNMS surveys. The NFCS and the NHANES exclude active-duty military people and persons in institutions, specifically hospitals, homes for the aged, convents, monasteries, and penal and mental institutions. Differences in how the agencies interpret what constitutes an institution do exist and can lead to differences in survey data.

Native Americans, homeless people, and residents

Table 3. Coverage of selected population groups by federal monitoring activities*

Population, year	Population (×1000)	NFCS	NHANES	Ped NSS†	Preg NSS†	NHIS	NMIHS	HDS
Civilian, noninstitutionalized, 1986[43]	235,661	XX	XX	XX	XX	XX		XX
Institutionalized‡ 1980[43]	2,492						X	
College dormitories, 1980[43]	1,994		X					
Military (in U.S.), 1986[43]	1,836							
White, 1986[43]	204,301	XX	XX	X	X	X	X	XX
Black, 1986[43]	29,306	X	X	X	X	X	X	X
Hispanic, 1986[43]	18,091	X	X	X	X	X	X	X
Asian, 1980[44]	3,726	X	X	X	X			X
Native Americans, 1980[45]	1,418	X		X	X			
Homeless, 1984[46]	250–350							

* NFCS, Nationwide Food Consumption Survey; NHANES, National Health and Nutrition Examination Survey; PedNSS, Pediatric Nutrition Surveillance System; PregNSS, Pregnancy Nutrition Surveillance System; NHIS, National Health Interview Survey; NMIHS, National Maternal and Infant Health Survey; HDS, Health and Diet Study. XX indicates coverage adequate for national population estimates; X indicates population surveyed but population estimates cannot be calculated.
† Convenience population from participating states.
‡ Excludes dormitories, military quarters, and boarding houses.

of some states are excluded from some surveys. Many national surveys exclude Native Americans living on reservations. However, the design of the 1987–88 NFCS and CSFII included reservations, but not enough Native Americans were sampled to permit separate estimates. Homeless people (those who do not have an address) are excluded from surveys because lists of addresses within census tracts are used as the basic unit for sampling. The core surveys also differ in whether the sampling frame is restricted to the 48 conterminous states (as is the case in NFCS and CSFII) or whether all 50 states are included (as is the case with NHANES). One way to remedy these deficiencies may be to conduct special surveys in these excluded groups or geographic areas. Such surveys have been done occasionally, for example, USDA special surveys in Alaska[48,49] and Hawaii[50,51] and on homeless people.[52]

Small-area Data. There has been an increasing demand by states, counties, and cities for federal surveys to provide data on their geographic areas. The federal surveys are designed to provide information about the dietary, nutritional, and health characteristics of the country and by four regions of the country (Northeast, North Central, South, and West) as defined by the Census Bureau. The primary sampling units are geographic areas such as counties that are grouped (or stratified, to use the statistical term) by characteristics such as urbanization and income. Areas are randomly selected within regions to provide the most representative sample while minimizing operational costs. Some areas are sufficiently populous to always fall into the samples; New York and Los Angeles, for example. However, although several hundred or thousand interviews or examinations may be performed in a city or state, the results are not necessarily representative of that city or state.

Recognizing the data needs of smaller geographic areas, the Division of Nutrition at CDC has worked with states to develop surveillance activities that use data already at hand. These activities include the Pediatric Nutrition Surveillance System (PedNSS), the Pregnancy Nutrition Surveillance System (PregNSS), and the Surveillance of Severe Pediatric Undernutrition (SSPUN). The target populations for PedNSS and PregNSS consist of a convenience sample of low-income children and pregnant women, respectively, who participate in publicly funded health, nutrition, and food assistance programs. Children meeting a specified case definition for severe undernutrition from a variety of settings, including hospitals, comprise the target population for SSPUN.

In 1973 CDC began working with five states to develop the PedNSS for the continuous monitoring of the nutritional status of low-income, high-risk infants and children from birth to age 17 y. Over the years the program has expanded and in 1987, 36 states plus the District of Columbia and Puerto Rico participated in the program. Information is collected on nutritional status indicators, such as anthropometry (birth weight, height, and weight) and hematology (hemoglobin and hematocrit). Estimates of the prevalences of low height-for-age, low and high weight-for-height, anemia, low birth weight, and trends in the prevalences of these indicators categorized by age, sex, and ethnicity are determined.[53–55]

PregNSS was started in 1979. In 1987, 15 states and the District of Columbia participated in the system, submitting approximately 86,850 records to CDC. The emphasis of PregNSS is to quantify and to track prevalent preventable nutrition-related problems (pregravid under- or overweight and anemia) and behavioral risk factors (smoking) among high-risk prenatal populations for the targeting of intervention efforts.

The SSPUN is a new surveillance activity at CDC that began in 1987. The goal of this effort is to identify preschool children (aged 0–5 y) with severe undernutrition and the etiologies and risk factors associated with this problem. Four states, namely Florida, Louisiana, Massachusetts, and Mississippi, have been funded to demonstrate the feasibility of SSPUN. The nutrition status indicators include height, weight, birth weight, and hemoglobin and/or hematocrit. The etiological categories being investigated include antenatal factors, chronic organic disease, child abuse and/or neglect, nonorganic etiology, and access to food programs.

Other innovative ways need to be explored to help smaller areas meet their needs for information about the nutritional status and health of their residents. One approach has been to provide software that permits the user to make synthetic estimates of the prevalence of selected diseases and indicators of malnutrition by using data from the NHANES II and population characteristics in the small area (M.G. Kovar, C. Weinberg, and C. E. Woteki, unpublished observations, 1986). The underlying assumptions in these programs are that the distribution of the characteristic is related to age, sex, and race and that it will be the same as in the national sample.

Timeliness. National surveys require large sample sizes and relatively long periods of time for data collection, resulting in many years to produce reports and public use data tapes of the survey findings. Over the past 5 y, the time required to process, analyze, and release reports and data tapes has been shortened. This improvement can be partially attributed to the introduction of automation into survey operations, for example, an automated system for assigning codes to food items. CSFII (1985) clearly demonstrates the improved capacity to process and publish survey results. Data collection for the first day of food intake of CSFII was completed in June 1985, a report of the food and nutrient intakes was published in November 1985,[56] and the documented public-use data tapes were available a few weeks later. To facilitate the timely release of the dietary data collected in NHANES III, an interactive computerized system will be used by dietary interviewers to obtain information on individual 24-h food intakes. With this system food coding will be completely automated. Both USDA and NCHS plan to continue their concerted efforts for faster data release and publication.

The nutrition surveillance system at CDC is known for its timely publication of data. For PedNSS the prevalence estimates of nutrition-related problems are reported back to the participating states monthly, quarterly, and annually. PregNSS data are reported to states annually. Findings of both PregNSS and PedNSS are published in the annual summary report, *Nutrition Surveillance*.[57] At the state and local levels this feedback is used in client follow-up, health resource allocation, and program planning, management and evaluation.

Policy Analysis. As discussed earlier, the *raison d'etre* for national nutrition surveys is primarily to provide information for policy decisions and only secondarily to contribute to research. The information provided by population surveys, vital records, special surveys, and surveillance systems contributes to the knowledge base used by decision makers when considering changes in federal programs and policies. For example, dietary and nutritional status data can be used to examine the need for changes in food fortification policies as well as for targeting food assistance programs to those groups most in need or developing new intervention strategies. The data also can be used to assess the relationships of diet and health and are useful to regulatory agencies evaluating health messages on food labels.

Much of the policy-related analysis is performed by the agencies charged with the regulatory or program responsibility. The agencies that conduct the large national surveys may not be aware of the decisions that are in the process of being made and, therefore, may not provide the data in the way most relevant to the decision being contemplated.

As the report of the Joint Nutrition Monitoring Evaluation Committee recognized,[41] there needs to be improved communication between agencies responsible for policy decisions and those responsible for nutrition monitoring surveys so that the system can be more responsive to policy needs. However, national surveys can never replace well-designed and well-conducted program evaluations.

Integrating the Information. One of the goals of NNMS is to evaluate the findings of the myriad data sources and reach some conclusions about the nutritional status of the population. To do this, an ad hoc committee, the Joint Nutrition Monitoring Evaluation Committee, was established. Its report in 1986 was the first time that data from several NNMS surveys and surveillance systems were brought together and analyzed in a systematic fashion. A second ad hoc expert panel is preparing the next report of this type, which is due for release in 1989. If this function is to continue on a regular basis as proposed in the Operational Plan, a specific allocation of resources must be part of the operational plans and budgets of DHHS and USDA.

Future Directions. To meet the goals of the NNMS, federal surveys and surveillance activities designed to meet the information needs of the sponsoring agencies are being knit into a network that yields a more comprehensive picture of the nutritional and health status of the total population and specific subgroups. To accomplish these goals, future federal activities need to emphasize improved coverage of populations considered to be at risk for nutritional problems and improved temporal coverage of the general population. Increased use of linked files may prove beneficial for enhancing population coverage and assessing program coverage.[58] The information provided by federal agencies must be timely, usable, and useful for making policy decisions, evaluating programs, and setting research priorities.

The authors thank L. Meyers, R. Rizek, F. Wong, and E. Yetley for their careful critique and thoughtful contributions to this chapter.

References

1. J.B. Mason, J.-P. Habicht, H. Tabatabai, and V. Valverde (1984) *Nutritional Surveillance*, World Health Organization, Geneva.
2. U.S. Department of Health and Human Services, Interagency Committee on Nutrition Monitoring (1988) *Announcement of Committee Formation.* 53 FR 26505 no. 134, U.S. Government Printing Office, Washington, DC.
3. G.L. Ostenso (1984) National Nutrition Monitoring System: a historical perspective. *J. Am. Diet. Assoc.* 84:1181–1185.
4. H.K. Stiebeling, D. Monroe, C.M. Coons, E.F. Phipard, and F. Clark (1941) *Family Food Consumption and Dietary Levels Five Regions.* Consumer Purchases Study. USDA Miscellaneous Publication no. 405, U.S. Government Printing Office, Washington, DC.
5. A.F. Morgan (1959) *Nutritional Status U.S.A.* California Agriculture Experimental Station Bulletin 769. University of California, Berkeley.
6. J.L. Kelsay (1969) A compendium of nutritional status and dietary evaluation studies conducted in the United States, 1957–1967. *J. Nutr.* 99:123–166.
7. U.S. Department of Health, Education and Welfare (1972) *Ten-State Nutrition Survey 1968–1970.* DHEW Publication nos. (HSM)

72-8130–72-8133, U.S. Government Printing Office, Washington, DC.

8. D. Porter (1987) *A National Nutrition Monitoring System: Brief Background and Bill Review*, CRS Report for Congress no. 87-419SPR, Congressional Research Service, Library of Congress, Washington, DC.

9. S.O. Welsh and R.M. Marston (1982) Review of trends in food use in the United States, 1909 to 1980. *J. Am. Diet. Assoc.* 81: 120–125.

10. J.A.T. Pennington (1983) Revision of the Total Diet Study food list and diets. *J. Am. Diet. Assoc.* 82:166–173.

11. U.S. Department of Agriculture (1972) *Food and Nutrient Intake of Individuals in the United States*. HFCS Report no. 11, U.S. Government Printing Office, Washington, DC.

12. U.S. Department of Agriculture (1972) *Food Consumption of Households in the United States: Seasons and Year 1965–66*. HFCS Report no. 12, U.S. Government Printing Office, Washington, DC.

13. U.S. Department of Agriculture (1983) *Food Consumption: Households in the United States, Seasons and Year, 1977–78*. Report no. H-6, U.S. Government Printing Office, Washington, DC.

14. National Center for Health Statistics (1987) *The Supplement on Aging to the 1984 National Interview Survey*. Vital and Health Statistics, series 1, no. 21, DHHS Publication no. (PHS) 87-1323. U.S. Government Printing Office, Washington, DC.

15. National Center for Health Statistics (1988) *Health Promotion and Disease Prevention: United States, 1985*. Vital and Health Statistics, series 10, no. 163, DHHS Publication no. (PHS) 88-1591. U.S. Government Printing Office, Washington, DC.

16. B.H. Schucker, K. Bailey, J.T. Heimbach, et al. (1987) Change in public perspective on cholesterol and heart disease: results from two national surveys. *JAMA* 258:3527–3531.

17. J.T. Heimbach (1987) Risk avoidance in consumer approaches to diet and health. *Clin. Nutr.* 6:159–162.

18. E.M. Gentry, W.D. Kalsbeek, G.C. Hogelin, et al. (1985) The behavioral risk factor analysis surveys: II Design, methods and estimates from combined state data. *Am. J. Prev. Med.* 1(6):9–14.

19. E.M. Gentry, J.T. Jones, J.C. Hogelin, et al. (1987) *Behavioral Risk Factor Surveillance System-Operations Manual*, Centers for Disease Control, Atlanta.

20. Field Services Branch, Division of Nutrition (1987) *Behavioral Risk Factor Surveillance System-Computer Assisted Telephone Interviewing System—Reference Manual*, Centers for Disease Control, Atlanta.

21. Centers for Disease Control (1987) Behavioral risk factor surveillance-selected states 1986. *MMWR* 36:252–254.

22. R.L. Remmington, M.Y. Smith, R.F. Anda, D.F. Williamson, E.M. Gentry, and G.C. Hogelin (1988) Design, characteristics and usefulness of state-based risk factor surveillance, 1981–1986. *Public Health Rep.* 103:366–375.

23. M.L. Stewart, J.T. McDonald, A.S. Levy, R.E. Schucker, and D.P. Henderson (1985) Vitamin/mineral supplement use: a telephone survey of adults in the United States. *J. Am. Diet. Assoc.* 85: 1585–1590.

24. A.S. Levy and R.E. Schucker (1987) Patterns of nutrient intake among dietary supplement users: attitudinal and behavioral correlates. *J. Am. Diet. Assoc.* 87:754–760.

25. U.S. Department of Agriculture (1984) *Nutrient Intakes: Individuals in 48 States, Year 1977–78*. NFCS 1977–78 Report no. I-2, U.S. Government Printing Office, Washington, DC.

26. U.S. Department of Agriculture (1987) *CSFII: Women 19–50 Years and Their Children 1–5 Years, 1 Day, 1986*. NFCS, CSFII Report no. 86-1, U.S. Government Printing Office, Washington, DC.

27. F.N. Hepburn (1982) The USDA National Nutrient Data Bank. *Am. J. Clin. Nutr.* 35:1297–1301.

28. National Center for Health Statistics (1973) *Plan and Operation of the Health and Nutrition Examination Survey, United States, 1971–1973. Part A—Development, plan, and operation*, Vital and Health Statistics, series 1, no. 10a, DHEW Publication no. (PHS) 79-1310. U.S. Government Printing Office, Washington, DC.

29. National Center for Health Statistics (1977) *Plan and Operation of the Health and Nutrition Examination Survey, United States, 1971–1973. Part B—Data Collection Forms of the Survey*, Vital and Health Statistics, series 1, no. 10b, DHEW Publication no. (PHS) 79-1310. U.S. Government Printing Office, Washington, DC.

30. National Center for Health Statistics (1981) *Plan and Operation of the Second National Health and Nutrition Examination Survey, 1976–80*. Vital and Health Statistics, series 1, no. 15, DHHS Publication no. (PHS) 81-1317. U.S. Government Printing Office, Washington, DC.

31. C.E. Woteki, R.R. Briefel, and R. Kuczmarski (1988) Contributions of the National Center for Health Statistics. *Am. J. Clin. Nutr.* 47: 320–328.

32. National Center for Health Statistics (1978) *Plan and Operation of the HANES I Augmentation Survey of Adults 25–74 Years, United States, 1974–1975*. Vital and Health Statistics, series 1, no. 14, DHEW Publication no. (PHS) 78-1314. U.S. Government Printing Office, Washington, DC.

33. National Center for Health Statistics (1985) *Plan and Operation of the Hispanic Health and Nutrition Examination Survey, 1982–84*. Vital and Health Statistics, series 1, no. 19, DHHS Publication no. (PHS) 85-1321. U.S. Government Printing Office, Washington, DC.

34. National Center for Health Statistics (1983) *Dietary Intake Source Data: United States, 1976–80*. Vital and Health Statistics, series 11, no. 231, DHHS Publication no. (PHS) 83-1681. U.S. Government Printing Office, Washington, DC.

35. National Center for Health Statistics (1987) *Anthropometric Reference Data and Prevalence of Overweight, United States, 1976–80*. Vital and Health Statistics, series 11, no. 238, DHHS Publication no. (PHS) 87-1688. U.S. Government Printing Office, Washington, DC.

36. National Center for Health Statistics (1987) *Plan and Operation of the NHANES I Epidemiologic Followup Study 1982–84*. Vital and Health Statistics, series I, no. 22, DHHS Publication no. (PHS) 87-1324. U.S. Government Printing Office, Washington, DC.

37. J.H. Madans, J.C. Kleinman, C.S. Cox, et al. (1986) 10 Years after NHANES I: report of initial followup, 1982–84. *Public Health Rep.* 101:465–473.

38. National Center for Health Statistics (1986) *Maternal Weight Gain and the Outcome of Pregnancy, United States, 1980*. Vital and Health Statistics, series 21, no. 44, DHHS Publication no. (PHS) 86-1922, U.S. Government Printing Office, Washington, DC.

39. National Center for Health Statistics (1988) *Health, United States, 1987*. DHHS Publication no. (PHS) 88-1232, U.S. Government Printing Office, Washington, DC.

40. Food and Nutrition Board, National Research Council (1984) *National Survey Data on Food Consumption: Uses and Recommendations*, National Academy Press, Washington, DC.

41. U.S. Department of Health and Human Services and U.S. Department of Agriculture (1986) *Nutrition Monitoring in the United States: A Progress Report from the Joint Nutrition Monitoring Evaluation Committee*. DHHS Publication no. (PHS) 86-1255, U.S. Government Printing Office, Washington, DC.

42. T.M. Smeeding and B.B. Torrey (1988) Poor children in rich countries. *Science* 242:873–877.

43. U.S. Bureau of the Census (1987) *Statistical Abstract of the United States: 1988*, 108th ed., U.S. Government Printing Office, Washington, DC.

44. U.S. Bureau of the Census (1983) *General Social and Economic Characteristics, United States Summary*. PC80-1-C1, U.S. Government Printing Office, Washington, DC.

45. Bureau of Indian Affairs (1988) *American Indians Today*, U.S. Government Printing Office, Washington, DC.

46. U.S. Department of Housing and Urban Development (1984) *A Report to the Secretary on the Homeless and Emergency Shelters,* U.S. Government Printing Office, Washington, DC.

47. A. Chu and J. Waksberg (1986) *NHANES III Methods Research Evaluation of Task 4 Investigation of the Feasibility of Producing Statistics for the U.S. Oriental Population in NHANES III,* Westat, Rockville, MD.

48. U.S. Department of Agriculture (1981) *Food Consumption and Dietary Levels of Households in Alaska, Winter 1978.* Science and Education Administration Preliminary Report no. 7, U.S. Government Printing Office, Washington, DC.

49. U.S. Department of Agriculture (1981) *Food and Nutrient Intakes of Individuals in 1 Day in Winter 1978.* Science and Education Administration Preliminary Report no. 6, U.S. Government Printing Office, Washington, DC.

50. U.S. Department of Agriculture (1981) *Food Consumption and Dietary Levels of Households in Hawaii, Winter 1978.* Science and Education Administration Preliminary Report no. 4, U.S. Government Printing Office, Washington, DC.

51. U.S. Department of Agriculture (1981) *Food and Nutrient Intakes of Individuals in 1 Day in Hawaii, Winter 1978.* Science and Education Administration Preliminary Report no. 5, U.S. Government Printing Office, Washington, DC.

52. M.R. Burt and B.E. Cohen (1988) *Feeding the Homeless: Does the Prepared Meals Provision Help?,* vol. 1 and 2, Food and Nutrition Service, Arlington, VA.

53. Centers for Disease Control (1987) Nutritional status of minority children—United States 1986. *MMWR* 36:336–369.

54. R. Yip, N.J. Binkin, R. Fleshood, and F.L. Trowbridge (1987) Declining prevalence of anemia among low-income children in the United States. *JAMA* 258:1619–1623.

55. R.E. Peck, J.S. Marks, M.J. Dibley, S. Lee, and F.L. Trowbridge (1987) Birth weight and subsequent growth among Navajo children. *Public Health Rep.* 102:500–507.

56. U.S. Department of Agriculture (1985) *Nationwide Food Consumption Survey: Continuing Survey of Food Intakes by Individuals, Women 19–50 Years and Their Children 1–5 Years, 1 Day, 1985.* NFCS, CSFII Report no. 85-1, U.S. Government Printing Office, Washington, DC.

57. Centers for Disease Control (in press). *Nutrition Surveillance 1984,* U.S. Government Printing Office, Washington, DC.

58. P.A. Buescher (In press) *Linking Administrative Data Files: Research and Policy Applications in a State Government Setting,* Proceedings of the American Statistical Association, American Statistical Association, Alexandria, VA.

Chapter 51   Gary R. Beecher and Ruth H. Matthews

....

Nutrient Composition of Foods

The nutrient content of foods has been tabulated for many decades. In the United States W. O. Atwater initiated the formal practice of publishing the composition of foods as an integral part of his research on energy metabolism.[1-3] Since the turn of the century, there have been many publications that reported the composition of foods (see Vanderveen and Pennington[4] for a historical listing). More recently the accessibility of computers, both personal and centralized systems, has stimulated the tabulation of the composition of foods on such media as computer tapes and disks.

Food composition data are used in many ways by a wide variety of professionals.[4,5] The more common uses include planning and evaluating menus, establishing nutritional adequacy of diets, evaluating diet-disease relationships, and developing regulatory and other government policies. Several additional uses of these data have been discussed and more will be developed as the relationship among foods, nutrients, and health is further elucidated.

Food composition is an all-inclusive term. However, within the context of this review, only components of foods considered to be essential nutrients that are discussed in the most recent Recommended Dietary Allowances (RDA)[6] will be highlighted. Food components such as pesticide residues and selected contaminants are monitored as part of the U.S. Food and Drug Administration's Total Diet Study. The resulting data are tabulated in periodic reports.[7] Factors such as the introduction of new foods, changes in food production and processing practices, food preparation procedures, and the development of new analytic techniques contribute to the obsolescence of food composition data and create the need for new and updated information. This review presents the state of knowledge concerning food composition and the associated state of analytic methodology as of 1989.

Forms of Food Composition Information

Scientists at the U.S. Department of Agriculture (USDA) have been collating and disseminating information on the composition of foods for many years. The most popular current publications are listed in Table 1.

Agriculture Handbook No. 8, Composition of Foods: Raw, Processed, Prepared, serves as the basic reference on food composition. A complete, extensive revision of this handbook has been underway since 1975. New composition data from nationwide sampling studies have been generated on the most important foods in the U.S. diet by USDA and its contractors and incorporated into the revisions. The revision utilizes a looseleaf format to ease future updating and to allow space for the inclusion of additional nutrients and food items. Each page contains the nutrient profile for a single food item. Data are presented for 100 g edible food, for two common measures, and for the edible portion of one pound as purchased. Values are provided for refuse, energy, components of proximate composition, fiber, nine elements, nine vitamins, individual fatty acids, cholesterol, total phytosterols, and 18 amino acids. To provide users with estimates of variability of the nutrient data, the standard error of the mean (for 100 g) and the number of samples on which the values are based are given in each table. To expedite the release of revised information, the revision is being published section by section according to food groups. Thus far, 19 sections have been published.[8-26] The remaining three sections will be published in the near future. Annual updates were initiated in 1989.

Home and Garden Bulletin No. 72[27] provides nutrient data for >900 commonly consumed food items. Data are presented in common household units, e.g., cups, ounces, and quarts. Values are included for water; energy; protein; fat; total saturated, mono-unsaturated, and polyunsaturated fatty acids; cho-

Table 1. USDA food composition publications*

USDA Handbook No. 8, *Composition of Foods, Raw, Processed, Prepared* (1963)
USDA Handbook No. 8, *Composition of Foods . . . Raw, Processed, Prepared,* Revised sections

8-1	*Dairy and Egg Products*	1976
8-2	*Spices and Herbs*	1977
8-3	*Baby Foods*	1978
8-4	*Fats and Oils*	1979
8-5	*Poultry Products*	1979
8-6	*Soups, Sauces and Gravies*	1980
8-7	*Sausages and Luncheon Meats*	1980
8-8	*Breakfast Cereals*	1982
8-9	*Fruits and Fruit Juices*	1982
8-10	*Pork Products*	1983
8-11	*Vegetable and Vegetable Products*	1984
8-12	*Nut and Seed Products*	1984
8-13	*Beef Products*	1986
8-14	*Beverages*	1986
8-15	*Finfish and Shellfish Products*	1987
8-16	*Legumes and Legume Products*	1986
8-17	*Lamb, Veal and Game Products*	1989
8-18	*Baked Products*	1990, projected
8-19	*Snacks and Sweets*	1990, projected
8-20	*Cereal Grains and Pastas*	1989
8-21	*Fast Foods*	1988
8-22	*Mixed Dishes*	1990, projected

Yearly supplements beginning in 1989
Home and Garden Bulletin No. 72
    Nutritive Value of Foods   1985
Home Economics Research Report
    No. 45 *Iron Content of Food*   1983
    No. 48 *Sugar Content of Selected Foods*   1987
Provisional tables
    Fatty Acid and Cholesterol Content of Selected Foods   1988
    Omega-3 Fatty Acids and Other Fat Components in Selected Foods   1988
    Vitamin K Content of Selected Foods   1987
    Stearic Acid, Total Fat and Other Fatty Acids in Selected Foods   1988
    Dietary Fiber Content of Selected Foods   1988
    Amino Acids in Fruits and Vegetables   1983
    Nutrient Content of Bakery Foods and Related Items   1981
    Percent Retention of Nutrients in Food Preparation   1984

* USDA Handbooks and revised sections, Home and Garden Bulletin, and Home Economics Research Reports are available from National Technical Information Service, 5285 Port Royal Road, Springfield, VA 22161. Provisional tables are available from Human Nutrition Information Service, Room 315, Federal Building, 6505 Belcrest Road, Hyattsville, MD, 20782.

lesterol; carbohydrates; calcium; phosphorus; iron; potassium; sodium; vitamin A; thiamin; riboflavin; niacin; and ascorbic acid.

Home Economics Research Reports (HERR) and provisional tables provide food composition data to users on a nutrient-by-nutrient basis. The data in HERR publications and provisional tables represent the compilation of values for nutrients that have not been reported in other food composition tables and

that are the most current. Factors that contribute to the publication of these tables include improved analytic methodology, recent sampling and analysis of a substantial number of foods, and user demand for specific nutrient data, i.e., n−3 fatty acids. These tables are subject to frequent updates, and data from these tables are incorporated into handbook revisions and data-tape updates.

Food composition data also are made available from USDA in the form of computer tapes and diskettes. Table 2 is a tabulation of several of the databases available on these media; a description of all available databases was published.[28]

USDA Nutrient Database for Standard Reference (Table 2) is periodically updated and incorporates the data published in the revised sections of Agriculture Handbook No. 8. Data from the 1963 edition are included for food groups for which revision is incomplete. Values not available from the handbook were imputed and included in the database.[29] Supporting files to be used with the database also appear on the tape. These files include the database format, a list of food descriptors and item numbers that can be used as a coding manual, and a file that links the food codes used in the 1963 Agriculture Handbook No. 8 to codes used in the updated sections of Handbook No. 8.

USDA Nutrient Database for Standard Reference for Microcomputers is a floppy-disk version of the *USDA Nutrient Database for Standard Reference.* It was created for use on a microcomputer and thus was designed to minimize the data storage requirement while providing all information on the tape version of the file. Supporting files also are included on the disk. An abbreviated version of this database is also available on disk. The disk is limited to 21 food components, and nutrient values are reported for 100-g amounts of edible portions of the food item.

USDA Nutrient Database for Individual Food Intake Surveys (Table 2) is a series of databases developed for use by USDA in the Nationwide Food Consumption Surveys and the Continuing Survey of Food Intakes by Individuals (CSFII).[30] These databases include a primary nutrient data set, a recipe file, and a table of retention factors that are linked together by a recipe-calculation program.[31] Most of the data in the primary nutrient data set were from the most recent version of the *USDA Nutrient Database for Standard Reference* (Table 3). If analytic data were not available, values were imputed from other forms of the foods or were estimated from data for similar foods (R.H. Matthews and D.B. Haytourtz, unpublished observations, 1989). The date and source for each nutrient value in the primary data set are given.

The recipe file contains >4,400 items; approximately half are multicomponent recipes used to gen-

Table 2. USDA food composition tapes and diskettes*

Computer tapes†
  USDA Nutrient Database for Standard Reference Release,
    8, 1989
  USDA Nutrient Database for Individual Intake Surveys,
    release 2.1, 1987
  Data Set 72-1 Nutritive Values of Foods, as in Home and
    Garden Bulletin No. 72, release 3, 1985
Diskettes‡
  USDA Nutrient Database for Standard Reference, release
    8, for microcomputers
  Data Set 72-1, Nutritive Values of Food, as in Home and
    Garden Bulletin No. 72, revised, 1985

* Tapes and diskettes are available from National Technical Information Service, 5285 Port Royal Road, Springfield, VA 22161. Additional information and latest releases of these data sets are described in reference 27.
  † Format is 9-track tape, 1,600 or 6,250 BPI, in ASCII or EBCDIC format.
  ‡ Diskettes are 5.25- or 3.5-inch floppy disks formatted for IBM-PC; data sets can be formatted in ASCII, data-base management systems, i.e., dBase III, or spreadsheet programs, i.e., Lotus 1-2-3.

erate data for the CSFII. Recipes usually are selected from the most popular cookbooks, for example, *Better Homes and Gardens New Cookbook*,[34] and are evaluated by food specialists on the Human Nutrition Information Service (HNIS) staff. Typically, the recipe that most closely represents the mixed dish or food is chosen. When a single recipe is not representative of a food or mixed dish, recipes are combined or specialty and regional cookbooks are consulted, e.g., *Southern Living—Annual Recipes*.[35] Recipes are continually reviewed and modified by staffs at HNIS and the National Center for Health Statistics to improve representativeness. An example of such a modification is the substitution of tuna packed in water for tuna packed in oil to coincide with trends indicated by data from nutrition and food consumption surveys. New and modified recipes are introduced at the beginning of each food and/or nutrition survey or survey cycle.

The table of nutrient-retention factors contains factors for calculating nutrient retention of 18 vitamins and minerals during cooking and food preparation. This table is based on a series of published factors[36,37] but also contains factors for several additional categories of foods and cooking methods that were determined specifically for this table. The factors used for the calculation of nutrient amounts were developed according to the procedure discussed by Murphy et al.[38]

The recipe calculation program utilizes these three databases (primary nutrient data set, recipe file, and retention-factor table) to generate data for the CSFII database.[31] The calculation procedures involve the following steps:

1. Determine the weight (g) of each ingredient and subtract the weight of any inedible part.
2. Calculate the nutrient amount in the specified weight of each ingredient.
3. Apply retention factors to vitamin and mineral values where losses may occur during cooking.
4. Calculate total uncooked weight of recipe by summing weights of all ingredients.
5. Calculate nutrient amount in total recipe by summing nutrient values for all ingredients.
6. Adjust total nutrient values to account for changes in moisture and fat during cooking.
7. Convert nutrient values for total recipe to values for 100 g.

A recent evaluation of methods to calculate the nutrient composition of recipes indicated that this method computed values for food constituents that were generally higher than the other three models tested.[39] The method also allows flexibility when recipes are coded and is applicable for both raw and cooked ingredients. This recipe calculation approach was used to generate a database that was used for the 1985–1986 CSFII and the Hispanic Health and Nutrition Examination Survey (HHANES). It is currently being used to generate a database for the 1987–1988 National Food Consumption Survey and the Third National Health and Nutrition Examination Survey, which are in progress.

Table 3. Source of data in primary data set of CSFII database*

Nutrient	Number of food items contributing 80% of nutrient intake†	Number of food items containing imputed values	Number of food items containing label-claim values
Protein	150	6	0
Dietary fiber	120	46	0
Fat	107	3	0
Cholesterol	49	4	0
Vitamin B-6	175	23	20
Thiamin	168	5	17
Riboflavin	165	5	15
Niacin	159	9	17
Folacin	129	20	14
Vitamin E	100	50	0
Vitamin A	60	5	9
Vitamin B-12	58	9	5
Carotene	33	0	0
Iron	217	21	18
Copper	209	30	0
Magnesium	187	27	0
Phosphorus	180	5	0
Zinc	169	20	6
Potassium	159	5	0

* Adapted from Hepburn.[32]
† Calculated from 4-d food consumption data for 1,088 women (weighted) in the 1985 *Continuing Survey of Food Intakes by Individuals*.[33]

Data Set 72-1 contains the data published as Table 2 of Home and Garden Bulletin No. 72 revised in 1985 (Table 2). Data are given for 20 components in >950 foods in terms of household measures. It is available as a tape or a diskette.

A large number of universities and most large food companies have food composition databases and associated computerized systems to support research, menu planning, food preparation, and associated activities. Many small businesses also developed microcomputer systems capable of diet analysis and/or menu planning. Nearly all of these systems utilized Agriculture Handbook No. 8, its revised sections, or *USDA Nutrient Database for Standard Reference* as the basis for their databases. A directory of university and commercial databases is published annually.[40] In addition, the Food and Nutrition Information Center (National Agricultural Library, Beltsville, MD) maintains a collection of commercial microcomputer software programs that are oriented toward diet analysis.[29]

Many countries in all parts of the world have active programs in the compilation of food composition information. The International Network of Food Data Systems (INFOODS) maintains an international directory of food composition tables and a list of other international activities related to food composition. This information can be obtained through the INFOODS Secretariat, Room N52-457, Massachusetts Institute of Technology, 77 Massachusetts Avenue, Cambridge, MA 02139.

State of Knowledge of Food Composition

The state of knowledge of the composition of foods has been reviewed.[41,42] The results of a recent evaluation by the Nutrient Data Research Branch, HNIS, USDA, are shown in Appendixes 1–5. These data resulted from research in several disciplines related to food processing and production and from a concentrated effort by several government agencies to generate food composition data. Careful examination of the table shows that there is a considerable amount of food composition information available for commodities.

Nonetheless, there is a lack of composition information for several food groups and for several categories of nutrients. Only limited data exist for those food groups consisting of highly processed or manufactured foods, i.e., baked products, snack foods, etc. (*see* Appendixes 1–5). Changes in the lifestyle of Americans have resulted in the proliferation of convenience and prepared foods (fast foods, frozen meals and entrees, restaurant food, etc.) for which limited composition data are available. In the case of entire categories of components, i.e., several trace and subtrace minerals, biological effects and require-

ments only recently were described and as a result data for these components in foods are very limited (Appendix 5). For some nutrients, lack of data can be attributed to the inadequacy of accurate, precise, and inexpensive analytic methods, e.g., folic acid, pantothenic acid (Appendix 4), vitamin A (Appendix 4), other sterols (Appendix 3). For a few nutrients, e.g., sugars, analytic methods are adequate and as a result, foods for which data are inadequate must be analyzed by these methods (Appendix 2). Ongoing efforts are needed to continue to improve the extent and quality of food composition information.

Adequacy of Food Composition Information

The adequacy, more correctly the inadequacy, of food composition data is often discussed. Until recently, there was no definitive measure of the state of these data. Hepburn[32] tabulated the number of important food items containing imputed and label-claim values in the primary data set of the 1985 CSFII Database (Table 3). These observations indicate that for many nutrients a high proportion of the data is derived from analytic values, e.g., protein, fat, and phosphorus. On the other hand, several nutrients for many important foods have values that were imputed or that were taken from label-claim values. Imputed values are derived from analytic values for similar foods and thus may have an inherent error.[43] Label-claim values establish limits (usually lower limits) of a nutrient in a food and as a result may underestimate the amount of a nutrient in the food. For nutrients with a large number of imputed values, inexpensive analytic methods usually are not available and the assay of foods is expensive. As a result, few data are generated. Development of analytic methods and extensive food sampling for these nutrients are high priorities.[29]

The impact of precision of food composition data on the variability of the content of a 1-d diet was discussed by Beaton.[44] Even though coefficients of variation (CV) for food composition data range as high as 30%, when these data were used to calculate 1,000 theoretical 1-d diets, assuming random variation, the error term in a 1-d–intake estimate was remarkably low (generally ≤10% CV). If one assumes that the CVs for food composition data are random, then statistical theory suggests that as more items of food are included in the diet, the variance of the nutrient content of the mixed diet will decrease. Beaton[44] suggested that although this approach is valid for assessing dietary intake of large groups or populations, it is not adequate for the accurate calculation of nutrient intakes of individuals. These observations suggest that systematic bias (accuracy) in food composition data may be of much greater concern than random variation.

An important aspect of all research that utilizes food composition data is accurate and complete documentation of the database or data tables that are used. Such documentation is relatively easy when USDA databases are used because each release of a data tape or diskette is identified with a version number. Similarly, data tables also are identified with specific numbers. When other databases (university, industry, or commercial) are used, the specific release or version may not be obvious. Nonetheless, every attempt should be made to obtain and report this information so that interested parties can use exactly the same database to perform diet calculations or be able to discern differences in the data.

Improvement of Food Composition Data

Because analytic values for several nutrients are missing (Table 3) and because the composition of foods may change as a result of modifications in food formulations and the introduction of new foods, improvement of food composition data is an important aspect of the diet–public health arena.[45] Quantification of all of the food components important to human health in all available foods is an immense task. A conservative estimate is that about one million analyses would be required to quantify a reasonable number of components in a few representative samples of each generic food available in the United States.[42] Therefore, it is important to establish priorities for both nutrients and foods to systematically improve food composition information.

Selection of Nutrients for Analysis

Three factors appear useful in establishing priorities for the analysis of specific food components. These factors include knowledge of food composition data, adequacy of analytic methodology, and involvement of a nutrient in a current public health problem in the United States (Figure 1). Nutrients that meet all three criteria (Region 1, Figure 1) should be given the highest priority for analysis. For nutrients that meet only the criteria of inadequate data and public health problems (Region 2, Figure 1), improvement of the measurement system must precede large-scale food-analysis studies before the highest-quality data can be accumulated.

The principal nutrition-related health problems of Americans are the major chronic diseases: coronary heart disease, cancer, hypertension, stroke, diabetes, and obesity.[46] Several food components have been associated with current public health issues.[45] These components include food energy, total fat, saturated fatty acids, cholesterol, alcohol, iron, calcium, and

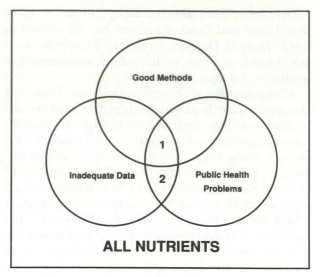

Figure 1. Factors used in the selection of nutrients for analysis. Region 1 represents nutrients for which it is appropriate to generate food composition data. Region 2 represents nutrients that should receive high-priority research on analytic methodology. Adapted from Beecher and Vanderslice.[42]

sodium. This group of nutrients should be given highest priority in terms of assessing the adequacy of analytic methodology and food composition data. Another group of nutrients (dietary fiber, vitamin A, carotenes, folacin, vitamin B-6, vitamin C, potassium, zinc, and fluoride) was identified as having potential association with public health issues and requires further study.[45] For many of the components in this group, acceptable analytic methods for quantifying amounts in foods are not available (Tables 4 and 5). Therefore, improvement of measurement systems must be of highest priority.

Valid analytical procedures are essential for reliable nutrient analysis of foods. The state of methodology for the analysis of nutrients in foods is tabulated in Table 5. The boundary between acceptable and unacceptable methods lies between substantial and conflicting states of methodology. Thus, if appropriate methods are used by trained analysts, values will probably be correct for nutritionally significant amounts of those nutrients listed as having adequate and substantial methodologies. For a few of the nutrients in the conflicting and lacking categories, reliable values may be obtained if extreme care is exercised by the analyst. However, for most of the nutrients in these categories, it is doubtful that valid results can be obtained during routine analysis.

Several factors were used to classify the state of methodology for each nutrient (Table 5). The criterion given the greatest weight was accuracy. An analytical method should yield a value within 10% of the true value when a nutrient is present at nutritionally significant amounts (>5% of the RDA per standard serving or daily intake). Most methods used to quan-

Table 4. State of development of methods for analysis of nutrients in foods

Nutrient category	Adequate	Substantial	Conflicting	Lacking
Carbohydrates, fiber, and sugars		Individual sugars Fiber (AOAC) Starch	Fiber components	
Energy	Bomb calorimetry		Calculated	
Lipids		Cholesterol Fat (total) Fatty acids (common)	Sterols Fatty acids (isomers)	
Mineral nutrients	Calcium Copper Magnesium Phosphorus Potassium Sodium Zinc	Iron Selenium	Arsenic Chromium Fluorine Iodine Manganese	Boron Cobalt Molybdenum Silicon Tin Vanadium Organic species
Proteins and amino acids	Nitrogen (total)	Amino acids (most)	Amino acids (some) Protein (total)	
Vitamins		Niacin Riboflavin Thiamin Vitamin B-6 Vitamin E	Carotenoids (pro-vitamin A) Vitamin A Vitamin B-12 Vitamin C Vitamin D Pantothenic acid	Biotin Folacin Vitamin K
Other			Phytate	Carotenoids (non-vitamin A)

tify nutrients in foods are field methods developed to provide results with reasonable accuracy and precision in a relatively short time. These methods must be validated with materials (standard reference materials, SRMs) in which the amount of nutrient is measured by use of techniques that are highly accurate and precise. Such definitive methods often take a long time to execute. Once a field method has been validated and an ongoing analytical quality control program established, routine nutrient composition data can be generated. The National Institute of Standards and Technology (formerly the National Bureau of Standards) produces a large number of SRMs; however, only a few have matrices similar to foods and only the amounts of inorganic nutrients have been certified.[47] Research efforts are being directed toward developing reference materials with matrices similar to foods and with certified values for many nutrients but especially for organic nutrients.[48,49] Analytic methods are often inaccurate for several reasons, including presence of interfering compounds, loss or destruction of the component of interest during extraction and sample preparation, and lack of specificity for the component occurring among closely related molecular species. Development and application of appropriate SRMs will overcome many of these problems and contribute greatly to the improvement of accuracy in food analysis.

Analyses of identical samples by several laboratories often show unacceptably large variations

Table 5. Description of methodology states

Factors	Adequate	Substantial	Conflicting	Lacking
Accuracy	Excellent	Good	Fair	Poor
Speed of analysis	Fast	Moderate	Slow	Slow
Cost per analysis	Modest (<$100)	Modest to high	High	?
Development needs	— — —	Method modification Extraction procedure Applications	Method development and/or modification Extraction procedure Applications	Method development Extraction procedure Applications

among laboratories.[50] Most nutrient composition tables and databases are compiled from data generated by different laboratories. As a result any interlaboratory variation will contribute to the variability of the compiled data. The appropriate use of quality control samples and the development and use of SRMs should reduce this variation and improve the quality of nutrient composition data.

Precision is also an important consideration in the evaluation of an analytic method. Common sense must be applied during the evaluation of analytical precision in nutrient analysis. The method must be sufficiently precise to yield credible nutrient composition information, and at the same time some imprecision must be tolerated in the interest of time and economics. With pure standards the maximum acceptable relative standard deviation (RSD) should range between 5% and 10%; attempts to obtain RSDs of ≤1% are probably impractical uses of resources. For nutrient analysis of foods, acceptable precision should be tempered by the amount of a nutrient in a food. Precision is generally lower when the component is present in small amounts. RSDs in the range of 10–15% are probably adequate for most nutrients. For those that occur at low amounts (5–30% RDA per serving), precision criteria should be relaxed by some predetermined standard.[41]

Modifications required to improve existing nutrient analysis methods are tabulated in Table 5. Changes to move a method from the substantial to the adequate category may require only minor modifications of the extraction and quantitation steps and/or application of the method to additional food groups. Changes, however, required to recategorize an unacceptable (conflicting or lacking) method as acceptable (adequate or substantial) may require extensive method modification or development, improvement of extraction and sample-preparation procedures, and application of the new method to several different food groups.

The state of knowledge and adequacy of food composition data were discussed in an earlier section of this chapter. Another important consideration is the quality of the analytic data that currently exist for a nutrient. The concept of quality indices for food composition data sets was first described by Exler[51] for iron in foods. It was later expanded and applied to selenium and copper.[52-54] Data quality indices provide indicators of the degree of confidence with which food composition data can be used. The process involves scoring a data set for each food for the following criteria: number of samples analyzed, analytic method utilized, sample-handling procedures and documentation, adequacy of sampling plan, and analytical quality control program. Each criterion is scored separately and the scores are combined to give an overall quality index for that component in a food.[52] In this manner highly reliable data can be distinguished from data requiring improvement, and food-analysis priorities can be established accordingly. Such a program is currently in progress for improving the selenium data of foods.

Selection of Foods for Analysis

A conceptual approach to establishing priorities for analysis of foods for nutrients is shown in Figure 2. Three factors are important in establishing these priorities. They are knowledge of the adequacy of food composition data, significant contribution of nutrient in the food to diet, and availability of data for foods as eaten. Foods that meet all three criteria (Region 1, Figure 2) should be given highest priority for analysis. Some foods may meet only the criteria of inadequate data and availability of data for foods as eaten (Region 2, Figure 2). These might be selected foods that are not significant contributors of a nutrient to the diet but for which some data are required, i.e., specialty foods, foods containing high concentrations of nutrient, etc.

Recent research demonstrated that a small-to-modest number of foods are the major contributors of a nutrient to the diet (Table 3).[53-56] Data from these studies indicate that from 30 to slightly >200 food entries (Table 3) or from 12 to 36 food groups contribute 80% of the nutrients to the diet.[53-56] These are the foods that deserve most attention in terms of assuring that databases and food tables contain the highest-quality and most-recent data. Foods on these lists also must be monitored for changes in nutrient content brought about by modifications in food production, processing, and marketing. For example, reduction of the fat trim on retail beef during the mid 1980s prompted a nationwide survey of retail beef. Results from this study indicated that steaks and roasts contained 25% less trim fat than was reported in food composition tables.[57] Use of the earlier data in nationwide surveys may have overestimated fat consumption for the population groups surveyed. The modification of other foods and the application of new technologies can be expected as consumers become more aware of diet-health relationships and create a demand for foods to meet these goals.

In view of the above discussion, foods that are major contributors of nutrients to the diet and that have imputed values (Table 3) or for which there is a dearth of analytic values (Appendixes 1–5) should be given highest priority for analysis. At a somewhat lower priority are those foods that are major contributors and for which there are inadequate data or data that were assigned low confidence codes.[51,53,54] Foods that fit into other categories should be analyzed only if there are obvious reasons and if resources are sufficient to accomplish the sampling and analysis.

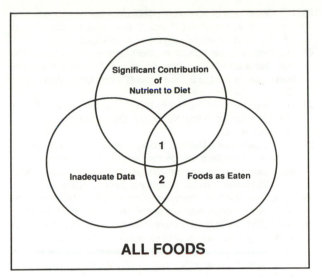

Figure 2. Factors used in the selection of foods for nutrient analysis. Region 1 represents foods for which it is appropriate to conduct large-scale sampling and analysis. Region 2 represents foods for which some data may be required (high concentration of nutrient, specialty food, etc.).

Analysis of nutrients in foods as eaten provides the most meaningful data on the composition of foods applicable to diet-health relationships. This concept permits a very direct approach to sampling, preparation, and analysis of many foods. However, some food items are made from complex recipes. Because of the difficulty in selecting and sampling representative foods of this type, it is often advantageous to calculate the composition of such foods from typical recipes, i.e., recipes selected from the most popular cookbooks.[34] These procedures not only require composition information but also must utilize nutrient retention data. Thus, for those foods that are basic to recipes and mixed dishes, composition data for both the raw and cooked forms are needed.

Representative sampling of foods is a complex task in a country as large as the United States and with as diverse a population and food supply. The primary objective of sampling for food composition should be to obtain accurate estimates of the nutrient composition of foods providing the majority of a nutrient or nutrients in the diet of the U.S. population. Sampling designs based on this objective were described for beef and fast-food chicken.[57–59] In general, the country was divided into five geographical regions. Two or three major metropolitan areas within each region were selected based upon population density and supermarket sales volume; within each city the leading supermarket chains or fast-food chains were chosen to account for at least one-third (in most cities more than one-half) of the grocery or product sales. Representative stores were selected randomly. Food samples were purchased during periods of normal product turnover, shipped to appropriate laborato-

ries, and analyzed for selected nutrients. Data from nationwide sampling studies permitted identification and evaluation of the major sources of variation in the nutrient composition of a food. As an example, fat content of ground beef (all types of ground beef combined) was significantly higher (25.0 vs. 20.7 g/ 100 g) for the North Central region of the United States than for the other four regions from which samples were purchased.[58] On the other hand, data from a nationwide sampling of fast-food fried chicken indicated that recipe for preparation and anatomical source of the meat (breast vs. thigh) contributed significant variation to the nutrient data.[59,60] Factors such as geographical source of the sample and, for most nutrients, commerical brand contributed insignificant ($p > 0.05$) variation to the data.[59,60] An insufficient number of nationwide sampling studies have been conducted and statistically evaluated to allow determination of the major sources of variation of the nutrient content of foods. Nonetheless, nutrient data from such studies are the most representative of foods consumed in the United States.

Summary

Food composition data are collated and tabulated in the form of handbooks, computer tapes, and diskettes. Substantial analytical data are available for many nutrients in many foods. For those nutrients that have been implicated in public health problems and for new highly processed foods, analytical data are less extensive and in many cases absent. The improvement of food composition data requires establishing priorities for the identification of nutrients to be quantified and the selection of foods that should be extensively sampled and analyzed. The collaboration of several federal and state agencies, food and production trade associations, universities, and food processors has greatly contributed to the present knowledge of food composition. Expansion of this collaboration in the future will improve the extent and recency of food composition information.

References

1. W.O. Atwater and C.D. Wood (1896) *The Chemical Composition of American Food Materials.* USDA Bulletin no. 28, U.S. Government Printing Office, Washington, DC.
2. W.O. Atwater and A.P. Bryant (1899) *The Chemical Composition of American Food Materials.* USDA Bulletin no. 28, U.S. Government Printing Office, Washington, DC.
3. W.O. Atwater and A.P. Bryant (1906) *The Chemical Composition of American Food Materials.* USDA Bulletin no. 28, U.S. Government Printing Office, Washington, DC.
4. J.E. Vanderveen and J.A.T. Pennington (1983) Use of food composition data by governments. *Food Nutr. Bull.* 5(2):40–45.
5. C.T. Windham, R.G. Hansen, B.W. Wyse, and A.W. Sorenson (1983) Uses of nutrient data bases for identifying nutritional rela-

tionships to public health and nutrition education in the United States. *Food Nutr. Bull.* 5(2):46–53.

6. National Research Council (1989) *Recommended Dietary Allowances,* 10th ed., National Academy Press, Washington, DC.

7. J.A.T. Pennington and E.L. Gunderson (1987) History of the Food and Drug Administration's Total Diet Study—1961 to 1987. *J. Assoc. Off. Anal. Chem.* 70:772–782.

8. U.S. Department of Agriculture (1976) *Composition of Foods: Dairy and Egg Products—Raw, Processed, Prepared.* Agriculture Handbook no. 8-1, U.S. Government Printing Office, Washington, DC.

9. U.S. Department of Agriculture (1977) *Composition of Foods: Spices and Herbs—Raw, Processed, Prepared.* Agriculture Handbook no. 8-2, U.S. Government Printing Office, Washington, DC.

10. U.S. Department of Agriculture (1978) *Composition of Foods: Baby Foods—Raw, Processed, Prepared.* Agriculture Handbook no. 8-3, U.S. Government Printing Office, Washington, DC.

11. U.S. Department of Agriculture (1979) *Composition of Foods: Fats and Oils—Raw, Processed, Prepared.* Agriculture Handbook no. 8-4, U.S. Government Printing Office, Washington, DC.

12. U.S. Department of Agriculture (1979) *Composition of Foods: Poultry Products—Raw, Processed, Prepared.* Agriculture Handbook no. 8-5, U.S. Government Printing Office, Washington, DC.

13. U.S. Department of Agriculture (1980) *Composition of Foods: Soups, Sauces and Gravies—Raw, Processed, Prepared.* Agriculture Handbook no. 8-6, U.S. Government Printing Office, Washington, DC.

14. U.S. Department of Agriculture (1980) *Composition of Foods: Sausages and Luncheon Meats—Raw, Processed, Prepared.* Agriculture Handbook no. 8-7, U.S. Government Printing Office, Washington, DC.

15. U.S. Department of Agriculture (1982) *Composition of Foods: Breakfast Cereals—Raw, Processed, Prepared.* Agriculture Handbook no. 8-8, U.S. Government Printing Office, Washington, DC.

16. U.S. Department of Agriculture (1982) *Composition of Foods: Fruits and Fruit Juices—Raw, Processed, Prepared.* Agriculture Handbook no. 8-9 U.S. Government Printing Office, Washington, DC.

17. U.S. Department of Agriculture (1983) *Composition of Foods: Pork Products—Raw, Processed, Prepared.* Agriculture Handbook no. 8-10, U.S. Government Printing Office, Washington, DC.

18. U.S. Department of Agriculture (1984) *Composition of Foods: Vegetable and Vegetable Products—Raw, Processed, Prepared.* Agriculture Handbook no. 8-11, U.S. Government Printing Office, Washington, DC.

19. U.S. Department of Agriculture (1984) *Composition of Foods: Nut and Seed Products—Raw, Processed, Prepared.* Agriculture Handbook no. 8-12, U.S. Government Printing Office, Washington, DC.

20. U.S. Department of Agriculture (1986) *Composition of Foods: Beef Products—Raw, Processed, Prepared.* Agriculture Handbook no. 8-13, U.S. Government Printing Office, Washington, DC.

21. U.S. Department of Agriculture (1986) *Composition of Foods: Beverages—Raw, Processed, Prepared.* Agriculture Handbook no. 8-14, U.S. Government Printing Office, Washington, DC.

22. U.S. Department of Agriculture (1987) *Composition of Foods: Finfish and Shell Fish Products—Raw, Processed, Prepared.* Agriculture Handbook no. 8-15, U.S. Government Printing Office, Washington, DC.

23. U.S. Department of Agriculture (1986) *Composition of Foods: Legumes and Legume Products—Raw, Processed, Prepared.* Agriculture Handbook no. 8-16, U.S. Government Printing Office, Washington, DC.

24. U.S. Department of Agriculture (1989) *Composition of Foods: Lamb, Veal and Game—Raw, Processed, Prepared.* Agriculture Handbook no. 8-17, U.S. Government Printing Office, Washington, DC.

25. U.S. Department of Agriculture (1988) *Composition of Foods: Fast Foods—Raw, Processed, Prepared.* Agriculture Handbook no. 8-21, U.S. Government Printing Office, Washington, DC.

26. U.S. Department of Agriculture (1989) *Composition of Foods: Cereal Grains and Pasta—Raw, Processed, Prepared.* Agriculture Handbook no. 8-20, U.S. Government Printing Office, Washington, DC.

27. U.S. Department of Agriculture (1985) *Nutritive Value of Foods.* Home and Garden Bulletin No. 72, U.S. Government Printing Office, Washington, DC.

28. Nutrition Monitoring Division, Survey Statistics Branch (1989) *Machine Readable Data sets on the Composition of Foods and Results from Food Composition Surveys.* HNIS Administrative Report no. 378, Human Nutrition Information Service, Hyattsville, MD.

29. Food and Nutrition Information Center (1988) *Microcomputer Software Collection,* National Agriculture Library, Beltsville, MD.

30. B.P. Perloff (1988) Development of the Continuing Survey of Food Intakes by Individuals (CSFII) database. In: *Proceedings of the 12th National Nutrient Data Bank Conference* (L.S. Hicks, D.B. Reed, and P. Pillow, eds.), pp. 25–30, The Cbord Group, Inc., Ithaca, NY.

31. B.P. Perloff (1986) Recipe calculations for NFCS database. In: *Proceedings of the 10th National Nutrient Data Bank Conference* (S. Murphy and D. Rauchwarter, eds.), pp. 11–21, National Technical Information Service, Springfield, VA.

32. F.N. Hepburn (1988) HNIS-USDA update. In: *Proceedings of the 12th National Nutrient Data Bank Conference* (L.S. Hicks, D.B. Reed, and P. Pillow, eds.), pp. 31–33, The Cbord Group, Inc., Ithaca, NY.

33. Human Nutrition Information Service (1987) *Nationwide Food Consumption Survey, Continuing Survey of Food Intakes by Individuals, Women 19–50 Years and Their Children 1–5 Years, 4 Days.* NFCS, CSFII Report no. 85-4, HNIS, Hyattsville, MD.

34. S. Granseth, ed. (1981) *Better Homes and Gardens New Cookbook,* 9th ed., Meredith Corporation, Des Moines, IA.

35. A.H. Harvey, ed. (1988) *Southern Living—Annual Recipes,* Oxford House, Birmingham, AL.

36. Nutrition Monitoring Division, Nutrient Data Research Branch (1984) *Provisional Table on Percent Retention of Nutrients in Food Preparation.* Human Nutrition Information Service, Hyattsville, MD.

37. Nutrition Monitoring Division (1988) *Conserving Nutrients in Foods.* HNIS Administrative Report no. 384, Human Nutrition Information Service, Hyattsville, MD.

38. E.W. Murphy, P.E. Criner, and B.C. Gray (1975) Comparison of methods for calculating retentions of nutrients in cooked foods. *J. Agric. Food Chem.* 23:1153–1157.

39. P.M. Powers and L.W. Hoover (1989) Calculating the nutrient composition of recipes with computers. *J. Am. Diet. Assoc.* 89:224–232.

40. L. Hoover (1989) *Nutrient Data Bank Directory,* 8th ed., Curators of the University of Missouri, Columbia, MO.

41. K.K. Stewart (1981) Nutrient analyses of food: a review and a strategy for the future. In: *Beltsville Symposia in Agricultural Research IV Human Nutrition Research* (G.R. Beecher, ed.), pp. 209–224, Allanheld, Osmun Publishers, Totowa, NJ.

42. G.R. Beecher and J.T. Vanderslice (1984) Determination of nutrients in foods: factors that must be considered. In: *Modern Methods of Food Analysis* (K.K. Stewart and J.R. Whitaker, eds.), pp. 29–55, AVI Publishing Company, Inc., Westport, CT.

43. J.A.T. Pennington, S.P. Murphy, W.M. Rand, and J.C. Klensin (in press) *Compiling Data for Food Composition Databases,* United Nations University, Tokyo.

44. G.H. Beaton (1986) New approaches to the national assessment of population dietary data. In: *Proceedings of the 10th National Nutrient Data Bank Conference* (S. Murphy and D. Rauchwarter, eds.), pp. 137–159, National Technical Information Service, Springfield, VA.

45. U.S. Department of Health and Human Services (1989) *Nutrition*

Monitoring in the United States, An Update Report on Nutrition Monitoring. DHHS Publication no. (PHS)89-1255, U.S. Government Printing Office, Washington, DC.

46. U.S. Department of Health and Human Services (1988) *The Surgeon General's Report on Nutrition and Health.* DHHS (PHS) Publication no. 88-50210, U.S. Government Printing Office, Washington, DC.

47. R.W. Seward, ed. (1988) *NBS Standard Reference Materials Catalog, 1988–1989.* NBS Special Publication 260, U.S. Government Printing Office, Washington, DC.

48. J.T. Tanner, J.S. Smith, G. Angyal, et al. (1987) The search for organic nutrient standards. *Fresenius Z. Anal. Chem.* 326:696–698.

49. W. Wolf and N.J. Miller-Ihli (1987) Characterization of a mixed diet reference material (NBS RM 8431) for inorganic elements and selected organic nutrients. *Fresenius Z. Anal. Chem.* 326:702–704.

50. E.R. Elkins (1985) Quality assurance and check sample program in the food industry. In: *Biological Reference Materials: Availability, Uses, and Need for Validation of Nutrient Measurement* (W.R. Wolf, ed.), pp. 229–237, John Wiley and Sons, New York.

51. J. Exler (1983) *Iron Content of Foods.* Home Economics Research Report no. 45, U.S. Department of Agriculture, Human Nutrition Information Service, Hyattsville, MD.

52. J.M. Holden, A. Schubert, W. Wolf, and G.R. Beecher (1987) A system for evaluating the quality of published nutrient data: selenium, a test case. In: *Food Composition Data: A User's Perspective* (W.M. Rand, C.T. Windham, B. Wyse, and V.R. Young, eds.), pp. 177–193, United Nations University, Tokyo.

53. A. Schubert, J.M. Holden, and W.R. Wolf (1987) Selenium content of a core group of foods based on a critical evaluation of published analytical data. *J. Am. Diet. Assoc.* 87:285–299.

54. D.G. Lurie, J.M. Holden, A. Schubert, W.R. Wolf, and N.J. Miller-Ihli (in press) The copper content of foods based on a critical evaluation of published analytical data. *J. Food Comp. Anal.*

55. G. Block, C.M. Dresser, A.M. Hartman, and M.D. Carroll (1985) Nutrient sources in the American diet: quantitative data from the NHANES II survey. I. Vitamins and minerals. *Am. J. Epidemiol.* 122:13–26.

56. G. Block, C.M. Dresser, A.M. Hartman, and M.D. Carroll (1985) Nutrient sources in the American diet: quantitative data from the NHANES II survey. II. Macronutrients and fats. *Am. J. Epidemiol.* 122:27–40.

57. J.W. Savell, H.R. Cross, D.S. Hale, and L. Beasley (1988) National Beef Market Basket Survey. *Meat Research Brief,* Texas A&M University, College Station, TX.

58. J.M. Holden, E. Lanza, and W.R. Wolf (1986) Nutrient composition of retail ground beef. *J. Agric. Food Chem.* 34:302–308.

59. B.W. Li, J.M. Holden, S.G. Brownlee, and S.G. Korth (1987) A nationwide sampling of fast-food fried chicken: starch and moisture content. *J. Am. Diet. Assoc.* 87:740–743.

60. J.A. Bowers, J.A. Craig, T.J. Tucker, J.M. Holden, and L.P. Posati (1987) Vitamin and proximate composition of fast-food fried chicken. *J. Am. Diet. Assoc.* 87:736–739.

Appendix 1. State of knowledge of the protein and amino acid composition of foods*

	Total protein	Cystine and methionine	Trypto-phan	All other common amino acids†
Baby foods	●	□	□	□
Baked products				
Bread	●	□	□	●
Sweet goods	●	□	□	□
Cookies and crackers	●	□	□	□
Beverages	*	*	*	*
Breakfast cereals	●	○	○	○
Candies	○	○	○	○
Cereal grains				
Whole	●	●	●	●
Flour	●	●	●	●
Pasta	●	●	●	●
Dairy products	●	●	●	●
Eggs and egg products	●	●	●	●
Fast foods	●	○	○	○
Fats and oils	*	*	*	*
Fish and shellfish				
Raw	●	●	●	●
Cooked	□	□	□	□
Frozen dinners	□	○	○	○
Fruits				
Raw	●	○	○	○
Cooked	□	○	○	○
Frozen or canned	●	○	○	○
Infant formula	●	●	●	●
Institutional food	○	○	○	○
Legumes				
Raw	●	●	●	●
Cooked	●	●	●	●
Processed	●	●	●	●
Meat				
Beef	●	●	●	●
Lamb	●	●	●	●
Pork	●	●	●	●
Sausages	●	○	○	○
Veal	●	●	●	●
Mixed dishes				
Commercial	●	○	○	○
Home prepared	□	○	○	○
Nuts and seeds	●	□	□	□
Poultry	●	●	●	●
Restaurant food	○	○	○	○
Snack foods	□	○	○	○
Soups	●	○	○	○
Vegetables				
Raw	●	○	○	○
Cooked	●	○	○	○
Frozen	●	○	○	○
Canned	●	○	○	○

* ○ Few or no data, □ inadequate data, ● substantial data, * not applicable.

† Includes alanine, arginine, aspartate, glutamate, glycine, histidine, isoleucine, leucine, lysine, proline, serine, threonine, tyrosine, and valine.

Appendix 2. State of knowledge of the carbohydrate composition of foods*

	Individual sugars	Starch	Dietary fiber
Baby foods	○	○	□
Baked products			
Bread	○	□	□
Sweet goods	○	□	□
Cookies and crackers	○	□	□
Beverages	□	*	*
Breakfast cereals	●	□	●
Candies	□	○	○
Cereal grains			
Whole	□	□	□
Flour	□	□	□
Pasta	□	□	□
Dairy products	●	*	*
Eggs and egg products	*	*	*
Fast foods	○	○	□
Fats and oils	*	*	*
Fish and shellfish			
Raw	*	*	*
Cooked	*	*	*
Frozen dinners	○	○	□
Fruits			
Raw	●	○	□
Cooked	□	○	□
Frozen or canned	□	○	□
Infant formula	○	○	○
Institutional food	□	□	□
Legumes			
Raw	□	□	□
Cooked	□	□	□
Processed	□	□	□
Meat			
Beef	*	*	*
Lamb	*	*	*
Pork	*	*	*
Sausage	*	*	*
Veal	*	*	*
Mixed dishes			
Commercial	○	○	□
Home prepared	○	○	□
Nuts and seeds	□	□	□
Poultry	*	*	*
Restaurant food	□	□	□
Snack foods	□	○	□
Soups	○	○	○
Vegetables			
Raw	□	●	□
Cooked	□	□	□
Frozen	□	□	□
Canned	□	□	□

* ○ Few or no data, □ inadequate data, ● substantial data, * not applicable.

Appendix 3. State of knowledge of the lipid composition of foods*

	Total fat	Fatty acids	Choles-terol	Other sterols	Trans fatty acids		Total fat	Fatty acids	Choles-terol	Other sterols	Trans fatty acids
Baby foods	●	□	□	○	○	Infant formula	□	□	○	○	○
Baked products						Institutional food	□	□	□	□	○
Bread	●	□	○	○	□	Legumes					
Sweet goods	●	□	○	○	□	Raw	●	□	*	□	*
Cookies and crackers	●	□	○	○	□	Cooked	●	□	*	○	*
Beverages	○	○	*	*	*	Processed	□	□	*	○	*
Breakfast cereals	●	□	○	○	○	Meat					
Candies	□	□	□	□	□	Beef	□	●	●	*	*
Cereal grains						Lamb	□	●	●	*	*
Whole	□	●	*	□	*	Pork	●	●	●	*	*
Flour	□	●	*	□	*	Sausage	●	●	●	*	*
Pasta	□	□	*	○	*	Veal	●	●	□	*	*
Dairy products	●	●	●	*	*	Mixed dishes					
Eggs and egg products	●	●	●	*	*	Commercial	□	□	□	□	○
Fast foods	●	□	□	□	□	Home prepared	□	□	□	○	○
Fats and oils	●	●	●	□	●	Nuts and seeds	●	●	*	□	*
Fish and shellfish						Poultry	●	●	●	*	*
Raw	●	●	●	□	○	Restaurant food	○	○	○	○	○
Cooked	●	●	●	○	○	Snack foods	●	□	□	○	□
Frozen dinners	□	□	□	○	○	Soups	●	□	□	□	○
Fruits						Vegetables					
Raw	●	□	*	□	*	Raw	□	□	*	□	*
Cooked	○	○	*	○	*	Cooked	□	○	*	○	*
Frozen or canned	●	○	*	○	*	Frozen	●	○	*	○	*
						Canned	●	○	*	○	*

* ○ Few or no data, □ inadequate data, ● substantial data, * not applicable.

Appendix 4. State of knowledge of the vitamin composition of foods*

	Vitamin A	Thiamin	Riboflavin	Vitamin B-6	Vitamin C	Niacin	Vitamin B-12	Folacin	Vitamin D	Vitamin E	Pantothenic acid
Baby foods	●	●	●	□	●	●	□	□	*	□	○
Baked products											
Bread	*	●	●	●	*	●	*	□	*	□	□
Sweet goods	□	●	●	□	*	●	□	□	*	□	□
Cookies and crackers	□	●	●	●	*	●	□	□	*	□	□
Beverages	□	□	□	□	□	□	*	□	*	*	□
Breakfast cereals	□	□	□	□	□	□	□	□	□	□	□
Candies	□	□	□	□	□	□	○	□	*	○	□
Cereal grains											
Whole	□	●	●	●	*	●	*	●	*	□	●
Flour	*	●	●	●	*	●	*	●	*	□	●
Pasta	*	●	●	●	*	●	*	●	*	○	●
Dairy products	●	●	●	●	●	●	●	□	●	□	●
Eggs and egg products	□	●	●	●	*	●	●	□	□	□	●
Fast foods	●	●	●	□	□	●	□	○	○	□	○
Fats and oils	□	*	*	*	*	*	*	*	□	□	*
Fish and shellfish											
Raw	□	□	□	□	*	□	□	□	□	□	□
Cooked	○	○	○	○	*	○	○	□	□	□	□
Frozen dinners	□	●	●	○	□	●	○	○	*	○	○
Fruits											
Raw	●	●	●	●	●	●	*	□	*	○	□
Cooked	□	□	□	□	□	□	*	□	*	○	□
Frozen or canned	●	●	*	□	●	●	*	□	*	○	□
Infant formula	○	○	○	○	○	○	○	○	○	○	○
Institutional food	○	○	○	○	○	○	○	○	○	□	○
Legumes											
Raw	□	●	●	□	*	●	*	●	*	●	●
Cooked	○	●	●	□	*	●	*	●	*	●	●
Processed	□	□	□	○	□	□	*	○	*	□	○

Appendix 4. (*Continued*)

	Vitamin A	Thiamin	Riboflavin	Vitamin B-6	Vitamin C	Niacin	Vitamin B-12	Folacin	Vitamin D	Vitamin E	Pantothenic acid
Meat											
Beef	●	●	●	●	*	●	●	□	□	□	□
Lamb	□	●	●	□	*	●	●	□	□	□	□
Pork	□	●	●	●	*	●	●	□	□	□	□
Sausage	□	●	●	●	●	●	●	□	□	○	□
Veal	□	●	●	●	*	●	●	●	□	□	□
Mixed dishes											
Commercial	□	●	●	□	□	●	□	□	○	□	○
Home prepared	□	□	□	□	□	□	□	○	○	○	○
Nuts and seeds	□	□	□	□	□	□	*	*	□	□	□
Poultry	□	●	●	□	*	●	□	□	□	□	□
Restaurant food	○	○	○	○	○	○	○	○	○	○	○
Snack foods	□	□	□	□	○	□	*	□	□	□	□
Soups	●	●	●	□	●	●	□	○	*	○	□
Vegetables											
Raw	●	●	●	□	●	●	*	□	*	□	○
Cooked	□	□	□	□	□	□	*	□	*	□	○
Frozen	●	●	●	○	●	●	*	□	*	○	□
Canned	●	●	●	○	●	●	*	□	*	○	□

* ○ Few or no data, □ inadequate data, ● substantial data, * not applicable.

Appendix 5. State of knowledge of the mineral composition of foods*

	Calcium	Iron	Phosphorus	Sodium	Magnesium	Potassium	Zinc	Copper	Manganese	Boron, chromium, fluorine, iodine, and selenium	Cobalt, nickel, silicon, tin, and vanadium
Baby foods	●	●	●	●	□	●	□	□	○	○	○
Baked products											
Bread	●	●	●	●	●	●	●	●	□	○	○
Sweet goods	●	●	●	●	●	●	●	□	□	○	○
Cookies and crackers	●	●	●	●	●	●	●	●	□	○	○
Beverages	□	□	□	□	□	□	□	□	○	○	○
Breakfast cereals	●	□	●	●	●	●	●	●	□	○	○
Candies	□	□	□	□	□	□	□	□	○	○	○
Cereal grains											
Whole	●	●	●	●	●	●	●	●	●	○	○
Flour	●	●	●	●	●	●	●	●	●	○	○
Pasta	●	●	●	●	●	●	●	●	●	○	○
Dairy products	●	●	●	●	●	●	●	●	□	○	○
Eggs and egg products	●	●	●	□	●	●	●	□	□	○	○
Fast foods	●	●	●	●	●	●	●	●	□	○	○
Fats and oils	○	○	○	○	○	○	□	□	*	*	*
Fish and shellfish											
Raw	●	●	●	●	●	●	●	●	●	○	○
Cooked	○	○	○	○	○	○	○	○	○	○	○
Frozen dinners	□	□	□	□	□	□	□	□	○	○	○
Fruits											
Raw	●	●	●	●	●	●	□	□	□	○	○
Cooked	□	○	○	○	○	□	○	○	○	○	○
Frozen or canned	●	●	●	●	●	●	□	□	○	○	○
Infant formula	□	□	□	□	□	□	○	○	○	○	○
Institutional food	○	○	○	○	○	○	○	○	○	○	○
Legumes											
Raw	●	●	●	●	●	●	●	●	●	○	○
Cooked	●	●	●	●	●	●	●	●	●	○	○
Processed	□	□	□	□	□	□	○	○	○	○	○

Appendix 5. (*Continued*)

	Calcium	Iron	Phosphorus	Sodium	Mag-nesium	Potas-sium	Zinc	Copper	Manga-nese	Boron, chromium, fluorine, iodine, and selenium	Cobalt, nickel, silicon, tin, and vanadium
Meat											
Beef	●	●	□	●	●	●	●	●	●	○	○
Lamb	●	●	●	●	●	●	●	●	□	○	○
Pork	●	●	●	●	●	●	●	●	●	○	○
Sausage	●	●	●	●	●	●	●	●	□	○	○
Veal	●	●	●	●	●	●	●	●	□	○	○
Mixed dishes											
Commercial	●	●	●	●	●	●	□	□	○	○	○
Home prepared	□	□	□	□	□	□	○	○	○	○	○
Nuts and seeds	●	●	●	●	●	●	●	●	●	○	○
Poultry	●	●	●	●	●	●	●	●	●	○	○
Restaurant food	○	○	○	○	○	○	○	○	○	○	○
Snack foods	□	□	○	●	○	○	○	○	○	○	○
Soups	●	●	●	●	●	●	●	●	○	○	○
Vegetables											
Raw	□	□	□	□	□	□	□	□	□	○	○
Cooked	□	□	□	□	□	□	○	○	○	○	○
Frozen	●	●	●	●	●	●	●	●	○	○	○
Canned	●	●	●	●	●	●	●	●	○	○	○

* ○ Few or no data, □ inadequate data, ● substantial data, * not applicable.

Chapter 52

Marvin E. Ament

Enteral and Parenteral Nutrition

Every patient hospitalized for major surgery or with a serious medical problem should be screened for nutritional status. If patients are found to be nutritionally compromised, they should be given nutritional support throughout the hospitalization. If the patient is moderately to severely depleted and surgery can be postponed for 10–14 d, then nutritional support should be given to reverse as soon as possible the nutritional deficit. If surgery cannot be postponed, parenteral support may be started in the immediate postoperative period. In the medical patient this is not a consideration.

Nutritional Assessment

The best way to determine if a patient is malnourished is by taking a complete nutritional history and doing a thorough physical examination.[1,2] The history and physical examination are the two most important tools that an experienced clinician can use in judging whether a patient is malnourished or has a potential for complications that may arise secondary to the patient's nutritional status.[3,4] A limited number of laboratory tests and measurements of body composition are of value in assessing a patient's nutritional status.

History. The most important question to ask the patient is whether there has been a recent change in weight and, if so, how much weight was gained or lost during the past month, 6 mo, or 1 y, and if the weight change was voluntary or involuntary. The patient should be questioned about the presence or absence of diarrhea because diarrhea, if chronic and voluminous, may be associated with major loss of electrolytes and trace metals. Questions should be asked to determine if there are factors that may impair selection, preparation, ingestion, digestion, absorption, and excretion of nutrients in food and liquids. Such factors include chronic diseases affecting nutrient utilization, e.g., diabetes mellitus, pancreatitis,

or malabsorption. The interviewer should determine if the patient has had surgical resection of the digestive tract or accessory organs of digestion, such as the pancreas. A history of any allergies or recognized intolerances to foods should be taken to avoid any problems in the postoperative period when feeding is reintroduced. The use of medications should be determined to learn if they are essential and if they can be given by the parenteral route. Some medications may cause gastritis and lead to abdominal pain, nausea, or anorexia and should be recognized before surgery. The physician should determine if the patient has chewing or swallowing difficulties that would interfere with the patient's ability to eat in the postoperative period. Information on the patient's usual bowel habits before surgery also may be used as a baseline for comparison in the postoperative period.

Physical Examination. Careful observation of the patient's appearance obviously can add to the evaluation of the patient's nutritional adequacy,[4] depending upon the experience and skill of the clinician. The diagnosis of frank malnutrition often is obvious and does not need to be deferred until laboratory tests are available for confirmation. Some patients present with a skeleton-like appearance of severe protein-calorie malnutrition (marasmus) or a bloated edematous appearance of kwashiorkor. In such instances clinicians can easily recognize the presence of the two types of malnutrition; severe wasting of the subcutaneous fat stores and skeletal protein are acutely evident. There are obviously intermediate forms of malnutrition that occur and are related to inadequate or excessive intake of different nutrients and that are not so easily defined. A review of systems also should be carried out to establish the degree of function of each of the body's systems as it relates to nutritional status.

The two most important anthropometric determinations for assessing nutritional status and for predicting energy and protein needs are height and weight. A history of weight loss generally is considered significant. Weight loss and body weight reveal what stores of energy and nutrients the patient has. Unexplained weight loss often is the first sign of an illness or disease. A rapid weight loss of 10% of usual adult weight is considered significant, a decline of 20% is viewed as critical or premorbid, and a weight loss of ≥30% is considered near lethal. Weight loss that occurs rapidly is of much greater immediate importance than weight loss that occurs gradually over time.

Ascites, pleural effusion, subcutaneous emphysema, and generalized edema all may affect body weight and overall appearance. A body weight that changes by >0.5 kg/d indicates fluid shifts, and a 1-L fluid shift can equal ~1 kg. Patients who suffer severe traumatic injury to the abdomen may require major fluid restoration that can result in invalidation of weight information given by the patient. On the other hand, traumatic injuries may contraindicate weighing the patient. Awareness of average weight for the patient's height, age, and sex is useful in placing patients on a scale of depletion, adequate nutrition, or obesity.

Although assigning an ideal body weight for any person is difficult at best, if not impossible to do, it is desirable to view weight in relationship to unusual leanness or notable obesity. Underweight and overweight are defined as weights that are greater or less than 10% below or above average for height and sex of the individual.

Body stores of fat can be assessed by measuring skinfold thickness. Body stores of protein can be assessed by measuring the mid-upper-arm circumference. These measurements are better used for sequential studies than taken as single, isolated determinants. They are not commonly used by most people doing practical clinical nutrition,[5,6] but they are of some value in providing a gross analysis of insufficient, adequate, or excessive provision of nutritional support of chronically ill patients who cannot be weighed.

Measures of Visceral Protein Compartment

Four proteins may be evaluated in assessing visceral protein mass and adequacy of protein provision to support necessary hepatic synthesis of circulating proteins. They are serum albumin, transferrin, thyroxin-binding prealbumin, and retinol-binding protein.[7,8,9] Concentrations of these proteins, as well as total lymphocyte count, have been correlated with morbidity and mortality.

Low serum albumin concentration is a frequently cited indicator of malnutrition. However, serum albumin can be affected by a number of factors: hydration state or blood loss; albumin infusions; renal or hepatic compromise; ongoing protein losses from wounds, burns, drainage tubes, or the gut; trauma, burns, surgery, and stress; steroid administration; and age.[8] Low concentrations of albumin, transferrin, prealbumin, and other proteins may be related to metabolic changes characteristic of stress and illness as well as to the depletion of visceral protein mass or protein synthesizing ability. Very low albumin concentrations are recognized to be associated with pronounced malnutrition, in particular marasmus-kwashiorkor, and are, therefore, of some importance in determining nutritional adequacy. Albumin concentrations may be of greater value in interpreting the significance of malnutrition in nonstressed than in stressed patients. Albumin has a half-life of ~14–19 d, which limits its usefulness in evaluating response to nutritional therapy. The visceral proteins with shorter half-lives are better markers of the adequacy of nutrient provision.

Transferrin, a circulating protein involved in iron transport, has a half-life of 8–10 d and a small extracellular pool as opposed to the large body pool of albumin. Transferrin can be estimated from total iron-binding capacity. However, there are a number of conditions that can affect its concentration. Elevated concentrations may be seen in iron deficiency, in acute hepatitis, in pregnancy, or with the use of oral contraceptives. Low concentrations are found in severe liver disease and protein-losing states. On the other hand, iron-binding capacity may decrease in marked bacterial infection.[9]

Thyroxin-binding prealbumin and retinol-binding protein, because of their short half-lives of 1–2 d for prealbumin and 10 h for retinol-binding protein, are much more sensitive indicators of protein synthesis. Prealbumin appears to be a very useful tool for assessing the body's protein status because it is not affected as greatly as transferrin is by exogenous factors. Within 4 d of repletion of the caloric and protein needs of a patient, the prealbumin can show a significant rise. Similarly, if nutritional support is less than adequate, the prealbumin may remain the same or decrease. By obtaining serial prealbumin concentrations the clinician can determine the success or failure of a particular regime. In our service we typically obtain a baseline prealbumin value and then determine prealbumin concentration again 4 d after full caloric and protein support are begun. Adjustments in nutritional support are made taking into account changes in prealbumin. If prealbumin concentration fails to increase we adjust our caloric support upward by 10%. If prealbumin shows an increase we do not change the level of support.

Immune Response and Nutrition

Malnourished patients are known to have increased rates of infection. When immunity is compromised, there is a reduced response from the complex system designed to aid the body in defending itself against invading organisms. The use of cutaneous hypersensitivity testing has not been used widely because of the technical, disease-specific, and iatrogenic factors that can alter the cutaneous response to test antigens.[10] However, immune response can be changed by nutrient adequacy. Energy and protein are among the factors necessary for the activity of cell-mediated immunity. Estimating the optimal condition for this function is difficult at present and beyond the scope of just doing simple skin antigen-recall tests. Total lymphocyte counts may be used to indicate the body's ability to combat invasive organisms and to assess the adequacy of protein provided and may be of value in screening nonseptic patients. Because the counts are so radically altered in septic patients or in patients treated with adrenocorticosteroids or chemotherapeutic agents, their usefulness can be questioned. We advise following the lymphocyte count in the nonseptic patient as a sign of the adequacy of parenteral support. Lymphocyte count will increase or decrease depending on the nutritional status of the patient: if anabolic, it will increase and if catabolic, it will decrease.

Measurement of Somatic Proteins

Nitrogen balance and creatinine-height index have been used to determine adequacy of protein supply and maintenance of lean body mass. Of the two techniques, nitrogen balance is superior. The estimation of nitrogen balance can be made by deducting the quantity of urea nitrogen lost daily in the urine and the nitrogen intake from enteral and/or parenteral sources. Nitrogen balance can then be calculated as follows: nitrogen balance equals nitrogen intake minus nitrogen excretion (which equals the protein intake divided by 6.25 minus the 24-h urine urea nitrogen plus estimated loss in stool). The accuracy of such studies depends a great deal on the completeness of urine collections as well as on careful measurement of the amount of protein administered. As a practical measure such studies are rarely done in clinical settings because of difficulties encountered in collecting 24-h urine samples. Following the prealbumin determinations serially is easier and gives similar information.

Determination of Nutrient Needs for Nutritional Support

Before specialized nutritional support through either the enteral or parenteral route is started, the clinician must determine the total energy needs of the patient; distribution of energy from carbohydrate, protein, and fat; and requirement for fluids, vitamins, minerals, and trace minerals. These determinations are based on the knowledge of the patient's prior nutritional status, requirements during the critical period, and awareness of the special changes caused by the illness. In the immediate postoperative period patients are in a physiologic state of stress as a result of surgery. The body's reactions to stress are regulated by the central nervous system, are sympathetically mediated, and result in elevations in antidiuretic hormone, adrenocorticotropic hormone, catecholamines, insulin, and growth hormone. The level of stress can be categorized by defining the severity of surgery and by stratifying the metabolic aberrations in response to stress.[11,12] Such an outline for clinical use has been established. It is based on urea nitrogen loss, plasma glucagon and glucose, and various plasma organic acids.

In starvation, liver glycogen reserves rapidly decrease. Liver glycogen is used first as the preferred energy source and usually is depleted within 24 h. Gluconeogenesis is activated simultaneously, and body stores of fat and protein provide energy during early starvation. After several weeks of starvation, adaptation to this state occurs, and the brain utilizes increasing quantities of ketones for energy. The transition from protein catabolism to lipid catabolism follows with resulting sparing of protein breakdown.

In contrast, the stress that follows surgery results in an increase in metabolic rate; hyperglycemia exists although use of glucose for energy is impaired. Endogenous fat deposits are not used in early or mild surgical stress. Protein catabolism occurs and is a major source of energy. Protein from lean body mass and eventually from visceral protein becomes a significant energy substrate. Protein is depleted both indirectly via gluconeogenesis and directly as peripheral muscle stores of the branched-chain amino acids (BCAAs) are converted to energy sources.[13-15] The classic characteristics of the surgical patient in the immediate postoperative period are hypermetabolism, hypercatabolism with negative nitrogen balance, hyperglycemia, and altered energy substrate utilization with increased usage of the BCAAs from muscle tissue.

Energy Requirements

After illness or surgery, energy needs may be increased because the metabolic rate may be driven upward by the response to stress. Energy requirements are assessed in a variety of ways. Indirect or direct calorimetry is used to determine energy consumption.[16] Such sophisticated tools are not usually available; in practice it is most common to estimate rather than measure energy requirements of patients after surgery.

Predicted Energy Requirements

The current practice is to provide calories adequate to meet energy needs during the critical period at a level that facilitates maintenance of present body weight and lean body mass. Repletion to previous usual weight, if weight loss has occurred, is deferred until after the resolution of the critical period. Overfeeding, with its associated complication of fluid overload, increased CO_2 production, and aberrations of hepatic enzyme function should be avoided. In the critically ill patient the goal should be to provide energy sufficient to maintain weight and optimal metabolic function at basal energy expenditure (BEE) or resting energy expenditure (REE). Because the BEE and REE vary by <5%, they may be considered equivalent in a clinical situation.

In addition to BEE or REE, estimation of energy needs must be increased to reflect energy required for physical activity and any anticipated hypermetabolic response to illness or injury. A set of factors is used to predict increased energy needs required in various activities and degrees of injury. These factors are used in the following manner: BEE (or REE) multiplied by activity factor multiplied by injury factor equals TEE (total energy expenditure). The activity factors suggested are 1.2 for the bedridden patient and 1.3 for the ambulatory, hospitalized patient, and the injury factors suggested are 1.2 for surgery (minor surgery), 1.35 for trauma (skeletal or blood trauma), 1.6 for sepsis (severe sepsis), and 2.1 for burns. Patients with thermal (burn) injuries have the longest duration of increased energy needs. Metabolic rate also is elevated by the presence of fever, with ~13% per degree of temperature (°C) elevation from normal. For the typical surgical patient we estimate needs to be in the range of 40–45 $kcal \cdot kg^{-1} \cdot d^{-1}$. This amount includes basal requirement plus energy required to meet the needs of surgical recovery.

Measured Energy Expenditure

Investigators recorded energy expenditure during seven basic activities in intensive care units.[17] The highest oxygen consumption was recorded during chest physical therapy and was 32% above REE values. The lowest values for oxygen consumption occur during sleep and were 9% less than REE.[17] Indirect calorimetry can be used with both the critically and the noncritically ill patient to determine energy expenditure by the measurement of respiratory gas exchange. By utilizing this technique, physicians can determine not only the energy consumed but the proportion of carbohydrate, fat, and protein providing the fuel for energy expenditure. Determination of the latter requires a 24-h urine collection to analyze for nitrogen excretion.[18] Indirect calorimetric measurements combined with urinary nitrogen values can be used to adjust nutritional support, to provide adequate calories, and to determine which nutrients are being used. Overfeeding in terms of total energy consumption and/or percent of carbohydrates has been implicated in precipitating respiratory failure and prolonged weaning in patients on ventilators, because of excessive CO_2 production resulting from carbohydrates.[19] Additionally, excessive calories may result in lipogenesis, which is also associated with an increase in CO_2 production.[20,21] It is prudent to provide a caloric intake of 10–30% above REE to all but the paralyzed or comatose patient. In critically ill patients who have CO_2 retention on or off ventilators, it is wise not to provide excess calories and to use as much fat as is tolerated as an energy source.[21,22]

Carbohydrate Requirements

During stress, carbohydrate metabolism changes dramatically. Hyperglycemia is one of the responses to stress. Primary utilization of glucose as an energy substrate changes to catabolism of peripheral muscle and subsequent increased usage of the BCAAs for energy. During very severe stress, lipolysis occurs with mobilization of triglycerides as potential energy substrates via ketone production. Despite very high levels of circulating glucose, the respiratory quotients of severely injured or traumatized patients suggest the dependence on fat as the major energy substrate.[23] However, during prolonged periods of stress, energy derived from fat also is impaired. Proteolysis, therefore, begins to occur with severe and often catastrophic results.

Under normal circumstances the body can oxidize glucose at the rate of 2–4 $mg \cdot kg^{-1} \cdot min^{-1}$. This rate is independent of elevations of serum concentrations of either glucose or insulin. During severe stress the oxidation rate of glucose is only slightly greater at 3–5 $mg \cdot kg^{-1} \cdot min^{-1}$. Administration at >4–5 $mg \cdot kg^{-1} \cdot min^{-1}$ exceeds the body's ability to oxidize and use it as an energy source. Synthesis of fat from unused glucose may increase CO_2 production, impairing the process of weaning if the patient is ventilator dependent. The provision of energy in excess of need may actually cause a rise in energy expenditure of 1 kcal for every 5 kcal beyond requirements.

D-Glucose is the most common form of carbohydrate used for intravenous infusion. D-Glucose monohydrate in solution has a caloric value of 3.4 kcal/g. Other carbohydrate sources for intravenous use include glycerol, sorbitol, maltose, fructose, and xylitol, but they are rarely used. Glycerol is used to reduce the osmolarity in intravenous fat emulsions. In central venous total parenteral nutrition (TPN), dextrose concentrations from 10% to 35% may be used. In peripheral TPN, dextrose concentration is limited to 10%.

Protein Requirements

Protein requirements in critical illness, after trauma, or in the postoperative period are increased. Additional protein is needed for synthesis of acute-phase proteins within the body, for wound repair, or to replace protein loss in drainage or exudate. Protein metabolism also occurs as energy needs are met by utilization of BCAAs from skeletal muscles. Urinary nitrogen excretion increases in the stressed or postoperative state. Hence, protein needs are elevated because of both increased losses and increased usage for synthesis, repair, and energy. Recommendations for the quantity of protein to be provided in critical illness or postoperatively vary rather widely.[23] Shils[24] suggested a range of 1.2–1.5 $g \cdot kg^{-1} \cdot d^{-1}$, with ongoing monitoring of urinary nitrogen and nitrogen balance for assessment of protein tolerance and adequacy. In healthy individuals 0.4 $g \cdot kg^{-1} \cdot d^{-1}$ is the minimal amount of protein necessary to sustain positive nitrogen balance; 0.8–1.0 $g \cdot kg^{-1} \cdot d^{-1}$ is more than adequate in most patients.[25] Cerra et al.'s[26] estimate of proteins in stress is 2 g/kg for multiple trauma and is 2.5 g/kg for sepsis. In patients with sepsis, they do not recommend any fat as an energy source. In the seriously ill patient it is necessary to match energy and protein requirements as accurately as possible. Alterations that lower the ratio of nonprotein calories (in kcal) to grams nitrogen have been suggested. Some investigators suggested ratios of 80–100 to 1 in severe stress.[27] However, in periods of severe stress multiple organ failure often occurs along with renal compromise thus preventing the administration of the necessary amount of protein. High protein intake can cause an elevated ventilatory response to CO_2. High-concentration BCAA solutions are believed by some to be superior for the management of patients with moderate to severe stress because they spare the breakdown of muscle protein. However, this topic is controversial.

Fat Requirements

Adults who receive parenteral dextrose and amino acids but no fat develop biochemical essential fatty acid deficiency by the end of the second week.[28] By the end of the seventh week, all patients have clinical essential fatty acid deficiency. If parenteral nutrition solutions containing only dextrose and amino acids are administered, patients typically develop fatty liver and cholestasis and have increased CO_2 production. Intravenous lipid emulsions increasingly are being used to replace some of the carbohydrate calories. Lipid emulsions currently available are primarily from vegetable oils, generally soy or a combination of soy and safflower, and for the most part are composed of long-chain triglycerides (LCT). Complications from the use of intravenous LCT infusions include hyperlipidemia, impaired alveolar diffusion capacity, and reduced function of the reticuloendothelial system. Intravenous fat emulsions can be used to provide calories and essential fatty acids or may be used only to prevent essential fatty acid deficiency. If peripheral parenteral nutrition is used, these lipid emulsions should be used to the maximum amount allowable to ensure that the patient's energy requirements are being provided.

Vitamin Requirements

In reviewing needs for nutrients in critical-care situations in patients receiving only parenteral support, common sense dictates that the known needs are considered first and recommendations for unusual requirements second. Although the recommended dietary allowances (RDA) do not take into account elevated requirements that may occur as a result of sepsis, injury, surgery, or trauma, selected products used for enteral support can be evaluated according to the amount required to meet the RDA.[29] This evaluation can serve as a starting point for determining whether further supplementation is indicated. The goal of nutritional support is to provide quantities of vitamins and minerals that at least meet recommendations for maintenance.[30] Beyond maintenance requirements, little of a definitive nature is known regarding the need for increased amounts of either vitamins or minerals during critical illness or injury except for those nutrients involved in wound repair. The major minerals (calcium, phosphorus, and magnesium) typically are provided in standard parenteral preparations as are the electrolytes, sodium, potassium, and chloride. Trace elements include iron, zinc, copper, manganese, chromium, iodine, selenium, and molybdenum. Deficiency states for these trace elements are unlikely to occur during illnesses of brief duration unless conditions exist in which stores are readily depleted, such as in severe malnutrition or chronic malabsorption syndromes.[31,32] Deficiency states can develop in patients receiving long-term parenteral support. Trace elements also can be toxic in excess, and care is required in making certain patients are neither under- nor overdosed.

Fluid Requirements

Many factors affect fluid balance. Equilibrium is achieved between intake and output when all sources of intake (oral, enteral, intravenous fluid and medications, and parenteral infusions) and losses (urine, stool, drainages, fistulas, emesis, respiration, and expiration) are considered. Under normal circumstances an estimate of fluid needs for an adult is expressed as mL/kcal energy intake. Renal compromise, congestive heart failure, and progression of ascites are a few of the conditions that require careful monitoring of fluid status and possible restriction of intake. Changes in spacing of fluid are common in the critically ill patient and make estimates of weight and fluid balances difficult. Fluid management must be responsive to electrolyte balance and hemodynamic variables for optimal functioning of all organs and systems. It is critically important that insensible losses are calculated each day a patient receives parenteral support to determine if the patient is in fluid balance.

Indications for Parenteral Nutrition

The enteral route of administration of nutrients is always preferred. The parenteral route is indicated when the enteral route is inadequate because of short-bowel syndrome, malabsorption syndromes, long-bone fractures, or major burns. Enteral nutrition should be avoided in cases of enterocutaneous fistulas (unless the fistula is distal in the small bowel), severe pancreatitis, acute inflammatory bowel disease with severe diarrhea, gastrointestinal obstruction, paralytic ileus, short-bowel syndrome, and severe malabsorption. Enteral nutrition may be hazardous in patients with inadequate gag reflex and in partial upper-bowel obstruction if an enteric tube cannot be passed beyond the pylorus, because the risk of reflux and aspiration in this situation is high. Conditions that commonly require parenteral nutrition include gastrointestinal dysmotility syndromes; Crohn's disease, chronic pancreatitis with ileus, and hemorrhagic pancreatitis; complications of gastrointestinal surgery, such as fistulas, paralytic ileus, abdominal abscess, and peritonitis in gastric outlet obstruction; oncologic and immunologic therapy, such as bone marrow transplantation; critical illness, such as sepsis, respiratory failure, trauma, acute renal failure, liver failure, and pulmonary disease requiring ventilation; and complications of thoracic or pleurovascular surgeries affecting gastrointestinal function. In urologic-surgery patients, parenteral nutrition is used commonly for patients who develop postoperative fistulas, pro-

longed ileus, and chronic diarrhea secondary to bowel resection and reanastomosis and radiation therapy.

Establishing Therapeutic Objectives

The objective of nutritional support is to maintain or replete lean body mass, thereby avoiding consequences of malnutrition. It is important in promoting wound healing, reducing susceptibility to infection, and reducing duration of hospitalization and convalescence from illness. There are times when the treatment of the critical condition takes priority over nutritional support. In such cases it is probably wisest to withhold nutritional support until the acute episode is corrected, because provision of complicated therapy when the utilization of exogenous nutrients is hindered by the hormonal milieu (as in acute injury) may do more harm than benefit. The first priority in acute situations is to moderate the injury component of the illness; second, to temper the endocrinologic response to injury so that the patient's tolerance and utilization of exogenous nutrients is improved; and third, to provide substrate required for energy. In some patients, it may be appropriate to use suboptimal nutrition support. There may be patients whose tolerance or utilization of nutrients is unpredictable but is likely to be impaired, and very low dosages or restricted quantities of certain nutrients may be prescribed.

Monitoring the Patient on Total Parenteral Nutrition

Nutritional requirements for parenteral nutrition are the net sum of the normal requirements in health as defined by the minimal daily requirements and the Recommended Dietary Allowance for all nutrients, the requirements for correction of preexisting deficits occurring as a result of disease or lack of adequate intake, and the requirements for replacement of continuous extraneous losses.

Patients receiving total parenteral nutrition should be weighed daily when possible and all their intakes and outputs should be recorded. At the end of each day it should be determined if the patients are receiving the proper amount of fluid and the calories ordered. Laboratory tests to establish the adequacy of the support should be done. Serum electrolytes, calcium, magnesium, and phosphorus should be determined on the first day to establish the adequacy of mineral support. Once adequacy is established, the patients should be rechecked daily for 2 additional days. If the electrolytes are stable on the third day, the patients then may be checked every other day for 1 wk. After the second week on parenteral support, the patients need to be checked only weekly. Complete blood counts may be done once or twice per week.

Complications from parenteral nutrition are not common. They fall into three categories: mechanical, relating to placement of the central venous catheter; septic, related to contamination of the catheter; and metabolic, relating to the solutions administered. The complication rates are inversely proportional to the care and attention provided in maintaining catheters and peripheral lines and time spent ensuring nutritional requirements are being provided.

References

1. R.A. Pettigrew, P.M. Charlesworth, R.W. Farmilo, et al. (1984) Assessment of nutritional depletion and immune competence: a comparison of clinical examination and objective measurements. *JPEN* 8:21–24.

2. A.S. Detsky, J.P. Bauer, R.A. Mendelson, et al. (1984) Evaluating the accuracy of nutritional assessment techniques applied to hospitalized patients: methodology and comparisons. *JPEN* 8:153–159.

3. G.P. Buzby and J.L. Mullen (1984) Enteral and tube feeding. In: *Nutritional Assessment* (J.L. Rombeau and M.D. Caldwell, eds.), pp. 127–147, W.B. Saunders Company, Philadelphia.

4. J.P. Baker, A.S. Detsky, D.E. Wesson, et al. (1982) Nutritional assessment: a comparison of clinical judgment and objective measurement. *N. Engl. J. Med.* 306:969–972.

5. J.P. Grant (1986) Nutritional assessment in clinical practice. *Nutr. Clin. Pract.* 1:3.

6. A.R. Frisancho (1974) Triceps skin fold and upper arm muscle size norms for assessment of nutritional status. *Am. J. Clin. Nutr.* 27:1052–1058.

7. M.F. Burritt and C.F. Anderson (1984) Laboratory assessment of nutritional status. *Hum. Pathol.* 15:130–133.

8. A.R. Forse and H.M. Shizgal (1980) Serum albumin and nutritional status. *JPEN* 4:450–454.

9. A.M. Roza, D. Tuitt, and H.M. Shizgal (1984) Transferrin—a poor measure of nutritional status. *JPEN* 8:523–528.

10. P. Twomey, D. Ziegler, and J. Rombeau (1982) Utility of skin testing in nutritional assessment: a critical review. *JPEN* 6:50–58.

11. J.E. Fischer (1980) Nutritional support in the seriously ill patient. *Curr. Probl. Surg.* 17:465–532.

12. J. Hassett, F. Cerra, J. Siegel, et al. (1982) Multiple system organ failure: mechanism and therapy. *Surg. Annu.* 14:25–72.

13. F.B. Cerra, D. Upson, R. Angelico, et al. (1982) Branched chains support postoperative protein synthesis. *Surgery* 92:192–199.

14. G.L. Hill and J. Church (1984) Energy and protein requirements of general surgical patients requiring intravenous nutrition. *Br. J. Surg.* 71:1–8.

15. J.M. Kinney and D.H. Elwyn (1983) Protein metabolism and injury. *Annu. Rev. Nutr.* 3:433–466.

16. C. Weissman, M. Kemper, J. Askanazi, et al. (1986) Resting metabolic rate of the critically ill patient: measured versus predicted. *J. Anesthesiol.* 64:673–680.

17. C. Weissman, M. Kemper, M.C. Damask, et al. (1984) Effect of routine intensive care interactions on metabolic rate. *Chest* 86: 815–819.

18. J.B. Weir (1949) New methods for calculating metabolic rate with special reference to protein metabolism. *J. Physiol.* 109:1–9.

19. S. Goldstein, J. Askanazi, B. Thomashow, et al. (1985) Metabolic demand, ventilation and muscle function during repletion of malnourished COPD and surgical patients. *Anesthesiology* 63:A276.

20. J. Askanazi, C. Weissman, P.A. LaSala, et al. (1984) Effect of protein intake on ventilatory drive. *Anesthesiology* 60:106–110.

21. D.S. Dark, S.K. Pingleton, and G.R. Kerby. (1985) Hypercapnea during weaning: a complication of nutritional support. *Chest* 88: 141–143.

22. J.P. Baker, A.S. Detsky, S. Steward, et al. (1984) Randomized trial of total parenteral nutrition in critically ill patients: metabolic effects of varying glucose-lipid ratios as the energy source. *Gastroenterology* 87:53–59.

23. D.H. Elwyn (1980) Nutritional requirements of adult surgical patients. *Crit. Care Med.* 8:9–20.

24. M.E. Shils (1988) Enteral (tube) and parenteral nutrition support. In: *Modern Nutrition in Health and Disease* (M.E. Shils and V.R. Young, eds.), pp. 1023–1066, Lea and Febiger, Philadelphia.

25. G.H. Anderson, D.G. Patel, and K.N. Jeejeebhoy (1974) Design and evaluation of nitrogen balance and blood aminograms of an amino acid mixture for total parenteral nutrition of adults with gastrointestinal disease. *J. Clin. Invest.* 53:904–912.

26. F.B. Cerra, N.K. Cheung, J.E. Fischer, et al. (1985) Disease-specific amino acid infusion (F080) in hepatic encephalopathy: a prospective, randomized, double-blind trial. *JPEN* 9:288–295.

27. M.F. Brennan, F.C. Cerra, J.M. Daly, et al. (1986) Report of a research workshop: branched-chain amino acids in stress and injury. *JPEN* 10:446–452.

28. J.D. Wene, W.E. Connor, and L. DenBesten (1975) The development of essential fatty acid deficiency in healthy men fed fat-free diets intravenously and orally. *J. Clin. Invest.* 56:127–134.

29. National Research Council (1989) *Recommended Dietary Allowances,* 10th ed, National Academy Press, Washington, DC.

30. American Medical Association (1979) Multivitamin preparations for parenteral use: a statement by the Nutrition Advisory Group. *JPEN* 3:258–262.

31. American Medical Association (1979) Guidelines for essential trace element preparations for parenteral use. *JAMA* 251:241–244.

32. D.R. Antonenko (1983) Vitamins and minerals. In: *Nutrition and Metabolism in the Surgical Patient* (J.R. Kirkpatrick, ed.), pp. 163–197, Futura, Mt. Kisco, NY.

Nutrient-drug Interactions

The distinction between chemicals ingested as micronutrients and as drugs often is not clearly drawn. Recent examples of toxic syndromes resulting from the overly enthusiastic use of vitamins[1] and amino acids[2] as "health supplements" remind us that the traditional emphasis on the importance of balance in nutrition continues to be valid. The purpose of this brief review is to outline the types of interactions that can take place between drugs and nutrients, with emphasis on those of clinical relevance. Occasionally, comments also will be made about animal studies and theoretical considerations. Because of both space limitations and the availability of several books and symposia on this general area,[3,4] references for the most part will be to other reviews of specific topics rather than to the primary-source articles. It is hoped that this approach will be most beneficial to students and clinicians alike.

There are a number of important areas that cannot be reviewed in an article of this size and have been dealt with elsewhere. These include the effects on nutritional status of drugs that are antimetabolites and that are used for cancer chemotherapy and of antibiotics that are relatively selective vitamin antagonists for microorganisms.[5] Limited reference will be made to the topics of interactions among drugs, nutrition, and alcohol[6,7] and electrolyte imbalances induced by diuretics and laxatives.[5] Appetite-stimulant and appetite-suppressive effects of drugs, an important area of great pharmacological interest in the management of eating disorders,[5,8] will not be covered here.

Nutrients have been shown to interact with virtually every aspect of drug availability and action. Such effects can range from simple physical alteration of drug absorption to specific influences on the metabolic site of drug effect. Many of the nutrient-drug interactions that were described in the past have proven to have little clinical relevance under normal conditions. What should be kept in mind, however,

is that careful observation and history taking must be combined with a high index of suspicion if such interactions are to be detected outside the setting of a truly attention-getting clinical disaster. A working familiarity with the general details of drug availability, action, and disposal is necessary to appreciate the full range of possible interactions with nutrients that can take place in an individual patient.[9] That individuals may have dietary peculiarities is commonly acknowledged by every medical student who asks hypertensive patients whether they ingest large quantities of licorice,[10] which can increase blood pressure because it contains a component with mineralocorticoid activity in humans. It is hoped that this review will help to acquaint the reader with additional examples of how dietary components can alter the response to and need for drug therapy as well as the general pharmacological principles involved.

Physical Nutrient-drug Interactions

Chemicals that enter the gastrointestinal tract together may combine in a way that markedly alters their absorption; some examples are listed in Table 1. Although emphasis has been on the reduced bioavailability of the more important or limited member of a pair of complexing molecules, there may be additional effects. The complexing of tetracyclines with di- and trivalent cations was the topic of a number of publications,[11] but this class of antibiotics is rarely prescribed for serious illnesses and usually is not used in high doses for a duration sufficient for there to be a clinical effect on iron or calcium balance. The excessive use of antacids, however, was found occasionally to cause clinically significant phosphate depletion by forming insoluble aluminum or magnesium phosphates.[12] A similar loss of dietary heavy metals occurs with the chronic ingestion of large quantities of plant-derived phytates, which are poly-

Table 1. Physical interactions between nutrients and drugs

Agents	Effects
Tetracyclines, phytates	Bind heavy metals into nonabsorbed complexes
Neomycin, cholestyramine	Bind bile acids and lower lipid-soluble vitamins
Mineral oil	Dissolves and removes lipophilic drugs and vitamins
Antacids (aluminum or magnesium)	Form insoluble phosphates
Body fat	Slows absorption of injected drugs and may increase volume of distribution of lipophilic drugs

hydroxy inositol derivatives that bind metals with a high affinity. Additional interactions of this type have been described.[13]

The interaction of neomycin with bile salts to form nonabsorbable precipitates is of use in hypercholesterolemia and is enjoying a renewed popularity in combination with the newly available cholesterol-synthesis inhibitors, such as mevinolin.[14] By causing a selective malabsorption of bile salts, neomycin enhances sterol excretion and helps reduce the body's cholesterol pool, but the absorption of other lipophilic compounds, including vitamins and drugs, is also reduced. Similar effects were noted with cholestyramine and other bile acid–binding resins, which can have the additional effect of binding other acidic drugs. It was shown years ago that the ingestion of mineral oil, frequently used by elderly people to aid bowel function, also will impair the absorption of lipid-soluble vitamins.[15] A further example of this type of interaction may evolve from the current emphasis on increasing the intake of bran and other vegetable polymers. Although several reported interactions between drugs and bran were shown to be of little clinical relevance,[16,17] there are suggestions that brans from different plant sources may have different properties. Such a possibility should be kept in mind by clinicians when faced with the apparent lack of absorption of a drug by a patient. An additional setting in which nutrient-drug incompatibility is often overlooked is in the tube-fed formula diets administered to many elderly, debilitated patients.[18]

Although a lowering of drug absorption by food is frequently considered, there are many examples where lipophilic drugs are more completely absorbed when ingested with a fatty meal.[19] This effect may be due to increased uptake in lipid micelles or to better solubilization in the presence of the increased concentration of bile salts and lecithins in the duodenum in the presence of fat. Delayed gastric emptying by fatty food can lead to increased dispersion of granular drug preparations as well as greater absorption of drugs from the stomach. In addition, drugs that are slowly removed from the duodenum by saturable transport processes may be more completely absorbed there if their exit from the stomach is more gradual.[19]

Metabolic Nutrient-drug Interactions

The effects of both specific nutrients and general nutritional status on drug bioavailability (summarized in Table 2) begin in the gastrointestinal tract itself. A number of examples were described in which the intestinal metabolism or absorption of drugs that are amino acid derivatives (e.g., methyl-dopa and L-dopa) was influenced by dietary protein.[18] It is also becoming more widely appreciated that intestinal bacteria metabolize a variety of drugs in addition to the well-known examples of L-dopa and sulfasalazine. The latter drug is delivered to its site of action, the colon, in prodrug form and is then cleaved by bacteria to an active drug (5-aminosalicylic acid), which is useful in treating inflammatory bowel disease.[20] The overall importance of drug metabolism by intestinal bacteria has not received a great deal of emphasis, because it has been difficult to demonstrate significant, sustained changes in the human intestinal flora via realistically achievable dietary manipulations. The most common event revealing this process clinically is the administration of an antibiotic to a patient on a stable dose of another drug, which then becomes a toxic or ineffective dose.[21]

Despite the general resilience of intestinal flora to dietary changes, it is possible that drastic or unusual dietary maneuvers, such as going on a formula-diet regimen or consuming large doses of fish oils high in unsaturated fatty acids, could alter the intestinal flora in a metabolically important way. In addition, the absorption and bacterial metabolism of a number of drugs has been found to depend upon the intes-

Table 2. Dietary factors affecting drug disposition and metabolism

- Dietary protein intake has effects on plasma albumin concentrations, drug-metabolizing enzymes in gut and liver, and gastrointestinal bacteria.
- Meal composition can alter intestinal activity and blood flow to accelerate or retard drug absorption or metabolism.
- Nutritional status also affects renal and biliary drug clearance rates and can cause specific changes in drug action or toxicity.

tinal transit time, which can be influenced by spicy or irritating foods, dietary fiber, and other food components.[18] Although one would not expect a marked change to take place over a prolonged period in fairly healthy patients, a large number of patients with acquired immunodeficiency syndrome (AIDS) have markedly reduced transit times and generally poor bioavailability of orally administered drugs.[22] Intermittent reductions in drug absorption may cause erratic plasma concentrations of drugs that are rapidly metabolized and that need to be kept at a fairly constant therapeutic concentration (e.g., drugs for treating cardiac arrythmias). Finally, the gastrointestinal tract itself has been shown to initiate the first-pass metabolism of a number of drugs.[23] Such drugs are subjected to a large degree of metabolic removal when they pass through the liver. These processes may be influenced not only by dietary protein, but also by the dietary fats that eventually determine the types of fatty acids making up the membrane phospholipid environment of the drug-metabolizing enzymes.

Dietary protein also has been shown to influence splanchnic blood flow, which can be important for drugs that have a first-pass effect. The amount of blood flow and the rapidity of drug absorption can determine what portion of the drug escapes first-pass metabolism via intrahepatic shunting or saturation of removal pathways.[24] Dietary protein also has important effects on the amounts and activities of drug-metabolizing enzymes in both the intestine and the liver.[25,26] Interestingly, previous studies showed little effect of dietary carbohydrate or fat on the removal of drugs by these enzymes.[27] However, the types of fat studied did not include fish oils, which currently are receiving a great deal of attention because of their potential benefits in cardiovascular disease.[28,29] Because fish oils induce peroxisome proliferation in rodents and alter the oxidation of fatty acids in addition to prolonging the bleeding time in humans,[28] it will be surprising if they are not eventually found to have clinically important interactions with a number of drugs. None has yet been reported, probably because clinical studies with these lipids are still at an early stage.

Other food components that are substrates of the drug-metabolizing enzymes can also influence enzyme activity by inducing the formation of increased amounts of enzyme. This effect has been noted for indoles present in cabbage and brussels sprouts as well as for charcoal-broiled meats[18] but is probably also true for other vegetables and smoked or preserved meats containing large amounts of chemicals that are metabolized by the cytochrome P-450 enzymes.

The effects of nutrients on drug-metabolizing en-zymes mentioned so far have not been specific for particular drugs. However, different members of cytochrome P-450 enzymes (the major family of enzymes responsible for drug removal from the body) act on different types of drugs and also have specific interactions with various nutrients.[26,30] As a result, particular drug-nutrient interactions were noted in which the drug stimulated or blocked the production of hormones or active forms of vitamins in the body. Examples include the reduction in availability of vitamins D and K by diphenylhydantoin and a number of other drugs, which, in turn, resulted in lowering of calcium absorption or in a bleeding diathesis.[5,18]

Interactions in Nutrient-drug Disposition

Although the specific action of certain drugs to increase or decrease appetite was mentioned above, the nonspecific adverse effects of many drug therapies on food ingestion by patients often are not appreciated. In hospitals the dietary or nursing staff can follow this situation carefully, but it is difficult to do so for outpatients. Effects can vary from inducing a bad taste in the mouth that makes all food unpalatable, to nausea, a feeling of early satiety, or other gastrointestinal discomfort. In most patients the result is merely noncompliance with a drug regimen; in others (particularly debilitated or elderly patients) there may be significant adverse effects on nutritional status.

Drug disposition in patients markedly above or below average in body fat can differ in important ways. The most obvious example would be in the administration of drugs by injection. In a cachectic patient, a subcutaneously administered drug, such as heparin, may be absorbed more rapidly and completely than normal. On the other hand, if drugs intended for intramuscular injection are injected into fat instead, they will be absorbed in a very delayed manner, if at all. Most intravenously administered drugs are given on a body-weight basis. It is important that lean body weight be used to determine the appropriate dose for drugs that do not distribute into adipose tissue to avoid overdosage. On the other hand, large amounts of very lipid-soluble drugs or toxins may be partitioned into the body fat of obese patients, thus requiring a prolonged period for removal.

The degree to which different drugs are protein bound in the plasma varies from low to nearly complete. The degree of binding is important for the metabolic removal of drugs because it is the unbound fraction that is accessible to further metabolism.[9] Such binding takes place to a great extent to albumin, although a number of lipophilic drugs and vitamins are transported by lipoproteins or other special carrier proteins. A relative deficiency of protein may result in a lowering of plasma albumin,[5] which often occurs in the catabolic postoperative state as well as with dietary inadequacy or severe malabsorption. This problem is being encountered with increasing frequency in patients with AIDS.[22] Lower plasma albumin concentrations influence the disposition of many drugs, but the degree and clinical importance of this effect vary considerably. For example, in children with protein-calorie malnutrition, penicillins are excreted more slowly because of lower renal elimination,[31] whereas other drugs are metabolized more slowly by the liver.[32] There have been suggestions that the postprandial increase in plasma free fatty acids can transiently displace drugs bound to albumin, but clinically important examples of such displacement have not been widely discussed.[25] The process of drugs displacing other drugs or endogenous metabolites from albumin, on the other hand, is frequently an important interaction and could result in the more rapid elimination of particular vitamins or other nutrients from the plasma.

Specific Nutrient-drug Interactions

A number of unexpected interactions between food items and drugs have been described. Examples of these interactions are given in Table 3. One of the best known of these involves the precipitation of a hypertensive-hyperadrenergic crisis by the ingestion of foods containing tyramine (including matured cheeses and red wine) or other sympathomimetic amines during therapy with drugs that are monoamine oxidase inhibitors (MAOI).[33] Use of the most potent MAOI drugs is now limited largely to psychiatry. The dietary precautions regarding MAOIs were reviewed.[8,33] Occasional patients, however, experience such reactions with drugs such as isoniazid, which usually have weak MAOI activity.[34]

Lithium is now commonly used for manic-depressive disorders, and it has been appreciated for some time that sodium intake strongly influences lithium excretion. Sodium restriction of patients taking lithium causes lithium accumulation and toxicity, whereas increased sodium intake leads to enhanced urinary lithium loss.[9] It was reported recently that the renal effects of caffeine also increase lithium excretion, and a cessation of coffee drinking in patients on lithium therapy resulted in decreased lithium excretion and increased toxicity, with an apparently paradoxical increase in tremulousness.[35]

Although the many interactions of alcohol, drugs, and nutrients are reviewed elsewhere,[6-8] an interaction pertinent to the present discussion is the flushing reaction that occurs in response to alcohol ingestion in persons taking disulfiram (Antabuse®)

Table 3. Specific nutrient-drug interactions

Action	Drugs	Nutrient item
Inhibited nutrient metabolism	Monoamine oxidase inhibitors	Sympathomimetic amines
	Disulfiram	Ethanol
Increased drug loss	Lithium	Sodium, caffeine
Reversed drug effect	Diuretics	Sodium
Increased nutrient loss	n−3 fatty acids	Vitamin E
	Diphenylhydantoin	Vitamin D
Drug-nutrient antagonism	Coumadin drugs	Vitamin K

or related drugs.[36] These drugs are aldehyde dehydrogenase inhibitors, and the accumulation of acetaldehyde in the body when ethanol is consumed causes flushing, nausea, and various degrees of chest and abdominal discomfort. The syndrome is sufficiently unpleasant so that disulfiram is used in the aversion treatment of alcoholics, but similar symptoms have been reported with a number of other drugs,[9] particularly metronidazole and chlorpropamide. Metronidazole often is prescribed for patients with trichomonal vaginitis or prostatitis and their sex partners, and the asymptomatic partner may be unaware of the frightening consequences of ingesting alcohol while taking the drug.

Humans receive a substantial supply of vitamin K via synthesis by their intestinal flora. Patients with poor dietary intakes and who are on prolonged antibiotic therapy may develop vitamin K deficiency and a bleeding diathesis.[37] Changes in these two natural sources have precipitated both over- and undertreatment of patients on vitamin K–antagonist anticoagulants (e.g., Warfarin®). The absorption, plasma binding, and metabolism of Warfarin® can be influenced by many other drugs to produce clinically serious effects, and these drug-drug interactions are widely appreciated.[9] Because patients often are on such anticoagulants for years, it is important that drastic changes in vitamin K availability be avoided. Occasionally, patients may not be aware that they are taking vitamin K supplements (as in enteric formula feedings) that can antagonize the effects of the anticoagulant drug.[18]

Marine oils containing n−3 fatty acids are the subject of a great deal of current medical research, especially in regard to their possible antiatherosclerotic and antithrombotic effects.[28] The interaction of these nutrients (which are often studied in pharmacologic doses) with drugs is as yet unknown, but there is some concern about the oxidant stress exerted in vivo by such supplements. The classical way to induce vitamin E deficiency in animals, for instance, is to feed high amounts of such polyunsaturated fatty acids without antioxidants, including tocopherols.[38] In fact, asymptomatic yellow-fat disease (caused by lipid peroxidation in vivo) was noted in animals receiving a diet with a high fish content while receiving vitamin E supplements.[39] Vitamin E deficiency has not been noted in studies in which unrefined fish oils were fed to humans but recently was seen in studies where highly purified n−3 polyunsaturated fatty acids were given.[40] Although the occurrence of vitamin E deficiency is viewed as an adverse effect in some settings, some workers are trying to take advantage of the vitamin E depletion in circulating erythrocytes resulting from dosing with fish oils to cure malaria by oxidative destruction of the parasites in the blood. This effect was first noted in mice 30 years ago[41] and was largely forgotten until recently.[42]

Final examples of nutrient-drug interactions involve the basic roles of sodium handling by the body in the development of hypertension and congestive heart failure and of potassium in regulating the electrical activity of cells. It is by now widely appreciated from both population studies and clinical trials that excessive sodium ingestion leads to blood pressure elevation in susceptible individuals.[43] Diuretics are widely used to enhance sodium excretion in patients with hypertension as well as in those with cardiac dysfunction associated with renal underperfusion and sodium retention (heart failure, with resultant edema formation). Patients in whom heart failure has been well compensated and others with histories of good blood pressure control often are seen in emergency rooms during certain holiday seasons because of acute clinical deterioration from a high intake of heavily salted preserved meat products (in the southern United States, country ham). Similarly, the basis for taking digitalis preparations to improve cardiac contractility involves inhibition of the Na^+-K^+ pump.[9] Patients taking diuretics or having prolonged episodes of diarrhea without adequate dietary replacement can have potassium losses sufficient to cause digitalis toxicity.[9] If dietary potassium via intake of fruits and vegetables is inadequate, potassium supplements frequently are prescribed.

Summary

Optimal pharmacologic therapy depends upon the predictable delivery and action of a prescribed drug. To assure this, one must take into account several aspects of the patient's general nutritional status as well as be aware of nutrient-drug interactions. These interactions range from physical nutrient-drug complexing causing altered drug and nutrient absorption to effects on the disposition, metabolism, and site of action of drugs. Drugs affect nutritional status, alter nutrient requirements, and antagonize the actions of vitamins. Specific nutrient-drug interactions can be clinically relevant and involve both nutrient-induced drug toxicity or ineffectiveness and drug-induced nutrient depletion.

Diet and other nonpharmacological therapies for a number of common diseases, such as hypertension and cardiovascular disease, have been emphasized recently. As patients with multiple medical problems increasingly use these types of therapeutic interventions, clinicians will need to become more aware of nutrient-drug interactions.

This work was supported in part by a grant from the National Institutes of Health (HL-35380). Dr. Knapp is an Established Investigator of the American Heart Association.

References

1. H. Schaumberg, J. Kaplan, A. Windebank, et al. (1983) Sensory neuropathy from pyridoxine abuse. A new megavitamin syndrome. *N. Engl. J. Med.* 309:445–448.
2. Anonymous (1990) The clinical spectrum of the eosinophilia-myalgia-syndrome (EMS) in California. *Morbid. Mortal. Weekly Rep.* 39:89–91.
3. J.N. Hathcock and J. Coon, eds. (1978) *Nutrition and Drug Interrelations.* Academic Press, New York.
4. J.N. Hathcock, ed. (1982) *Nutritional Toxicology.* Academic Press, New York.
5. D.A. Roe (1984) Nutrient and drug interactions. *Nutr. Rev.* 42:141–154.
6. H.K. Seitz (1985) Alcohol effects on drug-nutrient interactions. *Drug. Nutr. Interact.* 4:143–163.
7. F.A. Sexias (1975) Alcohol and its drug interactions. *Ann. Intern. Med.* 83:86–92.
8. G.E. Gray (1989) Nutritional aspects of psychiatric disorders. *J. Am. Diet. Assoc.* 89:1492–1498.
9. A.G. Gilman, L.S. Goodman, T.W. Rall, and F. Murad, eds. (1985) *The Pharmacological Basis of Theraputics.* 7th ed. Macmillan, New York.
10. M.T. Epstein, E.A. Espiner, R.A. Donald, et al. (1977) Effects of eating licorice on the renin-angiotensin-aldosterone axis in normal subjects. *Br. Med. J.* 1:488–490.
11. P.J. Neuvonen (1976) Interactions with the absorption of tetracyclines. *Drugs* 11:45–54.
12. L.R. Baker, P. Ackrill, W.R. Cattell, et al. (1974) Iatrogenic osteomalacia and myopathy due to phosphate depletion. *Br. Med. J.* 3:150–152.
13. P.G. Welling (1977) Influence of food and diet on gastrointestinal drug absorption: a review. *J. Pharmacokinet. Biopharm.* 5:291–334.
14. R.D. Illingworth (1987) Lipid-lowering drugs: an overview of indications and optimum therapeutic use. *Drugs* 33:259–279.
15. J.W. Morgan (1941) The harmful effects of mineral oil (liquid petrolatum) purgatives. *JAMA* 117:1135–1136.
16. M.N. Woods and J.A. Ingelfinger (1979) Lack of effect of bran on digoxin absorption. *Clin. Pharmacol. Ther.* 26:21–23.
17. H. Kasper, W. Zilly, H. Fassl, et al. (1979) The effect of dietary fiber on postprandial serum digoxin concentrations in man. *Am. J. Clin. Nutr.* 32:2436–2438.
18. D.A. Roe (1984) Therapeutic significance of drug-nutrient interactions in the elderly. *Pharmacol. Rev.* 36:109S–122S.
19. A. Melander (1978) Influence of food on the bioavailability of drugs. *Clin. Pharmacokinet.* 3:337–351.

20. M.A. Peppercorn and P. Goldman (1972) The role of intestinal bacteria in the metabolism of salicylazosulfapyridine. *J. Pharmacol. Exp. Ther.* 181:555–562.

21. K. Hartiala (1973) Metabolism of hormones, drugs and other substances by the gut. *Physiol. Rev.* 53:496–534.

22. J.S. Gillin, M. Shike, N. Alcock, et al. (1985) Malabsorption and mucosal abnormalities of the small intestine in the acquired immunodeficiency syndrome. *Ann. Intern. Med.* 102:619–622.

23. C.F. George (1981) Drug metabolism by the gastrointestinal mucosa. *Clin. Pharmacokinet.* 6:259–274.

24. P.A. Routledge and D.G. Shand (1979) Presystemic drug elimination. *Annu. Rev. Pharmacol. Toxicol.* 19:447–468.

25. J.N. Hathcock (1985) Metabolic mechanisms of drug-nutrient interactions. *Fed. Proc.* 44:124–129.

26. F.P. Guengerich (1984) Effects of nutritive factors on metabolic processes involving bioactivation and detoxification of chemicals. *Annu. Rev. Nutr.* 4:207–231.

27. K.E. Anderson, A.H. Conney, and A. Kappas (1979) Nutrition and oxidative metabolism in man: relative influence of dietary lipids, carbohydrate and protein. *Clin. Pharmacol. Ther.* 26:493–501.

28. C. von Schacky (1987) Prophylaxis of arteriosclerosis with marine omega-3 fatty acids: a comprehensive strategy. *Ann. Intern. Med.* 107:215–221.

29. H.R. Knapp (1989) Omega-3 fatty acids, endogenous prostaglandins and blood pressure regulation in humans. *Nutr. Rev.* 47:301–313.

30. T.C. Campbell and J.R. Hayes (1974) Role of nutrition in the drug metabolizing enzyme system. *Pharmacol. Rev.* 26:171–197.

31. N. Buchanan, R. Robinson, H.J. Koornhof, and C. Eyeberg (1979) Penicillin pharmacokinetics in kwashiorkor. *Am. J. Clin. Nutr.* 32:2233–2236.

32. R.K. Narang, S. Mehta, and V.S. Mathur (1977) Pharmacokinetic study of antipyrine in malnourished children. *Am. J. Clin. Nutr.* 30:1979–1982.

33. B.J. McCabe (1986) Dietary tyramine and other pressor amines in MAOI regimens: a review. *J. Am. Diet. Assoc.* 86:1059–1065.

34. C.K. Smith and D.T. Durack (1978) Isoniazid and reaction to cheese. *Ann. Intern. Med.* 88:520–521.

35. J.W. Jefferson (1988) Lithium tremor and caffeine intake: two cases of drinking less and shaking more. *J. Clin. Psychiatry* 49:72–76.

36. J. Hald and E. Jacobsen (1948) A drug sensitizing the organism to ethyl alcohol. Lancet 2:1001–1004.

37. J.E. Ansell, R. Kuman, and D. Deykin (1977) The spectrum of vitamin K deficiency. *JAMA* 238:40–42.

38. H. Dam (1962) Interrelations between vitamin E and polyunsaturated fatty acids in animals. In: *Vitamins and Hormones,* vol. 20 (R.S. Harris and I.G. Wool, eds.), pp. 527–540, Academic Press, Orlando, FL.

39. A. Ruiter, A.W. Jongbloed, C.M. van Gent, L.H. Danse, and S.H. Metz (1978) The influence of dietary mackerel oil on the condition of organs and on blood lipid composition in the growing young pig. *Am. J. Clin. Nutr.* 31:2159–2166.

40. T.A. Sanders (in press) Effects of n−3 polyunsaturated fatty acids on plasma lipids and lipoproteins. In: A.P. Simopoulos, ed. *II International Conference on the Health Effects of n−3 Fatty Acids in Seafoods.* Karger, Basel.

41. D.G. Godfrey (1957) Antiparasitic action of dietary cod liver oil upon *Plasmodium berghei* and its reversal by vitamin E. *Exp. Parasitol.* 6:555–565.

42. O.A. Levander, A.L. Ager, V.C. Morris, et al. (1989) Menhaden fish oil and a vitamin E–deficient diet: protection against chloroquin-resistant malaria in mice. *Am. J. Clin. Nutr.* 50:1237–1239.

43. F.C. Luft (1989) Salt and hypertension: recent advances and perspectives. *J. Lab. Clin. Med.* 114:215–221.

Chapter 54

Chapter *54*   Mack C. Mitchell

Alcohol

Alcoholic beverages constitute a small but significant source of calories in the diets of American adults. Dietary surveys estimated that in the general population 4–6% of ingested calories are derived from the ethanol in alcoholic beverages.[1] Alcoholics and other heavy drinkers may consume >50% of their daily calories as ethanol.

Ethanol is unique among dietary calorie sources, because in addition to contributing to energy requirements, it has potent pharmacologic and biochemical properties that may affect other aspects of nutrition and metabolism. This chapter will examine the caloric value of ethanol, including its efficacy as a source of energy, how it affects intermediary metabolism, and its effects on the absorption and utilization of micronutrients such as vitamins and trace minerals.

Caloric Value of Ethanol

Metabolism. After complete combustion in a bomb calorimeter, ethanol yields a theoretical caloric value of 7.1 kcal/g. After ingestion ethanol is almost completely absorbed from the upper gastrointestinal tract into the portal circulation. Over 90% of ingested ethanol is metabolized in the liver through sequential oxidation first to acetaldehyde and subsequently to acetate, which then enters the tricarboxylic acid (TCA) cycle. Although there are several enzymes that can metabolize ethanol to acetaldehyde, quantitatively alcohol dehydrogenase (ADH) is the most important. The isoenzymes of ADH can be divided into three classes, although the class I enzymes are most important for metabolism of the usual concentrations of ethanol.[2] These isoenzymes not only are under genetic control but also can be regulated by hormones, nutritional status, and other variables. Several comprehensive reviews of this subject were published.[2–5] During ADH-mediated oxidation of ethanol, 1 mol pyridine nucleotide, NAD^+, is reduced to NADH for each 1 mol ethanol oxidized to acetaldehyde. These reducing equivalents are shuttled into the mitochondria and enter the electron-transport chain providing energy for synthesis of ATP.

After the oxidation of ethanol, which occurs primarily in the cytosol, the acetaldehyde formed is transported into the mitochondrion where it is oxidized to acetate by aldehyde dehydrogenase (ALDH). This enzyme exists in several forms that differ in the affinity for acetaldehyde and NAD^+. The hepatic concentrations of acetaldehyde during ethanol oxidation are sufficiently low that the low K_m-mitochondrial enzyme is quantitatively more important in metabolism. Acetaldehyde oxidation by ALDH also generates reducing equivalents for ATP synthesis. Most of the acetate formed from acetaldehyde is exported out of the liver and is metabolized in extrahepatic tissues.

In addition to the ADH pathway for ethanol oxidation, there exists a microsomal mixed-function oxidase that can oxidize ethanol to acetaldehyde.[6] This enzyme has a higher K_m ($\sim$10-fold) than does ADH, but unlike ADH it can be induced by chronic ethanol ingestion. For these reasons it may contribute to overall ethanol oxidation, particularly at high concentrations or after chronic ingestion. Mixed-function oxidases including the microsomal ethanol-oxidizing system (MEOS) utilize the reduced pyridine nucleotide (NADPH) as a cofactor so that energy equivalents are consumed rather than generated during substrate oxidation. In the case of ethanol oxidation by this route, 2 mol NADPH are oxidized for each 1 mol ethanol oxidized to acetaldehyde. As discussed later in this section, this difference in metabolic pathways may account for some of the dose-related differences in the caloric value of ethanol.[7]

Balance Studies. Studies in animals and in humans have demonstrated that ethanol yields close to its theoretical maximum after low doses (<30% of total calories). The classical studies of Atwater and Benedict[8] and more recently those of Reinus et al.[9] did not observe increased oxygen consumption or thermogenesis or a hypermetabolic state during consumption of low doses of ethanol. Consistent with these findings are dietary surveys showing a positive correlation between alcohol consumption and body weight.[1]

By contrast, at higher doses of ethanol the theoretical caloric value may not be achieved. Indeed, subjects given 50% of calories as ethanol lost weight and were in negative nitrogen balance during the time of ingestion of large amounts of ethanol.[9-11] The mechanism for the observed inefficient caloric utilization of large doses of ethanol is a subject of controversy. Pirola and Lieber[7] attributed this incomplete utilization to metabolism of ethanol via MEOS at high concentrations of ethanol. This step requires energy for ethanol oxidation and consumes rather than generates reducing equivalents. Subsequent metabolism of the carbon skeleton continues normally.

Reinus et al.[9] re-examined this hypothesis with direct and indirect calorimetry during continuous intragastric infusion of diets containing ≤55% of calories as ethanol. These elegant studies did not provide support for inefficient utilization of ethanol as an energy source. In fact, subjects maintained positive energy balance when given ethanol as 30% or 55% of calories. Nonetheless, subjects lost weight during periods of ethanol infusion. Weight loss occurred in subjects in the absence of measurable blood ethanol concentrations and was associated with negative balances of nitrogen, sodium, potassium, phosphorus, and fluid. Urinary excretion of 3-methylhistidine was increased during ethanol infusion, suggesting increased catabolism of skeletal muscle proteins. There was also a small loss in the protein-derived component of energy balance. In some subjects additional urinary and respiratory losses of ethanol occurred when the maximal metabolic capacity of the liver for ethanol was exceeded, accounting for 4% of total energy intake. These sources of caloric loss often are not accounted for during intermittent consumption of alcohol that results in significant blood alcohol concentrations. Thus, although ethanol itself may be completely oxidized and calorically efficient as a fuel, ingestion of large amounts of ethanol may indirectly impair other components of metabolism.

Effects on Energy Metabolism. High concentrations of ethanol may impair mitochondrial function and reduce the capacity of the liver to synthesize ATP.[12-14] Numerous studies demonstrated that hepatic ATP content is lower in chronic ethanol-fed animals.[13-16] Such decreases could be due to increased

ATP-ase activity or to decreased synthesis of ATP. Although one study reported increased ATP-ase activity,[16] the majority of the evidence favors decreased synthesis as the explanation for lower hepatic ATP content.[12-14] The catalytic activity of the ATP-synthetase complex is decreased in ethanol-fed rodents, whereas ATP-P_i exchange appears to be unaffected.[13,14]

The greater chemical reactivity of acetaldehyde compared with ethanol led to the hypothesis that acetaldehyde might be responsible for the adverse effects of ethanol on mitochondrial function and energy metabolism. High concentrations of acetaldehyde inhibit both oxidative phosphorylation and ATP-P_i exchange in isolated mitochondria.[17,18] Of interest is the observation that the toxic effects of acetaldehyde could be prevented by cysteine in vitro.[18] However, the concentrations of acetaldehyde required to produce these effects exceed those normally encountered during ethanol metabolism.

An alternate hypothesis to explain decreased ATP concentrations suggests that acetate formed from acetaldehyde oxidation increases adenine nucleotide turnover because 2 mol ATP are required for each 1 mol acetate converted to acetyl CoA.[19] Regardless of the mechanism the net effect is decreased hepatic content of ATP after chronic but not acute ethanol ingestion.

Effects of Ethanol on Intermediary Metabolism

Most studies of the effects of ethanol on carbohydrate and lipid metabolism focused on acute effects seen with single large doses of ethanol. Under these conditions the principal changes are due to large shifts in the hepatic redox state that result from metabolism of ethanol. As mentioned, ADH-catalyzed oxidation of ethanol to acetaldehyde and acetate converts 2 mol NAD^+ to NADH. Considering that an average cocktail contains 0.2–0.3 mol ethanol (12–15 g; molecular weight of ethanol, 46), one can easily appreciate the reductive stress imposed by ethanol oxidation. Oxidation of ethanol takes precedence over other metabolic pathways in the liver, so that the redox state shifts to favor those reactions requiring NADH as a cofactor. Under some conditions, such as starvation, the reoxidation of NADH may even limit the rate of ethanol oxidation, although in general, the activity of ADH is rate limiting.[2,20]

Carbohydrate Metabolism. Oxidation of ethanol in the fasting state may drastically affect glucose homeostasis, leading to hypoglycemia. Hypoglycemia develops in fasted or malnourished subjects after ingestion of a large ethanol load or in children (after accidental poisoning), who seem to be more susceptible.[20] The mechanism is probably multifactorial. Impairment of gluconeogenesis occurs because of redox shifts that favor conversion of phosphoenolpyruvate to pyruvate and pyruvate to lactate. In addition, excess NADH resulting from ethanol oxidation suppresses the activity of the TCA cycle and prevents α-ketoglutarate and oxaloacetate (derived from amino acids) from being used as substrates in gluconeogenesis. Furthermore, the expected release of glycerol from adipose tissue is attenuated by ethanol. Alcohol also favors formation of α-glycerophosphate from glucose because of the increased NADH-to-NAD$^+$ ratio. The increase in α-glycerophosphate, in turn, may inhibit catabolism of glycerol. In certain individuals attenuated release of growth hormone and corticosteroid hormones may also contribute to hypoglycemia.[20]

In well-fed subjects, acute ingestion of ethanol enhances hepatic glycogenolysis, which is probably mediated through epinephrine release.[20] Other effects on carbohydrate metabolism include inhibition of the conversion of UDP-galactose to UDP-glucose, a reaction that is inhibited by an increased NADH-to-NAD$^+$ ratio.[20] This latter reaction is a necessary step in synthesis of UDP-glucuronic acid, a cofactor for glucuronidation of some drugs, such as acetaminophen.

Lipid Metabolism. Fatty infiltration of the liver is a common finding in alcoholics but may also occur in healthy subjects consuming large amounts of ethanol within 1–2 wk.[21] Similarly, administration of single large doses of ethanol to rats results in biochemically detectable increases in hepatic triglycerides. The pathogenesis of alcoholic fatty liver is also multifactorial and like hypoglycemia is due, in part, to the marked redox shifts that accompany ethanol metabolism. Because of the obligatory requirement for ethanol oxidation in the liver, ethanol replaces fatty acids as the preferred fuel source in mitochondria. In addition, acetaldehyde may inhibit certain enzymes in the TCA cycle. With decreased TCA-cycle activity, fatty acid oxidation is slowed. Excess NADH also favors lipogenesis (which requires NADPH for fatty acid synthesis from acetyl-CoA).

Dietary fat content greatly influences the source of hepatic fat in animals fed diets containing 35% of calories as ethanol. When dietary fat content is high (>30% of calories), most of the hepatic triglycerides are of exogenous origin, whereas low dietary fat (≤5% of calories) results in accumulation of endogenously synthesized triglycerides.[22] This shift from endogenous to exogenous fat accumulation with increasing dietary fat probably reflects a greater effect of ethanol in decreasing fatty acid oxidation compared with effects on fatty acid synthesis. Alternatively, this shift could be explained by variation in the carbohydrate content of the diet, because high-carbohydrate loads stimulate endogenous fat synthesis.

Lipoprotein release from the liver is enhanced by acute alcohol administration, although it may be decreased once cirrhosis develops. The effects of alcohol ingestion on serum lipoprotein profiles have been investigated extensively because of observed decreases in risk of coronary heart disease in moderate drinkers.[23,24] Positive correlations between alcohol consumption and serum high-density lipoprotein (HDL) cholesterol concentrations were reported in many studies.[25] Controlled experiments in which alcohol was administered to human volunteers also resulted in increases in serum HDL cholesterol concentrations and suggested a causal effect on serum lipoprotein concentrations.[26,27] The results of alcohol consumption on subfractions of HDL cholesterol (HDL$_2$ and HDL$_3$) are conflicting. In some studies HDL$_2$, the putative atherogenic protective fraction, and HDL$_3$ are increased by alcohol, whereas in others only fraction HDL$_3$ is increased.[27,28] Some of the discrepancies may be explained by differences in quantity of alcohol consumed. Hojacki et al.[29] reported that HDL$_2$ concentrations and HDL$_2$-HDL$_3$ ratios were increased in squirrel monkeys fed 12% of calories as ethanol, whereas higher ethanol doses (24% and 36% of calories) increased HDL$_3$ and LDL concentrations and decreased the ratio of HDL$_2$ to HDL$_3$.

The mechanism by which alcohol affects HDL concentrations remains unknown. Apolipoprotein A-I and A-II concentrations are increased by moderate alcohol consumption, whereas apoprotein B concentrations are decreased.[26] In subhuman primates, apoprotein B concentrations (low-density lipoprotein) increase with increasing ethanol dose, whereas in human alcoholics they may be lower.[30] The effects of ethanol on very-low-density–lipoprotein synthesis in humans are less well characterized.

Protein and Amino Acid Metabolism. Large doses of ethanol appear to inhibit protein synthesis in the brain, but the effects on hepatic protein synthesis are less clear. Ethanol inhibits albumin synthesis in the isolated perfused liver,[28] whereas the reported effects of ethanol on protein synthesis in vivo have been conflicting. Long-term ethanol feeding was shown to inhibit the release of export proteins from the liver resulting in accumulation of these proteins within hepatocytes.[30] This finding may explain, in part, some of the increase in liver size that is not due to fat accumulation in alcohol-fed animals. The mechanism for decreased excretion of export proteins is unproven but may be due to impairment in microtubular assembly and function.[30]

Although there is little direct effect of ethanol on protein synthesis, there are appreciable effects on amino acid metabolism. Intestinal absorption and transport of isoleucine, arginine, and methionine are impaired by high concentrations (3–10%) of ethanol. The results on hepatic uptake and transport are conflicting. Some studies using cultured hepatocytes showed increases in transport of amino acids by the A system whereas others reported decreases.[31] Branched-chain amino acids and α-amino-N-butyric acid (AANB) are increased in the plasma of alcoholics and chronically ethanol-fed rats.[32] The increase in AANB relative to leucine may serve as a marker for alcoholism or heavy drinking. Although the mechanism for the increase in AANB is uncertain, increased transsulfuration of methionine to cysteine, a metabolic pathway that produces α-ketobutyrate (the keto acid analogue of AANB), could account for the increase in AANB.

Presently, the stimulus for increased plasma AANB and/or transsulfuration of methionine is unknown. One hypothesis is that AANB increases because of increased hepatic requirements for glutathione.[33] Dietary requirements for methionine are known to be elevated in ethanol-fed rats presumably because of its lipotropic properties. However, because cysteine is rate limiting in glutathione synthesis, the increase in AANB may reflect an increased hepatic requirement for methionine-derived cysteine as a precursor for glutathione synthesis. Increased glutathione synthesis would be an alternative explanation for the reported increase in methionine utilization during ethanol feeding.

Effects of Ethanol on Micronutrients

Alcoholics are frequently deficient in both water- and fat-soluble vitamins. Certainly poor intake of vitamins is a primary cause for deficiencies, but ethanol can affect the absorption, storage, metabolism, and excretion of vitamins as well. This section will illustrate how ethanol affects each of these processes.

Folate. Folic acid deficiency is perhaps the most common vitamin deficiency encountered in alcoholics. At the time of admission to hospital, jejunal absorption of folate was found to be decreased in alcoholics, but absorption improved on an adequate diet supplemented with folate.[34] Both alcohol ingestion and folate-deficient diets appear to contribute to folic acid deficiency in alcoholics, because folate absorption was shown to improve when dietary folate supplements were given despite continued alcohol consumption.[34] Alterations in hepatic uptake or storage of folate are other potential mechanisms by which ethanol could cause deficiency. Hepatic uptake of folate appears to be decreased by acute ethanol administration, whereas conflicting results have been obtained on hepatic storage of folic acid. The polyglutamylated forms of the vitamin cannot be utilized easily for DNA synthesis or in other enzymatic reactions. In rats, alcohol treatment for 3 d increased the polyglutamylated form of the vitamin, whereas in monkeys no such increase was noted after 4 y of alcohol feeding.[35] Urinary excretion was reported to be increased by alcohol both in rats and in humans. Although all of these mechanisms may contribute to folate deficiency, decreased absorption appears to be quantitatively the most important.

Thiamin. As with folate, alcohol impairs absorption of thiamin. Hoyumpa et al.[36] found that active transport of thiamin across the intestinal mucosa is inhibited by ethanol, whereas passive transport is unimpaired. The impaired absorption may be secondary to decreased $Na,^+K^+$-ATPase activity in enterocytes. Impaired absorption occurs only in the presence of ethanol and is not observed after chronic administration or withdrawal.

Pyridoxine. Pyridoxine absorption is primarily passive and is affected only by very high concentrations of ethanol. Once absorbed, pyridoxine is taken up by the liver where it is phosphorylated to pyridoxal-5-phosphate (PLP) and stored. Hepatic accumulation of PLP is markedly decreased by ethanol and seems to be due to accelerated degradation of PLP caused by acetaldehyde.[37] Urinary loss of pyridoxine is also accelerated by ethanol and results in very low levels of both pyridoxine and PLP in plasma of alcoholics, particularly those with liver disease.

Vitamin A. Vitamin A is absorbed from the intestine by transport with chylomicrons. This process is not affected by ethanol. Like pyridoxine, however, hepatic storage of vitamin A is reduced by ethanol.[38] Cumulative liver injury seems to reduce vitamin A storage because hepatic levels are lower in persons with alcoholic cirrhosis than in those with only fatty infiltration. However, even the latter group has lower concentrations than do those with viral hepatitis. One possible mechanism for this effect is increased microsomal metabolism to retinoic acid because of induction of vitamin A–metabolizing enzymes by ethanol.

Zinc. Patients with alcoholic liver disease are frequently zinc deficient.[39] Ethanol impairs absorption of zinc in experimental animals, but poor intake is probably quantitatively more important. Zinc intake is highly correlated with protein intake and is generally low in alcoholics, particularly those with advanced liver disease. Increased urinary excretion of zinc was also observed in persons with alcoholic cirrhosis. Recent studies focused on the possibility that low plasma zinc concentrations may be due to increased hepatic production of interleukin by Kupffer cells stimulated by ethanol or its metabolites.

Selenium. Plasma concentrations of selenium are slightly decreased as are vitamin E concentrations in alcoholics. Some investigators speculated that these decreases may predispose alcoholics to lipid peroxidation, although direct evidence for this theory is lacking. The mechanism underlying the deficiencies is unclear.

Summary

The interactions between alcohol and nutrition are complex. Most evidence suggests that ethanol provides an efficient source of calories, although heavy consumption causes weight loss. In this context weight loss is probably due to accelerated breakdown of body proteins with negative balances of nitrogen and water. The in vitro effects of ethanol on mitochondrial energy metabolism may also play a role in the loss of weight, although this suggestion remains unproven. Intermediary metabolism of carbohydrates and lipids is altered by alcohol consumption. In general, most of the changes are due to increase in the NADH-to-NAD$^+$ ratio resulting from metabolism of ethanol by alcohol dehydrogenases. As a consequence, fatty infiltration of the liver occurs but is reversible with abstinence. Moderate consumption of alcohol increases serum HDL concentrations, which may explain in part the decrease in risk of coronary heart disease in moderate drinkers. Alcoholics are frequently malnourished and are often deficient in vitamins and trace elements. Alcohol ingestion affects vitamin metabolism by impairing absorption, storage, and metabolism and/or increasing excretion.

References

1. M.C. Mitchell and H.F. Herlong (1986) Alcohol and nutrition: caloric value, bioenergetics, and relationship to liver damage. *Annu. Rev. Nutr.* 6:457–474.

2. W.F. Bosron and T.K. Li (1986) Genetic polymorphism of human liver alcohol and aldehyde dehydrogenase and their relationship to alcohol metabolism and alcoholism. *Hepatology* 6:502–510.

3. E. Mezey (1983) Effects of hormones on ethanol metabolism. In: *Ethanol Tolerance and Dependence: Endocrinologic Aspects* (T.J. Cicero, ed.), pp. 190–200, U.S. Department of Health and Human Services, Rockville, MD.

4. D.H. Van Thiel, J.S. Gavaler, E. Rosenblum, and R.E. Tarter (1989) Ethanol, its metabolism and hepatotoxicity as well as its gonadal effects. *Pharmacol. Ther.* 41:27–48.

5. L.A. Pohorecky and J. Brick (1988) Pharmacology of ethanol. *Pharmacol. Ther.* 56:335–427.

6. C.S. Lieber and L.M. DeCarli (1968) Ethanol oxidation by hepatic microsomes: adaptive increase after ethanol feeding. *Science* 162: 917–918.

7. R.C. Pirola and C.S. Lieber (1976) Hypothesis: energy wastage in alcoholism and drug abuse: possible role of hepatic microsomal enzymes. *Am. J. Clin. Nutr.* 29:90–93.

8. W.D. Atwater and F.G. Benedict (1902) An experimental inquiry regarding the nutritive value of alcohol. *Mem. Natl. Acad. Sci.* 8: 235–397.

9. J.F. Reinus, S.B. Heymsfield, R. Wiskind, K. Casper, and J.T. Galambos (1989) Ethanol: relative fuel value and metabolic effects *in vivo. Metabolism* 38:125–135.

10. R.C. Pirola and C.S. Lieber (1972) The energy cost of the metabolism of drugs, including ethanol. *Pharmacology* 7:185–196.

11. J.T. McDonald and S. Morgan (1976) Wine versus ethanol in human nutrition. I. Nitrogen and caloric balance. *Am. J. Clin. Nutr.* 29: 1093–1103.

12. W.S. Thayer and E. Rubin (1981) Molecular alterations in the respiratory chain of rat liver after chronic ethanol consumption. *J. Biol. Chem.* 256:6090–6097.

13. R.E. Bottenus, P.I. Spach, S. Filus, and C.C. Cunningham (1982) Effect of chronic ethanol feeding on energy linked processes associated with oxidative phosphorylation: proton translocation and ATP-P$_i$ exchange. *Biochem. Biophys. Res. Commun.* 105:1368–1378.

14. P.I. Spach, R.E. Bottenus, and C.C. Cunningham (1982) Control of adenine nucleotide metabolism in hepatic mitochondria from rats with ethanol-induced fatty liver. *Biochem. J.* 202:445–452.

15. E. Gordon (1971) ATP metabolism in an ethanol-induced fatty liver. *Biochem. Pharmacol.* 26:1229–1234.

16. Y. Israel, L. Videla, and J. Bernstein (1975) Liver hypermetabolic state after chronic ethanol consumption. *Fed. Proc.* 34:2052–2059.

17. A.I. Cederbaum, C.S. Lieber, and E. Rubin (1974) The effect of acetaldehyde on mitochondrial function. *Arch. Biochem. Biophys.* 161:26–39.

18. A.I. Cederbaum and E. Rubin (1976) Protective effect of cysteine on the inhibition of mitochondrial functions by acetaldehyde. *Biochem. Pharmacol.* 25:963–973.

19. J.G. Puig and I.H. Fox (1984) Ethanol-induced activation of adenine nucleotide turnover. Evidence for a role of acetate. *J. Clin. Invest.* 74:936–941.

20. C.S. Lieber, ed. (1982) *Medical Disorders of Alcoholism*, W.B. Saunders Co., Philadelphia.

21. C.S. Lieber, D.P. Jones, and L.M. DeCarli (1965) Effects of prolonged ethanol intake: production of fatty liver despite adequate diets. *J. Clin. Invest.* 44:1009–1021.

22. C.S. Lieber, N. Spreitz, and L.M. DeCarli (1966) Role of dietary, adipose, and endogenously synthesized fatty acids in the pathogenesis of the alcoholic fatty liver. *J. Clin. Invest.* 45:51–62.

23. A.L. Klatsky, G.D. Friedman, and A.B. Siegelaub (1981) Alcohol and mortality; a ten-year Kaiser-Permanente experience. *Ann. Intern. Med.* 95:139–145.

24. T. Gorden and W.B. Kannel (1983) Drinking habits and cardiovascular disease: the Framingham Study. *Am. Heart J.* 105:667–673.

25. R.D. Moore and T.A. Pearson (1986) Moderate alcohol consumption and coronary artery disease: a review. *Medicine* 65:242–267.

26. R.D. Moore, C.R. Smith, P.O. Kwiterovich, and T.A. Pearson (1988) Effect of low-dose alcohol use versus abstention on apolipoproteins A-I and B. *Am. J. Med.* 84:884–890.

27. W.L. Haskell, C. Camargo, P.T. Williams, et al. (1984) The effect

of cessation and resumption of alcohol intake upon high density lipoprotein subfractions. *N. Engl. J. Med.* 30:805–810.

28. M.A. Rothschild, M. Oratz, J. Mongelli, and S.S. Schreiber (1971) Alcohol-induced depression of albumin synthesis: revival by tryptophan. *J. Clin. Invest.* 50:1812–1818.

29. J.L. Hojacki, J.E. Cluette-Brown, J.J. Mulligan, et al. (1988) Effect of ethanol dose on low density lipoproteins and high density lipoprotein fractions. *Alcoholism Clin. Exp. Res.* 12:129–154.

30. E. Baraona, M.A. Leo, S.A. Borowsky, and C.S. Lieber (1975) Alcoholic hepatomegaly: accumulation of protein in the liver. *Science* 190:794–795.

31. M.C. Mitchell and E. Mezey (1987) Ethanol and amino acid uptake by hepatocytes. *Hepatology* 7:310–312.

32. S. Shaw and C.S. Lieber (1980) Increased hepatic production of alpha amino-n-butyric acid after chronic alcohol consumption in rats and baboons. *Gastroenterology* 78:108–113.

33. J.L. Pierson and M.C. Mitchell (1986) Increased hepatic efflux of

glutathione after chronic ethanol feeding. *Biochem. Pharmacol.* 35:1533–1537.

34. C.H. Halsted, E.A. Robles, and E. Mezey (1971) Decreased jejunal uptake of labelled folic acid (^{3}H-PGA) in alcoholic patients. Roles of alcohol and nutrition. *N. Engl. J. Med.* 285:701–706.

35. T. Tamura and C.H. Halsted (1983) Folate turnover in chronically alcoholic monkeys. *J. Lab. Clin. Med.* 101:623–628.

36. A.M. Hoyumpa, S.G. Nichols, F.A. Wilson, and S. Schenker (1977) Effect of ethanol on intestinal (Na,K) ATPase and intestinal thiamine transport in rats. *J. Lab. Clin. Med.* 90:1086–1095.

37. R.L. Veitch, L. Lumeng, and T.K. Li (1975) Vitamin B_6 metabolism in chronic alcohol abuse. The effect of ethanol oxidation on hepatic pyridoxal-5-phosphate metabolism. *J. Clin. Invest.* 55:1026–1032.

38. M.A. Leo and C.S. Lieber (1982) Hepatic vitamin A depletion in alcoholic liver injury. *N. Engl. J. Med.* 37:597–601.

39. C.J. McClain, D.R. Antonow, D.A. Cohen, and S.I. Shedlofsky (1986) Zinc metabolism in alcoholic liver disease. *Alcoholism Clin. Exp. Res.* 6:582–589.

Chapter 55   Adria R. Sherman and Nora A. Hallquist

Immunity

The study of nutrition and immunology is in its early stages and is progressing rapidly. This chapter presents selected current information regarding nutrition and immunity.

The immune system, which includes cells of the thymus, lymph nodes, spleen, and bone marrow, is one of the most complex systems in the body, second only to the nervous system. It is highly interactive with itself and with every other system in the body, yet it does not have an organ of central control. The complex interactive nature of the immune system allows it to recognize and attack what is foreign and to recognize and preserve what is self. The immune system uses the lymphatic and circulatory systems as its highways through the body. Specific and nonspecific cellular patrols travel through the lymphatic and circulatory systems leaving some stationary cellular patrols in various organs. Cellular patrols that are specific for an invading foreign substance, or antigen, have been previously exposed to and sensitized by that antigen and will defend the body against the antigen. Cellular patrols that are nonspecific will defend the body against any invading antigen that is perceived as nonself.

When the host encounters a bacterial, viral, or chemical antigen, the first line of defense is the skin. Skin functions very well as a barrier. For example, consider the increased susceptibility to infection in burn patients where the skin is severed or removed. Body openings or orifices including the gastrointestinal (GI) tract, genitourinary tract, and respiratory tract are guarded against antigenic attack by the mucosa. The mucosa protects against invasion with powerful proteolytic enzymes and secretory antibodies that can immobilize and/or destroy invading antigens. The GI tract also is well protected from attack by antigens in ingested food. Included in the immune system of the GI tract is a system of lymph nodes called Peyer's patches, which contain many B cells that secrete immunoglobulin A, the class of antibody that protects against parasitic and microbial invasion. Peyer's patches also contain other immune cells, such as macrophages, T cells, and natural killer cells.

When bacteria successfully enter the body, they rapidly reproduce by using nutrients supplied by the host to proliferate and thrive. Just as rapidly, circulating components of the immune system identify the presence of invaders. Nonspecific blood-borne lymphocyte patrols called neutrophils, or polymorphonuclear leukocytes, immediately attack and phagocytize, or engulf, the invading bacteria. Phagocytosis is initiated with an energetic burst of cellular respiration, which includes increased oxygen uptake, increased hexose-monophosphate-shunt activity, and production of oxygen radicals, such as hydrogen peroxide, to kill bacteria. These cellular metabolic changes can be measured to determine the capacity of an immune cell to phagocytize and kill bacteria. Neutrophils signal for help from other immunologic cells by a process called chemotaxis, which is the chemical attraction of cells by substances released from the neutrophils. The next lymphocytes to arrive on the scene by chemoattraction are the macrophages. Macrophages engulf and kill bacteria while secreting a number of products that stimulate the immune system. Some of these macrophage-secreted products are macrophage activating factor, interferons, interleukins, and prostaglandins. Macrophages also process antigens on the surface of engulfed bacteria and present the antigens to T and B lymphocytes so that they can recognize and initiate specific attacks against the bacteria.

When activated, B lymphocytes (B cells) differentiate and mature into plasma cells that produce numerous antibodies that display a molecular mirror image of the tertiary structure of the macrophage-presented bacterial antigen. Antigens are usually foreign harmful chemical or biological substances that induce the formation of antibodies. Antibodies, also called immunoglobulins, are molecules that are produced by B cells in response to a specific antigen invasion and that combine with the antigen to form a complex. The antigen-antibody complex is removed by cells of the immune system. Humoral immunity is immunologic defense that protects the body against bacteria and toxins by circulating cell-derived components, primarily antibodies. Antibodies travel through the blood and attach, like a lock and key, to antigens on the multiplying bacteria. An antibody coating makes the bacteria more susceptible to attachment (opsonization) and phagocytosis by macrophages. The antigen-antibody complex also initiates another process that destroys the bacteria through the complement system, which is a cascade of serum proteins that are sequentially activated. Some of the B cells do not mature into plasma cells but are stored as memory B cells for response to future invasion by the same bacteria. Memory B cells are activated in a specific manner and at an accelerated rate if the same bacterium reenters the body. In fact, many bacteria are killed by antibodies from memory B cells that halt an invasion before the host shows clinical symptoms of infection.

The functional capacity of humoral immunity is assessed by measuring antibody production by B cells with a plaque-formation assay. Two types of antibodies are commonly measured by this assay. Immunoglobulin M (IgM) is produced upon first exposure of the host to an antigen; this reaction is called the primary (nonsensitized) response. Immunoglobulin G (IgG) is produced upon second or continued exposure of the host to an antigen and is called the secondary (sensitized) response. Other immunoglobulins include IgA, IgE, and IgD. IgA, which is abundant in secretions such as saliva and tracheobronchial secretions, protects against initial invasion by antigens. IgE is located on basophils and mast cells and is thought to be involved in protection against parasites and allergic responses. The biological function of IgD is not well known, but it may play a role in antigen-triggered lymphocyte differentiation. A second way of measuring functional capacity of humoral immunity is by assessing the ability of B cells to proliferate or blast transform when stimulated by a plant mitogen, such as lipopolysaccharide (LPS).

Cell-mediated immunity is immunologic defense that includes any immune response that is mediated by cells of the immune system rather than by antibodies. T cells or T lymphocytes and other lymphocytes of the immune system, such as natural killer (NK) cells, protect the body against viral and bacterial

infection or tumor growth. T cells and NK cells recognize virus-invaded or cancerous host cells as altered self. The stimulated response is either specific or nonspecific depending on whether the body has been exposed to that antigen in the past. In cell-mediated immunity the immune system kills by direct cell-to-cell contact. It is postulated that immune cells destroy virus-infected or cancerous cells by creating holes in the infected cells with chemicals produced by the immune cell. At the same time lymphocytes secrete lymphokines that mediate the activity of these lymphocytes, other lymphocytes, and the immune system as a whole. Examples of lymphokines include interferons, interleukins, and tumor necrosis factor.

T cells mature in the thymus into subpopulations of cells that have surface markers that are associated with specific T-cell functions. T helper cells are the primary coordinators of a battle against infection and activate macrophages, B cells, and T cells. Some antigens are T-helper-cell dependent; that is, T helper cells are necessary for the production of antibodies by B cells. T cytotoxic cells kill infectious cells by a process called cytotoxicity. To achieve balance in the killing process, T suppressor cells slow down and stop the battle by secreting deactivating or suppressor factors. Delayed hypersensitivity responses, such as allergic reactions of the skin, involve T-D cells. Skin reactions are relatively easy to test; therefore, delayed hypersensitivity is a convenient clinical measurement of the functional capacity of cell-mediated immunity. Another common measurement of the functioning capacity of cellular immunity is the stimulation of T cells to blast transform and function as activated T cells. Concanavalin A (Con A) and phytohemagglutinin (PHA) are plant mitogens that cause the blastogenesis of T cells.

Numerous substances are synthesized and secreted by immune cells. These substances mediate immune responses by activating or suppressing specific or general functions of immune cells. The concentration and activity of immunologic mediators may be altered in animals with abnormal nutrient status. Some examples include interferon and interleukin 2, which activate NK cells; interleukin 1, which activates T cells to produce interleukin 2 and causes fever; chemotactic factors, which chemically attract immune cells to a specific location; and prostaglandins, which are derived from membrane fatty acids and mediate local immune responses in a hormone-like manner.

Immunity involves metabolic processes, such as cell proliferation, cell differentiation, synthesis, and secretion of immunologic mediators; receptor recognition and binding; and the specific functions of each immune cell. Theoretically, altered nutritional status could precipitate breakdown of immune function wherever nutrients are involved in any of these cellular functions. Reviewed here are selected studies using animal models and human subjects that have contributed to our knowledge of nutrient-immunity interactions in the areas of generalized malnutrition and iron, zinc, copper, selenium, vitamin E, vitamin A, β-carotene, and vitamin C malnutrition.

Malnutrition

For some time it has been known that malnourished individuals are more susceptible to infections. For example, morbidity and mortality associated with protein-calorie malnutrition (PCM) often are caused by adverse effects of PCM on immune responses, but the type of effect depends on the severity and duration of the PCM.

Lymphopenia and a distorted proportion of B- and T-cell subpopulations were reported by Chandra[1] in children with PCM. The number of total circulating T cells was reduced in malnourished children, and the ratio of T helper cells to T cytotoxic cells decreased. The decreased number of total T cells was associated with decreased maturation of T cells. IgA-producing B cells and null cells, which have cytotoxic function but no T- or B-cell markers, increased in malnourished children compared with well-nourished control children.[1] In contrast to children, adults with marasmus showed no differences in lymphocyte number or proportion.[2]

Rats fed a protein-deficient diet for 3 wk and experimentally stimulated by intraperitoneal injection with glycogen showed increased chemotactic response of macrophages to an artificial chemotactic factor and decreased chemotactic response of macrophages to peritoneal fluid containing natural chemotactic factors.[3] These results suggested that macrophages from protein-deficient rats were able to respond to chemotactic factors, but de novo synthesis of chemotactic factors in the peritoneum decreased. Both responses returned to normal after 1 wk of protein repletion. Paswell et al.[4] reported that protein-deficient mice had decreased clearance of carbon by macrophages, which is a measurement of decreased phagocytic capacity. Whereas changes in metabolic processes associated with bactericidal activity of macrophages, such as decreased oxygen consumption and hexose-monophosphate-shunt activity, also were observed in protein-deficient rats, these changes did not affect overall bactericidal capacity.[3] Decreased migration toward bacterial chemotactic factors, decreased bactericidal activity, and increased hexose monophosphate shunt activity of macrophages were found in children with PCM.[5]

Impaired antibody production towards antigens used in vaccinations is well documented during PCM. However, different types of antibodies and primary and secondary humoral responses are affected to different degrees. Production of IgG but not IgM by B cells in response to tetanus toxoid was decreased in mice weaned to a protein-deficient diet.[6] In addition, the secondary antibody response to infection decreased even after transfer to a normal diet at first immunization.[7] Decreased production and affinity of antibody after repeated immunization with human serum transferrin was reported in 2–3-mo-old Ajax mice fed a protein-deficient diet.[4] In malnourished Indian children, the affinity of antibody to tetanus toxoid was reduced, especially after primary immunization.[8] In undernourished but not severely malnourished Nigerian children antibody response to tetanus toxoid was normal after routine infant immunization programs.[9] These results confirm that the severity of the PCM is an important factor in humoral immunity and provide support for the efficacy of immunizing moderately undernourished children.

Filteau et al.[10] demonstrated a decreased primary immunoglobulin response to trinitrophenylated *Brucella abortus* (TNP-BA), a T-independent antigen, and sheep red blood cells (sRBC), a T-dependent antigen, in food-restricted *CBA/J* mice such that 30% of weaning weight was lost in 14 d as compared with mice fed ad libitum. These investigators also found that the antibody response to both antigens improved with administration of triiodothyronine, a thyroid hormone that increases metabolism. Food-restricted mice showed diminished delayed hypersensitivity response to sRBC antigen that was not improved by triiodothyronine administration, suggesting that triiodothyronine enhances humoral B-cell responses but not cell-mediated T-cell responses. The authors suggested that therapeutic hormonal treatment could be used to improve antibody response to vaccination and subsequent exposure to antigen in malnourished individuals.

Other cell-mediated immune responses are altered during PCM. In 12 patients with recent weight loss to <85% of standard weight-height ratio but without decreased serum proteins (<30 g/L), cellular immunity was slightly impaired as indicated by decreased subcutaneous delayed hypersensitivity, peripheral lymphocyte count, and B- and T-lymphocyte blastogenesis.[2] However, cellular immunity was severely impaired in 18 patients with weight loss and decreased serum proteins when evaluated by decreased subcutaneous delayed hypersensitivity and T-lymphocyte blastogenesis. Nutritional repletion by intravenous hyperalimentation of these patients for 18 d restored T-cell responses.[11]

Interleukin 1 (IL1), also called leukocyte endogenous mediator, decreased in critically ill protein-malnourished patients.[12] Decreased ability to synthesize IL1 as indicated by the rat bioassay method correlated with an increased risk of dying during hospitalization. Increased intravenous nutritional support with both protein and calories correlated with increased ability to synthesize IL1. Critically ill patients who received parenteral nutrition with increased protein and calories survived longer. These workers[12] suggested that the ability to produce IL1 is an early marker for improved survival.

Taken together these studies show that different types of PCM alter humoral and cell-mediated immunologic responses differently and that restoration of immunity is possible with repletion of nutritional status.

Zinc

Zinc deficiency may occur in malnutrition, gastrointestinal disorders, renal diseases, diabetes, alcoholism, cancer, and chronic infection. Because zinc deficiency can result from both dietary deficiency and a variety of clinical states, it occurs across a wide range of population groups. In humans zinc deficiency causes growth retardation, anemia, hypogonadism, hepatosplenomegaly, rough dry skin, mental lethargy, and geophagia.[13] The relationship between zinc nutrition and immunity has been studied extensively, and immune response was proposed as a possible indication of dietary zinc requirement.

The requirement for zinc is not the same for various physiologic and immunologic responses. In mice fed increasing amounts of zinc (0.9–40.4 μg Zn/g diet) for 28 d postweaning, maximum serum concentrations were obtained at 3.4 μg Zn/g diet, and maximum carcass growth required 5.4 μg Zn/g diet.[14] However, optimal immunologic defense by NK cells against tumors required the highest amount of zinc fed (40 μg/g diet).

The humoral response of antibody production by B cells is reduced during zinc deficiency. Decreased antibody production also was associated with increased pneumonia, conjunctivitis, and infection with Candida albicans in patients suffering from acrodermatitis enteropathica.[15] IgM and IgG production in response to both T-cell–dependent and T-cell–independent antigens decreased in rat pups whose dams were fed a marginally zinc-deficient diet (1.6 μg Zn/g diet) on days 5–17 postpartum.[16] Marginal zinc deficiency during suckling did not lead to permanent impairment of antibody response because 2 wk of repletion with zinc restored antibody titers to normal. In slightly older mice fed a zinc-deficient diet (0.6–1.6 μg Zn/g diet) for 6 wks postweaning,

decreased antibody production to T-cell–dependent antigens but not T-cell–independent antigens was found, suggesting that T helper cells were not functioning in their capacity as mediators of antibody production by B cells.[17–19] Fraker et al.[19] also reported that zinc-deficient young adult mice are capable of restoring T-cell–dependent antibody-mediated immune responses upon nutritional repletion.

Altered cell-mediated immune response in zinc deficiency also is well documented. Seven-week-old mice fed a zinc-deficient diet for 1 mo demonstrated a reduced delayed hypersensitivity response to both cutaneous and subcutaneous application of dinitrofluorobenzene antigen.[20] Zinc repletion for 3 wk repaired the abnormal delayed hypersensitivity response.

Proliferation of T cells in response to PHA stimulation was depressed in zinc-deficient mice.[21] Addition of macrophages from mice fed adequate zinc to T-cell cultures from zinc-deficient mice corrected the T-cell response. T-cell response also was normalized by addition of increasing proportions of macrophages from zinc-deficient mice. These results suggest that the functional defect during zinc deficiency is due to the regulatory role of macrophages. The function of T cells also appears to be reduced in zinc deficiency. Decreased thymus weight was found in mice fed a zinc-deficient diet (0.5 μg Zn/g diet) for 4 wk.[17] Because T cells mature in the thymus, T-cell number and function are affected by decreased thymus weight. In children with acrodermatitis enteropathica, an inherited zinc-deficiency disease, T-lymphocyte response to PHA decreased.[15] In addition, delayed-hypersensitivity skin tests were negative in 7 of 10 children who had low plasma zinc concentrations. Upon administration of 5–10 mg zinc/kg body weight (as zinc sulfate), plasma zinc concentrations returned to normal, lymphocyte response improved, and 8 of the 10 children showed a positive delayed-hypersensitivity skin test. In another study an adult patient with zinc deficiency showed lymphopenia, decreased response of T cells to PHA, increased ratio of T suppressor cells to T helper cells, decreased NK cell cytotoxicity, and increased macrophage cytotoxicity. Intravenous zinc repletion with 12 mg zinc chloride/d improved all immunologic responses tested.[22]

T-killer-cell and NK-cell activity decreased in several strains of mice fed a zinc-deficient diet.[23] Decreased NK-cell activity also was seen in patients with zinc deficiency found after total parenteral nutrition deficient in zinc.[22] Because T killer cells and NK cells function in cell-mediated immunity against tumors, zinc status may be an important factor in the capacity to fight cancer.

Immunity against parasites is another area of immunologic defense that is altered during zinc deficiency. In mice fed a zinc-deficient diet for 8 d and infected with *Trypanosoma cruzi*, an indigenous South American parasite that causes Chagas' disease, the blood contained 20 times more parasites than blood of control mice when tested 15 d later.[24] By 22 d postinfection, 80% of the zinc-deficient mice had died. Zinc deficiency also decreased the rapid production of oxygen radicals in macrophages of mice with *Trypanosoma cruzi*. Oxygen-radical production is the initial response of phagocytes necessary to eliminate pathogens.[25] When physiological concentrations of zinc were provided in vitro for 30 min, zinc-deficient macrophages were able to kill parasites normally.[24] These data suggest that zinc is critical to oxygen-radical production.

Another important facet of the immune response is the memory capability of immunologic cells. DePasquale-Jardieu and Fraker[26] found that the secondary response to sRBC antigens decreased 43% in mice fed a zinc-deficient diet for 28 d postimmunization as compared with mice fed a control diet. Transfer of zinc-deficient spleen cells to irradiated control mice did not restore the response, and repletion with adequate dietary zinc for 4 wk only partially restored the memory response, confirming that memory cells were destroyed by zinc deficiency.[26] The secondary response that protects the host after primary vaccination functions through memory cells. Possibly zinc-deficient malnourished infants should not be vaccinated until their zinc status has been improved.

Evidence suggests that the damage caused by zinc deficiency to immunocompetence can be reversed, even before body weight is regained.[15,16,20,22] However, after a moderate zinc deficiency in pregnant mice (5 mg Zn/kg diet), repletion of pups postpartum did not completely restore IgM antibody-mediated response to sRBC inoculation in 6–10-wk-old offspring, and decreased antibody-mediated response persisted into the second and third generations.[27]

Zinc supplementation causes immunostimulation in vitro. The proliferative response of T cells to interleukin 2 (IL2) is enhanced by addition of zinc (0.10–0.015 mmol/L) to the culture medium.[28] Zinc also was shown to enhance the IL1-stimulated blastogenic response of T cells that were previously stimulated in vitro by suboptimal concentrations of PHA.

Recently zinc supplementation was reported to improve the depressed immune system of aged animals. In vitro supplementation with zinc (200 μmol/L) of spleen cells from 24-mo-old mice enhanced the production of antibody to sRBC, a T-dependent antigen.[29] The immunostimulatory effect was positively correlated with increased production of IL1 but not of IL2. In zinc-supplemented cultures (200 μmol Zn/L), activation with Con A enhanced T-cell production of B-cell–stimulating factor, which promotes antibody formation.[30] In vitro zinc supplementation was most effective within the first 24 h of stimulation of cells and was inhibitory if supplemented later. These results demonstrate that in vitro techniques have limited capacity and may not be relevant to the in vivo situation.

Measurements of zinc and immune status in unsupplemented elderly patients were evaluated by Bogden et al.[31] Dietary zinc was below the RDA in 90% of 100 elderly subjects tested. Delayed hypersensitivity response to seven skin antigens was nonexistent in 41% of the subjects and correlated highly with plasma zinc concentration. Because humoral and cell-mediated immune responses are depressed during zinc deficiency, zinc status may play a significant role in decreased immunocompetence and increased infectious illness of elderly people.

Iron

Much has been learned about iron deficiency and immune response in recent years, but some conflicting conclusions are readily apparent in the literature. Some of the conflicting literature is explained by variation in methodologies, differences in subject populations studied, and presence of other health and nutritional problems.

In 20 South African children with iron deficiency anemia, baseline concentrations of serum immunoglobulin and salivary IgA concentrations were normal and adequate antibody was produced in tetanus-toxoid stimulation.[32] The concentration of serum complement was within the normal range. Total lymphocyte number and subcutaneous delayed hypersensitivity were decreased whereas opsonization was normal.

Neutrophils of iron-deficient children did not show abnormal bactericidal metabolism by measurements of nitroblue tetrazolium (NBT) dye reduction, although bactericidal capacity and chemotactic activity of neutrophils were decreased.[32] NBT dye reduction reflects the capacity of phagocytes to generate an oxidative burst, which is a prerequisite to phagocytic killing and is dependent on the iron-containing cytochrome b. In contrast, Chandra[33] found that NBT dye reduction decreased in neutrophils of 12 Indian children aged 1–8 y with iron-deficiency anemia and normal serum vitamin B-12 and folate concentrations. Bactericidal capacity also decreased. However, opsonic activity and phagocytic engulfment were similar between the iron-deficient and age-matched control groups. Parenteral repletion with iron for 4–7 d normalized the oxidative burst capacity.[33] In another study, when 50 children with iron-deficiency anemia who were not malnourished and were not infectious were tested, the magnitude of the oxidative burst was unaltered when determined by NBT dye reduction assay but decreased when determined by hexose-monophosphate-shunt activity, a more quantitative assay than the NBT dye reduction assay.[34] Bactericidal capacity also decreased.[34] Kochanowski and Sherman[35] showed that phagocytic activity decreased in neonatal iron-deficient rats as indicated by NBT reduction, whereas the percentage of phagocytes in peripheral blood increased. This finding suggests that in iron deficiency there is a population of dysfunctional phagocytes. In 10 Chilean infants aged 6–23 mo with iron-deficiency anemia and no infectious illness or PCM, phagocytosis was unimpaired but bactericidal capacity decreased.[36] Oral repletion with a ferrous sulfate–ascorbic acid preparation did not restore bactericidal capacity in 3–4 d. However, bactericidal capacity returned to normal in 15 d, suggesting that iron is required during maturation of neutrophils.

The capacity of neutrophils to kill bacteria is decreased in iron deficiency and repletion of iron corrects neutrophil function. Myeloperoxidase, an iron-containing enzyme that destroys certain organisms by oxidative mechanisms, was either normal[34] or decreased[37] in iron deficiency. Defective myeloperoxidase may contribute to the defect in bactericidal capacity of phagocytes during iron deficiency.

With respect to humoral immunity, iron-deficient children demonstrated normal or elevated basal and stimulated antibody response to diphtheria and tetanus-toxoid antigen with no increase in number of B lymphocytes.[38] This finding suggests that production of antibodies to specific antigens may not be impaired. In contrast, when antibody formation to a specific antigenic challenge of sRBC was measured using the highly sensitive plaque assay in a neonatal rat model where iron was the only variable, antibody production was decreased in pups whose dams were fed an iron-deficient diet throughout gestation and lactation.[39] Dietary repletion of pups improved iron status but did not significantly increase IgM and IgG antibody production. Maternal iron deficiency resulted in irreversible impairment of humoral immunity even after short-term repletion that repaired iron deficiency completely. Discrepancy in these findings may be due to the different species, children vs. rat pups, or the dependence of B-cell response to sRBC on T helper cells and the independence of B-cell response to tetanus toxoid on T helper cells. Iron deficiency appears to have a detrimental effect on T-helper-cell function.

Cellular immunity is impaired in animals and humans during iron deficiency. Cellularity of key immune tissues, such as spleen and thymus, was found to be markedly decreased in iron-deficient neonatal rats[40] and is not easily repaired by iron repletion.[39] These observations provide a possible explanation for impaired cell-mediated immunity reported in iron deficiency. Splenic lymphocytes from mice with iron-deficiency anemia showed decreased T-cell blastogenic response to Con A and PHA and decreased B-cell blastogenic response to LPS.[41] Dietary repletion with iron restored the blastogenic response to normal within 10 d. Lymphocytes from humans with iron-deficiency anemia[42] or with iron-deficiency anemia and rheumatoid arthritis[43] show a decreased blastogenic response upon stimulation with phytomitogens. Blastogenic response to PHA and *Candida* was below normal in iron-deficient children.[32,44] Studies by Joynson et al.[45] confirmed the decreased lymphocyte transformation and depressed delayed hypersensitivity response in 12 adults with iron-deficiency anemia. An investigation of anemic pregnant women in their third trimester showed decreased percentage of B and T lymphocytes, unchanged PHA-induced T-lymphocyte transformation, and significantly elevated serum IgG concentration.[46] The decreased response of T cells to PHA stimulation in children but not in pregnant women may be due to the already depressed T-cell response present in pregnant women. Complications of iron-deficiency anemia during pregnancy may not further influence or decrease T-cell blastogenic response. Iron is required as a cofactor for ribonucleotide reductase, which is necessary for DNA synthesis. Decreased proliferation may be due to a reduction in ribonucleotide reductase activity causing decreased DNA synthesis. In addition, iron could be essential for the differentiation of a common precursor cell. Further study is required to define the mechanism whereby iron impairs blastogenesis of T and B cells.

Decreased NK-cell cytotoxicity towards the YAC-1 tumor cell line was reported in 21-d-old rat pups whose dams were fed an iron-deficient diet throughout gestation and lactation.[47] In response to in vivo stimulation by allogenic tumor cells, spleen and peritoneal cells of 61-d-old mice with iron deficiency showed decreased capacity to kill tumor cells in vitro.[48] It was speculated that iron deficiency causes decreased sensitivity of effector cells, decreased number of effector cells that are capable of becoming cytotoxic, and/or decreased functional capacity of effector cells to kill once activated.

Alterations in immune mediators may cause some

of the decrease in humoral and cell-mediated immunity. Decreased production of macrophage inhibitory factor was demonstrated in adults with iron-deficiency anemia.[45]

Interferon is a cytokine produced by macrophages that activates the cytolytic response of NK cells toward tumor cells or virus-infected cells. When interferon was added in vitro to NK cells of vaccinia-virus–stimulated rat pups whose dams were fed an iron-deficient diet throughout gestation and lactation, NK-cell cytotoxicity was not restored to control values.[49] Unstimulated NK cells from postweaning rat pups fed an iron-deficient diet for 6 wk were able to respond to added allogenic macrophage-produced interferon, but NK-cell cytotoxicity was not increased to control values.[50] Considering these data, it appears that the functional capacity of interferon as a mediator of cellular immunity is altered during iron deficiency.

IL1 production by iron-deficient rat peritoneal cells is impaired.[51] IL1 is produced by activated macrophages, causes a febrile response, and intensifies the activity of T helper cells to produce IL2. IL2 along with mitogens increased transferrin receptor expression on the surface of T cells and enhanced the blastogenic response of T cells.[52] If IL1 was decreased during iron deficiency, possibly IL2 was decreased, because IL1 causes T cells to produce IL2, and abnormal cellular immunologic responses occurred.

Transferrin is the primary carrier protein for iron in the serum. Transferrin receptors are expressed on macrophages at different stages of immunologic activation.[53] The role of transferrin receptor in immunity is an unknown piece in the puzzling effects of iron deficiency on immune function.

Iron overload also has been associated with altered immune function although only a few definitive studies have been undertaken in this area. Occasional reports that repletion with iron supplements was associated with infection and death in malnourished children have appeared. In 1970, 13 of 40 children between the ages of 1–5 y died during iron and protein repletion.[54] In 71 iron-deficient adult Somali nomads, daily doses of 900 mg oral ferrous sulfate for 1 mo caused increased infectious diseases, including malaria, brucellosis, and tuberculosis, when compared with 67 iron-deficient Somali nomads fed a placebo.[55] However, iron overload during chronic iron-overload diseases, such as idiopathic hemachromatosis, sickle cell anemia, and thalassemia, has not been directly implicated in increased risk of infection in humans.[56]

In one recent study of iron-overloaded patients undergoing dialysis, phagocytosis and killing capacity of blood neutrophils were reduced.[57] Reduced function of neutrophils and increased virulence of *Yersinia enterocolitica* with iron overload both contribute to high frequency of *Yersinia* infections.

Hyperferremia with increased transferrin saturation along with granulocytopenia and fever was demonstrated in cancer patients 1–15 d after chemotherapy.[58] Increased transferrin saturation was associated with increased in vitro growth of *Escherichia coli* and *Staphylococcus aureus* in culture media when fresh serum that was 95% iron-saturated transferrin from human volunteers was added.[58]

NK-cell cytotoxicity against K562 target cells decreased in patients with β-thalassemia major who were iron overloaded as a consequence of chronic transfusion therapy.[59] Therefore, natural immunity against tumors can be altered by iron overload.

Considerable evidence has accumulated showing that iron deficiency impairs humoral and cellular immune responses, leading to increased susceptibility to infection. Altered immune function sometimes but not always can be repaired with iron treatment to improve iron status. On the other side of the spectrum, iron overload also impairs immune responses and may be responsible for some disease processes. The mechanism for this apparent paradox is not known. Additional research is needed to elucidate the specific roles of iron in the immune response.

Copper

It has been demonstrated that copper deficiency depresses the immune system, but the exact biochemical roles of copper in immunity have not been delineated. A variety of immune functions were assessed by Koller et al.[60] to measure immune function in copper deficiency. When copper was omitted from the diet of rats 8 wk postweaning, thymus weight, IgG production in response to keyhole limpet hemocyanin (KLH) antigen, and NK-cell cytotoxicity decreased.[60] Dietary copper amount did not significantly affect delayed hypersensitivity response nor level of prostaglandin E_2 (PGE_2),[60] which plays a role in immunoregulation. Decreased thymus weight also did not significantly affect the delayed hypersensitivity measurement of T-cell function. Because KLH is a T-cell–dependent antigen, impaired function of either B cells or T helper cells could have decreased antibody titer. Decreased NK-cell activity may explain in part the increased incidence of extrahepatic tumors seen in rats fed a copper-deficient diet (1 mg Cu/kg diet) as compared with rats fed excess copper (800 mg Cu/kg diet) and treated with the carcinogens acetylaminofluorene and dimethylnitrosamine.[61] Decreased NK-cell activity was not due to the immunosuppressive effects of PGE_2.

In a study to determine the copper requirement of mice, pups from dams that received diets severely or marginally deficient in copper (0.5, 1, 2, or 6 mg Cu/kg diet) were weaned to their dam's diet at age 4 wk and killed at age 8 wk.[62] Diets containing ≤1 mg Cu/kg diet caused thymic atrophy, splenomegaly, and cardiomegaly. Males were more severely affected than females. Spleen cells of the copper-depleted groups responded less to LPS injection than did the control group. A dose-related reduction in splenic T-cell subpopulations was noted in the 0.5 and 1.0 mg Zn/kg diet groups.

Copper supplementation in species at risk appears to enhance immunocompetence. Scottish Blackface lambs, which have a genetic tendency towards low copper status, were more susceptible to bacterial infections causing increased mortality.[63] Copper supplementation in lambs at age 6 wk increased survival rates. Copper supplementation markedly reduced incidence of lower respiratory tract infection in infants recovering from marasmus with associated copper deficiency.[64] Supplementation with copper was suggested when infants were refed with a milk-based diet during recovery from marasmus.

Selenium

Selenium functions as a cofactor of glutathione peroxidase (GPx), an enzyme involved in cellular antioxidation. Selenium deficiency results in suppressed humoral and cell-mediated immune responses. Selenium was found to be required in the synthesis of lipoxygenase-derived eicosanoids, such as leukotrienes.[65]

GPx protects the phagocytic function of neutrophils from peroxide damage. Selenium deficiency results in decreased GPx activity and increased release of hydrogen peroxide in rat granulocytes caused by the inability of GPx-deficient granulocytes to metabolize hydrogen peroxide.[66] The inability to metabolize hydrogen peroxide results in destruction of the superoxide-generating system as demonstrated by an inability of the superoxide-generation system to stimulate the hexose monophosphate shunt.[67] The oxidative burst and superoxide-generating system that are necessary for the cytotoxic function of neutrophils was decreased in rats fed a selenium-deficient diet for 12–15 wk.[67] Phagocytosis of yeast by neutrophils of rats fed a selenium-deficient diet for 5 wk was not altered but fungicidal capacity decreased.[68]

Selenium deficiency also affects antibody production. IgG but not IgM titers to sRBC antigen decreased in mice fed a selenium-deficient diet for 4 wk. A selenium-deficient diet during gestation, lactation, and 4 wk postweaning resulted in reduced IgM and IgG

titers to sRBC in mice.[69] Taken together these data suggested that first-generation selenium deficiency resulted in decreased secondary antibody response and second-generation selenium deficiency resulted in decreased primary and secondary antibody response.

Selenium supplementation was found to have an immunostimulatory effect. Selenium supplementation in drinking water (2.5 mg/L ad libitum) of mice during malaria vaccination conferred a significantly higher survival rate when mice were challenged with *Plasmodium berghei*.[70] IgM but not IgG titers in response to sRBC antigen increased in growing mice fed diet supplemented with selenium,[71] although the increase was not as great in 247-day-old mice.[72] An increased number of antibody-forming cells seen in mice fed supplemental selenium for 10 wk may cause increased antibody titers.[73] Low levels of selenium supplementation did not increase antibody titers to salmonella vaccine, and high levels of selenium supplementation increased antibody titers only slightly.[74] Selenium-deficient lambs responded with increased GPx activity to low levels of supplemental selenium (5 mg selenium) or high levels of supplemental selenium (50 mg selenium) when selenium was injected subcutaneously.[74]

Experimental evidence suggests that low-level selenium supplementation has an antitumor effect. Ten weeks of low-level selenium supplementation (0.5 or 2.0 μg/L) in drinking water resulted in enhanced NK-cell cytotoxicity in rats, whereas high-level selenium supplementation (5.0 μg/L) in drinking water did not.[75,76]

Alterations in the production of soluble mediators of the immune response have resulted from selenium supplementation. In vitro supplementation of low amounts of selenium (0.1–10 μmol/L sodium selenite, sodium selenate, or selenium dioxide) increased production of interferon by human peripheral lymphocytes, and in vitro supplementation of high amounts of selenium (0.1 mmol/L) decreased production of interferon by human peripheral lymphocytes.[77] After drinking water of rats was supplemented with 0.5, 2.0, or 5.0 μg/L selenium for 10 wk, in vitro production of PGE_2 by rat peritoneal macrophages was reduced, although production of IL1 was not altered.[75] The immunostimulatory effects of supplemental selenium could be due to the protection of cellular integrity by preserving the function of GPx as an antioxidant.

GPx and vitamin E both function as antioxidants, and a combined selenium–vitamin E deficiency alters immunologic responses. In rats fed diets deficient in selenium and vitamin E for 5 wk, resistance to bacterial challenge was decreased as demonstrated by increased mortality and reduced GPx activity.[78] Rats fed a selenium-deficient diet for 4–6 wk demonstrated lower GPx activity of peritoneal neutrophils, peritoneal macrophages, and alveolar macrophages.[79] When these rats were fed diets deficient in selenium and α-tocopherol, higher GPx activity was seen in peritoneal neutrophils and peritoneal macrophages. However no greater activity was observed in alveolar macrophages than that caused by selenium deficiency alone.

Selenium–vitamin E deficiency also alters cell-mediated immunity. Decreased blastogenic response to B- and T-cell mitogens including Con A, PHA, pokeweed mitogen, streptolysin O, and LPS was found in lymphocytes from dogs, mice, and rats fed diets deficient in selenium and vitamin E.[80-82] Mice fed selenium- and/or vitamin E–deficient diets for 8 wk showed decreased cytotoxic function of NK cells against tumor cells; antibody-dependent cell-mediated cytotoxicity was unaltered by either or both deficiencies.[83]

Vitamin E

Vitamin E deficiency has not been reported in humans except in premature infants placed in an oxidative environment to enhance respiration. Supplemental vitamin E, between 50 and 200 mg α-tocopherol/kg diet, was reported to be immunostimulatory. Immunostimulation by vitamin E may be related to the effects of vitamin E as an antioxidant in the protection of cell membrane integrity.

The amount of dietary vitamin E needed to provide optimal immune response of T- and B-cell blastogenesis was greater than the amount of vitamin E needed for other measured responses of vitamin E status, such as body and organ weight gain, prevention of muscle myopathy, and prevention of red blood cell hemolysis.[84] Weanling spontaneously hypertensive rats were fed diets containing 0, 7.5, 15, 50, 200, and 1000 mg all-rac-α-tocopheryl acetate/kg diet for 8–10 wk. As dietary tocopherol increased so did concentrations of tocopherol in plasma and testes. Elevated plasma pyruvate kinase concentrations, indicating muscle degeneration, were prevented with 15 mg tocopherol/kg diet. Peroxidative hemolysis of red blood cells was prevented with 50 mg tocopherol/kg diet. Elevated platelet count was reduced by 200 mg tocopherol/kg diet. Stimulation of proliferation of splenic lymphocytes by the B-cell mitogen, LPS, and the T-cell mitogens, Con A and PHA, was maximal when dietary tocopherol was between 50 and 200 mg tocopherol/kg diet. Feeding 1000 mg tocopherol/kg diet did not further stimulate the proliferation of lymphocytes.[84] A different ex-

perimental approach of daily intraperitoneal injection with increasing amounts of all-rac-α-tocopherol in 7–10-wk-old mice increased B- and T-lymphocyte proliferation in response to Con A, PHA, and LPS. The B- and T-cell proliferative responses were inhibited when the dose injected became equivalent to 280–560 mg tocopherol/kg diet.[85]

Humoral response to vitamin E supplementation was studied in lambs to determine causes of livestock diseases. All-rac-α-tocopheryl acetate was fed at 33, 121, 276, 396, or 496 mg tocopherol/kg diet for 3 wk before primary immunization with KLH antigen.[86] Secondary immunization was done 3 wk after primary immunization. At the highest amount of dietary tocopherol, KLH increased antibody titer after primary immunization but not after secondary immunization.

In 10 patients on maintenance hemodialysis, peripheral blood mononuclear cells (PBMC) were deficient in vitamin E and showed increased membrane lipid peroxidation.[87] Fifteen days of parenteral supplementation with 300 mg α-tocopheryl acetate resulted in less lipid peroxidation, although no increase was seen in vitamin E concentrations of PBMC. NK-cell cytotoxicity and blastogenesis of PBMC to PHA were not influenced by treatment with vitamin E. These results are intriguing because cytotoxicity and blastogenesis are both dependent on cell membrane integrity. T-helper-cell number was unchanged by vitamin E treatment. However, T suppressor and T cytotoxic cell number decreased after vitamin E supplementation.[87]

To investigate the effects of supplemental vitamin E on phagocytosis and cell-mediated immunity, men and boys were supplemented with daily megadoses of 300 mg dl-α-tocopheryl acetate for 3 wk.[88] Decreased bactericidal activity of leukocytes and mitogen-induced lymphocyte proliferation were found, but delayed hypersensitivity was not affected by high concentrations of vitamin E.

One hypothesis for the mechanism of action of vitamin E in immunostimulation is that vitamin E inhibits prostaglandin synthesis. Prostaglandins are immunosuppressive especially toward T-cell activity. As the amount of dietary vitamin E was increased, the normal suppression of T-cell function was removed because of decreased prostaglandin synthesis.[89] For example, aged (24 mo) and young (3 mo) mice were fed a diet containing 30 or 500 mg dl-α-tocopheryl acetate/kg diet for 6 wk. Vitamin E supplementation enhanced delayed hypersensitivity to dinitrofluorobenzene and blastogenic response to Con A and LPS in aged mice. Aged mice supplemented with vitamin E had lower concentrations of PGE_2 than did young or old control mice.[89] Therefore, enhancement of immune response by vitamin E appeared to be mediated by suppression of PGE$_2$ synthesis. Vitamin E supplementation also increased the normally diminished IL2 activity seen in aged mice.

In summary, supplemental amounts of vitamin E appear to have stimulatory effects on a number of immune responses studied experimentally. The role of vitamin E in immunity as an antioxidant and on modulation of the immune response by eicosanoids and lymphokines needs further exploration. In addition, the pharmacological use of vitamin E requires more study.

Vitamin A and Carotenoids

The involvement of β-carotene and vitamin A in the initiation and progression of cancer and on immunological indices has been investigated. Effects of dietary vitamin A on immune function also have been investigated.

Carotenoids appear to have effects on immunity separate from vitamin A effects. In rats fed diets containing supplemental (20 mg/g) β-carotene or another carotenoid, canthaxanthin, for up to 66 wk, blastogenic responses of T and B lymphocytes to Con A, PHA, and LPS increased.[90] Because canthaxanthin cannot be converted to vitamin A, enhancement of immune response was attributed to a carotenoid effect.

β-carotene or its retinol derivatives also can be effective in immunity against tumors. When male rats were fed 0 or 100 mg β-carotene or retinoic acid/kg diet for 22 wk postinjection into salivary glands with dimethylbenzanthracene, the incidence in salivary gland tumors was reduced in rats fed β-carotene.[91] Retinoic acid had no effect on tumor incidence. When BALB/c mice were fed 120 μg β-carotene/d for 9 d and 10^7 BALB/c Meth A fibrosarcoma cells were implanted subcutaneously, the syngeneic tumor was rejected compared with tumors in unsupplemented controls.[92] However, when 10^7 BALB/c Meth 1 fibrosarcoma cells were implanted subcutaneously under the same conditions, there was no significant difference in rejection between β-carotene–supplemented rats and unsupplemented controls, suggesting that rejection of tumors may be specific to tumor antigens.

Smith and Hayes[93] investigated the effects of vitamin A deficiency on humoral immune responses. Mice were fed a vitamin A–deficient diet from weaning to age 6 or 8 wk and were tested for immunoglobulin response to KLH antigen. IgG1 and IgG3 titers were severely diminished at both ages. IgM was not yet affected at age 6 wk; however, vitamin A–deficient mice produced 30% less IgM at age 8 wk

compared with controls. Decreased antibody titers were attributed to decreased number of plasma cells producing antibody because the rate of antibody production per cell was not affected by dietary vitamin A. The authors hypothesized that vitamin A deficiency decreased the response of T helper cells, thereby decreasing secretion of interleukins that promote clonal expansion of B cells and intensify the immune response.

Cellular immunity and resistance to tumors are altered in mice supplemented with retinal palmitate.[94] Proliferative response to Con A and LPS increased with increasing doses of retinyl palmitate up to 150 d of treatment. IL2 and interferon released in response to stimulation with Con A increased with increasing dose of retinyl palmitate up to day 150 of treatment. Tumor rejection increased when three types of transplantable tumors were introduced to mice on days 75 and 150 of treatment, demonstrating that vitamin A has an antitumorigenic effect.

The cell surface is considered the primary target for phenotypic expression of carcinogenesis and can be monitored by lectin-induced agglutination. Vitamin A and vitamin A analogues reduced in vitro Con A-induced agglutination of human erythrocytes by direct action on the cell membrane.[95]

Because vitamin A was shown to inhibit the growth and development of neoplastic cells, much work has been done with NK-cell activity in response to dietary vitamin A concentrations. NK-cell activity is increased in wild-type BALB/c mice after intragastric feedings of 20 μg retinyl palmitate/d; however, athymic BALB/c nu/nu (nude) mice exhibited no change in NK-cell activity in response to vitamin A supplementation.[96] Because nude mice do not have T cells, the results suggested that vitamin A affected T-helper-cell function with respect to NK-cell activation. Dietary supplementation with retinyl palmitate (0, 200, 500, and 1000 IU/d) showed a dose-dependent increase in NK-cell activity after 50 d of supplementation.[97] An increase in the number of splenic large granular lymphocytes, a population of cells that includes NK cells, also was found.[97]

Macrophages have cytotoxic capability in destroying tumors. Watson et al.[98] demonstrated that treatment of adult BALB/c mice with retinyl palmitate during tumor promotion increased the number and cytotoxic capacity of macrophages in response to initiation of mammary tumor by dimethylbenzanthracene and promotion of tumors by tetradecanoylphorbol acetate.[98]

To date, considerable evidence has accumulated showing that vitamin A deficiency decreased antibody response, whereas vitamin A supplementation increased proliferative and cytotoxic responses to T cells, NK cells, and macrophages. Further research on the mechanisms by which vitamin A alters immunocompetence is needed.

Vitamin C

Ascorbic acid is an antioxidant or free-radical scavenger and may have effects on immune function similar to those of selenium and vitamin E. However, the antioxidant effects of vitamin C on immunity have not been investigated. Ascorbic acid has been investigated with respect to other aspects of immune function.

Vitamin C deficiency had no effect on blastogenic response of T cells to PHA, and percentage of T helper cells and percentage of T suppressor cells were similar in human volunteers.[99] Vitamin C deficiency also did not impair blastogenic response of B cells to LPS or of T cells to Con A in guinea pigs fed a diet containing 0.2 g/kg as compared with guinea pigs fed a diet containing 10.0 g/kg.[100]

In the presence of serum complement, specifically C'3, carrier-mediated active transport of ascorbic acid was inhibited.[101] Metabolic consequences of reduced ascorbate transport inhibition are unknown. However, in disease states where the complement system is activated, cells may not acquire enough vitamin C for normal functioning.

Supplemental vitamin C does not affect humoral immunity, but it does enhance cell-mediated immunity. Young adult mice that were immunized with sRBC antigen after 9–67 d supplementation with ascorbic acid showed anti-sRBC antibody production similar to that of unsupplemented mice.[102] In the same mice, blastogenic response to LPS, a B-cell mitogen, was not significantly different, but blastogenic response to Con A, a T-cell mitogen, was increased in mice fed supplemental vitamin C.[102] In human volunteers fed large doses of ascorbic acid, concentrations of IgG, IgM, IgA, C'3, and C'4 in the serum were unchanged.[103] However, T-cell blastogenic response to Con A and PHA was increased in blood lymphocytes.

When vitamin C was added in vitro to PHA- or Con A-stimulated cultures of human peripheral lymphocytes, a dose-dependent inhibitory effect was seen.[104] The greatest inhibition occurred as ascorbic acid or dehydroascorbic acid concentrations increased from 0.5 to 5.0 mmol/L. Physiological concentration of ascorbic acid in leukocytes is 1–3 mmol/L.

To determine if ascorbic acid supplementation has an immunostimulatory effect on human cells exposed to influenza virus, responsiveness of peripheral blood monocytes and macrophages to PHA was tested. Influenza virus depressed blastogenic response of monocytes and macrophages to PHA.[105] Ascorbic acid added in vitro enhanced blastogenic response of monocytes and macrophages to PHA and counteracted the depressed blastogenic response of cells exposed to influenza virus. Increased responsiveness of cellular immunity may underlie the decreased symptoms and severity of the common cold seen during vitamin C supplementation.

Vitamin C is known to detoxify histamine. Because histamine has immunosuppressive effects on the immune system by activating T suppressor cells, addition of ascorbic acid may enhance immune responses. Oh and Nakano[106] found that low concentrations of ascorbic acid added in vitro enhanced Con A-dependent lymphocyte blastogenesis by inhibiting histidine decarboxylase and, therefore, the production of histamine.

Because vitamin C is commonly taken as a supplement by individuals seeking protection from colds, investigation of the effects of vitamin C on immune function needs further study.

Conclusion

Study of nutritional status and the immune response is very new, and our understanding of the mechanisms involved is far from complete. For each of the nutrients reviewed, evidence has accumulated that dietary alterations in the nutrient alters immunity and/or susceptibility to infection and/or cancer. What is still in its infancy is elucidation of how the nutrient is functioning in immunity. Whether immune function requires heretofore unrecognized roles for nutrients at the molecular-biochemical level remains to be determined.

References

1. R.K. Chandra (1979) T and B lymphocytes and leukocyte terminal deoxynucleotide-transferase in energy-protein malnutrition. *Acta Pediatr. Scand.* 68:841–845.
2. B.R. Bristrian, M. Sherman, G.L. Blackburn, R. Marshall, and C. Shaw (1977) Cellular immunity in adult marasmus. *Arch. Intern. Med.* 137:1408–1411.
3. G.T. Keush, S.D. Douglas, G. Hammer, and K. Braden (1978) Antibacterial function of macrophages in experimental protein-calorie malnutrition. II. Cellular and humoral factors for chemotaxis, phagocytosis, and intracellular bactericidal activity. *J. Infect. Dis.* 138:134–142.
4. J.H. Paswell, M.W. Steward, and J.F. Soothill (1974) The effects of protein malnutrition on macrophage function and the amount and affinity of antibody response. *Clin. Exp. Immunol.* 17:491–495.
5. K. Shopfer and S.D. Douglas (1976) Neutrophil function in children with kwashiorkor. *J. Lab. Clin. Med.* 88:450–461.
6. P. Price and R.G. Bell (1976) The response of protein-deficient mice to tetanus toxoid: effects of antigen dose, adjuvants, period

of deprovation and age on antibody production. *Immunology* 31:953–956.

7. P. Price and R.G. Bell (1977) The effects of nutritional rehabilitation on antibody production in protein-deficient mice. *Immunology* 32:65–74.

8. R.K. Chandra, S. Chandra, and S. Gupta (1984) Antibody affinity and immune complexes after immunization with tetanus toxoid in protein-energy malnutrition. *Am. J. Clin. Nutr.* 40:131–134.

9. B.R. Kirkwood and H.M. Gilles (1986) The immune response to vaccination in undernourished and well-nourished Nigerian children. *Ann. Trop. Med. Parasitol.* 80:537–544.

10. S.M. Filteau, E. Berdusco, K.J. Perry, and B. Woodward (1987) The effect of triiodothyronine on evanescent delayed hypersensitivity to sheep red blood cells and on the primary antibody response to trinitrophenylated *Brucella abortus* in severely undernourished weanling mice. *Int. J. Immunopharmacol.* 9:811–816.

11. D.K. Law, S.J. Dudrick, and N.I. Abdou (1973) Effects of nutrition repletion. *Ann. Intern. Med.* 79:545–550.

12. R.A. Keenan, L.L. Moldawer, R.D. Yang, I. Kawamura, G.L. Blackburn, and B.R. Bistrain (1982) An altered response by peritoneal leukocytes to synthesize or release leukocyte endogenous mediator in critically ill, protein-malnourished patients. *J. Lab. Clin. Med.* 100:844–857.

13. A.S. Prasad (1984) Discovery and importance of zinc in human nutrition. *Fed. Proc.* 43:2829–2834.

14. M.J. Bunk, J.E. Galvin, Y. Young, A.M. Dnistrian, and W.S. Blaner (1987) Relationship of cytotoxic activity of natural killer cells to growth rates and serum zinc levels of female RIII mice fed zinc. *Nutr. Cancer* 10:79–87.

15. R.K. Chandra (1980) Acrodermatitis enteropathica: zinc levels and cell-mediated immunity. *Pediatrics* 66:789–791.

16. P.J. Fraker, K. Hildebrandt, and R.W. Luecke (1984) Alteration of antibody mediated responses of suckling mice to T-cell-dependent and independent antigens by maternal marginal zinc deficiency: restoration of responsivity by nutritional repletion. *J. Nutr.* 114:170–179.

17. P.J. Fraker, S.M. Haas, and R.W. Luecke (1977) Effect of zinc deficiency on the immune response of the young adult A/J mouse. *J. Nutr.* 107:1889–1895.

18. P.J. Fraker, M.E. Gershwin, R.A. Good, and A. Prasad (1986) Interrelationships between zinc and immune function. *Fed. Proc.* 45:1474–1479.

19. P.J. Fraker, P. DePasquale-Jardieu, C.M. Zwickl, and R.W. Luecke (1978) Regeneration of T-helper cell function in zinc-deficient adult mice. *Proc. Natl. Acad. Sci. USA* 75:5660–5664.

20. P.J. Fraker, C.M. Zwickl, and R.W. Luecke (1982) Delayed type hypersensitivity in zinc deficient adult mice: impairment and restoration of responsivity to dinitrofluorobenzene. *J. Nutr.* 112:309–313.

21. S.J. James, M. Swendseid, and T. Makinodan (1987) Macrophage-mediated depression of T-cell proliferation in zinc-deficient mice. *J. Nutr.* 117:1982–1988.

22. J.I. Allen, R.T. Perri, C.J. McClain, and N.E. Kay (1983) Alterations in human natural killer cell activity and monocyte cytotoxicity induced by zinc deficiency. *J. Lab. Clin. Med.* 102:577–589.

23. G. Fernandes, M. Nair, K. Onoe, T. Tanaka, R. Floyd, and R.A. Good (1979) Impairment of cell-mediated immunity functions by dietary zinc deficiency in mice. *Proc. Natl. Acad. Sci. USA* 76:457–461.

24. P.J. Fraker, R. Caruso, and F. Kierszenvaum (1982) Alteration of the immune and nutritional status of mice by synergy between zinc deficiency and infection with *Trypanosoma cruzi. J. Nutr.* 112:1224–1229.

25. S.J. Weiss and A.F. LoBuglio (1982) Biology of disease: phago-cyte-generated oxygen metabolites and cellular injury. *Lab. Invest.* 47:5–17.

26. P. DePasquale-Jardieu and P.J. Fraker (1984) Interference in the development of a secondary immune response in mice by zinc deprivation: persistence of effect. *J. Nutr.* 114:1762–1769.

27. R.S. Beach, M.E. Gershwin, and L.S. Hurley (1982) Gestational zinc deprivation in mice: persistence of immunodeficiency for three generations. *Science* 218:469–471.

28. R.A. Winchurch (1988) Activation of thymocyte responses to interleukin 1 by zinc. *Clin. Immunol. Immunopathol.* 47:174–180.

29. R.A. Winchurch, J. Togo, and W.H. Alder (1987) Supplemental zinc ($Zn+^2$) restores antibody formation in cultures of aged spleen cells. II. Effect on mediator production. *Eur. J. Immunol.* 17:127–132.

30. C.L. Reardon and D.O. Lucas (1987) Heavy-metal mitogenesis: Zn^{++} and Hg^{++} induce cellular cytotoxicity and interferon production in murine T lymphocytes. *Immunobiology* 175:455–469.

31. L.D. Bogden, J.M. Oleske, E.M. Munves, et al. (1987) Zinc and immunocompetence in the elderly: baseline data on zinc nutriture and immunity in unsupplemented subjects. *Am. J. Clin. Nutr.* 46:101–109.

32. L.G. MacDougall, R. Anderson, G.M. McNab, and J. Katz (1975) The immune response in iron-deficient children: impaired cellular defense mechanisms with altered humoral components. *J. Pediatr.* 86:833–843.

33. R.K. Chandra (1973) Reduced bactericidal capacity of poly-morphs in iron deficiency. *Arch. Dis. Child.* 48:864–866.

34. S. Yetgin, C. Altay, G. Ciliv, and Y. Laleli (1979) Myeloperoxidase activity and bactericidal function of PMN in iron deficiency. *Acta Haematol.* 61:10–14.

35. B.A. Kochanowski and A.R. Sherman (1984) Phagocytosis and lysozyme activity in granulocytes from iron-deficient rat dams and pups. *Nutr. Res.* 4:511–520.

36. T. Walter, S. Arredondo, M. Arevalo, and A. Stekel (1986) Effect of iron therapy on phagocytosis and bactericidal activity in neutrophils of iron-deficient infants. *Am. J. Clin. Nutr.* 44:877–882.

37. J.S. Prasad (1979) Leukocyte function in iron-deficiency anemia. *Am. J. Clin. Nutr.* 32:550–552.

38. K. Bagchi, M. Mohanram, and V. Reddy (1980) Humoral immune response in children with iron-deficiency anaemia. *Br. Med. J.* 280:1249–1251.

39. B.A. Kochanowski and A.R. Sherman (1985) Decreased antibody formation in iron-deficient rat pups—effect of iron repletion. *Am. J. Clin. Nutr.* 41:278–284.

40. B.A. Kochanowski and A.R. Sherman (1982) Cellular growth in iron-deficient rat pups. *Growth* 46:126–134.

41. S. Kubividila, K.M. Nauss, S. Baliga, and R.M. Suskind (1983) Impairment of blastogenic response of splenic lymphocytes from iron-deficient mice: in vivo repletion. *Am. J. Clin. Nutr.* 37:15–25.

42. B. Sawitsky, R. Kanter, and A. Sawitsky (1976) Lymphocyte response to phytomitogens in iron deficiency. *Am. J. Med. Sci.* 272:153–160.

43. R.J. Polson, A. Bombford, H. Berry, and R. Williams (1988) Phytohemagglutinin induced proliferation of lymphocytes from patients with rheumatoid arthritis and iron deficiency. *Ann. Rheum. Dis.* 47:570–575.

44. R.K. Chandra and A.K. Saraya (1975) Impaired immunocompetence associated with iron deficiency. *J. Pediatr.* 86:899–902.

45. D.H.M. Joynson, D.M. Walker, A. Jacobs, and A.E. Dolby (1972) Defect of cell-mediated immunity in patients with iron deficiency anaemia. *Lancet* 2:1058–1059.

46. K. Prema, B.A. Ramalakshmi, E. Madhavapeddi, and S. Babu (1982) Immune status of anaemic pregnant women. *Br. J. Obstet. Gynaecol.* 89:222–225.

47. A.R. Sherman and J.F. Lockwood (1987) Impaired natural killer cell activity in iron-deficient rat pups. *J. Nutr.* 117:567–571.

48. S.R. Kuvibidila, B.S. Baliga, and R.M. Suskind (1983) The effect of iron-deficiency anemia in cytolytic activity of mice spleen and peritoneal cells against allogenic tumor cells. *Am. J. Clin. Nutr.* 38:238–244.

49. J.F. Lockwood and A.R. Sherman (1988) Spleen natural killer cells from iron-deficient rat pups manifest an altered ability to be stimulated by interferon. *J. Nutr.* 118:1558–1563.

50. N.A. Hallquist and A.R. Sherman (1989) Effect of iron deficiency on the stimulation of natural killer cells by macrophage-produced interferon. *Nutr. Res.* 9:283–292.

51. L. Helyar and A.R. Sherman (1987) Iron deficiency and interleukin 1 production by rat leukocytes. *Am. J. Clin. Nutr.* 46:346–352.

52. E. Pelosi-Testa, P. Samoggia, G. Giannella, et al. (1988) Mechanisms underlying T-lymphocyte activation: mitogen initiates and IL-2 amplifies the expression of receptors via intracellular iron level. *Immunology* 64:273–279.

53. T.A. Hamilton, J.E. Weiel, and D.O. Adams (1984) Expression of the transferrin receptor in murine peritoneal macrophages is modulated in the different stages of activation. *J. Immunol.* 132:2285–2290.

54. H. McFarlane, S. Reddy, K.J. Adcock, H. Adeshina, A.R. Cooke, and J. Akene (1970) Immunity, transferrin, and survival in kwashiorkor. *Br. Med. J.* 4:268–270.

55. M.J. Murray, A.B. Murray, M.B. Murray, and C.J. Murray (1978) The adverse effects of iron repletion on the course of certain infections. *Br. Med. J.* 2:1113–1115.

56. C. Hershko, T.E.A. Peto, and D.J. Weatherall (1988) Iron and infection. *Br. Med. J.* 296:660–664.

57. B. Cantinieux, J. Boelaert, C. Hariga, and P. Fondu (1988) Impaired neutrophil defense against *Yersinia enterocolitica* in patients with iron overload who are undergoing dialysis. *J. Lab. Clin. Med.* 111:524–528.

58. V.R. Gordeuk, G.M. Brittenham, G.D. McLaren, and P.J. Spagnulo (1986) Hyperferremia in immunosuppressed patients with acute nonlymphocytic leukemia and the risk of infection. *J. Lab. Clin. Med.* 108:466–472.

59. A.N. Akbar, P.A. Fitzgerald-Bocarsly, M. deSusa, P.J. Gardina, M.W. Hilgartner, and R.W. Grady (1986) Decreased natural killer cell activity in thalassemia major: a possible consequence of iron overload. *J. Immunol.* 136:1635–1640.

60. L.D. Koller, S.A. Mulhern, N.C. Frankel, M.G. Stevens, and J.R. Williams (1987) Immune dysfunction in rats fed a diet deficient in copper. *Am. J. Clin. Nutr.* 45:997–1006.

61. W.W. Carelton and P.S. Price (1983) Dietary copper and the induction of neoplasms in the rat by acetylaminofluorene and dimethylnitrosamine. *Food Cosmet. Toxicol.* 11:827–840.

62. S.A. Mulhern and L.D. Koller (1988) Severe or marginal copper deficiency results in a graded reduction in immune status in mice. *J. Nutr.* 118:1041–1047.

63. N.F. Suttle and D.G. Jones (1986) Copper and disease resistance in sheep: a rare natural confirmation of interaction between a specific nutrient and infection. *Proc. Nutr. Soc.* 45:317–325.

64. C. Castollo-Duran, M. Fisberg, A. Vanlenzuela, J.I. Egana, and R. Uauay. (1983) Controlled trial of copper supplementation during the recovery from marasmus. *Am. J. Clin. Nutr.* 37:898–902.

65. R.W. Bryant and J.M. Barley (1980) Altered lipoxygenase metabolism and decreased glutathione peroxidase activity in platelets from selenium deficient rats. *Biochem. Biophys. Res. Commun.* 92:268–276.

66. S.S. Baker and H.J. Cohen (1984) Increased sensitivity to H_2O_2 in glutathione peroxidase-deficient rat granulocytes. *J. Nutr.* 114:2003–2009.

67. S.S. Baker and H.J. Cohen (1983) Altered oxidative metabolism in selenium-deficient rat granulocytes. *J. Immunol.* 130:2856–2860.

68. R.E. Serfass and H.E. Ganther (1975) Defective microbicidal activity in glutathione peroxidase-deficient neutrophils of selenium-deficient rats. *Nature* 255:640–641.

69. S.A. Mulhern, G.L. Taylor, L.E. Magruder, and A.R. Vessey (1985) Deficient levels of dietary selenium suppress the antibody response in first and second generation mice. *Nutr. Res.* 5:201–210.

70. R.S. Desowitz and J.W. Barnwell (1980) Effect of selenium and dimethyl dioctadecyl ammonium bromide on the vaccine-induced immunity of Swiss-Webster mice against malaria (*Plasmodium berghei*). *Infect. Immunol.* 27:87–89.

71. J.E. Spallholz, J.L. Martin, M.L. Gerlach, and R.H. Heinzerling (1973) Immunologic response of mice fed diets supplemented with selenite selenium. *Proc. Soc. Exp. Biol. Med.* 143:685.

72. J. Shackelford and J.L. Martin (1980) Antibody response of mature male mice after drinking water supplemented with selenium. *Fed. Proc.* 39:339.

73. L.D. Koller, N. Isaacson-Kerkvliet, J.H. Exon, J.A. Bauner, and N.M. Patton (1979) Synergism of methylmercury and selenium producing enhanced antibody formation in mice. *Arch. Environ. Health* 34:248–252.

74. J.M. Finch and R.J. Turnes (1986) Selenium supplementation in lambs: effects on antibody responses to salmonella vaccine. *Vet. Rec.* 199:430–431.

75. L.D. Koller, J.H. Exon, P.A. Talcott, C.A. Osborne, and G.M. Henningsen (1986) Immune responses in rats supplemented with selenium. *Clin. Exp. Immunol.* 63:570–576.

76. P.A. Talcott, J.H. Exon, and L.D. Koller (1985) Alteration of natural killer cell-mediated cytotoxicity in rats treated with selenium, diethylnitrosamine and ethylnitrosourea. *Cancer Lett.* 23:313–322.

77. R.R. Watson, S. Moriguchi, B. McRae, L. Tobin, J.C. Mayberry, and D. Lucas (1986) Effects of selenium in vitro on human T-lymphocyte functions and K-562 tumor cell growth. *J. Leukocyte Biol.* 39:447–457.

78. R.E. Serfass, R.D. Hinsdill, and H.E. Ganther (1974) Protective effect of selenium on salmonella infection: relation to glutathione peroxidase and superoxide dismutase activities of phagocytes. *Fed. Proc.* 33:694(abstr.).

79. R.E. Serfass and H.E. Ganther (1976) Effects of dietary selenium and tocopherol on glutathione peroxidase and superoxide dismutase activities in rat phagocytes. *Life Sci.* 19:1139–1144.

80. B.E. Sheffy and R.D. Schultz (1978) III. Nutrition and the immune response. *Cornell Vet.* 68(suppl. 7):48–61.

81. M.L. Eskew, R.W. Scholz, C.C. Reddy, D.A. Todhunter, and A. Zarkower (1985) Effects of vitamin E and selenium deficiencies on rat immune function. *Immunology* 54:173–180.

82. M.J. Parnham, J. Winkelman, and S. Leyck (1983) Macrophage, lymphocyte and chronic inflammatory responses in selenium deficient rodents. Association with decreased glutathione peroxidase activity. *Int. J. Immunopharmacol.* 5:455–461.

83. H.C. Meeker, M.L. Eskew, W. Scheuchenzuber, R.W. Scholz, and A. Zarkower (1985) Antioxidant effects on cell-mediated immunity. *J. Leukocyte Biol.* 38:451–458.

84. A. Bendich, E. Gabriel, and L.J. Machlin (1986) Dietary vitamin E requirement for optimum immune responses in the rat. *J. Nutr.* 116:675–681.

85. T. Yasunaga, H. Kato, K. Ohgaki, T. Inamoto, and Y. Hikasa (1982) Effect of vitamin E as an immunopotentiation agent for mice at optimal dosage and its toxicity at high dosage. *J. Nutr.* 112:1075–1084.

86. K.A. Ritacco, C.F. Nockles, and R.P. Ellis (1986) The influence of supplemental vitamins A and E on ovine humoral immune response. *Proc. Soc. Exp. Biol. Med.* 182:393–398.

87. M. Taccone-Gallucci, O. Giardini, C. Ausiello, et al. (1986) Vitamin

E supplementation in hemodialysis patients: effects on peripheral blood mononuclear cells lipid peroxidation and immune response. *Clin. Nephrol.* 25:81–86.

88. J.S. Prasad (1980) Effect of vitamin E supplementation on leukocyte function. *Am. J. Clin. Nutr.* 33:606–608.

89. S.N. Meydani, M. Meydani, C.P. Verdon, A.A. Shapiro, J.B. Blumberg, and K.C. Hayes (1986) Vitamin E supplementation suppresses prostaglandin E$_2$ synthesis and enhances the immune response of aged mice. *Mech. Ageing Dev.* 34:191–201.

90. A. Bendich and S.S. Shapiro (1986) Effect of beta-carotene and canthaxanthin on the immune response of the rat. *J. Nutr.* 116: 2254–2262.

91. B.S. Alam, S.Q. Alam, J.C. Weir, and W.A. Gibson (1984) Chemoprotective effects of beta-carotene and 13-cis-retinoic acid on salavary gland tumors. *Nutr. Cancer* 6:4–12.

92. Y. Tomita, K. Humeno, K. Nomoto, H. Endo, and T. Hirohata (1987) Augmentation of tumor immunity against syngeneic tumors in mice by beta-carotene. *JNCI* 78:679–681.

93. S.M. Smith and C.E. Hayes (1987) Contrasting impairments in IgM and IgG responses of vitamin A-deficient mice. *Proc. Natl. Acad. Sci. USA* 84:5878–5882.

94. G. Forni, S.C. Sola, M. Giovarelli, A. Santoni, P. Martinetto, and D. Vietti (1986) Effect of prolonged administration of low doses on dietary retinoids on cell-mediated immunity in the growth of transplantable tumors in mice. *JNCI* 76:527–533.

95. B.S. Rao (1986) Effect of vitamin A analogues on concanavalin-induced agglutination of erythrocytes. *Biochem. Int.* 13:721–727.

96. L.D. Fraker, S.A. Halter, and J.T. Forbes (1986) Effects of orally administered retinol on natural killer cell activity in wild type BALB/c and congenitally athymic BALB/c mice. *Cancer Immunol. Immunother.* 21:114–118.

97. A. Santoni, A.C. Sola, S. Giovarelli, P. Martinetto, D. Vietti, and G. Forni (1986) Modulation of natural killer cell activity in mice by prolonged administration of various doses of dietary retinoids. *Nat. Immun. Cell Growth Regul.* 5:259–266.

98. R.R. Watson, S. Moriguchi, and H.L. Gensler (1987) Effects of dietary retinyl palmitate and selenium on tumoricidal capacity of macrophages in mice undergoing tumor promotion. *Cancer Lett.* 36:181–187.

99. N.E. Kay, D.E. Holloway, S.W. Hutton, N.D. Bone, and W.C. Duane (1982) Human T-cell function in experimental ascorbic acid deficiency and spontaneous scurvy. *Am. J. Clin. Nutr.* 36: 127–130.

100. A. Bendich, P. D'Apolito, E. Gabriel, and L.J. Machlin (1984) Interaction of dietary vitamin C and vitamin E on guinea pig immune responses to mitogens. *J. Nutr.* 114:1588–1593.

101. H. Padh and J.J. Aleo (1987) Activation of serum complement leads to inhibition of ascorbic acid transport. *Proc. Soc. Exp. Biol. Med.* 185:153–157.

102. B.V. Siegel and J.I. Morton (1979) Vitamin C and the immune response. *Experimentia* 33:393–395.

103. R. Anderson, R. Oosthuizen, R. Maritz, A. Theron, and A.J. Van Rensburg (1980) The effects of increasing weekly doses of ascorbate on certain cellular and humoral immune functions in normal volunteers. *Am. J. Clin. Nutr.* 33:71–76.

104. I. Ramirez, E. Richie, Y. Wang, and J. Van Eys (1980) Effect of ascorbic acid in vitro on lymphocyte reactivity to mitogens. *J. Nutr.* 110:2207–2215.

105. J.P. Manzella and N.J. Roberts (1979) Human macrophage and lymphocyte responses to mitogen stimulation after exposure to influenza virus, ascorbic acid, and hyperthermia. *J. Immunol.* 123:1940–1944.

106. C. Oh and K. Nakano (1988) Reversal by ascorbic acid of suppression by endogenous histamine of rat lymphocyte blastogenesis. *J. Nutr.* 118:639–644.

Chapter 56

David R. Bevan

Toxicants in Foods

The subject of toxicants in foods has been reviewed several times from a variety of perspectives.[1–6] In the previous edition of this volume, the emphasis was on toxicants produced by microorganisms.[7] These bacterial toxins and mycotoxins clearly are toxic to humans and animals and thus are of great concern. However, exposure to these toxicants can be minimized by preventing or eliminating contamination by the toxin-producing microorganisms. Other toxicants in foods are naturally occurring constituents of food or are produced during common processing and cooking procedures. Several classes of these toxicants for which some details of molecular mechanisms of toxicity are understood will be examined herein. The toxicity of these compounds generally has been evaluated in laboratory animals or in vitro. However, the impact of most of these toxicants on human health has not been assessed despite the potential for widespread exposure to some of these compounds. In this review particular consideration will be given to the mechanisms by which these toxicants in foods exert their toxicity. An understanding of these mechanisms may aid in assessing human health risks associated with exposure to these compounds and, in addition, may facilitate the evaluation of toxicity of other compounds contained in foods.

Alkenylbenzenes

Some of the alkenylbenzenes, which are found in spices, are carcinogenic.[8,9] Safrole (1-allyl-3,4-methylenedioxybenzene) (Figure 1) was the first alkenylbenzene that was shown to be a carcinogen; it acts as a weak hepatocarcinogen in rats and mice. It is a major component, as high as 93%, of the essential oil from sassafras trees (*Sassafras albidum*). Lesser amounts (1–10%) of safrole are found in essential oils from nutmeg, mace, ginger, cinnamon, and black pepper. Safrole was used in the United States to flavor root beer, although in 1960 it was banned from commercial use in foods.[9] Estragole (1-allyl-4-methoxybenzene) and methyleugenol (1-allyl-3,4-dimethoxybenzene) (Figure 1) have hepatocarcinogenic activities in rats and mice comparable to that of safrole. Estragole is a major constituent of oils from tarragon and sweet basil, and methyleugenol is a constituent of cloves, sweet bay, and lemongrass. A variety of other natural and synthetic alkenylbenzenes, such as myristicin, elemicin, and dill apiol, do not appear to be as potent carcinogens.[10]

Currently it is believed that chemical carcinogenesis may be initiated by the formation of a covalent addition product (adduct) between the carcinogen and DNA.[11] For carcinogens to act via this mechanism, they either must contain electrophilic moieties or be metabolized to contain them to allow for binding to nucleophilic groups in the DNA bases. Some studies of the metabolism of safrole and its relationship to carcinogenicity were concerned with metabolism at the allyl side chain vs. that at the methylenedioxy group.[12] The allylic moiety was metabolized to a 1'-hydroxy derivative and a 2',3'-epoxy derivative, whereas metabolism at the methylenedioxy group yielded catechols. Metabolism of safrole at the methylenedioxy group is proposed to produce a carbene intermediate that forms a complex with cytochrome P-450. It was suggested that the resultant changes in cytochrome P-450 activities could produce carcinogenicity through epigenetic mechanisms.[12] However, subsequent studies of alkenylbenzene carcinogenicity provided further association of metabolism of the allyl side chain with the development of cancer. For example, estragole, methyleugenol, and their 1'-hydroxy derivatives all are compounds that do not have a methylenedioxy group but they were carcinogenic in rats and mice.[10] The synthetic acetylenic derivative of estragole, 1'-hydroxy-2',3'-dehydroestragole, was even more potent as a carcinogen than these compounds. The 2',3'-oxides of safrole, estragole, eugenol, and 1'-hydroxysafrole were in-

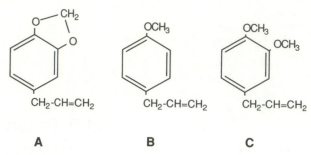

Figure 1. Alkenylbenzenes: safrole (A), estragole (B), and methyleugenol (C).

active in most of the bioassays and were only weakly carcinogenic in a skin-painting experiment, indicating that epoxidation inactivated rather than activated the compounds.[10] After administration of 1'-hydroxy-2',3'-dehydroestragole in vivo, adducts in liver were predominantly N^2-(2',3'-dehydroestragol-1'-yl)-deoxyguanosine.[13,14] Inhibition of sulfotransferase activity in animals decreased the formation of adducts and the carcinogenicity, from which it was inferred that an ultimate carcinogenic form was 1'-sulfooxy-2',3'-dehydroestragole.[14]

Amino Acid Analogues

L-Canavanine. L-Canavanine (Figure 2) is a guanidinoxy structural analogue of arginine. It is present in amounts of ~1.5% of the dry weight of alfalfa seeds and sprouts,[15] and it also is found in other legumes.[3]

L-Canavanine is toxic to many organisms;[16] its toxicity in man and monkeys is manifested as a systemic lupus erythematosus–like syndrome. This syndrome is characterized by an impairment of the immune system.[15] In the primate model, anemia may result from the production of antibodies to red blood cells. Additional abnormalities include lowered complement components in serum, antibodies to nuclear antigens, and antibodies to double-stranded DNA.[15]

One mechanism by which L-canavanine exerts its toxicity appears to originate from the substitution of L-canavanine for arginine in metabolic pathways.[15] In particular, arginine t-RNA can be charged with L-canavanine, and the analogue then is incorporated into proteins.[17] If histones contain L-canavanine, their interaction with DNA may be altered. Hence, an antibody response to nuclear antigens and double-stranded DNA can occur. A mechanism involving reactive oxygen species was invoked to explain the chromosome breakage that is seen in systemic lupus erythematosus.[2,15] In this disease phagocytic activity and its associated respiratory burst involving reactive oxygen species are thought to be increased in

response to complexes of antibodies with L-canavanine–containing proteins. In support of this hypothesis, superoxide dismutase protects against chromosome breakage in human lymphocyte cultures produced by serum from systemic lupus erythematosus patients.[18]

Hypoglycin. Hypoglycin (L-[methylenecyclopropyl]alanine) (Figure 3) is found in the fruit of the Jamaican ackee tree (*Blighia sapida*).[19] In fact, two related toxic compounds are present, hypoglycin A (hypoglycin) and hypoglycin B (γ-glutamylhypoglycin). In unripe fruit these compounds are present in the arillus that surrounds the seeds of the fruit. During ripening hypoglycin is translocated to the seeds. Thus, toxicity may occur when unripe fruit is consumed, because it is the arillus that is cooked and eaten.

The acute toxicity, measured as an LD_{50}, for hypoglycin ranges from 10 to 150 mg/kg, depending on species; for humans the LD_{50} is not known.[19] Symptoms of toxicity include severe hypoglycemia accompanied by depletion of liver glycogen, accumulation of fat in liver, elevated concentrations of free fatty acids in plasma, dicarboxylic aciduria, and organic acidemia.

Toxicity because of exposure to hypoglycin is caused principally by one of its in vivo metabolites. Hypoglycin is metabolized to methylenecyclopropylpyruvate, which in turn is converted to methylenecyclopropylacetyl-CoA (MCPA-CoA). MCPA-CoA inactivates several enzymes involved in catabolism. Included are the general acyl-CoA and butyryl-CoA dehydrogenases that catalyze the β-oxidation of fatty acids and isovaleryl-CoA, 2-methylbutyryl-CoA, and glutaryl-CoA dehydrogenases that are involved in catabolism of amino acids. MCPA-CoA functions as a suicide inhibitor of the general acyl-CoA dehydrogenase and is assumed to act via a similar mechanism in inhibiting the other dehydrogenases.[20] Specifically, the mechanism of inhibition appears to involve an abstraction of a proton from the 2 position of MCPA-CoA to produce a reactive carbanion that reacts with and covalently modifies the FAD cofactor associated with these enzymes.

Although a number of metabolic processes will be affected by inhibition of these enzymes, hypoglycin appears to produce its hypoglycemic effect principally through inhibition of gluconeogenesis. Normally, the β-oxidation of fatty acids stimulates gluconeogenesis by providing ATP, NADH, and acetyl-CoA, with the

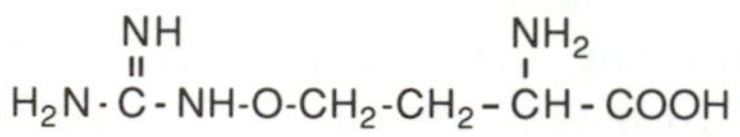

$$\overset{\text{NH}}{\underset{\|}{}} \qquad \overset{\text{NH}_2}{\underset{|}{}}$$
$$H_2N \cdot C \cdot NH\text{-}O\text{-}CH_2\text{-}CH_2\text{-}CH\text{-}COOH$$

Figure 2. L-Canavanine.

acetyl-CoA functioning as an allosteric effector of pyruvate carboxylase. Competitive inhibition of the activation of pyruvate carboxylase by the increased concentrations of isovaleryl-CoA, 2-methylbutyryl-CoA, glutaryl-CoA, and butyryl-CoA appears to be the principal mechanism by which toxicity is exerted.[19]

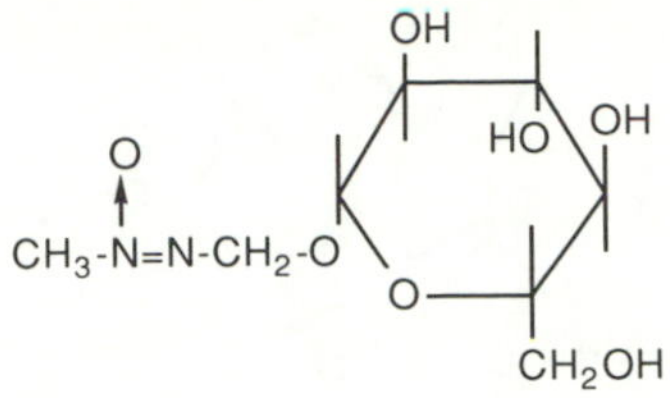

Glycosides

Cycasin. Cycasin (methylazoxymethanol-β-glucoside) (Figure 4) is a naturally occurring constituent of cycads.[8,21] The cycads are palm-like trees belonging to nine genera found mainly in tropical and subtropical climates.[22] Levels of cycasin as high as 2.3% were reported in nuts of cycads.[8]

Cycads have been used primarily as a source of food starch. Although it appears that cycads currently are used only occasionally as a food source, they were used more extensively in the past, especially in times of emergencies. The toxicity of cycads was established, and procedures were developed to reduce levels of cycasin. These procedures generally involve soaking pieces of seeds or stems in water to remove the cycasin.[21]

Studies of the toxicity of cycads originally were initiated because native Chamorro on the island of Guam, whose diet regularly included products of cycads, were observed to have an increased incidence of amyotrophic lateral sclerosis (ALS).[23] However, animal studies generally did not indicate neurological lesions as would be expected in ALS. Instead, the principal pathology was cancer.[24] It has now been demonstrated that cycasin is a carcinogen in many animal species (rats, mice, hamsters, guinea pigs, rabbits, and aquarium fish), with tumors being observed principally in liver, kidneys, and the intestinal tract.[8]

Studies of the mechanism of cycasin carcinogenicity revealed that a metabolite of cycasin, methylazoxymethanol (MAM), is the ultimate carcinogen.[25] From a variety of studies it was shown that MAM is produced from cycasin in vivo as a result of hydrolysis catalyzed by a β-glucosidase present in intestinal microflora. For example, cycasin was carcinogenic when given orally but not when given by injection.[8,26] In addition, cycasin was not carcinogenic in germ-free animals although it was carcinogenic after colonization of these animals with bacteria containing β-glucosidase.[27] As expected, MAM was carcinogenic

Figure 4. Cycasin.

regardless of the route of administration and in germ-free animals.[28] MAM acts as a methylating agent, and 7-methyldeoxyguanine was isolated from animals exposed to MAM.[29,30] Methylation of RNA also was observed.[30] Methyldiazonium hydroxide is believed to be the methyl donor, and both nonenzymatic and alcohol dehydrogenase–catalyzed pathways for its formation were proposed.[31,32]

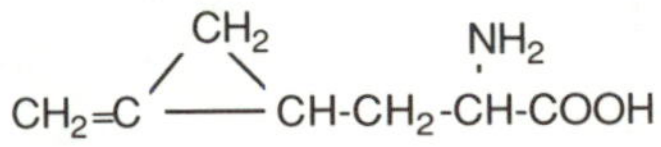

Neurotoxicity associated with exposure to cycasin is less clearly understood. MAM was shown to induce microencephaly in a number of animal species (rats, hamsters, ferrets, rabbits, cats, and dogs).[21,33] In addition, a neurological disorder characterized by locomotor difficulty, as would be expected in ALS, was induced in some species (mice, hamsters, and ferrets) by cycasin.[34] Mechanisms for this neurotoxicity have not yet been established.

Bracken Fern. Consumption of bracken fern (*Pteridium aquilinum*) has long been associated with toxicity in agricultural animals.[8,35,36] More recently, it was recognized that constituents of bracken fern are carcinogenic in farm and laboratory animals and hence are possible carcinogens in humans. Bracken fern grows best in temperate and midtropic zones, and it is one of the first plants to develop in the spring.[36] Bracken fern also is produced commercially in Japan, Canada, and the United States. Human exposures can be via consumption of bracken fern as greens or through milk and dairy products obtained from cows grazing on bracken fern.[36]

The symptoms of bracken fern toxicity differ among farm animals. For example, horses suffer from a thiamin deficiency that leads to anorexia and incoordination, and cows develop depressed bone marrow activity.[37] Bracken fern also is a carcinogen in cows, rats, mice, quail, hamsters, and guinea pigs.[35] The most frequent sites of tumor formation are the intestinal tract, urinary bladder, and upper alimentary tract.

Despite much research the components of bracken fern that are toxic and carcinogenic are not precisely known. In fact, the constituents leading to symptoms of toxicity in farm animals may be different from those producing carcinogenicity. Several difficulties have hindered identification of the toxic and carcinogenic components. That is, rats and mice do not

Figure 3. Hypoglycin.

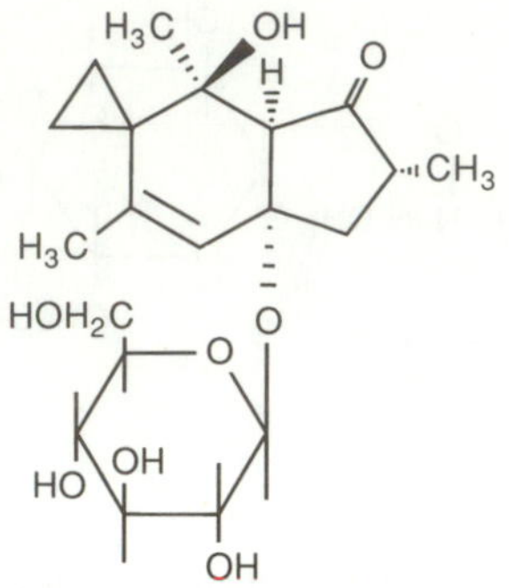

Figure 5. Ptaquiloside.

respond to bracken fern with an easily identifiable acute toxic response such as the hematological disorders in cattle. In addition, short-term mutagenicity tests have not proved reliable for identification of the carcinogenic components in bracken fern.[35] A variety of compounds have been isolated from bracken fern and tested for toxicity, carcinogenicity, and mutagenicity. These compounds include shikimic acid, pterosin, pteroside, pterolactam, tannin, and quercetin. However, none of these compounds is considered to be the principal active component of bracken fern, because none has consistently been found to be toxic, carcinogenic, or mutagenic when tested in a variety of systems.[8,35,36]

More recently, a glycoside denoted ptaquiloside (Figure 5) has been isolated from bracken fern, and this compound may make the greatest contribution to the toxicity and carcinogenicity.[38] Ptaquiloside is carcinogenic in female CD rats, and when administered to a female Holstein-Friesian calf, it induced hematological disorders characteristic of bracken fern toxicity.[39,40] The mechanism by which this compound exerts its toxicity is not yet established.

The carcinogenicity of bracken fern in humans cannot be assessed definitively. However, it normally is consumed after processing to remove the astringent taste, a procedure that involves boiling the bracken fern in water containing wood ash or sodium bicarbonate. Processing of bracken fern lowers but does not eliminate its carcinogenicity in experimental animals.[41] It was suggested that consumption of bracken fern may contribute to the high incidences of stomach and esophageal cancer in Japan.[42]

Cyanogenic Glycosides. Over 1000 species of plants are known to contain compounds that are classified as cyanogenic glycosides.[43] Hydrogen cyanide (HCN) is released when these compounds are treated with acid or with β-glucosidases that are found in the plants. The aglycones formed when HCN is released have not been identified in all cases but include a variety of α-hydroxynitriles. The toxicity of HCN results from inhibition of mitochondrial

respiration. Specifically, HCN inhibits the activity of cytochrome oxidase by binding to it.[44]

Cyanogenic glycosides have been found in cassava, some beans, stone fruits, and sorghum.[43] Amounts of cyanide in apricot kernels range from 12 to 177 mg/100 g, and amounts in lima beans range from 10 to 300 mg/100 g, depending on the strain of bean.[43,45,46] The amount of HCN released from cassava root was 38 mg/100 g, but amounts were reduced significantly during food preparation.[47] The lethal dose of HCN in humans ranges from 50 to 250 mg, so diets high in some plants could present a hazard because of HCN. In fact, reports of HCN poisoning in humans because of consumption of these plants have appeared.[46,48,49]

Vicine and Convicine. Consumption of broad (fava) beans (*Vicia faba*) by some humans results in a disease call favism, which is characterized by hemolysis and can result in jaundice and hemoglobinuria.[50] It is particularly prevalent among individuals living in the area of the Mediterranean Sea and in the Middle East. Favism results from a deficiency of glucose-6-phosphate dehydrogenase (G6PD) such that cells are unable to maintain concentrations of reduced glutathione (GSH) sufficient to protect against oxidative damage. It is estimated that G6PD deficiency affects ~100 million people in the world, with the incidence of the defect varying greatly among ethnic groups.[50,51]

The compounds in fava beans that appear to lead to favism are vicine and convicine (Figure 6).[50] These β-glycosides may be converted by β-glucosidases to their respective aglycones, divicine, and isouramil.[52] These compounds can exist in tautomeric forms as illustrated for isouramil (Figure 7). The aminoenol form is unstable and can autooxidize with the loss of electrons to produce reactive oxygen species. In individuals with a deficiency of G6PD, this oxidative stress exceeds the capacity of erythrocytes to repair oxidative damage and hemolytic anemia results.

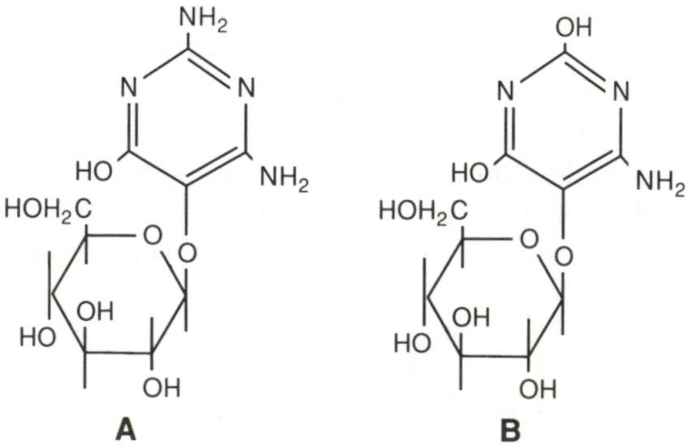

Figure 6. Vicine (A) and convicine (B).

Hydrazines

Edible mushrooms contain hydrazines or their precursors, and a variety of toxic phenomena, to be discussed below, have been attributed to these compounds.[8,53] Agaritine (β-N-[γ-L(+)glutamyl]-4-hydroxymethylphenylhydrazine) (Figure 8) is a hydrazide found in *Agaricus bisporus,* the common cultivated mushroom.[54] Concentrations of agaritine in fresh mushrooms are 0.04–0.3% of wet weight.[55] These concentrations decline with storage,[56] a factor that may contribute to variability in amounts found in mushrooms. Frozen mushrooms were reported to contain 0.033% agaritine, but the compound was not detected in canned mushrooms.[56] Agaritine is metabolized by γ-glutamyltranspeptidase in both mushrooms and mammalian systems to glutamate and 4-(hydroxymethyl)phenylhydrazine.[56,57]

Gyromitrin (acetaldehyde methylformylhydrazone) (Figure 8) is found in *Gyromitra esculenta,* one of the false morel mushrooms, at concentrations of ~50 mg/kg.[53] Also found in relatively large amounts are N-methyl-N-formylhydrazine (500 mg/kg) and methylhydrazine (14 mg/kg). Several other methylformylhydrazone derivatives also are found in small quantities (<3 mg/kg). Gyromitrin is converted to methylhydrazine via an N-methyl-N-formylhydrazine intermediate under conditions simulating the pH of the human stomach,[58] suggesting that humans may be exposed to large levels of methylhydrazine after consumption of this false morel.

Toxic effects of hydrazines include neurological disorders, hypoglycemia, immunotoxicity, and carcinogenesis.[59] Neurological disorders include convulsions, numbness, and neuronal degradation. The mechanisms by which hydrazines produce these neurological disorders are postulated to involve inhibition of pyridoxal phosphate–dependent enzymes as a result of hydrazone formation between a free amino group of hydrazines and the carbonyl group of pyridoxal phosphate.[60,61] Enzymes that are affected include glutamic acid decarboxylase, γ-aminobutyric acid (GABA) aminotransferase, and 5-hydroxytryptophan decarboxylase.[60–62] Hypoglycemia caused by hydrazines appears to involve a diminished capacity for gluconeogenesis possibly caused by inhibition of

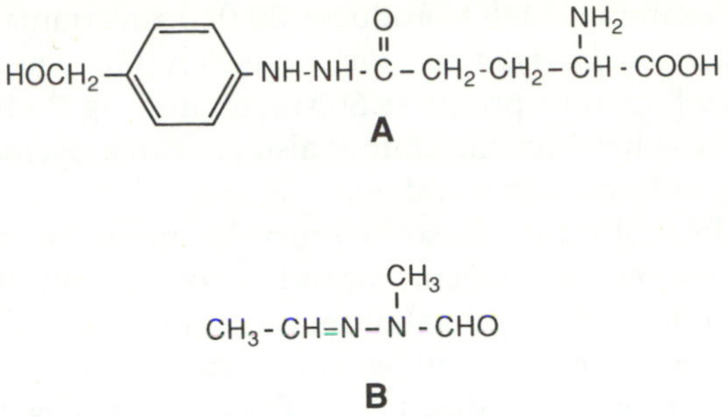

Figure 8. Agaritine (A) and gyromitrin (B).

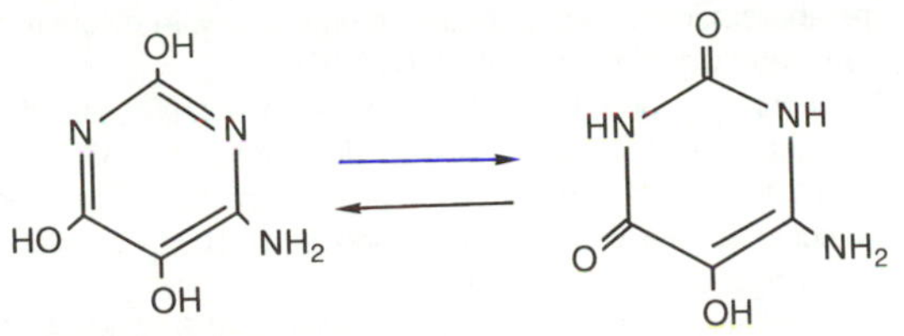

several enzymes associated with gluconeogenesis, including phosphoenolpyruvate carboxykinase, pyruvate dehydrogenase, and amino acid transaminases.[59] Immunotoxicity manifested as systemic lupus erythematosus, as described above for L-canavanine, also is associated with hydrazine exposure. The antibody response may result from binding of hydrazines to macromolecules, which allows them to function as haptens.[63,64] Alternatively, the compounds may act as adjuvants or immunostimulants.[65] Many hydrazines are carcinogenic, and these compounds may initiate carcinogenesis via alkylation of DNA.[59] An intermediate in metabolism of some hydrazines, including methylhydrazine, may be methylazomethanol, a compound similar to that associated with carcinogenicity of cycads.[66] Activation of agaritine is proposed to involve diazonium ion formation.[55,67] Mechanisms involving free radical reactions also were proposed to account for the alkylation reactions.[68]

Protein Pyrolysates

Sugimura and coworkers[1,69,70] initiated a series of experiments to investigate the formation of mutagens during cooking. To facilitate their experiments, they used the Ames test to screen samples for mutagenic activity. Initially, it was observed that extracts of grilled sardines and ground beef were mutagenic.[71] Analysis of pyrolysates of proteins, DNA, RNA, starch, and vegetable oil revealed that most of the mutagenic activity was associated with the protein extracts.[72,73] Metabolic activation was required for mutagenesis.[74] Pyrolysis of specific amino acids indicated that pyrolysates of tryptophan, glutamic acid, phenylalanine, and lysine contained mutagens.[69,74] The compounds responsible for mutagenic activity were isolated from pyrolysates and characterized. Structures of some of these compounds are illustrated in Figure 9 and can be recognized as heterocyclic amines.

The mutagenicity of these compounds is extremely high relative to that of some well-studied mutagens.

Figure 7. Tautomerism of isouramil.

For example, MelQ produces 30,000 revertants/μg in *Salmonella typhimurium* strain TA100, whereas benzo[a]pyrene produces 660 revertants/μg.[69] Many of these heterocyclic amines also are carcinogenic in rats and mice after oral administration.[75,76]

Metabolism of these heterocyclic amines to mutagenic and carcinogenic forms has been investigated. The initial step in metabolism is the formation of the hydroxyamino derivatives in a reaction catalyzed by mixed function oxidases.[70,74] Subsequent conjugation reactions involving *O*-acylation or *O*-sulfation produce the ultimate carcinogenic forms of these compounds. DNA adducts, which are thought to initiate carcinogenesis, have been characterized for a variety of these heterocyclic amines.[76–78]

Currently, it is difficult to assess human health risks associated with exposure to these compounds. Amounts of these compounds ranging from about 1 to 700 μg/kg have been isolated from broiled or fried meats.[79–82] Consequently, a large portion of the population is exposed to these potent mutagens, and it will be important to assess their contribution to carcinogenesis in humans.

Summary

This discussion of toxicants in foods illustrates the variety of naturally occurring food toxicants and the diverse mechanisms by which they can exert their toxicity. At the same time, some similarities are observed among mechanisms of toxicity. For example, toxic responses for the compounds discussed here included carcinogenesis, a systemic lupus erythematosus–like syndrome, hypoglycemia, hematological and neurological disorders, and inhibition of electron transport. However, metabolism of two of the classes of toxicants, alkenylbenzenes and compounds in protein pyrolysates, produces carcinogenic forms via conjugation reactions. Carcinogenesis by cycasin and hydrazines also involves structurally similar metabolites. The systemic lupus erythematosus–like syndrome caused by L-canavanine may result from changes in nuclear protein structure whereas that caused by hydrazines may result from changes in DNA structure, both of which may alter protein-DNA interactions. Another similarity in mechanisms of toxicity is the possible involvement of reactive oxygen species. This aspect of toxicants in foods was reviewed.[2]

It is difficult at this point to assess accurately the human health effects resulting from exposure to these and other toxicants in foods. Most diets probably would result in only low exposures to these compounds. However, cumulative exposure to a large number of compounds over an extended period of time could potentially represent a health hazard. An

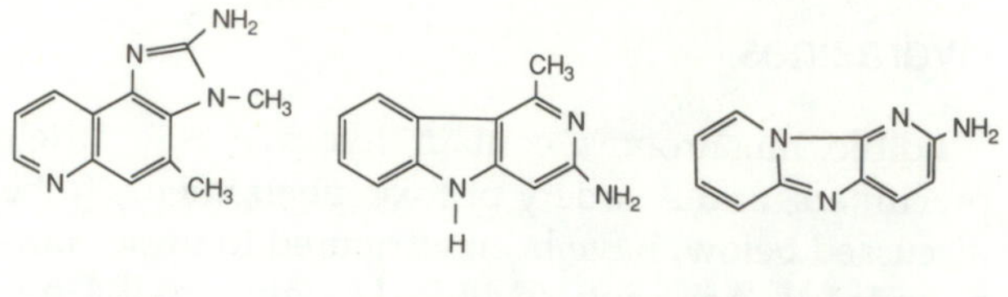

Figure 9. Representative heterocyclic amines isolated from protein pyrolysates. MelQ (2-amino-3,4-dimethylimidazo[4,5-f]quinoline), Trp-P-2 (3-amino-1-methyl-5H-pyrido[4,3-b]indole), and Glu-P-2 (2-aminodipyrido[1,2-a:3'2'-d]imidazole).

understanding of the mechanisms of toxicity, as discussed in this review, should assist in identifying potential toxicants in foods and in evaluating risks associated with exposure to them.

References

1. T. Sugimura (1982) Tumor initiators and promoters associated with ordinary foods. In: *Molecular Interrelations of Nutrition and Cancer* (M.S. Arnott, J. van Eys, and Y.-M. Wang, eds.), pp. 3–24, Raven Press, New York.
2. B.N. Ames (1983) Dietary carcinogens and anticarcinogens. *Science* 221:1256–1264.
3. C.S. Evans (1983) Naturally occurring food toxicants: toxic amino acids. In: *CRC Handbook of Naturally Occurring Food Toxicants* (M. Rechcigl, Jr., ed.), pp. 3–14, CRC Press, Boca Raton, FL.
4. C. Furihata and T. Matsushima (1986) Mutagens and carcinogens in foods. *Annu. Rev. Nutr.* 6:67–94.
5. D.Y. Lai and Y.-T. Woo (1987) Naturally occurring carcinogens: an overview. *J. Environ. Sci. Health* [C] 5:121–173.
6. P.M. Newberne (1988) Naturally occurring food-borne toxicants. In: *Modern Nutrition in Health and Disease*, 7th ed. (M. Shils and V.R. Young, eds.), pp. 685–697, Lea and Febiger, Philadelphia.
7. B. Wilson (1984) Toxicants occurring naturally in foods. In: *Present Knowledge in Nutrition*, 5th ed. (R.E. Olson, H.P. Broquist, C.O. Chichester, W.J. Darby, A.C. Kolbye, and R.M. Stalvey, eds.), pp. 819–839. The Nutrition Foundation, Washington, DC.
8. I. Hirano (1981) Natural carcinogenic products of plant origin. *CRC Crit. Rev. Toxicol.* 8:235–277.
9. J.A. Miller, E.C. Miller, and D.H. Phillips (1982) The metabolic activation and carcinogenicity of alkenylbenzenes that occur naturally in many spices. In: *Carcinogens and Mutagens in the Environment*, vol. 1 (H.F. Stitch, ed.), pp. 83–120, CRC Press, Boca Raton, FL.
10. E.C. Miller, A.B. Swanson, D.H. Phillips, T.L. Fletcher, A. Liem, and J.A. Miller (1983) Structure-activity studies of the carcinogenicities in the mouse and rat of some naturally occurring and synthetic alkenylbenzene derivatives related to safrole and estragole. *Cancer Res.* 43:1124–1134.
11. S.B. Oppenheimer (1985) *Cancer—A Biological and Clinical Introduction*, 2nd ed., pp. 28–38, Jones and Bartlett Publishers, Inc., Boston.
12. C. Ioannides, M. Delaforge, and D.V. Parke (1981) Safrole: its metabolism, carcinogenicity and interactions with cytochrome P-450. *Food Cosmet. Toxicol.* 19:657–666.
13. T.R. Fennell, U. Juhl, E.C. Miller, and J.A. Miller (1986) Identification and quantitation of hepatic DNA adducts formed in B6C3F$_1$ mice from 1'-hydroxy-2',3'-dehydroestragole: comparison of the adducts detected with the 1'-^{3}H-labelled carcinogen and by ^{32}P-postlabelling. *Carcinogenesis* 7:1881–1887.
14. T.R. Fennell, R.W. Wiseman, J.A. Miller, and E.C. Miller (1985) Major role of hepatic sulfotransferase activity in the metabolic ac-

tivation, DNA adduct formation, and carcinogenicity of 1'-hydroxy-2',3'-dehydroestragole in infant male C57BL/6J × C3H/HeJ F$_1$ mice. *Cancer Res.* 45:5310–5320.

15. M.R. Malinow, E.J. Bardana, B. Pirofsky, S. Craig, and P. Mc-Laughlin (1982) Systemic lupus erythematosus-like syndrome in monkeys fed alfalfa sprouts: role of a nonprotein amino acid. *Science* 216:415–417.

16. G.A. Rosenthal (1977) The biological effects and mode of action of L-canavanine, a structural analogue of L-arginine. *Q. Rev. Biol.* 52:155–178.

17. C.C. Allende and J.E. Allende (1964) Purification and substrate specificity of arginyl-ribonucleic acid synthetase from rat liver. *J. Biol. Chem.* 239:1102–1106.

18. I. Emerit, A.M. Michelson, A. Levy, J.P. Camus, and J. Emerit (1980) Chromosome-breaking agent of low molecular weight in human systemic lupus erythematosus. *Hum. Genet.* 55:341–344.

19. H.S.A. Sherratt (1986) Hypoglycin, the famous toxin of the unripe Jamaican ackee fruit. *Trends Pharmacol. Sci.* 7:186–191.

20. A. Wenz, C. Thorpe, and S. Ghisla (1981) Inactivation of general acyl-CoA dehydrogenase from pig kidney by a metabolite of hypoglycin A. *J. Biol. Chem.* 256:9809–9812.

21. H. Matsumoto (1983) Cycasin. In: *CRC Handbook of Naturally Occurring Food Toxicants* (M. Rechcigl, Jr., ed.), pp. 43–61, CRC Press, Boca Raton, FL.

22. M.R. Birdsey (1972) A brief description of the cycads. *Fed. Proc.* 31:1467–1469.

23. L.T. Kurland (1972) An appraisal of the neurotoxicity of cycad and the etiology of amyotrophic lateral sclerosis on Guam. *Fed. Proc.* 31:1540–1542.

24. G.L. Laqueur, O. Mickelsen, M.G. Whiting, and L.T. Kurland (1963) Carcinogenic properties of nuts from *Cycas circinalis* L. indigenous to Guam. *J. Natl. Cancer Inst.* 31:919–951.

25. H. Matsumoto and F.M. Strong (1963) The occurrence of methylazoxymethanol in *Cycas circinalis* L. *Arch. Biochem. Biophys.* 101:299–310.

26. M. Spatz, E.G. McDaniel, and G.L. Laqueur (1986) Cycasin excretion in conventional and germfree rats. *Proc. Soc. Exp. Biol. Med.* 121:417–422.

27. M. Spatz, D.W.E. Smith, E.G. McDaniel, and G.L. Laqueur (1967) Role of intestinal microorganisms in determining cycasin toxicity. *Proc. Soc. Exp. Biol. Med.* 124:691–697.

28. A. Kobayashi and H. Matsumoto (1965) Studies on methylazoxymethanol, the aglycone of cycasin. *Arch. Biochem. Biophys.* 110:373–380.

29. R.C. Shank and P.N. Magee (1967) Similarities between the biochemical actions of cycasin and dimethylnitrosamine. *Biochem. J.* 105:521–527.

30. Y. Nagata and H. Matsumoto (1969) Studies on methylazoxymethanol: methylation of nucleic acids in the fetal rat brain. *Proc. Soc. Exp. Biol. Med.* 132:383–385.

31. H. Druckrey and A. Lang (1972) Carcinogenicity of azoxymethane dependent on age in BD rats. *Fed. Proc.* 31:1482–1484.

32. E.C. Miller and J.A. Miller (1981) Searches for ultimate chemical carcinogens and their reactions with cellular macromolecules. In: *Accomplishments in Cancer Research 1980* (J.G. Fortner and J.E. Rhoads, eds.), pp. 63–98, Lippincott, Philadelphia.

33. R.K. Haddad, A. Rabe, and R. Dumas (1972) Comparison of effects of methylazoxymethanol acetate on development in different species. *Fed. Proc.* 31:1520–1523.

34. I. Hirono and C. Shibuya (1967) Induction of neurological disorder by cycasin in mice. *Nature* 216:1311–1312.

35. I. Hirono (1986) Carcinogenic principles isolated from bracken fern. *CRC Crit. Rev. Toxicol.* 17:1–22.

36. G.T. Bryan and A.M. Pamukcu (1982) Sources of carcinogens and mutagens in edible plants: production of urinary bladder and intestinal tumors by bracken fern (*Pteridium aquilinum*). In: *Car-cinogens and Mutagens in the Environment,* vol. 1 (H.F. Stich, ed.), pp. 75–82, CRC Press, Boca Raton, FL.

37. R.D. Radeleff (1970) *Veterinary Toxicology,* pp. 70–73, Lea and Febiger, Philadelphia.

38. I. Hirono, K. Yamada, H. Niwa, et al. (1984) Separation of carcinogenic fraction of bracken fern. *Cancer Lett.* 21:239–246.

39. I. Hirono, S. Aiso, T. Yamaji, et al. (1984) Carcinogenicity in rats of ptaquiloside isolated from bracken. *Gann* 75:833–836.

40. I. Hirono, Y. Kono, K. Takahashi, et al. (1984) Reproduction of acute bracken poisoning in a calf with ptaquiloside, a bracken constituent. *Vet. Rec.* 115:375–378.

41. I. Hirono, C. Shibuya, M. Shimizu, and K. Fushimi (1972) Carcinogenic activity of processed bracken used as human food. *J. Natl. Cancer Inst.* 48:1245–1250.

42. A.M. Pamukcu and J.M. Price (1969) Induction of intestinal and urinary bladder cancer in rats by feeding bracken fern (*Pteris aquilina*). *J. Natl. Cancer Inst.* 43:275–281.

43. D.K. Salunkhe and M.T. Wu (1977) Toxicants in plants and plant products. *CRC Crit. Rev. Food Sci. Nutr.* 9:265–324.

44. A.L. Lehninger (1970) *Biochemistry,* Worth Publishers, New York.

45. G.S. Stoewsand, J.L. Anderson, and R.C. Lamb (1975) Cyanide content of apricot kernels. *J. Food Sci.* 40:1107.

46. R.D. Montgomery (1965) The medical significance of cyanogen in plant foodstuffs. *Am. J. Clin. Nutr.* 17:103–113.

47. B.O. Osuntokun (1968) An ataxic neuropathy in Nigeria. *Brain* 91:215–248.

48. J.M. Kingsbury (1964) *Poisonous Plants of the United States and Canada,* Prentice-Hall, Englewood Cliffs, NJ.

49. J.W. Sayre and S. Kaymakcalan (1964) Cyanide poisoning from apricot seeds among children in Turkey. *N. Engl. J. Med.* 270:1113–1115.

50. M. Chevion, J. Mager, and G. Glaser (1983) Naturally occurring food toxicants: favism-producing agents. In: *CRC Handbook of Naturally Occurring Food Toxicants* (M. Rechcigl, Jr., ed.), pp. 63–79, CRC Press, Boca Raton, FL.

51. P.E. Carson (1960) Glucose-6-phosphate dehydrogenase deficiency in hemolytic anemia. *Fed. Proc.* 19:995–1006.

52. J. Mager, G. Glaser, A. Izak, S. Bien, and J. Noam (1965) Metabolic effects of pyrimidines derived from fava bean glycosides on human erythrocytes deficient in glucose-6-phosphate dehydrogenase. *Biochem. Biophys. Res. Commun.* 20:235–240.

53. B. Toth (1983) Carcinogens in edible mushrooms. In: *Carcinogens and Mutagens in the Environment,* vol. III (H.F. Stich, ed.), pp. 99–108, CRC Press, Boca Raton.

54. B. Levenberg (1960) Structure and enzymatic cleavage of agaritine, a new phenylhydrazine of L-glutamic acid isolated from agaricaceae. *J. Am. Chem. Soc.* 83:503–504.

55. A.E. Ross, D.L. Nagel, and B. Toth (1982) Evidence for the occurrence and formation of diazonium ions in the *Agaricus bisporus* mushroom and its extracts. *J. Agric. Food Chem.* 30:521–525.

56. A.E. Ross, D.L. Nagel, and B. Toth (1982) Occurrence, stability, and decomposition of β-N[γ-L(+)-glutamyl]-4-hydroxymethyl-phenylhydrazine (agaritine) from the mushroom *Agaricus bisporus.* *Food Chem. Toxicol.* 20:903–907.

57. H.J. Gigliotti and B. Levenberg (1964) Studies on the γ-glutamyltransferase of *Agaricus bisporus.* *J. Biol. Chem.* 239:2274–2284.

58. D. Nagel, L. Wallcave, B. Toth, and R. Kupper (1977) Formation of methylhydrazine from acetaldehyde N-methyl-N-formylhydrazone, a component of *Gyromitra esculenta.* *Cancer Res.* 37:3458–3460.

59. S.J. Moloney and R.A. Prough (1983) Biochemical toxicology of hydrazines. In: *Reviews in Biochemical Toxicology,* vol. 5 (E. Hodgson, J.R. Bend, and R.M. Philpot, eds.), pp. 313–348, Elsevier Biomedical, New York.

60. J.D. Wood and S.J. Peesker (1972) The effect on GABA metabolism in the brain of isonicotinic acid hydrazide and pyridoxine as

a function of time after administration. *J. Neurochem.* 19:1527–1537.

61. B. Dubnich, G.A. Lesson, and G.E. Phillips (1962) In vivo inhibition of serotonin synthesis in mouse brain by β-phenylethylhydrazine, an inhibitor of monoamine oxidase. *Biochem. Pharmacol.* 11:45–52.

62. J.D. Wood and D.E. Abrahams (1971) The comparative effects of various hydrazides on γ-aminobutyric acid and its metabolism. *J. Neurochem.* 18:1017–1025.

63. Y. Yamauchi, A. Litwan, L. Adams, H. Zimmer, and E.V. Hess (1975) Induction of antibodies to nuclear antigen in rabbits by immunization with hydralazine-human serum albumin conjugates. *J. Clin. Invest.* 56:958–969.

64. E.M. Tan (1974) Drug-induced autoimmune disease. *Fed. Proc.* 33:1894–1897.

65. R.T. Schoen and D.E. Trentham (1981) Drug-induced lupus: an adjuvant disease. *Am. J. Med.* 71:5–8.

66. H. Druckrey (1970) Production of colonic carcinomas by 1,2-dialkylhydrazines and azoalkanes. In: *Carcinoma of the Colon and Antecedent Epithelium* (W.J. Burdette, ed.), pp. 267–279, C.C. Thomas, Springfield, IL.

67. B. Toth, D. Nagel, and A. Ross (1982) Gastric tumorigenesis by a single dose of 4-(hydroxymethyl)benzenediazonium ion of *Agaricus bisporus. Br. J. Cancer* 46:417–422.

68. B. Kalyanaraman and B.K. Sinha (1985) Free radical-mediated activation of hydrazine derivatives. *Environ. Health Perspect.* 64:179–184.

69. T. Sugimura (1982) Mutagens, carcinogens, and tumor promoters in our daily food. *Cancer* 49:1970–1984.

70. T. Sugimura (1988) New environmental carcinogens in daily life. *Trends Pharmacol. Sci.* 9:205–209.

71. M. Nagao, M. Honda, Y. Seino, T. Yahagi, and T. Sugimura (1977) Mutagenicities of smoke condensates and the charred surface of fish and meat. *Cancer Lett.* 2:221–226.

72. M. Nagao, M. Honda, Y. Seino, Y. Yahagi, T. Kawachi, and T. Sugimura (1977) Mutagenicities of protein pyrolysates. *Cancer Lett.* 2:335–340.

73. M. Nagao, T. Yahagi, T. Kawachi, et al. (1977) Mutagens in foods, and especially pyrolysis products of protein. In: *Progress in Genetic Toxicology* (D. Scott, B.A. Bridges, and F.H. Sobels, eds.), pp. 259–264, Elsevier/North-Holland Biomedical Press, New York.

74. R. Kato (1986) Metabolic activation of mutagenic heterocyclic aromatic amines from protein pyrolysates. *CRC Crit. Rev. Toxicol.* 16:307–348.

75. S. Takayama, Y. Nakatsuru, H. Ohgaki, S. Sato, and T. Sugimura (1985) Carcinogenicity in rats of a mutagenic compound, 3-amino-1,4-dimethyl-5H-pyrido[4,3b]indole, from tryptophan pyrolysate. *Jpn. J. Cancer Res.* 76:815–817.

76. T. Sugimura (1986) Studies on environmental chemical carcinogenesis in Japan. *Science* 233:312–318.

77. Y. Hashimoto and K. Shudo (1985) Chemical modification of DNA with muta-carcinogens. I. 3-Amino-1-methyl-5H-pyrido[4,3b]indole and 2-amino-6-methyldipyrido[1,2-a:3′,2′-d]imidazole: metabolic activation and structure of the DNA adducts. *Environ. Health Perspect.* 62:209–214.

78. Y. Hashimoto and K. Shudo (1985) Chemical modification of DNA with muta-carcinogens. II. Base sequence-specific binding to DNA of 2-amino-6-methyl-dipyrido[1,2-a:3′,2′-d]imidazole (Glu-P-1). *Environ. Health Perspect.* 62:215–218.

79. K. Yamaguchi, K. Shudo, T. Okamoto, T. Sugimura, and T. Kosuge (1980) Presence of 3-amino-1,4-dimethyl-5H-pyrido[4,3b]indole in broiled beef. *Gann* 71:745–746.

80. Z. Yamaizume, T. Shiomi, H. Kasai, S. Nishimura, Y. Takahashi, M. Nagao, and T. Sugimura (1980) Detection of potent mutagens, Trp-P-1 and Trp-P-2, in broiled fish. *Cancer Lett.* 9:75–83.

81. T. Sugimura, M. Nagao, and K. Wakabayashi (1981) Mutagenic heterocyclic amines in cooked food. In: *Environmental Carcinogens: Selected Methods of Analysis,* vol. 4 (H. Egan, L. Fishbein, M. Castegnaro, I.K. O'Neill, and H. Bartsch, eds.), pp. 251–267, International Agency for Research on Cancer, Lyon.

82. T. Matsumoto, D. Yoshida, and H. Tomita (1981) Determination of mutagens, amino-α-carbolines in grilled foods and cigarette smoke condensate. *Cancer Lett.* 12:105–110.

Chapter 57

Genetics

It was not until the fourth edition of *Present Knowledge in Nutrition*, published in 1976, that chronic diseases were included.[1] That addition reflected a decline in the prevalence of acute diseases, primarily infectious and nutritional in origin, without a concomitant decline in chronic diseases, which in some cases had increased in prevalence especially in developed countries. Foremost among the factors causing the decline in acute diseases (which started over a half century before the first edition in 1953) were improved living conditions and better nutrition. New lifestyles, particularly the increase in smoking, contributed to an increase in the prevalence of some chronic diseases. With this change the role of genes in modifying nutritional requirements has become evident, as will be considered in the first two sections of this chapter.

Variation in nutritional requirements for at least some nutrients is approximately Gaussian with fairly large variances.[2] This variation is partly genetic in origin as is suggested by the correlation of plasma lipid concentrations between first-degree relatives but not between spouses.[3] Moreover, only a small number of genetic variants—each of which causes a different response to an environmental agent, such as the response in plasma cholesterol concentration when the amount of saturated fatty acids in the diet is changed by a fixed amount—is needed to obtain the Gaussian distribution.[4] Although genetic variants can account for those individuals with requirements at one end of the distribution, it may come as a surprise that other susceptibility-conferring genetic variants have attained high frequencies. Explanations for this phenomenon will be discussed in the third section.

In the final sections how recombinant DNA technology has greatly expanded our ability to discover many more genetic variants and the mechanisms by which some of these variants alter nutritional intakes and requirements will be discussed.

Unmasking Genetic Diseases

Research played an important role in unmasking the presence of genetic disease. The discovery of vitamins and other essential nutrients led to extensive educational efforts and public policies to assure that large segments of the population would receive an adequate supply. For example, the supplementation of milk with vitamin D vastly diminished vitamin D–deficiency rickets, but a few people developed rickets despite vitamin D intakes that were adequate for the vast majority. Iodizing table salt virtually eliminated goiter due to iodine deficiency, but some patients developed goiter despite adequate iodine intake. Researchers increasingly turned to the study of the residual disorders and soon found that genes played a decisive role.[5]

Other investigators uncovered specific causes of diseases, such as mental retardation, that previously had been lumped together in one broad category. The discovery in the 1930s that the urinary excretion of phenylketones (phenylketonuria or PKU) was associated with mental retardation was followed in the 1950s with the discovery that the high concentration of phenylalanine in the blood of phenylketonuric subjects could be reduced by lowering the amount of phenylalanine in the diet. In older infants and children this reduction was not accompanied by significant improvement in mental development. This finding led in the 1960s to screening of newborns and the prompt administration of low-phenylalanine diets to infants with persistent hyperphenylalaninemia. It is now apparent that lowering blood phenylalanine by dietary control prevents the retardation of PKU. However, the low-phenylalanine diet must be started promptly when the disease is diagnosed after neonatal screening and maintained at least until age 10 y.[6] Since the discovery of PKU, other genetic disorders were discovered that have outcomes that can be improved by dietary modification (such as galactosemia and some types of glycogen storage disease) or by blocking the absorption or enhancing the excretion of nutrients (as in familial hypercholesterolemia and Wilson's disease). The advent of recombinant DNA technology will lead to breakthroughs in many more diseases.

The Increasing Role of Genetics in Diseases

The increased availability of foods high in animal fat in developed countries is associated with higher rates of cardiovascular diseases, which increased in the United States from 1900 to ~1965,[7] making them the leading cause of death in many of these countries. In addition, the incidence of some cancers increased in the last 30 y (lung, colon, breast, and prostatic cancers) although others decreased (stomach, rectum, and cervix).[8] The increases cannot be explained entirely by better diagnosis or longer life span. One possibility is that those individuals who possess common genetic variants are not suited to the high intakes of certain nutrients that have occurred since World War II in many developed countries.

This hypothesis takes on added luster when one recognizes that the harmful effects of surfeit, of highly refined diets, or of cigarette smoking are not uniformly distributed. Why, for instance, do fewer than one-third of men aged 33–49 y in the highest quintile of plasma cholesterol manifest coronary artery disease within 20 y?[9] Why do no more than 5% of men aged 65–75 y who smoked most of their lives succumb to lung cancer?[10] The presence of genetic variants that increase susceptibility provides part of the answer.[11]

Frequency of Genetic Variants

The possibility that genetic variants (alleles) could attain sufficiently high frequency to account for common diseases seems a contradiction in terms. If alleles cause disease, how can they be passed from one generation to the next? If they cannot be passed from one generation to the next, how can they attain high frequency? New mutation does not occur at a rate high enough to account for common diseases.

Part of the answer lies in the changing conditions under which humans evolved. Fewer than 1% of all human generations have been born since the discovery of agriculture. Hunting-gathering characterized most of humans' evolution. Alleles that were advantageous or neutral for the hunter-gatherer but that are harmful in modern environments still will be present in fairly high frequency because selective mechanisms have not had time to remove them. Non-insulin-dependent diabetes may be due to the possession of alleles that provided selective reproductive advantage to hunter-gatherers perhaps by increasing

resistance to famine, which alternated with feasting. During the evolution of hunter-gatherers, such alleles would increase in frequency. In societies in which food is continuously abundant and available, these alleles may predispose to diabetes.[12]

Another part of the answer lies in the natural history of the common diseases in which genes play a role, most importantly cardiovascular disease and cancer. These diseases are relatively late in onset often occurring after people have had their children. Therefore, those who have genetic predispositions will have passed on the susceptibility-conferring alleles before the disease becomes manifest.

Another part lies in gene dosage. Some alleles are deleterious only when they are inherited from both parents. (The resulting disease is said to be recessive; affected individuals are homozygous for the deleterious allele.) Offspring inheriting one dose (heterozygotes) may have a reproductive advantage over individuals inheriting only the normal (wild-type) allele as well as over affected homozygotes. As a result, the frequency of heterozygotes in the population will increase up to the point when matings between heterozygotes occur with such frequency that the loss of affected homozygotes cancels out the homozygote advantage (balanced polymorphism). Such is the case for sickle cell anemia. For other autosomal-recessive disorders, heterozygotes for susceptibility-conferring alleles may develop milder, later-onset disease than affected homozygotes; such individuals propagate the allele before manifesting the disease.

Gene dosage also explains the high frequency of deficiency of the enzyme glucose-6-phosphate dehydrogenase (G6PD) in populations in which malaria is endemic. The G6PD gene is X linked. Therefore, affected males, who have only one X chromosome, have no normal G6PD to offset the deficiency. Females have two doses of X-chromosome genes although only one is active in any cell. The high frequency of G6PD deficiency alleles can be explained by the finding that the malaria parasite survives less well in the red blood cells of female heterozygotes than in male hemizygotes or normal females or males.[13]

Occasionally, a mutation leading to an allele capable of causing severe recessive disease will occur in one individual in a relatively small closed population. This allele can be passed in single dose to successive generations, resulting in its relatively high frequency. Eventually, matings between heterozygotes begin to limit the increase of the allele as affected homozygotes fail to survive long enough to reproduce. This founder effect may explain the high frequency of Tay Sachs disease in Jews from eastern Europe.

Finally, more than one allele at the same gene locus or alleles at more than one gene locus can cause or contribute to the occurrence of a single disease entity. If several alleles can each cause the same disease, then no one of them has to attain as high a frequency as if it were the only allele capable of causing the disease. The extent of genetic variation, or heterogeneity, is considerable. Two or more alleles have been found at about one-third of gene loci responsible for the synthesis of specific enzymes; the least common of the alleles at these loci occurs in at least 2% of the population.[14] These common sets of variants are called polymorphisms. There may be an even larger number of rare alleles. No fewer than 18 different alleles, each of which causes a defect in the low-density-lipoprotein receptor molecule, can result in hypercholesterolemia and heart disease.[15]

Role of Recombinant DNA Technology

Recombinant DNA techniques revealed even more polymorphisms than had previously been discovered. Because the relation between a polymorphism and the genes near it is constant, polymorphisms can be used to localize disease-related genes to specific regions of specific chromosomes. The finding that one form of a polymorphism is associated with the presence of a disease in a family more often than expected by chance suggests linkage between the polymorphism and the gene for the disease. The method requires the presence of multiple families in which the disease in question is inherited in Mendelian fashion and is present in more than one family member. Some individuals in each of the families must be heterozygotes for the polymorphisms being used to test for linkage. Localization of the genes for cystic fibrosis, bipolar affective disorder, and familial colon cancer has been accomplished. Once a gene is localized, recombinant DNA and other techniques can be used to identify the gene and determine its function. By use of this methodology, the Duchenne muscular dystrophy and retinoblastoma genes[11] and recently the cystic fibrosis gene[16] were identified.

Once a gene is identified, tests to discover asymptomatic individuals who are destined to manifest the disease later in life can be developed. If the pathogenesis of the disease is known, the occurrence of disease might be prevented or postponed by, for example, dietary modification. Tests can also discover heterozygote carriers of disease-causing or susceptibility-conferring alleles who are not themselves at risk but whose offspring may be. The tests also can be employed prenatally to discover whether the fetus is affected. Tests employing recombinant DNA techniques require only a tiny amount of DNA, which can be obtained any time after conception from any nucleated cell. Prediction of genetic risks for a wide range of diseases—both common and rare—soon will be possible.

Mechanisms Operating in Nutritional Disorders of Genetic Origin

The extent of genetic heterogeneity leads to the prediction that variants occur for at least some of the receptor and transport proteins and enzymes involved in metabolism and that some of these variants, at least when present in double (homozygous) dosage, could modify food preferences, nutrient requirements, or nutrient tolerances. With a few notable exceptions most of the genetic disorders discovered thus far are rare autosomal-recessive disorders. It should be recognized, however, that heterozygotes for rare alleles have relatively high frequencies. If a common allele has a frequency of p and a rare allele a frequency of q (such that $p + q = 1$), then the ratio of heterozygotes (frequency $2pq$) to affected homozygotes (frequency q^2) is $2p/q$. When q^2 equals 0.000001, heterozygotes will be 2000 times more frequent than affected heterozygotes and will occur with a frequency of 0.002.

Heterozygotes for alleles that cause severe disease in homozygotes may manifest growth disturbances or disease under some circumstances. Although they would be expected to have ~50% of the protein concentration of normal homozygotes, this amount may be inadequate when the protein (or enzyme) is the rate-limiting step in a transport or metabolic sequence, especially when the intake of the nutrient deviates from the normal mean. Heterozygotes for an allele with a product that impairs detoxification of a nutrient may be less tolerant of high intakes of the nutrient than normal homozygotes, whereas heterozygotes for an allele with a product that impairs absorption may require higher intakes than normal homozygotes require. Examples of variants that affect the various stages of nutrient utilization and excretion are given in this section.

Taste. The ability of people to taste certain substances varies widely. The threshold for tasting phenylthiocarbamide (PTC) and about 40 related compounds is determined by a single gene locus; the threshold may be modified by a second locus controlling a more general taste ability.[17] About one-third of whites are recessive, lacking the ability to taste PTC at concentrations easily tasted by heterozygotes and unaffected homozygotes, who cannot be distinguished. Among the compounds for which PTC tasters and nontasters differ are caffeine, saccharin, and potassium chloride. These differences are evident at concentrations of the substance used in beverages and foods. In each case, PTC tasters perceive the compounds as more bitter than do nontasters. PTC tasters also have a greater number of food dislikes than do nontasters but not in all categories of foods.

The lower threshold that tasters have to bitter substances, some of which may be poisonous, may have given tasters a selective evolutionary advantage in preagricultural populations. With the advent of agriculture and concomitantly with less reliance on wild plants, selection against nontasters may have been relaxed. Consistent with this hypothesis, the frequency of nontasters today is lower in primitive than in more-developed populations.[18] Some of the naturally occurring bitter compounds that PTC tasters dislike have antithyroid activity. The incidence of adenomatous goiter has been reported to be higher among nontasters than tasters (although the reverse may be true for other types of goiter). It is possible that by modifying food preferences, genetically determined differences in taste could alter susceptibility or resistance to chronic diseases for which foods play a modulating role, such as some cancers.

Digestion. Lactase production in adults is a dominant trait.[19] In populations in which unmodified milk is frequently ingested after weaning, the majority of adults have the trait and are lactose tolerant. In populations in which milk is fermented (thereby digesting the lactose) or not used as a food, most adults are lactose intolerant. They are homozygous for an allele at the lactase locus that is incapable of generating adequate amounts of functional lactase. The high frequency of the adult lactase allele in milk-drinking populations in North Africa and Arabia probably stems from the selective reproductive advantage it conferred when milk was a major source of calories. Its high frequency in Scandinavia, where diminished exposure to sunlight increases the risk of calcium deficiency, may result from the facilitation of calcium absorption by the digestion of lactose in milk. Inherited lactose intolerance is a frequently encountered cause of chronic gastrointestinal discomfort and diarrhea. However, fewer than one-third of lactose-intolerant individuals manifest symptoms after the ingestion of 240 mL of milk. Lactose-intolerant individuals tend to choose foods that do not contain lactose.

Approximately 1 in 2000 white infants is born with cystic fibrosis (CF), an autosomal-recessive disorder.[20] The gene for CF has been identified; it probably plays a role in chloride transport.[16] As a result of viscous pancreatic secretions secondary to the chloride-transport defect, the concentration of proteolytic enzymes in the gut of infants with CF is often diminished, resulting in malabsorption and consequent short stature. Growth can be improved by the administration of pancreatic enzymes, but thick respiratory secretions and recurrent lung infections remain major problems in the disease. Children with CF can become salt depleted in hot weather because of large losses of sodium chloride in sweat and other secretions.

Absorption. Most of the absorption of monosaccharides, amino acids, and several of the water-soluble vitamins depends on active transport; absorption occurs against a concentration gradient, requires energy, and reaches a maximum rate. The process often depends on the presence of specific proteins in intestinal mucosal cell membranes that are capable of binding the nutrient in question. Sometimes a few structurally similar nutrients are transported by the same system. Genetic variants in which the affinity of a transport protein for the nutrient or its ability to transport the nutrient is impaired have been found for glucose and galactose; the basic amino acids ornithine, lysine, arginine, and cystine; tryptophan and other neutral amino acids; folic acid, vitamin B-12; and biotin.[21] Some, but not all, of these transport systems operate by facilitating tubular reabsorption in the kidney as well as by facilitating absorption in the intestine. Consequently, a deficiency resulting from an intestinal absorption defect may be intensified by increased renal excretion.

For some nutrients, more than one system, each under independent genetic control, may be available, thereby moderating the effect of a defect in one system. There are at least two basic amino acid systems, one transporting only ornithine, arginine, and lysine and the other transporting cystine as well. Patients with cystinuria often develop kidney stones. Disease in patients with a defect in the other system, known as lysinuric protein intolerance, is partially due to decreased availability of ornithine for urea cycle activity with a consequent increase in blood ammonia.

Although disease does not always occur in homozygotes and heterozygotes for transport variants, it may appear when environmental factors, such as starvation, limit the availability of nutrients or interfere with absorption, as in the case of infectious gastroenteritis.[21,22] Most patients with Hartnup disorder, a defect in the transport of tryptophan and other neutral amino acids, are asymptomatic. When the availability of tryptophan is reduced they are prone to develop pellagra because of their inability to synthesize niacin from tryptophan.

Genetically determined increased absorption of nutrients also can lead to disease as is the case with primary hemochromatosis in which increased, potentially toxic amounts of iron are absorbed.[23] The basic defect is unknown, but failure of intestinal mucosal cells to block iron may result in increased iron absorption. The gene locus at which the hemochromatosis allele resides is closely linked to the histocompatability human leukocyte antigen A (HLA-A) locus on chromosome 6. As many as 1 in 400 people in the U.S. population are homozygotes for closely linked HLA-A alleles, suggesting that they could develop hemochromatosis. Clinically evident hemochromatosis is much less common. This finding can be explained by insufficient iron in the diet to cause toxicity, by occasional meiotic crossing over between the HLA-A and hemochromatosis loci, or by the contribution of other genetic and environmental factors. There is no evidence that heterozygotes, who may constitute 10% of the U.S. population, are at increased risk of iron toxicity. The high frequency of the allele may be due to a reproductive advantage conferred by increased iron absorption when dietary iron was scarce or fluctuated in abundance or, alternatively, to an advantage conferred by the closely linked HLA alleles.

Metabolism. In patients with some genetically determined defects of intermediary metabolism, certain nutrients ingested in normal amounts will prove to be toxic, whereas in other disorders nutrient deficiencies will develop at usual intakes.[24] Phenylketonuria and galactosemia are autosomal-recessive disorders in which failure to metabolize phenylalanine and galactose, respectively, results in mental retardation unless the intake of the substance is restricted. In type 1 glycogen storage disease, in which glucose cannot be utilized from glycogen because of defective glucose 6-phosphatase, life-threatening hypoglycemia and ketoacidosis can be prevented by the continuous or frequent feeding of glucose. In patients with orotic aciduria, uridine-5-phosphate cannot be synthesized from orotic acid. A dietary source of uridine can compensate for the defect. In some inherited metabolic defects, the enzyme that appears to be defective can be activated if large doses of cofactor, frequently a vitamin, is provided. Such is the case in one type of homocystinuria, which is responsive to pyridoxine, and in methylmalonic acidemia, which is responsive to vitamin B-12. In a few patients with PKU, the enzyme defect is not in phenylalanine hydroxylase, which converts phenylalanine to tyrosine, but in other enzymes that recycle or synthesize the biopterin cofactor (a folic acid metabolite).[25] Occasionally, malnourished chronic alcoholics develop the Wernicke-Korsakoff syndrome, which is known to result from thiamin deficiency. These individuals were found to have a variant form of transketolase that requires much larger amounts of thiamin to function than does the normal enzyme.[26]

As discussed earlier, G6PD deficiencies occur frequently in some populations. Over 300 variants of G6PD have been described and 10% of the world's population have a G6PD-deficient variant.[13] Males with variants in which enzyme activity is drastically reduced often develop neonatal jaundice and nonspherocytic hemolytic anemia. In most of the more common deficiencies, hemolysis is seen only after the ingestion of external agents that oxidize glutathione faster than it can be reduced by the NADPH generated from oxidation of glucose by G6PD in the pentose phosphate pathway. Hemolysis is triggered by a number of drugs as well as by fava beans, which are a popular food in parts of the world in which the frequency of G6PD deficiency is high. Elimination of fava beans from the diet reduces the frequency of hemolytic anemia in people with G6PD deficiency.

About 1 in 500 people is heterozygous for low-density-lipoprotein-receptor defects.[15] This accounts for ~5% of coronary artery disease in men under 60 y. Recessive disease occurs only about once in a million births and results in death from coronary artery disease by the third decade of life. As a result of the defect in heterozygotes, endogenous cholesterol synthesis is only partially inhibited, resulting in increased concentrations of plasma cholesterol. Cholesterol concentrations can be lowered by sequestering cholesterol in the gut or, more effectively, by inhibiting endogenous cholesterol synthesis.

Excretion. Failure to eliminate nonmetabolizable nutrients, such as trace metals, from the body at a rate equal to their absorption results in accumulations that can become harmful. Such is the case in Wilson's disease, an autosomal-recessive disorder in which decreased biliary excretion of copper leads to neurologic and hepatic problems.[27] The gene for the disease was localized to chromosome 13, but the basic defect has not been elucidated. The harmful consequences can be prevented by reducing copper intake and using chelators that bind copper in relatively innocuous complexes if not by increasing its excretion.[28]

Genetic defects can also result in excessive excretion. In nephrogenic diabetes insipidus, an X-linked disorder, the renal tubules are unresponsive to vasopressin and cannot, therefore, conserve water.[29] Dehydration results unless water intake is increased and solute load is reduced.

Summary and Conclusions

A large number of genetic variants that modify preferences, requirements, and tolerances for foods have been identified. With the application of recombinant DNA techniques many more will be discovered. Some of the known variants are common, at least in some populations, but most are rare. Some of these variants cause disease in heterozygotes, whereas others apparently cause disease only in homozygotes or hemizygotes. Disease in heterozygotes for some alleles may be milder and of later onset than in affected homozygotes. The explanation for why some people develop disease as a result of exposure to environmental agents, including foods, whereas others do not is likely to be at least partially genetic.

Treatment is possible for many genetic disorders in which nutritional requirements are altered. Outcomes can be improved by providing larger amounts of a nutrient to individuals who have an increased requirement or limiting the intake or otherwise reducing the toxicity of nutrients in those with reduced tolerance.

For some diseases, dietary modification is effective after clinical symptoms appear. For others only pre-symptomatic treatment is effective. Individuals at risk can be identified if there is a family history of the disorder, but for autosomal recessive disorders a history of disease in previous generations is unlikely. Public health approaches are an alternative. One approach involves modifying the diet of the entire population, as is currently being attempted in an effort to reduce coronary artery disease. This approach is justifiable only when the modification will not be harmful to anyone. The other involves screening, as is currently done to identify newborns with phenyl-ketonuria. Currently, screening tests are not available for many genetic disorders. The application of re-combinant DNA techniques promises to make many more tests available. The validity and reliability of new tests and the improvement of outcomes because of the prompt institution of therapy need to be demonstrated before any test or dietary modification is widely adopted.

References

1. R.E. Olson (1984) Foreword. In: *Present Knowledge in Nutrition*, 5th ed. (R.E. Olson, H.P. Broquist, C.O. Chichester, W.J. Darby, A.C. Kolbye, Jr., and R.M. Stalvey, eds.), pp. xvii–xviii, The Nutrition Foundation, Washington DC.

2. G.H. Beaton (1984) Variability of nutrient requirements in the human. In: *Genetic Factors in Nutrition* (A. Velazquez and H. Bourges, eds.), pp. 189–198, Academic Press, Orlando, FL.

3. G.A. Chase, P.O. Kwiterovich, Jr., and P.S. Bachorik (1979) The Columbia Population Study. II. Familial aggregation of plasma cholesterol and triglycerides. *Johns Hopkins Med. J.* 145:150–156.

4. D.F. Roberts (1985) Genetics and nutritional adaptation. In: *Nutritional Adaptation in Man* (K. Blaxter and J.C. Waterlow, eds.), pp. 45–58, John Libbey, London.

5. C.R. Scriver (in press) Changing heritability of nutritional disorders. In: *Genetic Variation in Nutrition* (A. Simopoulos and B. Childs, eds.), Karger, Basel.

6. N.A. Holtzman, R.A. Kronmal, W. van Doorninck, C. Azen, and R. Koch (1986) Effect of age at loss of dietary control on intellectual performance and behavior of children with phenylketonuria. *N. Engl. J. Med.* 314:593–598.

7. U.S. Department of Commerce (1975) *Historical Statistics of the United States. Colonial Times to 1970, Part I.* U.S. Government Printing Office, Washington DC.

8. National Cancer Institute (1988) *1987 Annual Cancer Statistics Review Including Cancer Trends: 1950–1985.* NIH Publication no. 88-2789, National Cancer Institute, Bethesda, MD.

9. W.B. Kannel and T. Gordon (1982) The search for an optimum serum cholesterol. *Lancet* 2:374–375.

10. R. Doll and A.B. Hill (1956) Lung cancer and other causes of death in relation to smoking. *Br. Med. J.* 2:1071–1081.

11. N.A. Holtzman (1989) *Proceed with Caution: Predicting Genetic Risks in the Recombinant DNA Era,* Johns Hopkins University Press, Baltimore.

12. J.V. Neel (1982) The thrifty genotype revisited. In: *The Genetics of Diabetes Mellitus* (J. Kobberling and R. Tattersall, eds.), pp. 283–293, Academic Press, London.

13. L. Luzzato (1986) Glucose-6-phosphate dehydrogenase deficiency and other genetic factors interacting with drugs. In: *Ethnic Differences in Reactions to Drugs and Xenobiotics* (W. Kalow, H.W. Goedde, and D.P. Agarwal, eds.), pp. 385–399, Alan R. Liss, New York.

14. H. Harris (1980) *The Principles of Human Biochemical Genetics,* 3rd ed. Elsevier, Amsterdam.

15. J.L. Goldstein and M.S. Brown (1989) Familial hypercholesterol-emia. In: *The Metabolic Basis of Inherited Disease,* 6th ed., vol. I (C.R. Scriver, A.L. Beaudet, W.S. Sly, and D. Valle, eds.), pp. 1215–1250, McGraw Hill, New York.

16. J.R. Riordan, J.R. Rommens, B. Kerem, et al. (1989) Identification of the cystic fibrosis gene: cloning and characterization of the complementary DNA. *Science* 245:1066–1073.

17. A. Drenowski (in press) Genetics of taste and smell. In: *Genetic Variation in Nutrition* (A. Simopoulos and B. Childs, eds.), Karger, Basel.

18. H. Kalmus (1971) Genetics of taste. In: *Handbook of Sensory Physiology,* vol. IV, part 2 (L.M. Beidler, ed.), pp. 165–179, Springer-Verlag, New York.

19. G. Flatz (1989) The genetic polymorphism of intestinal lactase activity in adult humans. In: *The Metabolic Basis of Inherited Disease,* 6th ed., vol. 2 (C.R. Scriver, A.L. Beaudet, W.S. Sly, and D. Valle, eds.), pp. 2999–3006, McGraw Hill, New York.

20. T.F. Boat, M.J. Welsh, and A.L. Beaudet (1989) Cystic fibrosis. In: *The Metabolic Basis of Inherited Disease,* 6th ed., vol. 2 (C.R. Scriber, A.L. Beaudet, W.S. Sly, and D. Valle, eds.), pp. 2649–2680, McGraw Hill, New York.

21. R.E. Hillman (1984) Genetics and intestinal absorption. In: *Genetic Factors in Nutrition* (A. Velazquez and H. Bourges, eds.), pp. 199–210, Academic Press, Orlando, FL.

22. C.R. Scriver (in press) Changing heritability of nutritional disorders. In: *Genetic Variation in Nutrition* (A. Simopoulos and B. Childs, eds.), Karger, Basel.

23. T.H. Bothwell, A.W. Charlton, and A.G. Motulsky (1989) Hemo-chromatosis. In: *The Metabolic Basis of Inherited Disease,* 6th ed., vol. I (C.R. Scriver, A.L. Beaudet, W.S. Sly, and D. Valle, eds.), pp. 1433–1462, McGraw Hill, New York.

24. N.A. Holtzman (1970) Dietary treatment of inborn errors of metabolism. *Ann. Rev. Med.* 21:335–356.

25. C.R. Scriver, S. Kaufman, and S.L.C. Woo (1989) The hyper-phenylalaninemias. In: *The Metabolic Basis of Inherited Disease,* 6th ed., vol. I (C.R. Scriver, A.L. Beaudet, W.S. Sly, and D. Valle, eds.), pp. 495–546, McGraw Hill, New York.

26. J.P. Blass and G.E. Gibson (1977) Abnormality of a thiamine-requiring enzyme in patients with Wernicke-Korsakoff syndrome. *N. Engl. J. Med.* 297:1367–1370.

27. D.M. Danks (1989) Disorders of copper transport. In: *The Metabolic Basis of Inherited Disease,* 6th ed., vol. I (C.R. Scriver, A.L. Beaudet, W.S. Sly, and D. Valle, eds.), pp. 1411–1431, McGraw Hill, New York.

28. I.H. Scheinberg, I. Sternlieb, M. Schulsky, and R.J. Stockert (1988) Penicillamine may detoxify copper in Wilson's disease. *Lancet* 2:95.

29. W.B. Reeves and T.E. Andreoli (1989) Nephrogenic diabetes in-sipidus. In: *The Metabolic Basis of Inherited Disease,* 6th ed., vol. 2 (C.R. Scriver, A.L. Beaudet, W.S. Sly, and D. Valle, eds.), pp. 1985–2011, McGraw Hill, New York.

Chapter 58

Dietary Standards and Dietary Guidelines

Many commentaries on dietary standards and a plethora of reports on dietary guidelines have appeared since the last edition of *Present Knowledge in Nutrition* was published. Until recently, the latest report on Recommended Dietary Allowances (RDA) of the Food and Nutrition Board (FNB) of the National Research Council of the National Academy of Sciences (NAS/NRC) was the ninth edition, which was published in 1980.[1] A tenth edition was completed in 1985 but publication was withheld by the NAS because the FNB refused to recognize, as the RDA Committee had, that dietary standards for meeting physiological needs for essential nutrients should not be influenced by public policy recommendations for disease prevention. The nature of the conflict that led to this 4-y delay was described clearly and succinctly by Pellett.[2] After much turmoil, the tenth edition was published late in 1989.[3] At this time, it is not possible to discuss modifications of the RDA since 1980.* My objectives here, therefore, will be to identify recent, pertinent publications on this subject, to comment on the limitations of dietary standards and new directions to overcome some of these limitations, and to discuss the importance of distinguishing clearly between dietary standards based on scientific evidence of physiological requirements for essential nutrients and dietary guidelines proposed as public health policy largely on the basis of inferences from epidemiologic studies of associations between diet and disease.

Recent Reports

The evolution of dietary standards including the RDA was described in recent reviews,[4-6] recommended intakes of nutrients around the world were summarized,[7] approaches to formulating dietary standards in the United Kingdom and the United States were compared,[8] presentations at a series of workshops on research in human nutrition that dealt in large measure with the RDA and dietary guidelines were published,[9] and criteria for assessing the nutritional adequacy of diets were evaluated critically.[10] These articles provide an extensive bibliography on dietary standards, their uses, and their limitations.

A new report on energy and protein requirements was published by the World Health and Food and Agriculture organizations and the United Nations University (WHO/FAO/UNU).[11] *Recommended Nutrient Intakes for Canadians* was revised.[12] The United Kingdom reprinted its 1979 Recommended Daily Intakes.[13] The Australian Department of Health has been publishing the background papers prepared by its experts as the basis for revising Recommended Dietary Intakes for Australians.[14-16] The latter provide much more information than is usually included in reports on dietary standards. Because the same literature is used by all national committees on dietary standards, and because average requirements for essential nutrients should be the same the world over, it would be much simpler than it now is to identify the reasons (selection of data, judgments, safety factors, bioavailability of nutrients from national foods) for differences among the various dietary standards[6] (allowances, safe intakes) if more national committees were to follow the Australian lead. Many of the problems encountered in using dietary standards to assess the risk of observed nutrient intakes being inadequate and the reasons for the confusion that exists between dietary standards and dietary guidelines were discussed in some of these[3-10] and other recent articles.[17-21]

---

* An appendix, added in proof, addresses differences between the 1989 RDA report and the 1980 and original 1985 reports.

Dietary Standards—What Are They?

Dietary standards, regardless of the name they go by—Recommended Dietary Allowances, Recommended Nutrient Intakes, Recommended Daily Amounts of Nutrients, Safe Intakes of Nutrients—are the average daily amounts of essential nutrients estimated on the basis of available scientific knowledge to be sufficiently high to meet the physiological needs of practically all healthy persons in a group with specified characteristics.[6] The recommended intakes of essential nutrients must, therefore, by definition exceed the requirements of almost all individuals in the group. The standards for food energy intake, in contrast, are average requirements of population groups. Thus, the energy requirements of about half the group will be below and about half will be above the recommended intake. However, individuals in a group with ready access to food will ordinarily meet their individual energy needs by adjusting their food intakes to match their energy expenditures. The original purpose of dietary standards was to serve as a reliable guide to the amounts of essential nutrients and energy that should be provided in diets for large groups of people to assure the nutritional health of all of the individuals in the specified group when the requirements of the individuals were not known.[22] Therefore, these distinctly different approaches for establishing recommended intakes for essential nutrients and energy were, and remain, most appropriate for planning nutritionally adequate diets. Problems with the RDA and dietary standards generally have arisen when the uses of the standards were extended beyond their original purpose.

Scientific Basis for Establishing Dietary Standards

The steps in establishing dietary standards are, first, to evaluate critically the literature on human requirements for each essential nutrient and to estimate average requirements for different age-sex groups; second, to estimate the variability of the requirements of individuals and to increase the average requirement by an amount sufficient to meet the needs of those with the highest requirements; and third, to estimate the efficiency of utilization of nutrients and their precursors (biological availability) from the foods usually consumed. Not only scientific knowledge but critical judgment is required in each of these steps. Differences in values proposed for allowances by different national committees and in the consistency among the values for different nutrients within the various individual sets of standards can result

from differences in judgment either between or within committees at any point in the process.

Average Requirements. There is not always agreement on the criteria for deciding when a requirement has been met. If the requirement is considered to be the minimum amount that will maintain normal physiological function and reduce the risk of impairment of health from nutritional inadequacy to essentially zero, we are left with questions such as, What is normal physiological function?, What is health?, and What degree of reserve or stores of the nutrient is adequate? Differences in judgment on such issues are to be expected.

The objective in establishing a requirement is to ensure that the body pool of the nutrient will be adequate to maintain normal physiological function even if intake falls below the estimated requirement for short periods of time. Knowledge of the size of the body pool and the rate of loss of the nutrient from the pool (turnover) makes it possible to estimate the time required for depletion of the pool if intake falls. Such information is available for few nutrients. For most it is necessary to depend upon indirect evidence of the adequacy of the pool size, such as maintenance of a satisfactory blood concentration, excretion of a high proportion of an administered dose in the urine, maintenance of zero balance in healthy individuals, maintenance of a biochemical function that can be measured without the use of invasive techniques, or the intake necessary to prevent or cure clinical signs.[23] However, even when the pool size and the rate of turnover of the nutrient can be measured, the question of the degree to which the pool can be depleted without impairment of physiological function or health still must be answered.

Estimates of pool size and rates of catabolism provide valuable information about the metabolic fate and potential storage of nutrients but not about requirements. In the United States and Canada, saturation of stores or the upper limit of metabolic losses was accepted as a guide to requirements and recommended allowances for ascorbic acid without considering the relationship between pool size and physiological function.[1,12] If such an approach were used for establishing allowances for retinol, for example, saturation of the pool would be associated with toxicity; if it were used for protein allowances, metabolic losses would increase steadily with increasing intake up to the point at which the protein allowance would represent the major source of energy. For explorers setting out on voyages exceeding 60 d with rations low in ascorbate, saturation of the ascorbate pool would be an appropriate criterion of need. It is difficult to understand why the recommended intake for individuals eating a basically adequate diet regularly should be that high (≥60 mg/d) when an intake of 30 mg/d will maintain a body pool of ascorbic acid of ≥600 mg and ensure prevention of clinical signs of scurvy even if ascorbic acid intake is zero for >3 wk.[24] Use of metabolic information as a substitute for judgment in setting the RDA for ascorbate and use of the RDA as a standard for the adequacy of intake of ascorbate have ensured that the prevalence of inadequate ascorbate intakes found in nutrition surveys will approach 40% in the adult male population,[10] an observation greatly at variance with the results of biochemical studies of ascorbate status.[25]

Individual Variability. The problem of individual variability in requirements was recognized before dietary allowances were established. Stiebling[26] originally proposed that the average requirement should be increased by 50% to cover individual variability. Pett et al.[27] proposed that, because requirements probably follow a Gaussian distribution, the appropriate increase to cover individuals with the highest requirements would be ≥3 standard deviations (SDs). Subsequently FAO and WHO committees proposed that the average requirement plus 2 SDs, a value that should cover the needs of 97.5% of the population, was an appropriate practical procedure for estimating safe intakes of essential nutrients.[28] In view of the tendency to use criteria for establishing average requirements that are generous in relation to intakes required to prevent clinical signs and in view of the ability of individuals to adjust to intakes somewhat below usual recommended intakes without evident adverse effects,[10] selection of 2 rather than 3 SDs seems reasonable. Judging from the low incidence of nutritional inadequacy detected among populations in which substantial numbers consume less than recommended intakes for one or more essential nutrients,[25] dietary standards established in this way are appropriate guides for formulation of nutritionally adequate diets for population groups.

Biological Availability. A dietary allowance, to be useful for planning diets, should be high enough to meet the requirement when the nutrient is provided by the usual selection of foods. If the nutrient is not readily released from foods during digestion or is not absorbed efficiently, the recommended intake must take this factor into account. Unfortunately, bioavailability of minerals and vitamins varies greatly from food to food, with the level of intake of the nutrient and with other dietary factors, such as fiber content. An estimate must be made from limited information for most nutrients of an average value for bioavailability of the nutrient from the major food sources in the diet.[9,28] The recommended intake is then increased to compensate for low availability. Differences in bioavailability can account for some major differences among the recommended intakes proposed by different national committees. In many Western nations where much of the iron, for example, is from meat with iron availability of ~20–25%, average availability of iron is estimated to be ~10%. In nations where most of the iron is from vegetable sources with iron availability of 2–8%, estimates of average iron availability may be as low as 3% and the recommended allowance two- to threefold higher. Recommended intakes of iron for women range from 14 mg/d in Canada to 32 mg/d in India largely on this basis.

The Allowance. The RDA and other dietary standards, thus, are set high enough to ensure that individuals with the highest requirements will be able to meet their nutritional needs if they consume an amount equal to the recommended intake from the usual supply of foods. The question still arises as to whether use of the FAO/WHO procedure does not represent failure to consider adequately the needs of the 2.5% of the population with the highest requirements, but this does not appear to be so. The most obvious reason is that committees on dietary standards tend to select the more generous of alternate values for average requirements and availability because moderate excesses of nutrients are not deleterious whereas even a small deficit can lead eventually to depletion and deficiency. This presumably accounts for the observation that allowances, once established, tend to decline as new information accumulates. No doubt there are differences in the reserves of individuals with the same intake whose requirements differ, but claims of health impairment occurring from intakes at the RDA level have not been substantiated.

Although the RDA and other dietary standards are recommended intakes for planning food supplies for population groups, they serve also as standards for the diets of individuals. It is not likely that any nutritional inadequacy will occur in individuals who consume amounts of nutrients equivalent to the RDA. On the other hand, even if the food supply for a population group provides amounts of nutrients in excess of the RDA and the average intake of the group exceeds the RDA, it cannot be assumed that all individuals in the group are consuming a nutritionally adequate diet. There is great individual variability in food consumption and food selection as well as in requirements; hence intakes of some nutrients by a proportion of the group may be inadequate even though average intake exceeds the RDA.[29]

RDA for some nutrients are evidently higher than they need to be as judged from differences among various national standards and from failure to detect biochemical changes indicative of inadequate intakes when these intakes are well below the RDA for a large proportion of the population. Although in Canada >40% of adults consume less than the RDA for ascorbic acid, low serum concentrations of the vitamin are found in only ~3% of the population.[10] Similar discrepancies between estimates of inadequacy based on intake and biochemical measurements are found in the United States for iron and calcium among women.[25] If allowances are set considerably above physiological needs, this is of little consequence for planning diets provided that nutrients are abundant in the food supply and the sources are not unduly expensive. However, if recommended intakes are used as standards for evaluating the adequacy of nutrient intakes and a large percentage of the population is judged to have an inadequate intake even though such a conclusion is not supported by clinical or biochemical observations, the dietary standard tends to fall into disrepute. When correspondence between the predicted and the observed incidence of nutritional inadequacy is poor, nutritionists should feel obligated to examine critically both the basis for the standard and the method used to assess the degree of inadequacy.

Uses of Dietary Standards

Dietary standards, like other technical standards, were developed for the use of professionals who are designing products. In the case of RDA the products include diet plans, nutrition education, and food and nutrition regulations. RDA are not guidelines for the consumer. Their original purpose was, as has already been emphasized, to serve as standards for planning and procuring food supplies for population groups, and they continue to serve satisfactorily for this purpose. They are equally satisfactory for other uses that are outgrowths of this primary use.

Food Guides. An early practical application of the RDA was to provide the basis for development of food guides for public nutrition education.[30] For this purpose, foods were separated into a limited number of groups according to the complement of nutrients they provided, and advice was given for selecting appropriate numbers of servings from a wide variety of foods in each food group. This grouping represented easily understood advice for selecting a diet that would contain the quantities of nutrients needed to meet the RDA by consuming a mixture of familiar foods in an amount that would provide less than the required intake of energy (calories).[31] It was a highly appropriate and successful use of the RDA.

Questions have arisen about the adequacy of in-

takes of several nutrients, especially calcium, iron, vitamin B-6, folate, magnesium, and zinc in diets based on the food guides, but measurements of nutritional status with respect to these nutrients have not provided convincing evidence of inadequacy of either the dietary guidance or the food supply.[25] It seems more likely that problems reported with these nutrients result from inappropriate food selection, inadequate food intake, or overestimation of the RDA. It is important, nonetheless, that the basis for both the RDA and the food guides be reviewed regularly as more accurate information about both nutrient requirements and food composition is obtained, as Guthrie[9] has stated, to ensure that the food guides are fulfilling their purpose effectively.

Food and Nutrition Regulations. The RDA also have been used by the Food and Drug Administration to develop a simplified standard for food labeling and food fortification. This standard, the U.S. RDA, consists of a set of single values—the highest RDA for any age group. It is, therefore, not a guide to appropriate intakes of nutrients for individuals other than young adult males. The main purpose of the U.S. RDA is to permit comparisons of the nutrient content of different foods by comparing food labels and to provide a guide for appropriate levels of fortification of foods when it is considered desirable. This is an appropriate use of the RDA for educating the public about the relative value of foods as sources of nutrients and for providing nutritional guidance for food manufacturers who are developing new food products.

Evaluating the Adequacy of Nutrient Intakes. Dietary standards were not designed for assessing the occurrence of nutritional inadequacy from estimates of nutrient intakes. They were obviously meant to be used to determine whether the diets of individuals or populations met the standard and to provide guidance in modifying the proportions of foods in the diet to correct apparent deficits. It was inevitable that reports providing information about the numbers of people consuming diets that failed to meet the standard would be published. Unfortunately, this information often was equated with the numbers of people consuming diets that are inadequate, but what was all too often overlooked was that that standard was set to exceed the requirements of most healthy persons. It should not be surprising that the numbers of individuals whose diets provided less than the RDA for some nutrients exceeded greatly the numbers identified by biochemical or clinical assessments as having inadequate intakes and that the RDA were therefore assumed to be unsatisfactory standards for evaluating the adequacy of nutrient intake.

RDA are not standards for identifying the point at which the nutrient intake of an individual becomes inadequate. If the habitual intake of an individual equals or exceeds the RDA, the risk of dietary inadequacy is remote. If the habitual intake is <50% of the RDA, the risk of dietary inadequacy is great. Because individuals whose requirements are high cannot be distinguished from those whose requirements are low, all that can be said when intake falls between these extremes is that the farther intake falls below the RDA, the greater is the risk of deficiency. When the RDA is used as a standard against which to evaluate the adequacy of nutrient intake of a population, the situation is even worse because variability among the intakes of individuals must also be taken into consideration. Hence, even if a population's average intake exceeds the RDA, a proportion may have low intake. Again, all that can be said is that the probability of deficiency occurring within the population rises the farther average intake falls below the RDA and that the probability is not zero even if average intake substantially exceeds the RDA.

This problem was recognized in the 1940s by Pett et al.[27] when dietary standards first were being developed. It is not, however, a shortcoming of dietary standards. It is not possible to assess the adequacy of the nutrient intake of an individual whose intake falls below the RDA without knowledge of that individual's requirements. It is possible, nevertheless, by use of a statistical approach, as is done in epidemiologic studies, to estimate the probability or risk of the intake of an individual being inadequate or the probability or risk of inadequate intakes occurring in a population for which the average intake is known. Little attention was given to the probability approach between the 1940s and the 1970s until Lorstad[32] and Beaton[33] began to apply it to the problem of assessing the incidence of nutritional inadequacy and FAO/WHO committees began to incorporate the concept into their reports. Beaton[18] discussed application of this approach extensively and reports of WHO/FAO/UNU[11] and NRC[21] committees elaborated on the procedure.

The principle is illustrated in Figure 1. The curve can be taken to represent the cumulative distribution of requirements assuming that requirements do not deviate appreciably from a Gaussian (normal) distribution. The vertical axis on the right indicates the probability of a given intake by an individual being inadequate, and that on the left indicates the expected prevalence of inadequate intakes in a population with a particular average intake. This approach permits a quantitative statement about the probability of intake being inadequate for an individual or of the probable incidence of inadequate intakes in a population if

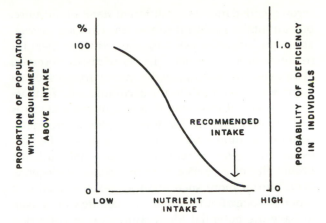

Figure 1. Cumulative plot of the distribution of nutrient requirements for a homogeneous population and the probability of intake being inadequate. (From an unpublished report by G.H. Beaton. Modified versions appear in references 10–12, 21, 28.)

average nutrient intake is known. It should be recognized that the reliability of the estimate depends upon the accuracy of the estimate of the average requirement and its variability and on the accuracy of the estimate of average intake. It also cannot be assumed that the estimate of risk applies to a particular individual, only that on the average it applies to individuals with a particular specified intake. This approach should, however, reduce the discrepancy between the proportion of individuals estimated to be at risk on the basis of biochemical and clinical measurements and the proportion estimated to be at risk on the basis of information on the distribution of intakes less than the RDA.[10] It also should provide a basis for assessing the reliability of values proposed for nutrient requirements from comparisons of the incidence of inadequate nutritional status observed in health surveys using biochemical and clinical indicators, with the incidence predicted from knowledge of the estimated requirements and the average intake of the population.[34]

Two or More Tiers of Dietary Standards

In 1977 at a conference of European nutrition societies, proposals were made for two or three levels of dietary standards. The idea behind this proposal was to have a diagnostic standard, the minimum requirement to meet physiological needs, for evaluating the nutritional adequacy of diets and a higher prescriptive standard for diet planning, public nutrition education, and public policy recommendations. Development of this proposal was described by Truswell.[7] Beaton[18,28] discussed favorably proposals by NRC and FAO/WHO committees to define different recommended intakes for different states of nutriture: one an intake sufficient to prevent clinically detectable signs of deficiency and one or more others for maintenance of specified levels of tissue reserves. With extensive and detailed dietary surveys such an approach could result in the accumulation of a massive amount of information about nutritional status that would be useful for assessing the appropriateness of nutrition policies, but it would still be necessary to assess, in relation to each standard, the probability of a particular intake being inadequate. With two or more such analyses, each related to a different state of nutriture, the procedure would seem to have the potential for creating greater confusion about uses of dietary standards than exists at present.

The problem of relating the different states of nutriture to meaningful differences in health status could become an exercise in ingenuity. One can envision having three levels of ascorbate nutriture based on different sizes of body pools with no criteria for distinguishing among them on the basis of altered physiological function. It would seem important first to establish one set of clearly defined and dependable criteria for average requirements and a set of recommended intakes that will ensure prevention of readily measurable functional impairment before attempting to subdivide the population into categories at different risk of impairment even if, for some nutrients, different degrees of physiological impairment can be related clearly to different levels of intake. Adoption of multiple RDA also could lead to the kind of morass into which we have fallen with respect to assessment of risk of developing chronic and degenerative diseases; by adjusting the criteria of risk upward or downward, the proportion of the population at risk can be adjusted to solve or create health problems.

The objective of proposals for multiple dietary standards is to provide a more comprehensive analysis of the nutritional status of a population, not to provide a better standard for planning or evaluating the adequacy of diets. This is a desirable objective. In fact, it is being done in the United States for iron nutrition. It is being done, however, by measuring two or more different biochemical indicators of adequacy of nutrient intake on statistical samples of the population;[25] thus, direct measures of nutritional status are provided rather than indirect ones that depend upon the reliability of food intake measurements and estimates of food composition as well as on the probability of a given intake being associated with a specified reserve of the nutrient. Making multiple measures of the inadequacy of nutrient intake seems to be a more appropriate approach than multiple dietary standards. It is important, nonetheless,

for committees dealing with dietary standards to report their estimates of average requirements as well as their estimates of recommended nutrient intakes and to specify clearly the nature of the risk associated with intakes below those recommended. It would then be easier to identify the reasons for discrepancies among the various recommendations.

A procedure based on the concept of nutrient density (units of nutrient/1000 kcal) has been proposed as an alternative dietary standard for assessing the nutritional quality of foods and diets.[35,36] It is presented as a standard for ensuring that a diet providing the amount of energy needed will contain quantities of nutrients that will meet all essential nutrient requirements. The usual practice for developing a nutrient-density standard is, for each age group, to divide the RDA for each nutrient by the average energy allowance and multiply by 1000 to obtain a measure of the amount of nutrient needed per 1000 kcal of energy needed. For thiamin, riboflavin, and niacin the same value is obtained for all age groups because the RDA for these nutrients are calculated on the basis of requirement per 1000 kcal of energy; for some others the discrepancies are not great, but for still others, such as protein, calcium, ascorbic acid, folate, and iron, differences among the values for different age groups are quite large. Therefore, to obtain a set of single-value nutrient allowances for evaluation of the nutritional quality of foods and diets and to ensure that each allowance will be high enough for all age groups (a major advantage claimed for this procedure), it is necessary to select RDA values toward the upper end of the range observed for the different age groups. The nutrient-density values for individual foods or diets can then be compared with the standard to determine the contribution the food or diet makes to the RDA for essential nutrients in relation to its contribution to the average caloric requirement. If, for example, the single-value allowance for ascorbic acid is 30 mg/1000 kcal, consuming a diet containing that proportion of ascorbic acid should ensure that the RDA for ascorbic acid for any age group will be met.

The nutrient density procedure is based on assumptions about RDA that differ from the principles on which RDA are established. The assumption that nutrients are required in proportion to calories is not accepted for nutrients other than thiamin, riboflavin, and niacin, and for the latter two the evidence for the assumption is tenuous. In addition, RDA are designed to cover the essential nutrient needs of individuals with the highest requirements, whereas RDA for energy are group averages; therefore, if energy needs are low, as for elderly people, or intakes are low, as for persons on reducing diets, nutrient density of diets needed to meet the RDA will have to be higher than the standard. The reverse will be the case for individuals with high energy expenditure. Beaton[10] elaborated more fully on the problems encountered in attempting to establish appropriate standards based on the nutrient-density concept.

The concept does, nevertheless, provide a simple procedure for comparing the nutrient contributions of foods that provide about the same amounts of calories per serving or per unit weight. However, in comparing the nutritive values of foods for which serving sizes differ greatly, it is important to realize that a food with high nutrient density contributes very little to the diet if the amount ordinarily consumed provides only a small number of calories daily.

Dietary Guidelines

Dietary guidelines are not a new and novel development in the fields of nutrition and public health. They have been a part of health policy for over 100 y. Recommendations for appropriate intakes of energy sources and protein in the 19th century were based, with very few exceptions, more on observations on the dietary patterns of healthy segments of the population than on experimental measurements of need. The British recommendation in 1918 that diets of children should contain a substantial proportion of milk and that of the League of Nations in the 1930s for inclusion of protective foods (milk, leafy vegetables, fish, meat, and eggs) in all diets represented advice for the public.[4] In fact, no clear distinction between such dietary guidelines and dietary standards, such as the RDA, was made until the 1940s, when the need to provide a reliable scientific basis for dietary guidelines for the public was recognized.[4]

Guidelines for healthful diets and guidelines for disease prevention are components of public health policy. They represent advice for the public that may be instituted, not only on scientific grounds, but for a variety of reasons including political considerations. RDA and similar dietary standards are not dietary guidelines. They are reference standards for levels of intake of essential nutrients needed on the basis of the available scientific evidence to ensure nutritional adequacy, and they are designed for use by organizations and agencies that provide dietary advice for the public. RDA have been criticized because they do not include recommendations for appropriate intakes of fat, carbohydrate, and fiber and because they do not deal with associations between diet and chronic and degenerative diseases and other public health issues. These criticisms arise from failure to recognize the distinctly different purposes of dietary standards and dietary guidelines.

Use of the term Recommended Dietary Allowances for the U.S. dietary standard has contributed to confusion about their purpose and uses. Terms such as recommended nutrient intakes and safe intakes do not have quite the same connotation of appropriate or desirable intake as do RDA, but they are not entirely free of it. Although the RDA for protein for adults, for example, is $0.8 \text{ g} \cdot \text{kg body wt}^{-1} \cdot \text{d}^{-1}$, it is doubtful that such a low intake is ever recommended except for patients whose protein intake must be restricted. It represents an intake sufficient to prevent impairment of health from protein inadequacy but the usual guideline, for reasons other than avoidance of inadequate intakes, is for 10–15% of calories from protein. It was the failure of the recent FNB to recognize this distinction that led to the controversy over the 10th edition of the RDA.[2,18]

Development of Dietary Guidelines. The early development of dietary guidelines was described in articles on the evolution of dietary standards,[4-6] and development by the USDA of food guides for selection of a nutritionally adequate diet—the major dietary guidelines for the American public during this century—was described by Hertzler and Anderson.[30] In the 1950s, after the health of the populations of industrialized nations had improved immensely, life expectancy had increased, and chronic and degenerative diseases had become the major causes of death, observations suggesting that the incidence of some of these diseases might be influenced by certain dietary constituents began to attract attention. During this period experimental observations that blood lipid concentrations could be influenced by diet and epidemiologic observations of associations between the amounts and types of fat consumed and mortality from heart disease led the American Heart Association to propose dietary guidelines for reducing the incidence of heart attacks. This was the beginning of a proliferation of new dietary guidelines for disease prevention by a variety of professional organizations and national committees that has increased in intensity in recent years. Summaries of at least 30 sets of such guidelines were published by 1986.[5,37,38] Since then two large reports on diet and chronic and degenerative diseases, one from the Surgeon General[39] the other from a National Research Council committee,[40] reiterated most of the dietary recommendations proposed previously and provided compilations of much of the information used as the basis for these recommendations.

Although some of these sets of guidelines include recommendations for maintaining intakes of essential nutrients (such as calcium, iron, and fluoride[40]) that are in accord with the RDA, their primary and often exclusive focus is on prevention of chronic and degenerative diseases and disorders, especially ischemic heart disease, hypertension, and cancer, by modifying dietary intakes of fats, carbohydrates, cholesterol, sodium, and fiber, which are nutrients and food constituents that, with the exception of sodium, are not covered in detail in RDA publications. The recommendations for disease prevention did not follow procedures used in formulating dietary standards, in which the scientific literature bearing on the subject was evaluated critically by a committee not involved in establishing public policy. Interpretations of the literature were prepared mainly by committees making public policy recommendations.

These distinctly different approaches for developing dietary standards and dietary guidelines should be recognized by those involved in instituting educational programs based on the guidelines. There should also be greater awareness of the extent of differences of opinion over both the interpretation of the evidence on which the guidelines are based and the appropriateness of the public policy itself than is readily apparent. This is not the place to discuss the extent of these differences in detail, but it can be illustrated by a few examples. The rationale for guidelines for prevention of heart disease published by the American Heart Association[41] was severely criticized by Reiser,[42] and the procedures and conclusions of the NIH Consensus Conference on Coronary Heart Disease similarly were criticized by Olson,[43] Ahrens,[44] and Oliver.[45] The recent extensive reports on diet and disease prevention[39,40] were prepared after the various dietary guidelines on the subject were proposed, and the organizations publishing them were involved in promoting such guidelines. The extensive literature on diet and heart disease also was evaluated critically by Smith and Pinckney[46] who, in a similarly comprehensive report, came to conclusions that were quite different from the previous two organizations about diet-disease relationships but were in accord with many critiques published over the past two decades. In a recent analysis of the basis for the policy represented by dietary guidelines for disease prevention, Moore[47] differed strongly with the conclusions of the American Heart Association and the National Heart, Lung and Blood Institute.

The major reason for citing these conflicting views is to emphasize that the scientific issues underlying control of chronic and degenerative diseases and the role of diet in such control have not been resolved. Many of the guidelines for disease prevention have been modified from time to time since they were first proposed and, with the pace of current advances in understanding the genetic and biochemical bases for these major diseases, reconsideration of such public policy recommendations will be ongoing. The risk of creating unnecessary apprehension about food and diet and, as Beaton[18] cautioned in the words of McCollum, of attributing extravagant values to nutrients should be kept clearly in mind.

Dietary Guidelines for Health. Two dietary guidelines for health are universally accepted. These are to consume a nutritionally adequate diet composed of a wide variety of foods and to consume food sources of energy in moderation in order to maintain appropriate body weight. The U.S. Departments of Agriculture and Health and Human Services, in their efforts to provide balanced dietary guidance for the public during the period when dietary recommendations for disease prevention were beginning to proliferate, included these as their first two guidelines.[48] Scientific evidence to support these recommendations was considered incontrovertible by the FNB when it undertook in 1980 to assess the adequacy of scientific knowledge for formulating dietary guidelines.[49] The USDA/HHS guidelines[48] also include advice to avoid too much fat, saturated fat, cholesterol, sugar, and sodium; to eat foods with adequate starch and fiber; and to use alcoholic beverages only in moderation. These additional guidelines strike a compromise between those for disease prevention and general guidelines for health but are presented without a strong implication that they will prevent chronic and degenerative diseases. They can be supported on general nutritional principles except for the advice on cholesterol, which is essentially therapeutic. Like most recent guidelines, they are oversimplifications and tend to shift attention away from the central role of nutrition for maintenance of health at each of the stages of life by focusing too much on guidance for overweight, middle-aged males.

There is a need for dietary guidance beyond these current guidelines that will provide perspective and reassurance for the public about diet and health and particularly beyond the guidelines for disease prevention, which seem designed to create fear and apprehension by implying that mortality from chronic and degenerative diseases is the only meaningful measure of nutritional health. This approach undermines balance in nutrition education by encouraging the belief that there are good foods (which will prevent disease) and bad foods (which will promote disease) instead of emphasizing the importance of diet as a whole in maintaining health.

To provide the perspective needed in presenting dietary guidance, the approach of the 1979 Surgeon General's report *Healthy People*[50] has great merit.

Improvements in the state of health of Americans of different ages during this century are described, the nature of current problems of each age group is presented, and, with a few notable exceptions having to do mainly with diet and disease, probable solutions and their limitations are discussed realistically.

At least three types of reports are needed to resolve the conflicts that have arisen during the past 15 y over dietary standards and guidelines. The first is a dietary standard such as RDA, perhaps with a new name to indicate the purpose of the standard more clearly. The RDA report presently serves quite well as a guide to both physiological needs for essential nutrients and the appropriate uses of the RDA by public health professionals and policy makers. The second is an expanded set of dietary guidelines for health of the type developed by USDA/HHS but which, using the approach of the previous Surgeon General's report,[50] describes objectively and in perspective the nutritional and dietary problems encountered at each stage of life with balanced advice about the merit and limitations of diet in solving these problems. The third type is a report on associations between diet and disease, prepared by scientists who are not advocates of specific public health policies, in which each major chronic and degenerative disease and disorder is discussed as a complex entity and what is known and what is controversial about the role of diet in its etiology and treatment are described factually and with a minimum of inference. With a set of reports such as these, it might just be possible to reduce the confrontational and advocacy approaches currently in vogue and to develop appropriate public health and nutrition programs on the basis of established scientific knowledge and objective discussion.

References

1. Food and Nutrition Board (1980) *Recommended Dietary Allowances,* 9th ed., National Academy Press, Washington, DC.
2. P.L. Pellett (1988) The RDA controversy revisited. *Ecol. Food Nutr.* 21:315–320.
3. Food and Nutrition Board (1989) *Recommended Dietary Allowances,* 10th ed., National Academy Press, Washington, DC.
4. A.E. Harper (1985) Origin of recommended dietary allowances—an historic overview. *Am. J. Clin. Nutr.* 41:140–148.
5. A.S. Truswell (1987) Evolution of dietary recommendations, goals, and guidelines. *Am. J. Clin. Nutr.* 45:1060–1072.
6. A.E. Harper (1987) Evolution of recommended dietary allowances—new directions? *Annu. Rev. Nutr.* 7:509–537.
7. A.S. Truswell (1983) Recommended dietary intakes around the world. *Nutr. Abstr. Rev.* 53:939–1015, 1085–1119.
8. A.F. Walker, J.V.G.A. Durnin, J.C. Waterlow, A.E. Harper, C.J. Bates, R. Wenlock, and D. Buss (1987) RDAs—are changes necessary? (6 articles) *Chem. Ind.* 16(Aug. 17):542–564.
9. A.R. Doberenz, J.A. Milner, and B.S. Schweigert, eds. (1986) *Food and Agricultural Research Opportunities to Improve Nutrition,* University of Delaware, Newark, DE.
10. G.H. Beaton (1988) Criteria of an adequate diet. In: *Modern Nutrition in Health and Disease* (M.E. Shils and V.R. Young, eds.), pp. 649–665, Lea and Febiger, Philadelphia.
11. FAO/WHO/UNU (1985) *Energy and Protein Requirements,* WHO Technical Report Series 724, World Health Organization, Geneva.
12. Department of National Health and Welfare (Canada) (1983) *Recommended Nutrient Intakes for Canadians,* Canadian Government Publishing Centre, Ottawa.
13. Department of Health and Social Security (U.K.) (1985) *Recommended Daily Amounts of Food Energy and Nutrients for Groups of People in the United Kingdom,* Her Majesty's Stationery Office, London.
14. N. Palmer, I.H.E. Rutishauser, I.E. Dreosti, R.M. English, J. Bullock, and A.S. Truswell (1982) Recommended dietary intakes for use in Australia (6 articles, Commonwealth Department of Health). *J. Food Nutr.* 39:157–192.
15. N. Palmer, B. Wood, I.H.E. Rutishauser, I.E. Dreosti, R.M. English, and A.S. Truswell (1985) Recommended dietary intakes for use in Australia (6 articles, Commonwealth Department of Health). *J. Food Nutr.* 41:109–154.
16. N. Palmer, I.H.E. Rutishauser, I.E. Dreosti, B.E.C. Nordin, and H.P. Roeser (1986) Further recommendations for dietary intakes for use in Australia (5 articles, Commonwealth Department of Health). *J. Food Nutr.* 42:47–92.
17. W.R. Bidlack and C.H. Smith (1988) Nutritional requirements of the aged. *CRC Crit. Rev. Food Sci Nutr.* 27:189–218.
18. G.H. Beaton (1986) Toward harmonization of dietary, biochemical and clinical assessments: the meanings of nutritional status and requirements. *Nutr. Rev.* 44:349–358.
19. H. Draper (1987) Micronutrients and cancer prevention: are the RDAs adequate? *Free Radic. Biol. Med.* 3:203–207.
20. H. Draper (1988) Nutrients as nutrients and nutrients as prophylactic drugs. *J. Nutr.* 118:1420–1421.
21. National Research Council (1985) *Nutrient Adequacy: Assessment Using Food Consumption Surveys,* National Academy Press, Washington, DC.
22. American Dietetic Association (1941) Recommended allowances for the various dietary essentials. *J. Am. Diet. Assoc.* 17:565–567.
23. A.E. Harper (1978) Nutritional requirements and dietary allowances. *Compr. Ther.* 10:10–17.
24. J.A. Olson and R.E. Hodges (1987) Recommended dietary intakes (RDI) of vitamin C in humans. *Am. J. Clin. Nutr.* 45:693–703.
25. USDA/HHS (1986) *Nutrition Monitoring in the United States—A Report from the Joint Nutrition Monitoring Evaluation Committee.* DHHS Publication no. (PHS) 86-1255, U.S. Government Printing Office, Washington, DC.
26. H.K. Stiebling (1933) *Food Budgets for Nutrition and Production Programs.* USDA Miscellaneous publication no. 183, U.S. Government Printing Office, Washington, DC.
27. L.B. Pett, C.A. Morrell, and F.W. Hanley (1945) The development of dietary standards. *Can. J. Public Health* 36:232–239.
28. G.H. Beaton (1988) Nutrient requirements and population data. *Proc. Nutr. Soc.* 47:63–78.
29. A.E. Harper (1974) Recommended dietary allowances: are they what we think they are? *J. Am. Diet. Assoc.* 64:151–156.
30. A.A. Hertzler and H.L. Anderson (1974) Food guides in the United States. *J. Am. Diet. Assoc.* 64:19–28.
31. L. Page and E.F. Phipard (1957) *Essential of an Adequate Diet.* Home Economics Research Report no. 3, USDA/Agricultural Research Service, U.S. Government Printing Office, Washington, DC.
32. M.H. Lorstad (1971) Recommended intake and its relation to nutrient deficiency. *FAO Nutr. Newslett.* 9:18–24.
33. G.H. Beaton (1972) *The Use of Nutritional Requirements and Allowances.* Proceedings of the Western Hemisphere Nutrition Congress III, pp. 356–363, Futura, Mount Kisco, NY.

34. G.H. Beaton and A. Chery (1989) Protein requirements of infants: A reexamination of concepts and approaches. *Am. J. Clin. Nutr.* 48:1403–1412.

35. R.G. Hansen and B.W. Wyse (1980) Expression of nutrient allowances per 1000 kilocalories. *J. Am. Diet. Assoc.* 76:223–227.

36. A. Wretlind (1982) Standards for nutritional adequacy of the diet: European and WHO/FAO viewpoints. *Am. J. Clin. Nutr.* 36:366–375.

37. T.P. O'Connor and T.C. Campbell (1986) Dietary guidelines. In: *Dietary Fat and Cancer* (C. Ip, D.F. Birt, A.E. Rogers, and C. Mettlin, eds.), pp. 731–771, Alan R. Liss, New York.

38. K. McNutt (1980) Dietary advice to the public: 1957–1980. *Nutr. Rev.* 38:353–360.

39. *U.S. Department of Health and Human Services* (1988) *The Surgeon General's Report on Nutrition and Health.* DHHS (PHS) Publication no. 88-50210, U.S. Government Printing Office, Washington, DC.

40. National Research Council (1989) *Diet and Health Implications for Reducing Chronic Disease Risk*, National Academy Press, Washington, DC.

41. S.M. Grundy et al. (1982) Rationale of the diet-heart statement of the American Heart Association. *Circulation* 65:839A–854A.

42. R. Reiser (1984) A commentary on the rationale of the diet-heart statement of the American Heart Association. *Am. J. Clin. Nutr.* 40:654–658.

43. R.E. Olson (1986) Mass intervention vs screening and selective intervention for prevention of coronary heart disease. *JAMA* 255: 2204–2207.

44. E.H. Ahrens, Jr. (1985) The diet-heart question in 1985: has it really been settled? *Lancet* 1:1085–1087.

45. M.F. Oliver (1986) Prevention of coronary heart disease—propaganda, promises, problems and prospects. *Circulation* 73:1–9.

46. R.L. Smith and E.R. Pinckney (1988) *Diet, Blood Cholesterol and Coronary Heart Disease: A Critical Review of the Literature*, Vector Enterprises, Inc., Santa Monica, CA.

47. T.J. Moore (1989) The cholesterol myth. *Atlantic Monthly* September: 37–70.

48. USDA/US DHHS (1985) *Nutrition and Your Health: Dietary Guidelines for Americans*, 2nd ed. Home and Garden Bulletin no. 232, U.S. Government Printing Office, Washington, DC.

49. National Research Council (1980) *Toward Healthful Diets*, National Academy Press, Washington, DC.

50. US DHEW (1979) *Healthy People: The Surgeon General's Report on Health Promotion and Disease Prevention.* DHEW (PHS) 017-001-00416-2, U.S. Government Printing Office, Washington, DC.

Appendix (The 1985–89 RDA)

The 10th edition of the RDA,[1] scheduled for publication in 1985, was released by the NAS/NRC in October 1989. The draft manuscript prepared by the RDA Committee in 1985 was completed, according to the preface, by a subcommittee of the Food and Nutrition Board (FNB) appointed in 1987. From the title page and comments in the text, it appears that the subcommittee took both responsibility and credit for the published version. The subcommittee appears to have adopted in principle most of the changes proposed by the 1980–85 RDA Committee,[2–7] but it should be no surprise, in view of the refusal of the FNB to accept the reductions recommended in the RDA values for vitamins A and C,[8–10] that the sections on these two nutrients[5,6] were modified considerably to justify retention of the higher 1980 values. Members of the 1980–85 RDA Committee, chaired by the late Dr. Henry Kamin, should take great satisfaction from the fact that, with these two exceptions in which policy issues were involved, their scientific judgment was upheld in the final report. It should be particularly gratifying when the reason given by the NAS for suspending publication of their report was that "the committee and the reviewers were unable to agree on the interpretation of scientific data on several of the nutrients."

RDA for vitamins A, D, E, and C; thiamin; riboflavin; calcium; phosphorus; and iodine remain essentially unchanged in the 10th edition, except that the value of 1200 mg/d for calcium for adolescents is now extended through age 24 y. Some minor changes in the table of allowances are undoubtedly due to replacement of the reference body weight values for adult males and females with the higher, actual median body weights of the U.S. population. Although RDA for most nutrients for adult females are proportionately lower than those for males because of body-weight differences, the RDA for calcium, iodine, and vitamins C and B-12 were not similarly adjusted.

RDA for vitamin K and selenium were included in the table of allowances for the first time.

The most significant changes in the 10th edition are reductions in many of the RDA for vitamins B-6 and B-12, folate, iron, and zinc, changes similar to, but not always identical with, those proposed by the 1980–85 RDA Committee. Some of the RDA for protein and magnesium also were reduced.

RDA for protein for adults remain unaltered except that the inordinately high addition of 30 g protein/ d during pregnancy[11] recommended in the last two editions was lowered to a more realistic 10 g/d. Protein allowances for children aged 1–6 y were reduced by 20–30%, to bring them into line with the safe intakes of milk or egg proteins recently proposed by FAO/WHO.[12] The low value of 1.23 g·kg body wt^{-1}·d^{-1} for young children (1–3 y) is considerably below that proposed by the 1980–85 committee. It is based on the assumption that the quality of the mixed proteins of typical U.S. diets is as high as that of the reference milk or egg proteins, an assumption the FAO/WHO/UNU committee[12] concluded does not apply to children whose diets include a high proportion of foods of plant origin (cereals and vegetables).

RDA for folate were reduced by ≥50% for all age groups above infancy. More accurate estimates of the folate content of diets and of the bioavailability of folates from foods provided the basis for this revision proposed by the 1980–85 committee.[2] The situation is similar for vitamin B-12, with reductions of 35% in the RDA for adults and greater reductions in the recommendations for children. The accumulated evidence from a variety of sources supports the conclusion that these amounts will maintain adequate body reserves.[3] RDA for vitamin B-6 for children and adult males were reduced modestly and for adult females by ~20–25%. The downward shift, based on evidence that ~20% less vitamin B-6 is required per gram of protein consumed than was previously thought necessary,[11] is less than was proposed by the 1980–85 RDA Committee.

RDA for iron for young children were reduced by 50%, for adolescent males by 35%, and for adult females by 17%. These values are almost identical with those proposed by the 1980–85 Committee based on evidence that individuals will maintain an iron store three to five times the 100-mg store at which evidence of iron deficiency begins to appear.[4] RDA for zinc for females over the age of 10 y were reduced by 30%. For males the values remain unchanged, but because reference body weights are now 10% higher, the current RDA represent a decrease of ~10% for those >24 y of age. Although these modifications are not identical with those proposed by the 1980–85 RDA Committee, the direction is the same. It does seem anomalous that the RDA for zinc of 10 mg/d for the 13 kg, 1–3-y age group is the same as that for the 28 kg, 7–10-y age group when a downward adjustment was made for females on the basis of their body weights being lower than those of males. RDA for magnesium for children are 30–45% lower than previous values and for females generally are ~7% lower.

Most of these changes bring the RDA more into line with FAO/WHO dietary standards and increase consistency among the values for RDA. In addition, the new values should reduce concern over the high proportion of intakes of iron, vitamin B-6, folate, magnesium, and zinc that are reported to be low in the United States in relation to RDA despite the sparsity of evidence that nutritional status is impaired by current intakes of these nutrients.[13]

The 10th edition of the RDA remains, as previous editions have always been, an excellent source of information and literature citations on human requirements for nutrients. When there was obviously so much agreement between the FNB and the 1980–85 RDA Committee, it seems unfortunate that the FNB was so inflexible in its stand on RDA for vitamins A and C.[10,14] The RDA for these nutrients remain above the FAO/WHO standards, no health problems have been encountered in the United States with re-

spect to either of them,[13] and critical evaluation of information on requirements for these led the 1980–85 RDA Committee to conclude that RDA much closer to the international safe intakes were appropriate.[5,6] In addition, although the FNB previously suggested that RDA for vitamins A and C should not be lowered because these nutrients might protect against cancer,[8–10] the evidence for this claim is all but dismissed in the sections on these vitamins in the 10th edition.

The impasse created by resistance of the FNB to the proposal to lower RDA has created a schism within the nutrition community that is not yet healed, has delayed publication of the 10th edition for 4 y, and has cost an immense amount of time and money in converting the original draft prepared by the 1980–85 RDA Committee into a report of a subcommittee of the board. The delay in publication has, however, had one beneficial outcome. Teachers of nutrition have been provided with materials for an enlightening series of seminars for graduate students based on critical comparisons of the six articles on Recommended Dietary Intakes published by members of the 1980–85 RDA Committee[2–7] with the modified versions prepared for the 10th edition[1] by the FNB subcommittee and its staff.

References

1. National Research Council (1989) *Recommended Dietary Allowances*, 10th ed., National Academy Press, Washington, DC.
2. V. Herbert (1987) Recommended dietary intakes (RDI) of folate in humans. *Am. J. Clin. Nutr.* 45:661–670.
3. V. Herbert (1987) Recommended dietary intakes (RDI) of vitamin B-12 in humans. *Am. J. Clin. Nutr.* 45:671–678.
4. V. Herbert (1987) Recommended dietary intakes (RDI) of iron in humans. *Am. J. Clin. Nutr.* 45:679–686.
5. J.A. Olson (1987) Recommended dietary intakes (RDI) of vitamin K in humans. *Am. J. Clin. Nutr.* 45:687–692.
6. J.A. Olson and R.E. Hodges (1987) Recommended dietary intakes (RDI) of vitamin C in humans. *Am. J. Clin. Nutr.* 45:693–703.
7. J.A. Olson (1987) Recommended dietary intakes (RDI) of vitamin A in humans. *Am. J. Clin. Nutr.* 45:704–716.
8. P.L. Pellett (1988) The RDA controversy. *Ecol. Food Nutr.* 21: 315–320.
9. J.A. Olson (1987) Should RDA values be tailored to meet the needs of their users? *J. Nutr.* 117:220–222.
10. V. Herbert (1987) The 1986 Herman Award Lecture. Nutrition science as a continually unfolding story: the folate and vitamin B-12 paradigm. *Am. J. Clin. Nutr.* 46:387–402.
11. National Research Council (1980) *Recommended Dietary Allowances*, 9th ed., National Academy Press, Washington, DC.
12. FAO/WHO/UNU (1985) *Energy and Protein Requirements*, WHO Technical Report Series 724, World Health Organization, Geneva.
13. USDA/USDHHS (1986) *Nutrition Monitoring in the United States— A Report from the Nutrition Monitoring Evaluation Committee.* DHHS Publication no. (PHS) 86-1255, U.S. Government Printing Office, Washington, DC.
14. P.L. Pellett (1986) Commentary: The RDA controversy. *Ecol. Food Nutr.* 18:277–285.

Chapter 59

Robert E. Olson

Evolution of Nutrition Research

Each science has its historical roots as well as a current presence and the promise of future discoveries. The early history of nutrition science is well described by Todhunter[1] in her chapter " 'Historical Landmarks' in Nutrition" in the fifth edition of *Present Knowledge in Nutrition*. It is clear that roots of nutrition science are imbedded in both medicine and in chemistry.[2] It also is clear that nutrition science is a field and not a discipline, to which many scientific specialists have made and will continue to make important contributions.

The Role of Physicians

It was recognized by Hippocrates in the fourth century before Christ that food was a source of body energy and heat. In his mini-textbook of medicine, Hippocrates gives 25 injunctions about diet and nutrition that reflect in many ways the dietary guidelines that are in place today. The classical vitamin-deficiency diseases in man, namely, scurvy, rickets, pellagra, beri-beri, and xerophthalmia, all were described first by physicians as diseases of unknown etiology. Scurvy was observed during the crusades and on voyages to the New World. The recovery of British sailors from scurvy upon reaching tropical ports led to the view that the cure was dietary, possibly due to a component of citrus fruits. In 1747 James Lind, a British Naval Medical Officer aboard the frigate Salisbury, carried out the first controlled clinical investigation in which he showed that citrus fruit could cure scurvy whereas other supplements could not. In 1907 scurvy was produced experimentally in guinea pigs by Holst and Frolich, but vitamin C was not isolated until 1920 independently by Albert Szent-Gyorgyi in Hungary and Charles Glenn King in the United States.

Beri-beri was described in the oriental medical literature about the time of Christ. A Dutch physician

reported the disease in persons in Java (Indonesia) in 1642, and in 1890 the Dutch government, alarmed by the prevalence of the disease in its Far East colony, dispatched a commission from Holland to Java headed by Christian Eijkman, who demonstrated in chickens that polished rice produced a polyneuritis that resembled beri-beri and that rice bran would cure the disease in both chickens and humans.

Rickets was first described by Frances Glisson, an English physician in London, in 1650, and cod liver oil was used empirically by John Darby at the Manchester Infirmary in 1789. Pellagra was first described by Gaspa Casal, physician to Phillip V of Spain, in 1735, and xerophthalmia was first described by David Livingstone, a Scottish medical missionary in Africa, in 1850. Experimental models for these diseases were developed many decades later.

The Role of Chemists

In parallel with these developments, during the 18th century Lavoisier and Laplace showed that animal respiration was a chemical process that resulted in the consumption of oxygen and the production of carbon dioxide.[3] These discoveries laid the foundation for the measurement of energy requirements and the determination of the caloric value of foods. Calorimetry was pioneered by Liebig in 1824, and his students (Voit, Atwater, and Benedict) applied these principles of direct calorimetry to measure the energy content of individual foods and the energy exchange in whole animals including humans.

Because of the dominance of Pasteur and the bacteriologists in the 19th century, it was difficult for early investigators of deficiency diseases to draw the conclusion that they had discovered a disease caused by lack of a protective chemical substance rather than the presence of a toxic chemical. Nonetheless, it was Frederick Hopkins[4] at the University of Cambridge in England who first demonstrated a deficiency disease in animals. He purified all the macronutrients of milk, including the ash, and showed that weanling rats could not grow on such a ration. When a small supplement of whole milk, equivalent to <3% of calories, was added to such purified diets, the rats grew at a miraculous rate. He concluded that "no animal can live upon a mixture of pure protein, fat and carbohydrate and even when the necessary inorganic material is carefully supplied the animal cannot flourish." The animal body is adjusted to live either upon plant tissues or tissues of other animals, and these tissues contain countless substances other than protein, carbohydrates, and fats. He called the factors active in promoting growth from milk "accessory food factors." It was Casimir Funk who unknowingly isolated nicotinic acid when he was looking for thiamin and who coined the term *vitamines* (life-giving amines) for these accessory food factors.

After Hopkins, biochemists in many parts of the world were able in a space of 25 y to identify, isolate, characterize, and, for the most part, synthesize the 13 vitamins we recognize today as essential for humans. This was the time when nutrition science was the principal concern of biochemists. By developing methods of isolating these trace organic compounds and testing them in deficient microorganisms or animals for biological activity, they made rapid progress in characterizing the vitamins.

The Advent of Enzymology

Enzymology became an integral part of biology in 1835 with the discoveries of the Swedish chemist Berzelius, who recognized that a number of biological extracts including saliva, gastric juice, and malt extract could break down carbohydrates and proteins to their component parts.[5] Berzelius further suggested that far from being a vital force, these substances might be catalysts for the digestion of macronutrients. By 1874 it was recognized by Kuhne that these ferments (which he called enzymes) could direct chemical reactions along particular paths and hence accelerate reaction rates. Although it was discovered that heating the biological extracts would destroy enzyme activity, the conclusion that the enzymes were in fact proteins was not accepted until Sumner[6] isolated urease from jack beans in 1926 and showed that it was a crystalline protein. Since then, hundreds of enzymes have been isolated and many crystallized. Each enzyme proved to be a distinct and unique protein.

In 1932 Warburg and Christian[7] identified the vitamin riboflavin as part of the coenzyme flavin mononucleotide, which in turn was required for the activity of the enzyme glucose-6-phosphate dehydrogenase. This discovery created a new linkage between nutrition and enzymology and resulted in the identification of all the vitamins of the B complex as precursors of coenzymes in animal and plant tissues. In contrast, the fat-soluble vitamins were identified as catalysts for synthesis or modification of proteins with highly differentiated biological activities.[8] Examples are prothrombin and other vitamin K–dependent proteins, vitamin D transport proteins, rhodopsin, and glycosyl transferase enzymes (vitamin A).

The development of enzymology in the first half of this century gave a great impetus to nutrition science as investigators began to study enzyme activity as a function of nutritional status. It became obvious in these studies that not only vitamins played a role in controlling enzyme activity, but the trace minerals did also. Iron, zinc, copper, manganese, molybdenum, and selenium were soon determined to be required for the synthesis of biologically active amino acids and proteins. Iodine was found to be a component of thyroxin. Iron was shown to be an essential component of hemoglobin, myoglobin, and a variety of cytochromes. Zinc also was found to be a component of dehydrogenases, carbonic anhydrase, and an array of digestive enzymes. Copper is a component of cytochrome oxidase, lysyl oxidase, ceruloplasmin, superoxide dismutase, tyrosinase, and dopamine-β-hydroxylase. Selenium is an intrinsic part of the enzyme glutathione peroxidase and of the enzymes glycine reductase, formate dehydrogenase, and xanthine dehydrogenase in anaerobic microorganisms. Manganese is a component of a number of manganoproteins, including glycosyl transferases, pyruvate carboxylase, and mitochondrial superoxide dismutase.

The Introduction of Isotopic Tracers

The advent of isotopic tracers after World War II provided another impetus to research in biochemistry and nutrition. The availability of isotopic atoms to trace both minerals and organic compounds in the animal body and thus to measure the turnover of body constituents was an important development. In fact it was with heavy hydrogen and heavy nitrogen (i.e., deuterium and ^{15}N) that Rudolph Schoenheimer carried out his pioneering studies at Columbia University in the 1930s, which led to a new concept described in his classic monograph "The Dynamic State of Body Constituents."[9] His work provided evidence that fats and proteins were in a state of constant turnover involving synthesis and degradation from and to fatty acids and amino acids, respectively.

Progress in Lipid Research

In 1823 Chevreul in Paris established the structure of the triglycerides and described the properties of a large number of animal and vegetable fats. McCollum and Simmonds[10] showed in 1920 that both animal and vegetable fats contained vitamin A activity, and Mellanby[11] showed that cod liver oil contained both vitamin A and vitamin D activity. It was Burr and Burr[12] in 1929 who first reported that polyunsaturated fatty acids were essential for normal nutrition in rats.

In more recent times, improvements in methods for characterizing fats and fatty acids by gas chromatography, high-pressure liquid chromatography, and mass spectrometry coupled to gas chromatography have led to the characterization of not only the common fatty acids but also trace products of arachidonate metabolism. These products include prostaglandins, thromboxanes, prostacyclins, and leukotrienes, all of which have remarkable physiological activities.[13] Because these products are derived from essential fatty acids, that relationship provides an opportunity to study the role of nutrients in the formation of eicosanoids. Platelet aggregation and even coagulation are associated with these trace metabolites of essential fatty acids. Currently the biological effects of the polyunsaturated fatty acids of the n−3 and n−6 series are under intensive investigation.

The Present Supremacy of Molecular Biology

At the present time molecular biologists dominate the field of biochemistry and are providing new technologies for application in nutrition science. Beginning with the discovery of the structure of DNA by Watson and Crick[14] in 1953 and the elucidation of the genetic code, advances in our understanding of gene structure and regulation of gene expression have led to an explosion of new knowledge about biochemical genetics. Through the use of restriction enzymes discovered by Nathans and Smith[15] at Johns Hopkins University, it has been possible to introduce genetic material into plasmids of bacteria, which amplify the gene number and make possible the production of novel mammalian products in bacterial systems, such as hormones, cytokines, and coagulation proteins. Cloning genes has now become a routine procedure in biochemical laboratories. This new knowledge has led to the hope that genetic engineering can be effected in human subjects to correct genetic disorders by introducing the correct gene in a suitable vector.

It is clear that the application of molecular biology to nutritional problems will cast new light on the function of nutrients and the regulation of metabolism. Molecular biology already has made important contributions to nutrition science. For example, it was shown by Goodrich[16] at Case Western Reserve that nutrients in the diet can affect the gene expression of a series of enzymes concerned with fatty acid synthesis and oxidation. The pathway from nutrient to genome is not clear, but it is becoming more certain that many nutrients can affect gene expression. This is well illustrated by the recent finding that the receptors for active vitamin A (retinoic acid) and active vitamin D (1,25-dihydroxycholecalciferol) belong to the superfamily of steroid receptors that interact directly with the genome to affect gene expression.[17]

Reductionism vs. Integration of New Knowledge

Some nutrition scientists are concerned about the present devotion of biology to scientific reductionism, the reduction of a phenomenon to its simplest elements. In the case of biochemistry, reductionism connotes the study of genes, macromolecules, and lipids to determine their structure and function at the subcellular level, usually without reference to their role in the total functioning of the organism. Integrationists in nutrition science, however, emphasize the importance of using new knowledge to account for the regulated metabolism of the intact organism. Both approaches are important. The vertical organization of nutrition science, from molecule to human, demands constant interaction between reduction and integration of scientific knowledge. It seems to me that in the field of clinical nutrition, where so much needs to be learned about the role of nutrients in increasing or decreasing disease susceptibility, both approaches are vital. In humans the genetics of the susceptibility of individuals to the common chronic diseases of coronary heart disease, cancer, diabetes, and hypertension is as important as the effects of diet and other environmental variables. Both effects are mediated through metabolic pathways that should provide an understanding of the mechanism of disease susceptibility.

The Challenge for Clinical Nutrition

Another frontier for the future is the expansion of knowledge about clinical nutrition. There was a period when clinical nutrition consisted principally of the evaluation of body composition and nutritional status. With the advent of new technologies (nuclear magnetic resonance, heavy isotopes, computer-aided tomography) for probing metabolism and with the advent of better technologies for feeding human beings by vein (i.e., total parenteral nutrition), new knowledge will be forthcoming about the pathophysiology of the chronic degenerative diseases that lead to multiple organ failure. I see much opportunity in the future for a better understanding of human metabolism, the pathophysiology of human disease, and the contributions that nutrition can make to human health. Nutrition scientists who study chronic diseases in humans or models thereof using cell biology, experimental nutrition, clinical nutrition, or epidemiology should be cautious in concluding that any one variable is the single cause of these complex chronic diseases. For example, serum cholesterol, long considered a risk factor for coronary heart disease, is made up of several cholesterol-containing lipoprotein fractions with variable effects on risk.

Some variables associated with a disease may, in fact, turn out to be one of many causes of the disease and some may turn out to be merely associated or epiphenomena. Dogmas usually develop when proof is not possible and only when circumstantial evidence is available. Such dogmas, in fact, may be inimical to progress. Far from shouting "Eureka!" we should be designing new experiments, applying new technologies, and rigorously testing existing hypotheses.

I believe that nutrition science has a great future. The corps of workers in the field will certainly change with the advent of new techniques and concepts. As with medicine, the scientific frontier of nutrition in the future may be even more distant from the activities of practitioners than is the case at present. So be it! With good communication all segments of the nutrition field will profit from a vigorous and productive research effort.

References

1. E.N. Todhunter (1984) "Historical landmarks" in nutrition. In: *Present Knowledge in Nutrition*, 5th ed. (R.E. Olson, H.P. Broquist, C.O. Chichester, W.J. Darby, A.C. Kolbye, Jr., and R.M. Stalvey, eds.), pp. 871–882, Nutrition Foundation, Washington, DC.
2. R.E. Olson (1978) Clinical nutrition, the interface between human ecology and internal medicine. *Nutr. Rev.* 36:161–178.
3. D. McKie (1952) *Antoine Lavoisier, the Founder of Modern Chemistry*, Constable, London.
4. F.G. Hopkins (1912) Feeding experiments illustrating the importance of accessory factors in normal dietaries. *J. Physiol.* 44:425–465.
5. M. Dixon and E.C. Webb (1964) *Enzymes*, 2nd ed., Academic Press, New York.
6. J.B. Sumner (1926) The isolation and crystallization of the enzyme urease. *J. Biol. Chem.* 69:435–441.
7. O. Warburg and W. Christian (1932) A new oxidation enzyme and its absorption spectrum. *Biochem. Z.* 254:438–458.
8. R.E. Olson (1965) The regulatory function of the fat-soluble vitamins. *Can. J. Biochem.* 43:1565–1573.
9. R. Schoenheimer (1942) *The Dynamic State of Body Constituents*, Harvard University Press, Cambridge, MA.
10. E.V. McCollum and N. Simmonds (1929) *The Newer Knowledge of Nutrition*, 4th ed., Macmillan, New York.
11. E. Mellanby (1950) *The Story of Nutrition Research. The Effect of Some Dietary Factors on Bones and the Nervous System*, Williams and Wilkins, Baltimore.
12. G.O. Burr and M.M. Burr (1929) A new deficiency disease produced by the rigid exclusion of fat from the diet. *J. Biol. Chem.* 82:345–367.
13. S. Bergstrom, H. Danielsson, and B. Samuelson (1964) The enzymatic formation of prostaglandin E_2 from arachidonic acid. *Biochim. Biophys. Acta* 90:207–210.
14. J.D. Watson and F.H.C. Crick (1953) A structure for desoxyribonucleic acid. *Nature* 171:737–738.
15. D. Nathans and H.O. Smith (1975) Restrictive endonucleases in the analysis and restructuring of DNA molecules. *Annu. Rev. Biochem.* 44:273–293.
16. A.G. Goodrich (1987) Dietary regulation of gene expression: enzymes involved in carbohydrate and lipid metabolism. *Annu. Rev. Nutr.* 7:157–185.
17. V. Giguere, E.S. Ong, P. Segui, and R.M. Evans (1987) Identification of a receptor for the morphogen retinoic acid. *Nature* 330:624–629.

Index